Women's Health Care

in **Advanced Practice Nursing**

Catherine Ingram Fogel, PhD, WHCNP-BC FAAN, is a professor and coordinator of the Women's Health Practice Area at the University of North Carolina at Chapel Hill School of Nursing. She is the author of several texts on women's health, including the award-winning *Women's Health Care* (Fogel & Woods, 1995) and has authored numerous research and clinical articles on women's health. For the past thirty years she has had a both a sustained research program and clinical practice with incarcerated women. Her research has increased nursing's awareness and understanding of the health problems of incarcerated women. Fogel is the principle investigator on one NIH funded and one CDC funded grant focusing on prevention of sexually transmitted infections and HIV in women; another NIH funded grant exploring the experiences of parenting from prison; and a CDC-funded grant to deliver an STI risk reduction intervention to HIV-infected women living in the Southeast.

Fogel is a member of the American Nurses Association, the Association for Women's Health, Obstetrics and Neonatal Nurses, and Sigma Theta Tau. She is a fellow of the American Academy of Nursing. She has been certified as a women's health care nurse practitioner since 1982. She received a North Carolina Community Service Award for her work with women prisoners and the 1993 AWHONN National Excellence in Clinical Practice Award.

Nancy Fugate Woods, PhD, RN, FAAN, is dean of the School of Nursing and professor in the Department of Family and Child Nursing at the University of Washington. Since the late 1970s, she has led a sustained program of research in the field of women's health. Her collaborative research has resulted in an improved understanding of women's transition to menopause, including hormonal and psychosocial factors as well as menstrual cycle symptoms. Her work has advanced nursing care for reproductive-aged and mid-life women and has provided women with a better understanding of their health. In 1989, Woods helped establish the first NIH-funded Center for Women's Health Research at the University of Washington.

Woods has served as president of the American Academy of Nursing, the North American Menopause Society, and the Society for Menstrual Cycle Research. She helped set research agendas as a member of the National Institutes of Health Women's Health Task Force and Office of Women's Health Research Advisory Council. Her honors include election to the Institute of Medicine of the National Academies and to the American Academy of Nursing. She received the American Nurses Foundation Distinguished Contribution to Nursing Research Award, and, in 2003, she received the Pathfinder Award from the Friends of the National Institute for Nursing Research. She earned a BS in nursing from the University of Wisconsin, Eau Claire, in 1968; an MN from the University of Washington in 1969; and a PhD in epidemiology from the University of North Carolina, Chapel Hill, in 1978. She has been awarded honorary doctoral degrees by the University of Pennsylvania, Haifa University, and Chiang Mai University.

Women's Health Care

in **Advanced Practice Nursing**

EDITORS   Catherine Ingram Fogel, PhD, RNC, FAAN
Nancy Fugate Woods, PhD, RN, FAAN

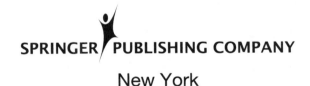

SPRINGER PUBLISHING COMPANY

New York

Springer Publishing Company, LLC
11 West 42nd Street
New York, NY 10036
www.springerpub.com

Acquisitions Editor: Allan Graubard
Production Editor: Julia Rosen
Cover design: Joanne E. Honigman
Composition: Apex Publishing, LLC

10 11 12 / 5 4 3

Library of Congress Cataloging-in-Publication Data

Women's health care in advanced practice nursing / [edited by] Catherine Ingram Fogel, Nancy Fugate Woods.
    p. ; cm.
    Includes bibliographical references and index.
    ISBN 978-0-8261-0235-5 (alk. paper)
  1. Women—Diseases—Nursing. 2. Women—Health and hygiene. I. Fogel, Catherine Ingram, 1941– II. Woods, Nancy Fugate.
    [DNLM: 1. Nursing Care. 2. Women's Health Services. 3. Health Promotion.
4. Nurse Practitioners. 5. Women's Health. WA 309 W87215 2008]

RT42.W66   2008
613'.04244—dc22   2007051945

Printed in the United States of America by Bang Printing.

Contents

PART I

Women and Their Lives

PART II

Frameworks for Practice

Chapter 9   **Well-Woman Assessment 185**

Donna W. Roberson and Catherine Ingram Fogel

Chapter 10   **Legal Issues in the Care of Women 195**

Diane K. Kjervik

PART III

Health Promotion

Chapter 11   **Healthy Practices: Nutrition. 205**

Betty Lucas

PART IV

Threats to Health and Health Problems

Contributors

Judith A. Berg, PhD, RNC, WHNP, FAAN, FAANP
Associate Professor
University of Arizona College of Nursing
Tucson, Arizona

Beth Perry Black, PhD, RN
Assistant Professor
University of North Carolina at Chapel Hill
School of Nursing
Chapel Hill, North Carolina

Eleanor F. Bond, PhD, RN, FAAN
Professor, Department of Biobehavioral
Nursing and Health Systems
Susan and Michael Cummings Term

Professor in Nursing
University of Washington School of Nursing
Seattle, Washington

Janet Cady, MN, ARNP
Pediatric Nurse Practitioner
Senior Lecturer
Department of Family and Child Nursing
University of Washington
Seattle, Washington

Pediatric Nurse Practitioner
High Point Medical Clinic
Medical Director
School-based Health Programs
Puget Sound Neighborhood Health Centers
Seattle, Washington

Jacquelyn C. Campbell, PhD, RN, FAAN
Anna D. Wolf Chair and Professor
Johns Hopkins University School of Nursing
Baltimore, Maryland

Phyllis L. Christianson, MN ARNP
Senior Lecturer, Biobehavioral Nursing
and Health Systems
University of Washington School of Nursing

Geriatric Care Specialist, Group Health Cooperative
Nursing Home Services
Seattle, Washington

Barbara B. Cochrane, PhD, RN, FAAN
Associate Professor, Family and Child Nursing
de Tornyay Term Professor, Healthy Aging

Director, de Tornyay Center, Healthy Aging
University of Washington
Seattle, Washington

Cheryl L. Cooke, PhD, MN, RN
Acting Assistant Professor
Nursing Program
University of Washington Bothell
Bothell, Washington

Susanna Garner Cunningham, BSN, PhD, FAAN, FAHA
Professor, Department of Biobehavioral
Nursing and Health Systems
University of Washington
Seattle, Washington

Anne Hopkins Fishel, PhD, MSN
Professor, School of Nursing
University of North Carolina at Chapel Hill
Chapel Hill, North Carolina

Holly B. Fontenot, RNC, MS, SANE
Clinical Instructor
William F. Connell School of Nursing
Boston College
Chestnut Hill, Massachusetts

Catherine Garner, DrPH, RN, FAAN
Provost/Dean
International University of Nursing

Chief Operating Officer
University of Medicine and Health Sciences
St. Kitts, West Indies

Allyssa Harris, RNC, MS
PhD candidate, Clinical Instructor
William F. Connell School of Nursing
Boston College
Chestnut Hill, Massachusetts

Joellen W. Hawkins, RNC, PhD, FAAN
Professor, William F. Connell School of Nursing
Boston College
Chestnut Hill, Massachusetts

Janet C. Horton, RN, MS, FNP
Family Nurse Practitioner
Cold Harbor Family Medicine
Mechanicsville, Virginia

Diane K. Kjervik, JD, RN, FAAN
Professor and Academic Division Chair
School of Nursing
University of North Carolina at Chapel Hill
Chapel Hill, North Carolina

Kären Landenburger, RN, PhD
Professor, University of Washington Tacoma
Tacoma, Washington

Cheryl A. Cahill Lawrence, RN, PhD
Amelia Peabody Professor of Nursing
MGH Institute of Health Professions
Boston, Massachusetts

Carol J. Leppa, PhD, RN
Professor, Nursing Program
University of Washington, Bothell
Bothell, Washington

Aileen MacLaren Loranger, RN, PhD
Clinical Assistant Professor
University of Washington, Seattle
School of Nursing
Family and Child Nursing
Seattle, Washington

Deitra Leonard Lowdermilk, PhD, RNC, FAAN
Clinical Professor Emerita
University of North Carolina at Chapel Hill
School of Nursing
Chapel Hill, North Carolina

Betty Lucas, MPH, RD, CD
Lecturer, Family and Child Nursing
University of Washington, School of Nursing
Seattle, Washington

Mona T. Lydon-Rochelle, PhD, MPH, CNM, RN
Associate Professor, Family and Child Nursing
University of Washington, Seattle
Seattle, Washington

Ellen Sullivan Mitchell, PhD
Associate Professor Emeritus
University of Washington, School of Nursing
Seattle, Washington

Merry-K. Moos, BSN, FNP, MPH, FAAN
Professor, School of Medicine
University of North Carolina at Chapel Hill
Chapel Hill, North Carolina

Shirley A. Murphy, RN, PhD, FAAN
Professor Emeritus
Psychosocial and Community Health Department
School of Nursing
University of Washington
Seattle, Washington

Ellen Olshansky, DNSc, RNC, FAAN
Professor and Director
Nursing Science Program
College of Health Sciences
University of California, Irvine
Irvine, California

Janet Primomo, PhD, RN
Associate Professor
University of Washington, Tacoma
Tacoma, Washington

Donna W. Roberson, PhD, WHCNP-BC
Associate Professor, School of Nursing
East Carolina University
Greenville, North Carolina

Kathleen J. Sawin, DNS, CPNP, FAAN
Professor and Joint Research Chair in the
Nursing of Children
Children's Hospital of Wisconsin and
College of Nursing
University of Wisconsin–Milwaukee
Milwaukee, Wisconsin

Anne H. Skelly, PhD, RN, CS, FAANP
Professor
University of North Carolina at Chapel Hill
Chapel Hill, North Carolina

Diana Taylor, RNP, PhD
Professor Emerita, School of Nursing
Research and Evaluation Director, Access through
Primary Care Initiate
University of California, San Francisco
San Francisco, California

Julie Smith Taylor, PhD, RN
Assistant Professor and Graduate Coordinator
UNCW School of Nursing
Wilmington, North Carolina

Debbie Ward, PhD, RN
Associate Professor
Psychosocial and Community Health
University of Washington, Seattle
Seattle, Washington

Heather M. Young, PhD, GNP, FAAN
Grace Phelps Distinguished Professor
Director of the John A. Hartford Center for Geriatric
Nursing Excellence and Director of Rural Health
Research Development
Ashland, Oregon

Women's health is inextricably linked to the context in which they live their lives. Only within the past few decades have researchers and clinicians acknowledged the importance of women's lived experiences for their well-being. The feminist movement of the 1960s and 1970s prompted critical analysis of women's health and its relationship to society, and of women's health care options. Together these social movements gave voice to women's increasing dissatisfaction with health services and prompted the creation of alternative services that reflected new values about women and allowed them to reclaim control over their bodies and assume responsibility for their own health. During this same period, the nursing profession, largely composed of women, began to recognize that many assumptions that had limited women's opportunities had also limited those of the nursing profession. As a result of the women's health movement, nurses began to address problems of sexism as they affected the nursing profession as well as the women who sought health care.

The 1980s saw a rapid development of nursing literature focusing on women's health problems, with some works examining women's health from a feminist perspective. Efforts of nurses over the next decades have culminated in redefining women's health as more than reproductive health, integrating a holistic view of biological, psychosocial, and cultural dimensions of health and well-being. Nurses have helped to change the way that health care is delivered to women, advocating for integrative models of services such as mind-body care and opportunities for women to participate actively in the decisions about their care, seen dramatically in the practice of nurse midwives and nurse practitioners who deliver women's primary care. Nurse theorists and scientists have also made significant contributions, expanding our understanding of women's experiences of their health across the life span and in response to specific threats to their health and developing and testing therapeutic interventions for health promotion and prevention and promoting recovery from illness. Finally, nursing educators have infused knowledge about women's health in undergraduate and graduate curricula, transforming the ungendered view of health to one that is tailored to the sex and gender differences that affect human health.

This text was written initially in 1980 to inform health professionals, especially practitioners of nursing, about the complex nature of women's health. Over nearly three decades, we have witnessed continuing progress in the development of knowledge to guide the practice of women's health care. Near the end of the first decade of the 21st century, we can celebrate the achievements of scientists and clinicians, in collaboration with women, who continue to transform how we think about and care for women's health. During the 1990s and the first decade of the 21st century, we have continued to see progress in the science and practice of women's health.

This 2008 revised edition provides a resource focusing on several dimensions of women's health in an effort to support the practices of students and practitioners in a wide range of clinical and community settings. As we have seen an increased emphasis on women's health in advanced practice in nursing, we have incorporated material that we believe will support nurse practitioners as well as nurses. We hope that this text will become a personal resource for nurses and for women who wish to learn more about their health, whatever their focus of practice or type of work.

In Part I, we focus on the connections between women's lives and women's health. This section begins with an examination of the paradoxical relationship between gender and health and the use of health services. Although women experience more sickness, especially chronic illness, and use health services more frequently than men, they experience a significant advantage: a longer life span. Biological and social dimensions of women's and men's lives differ and are likely to have important effects on health outcomes. Women have been engaged in providing health care for themselves and their families since the beginning of recorded history, yet only certain aspects of health care have come to be viewed as women's work. The stratification of our health care professions by gender, ethnicity, and social class influences who delivers health care and the circumstances of the practice. Women's bodies possess unique strengths and capabilities, such as childbirth and lactation, yet these unique characteristics are often the target for discrimination and the basis for sexist interpretations that affect women's lives. Revisionist thinking about women's development throughout the life span has influenced models for thinking about menarche, menstruation, menopause, and aging, yet these notions are only beginning to influence how clinicians are educated to care for women. Sexism and ageism both combine to damage women's chances for health, especially as they age.

Part II addresses frameworks for nursing practice with women. Conceptual frameworks for nursing practice that respect the complexity of women's health and reflect contemporary views of nursing practice provide a foundation for examining health assessment for well women and legal considerations in providing women's health care.

Part III focuses on health promotion for women. Nutrition and physical activity provide opportunities for women to promote their health and prevent many chronic diseases, including heart disease and cancers as discussed in the final section of the book. Mental health, including a sense of well-being along with problems such as depression, often has a life span impact, influencing not only a woman but her children. Sexual health care, fertility control, and preconceptional health care are addressed because each has a major influence on most women for a large portion of the life span, in particular the reproductive years.

Part IV addresses threats to health and health promotion strategies, including infertility, unintended pregnancy, high risk pregnancy, perimenstrual and perimenopausal symptoms and syndromes, reproductive surgery, substance abuse, violence, sexually transmitted infections, HIV/AIDS, cardiovascular disease, chronic illnesses, breast health problems, and disability. Taken together, these topics are likely to be the subject matter of many women's health care ventures.

We hope that discussion of these topics provides nurses and nurse practitioners as well as other health professionals with a contemporary view of women's health. We thank the many women in our lives who helped to bring this project to fruition, and we dedicate our work to them.

Acknowledgments

Dedicated to the memories of my mother, Elizabeth Barnes Fugate, who advocated for women's education and questioned authority, and to my friend, Marie Cowan, who was an extraordinary friend and role model for nurses.

In acknowledgment of the support I receive from special women in my life: my daughter Erin; my sisters, Sue, Jane, and Pat; my nieces Annie, Lizzy, and Susan; and my good friend Joan. Thanks to my husband, Jim Woods, who has supported my academic efforts and worked to advance the careers of many women in science.

Nancy Fugate Woods

This book is my thank you to all of the women I have worked with over the years, especially the incarcerated women who have shared so much of their lives with me and the students who have taught me more than I ever taught them.

None of this could have been done without the support and comfort my close circle of women friends and that of my husband, Mark Fogel, who has never faltered in his unconditional support of me.

Catherine Ingram Fogel

PART I

Women and Their Lives

Women and Their Health

Mona Lydon-Rochelle and
Nancy Fugate Woods

Our understanding of women's health—informed by research that extends from molecular events to behavioral, psychological, and societal phenomena—has emerged as one of the most exciting challenges of scientific inquiry at the beginning of the 21st century. The 20th century witnessed an increased understanding of issues associated with women's health and saw extraordinary improvements in the health and well-being of women in the United States resulting from research and innovative approaches to health care. Despite the progress, the health of women in the United States remains subject to wide disparities. These disparities among women overall are readily apparent when viewed through the lenses of race and ethnicity and age and are often further compounded for specific populations of women based on socioeconomic status. Recent trends in women's demographics—including educational attainment, employment status, family composition, reproduction, and access to health care—suggest an increasingly complex social context (Grason, Hutchins, & Silver, 1999). An understanding of women's health issues, if it is to be truly comprehensive, must not ignore such factors and trends.

In 2000, there were 141.1 million females of all ages in the United States, and women outnumbered men in every age group, from ages 25 and older (U.S. Census Bureau, 2000a). The first section of this chapter describes selected sociodemographic characteristics of women in the United States. Some of the most notable of these characteristics at the beginning of the 21st century are the changing racial and ethnic population. The second section presents selected measures of health status. These include mortality, morbidity, and health care access and utilization. Next, we discuss the complicated interplay between and steadily changing scientific knowledge regarding the areas of biology and environment. We conclude with an exploration of the future directions for women's health.

SOCIAL CONTEXT

To understand the health of women in the U.S. social context, we present the most recently available data on selected social characteristics of women, with a focus on the changing population demographics. Differences in the life circumstances of women are influenced through a number of pathways, many of which are not yet understood. Considering the health of women within their broad sociostructural environment is important in light of ethnicity and socioeconomic status, all of which impact women's health. Gender differences in some aspects of health status are presented when the differences are notable. Notably, data regarding women's health are limited and often are not available by important demographic characteristics. Race and ethnic variation is discussed when the data sources are available. We recognize the limitations of reporting demographics such as race and ethnicity, because definitions vary over time, and data are inconsistently available for small but growing populations. Further, reporting can obscure the diversity within and among subgroups of women. For example, the Asian and Pacific Islanders category includes over 25 heterogeneous groups, and no distinction is made in terms of their immigration status. Also, because detailed racial and ethnic information frequently is unavailable, and since socioeconomic status and cultures of ethnic and racial groups may vary dramatically with important health consequences, racial labeling may mask notable health differences and thus should be considered with caution. Finally, given the strong association between socioeconomic status as measured by family income, poverty threshold, or level of education and the health of women, differences are also noted when data permit.

Population Trends

Growth

Numerous demographic trends herald social changes in the early 21st century. In 2000, the female population was racially and ethnically diverse and was comprised of White (71.3%), Black (12.5%), Hispanic (11.5%), Asian and Pacific Islander (3.9%), and American Indian, Eskimo, and Aleutian (1%) (U.S. Census Bureau, 2000a). Population growth rates are higher among the Hispanic population than among White non-Hispanic or Black subgroups. Moreover, the growth of the Hispanic population is likely to continue, since Hispanic women comprise a large proportion of the population of reproductive age and have the highest fertility rates. In fact, by the year 2050, population projections indicate that Hispanic, Black, American Indian, and Asian adolescents will constitute 56% of the total adolescent population.

Immigration

The immigrants and refugees of the 21st century are not as well educated as the professionals of the 1950s and 1960s, since many immigrants now come from poverty-stricken countries such as Ethiopia or are survivors of war-ravaged nations such as Bosnia and Kosovo. Notably, descendants of these immigrants and refugees represent the largest segment of U.S. population growth, a trend that is predicted to continue. In 1999, 26.4 million foreign-born people resided in the United States, representing nearly 10% of the total U.S. population (Brittingham, 2000). Among the foreign-born population, 50.7% were born in Latin American, 27.1% were born in Asia, 16.1% were born in Europe, and the remaining 6.2% were from other areas of the world. The continuing influxes of immigrants contribute to growing diversity in the U.S. population. Regardless of the country of origin, all immigrants confront challenges such as linguistic differences and changes in financial status upon arriving in the United States. The process of immigration can affect health status and behaviors adversely through disruption of social networks; new exposure to racial and class-based discrimination; differential adverse environmental exposures; and adjustment to new language, culture, and values. For example, rates of smoking, alcohol, and illicit drug use tend to increase among Mexicans who immigrate to the United States. In contrast, foreign-born Mexican immigrant women are reported to have better birth outcomes than U.S.-born Mexican women, which may result from such protective factors as strong family support and cultural ties (Hajat, Lucas, & Kington, 2000).

Linguistic Differences

When immigrant women enter health care organizations, their level of English proficiency combined with the provider's potential lack of linguistically and culturally competent health care can lead to the underutilization of use health care services and unintended adverse health outcomes. Marked linguistic diversity exists among these populations. For example, among foreign-born Blacks, most of whom are from island nations such as the Dominican Republic, Haiti, Jamaica, and Trinidad, English proficiency is common. In contrast, more traditional Hispanic immigrants often have limited English proficiency. Similarly, Asian and Pacific Islander women, who emigrate from more than 20 countries, may speak one of more than 1,000 different languages.

Educational Attainment

Educational attainment is one of the most important influences on economic well-being among women and has a profound impact on women's health. Graduating from high school and college significantly improves women's health and well-being by increasing economic security and by providing the literacy skills necessary to navigate the health care system. Conversely, lacking a high school diploma may cause women to have lower earnings, greater difficulty in obtaining health care, and be more likely to engage in substance abuse and suffer from other adverse health consequences. Although the U.S. overall trends reflect a more educated population, significant differences in educational attainment persist with regard to gender and ethnicity or race. Persons with less than a high school education have death rates at least double those with education beyond high school. Nonetheless, the educational attainment of women indicates a dramatic improvement for a group that has historically been less educated, and these differences have been decreasing in recent years. In 1999, the Current Population Survey, a sample of 60,000 households from which data are collected by personal and telephone interviews, reported that, for women 25 to 29 years of age, educational attainment levels exceeded those of men (U.S. Census Bureau, 2000b). For example, 30% of women compared with 27% of men earned a bachelor's degree or higher. Despite the narrowing in educational attainment between women and men, persisting differences among ethnic or racial groups may contribute to restricted employment opportunities and decreased financial solvency for less-educated women. Among women 15 years and older, 34% of Whites, 32% of Blacks, 25% of non-White Hispanics, and 23% of Asians reported obtaining a high school education (U.S. Census Bureau, 2000c). The pattern differs dramatically among women reporting the completion of a bachelor's degree: 25% of Asians, 16% of Whites, 10% of Blacks, and 7% of Hispanics.

Employment

One of the striking social developments of the late 20th century was the dramatic increase in the proportion of women in the labor force. In 1950, one in three women participated in the labor force; however, by 1998, nearly three of every five women of working age were in the labor force (U.S. Census Bureau, 2000d). Among women age 16 and older, the labor force participation rate rose markedly from 40% in 1950 to 60% in 1998. Changes in labor force participation also varied by age. The major increase in labor force participation was among women ages 25 to 34; their rate rose from 34% in 1950 to 76% in 1998. Overall labor force participation growth rates among women are expected to slow, but participation of women will still increase at a faster rate than that of men. As a result, the share of women in the labor force is projected to grow from 46% in 1998 to 48% in 2008 (Fullerton, 1999). Currrent estimates from the U.S. Department of Labor, Bureau of Labor Statistics, are that 56.6% of women age 16 and older are employed; 72% of those age 25–54, 56.5% of those age 55–64, and 11% of those age 65 and older (U.S. Department of Labor, 2007, Table 1). The labor force participation rates of women have been increasing across age groups, except for young and older women. Regardless of gender, the Asian labor force is projected to increase most rapidly, and the Hispanic labor force is projected to be larger than the Black labor force due to faster population growth.

Employment can have beneficial or negative effects on the well-being of women. Previous research reports show inconsistent findings on how employment affects women's health. While some studies report an association between employment and good health as measured by self-esteem, perceived health, and physical functioning (Pugliesi, 1995; Ross & Mirowsky, 1995), others report that excessive strain is associated with poor health (Amick et al., 1998; Brett, Strogatz & Savitz, 1997; Savitz, Brett, Dole, & Tse, 1997). The increase in the percentages of women with children as well as two-parent families who are employed outside the home highlight the importance of child care issues and support systems for women faced with multiple responsibilities.

The United States is one of the few industrialized countries that does not provide paid maternity leave and health benefits guaranteed by law. Although the 1993 Family and Medical Leave Act (FMLA) guarantees unpaid leave to workers in businesses with 50 or more employees, the FMLA disproportionately excludes low-wage workers who often work in smaller businesses (Commission on Family and Medical Leave, 1996). For example, in 1996, nearly half of U.S. working women were not eligible for FMLA protection. Further, among workers eligible for family or medical leave, 64% reported that, although they needed leave, they could not take it because they needed the income. In 1996, the United States dramatically altered its welfare program with the passage of the Personal Responsibility and Work Reconciliation Act (PRWORA), which ended federal administration of welfare and replaced it with block grants to the states. This cash assistance program, known as Temporary Aid to Needy Families (TANF), imposes lifetime limits on benefits, more stringent work requirements, and a host of behavioral mandates. The PRWORA ended entitlement to child care for families that receive welfare and established the Child Care Development Fund block grant; however, the law did not require states to make child care available. Notably, sanctions penalize women for deviation from prescribed behaviors (i.e., mandated immunization, paternity identification, and family planning services) by cutting some or all of their benefits (Chavkin, 1999). Although no federal program is in place to follow women after they stop receiving TANF, state-specific studies have reported on women's subsequent employment and income (Heymann & Earle, 1999; Parrott, 1998; Regenstein, Meyer, & Hicks, 1998). Overall, most women report that they did not receive paid sick leave, paid vacation, or health benefits. The working conditions faced by mothers who had been on welfare previously are in part due to the their significant lower levels of education, which increases the likelihood of their having to work in poorer conditions, including part-time positions that lack benefits (U.S. Department of Health and Human Services, 1998). Essentially, women who leave TANF to work often need to work under conditions that prevent them from fulfilling their parental responsibilities.

Economic Status

Despite increases in income and declines in poverty in 1999, nearly 13% of U.S. women live in poverty (U.S. Census Bureau, 1999). Between 1998 and 1999, median household income increased 2.7 percent, to $40,800. For the first time, households in the United States have sustained five consecutive annual statistically significant increases in their real median income. In addition, the poverty rate fell for the third consecutive year, the lowest poverty rate since 1979. Although the number of poor dropped significantly, from 34.5 million poor in 1998 to 32.3 million poor in 1999, poverty

RACE/ETHNICITY	ALL PERSONS	FEMALE HOUSEHOLDER, NO SPOUSE PRESENT
White	10.5	37.0
Black	24.4	49.8
Asian	11.8	37.4
Hispanic	22.5	50.6
White, non-Hispanic	8.2	30.7

Percentage of People and Families in Poverty by Ethnicity or Race in the United States, 2003

Note. From *Health, United States, 2005* (Table 2, p. 130), by National Center for Health Statistics, 2005, Washington, DC: Author.

has immediate and lasting negative consequences on women's health. Household income inequalities persist by gender and household composition, with one-parent households headed by women experiencing the highest rates of poverty. Female-headed households are at an economic disadvantage relative to male-headed and married couple households, with ethnicity and race modifying the effect of poverty status (see Table 1.1). The real median earnings of men who worked full time, year-round increased by 1% between 1998 and 1999, their third straight annual increase (U.S. Census Bureau, 1999). In contrast, the comparable earnings for women remained unchanged. The combination led to a drop in the ratio of female-to-male earnings for full-time year-round workers to 72%, down from its all-time high of 74% first reached in 1996. This 25% wage gap between men and women is an important indicator of women's economic security, reflecting the economic hurdles women may face that can compromise their health and well-being.

In 1999, the Census Bureau began reporting income and poverty data for American Indians and Alaska Natives; however, given the relatively small sample size, data by gender are not provided. The 3-year average median household income of American Indians and Alaska Natives was $30,800, which was higher than that for Blacks, equal to the income estimate for Hispanics, and lower than the income estimate for Whites, non-Hispanic Whites, and Asians and Pacific Islanders (Weinberg, 2000).

Family Composition

Dramatic changes in family formation and marriage patterns have occurred since the mid-1960s, with increasing proportions of women and men postponing marriage, and also a significant increase in the per-

centage of people who never marry. According to the 1995 National Survey of Family Growth (NSFG), approximately 50% of women 25 to 39 years of age have had an unmarried cohabitation with a man at some time in their life (Abma, Chandra, Mosher, Peterson & Piccinino, 1997). While 57% of these cohabitations resulted in marriage, nearly one-third dissolved, and 10% were reported to have remained intact. Additionally, 30% of the population lives alone or in nonfamily combinations, which include friends, housemates, or partnerships outside legal marriage. An important change in marital status patterns has been the large increase in cohabitation among unmarried couples (Bramlett & Mosher, 2002). From 1990 to 1994, 39% of nonmarital births were to cohabiting couples. In 1998, among those between 25 and 34 years old, about 35% (14 million) had never been married, and among Blacks in this age group, 53% had never been married. Similarly, a substantial increase in the proportion of young women who delay marriage has occurred (Saluter, 1997). In 1994, the median age at first marriage among women was 25 years compared to 27 years among men. Notably, the proportion of married couples that identified the woman as the head of the household tripled from 1990 (7.4%) to 1998 (22.9%). Finally, 45% of women 65 years old and older were widowed.

Caregivers

In addition to contributing solely or significantly to their family's income through employment, many women are the main caregivers of children and aging parents. Given that women disproportionately carry the responsibility for family caregiving, they often put their own health at risk by struggling to meet the demands of both work and family care. According to the NSFG, women 14 to 44 years of age had 1.2 births per woman and were expected to finish their childbearing with an average of 2.2 children (Abma et al., 1997). Women also serve in the role of caregiver to older family members. For example, among noninstitutionalized people 70 years of age and older, 34% reported receiving help formally or informally from a caregiver with at least one activity of daily living. Seventy percent of the 12 million caregivers were women, and a large proportion are unpaid (National Center for Health Statistics, 1999a).

Reproductive Trends

Fertility

The fertility rate relates the number of births to the number of women of childbearing age. In 2002, the overall fertility rate was 64.8 per 1,000 women aged 15 to 44 years in the United States (Sutton, 2003). Fertility rates increased among non-Hispanic Black, non-Hispanic White, American Indian, and Puerto Rican women, whereas fertility rates declined among Asian or Pacific Islander, Mexican, and Cuban women (Ventura, Martin, Curtin, Mathews, & Park, 2000). Overall, fertility rates differed by ethnicity or race, with Hispanic (104.4), American Indian (70.7), and Black (71.0) women having higher fertility rates than White (64.6) and Asian or Pacific Islander (64.0) women.

Birth Rates

The birth rate fell to 14.0 per 1,000 population in 2002 from 14.3 in 2001 (Sutton, 2003). While birth rates among teenagers fell from 2% to 5%, rates for women in their 20s increased from 1% to 2% and for women in their 30s, from 2% to 4%. The proportion of multiple births continued to increase; higher-order multiple births (i.e., triplets, quadruplets) increased by 13%. The percentage of low–birth weight and preterm births increased, which were due in large part to the increases in multiple births.

Nonmarital Childbearing

After rising thirteen fold from 1940 through 1990, the rate of increase of nonmarital childbearing slowed during the 1990s. The birth rate among unmarried women increased between 1990 and 1994 from 43.8 births per 1,000 unmarried women aged 15 to 44 years to 46.9 and then declined (Ventura & Bachrach, 2000). Several key factors contributed to the rise in the number of nonmarital births through 1990, including increased birth rates and steep increases in the number of unmarried women of childbearing age. Also, the number of women of childbearing age (defined as between 15 and 44) increased substantially from the mid-1960s through the early 1990s—reflecting the impact of the baby boom. Further, increasing proportions of women

and men delayed marriage beginning in the 1960s, a trend that is not abating.

Contraception

According to the NSFG, among women who were 14 to 44 years of age, the leading method of contraception was female sterilization (18%), followed by the oral contraceptive pill (17%), the male condom (13%), and male sterilization (7%) (Abma et al., 1997). Three new contraceptive methods that were introduced between 1988 and 1995 were hormonal implants, hormonal injectables, and female condoms. Finally, the proportion of women who are voluntarily childless increased from 4.9% in 1982 to 6.6% in 1995; the percentage of women who were involuntary childless remained at 2%.

HEALTH EXPENDITURES

The United States continues to spend more on health care than any other industrialized country and health spending is increasing rapidly (National Center for Health Statistics, 2005). In 2003, national health care expenditures were an estimated $1.7 trillion. The expenditures for prescription drugs increased more rapidly than any other type of health expenditure. The United States continues to spend a larger proportion of its gross national product on health care than any other major industrialized country. The demographics of expenditures by type of care and source of funding continue to change. Much of the U.S. health care spending is directed to care for chronic diseases and conditions that reflect the aging population.

Major sources of payment for health care in the United States include the government and employers. The government was the primary payer for hospital and nursing home care, paying for about 60% of these services. Private insurers paid for almost half of physician services and prescription drugs. An estimated 18% of the population is uninsured (National Center for Health Statistics, 2005).

HEALTH STATUS INDICATORS

One of the simplest ways to understand health status across populations includes using data on mortality, morbidity, and health services access and utilization. The following health status indicators are selected primarily based on whether they had a marked impact on women's quality of life, functioning, or well-being; affected a large proportion of women or a subgroup of women; or reflected an important emerging health issue. When data are available and differences for key health conditions are notable, we provide prevalence or incidence estimates based on race and ethnicity and gender. Also, given the strong relationship between health and income, which is especially important for women who represent the majority of the poor in the United States, we report health measures by socioeconomic differences when the data are available.

Mortality

Life Expectancy and Mortality Patterns

Life expectancy is a key indicator of health status worldwide, and mortality is the measure of the most

COUNTRY	LIFE EXPECTANCY (YEARS)	RANK
Japan	84.9	1
Hong Kong	84.6	2
Switzerland	83.0	3
Sweden	82.9	4
Spain	82.9	4
Italy	82.8	6
Australia	82.4	7
Canada	82.2	8
Sweden	82.1	9
Israel	81.6	10
Austria	81.5	11
Finland	81.5	11
Norway	81.5	11
Germany	81.3	14
Singapore	81.1	15
Belgium	81.1	15
New Zealand	80.9	17
Netherlands	80.7	18
Greece	80.7	18
England and Wales	80.6	20
Portugal	80.3	21
Northern Ireland	80.1	22
Puerto Rico	80.0	23
Costa Rica	79.9	24
United States	79.8	25

Women's Life Expectancy at Birth for Selected Countries, 2001

Note. From *Health, United States 2005* (Table 26, p. 165), by National Center for Health Statistics, 2005, Washington, DC: Author.

serious women's health event. The life expectancy of U.S. women has nearly doubled since the turn of the 20th century, from 48 years in 1900 to a record high of 80 years in 2001 (Miniño, Arias, Kochanek, Murphy, & Smith, 2002; National Center for Health Statistics, 2005). Overall, women are expected to outlive men by an average of 5.7 years, and Whites are expected to outlive Blacks by an average of 6 years. White women continue to have the highest life expectancy at birth (80.8 years), followed by Black women (76.3 years), White men (75.7 years), and Black men (69.5 years) (National Center for Health Statistics, 2005; National Center for Health Statistics, 2006, Table 27). However, by age 65, these differences narrow and life expectancy was only 1.7 years longer for White women than for Black women and 1.8 years longer for White men than for Black men. Notably, at age 85, the life expectancy for Black persons was higher than for White persons. While some research reports that age misreporting may account for these findings, other research has suggested that Black persons who survive to the oldest ages may in fact be healthier than White persons (National Center for Health Statistics, 1999b). Although the United States has the highest health care expenditures as a percentage of gross domestic product than other developed countries, the life expectancy for women is lower in the United States than in 24 other developed countries (Anders & Poullier, 1999; see Table 1.2). Women from developed countries tend to live longer than men.

Causes of Death

In 1900, the leading causes of mortality among U.S. women included infectious diseases and pregnancy and childbirth. However, in the 20th century, significant progress was made toward increasing the years of life for most Americans, and regardless of ethnicity, race, or gender, Americans live longer than ever before. Presently, the chronic conditions of heart disease, cancer, and stroke account for 63% of U.S. women's deaths and are the leading causes of mortality for both women and men. Although women have a longer life expectancy than men, they do not necessarily live those extra years in good physical and mental health. Age-adjusted death rates per 1000,000 population according to cause of death are given in Table 1.3. Heart disease, malignant neoplasms, and chronic respiratory disease, liver disease, and diabetes mellitus claim a high proportion of women's lives. Human immunodeficiency virus (HIV) is claiming an increasing number of women's lives and is comparable to death rates from homicide. Unintentional injuries and suicides also account for a relatively high number of women's deaths.

Leading causes of death differ by demographic characteristics such as age, gender, race, marital status,

1.3 Age-Adjusted Death Rates per 100,000 Population for Selected Causes of Death for Women, 2003

CAUSE OF DEATH	AGE-ADJUSTED DEATH RATE FOR WOMEN PER 100,000 POPULATION
All causes	706.2
Diseases of the heart	190.3
Ischemic heart disease	127.2
Cerebrovascular diseases	52.3
Malignant neoplasms	160.9
Trachea, bronchus, and lung	41.3
Colon, rectum, and anus	16.2
Breast	25.3
Chronic lower respiratory diseases	37.8
Influenza and pneumonia	19.4
Chronic liver diseases and cirrhosis	6.0
Diabetes mellitus	22.5
HIV	2.4
Unintentional injuries	24.1
Motor vehicle–related injuries	9.3
Suicide	4.2
Homicide	2.6

Note. From *Health, United States, 2005* (Table 29, p. 170), by National Center for Health Statistics, 2005, Washington, DC: Author.

accidents ranked as the second leading cause of death. Stroke, the third leading cause of death for women, was fourth for men, and chronic obstructive pulmonary disease, the fourth leading cause for women, was fifth for men. While fifth in the leading causes of death among women, pneumonia and influenza was sixth among men. Alzheimer's disease, kidney disease, and septicemia were among the 10 leading causes of death for women but not for men; whereas suicide, chronic liver disease, and homicide were lead causes for men but not for women. The female patterns in leading causes of death also differed according to age. For example, for the age group 15 to 24 years, accidents were the leading cause of death, while malignant neoplasms ranked number one among women aged 25 to 64 and heart disease for women 65 years or older.

In 2000, age-adjusted death rates by marital status revealed that those who had never married had the highest mortality, followed by those who were divorced or widowed. In contrast, those who were married at the time of death had the lowest mortality. People who never married had a 70% higher death rate than the ever married. For each marital status group, women had lower death rates than men. Conversely, Black persons in each marital status group were more likely to die than White persons. Finally, for women and men alike, mortality was inversely associated with educational attainment; the average risk of death decreased markedly with increasing educational attainment.

Years of potential life lost before age 75 for selected causes of death provides an indicator of the impact of mortality on women's health. Table 1.4 provides estimates of years of life lost prior to age 75 according to various causes of death for women.

Morbidity

One of the simplest ways to compare health status across populations includes using health data on mortality, morbidity, and health services utilization. Morbidity is a generic measure that assesses the quantity of health in a given population, which is easy to interpret and compare across populations and time. Incidence of specific outcomes such as injuries, chronic conditions, mental illness, and activity limitations are summary measures of morbidity, which are presented in this section.

Injuries

In 1997, 34.4 million medically attended episodes of injury and poisoning were reported among the U.S. civilian noninstitutionalized population (Warner, Barnes, & Fingerhut, 2000). The age-adjusted injury and poisoning episode rate for women was 79% lower than the

and educational attainment. In 2000, 7 of the 10 leading causes of death were the same among U.S. women and men, although there were differences in ranking (Miniño et al., 2002). Heart disease was the number one killer of women, causing more than one-third of all deaths among women. However, heart disease usually occurred 10 years later in life for women than for men. While the heart disease mortality rate was two-thirds higher for Black women than White women, Hispanic, American Indian, and Asian and Pacific Islander women had lower rates than did White women. Except for American Indian women, lung cancer was the second most common cause of death and the leading cause of cancer-related death. American Indian women were unique in that they were the only group among whom

Years of Potential Life Lost Before Age 75 for Women According to Selected Causes of Death, 2003

CAUSE OF DEATH	AGE-ADJUSTED YEARS LOST
All causes	5,560.5
Diseases of the heart	739.5
Ischemic heart disease	415.0
Cerebrovascular diseases	183.0
Malignant neoplasms	1,477.3
Trachea, bronchus, lung	328.1
Colorectal	111.9
Breast	313.7
Chronic lower respiratory disease	169.9
Influenza and pneumonia	76.0
Chronic liver disease and cirrhosis	92.6
Diabetes mellitus	152.9
HIV	84.1
Unintentional injuries	624.6
Motor vehicle–related injuries	339.2
Suicide	136.6
Homicide	112.9

Note. From *Health, United States, 2005* (Table 20, p. 174), by National Center for Health Statistics, 2005, Washington, DC: Author.

rate for men. Falls were the only category of external causes for which the rate for women exceeded that for men (47.2 versus 37.6 per 1,000 persons, respectively). The higher rate of falls among women is likely due to the higher number of women who are older than 45 and especially 65 years and older, for whom the rate of falls for women was twice that for men.

Violence Against Women

Violence is a term that encompasses a broad range of maltreatment against women. Violence and abuse against women refers to the combination of the following five major components of such maltreatment: physical violence, sexual violence, threats of physical and/or sexual violence, stalking, and psychological/emotional abuse (Centers for Disease Control and Prevention, 2000a). Physical violence, sexual violence, and threats of physical and/or sexual violence comprise the narrower category of violence against women. Available data suggest that violence against women is a significant public health problem in the United States. Despite estimates that approximately 55% of women

have been physically assaulted or raped in their life time, a significant lack of reliable and consistent data are collected at the national and state levels. Law enforcement data indicate that 3,419 women died in 1998 as a result of homicide, and approximately one-third of these women were murdered by a spouse, ex-spouse, or boyfriend (Centers for Disease Control and Prevention, 2000a). Survey data collected during 1995–1996 suggests that 2.1 million women are physically assaulted or raped annually and that 1.5 million of these assaults or rapes were by a current or former intimate partner (Tjaden & Thoennes, 1998). In 1998, based on survey data from the Bureau of Justice Statistics' National Crime Victimization Survey, women were victims in nearly 900,000 violent crimes committed by an intimate partner. Although these data indicate the high prevalence of the problem, reporting of violence against women remains inconsistent. While some experts believe that studies overestimate the extent of violence against women, others believe that there is underestimation. To date, no national studies report on women who are immigrants, homeless, disabled, or in the military or other institutionalized situations, which may be populations at significantly greater risk of violence against women.

Emerging Infections

Infectious diseases continue to affect all people, regardless of gender, age, ethnic background, lifestyle, and socioeconomic status. They cause suffering and death and impose an enormous financial burden in the United States. Many infectious diseases have been conquered by modern interventions such as vaccines and antibiotics. New diseases are constantly emerging, including severe acute respiratory syndrome, Lyme disease, and hantavirus pulmonary syndrome; others reemerge in drug resistant forms, including malaria, tuberculosis, and bacterial pneumonias. Among women, populations of particular concern include pregnant women, immigrants, and refugees. For example, if a pregnant woman acquires an infection, it can increase the infant's risk of preterm delivery, low birth weight, long-term disability, or death. While many of these adverse birth outcomes could be prevented by prenatal care, access to and utilization of prenatal care is disparate by race and ethnicity and socioeconomic status. For example, infants born to American Indian and Black women have the highest neonatal death rates due to infectious diseases than any other group (Centers for Disease Control and Prevention, 2000b).

HIV

In 2000, the Centers for Disease Control and Prevention estimated that between 120,000 and 160,000 adult and adolescent females were living with HIV infection, including those with AIDS (Centers for Disease Control and Prevention, 2000c). Between 1992 and 1998, the number of persons living with AIDS increased in all groups as a result of the 1993 expanded AIDS case definition and, more recently, improved survival among those who have benefited from the new combination drug therapies. During that 6-year period, a growing proportion of women were living with AIDS, reflecting the ongoing trend in populations affected by the epidemic. In 1992, women accounted for 14% of persons living with AIDS; however, by 1998, the proportion had grown to 20%. Thus, in just over a decade, the proportion of all AIDS cases reported among adult and adolescent women more than tripled, from 7% in 1985 to 23% in 1999. The epidemic has increased most dramatically among Black and Hispanic women. Although Black and Hispanic women represent less than one-fourth of all U.S. women, they accounted for more than three-fourths (77%) of AIDS cases reported to date among women. In 1999, the incidence of AIDS for Black persons 13 years of age and older was 2.4 times the rate for Hispanics in the same age group, over 7 times the rate for American Indians or Alaska Natives, over 9 times the rate for non-Hispanic White people, and 20 times the rate for Asians or Pacific Islanders. Notably, the AIDS epidemic is far from over. Cases of HIV infection reported among 13- to 24-year-olds, of whom nearly 50% are female, are increasing for this age group who had reported recent high-risk behavior. (Table 1.5 includes data about the distribution of HIV/AIDS by race and Hispanic origin.)

Chronic Conditions

Chronic conditions are often debilitating and contribute significantly to key causes of death among women. There is a complex and long-term interplay between chronic conditions and health across a woman's life span. Although women live longer than men, women also experience greater morbidity at younger ages and utilize health services at higher rates than men. In 1995, the National Health Interview Survey (NHIS) reported that, as women progress from childbearing ages through menopause and to postmenopause years, the prevalence of chronic conditions increases, with an associated shift to conditions linked to environmental factors (National Center for Health Statistics, 1997). Overall, the pattern and magnitude of chronic conditions vary markedly by gender. Women were more likely to report arthritis, cataracts, orthopedic impairment, goiter or thyroid disease, diabetes, hypertension, varicose veins, chronic bronchitis, asthma, and chronic sinusitis; men were more likely to report visual impairment, hearing impairment, and heart disease.

The burden of chronic diseases occurs disproportionately among poor women. Chronic conditions are reported more frequently by low-income and less-educated women (Misra, 1999). Based on NHIS data, low income was correlated with the occurrence of

1.5 | Acquired Immunodeficiency Syndrome: Distribution by Sex, Age, Race, and Hispanic Origin

CHARACTERISTICS	NUMBER OF CASES DIAGNOSED IN 2003	PERCENT DISTRIBUTION
All persons	43,171	
Female, 13 years and older	11,498	26.6
Male, 13 years and older	31,614	73.2
Children, under 13 years	59	0.1
Not Hispanic or Latino: White	12,222	28.3
Black or African American	21,304	49.3
American Indian or Alaska Native	196	0.5
Asian or Pacific Islander	497	1.2
Hispanic or Latino	8,757	20.3

Note. From *Health, United States, 2005* (Table 52, p. 232), by National Center for Health Statistics, 2005, Washington, DC: Author.

diabetes, asthma, hypertension, and thyroid disease (National Center for Health Statistics, 1997). Additionally, the differences in chronic conditions by racial and ethnic populations can differ dramatically. For example, American Indians or Alaska Natives were three times more likely to have had diabetes and end-stage renal disease than Asians or Pacific Islanders and six times more likely to have had these conditions than Whites. Blacks were twice as likely as Asians or Pacific Islanders to have diabetes and end-stage renal disease and four times more likely to have these conditions than Whites (U.S. Department of Health and Human Services, 2000a). Similarly, breast cancer, which is the most common form of malignancy in U.S. women, has racial disparities. Although 12% to 29% more White women than Black women are diagnosed with breast cancer, Black women are 28% more likely than White women to die from the disease. Also, the 5-year breast cancer survival rate is 69% among Black women compared with 85% for White women. Table 1.6 displays the distribution of cancer by site and by race. Table 1.7 gives the incidence of selected chronic illnesses for women. Table 1.8 includes data about limitations related to

chronic illness, self-assessed health status, and severe psychological distress.

Mental Illness

Mental illnesses affect women and men differently. Scientists are only beginning to understand the contribution of various biological and psychosocial factors to mental health and mental illness in both women and men. Research on women's health—which has grown substantially in the last 20 years—helps to clarify the risk and protective factors for mental disorders in women and to improve women's mental health treatment outcomes. In the United States, nearly 12.4 million women (12.0%) and 6.4 million men (6.6%) are affected by a depressive disorder each year. Depressive disorders include major depression, dysthymic disorder (a less severe but more chronic form of depression), and bipolar disorder (manic-depressive illness). Notably, major depression is the leading cause of disease burden among females ages 5 and older worldwide. The first Surgeon General's report on mental health underscores the close relationship between mental and

1.6 | Age-Adjusted Cancer Incidence Rates for Selected Cancer Sites: Number of New Cases per 100,000 Population, 2002

CANCER SITE	WHITE	BLACK OR AFRICAN AMERICAN	AMERICAN INDIAN OR ALASKA NATIVE	ASIAN OR PACIFIC ISLANDER	HISPANIC OR LATINO	WHITE, NOT HISPANIC OR LATINO
Cancer, all sites	418.2	399.5	189.4	308.1	305.9	432.5
Lung/bronchus	49.9	54.3	*	28.4	21.6	52.7
Colon/rectum	44.2	43.2	54.2	40.7	30.3	44.3
Breast	135.8	119.3	47.9	97.4	88.5	144.2
Cervix	8.1	9.6	*	8.1	14.4	6.6
Corpus uteri	24.4	21.9	*	18.6	17.0	25.0
Ovary	14.0	9.4	*	11.6	13.1	14.0
Oral cavity	6.4	6.1	*	5.8	3.8	6.7
Stomach	4.9	9.6	*	10.8	9.9	4.1
Pancreas	9.6	15.2	*	8.7	9.8	9.4
Urinary bladder	10.0	8.2	*	3.1	6.0	10.5
Non-Hodgkins lymphoma	16.7	11.4	*	11.5	12.8	17.0
Leukemia	9.3	7.0	*	6.0	7.6	9.1

Note. From *Health, United States, 2005* (Table 52, pp. 234–236), by National Center for Health Statistics, 2005, Washington, DC: Author.
* = data not available.

Chronic Conditions Among Women 20 Years and Older: Percent of Population With Diagnosis, 1999–2002

CHRONIC CONDITION	PERCENT OF POPULATION
Diabetes	8.5
Diagnosed	6.3
Undiagnosed	2.2
Respiratory	
Asthma	5.0
Sinusitis	17.6
Hay fever	9.6
Pain conditions	
Severe headache or migraine	20.6
Low back pain	28.3
Neck pain	15.7
Vision and hearing limitations	
Trouble seeing, even with glasses or contacts	10.4
A lot of trouble hearing or deaf	2.4

Note. From *Heatlh, United States, 2005* (Tables 55, 56, 57, 58, and 59), by National Center for Health Statistics, 2005, Washington, DC: Author

Indicators of Health Status: Respondent-Assessed Health Status, Serious Psychological Distress, and Limitation of Activity Caused by Chronic Illness, 2002–2003

INDICATOR	PERCENTAGE OF WOMEN
Limitation of activity caused by chronic conditions	12.3
Self-assessed fair or poor health	9.5
Serious psychological distress	3.9

Note. From *Health, United States, 2005* (Tables 59, 60, and 61), by National Center for Health Statistics, 2005, Washington, DC: Author.

ment. Among all areas of health, the mental health field is beset by disparities in the availability of and access to services occurring by means of financial barriers and stigmatization. While women are more likely to be affected by Alzheimer's disease, depression, and panic disorders, men are more likely to be affected by attention deficit hyperactivity disorder, and both are equally likely to experience obsessive-compulsive disorders (U.S. Department of Health and Human Services, 1999). Although depression is not the only mental illness that affects women more often than men, it is significant due to its common occurrence, recurrence, and effect on functioning. The prevalence of depression among women has been reported to range from 6% to 11% for a 1-month risk of a major depressive episode, with a lifetime risk of major depression as high as 21% (Ruderman & O'Campo, 1999). Depression has been reported to be more common among Hispanic and Black women than among White women; however, most studies have not accounted for the important influence of income, education, and marital status. Further, data from a U.S. nationally representative sample on depression provided evidence that depression was more prevalent among those in lower socioeconomic strata, particularly women (Blazer, Kessler, McGonagle, & Swartz, 1994).

Anxiety disorders—which include panic disorder, obsessive-compulsive disorder, post-traumatic stress disorder, phobias, and generalized anxiety disorder—affect an estimated 13.3 percent of Americans ages 18 to 54 in a given year. Except for obsessive-compulsive disorder and social phobia, women outnumber men in each illness category. The main risk factor for developing Alzheimer's disease—a dementing brain disorder that leads to the loss of mental and physical functioning and eventually to death—is increased age. While the number of new cases of Alzheimer's disease is similar in older adult women and men, the number of existing cases is somewhat higher among women. Caregivers of people with Alzheimer's disease are usually wives and daughters, and the chronic stress often associated with the caregiving role can contribute to mental health problems. Because women in general are at greater risk for depression than men, and since caregivers are much more likely to suffer from depression than the average person, women caregivers of people with Alzheimer's disease may be particularly vulnerable to depression.

Eating Disorders

Eating disorders primarily affect women—90% of eating disorders are diagnosed among adolescent girls and young adult women. Eating disorders such as anorexia or bulimia may have potentially serious medical complications, yet they often go undetected and untreated.

physical health (U.S. Department of Health and Human Services, 1999). Mental disorders such as schizophrenia, depression and bipolar disorders, Alzheimer's disease, and obsessive compulsive disorders affect nearly one in five Americans each year. Nearly 70% of adults with a diagnosed mental disorder do not receive treat-

In fact, eating disorders have one of the highest death rates of any mental disorder among women. Although the prevalence of eating disorders is particularly difficult to measure because of the underlying denial and secretive nature of the behavior, the survey data suggest prevalence rates of 1% to 3% among the female population.

Activity Limitations

Women's quality of life is affected by their ability to carry out daily activities at work, at home, and in the community. Adverse health affects all aspects of women's lives, particularly their ability to engage in daily activities. Activity limitation due to a physical, mental, or emotional health problem is a broad measure of health functioning for women (see Table 1.8). In 1997, women were nearly twice as likely as men to report activity limitation (17% compared with 9%). Activity limitation due to chronic condition was substantially higher among women with lower family incomes.

Health Care Access and Utilization

Women in the United States obtain health care services through a variety of sources. Numerous factors affect women's access to health care services, including affordability and availability of services and whether women have information about how and why it is important to access and utilize such services. Given the consolidation of the health care system, the shift to managed care, and decreased public funding of health care and health-related programs, the changes in health care delivery have serious implications for women's health care utilization. Although women commonly enter the health care delivery system for pregnancy prevention or pregnancy-related services, these reproductive health services typically are provided separately from other aspects of women's health care. The number of health services organizations for women include private- and public-sector groups. For women, the fragmentation of care, lack of coordination of services, and discontinuities in the health care delivery system contribute to higher costs to individual women and both deficiencies and excesses in care (Clancy & Massion, 1992).

Access to health care is important for preventive care and for prompt treatment of illness and injuries. Indicators of health care access and utilization include use of preventive services, outpatient care, and inpatient care—all of which vary by health insurance status, poverty status, race, and ethnicity. Women's access to health care services is seriously compromised by inadequate health insurance, and women without health insurance generally cannot obtain appropriate health care. Despite the Healthy People 2010 objective that all people

in the United States have health insurance coverage, in 2000 nearly 15% of U.S. women were uninsured (U.S. Department of Health and Human Services, 2000b). While little is known about how women obtain basic health care in the United States, national survey data report that women are more likely than men to have a usual source of care, have more outpatient visits, have more hospital stays (even excluding maternity stays), use home health services, and to use nursing homes.

Publicly Funded Health Programs

The two major publicly funded health programs are Medicare and Medicaid. Medicare, which is funded by the federal government and reimburses the elderly and disabled for their health care, had 38.8 million enrollees and expenditures of $213 billion in 1998. In contrast, Medicaid, which is funded jointly by federal and state governments to provide health care for the poor, had 40.6 million recipients and spent $142 billion during the same time period. Although Medicaid eligibility and benefits vary by state, Medicare and Medicaid health care utilization and costs often vary dramatically by state. For example, Medicare payments per enrollee ranged from $3,800 in Vermont to more than $6,700 in Louisiana. Among the 40.6 million Medicaid recipients, 41.3% were White, 24% Black, 16% Hispanic, 2.5% Asian or Pacific Islander, and 1% American Indian or Alaskan Native.

Privately Funded Health Care

Approximately 70% of the U.S. population has private health insurance, most of which is obtained through the work place. As the health insurance marketplace continues to rapidly change as new types of managed care products emerge, the share of employee's total compensation for health insurance and the use of traditional fee-for-service medical care continues to decline markedly. For example, among employees of medium and large companies, 27% of participating full-time employees were in fee-for-service plans in 1997, down from 67% in 1991 (National Center for Health Statistics, 2000). Conversely, health maintenance enrollment has been steadily increasing and has doubled since 1993. Although women and men report similar levels of enrollment for private insurance, enrollment varies significantly by race and ethnicity and poverty status (see Table 1.9).

Prevention Services

Use of prevention services has substantial positive effects on the long-term health status of women who receive the services. The use of several different types of preventive services has been increasing; however, disparities in their use of these interventions according

Men's and Women's Health Insurance Status, 2003

CHARACTERISTICS	PERCENTAGE OF POPULATION WITH PRIVATE HEALTH INSURANCE	PERCENTAGE OF POPULATION WITH MEDICAID	PERCENTAGE OF POPULATION WITH NO HEALTH INSURANCE
Female	68.9	13.6	15.8
Male	69.0	10.9	17.7

Note. From *Health, United States, 2005* (Tables 132, 133, and 134), by National Center for Health Statistics, 2005, Washington, DC: Author.

to income and by race and ethnicity persist among all persons. The importance of promoting wellness and preventing illness among women involves screening for conditions such as breast cancer, cervical cancer, and colorectal cancer. Regular mammography screening for women aged 50 years and older is effective in reducing deaths from breast cancer. In 1998, 69% of women aged 50 years and older reported mammography screening in the previous 2-year period, up from 61% in 1994 (National Center for Health Statistics, 2000). Among women living below the poverty level, 53% reported recent screening compared with 72% of women with family income at or above poverty level. Additionally, the percentage of women 40 years of age and older who reported having a mammogram in the last 2 years was highest for non-Hispanic Whites (68.1%) and Blacks (65.9%), lower among Asian or Pacific Islanders (60.7%) and Hispanics (60.5%), and lowest for American Indians or Alaskan Natives (44.6%) (U.S. Department of Health and Human Services, 2000a). Similarly, although all groups of women increased their use of the Pap test, the percentage of women 18 years of age and older who reported having a Pap test within the previous 3 years differed by race and ethnicity. The reported prevalence was as follows: non-Hispanic Black women, 83%; non-Hispanic White women, 80%; Hispanic women, 74%; American Indian or Alaskan Native women, 72%; and Asian or Pacific Islander women, 67%. Finally, colorectal cancer is the third leading cause of cancer-related deaths among women after lung and breast cancer. Although early detection and treatment can substantially reduce the risks associated with colorectal cancer for people aged 50 and older, only 37.7% of women received colorectal cancer screening in 1999. (Table 1.10 includes data for the use of mammography and Pap smears according to selected characteristics.)

Outpatient Care

Important changes in the delivery of health care in the United States are driven in large part by the need to contain rising health care costs. One significant change has been a decline in the use of inpatient services and an increase in outpatient services such as outpatient surgery and hospice care. Most women obtain health services from private physicians; however, women also obtain reproductive health services and routine care from public-sector organizations and private organizations that are funded with public funds. Generally, publicly funded health services target women with low incomes or who are otherwise disadvantaged. In 1998, according to the National Ambulatory Medical Care Survey, women comprised 51% of the U.S. population but made 60.2% of all outpatient department visits relative to men, who made 39.8% of visits. Women of all ages made 32.9 visits per 100 persons per year, compared with 22.8 for men (Slusarcick & McCaig, 2000). Also, outpatient visit rates for Blacks (51.8 per 100 persons per year) were higher than for Whites (24.8), Asian and Pacific Islanders (22.1), and American Indians (7.9).

Although women frequently enter the health care delivery system with reproductive health concerns, they seldom benefit from primary care that is comprehensive and coordinated. Regardless of the type of provider or reason for accessing care, women's health care delivery in the United States remains fragmented. An estimated 80% of women report that they have a usual source of care, which is predominately in physician offices; however, the comprehensiveness of primary care content is poorly understood and varies by type of provider (Rosenblatt, Hart, & Gamliel, 1995). Among physician providers, family practitioners, general internists, and obstetrician-gynecologists provide the majority of basic health care to women; however, women may rely on multiple providers (Bartman & Weiss, 1993). For example, 33% of women aged 18 and older reported seeing an obstetrician-gynecologist and additional primary care provider for their regular care. Women who used two or more physicians for regular care were more likely to be younger, have private insurance, and have higher income than women who used only one physician. Also, these women were more likely to have more annual

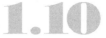 | Screening Services: Use of Mammography and Pap Smears by Selected Characteristics, 2003

CHARACTERISTICS	PERCENTAGE OF WOMEN HAVING MAMMOGRAM IN PAST 2 YEARS	PERCENTAGE OF WOMEN HAVING PAP SMEAR IN PAST 3 YEARS
Age		
18–44 years		83.9
45–64 years		81.3
65 and older		60.8
40–49	64.4	
50–64	76.2	
65–74	74.6	
75 and older	60.6	
Race		
White only	70.1	78.7
Black/African American	70.4	84.0
American Indian/Alaska Native only	63.1	84.8
Asian only	57.6	68.3
Native Hawaiian and other Pacific Islander only	*	*
Two or more races	65.3	81.6
Hispanic origin		
Hispanic or Latino	65.0	75.4
Not Hispanic or Latino	70.1	79.5
White only	70.5	79.3
Black or African American only	70.5	83.8
Poverty status		
Poor	55.4	70.5
Near poor	60.8	71.4
Not poor	74.3	83.0
Insurance status	Women 40–64 years	Women 18–64 years
Private insurance	76.3	87.0
Medicaid	63.5	82.8
Uninsured	41.5	66.6

Note. From *Health, United States, 2005* (Tables 86 and 87), by National Center for Health Statistics, 2005, Washington, DC: Author.
* = data not given.

visits and receive more clinical preventive services. Among women who relied on only one physician, 39% reported using a family practitioner or an internist, 16% used an obstetrician-gynecologist, 3% used a specialist, and 10% had no regular physician (Weisman, Cassard, & Plichta, 1995). Finally, despite estimates that over 100,000 advanced practice nurses deliver primary health care, less than 2% of women report using nonphysician providers as a regular source of care (Weisman et al., 1995). While approximately 7,000 midwives attended 7.4% of U.S. births in 1998, no data are available on the proportion of outpatient primary care that they provided (Ventura et al., 2000). Table 1.11 gives data related to women's use of outpatient services.

In 1996, an estimated 59,400 persons received hospice care in the United States. Hospice care is defined as a program of palliative and supportive care services that provides physical, psychological, social, and spiritual care for dying persons, their families, and loved ones. Findings from the 1996 National Home and Hospice Care Survey revealed significant differences in patient characteristics by gender (Haupt, 1998). For example, more patients were women (55%), and, among the patients who are 85 years of age or older, there was a higher proportion of women than men (27.8% vs. 13.4%). The differences in marital status between women and men were reflected in both their living arrangements and in their relationship to their primary caregivers. A significantly larger percentage of women than men lived alone (30% vs. 6%). While most men were cared for by a spouse, lived with family members, and had a primary care person with whom they lived, women were more likely to live alone or with non–family members. Notably, the primary caregiver of most women was a

relative other than a spouse—most often a child or child-in-law. Table 1.12 includes data related to women's use of hospice and home care services. There is a striking increase in the use of each service as women age. The most common admission diagnoses for home health care include malignant neoplasms; diabetes; disease of the nervous system and sense organs, circulatory, respiratory, and musculoskeletal systems; decubitus ulcers; and fractures. Primary admission diagnoses for hospice care include malignant neoplasms and diseases of the heart and respiratory system.

Inpatient Care

Hospitalization is dependent not only on a woman's medical condition, but also her ability to access and use ambulatory health care. Delaying or not receiving timely and appropriate care for chronic conditions and other

1.11 | Women's Use of Outpatient Services, 2003: Number of Visits per 100 Persons

AGE	ALL PLACES	PHYSICIAN'S OFFICES	HOSPITAL OUTPATIENT	HOSPITAL EMERGENCY DEPARTMENTS
Under 18 years	297	223	36	38
18–44 years	396	309	41	47
45–54 years	474	403	38	33
55–64 years	561	486	45	30
65–74 years	697	613	45	39
75 years and older	830	730	37	63

Note. From *Health, United States, 2005* (Table 88), by National Center for Health Statistics, 2005, Washington, DC: Author

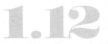 | Women's Use of Home Health Care, Hospice, and Nursing Home Services, 2000

AGE	HOME HEALTH CARE PATIENTS (NUMBER OF PATIENTS PER 10,000 POPULATION)	HOSPICE PATIENTS (NUMBER OF PATIENTS PER 10,000 POPULATION)	NURSING HOME RESIDENTS (NUMBER PER 1,000 POPULATION)
Total	61.8	4.3	54.6
Under 65 years	17.2	0.9	—
65–74 years	154.6	7.6	11.2
75–84 years	400.4	23.3	51.2
85 years and older	754.9	66.2	210.5

Note. From *Health, United States, 2005* (Tables 94, 95, and 102, pp. 322–324, 339), by National Center for Health Statistics, 2005, Washington, DC: Author.

health problems may lead to the development of more serious health conditions that require hospitalization. Utilization of inpatient services has declined, as has the number of beds in community hospitals. The National Hospital Discharge Survey is the principal source of national data on the characteristics of patients discharged from nonfederal short-stay hospitals. Hospital discharge rates are higher among poor persons than among those with higher family incomes. For example, in 1998, hospital discharge rates for the poor were double those for persons with family incomes above twice the poverty level (National Center for Health Statistics, 2000). Compared with men, women were hospitalized more frequently (1,385.3 vs. 934.7 per 10,000 population) but had shorter average lengths of stay (4.7 vs. 5.5 days per 20,000 population) (Hall & Popovic, 2000). The pattern of diagnoses and procedures varied between women and men in large part because of hospitalizations for pregnancy-related causes (including deliveries and diagnoses associated with pregnancy) (see Tables 1.13 and 1.14). Hysterectomy, the second most common major

operation, occurs in over 30% of women by age 60, with annual costs exceeding $5 billion.

In 1997, approximately 1.5 million elderly lived in nursing homes on an average day in the United States. As more people live to the oldest ages and because many debilitating illnesses such as diabetes, dementia, and osteoporosis increase with age, the number of elderly nursing home residents will continue to grow and issues surrounding long-term care will become increasingly important. According to findings from the 1997 National Nursing Home Survey, the majority of nursing home residents were White, widowed, and functionally dependent women (Gabrel, 2000). The leading admission diagnosis for elderly nursing home residents (both men and women) were diseases of the circulatory system, followed by mental disorders. However, the average length of time since admission for women (907 days) and unmarried persons (1,318 days) was longer than for men (761) or married persons (596 days). Table 1.13 includes information about women's use of nursing home care.

1.13 Rate of Discharges From Short-Stay Hospitals and Days of Care for Women by Age and Selected First-Listed Diagnosis, 2003

AGE AND FIRST-LISTED DIAGNOSIS	NUMBER OF CASES PER 1,000 POPULATION	DAYS OF CARE	AVERAGE LENGTH OF STAY (DAYS)
All ages	135.1	605.2	4.5
Under 18 years	42.2	190.9	4.5
Pneumonia	4.5		
Asthma	2.3		
Injuries and poisonings	3.6		
Fractures	1.1		
18–44 years	135.2	444.2	3.3
HIV infection	0.3		
Delivery	69.5		
Alcohol and drug	1.9		
Serious mental illness	6.0		
Diseases of the heart	1.8		
Intervertebral disc disorders	1.1		
Injuries and poisonings	4.8		
Fractures	1.0		
45–64 years	116.5	560.9	4.8
HIV infection	—		
Malignant neoplasms	6.4		
Diabetes	2.8		
Alcohol and drug	1.6		
Serious mental illness	5.4		

1.13 | Rate of Discharges From Short-Stay Hospitals and Days of Care for Women by Age and Selected First-Listed Diagnosis, 2003 (*continued*)

AGE AND FIRST-LISTED DIAGNOSIS	NUMBER OF CASES PER 1,000 POPULATION	DAYS OF CARE	AVERAGE LENGTH OF STAY (DAYS)
Diseases of the heart	14.1		
Cerebrovascular diseases	3.0		
Pneumonia	3.9		
Injuries and poisonings	8.8		
Fractures	2.0		
65–74 years	255.5	1,398.4	5.5
Malignant neoplasms	14.5		
Diabetes	5.1		
Serious mental illness	4.4		
Diseases of the heart	48.0		
Cerebrovascular diseases	11.1		
Pneumonia	11.8		
Osteoarthritis	13.2		
Injuries and poisonings	18.5		
Fractures of hip	2.8		
75 years and over	470.5	2,734.8	5.8
Malignant neoplasms	15.9		
Diabetes	6.2		
Serious mental illness	3.3		
Diseases of the heart	97.2		
Cerebrovascular diseases	24.5		
Pneumonia	29.7		
Osteoarthritis	10.6		
Injuries and poisonings	46.2		
Fracture of the hip	15.5		

Note. From *Health, United States, 2005* (Table 96, pp. 329–331, and Table 99, pp. 332–334), by National Center for Health Statistics, 2005, Washington, DC: Author.

Health Behaviors

All people engage in behaviors that are either helpful or harmful to themselves and others, with consequences to their health and well-being that will have both immediate and long-term effects. Many of these patterns of behavior are associated with morbidity and mortality. Exercising, not smoking, not using drugs, drinking alcohol in moderation, and good nutrition can improve or maintain women's general health and well-being and can also reduce the risk of selected morbidities and the consequences of such morbidities.

Physical Activity

The 1996 Surgeon General's report on physical activity and health reported that three-quarters of U.S. adults exercise during their leisure time (U.S. Department of Health and Human Services, 1996). Despite the implementation of the 1972 Title IX Education Amendment, which provides for equal opportunity for women in school sporting activities, one-third of women report no leisure-time physical activity. Women's multiple roles in the work place and at home compete with leisure-time physical activity.

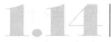 | Hospital Stays With at Least One Procedure, According to Age and Selected Procedures, 2002–2003

AGE AND PROCEDURE CATEGORY	NUMBER PER 10,000 POPULATION	NUMBER IN 1,000S
18 years and older	1076.2	12,199
Cardiac catheterization	42.2	
Insertion, replacement, removal, and revision of pacemaker leads or device	9.1	
Incision, excision, and occlusion of vessels	61.1	
Angiocardiography using contrast	35.8	
Operations on vessels of heart	25.4	
Diagnostic procedures on small intestine	47.8	
Diagnostic procedures on large intestine	28.3	
Diagnostic radiology	35.6	
Diagnostic ultrasound	32.2	
Joint replacement, lower extremity	39.3	
Reduction of fracture or dislocation	23.6	
Excision or destruction of intervertebral disc	12.9	
Cholecystectomy	24.4	
Lysis of peritoneal adhesions	24.1	
18–44 years		
Cesarean section and removal of fetus	191.0	5,757
Forceps, vacuum, and breech delivery	55.6	
Other procedures inducing or assisting delivery	399.5	
Dilation and curettage of uterus	7.1	
Total abdominal hysterectomy	36.5	
Vaginal hysterectomy	18.8	

Note. From *Health, United States, 2005* (Table 100, pp. 334–336), by National Center for Health Statistics, 2005, Washington, DC: Author

Women's participation in moderate-intensity activities of at least 30 minutes duration on most days of the week are associated with numerous health benefits, including decreased risk of cardiovascular disease, non–insulin-dependent diabetes mellitus, osteoporosis, obesity, and depression (Bowman & Spangler, 1997; Bryner, Toffle, Ulrich, & Yeater, 1997; Buckworth, Dishman, & Cureton, 1994; Manson et al., 1991). In contrast, unintended adverse health consequences can result from physical activity. For example, exercise undertaken incorrectly can lead to musculoskeletal injuries and metabolic abnormalities. Also, excessive exercise among girls during puberty can result in the "female athlete triad": disordered eating, amenorrhea, and osteoporosis (Jacobs Institute of Women's Health, 1998).

Nutrition

Given the established relationship between nutrition and health, the majority of health promotion behavior changes are nutrition related. The nutritional status of adult women is the culmination of nutrient intake, metabolism, and utilization over their life span. Research shows that women reporting dietary patterns that include fruits, vegetables, whole grains, low-fat dairy, and lean meats, as recommended by current dietary guidelines, have a lower risk of mortality and have associated improved health outcomes (Kant, Schatzkin, Graubard, & Schairer, 2000; Kant, Schatzkin, Harris, Ziegler, & Block, 1993). However, women's eating patterns are affected by numerous societal factors that reflect the cultural and socioeconomic landscape of the 21st century. These factors include increased employment outside the home, consumption of convenience foods, meals eaten away from home, single woman–headed households, and tobacco use (Johnson, 1996). For many reasons such as professional fulfillment, economic necessity, and TANF, women of all age groups are employed and thus burdened by the multiple responsibilities of employment, child care, and home management, which leaves minimal time and energy to prepare well-balanced, home-cooked meals for themselves and their families. Because nutrition is a modifiable factor for numerous chronic diseases, the Healthy People 2010 Nutritional Initiative includes objectives that concern weight gain, obesity, dietary intake, and nutrients (folate, calcium and iron), which directly impact women's health.

Sexual Activity

In 1995, approximately 50% of women aged 15 to 19 reported that they had ever had heterosexual intercourse, which was a decline from the 55% reported in 1990 (Abma et al., 1997). Among women 14 to 44 years of age, 20% reported that they had been forced by a man to have intercourse against their will at some time in their lives, and 35% of women who were divorced or separated reported they had been forced to have intercourse. Among unmarried women, 14% reported they had had four or more sexual partners between 1991 and 1995. These statistics provide health professionals with information about the potential risks of sexual exposure for women as they relate to sexually transmitted infections and violence.

Substance Abuse

Substance abuse may have a profound impact on the current and future health of women. Women who use illicit substances are more likely to have poor nutrition and serious morbidity and to have died from drug overdose, suicide, and violence. Further, studies report an increased risk of mental disorders, including major depression, anxiety disorders, and post-traumatic stress disorder (Kessler et al., 1997). Rates of substance use and choice of substance varies by gender, age, race and ethnicity, educational attainment, and poverty status. In 1998, lifetime and current rates of illicit substance abuse were lower for women than for men (National Center for Health Statistics, 2000). Notably, among women, the peak age for use of illicit substances occurs during the childbearing years of 18 to 35, whereas the lowest rates are reported among women 50 years and older. White women reported a greater lifetime use of any illicit drug, marijuana, cocaine, hallucinogenic, inhalant, and psychotherapeutic than Hispanic and non-Hispanic Black women (see Table 1.15)

In 1998, 62% of adults 18 years of age and older reported they were current drinkers, 22% reported they were lifetime abstainers, and 16% were former drinkers (National Center for Health Statistics, 2000). Although women were twice as likely as men to be lifetime abstainers, women appear to suffer more severe consequences than men do after shorter duration of less alcohol intake. Finally, among women of childbearing age, 21% report binge drinking.

Cigarette smoking is the major preventable cause of mortality among adult women and leads to an increased risk of cancer, heart disease, stroke, reproductive health problems, and pulmonary conditions. Once women start smoking, they continue to smoke for a number of reasons, including nicotine addiction, stress management, to combat depression, and weight management. Women are less likely to report smoking than men, with approximately one in four women reportedly smoking (see Table 1.16). In 1998, among women, the prevalence of smoking was highest among American Indian women (29%) and lowest among Hispanic women (14%) and Asian women (11%). Notably, except for among Hispanic women, the prevalence of smoking

1.15 | Use of Selected Substances in the Past Month by Women 12 Years and Older, 2003

CHARACTERISTICS	ANY ILLICIT DRUG	MARIJUANA	NONMEDICAL USE OF PSYCHOTHER-APEUTIC DRUG	ALCOHOL USE	BINGE ALCOHOL USE	HEAVY ALCOHOL USE
Age 12–17	6.5	4.4	2.6	18.3	10.1	**2.3**
Age 18 and older				55.2		**7.4**

Note. From *Health, United States, 2005* (Table 66, pp. 259–260, and Table 68, pp. 264–266), by National Center for Health Statistics, 2005, Washington, DC: Author.

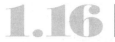 | Percentages of Women Who Are Current Cigarette Smokers According to Age and Race

AGE	ALL WOMEN	WHITE	BLACK OR AFRICAN AMERICAN
18–24 years	21.5	23.6	10.8
25–34 years	21.3	22.5	17.0
35–44 years	24.2	25.2	23.2
45–64 years	20.2	20.1	23.3
65 years and older	8.3	8.4	8.0

Note. From *Health, United States, 2005* (Table 63, p. 154), by National Center for Health Statistics, 2005, Washington, DC: Author

decreased markedly as women attained more education or were of higher socioeconomic status.

Overall, the profile of health-promoting behaviors for women shows that activity levels decrease with age and that only 34% of young adult women engage in regular physical activitity. Fat and carbohyrate intake remains relatively stable at 50% and 33% respectively across the lifespan, but total kilcalories taken in decreases with age. The proportion of women at a healthy weight (not overweight or obese) increases as women age (see Table 1.17).

Changing Biology and Environmental Factors

The last decade of the 20th century was a time of significant advances in women's health. Prompted by the feminist movement of the 1960s and 1970s, increasing attention to women's health brought changes in health services, such as freestanding birth centers, development of academic coursework in women's health for professionals and the general public, and advances in research about women's health. Each of these changes portends enhanced possibilities for women's health during the 21st century. The consequences of advanced understanding of women's health through research may be the most dramatic in the decades ahead.

The Human Genome

Research focused on the human genome has revealed new understandings about sex differences that may have profound implications for women's health. Not only have new insights about sex differences in the genetic bases for phenotypic differences between men and women revolutionized this field, but also some genetic discoveries have been made that may drive health consequences for women. An Institute of Medicine (2001) report, provides significant evidence that sex does matter. Being male or female is linked to differences in health and illness, and

these differences are influenced by genetic, physiological, environmental, and experiential factors. Although in many instances sex differences can be traced to effects of reproductive hormones, hormones are no longer a universal explanation for these differences. Research on understanding the human genome has provided us with a basis for learning about the molecular and cellular mechanisms that underlie sex-specific differences in phenotype. Many of these new understandings warrant further investigation. Sexual genotype (XX in females, XY in males) has effects far beyond elaboration of reproductive hormones. Genes on sex chromosomes can be expressed differently in females and males. Single or double copies of the genes, meiotic effects, X-chromosome inactivation, and genetic imprinting are a few of the phenomena involved. X-chromosome inactivation is the random silencing of one or the other X chromosome that takes place during early embryonic development. X inactivation, which occurs about the time of implantation, is a unique biochemical process in that it occurs only in females. Females inherit a paternally imprinted X chromosome, unlike males, who inherit only a maternally imprinted X chromosome. A subset of genes on the X chromosome may escape inactivation. As a result, females can get double doses of certain genes. The Y chromosome has a host of actively transcribed genes that are expressed throughout the male body but are absent from the female body.

Although the new biological discoveries are important to the understanding of women's health, it remains important to recall that these sex differences are not the same as gender differences. Sex differences refer to differences that are biologically driven, whereas gender refers to differences that are socially influenced: self-representation as male or female and social responses to one's phenotype. There are many differences between males and females in basic cellular biochemistries that can affect health, and many do not arise only because of hormonal differences between the sexes. Research is in

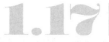

Health-Promoting Behaviors by Women According to Age, Activity Level, Calorie Intake, and Body Mass Index

AGE	INACTIVE %	SOME LEISURE TIME ACTIVITY %	REGULAR LEISURE TIME ACTIVITY %
18–44 years	34.9	31.1	34.0
45–54 years	36.5	31.1	32.4
55–64 years	41.9	30.4	27.6
65–74 years	48.0	26.6	25.4
75 years and older	63.7	22.0	14.3

	TOTAL KCALS	CARBOHYDRATE % OF KCALS	TOTAL FAT % OF KCALS	SATURATED FAT % OF KCALS
20–39 years	2,028	52.6	32.3	10.9
40–59 years	1,828	50.9	33.1	11.1
60–74 years	1,596	51.1	33.3	10.9

	HEALTHY WEIGHT % (BODY MASS INDEX 18.5–24)	OVERWEIGHT % (BODY MASS INDEX ≥ 25)	OBESE % (BODY MASS INDEX ≥ 30)
20–34 years	42.6	52.8	28.4
35–44 years	37.1	60.6	32.1
45–54 years	33.1	65.1	36.9
55–64 years	27.6	72.2	42.1
65–74 years	26.4	70.9	39.3
75 years and older	36.9	59.9	23.6

Note. From *Health, United States, 2005* (Tables 71, 72, and 73), by National Center for Health Statistics, 2005, Washington, DC: Author.

progress on the functions and effects of X-chromosome and Y-chromosome linked genes in somatic as well as germ cells. Mechanisms of influence of genetic sex differences in biological organization (cell, organ, organ system, and organism), effects of genes versus the effects of hormones, and sex differences across the life span remain to be fully understood.

Environments for Women's Health

Effects of women's environmental exposures on their health have gained scientific attention (Haynes et al., 2000). As a basis for its work, the Federal Interagency Working Group on Women's Health and the Environment of the Department of Health and Human Services defined *environment* to include the home, school, indoor and outdoor work places, public and private facilities and outdoor spaces, and health care services and recreational settings. Women's health can be affected by the products women use in these settings as well as by contact with physical, chemical, and biological toxicants in air, water, soil, food, and other organisms. In addition, lifestyle, substances ingested, and economic circumstances can influence health. There are multiple mechanisms by which environmental exposures can influence health. For example, environmental chemicals may increase or decrease signaling molecules by mimicking or blocking effector molecule signals that disrupt signal pathways.

How populations differ in their susceptibility and how susceptibility changes over time may be explained in part by focusing on the intersection of genetic and environmental influences—for example, understanding how environmental agents with estrogenic-like activity interact with genes. Study of endocrine disruptors and their potentially adverse health effects could contribute significantly to improving women's health through curtailment of environmental exposures. In addition, studies of genetic susceptibility to environmental exposures—for example, the NATZ gene, which determines slow acetylation among smokers and its effect on breast cancer—may help reduce risk if these biological indicators become readily available to women.

Finally, as we have come to appreciate the disparities in health experienced by many populations of women, we are beginning to understand the utility of the concept of gender disparities. Health disparities exist when there are differences in the incidence, prevalence, mortality, and burden of disease and other adverse health outcomes when compared to the general population. Sociocultural environments form the context for women's lives and have profound effects on their health and that of future generations. Critical intersection of gender, race, ethnicity, class, and age shape the environments that influence women's chances for health. Consequently, it is difficult to attribute gender disparities in health to biology, environments, physiology, or human experience. The intersection of gender with other characteristics often determines women's

■ Exposures to toxins
■ Social relations such as those linked to low social and economic status
■ Racism
■ Sexism
■ Heterosexism
■ Stress
■ Tobacco/alcohol/other substance use.

Sociocultural as well as physical and chemical environments thus form the context for women's lives and have profound effects on their health and that of future generations. It is therefore critical to consider women's health from an integrative perspective and to move beyond research describing the nature of women's health problems to that which engages women in the study of solutions to their health problems. Likewise, it is critical to consider both the individual experience of health as well as the community's health. A multilevel approach to health is important in order to institute the kinds of programs that are likely to be successful in improving women's chances for health.

GLOBALIZATION

A final important factor influencing women's health in this century is globalization. As economic forces move women into a global economy, some would point out that the world continues to be an unsafe place for girls and women. Meleis (2005) asserted that the gender divide compromises safety of women. Women are at risk for violence, rape, trafficking, and abuse. Their

mortality and injury rates reflect the limited definition of the nature and type of work they do. Conditions expose them to infections such as HIV/AIDS, pregnancy and birthing cycles, and unsafe abortions owing to inadequacy and inaccessibility of health services. She urges several urgent actions to enhance safe womanhood, not just safe motherhood. Among these are women's work, marriage, violence, reproductive rules, resources, and others. Education of young girls sets their horizons by determining their options for work. How work is defined limits consideration of the nature, burden of double and triple shifts, and hazards of work that are not currently considered in the economic and labor statistics or health studies. Marriage defines many women and obligates them to provide services and resources to husbands and families, as well as shoulder the burdens of multiple roles. Battering and abuse of girls and women, trafficking, and access to income through sex work all put women at great health risk, including for HIV/AIDS. Wars and terrorism increase women's chances of rape and burden. Pregnancy, birth, and motherhood also escalate the risk of poor health for women. Finally, health care services that are fragmented, inaccessible, and focused on disease rather than prevention and health promotion become a source of overload for women. The invisibility of women's health care issues on national and international agendas intensifies the risk for women.

Meleis proposes that a fundamental change is necessary in the conceptual framework for women's health. She recommends using a human rights framework that is guided by a focus on women's life situations and experiences as a starting point for considering health. Stigma, exploitation, and oppression are key concepts in understanding women's health. Second, she urges redefinition of women's work from employment to a multidimensional framework that includes the amount of energy, activity, and space occupied; the amount and quality of time; resources for their work; and the results, values, and meaning of their work. Third, she recommends development of policies that acknowledge women's perspectives, experiences, and life context as well as giving women a platform and advocacy to have their voices heard in the policy arena. Finally, Meleis recommends that societies consider women the center of the family and the community, expecting them to be the agents for continuity of values, gatekeepers, integrators, and guardians of social capital. This implies placing women's health at the forefront of foreign policy and international consciousness in war and peace.

THE FUTURE OF WOMEN'S HEALTH

Notable advances have been achieved in the scope and depth of women's health care research in the last century. However major challenges continue to emerge,

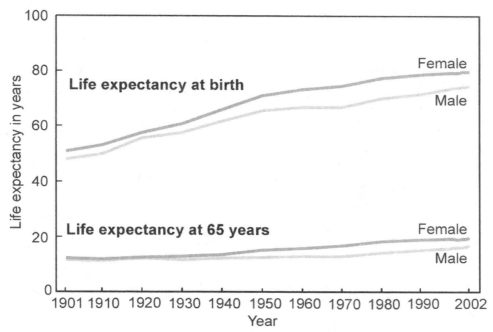

Figure 1.1 Life expectancy in years by year for women and men.
Source: National Center for Health Statistics, Health, United States (2005), Figure 26.

which are influenced by socioeconomic and environmental trends; genetic, hormonal, and biological determinants; globalization; and other social issues. Future and emerging issues for women's health in the 21st century will need to address the effects of demographic and sociocultural change on women's health and also focus on the impact of such changes on the health care system and the ability of women to access appropriate high quality care. The need to broaden research topics and to take into account populations that have been inadequately studied to date is essential. In general, although health care providers are committed to doing everything possible to promote women's health, the range of clinical and public health interventions are often limited, access to health care is inequitable, and the research evidence specific to women is quite incomplete. Therefore, when considering future directions in research, one should ask whether study results will advance the ability to improve women's health.

REFERENCES

Abma, J., Chandra, A., Mosher, W., Peterson, L., & Piccinino, L. (1997). Fertility, family planning, and women's health: New data from the 1995 National Survey of Family Growth. Series 23, No. 19. Hyattsville, MD: National Center for Health Statistics, Centers for Disease Control and Prevention, Public Health Service, U.S. Department of Health and Human Services.

Amick, B. C., Kawachi, I., Coakley, E. H., Lerner, D., Levine, S., & Colditz, G. A. (1998). Relationship of job strain and iso-strain to health status in a cohort of women in the United States. *Scandinavian Journal of Work Environment and Health, 24*(1), 54–61.

Anderson, G. F., & Poullier, J. P. (1999). Health spending, access, and outcomes: Trends in industrialized countries. *Health Affairs, 18*(3), 178–192.

Bartman, B. A., & Weiss, K. B. (1993). Women's primary care in the United States: A study of practice variation among physician specialties. *Journal of Women's Health, 2,* 261–268.

Blazer, D. G., Kessler, R. C., McGonagle, K. A., & Swartz, M. S. (1994). The prevalence and distribution of major depression in a national community sample: The National Comorbidity Survey. *American Journal of Psychiatry, 151*(7), 979–986.

Bowman, M. A., & Spangler, J. B. (1997). Osteoporosis in women. *Primary Care, 24*(1), 27–36.

Bramlett, M. D., & Mosher, W. D. (2002). Cohabitation, marriage, divorce, and remarriage in the United States. National Center for Health Statistics. *Vital and Health Statistics, 23*(22), 1–93.

Brett, K. M., Strogatz, D. S., & Savitz, D. A. (1997). Employment, job strain, and preterm delivery among women in North Carolina. *American Journal of Public Health, 87*(2), 199–204.

Brittingham, A. (2000). The foreign-born population in the United States. *Current Population Reports,* 1–6. U.S. Department of Commerce, U.S. Census Bureau.

Bryner, R. W., Toffle, R. C., Ulrich, I. H., & Yeater, R. A. (1997). The effects of exercise intensity on body composition, weight loss, and dietary composition in women. *Journal of the American College Nutrition, 16*(1), 68–73.

Buckworth, J., Dishman, R. K., Cureton, & K. J. (1994). Autonomic response of women with parental hypertension: Effects of physical activity and fitness. *Hypertension, 24*(5), 576–584.

Centers for Disease Control and Prevention. (2000a). Building data systems for monitoring and responding to violence against women: Recommendations from a workshop. *MMWR, 49*(RR-11).

Centers for Disease Control and Prevention. (2000b). *Preventing emerging infectious diseases: A strategy for the 21st century.* Atlanta, GA: U.S. Department of Health and Human Services.

Centers for Disease Control and Prevention. (2000c). *HIV/AIDS among U.S. women: Minority and young women at continuing risk.* Retrieved January 2006, from http://www.cdc.gov/hiv/pubs/facts/women.htm

Chavkin, W. (1999). What's a mother to do? Welfare, work, and family. *American Journal of Public Health, 89*(4), 477–479.

Clancy, C. M., & Massion, C. T. (1992). American women's health care: A patchwork quilt with gaps. *Journal of the American Medical Association, 268*(14), 1918–1920.

Commission on Family and Medical Leave. (1996). *A workable balance: Report to Congress on family and medical leave.* Washington, DC: U.S. Department of Labor.

Fullerton, H. N., (1999). The labor force projections to 2008: Steady growth and changing composition. *Monthly Labor Review, 122*(11), 19–32.

Gabrel, C. S. (2000). Characteristics of elderly nursing home current residents and discharges: Data from the 1997 National Home Survey. *Advance data from vital and health statistics,* No. 312. Hyattsville, MD: National Center for Health Statistics.

Grason, H. A., Hutchins, J. E., & Silver, G. B. (Eds.). (1999). *Charting a course for the future of women's and perinatal health: Vol. 1. Concepts, findings, and recommendations.* Baltimore: Women's and Children's Health Policy Center, Johns Hopkins School of Public Health.

Hajat, A., Lucas, J. B., & Kington, R. (2000). Health outcomes among Hispanic subgroups: United States, 1992–95. *Advance data from vital and health statistics,* No. 310. Hyattsville, MD: National Center for Health Statistics.

Hall, M. J., & Popovic, J. R. (2000). 1998 summary: National Hospital Discharge Survey. *Advance data from vital and health statistics,* No. 316. Hyattsville, MD: National Center for Health Statistics.

Haupt, B. J. (1998). Characteristics of hospice care users: Data from the 1996 National Home and Hospice Care Survey. *Advance data from vital and health statistics,* No. 299. Hyattsville, MD: National Center for Health Statistics.

Haynes, S. et al. (2000). Women's health and the environment: Innovations in science and policy. *Journal of Women's Health and Gender-Based Medicine, 3,* 245–272.

Heymann, S. J., & Earle, A. (1999). The impact of welfare reform on parents' ability to care for their children's health. *American Journal of Public Health, 89,* 502–505.

Institute of Medicine, Committee on Understanding the Biology of Sex and Gender Differences. (2001). *Exploring the biological contributions to human. Does sex matter?* Washington, DC: National Academy of Sciences.

Jacobs Institute of Women's Health. (1998). National Leadership Conference on Physical Activity and Women's Health. *Women's Health Issues, 8*(2), 69–97.

Johnson, R. K. (1996). Normal nutrition in premenopausal women. In D. A Krummel & P. M. Kris-Etherton (Eds.), *Nutrition in women's health.* Gaithersburg, MD: Aspen, 174–211.

Kant, A. K., Schatzkin, A., Graubard, B. I., & Schairer, C. (2000). A prospective study of diet quality and mortality in women. *Journal of the American Medical Association, 283*(16), 2109–2115.

Kant, A. K, Schatzkin, A., Harris, T. B., Ziegler, R., & Block, G. (1993). Dietary diversity and subsequent mortality in the First National Health and Nutrition Examination Survey epidemio-

logic follow-up study. *American Journal of Clinical Nutrition, 57*(3), 434–440.

Kessler, R. C., Crum, R. M., Warner, L. A., Nelson, C. B., Schulenberg, J., & Anthony, J. C. (1997). Lifetime co-occurrence of DSM-III-R alcohol abuse and dependence with other psychiatric disorders in the National Comorbidity Survey. *Archives of General Psychiatry, 54*(4), 313–321.

Manson, J. E., Rimm, E. B., Stampfer, M. J., Colditz, G. A., Willet, W. C., & Krowleski, A. S. (1991). Physical activity and incidence of non-insulin-dependent diabetes mellitus in women. *Lancet, 338,* 774–778.

Meleis, A. (2005). Safe womanhood is not safe motherhood: Policy implications. *Health Care for Women International, 26,* 464–471.

Miniño, A. M., Arias, E., Kochanek, K. D., Murphy, S. L., & Smith, B. L. (2002). Deaths: Final data for 2000. *National Vital Statistics Reports, 50*(15). Hyattsville, MD: National Center for Health Statistics.

Misra, D. (1999). Women's experience of chronic diseases. In H. A. Grason, J. E. Hutchins, & G. B. Silver (Eds.), *Charting a course for the future of women's and perinatal health: Vol. 2. Review of key issues* (pp. 137–146). Baltimore: Women's and Children's Health Policy Center, Johns Hopkins School of Public Health.

National Center for Health Statistics. (1997). Table 58. Number of selected reported chronic conditions per 1,000 persons, by sex and age: United States, 1995. *National Health Interview Survey, 10*(199), 79.

National Center for Health Statistics. (1999a). Life expectancy at single years of age, United States, 1997. *National Vital Statistics Reports, 47*(28).

National Center for Health Statistics. (1999b). *Health, United States, 1999 with Health and Aging Chartbook.* Hyattsville, MD: Author.

National Center for Health Statistics. (2000). Table 1. Live births, birth rates, and fertility rates, by race: United States, specified years 1940–55 and each year, 1960–98. *National Vital Statistics Report, 48*(3).

National Center for Health Statistics. (2005). *Health, United States, 2005 with Chartbook on Trends in the Health of Americans.* Hyattsville, MD: Author.

National Center for Health Statistics. (2006). *Health, United States, 2006 with chartbook on trends in the health of Americans.* Hyattsville, MD: Author.

Parrott, S. (1998). *Welfare recipients who find jobs: What do we know about their employment and earnings?* Washington, DC: Center on Budget and Policy Priorities.

Pugliesi, K. (1995). Work and well-being: Gender differences in the psychological consequences of employment. *Journal of Health and Social Behavior, 36*(1), 57–71.

Regenstein, M., Meyer, J. A., & Hicks, J. D. (1998). *Job prospects for welfare recipients: Employers speak out.* Washington, DC: Urban Institute.

Rosenblatt, R. A., Hart, G., & Gamliel, S. (1995). Identifying primary care disciplines by analyzing the diagnostic content of ambulatory care. *Journal of the American Board of Family Practice, 8*(1), 34–45.

Ross, C., & Mirowsky, J. (1995). Does employment affect health? *Journal of Health and Social Behavior, 36*(3), 230–243.

Ruderman, M., & O'Campo, P. (1999). Depression in women. In H. A. Grason, J. E. Hutchins, & G. B. Silver (Eds.), *Charting a course for the future of women's and perinatal health: Vol. 2. Review of key issues* (pp. 147–163). Baltimore: Women's and

Children's Health Policy Center, Johns Hopkins School of Public Health.

Saluter, A. F. (1997). Marital status and living arrangements. *Current Population Reports,* Series P20-484. Washington, DC: U.S. Government Printing Office.

Savitz, D. A., Brett, K. M., Dole, N., & Tse, C. K. (1997). Male and female occupation in relation to miscarriage and preterm delivery in central North Carolina. *Annals of Epidemiology, 7*(7), 509–516.

Slusarcick, A. L., & McCaig, L. F. (2000). National Hospital Ambulatory Medical Care Survey: 1998 outpatient department summary. *Advance data from vital and health statistics,* No. 317. Hyattsville, MD: National Center for Health Statistics.

Sutton, P. D. (2003). Births, marriages, divorces, and deaths: Provisional data for July–September 2002. *National Vital Statistics Reports, 51*(8). Hyattsville, MD: National Center for Health Statistics.

Tjaden, P., & Thoennes, N. (1998). *Prevalence, incidence and consequences of violence against women: Findings from the National Violence Against Women Survey—Research in brief.* Washington, DC: National Institute of Justice and Centers for Disease Control. NCJ 172837.

U.S. Census Bureau. (1999). *Money income in the United States.* Population Estimates Program. Washington, DC: U.S. Census Bureau, Population Division.

U.S. Census Bureau. (2000a). *Resident population estimates of the United States by sex, race, and Hispanic origin: April 1, 1990 to July 1, 1999, with short-term projection to October 1, 2000.* Population Estimates Program. Washington, DC: U.S. Census Bureau, Population Division.

U.S. Census Bureau. (2000b). *Educational attainment in the United States: Population characteristics, March 1999.* Washington, DC: U.S. Department of Commerce, Economics and Statistics Administration, http://www.census.gov/population/estimates/nation/intfile3-1.txt.

U.S. Census Bureau. (2000c). *Table 4: Educational attainment of the population 15 Years and over, by household relationship, age, sex, race, and Hispanic origin: March 1999,* http://www.census.gov/population/www/socdemo/education/p20-528.html.

U.S. Census Bureau. (2000d). *Employment status: Table 3. Employment status of the civilian noninstitutional population by age, sex, and race: Labor force statistics from the Current Population Survey.* Washington, DC: U.S. Census Bureau for the Bureau of Labor Statistics, http://www.bls.gov/cpsaatab.htm.

U.S. Department of Health and Human Services. (1996). *Physical activity and health: A report of the surgeon general.* Washington, DC: U.S. Government Printing Office.

U.S. Department of Health and Human Services. (1998). *Characteristics and financial circumstances of TANF recipients, July–September 1997.* Washington, DC: Author.

U.S. Department of Health and Human Services. (1999). *Mental health: A report of the surgeon general—Executive summary.* Rockville, MD: U.S. Department of Human Services, Substance Abuse and Mental Health Services Administration, Center for Mental Health Services, National Institutes of Health, National Institute of Mental Health.

U.S. Department of Health and Human Services. (2000a). *Data on health disparities.* Atlanta, GA: Centers for Disease Control and Prevention and National Center for Health Statistics.

U.S. Department of Health and Human Services. (2000b). *Tracking Healthy People 2010.* Washington, DC: U.S. Government Printing Office.

U.S. Department of Labor. (2007). Women in the labor force: A databook. Washington, DC: Author, U.S. Bureau of Labor Statistics.

Ventura, S. J., & Bachrach, C. A. (2000). Nonmarital childbearing in the United States, 1940–1999. *National Vital Statistics Reports, 48*(16). Hyattsville, MD: National Center for Health Statistics.

Ventura, S. J., Martin, J. A., Curtin, S. C., Mathews, T. J., & Park, M. M. (2000). Births: Final data for 1998. *National Vital Statistics Reports, 48*(3). Hyattsville, MD: National Center for Health Statistics.

Warner, M., Barnes, P. M., & Fingerhut, L. A. (2000). Injury and poisoning episodes and conditions: National Health Interview Survey, 1997. *Vital Health Statistics, 10*(202).

Weinberg, D. H. (2000, September 26). *Press briefing on 1999 income and poverty estimates.* Chief, Housing and Household Economic Statistics Division: U.S. Census Bureau.

Weisman, C. S., Cassard, S. D., & Plichta, S. D. (1995). Types of physicians used by women for regular health care: Implications for services received. *Journal of Women's Health,* 4, 40–416.

Women as Health Care Providers

Diana Taylor, Carol J. Leppa, and
Nancy Fugate Woods

HEALTH CARE SERVICES IN THE UNITED STATES

The delivery of health services is one of the largest industries in the United States, with about 13.5 million jobs or almost 10% of all U.S. jobs in 2004. More than half of all health care jobs are in hospitals and another one-third are in nursing and personal care facilities or physician offices (U.S. Department of Labor, 2007a). In 2004, about 40% of health service jobs were held by professional specialties such as physicians, nurses, dentists, pharmacists, social workers, physical and occupational therapists, dietitians and nutritionists, computer systems engineers, and speech language pathologists. Registered nurses accounted for 15% of these jobs in 2004. Almost one-third of the health service jobs are in the service, technical, or support categories that include psychiatric, home health, pharmacy, dental, medical, and nursing assistants; licensed practical nurses; dental hygienists; medical record and health information technicians; laboratory and radiology technicians; food service workers; and dispensing opticians. Another 20% of health service workers are in administrative support and management jobs.

Although the term *health care provider* has usually referred to people who provide care to patients, this term has been expanded to include the settings in which health services are provided. More than 545,000 establishments make up the health services industry with nine general segments: hospitals (public and private); nursing and residential care facilities; physician clinics/offices; home health care services; dental clinics/offices; other health practitioner offices/clinics (chiropractors, optometrists, podiatrists, occupational/physical therapists,

psychologists, speech/hearing therapists, nutritionists, alternative medicine practitioners); outpatient care centers (kidney dialysis centers, drug treatment clinics, mental health centers, rehab centers); medical and diagnostic laboratories; and other ambulatory health care services (ambulance and helicopter transport services, blood and organ banks, pacemaker monitoring services) (U.S. Department of Labor, 2007b).

Definitions of health care professionals and health care workers are rooted in history; their evolution is shaped by social, economic, and political forces. With the rapid and massive changes in the U.S. health care system, system redesign is occurring along with a redefinition of health care workers' roles. These changes are influenced by multiple determinants: the form of government, definitions of health, social values, costs, society's expectations for the health care system, and the political power of various players. In addition to external systems change, the health care work force must be engaged in and capable of setting bold aims, measuring progress, finding alternative designs for the work itself, and testing changes rapidly and informatively (Berwick, 2003; Jacox, 1997). Engaging the health care work force requires addressing the social values related to gender and work, which exert a major influence on who does what in health care.

WOMEN AS PAID HEALTH CARE PROVIDERS

One of the most striking developments of the post–World War II period has been the increase in women working outside the home. Worldwide, women now make up over one-third of the paid labor force and are concentrated in particular sectors of the economy such as service jobs. Despite equal opportunity laws, women have not achieved parity with men's earnings, and many continue to be crowded into female "employment ghettos," such as factories and hospitals.

Across the world, women provide the majority of paid health care. In the United States, women are over-represented in the health work force compared to the total population. In 2005, slightly more than half of the U.S. population was women (51%), yet they accounted for approximately 79% of workers across all health care settings (U.S. Census Bureau, 2006). In addition, the profession of medicine is becoming feminized as the number of women enrolled in medical school and residency programs has increased dramatically (Levinson & Lurie, 2004). As an example, in 2004, 8% of physicians age 65 and older were women, but almost half (47%) of all graduating medical students were women (American Medical Association, 2004). This phenomenon is not new. Bullough and Bullough (1975) described it 30 years ago, and Butter and colleagues (1985, 1987) elaborated on it in the 1980s. As we move into the 21st century, there continues to be an over-representation of women and women of color in the lowest paying and lowest status health occupations. Although women are making significant advances in the traditionally male occupations of medicine, dentistry, pharmacy, and some highly technical occupations, they continue to far outnumber men in the traditionally female occupations: nurse, occupational and physical therapist, dietitian/nutritionist, dental assistant/dental hygienist, nursing assistant, and health aide/technician. Overall, women earn 20% less than men working in health care occupations, and women physicians earn 61% of men physicians (U.S. Department of Labor, 2006b).

In addition to gender, the health work force does not match the ethnic or racial distribution of the U.S. population. At the turn of the 21st century, the racial distribution in the United States is as follows: 67.4% are non-Hispanic Whites; 12.2% are Black; 14.1% are of Hispanic origin; 4.2% are Asian and Pacific Islander; and less than 1% are American Indian, Eskimo, and Aleut. By 2050, these proportions will shift quite dramatically. Less than 53% will be non-Hispanic White; 15% Black; over 24% Hispanic origin; almost 9% Asian and Pacific Islander; and just over 1% American Indian, Eskimo, and Aleut (U.S. Census Bureau, 2006, 2007). Although national health work force data are limited, a California work force study (Ruzek, Bloor, Anderson, & Ngo, 1999) found that Hispanics were under-represented across all health care settings (hospitals, nursing facilities, health facilities, and medical offices); Asians and Pacific Islanders were over-represented in the nursing facility setting; and Whites, regardless of gender, constituted 67% of the professional occupations and 33%

of the nonprofessional occupations. While Asian-Pacific Islanders were similar to Whites, Blacks and Hispanics were over-represented in the nonprofessional occupations. For example, in health facilities, Blacks made up 8% of the professional occupations and 15% of the nonprofessional categories. However, health care provider ethnicity is complicated by health insurance status and access to ethnic provider status by patients with limited English language proficiency. In a study of 2,240 California primary care and specialist physicians, where the supply of Spanish-speaking physicians in California is relatively high (24%), the insurance status of Spanish-speaking patients with limited English language proficiency limits their access to the physicians (Yoon, Grumbach, & Bindman, 2004).

The statistics presented in Table 2.1 illustrate the status of women workers in selected paid health care occupations. Overall, Table 2.1 does not present new information. Many authors have compared the proportion of women in the health occupations and explored the gender hierarchies in the health labor force (Brown, 1982; Butter et al., 1985, 1987; Levinson & Lurie, 2004; Marieskind, 1980). The statistics are followed and updated annually by the federal government and reported in various government reports available to the public— for example, reports from the U.S. Census Bureau, the Department of Labor, the Bureau of Labor Statistics, and the Bureau of Health Professions. More recently, the federal government has focused on women workers through the establishment of a Women's Bureau of the Department of Labor and the National Center for Health Workforce Information and Analysis at the Health Resources and Service Administration's Bureau of Health Professions. There is a rising awareness of the need to collect and analyze data regarding the national, regional, and state differences of personnel working in the U.S. health care delivery system, including gender, class, and ethnic factors. The occupations listed in Table 2.1 are not all of those on which information is available, but they provide a good representation and clear picture of the continued disparity between women's and men's paid health care roles. The occupations are listed in order of median reported income for 2004 to 2006 (U.S. Department of Labor, 2006a, 2006c). Notably, the large numbers of nurse's aides and medical assistants, of which 90% or more are women, account for the majority of women in all health care occupations. Clearly, women are clustered in jobs and occupations that are lower in pay, lower in status, and less autonomous than the jobs of most men in the health care field (Butter et al., 1987; Doyal, 1995; Fisher, 1995).

A few decades ago, Navarro (1975) wrote that the occupational, class, and sex structure in the U.S. health work force reflected the structure seen in other economic sectors. He compared the distribution of health workers by class and sex with the distribution of workers in

| Women Workers in Selected Health Occupations, 2004–2006

HEALTH OCCUPATION	% OF WOMEN OF TOTAL	TOTAL WORKERS (IN 1,000S)	AVERAGE EARNINGS (IN DOLLARS)
Physicians	32.3	780	201,000
Dentists	22.5	164	129,920
Pharmacists	46.0	248	93,500
Physical therapists	68.9	177	68,050
Dental hygienists	97.1	143	62,430
Registered nurses	91.3	2,421	59,963
Nutritionists/dietitians	95.3	51	47,890
Radiology technicians	72.0	190	49,320
Clinical lab technicians	74.2	305	50,550
Licensed practical nurses	93.4	720	37,530
Dental assistants	96.1	259	26,630
Medical assistants	—	361	24,680
Nurses aides, psychiatric aides, home health aides	88.7	1,900	22,880

Note. Figures for the percentage of women of total and number of total workers are from "Resident Population by Sex, Race and Hispanic Origin Status: 2000–2004," in *Statistical Abstract of the United States, 2006* (Table 13), by U.S. Census Bureau, 2006, Washington, DC: Author. http://www.census.gov/prod/s005pubs/06statab/pop.pdf; *Statistical Abstract of the United States: 2007* (126th ed.), by U.S. Census Bureau, 2007, Washington, DC: Author. http://www.census.gov/statab/www; *Physician Characteristics and Distribution in the U.S.,* by American Medical Association, 2004, Chicago: Author; *Annual* Averages, by U.S. Department of Labor, Bureau of Labor Statistics, 2006, retrieved May 18, 2007, from http://www.dol.gov/wb/factsheets/20lead2006.htm; *Women in the Labor Force: A Databook 2006,* Report 996, by U.S. Department of Labor, Bureau of Labor Statistics, 2006, Washington, DC: Author. http://www.bls.gov/cps/wlf-databook2006.htm; and Occupation Employment Statistics, by U.S. Department of Labor, Bureau of Labor Statistics, 2006, Washington, DC: Author. http://www.bls.gov/oes/home.htm. Figures for average earnings are from *Annual Averages,* 2006; Women in the Labor Force: A Databook 2006, 2006; and *Occupation Employment Statistics,* 2006, for years 2005 to 2007.

other work force sectors. Ehrenreich (1975) commented that "the stratification with the U.S. health industry has been documented again and again—in tones ranging from academic resignation to feminist outrage" (p. 7). Thirty years later, we find more women represented in the professional occupations traditionally held by men but few men represented in the professional and support occupations largely held by women.

The stratification of the labor force in general is further explored in Table 2.2, which compares four health professions and makes projections for the future health professions work force composition in terms of numbers and gender. We follow this with a discussion of current social and economic trends that maintain this stratification. The occupations of medicine, dentistry, and pharmacy were chosen not only because they have the highest visibility and occupy the three top spots in terms of income in Table 2.1, but also because the data exist in current federal reports. Although it is true that, for male nurses, a change from 2.7% in 1970 to 5.8% in 1990 represents a greater than 100% increase such that in 1990 some 93,000 nurses were men, the effect on the profession as a whole

is minimal. Nursing remains a profession dominated by women (U.S. Department of Labor, 2005a).

The importance of Table 2.2 is its illustration of how the health labor force is changing. According to U.S. government reports and projections, all of the traditionally male health care occupations have experienced and will continue to experience dramatic increases in the percentage of women in their ranks. More women are enrolled in educational programs in the traditionally male health professions than in nursing education programs. In the past 30 years, the numbers of women enrolling in schools of medicine, dentistry, and pharmacy have increased by 30 to 40%, and the numbers of women enrolled in optometry programs has increased by 50%. During the same period, there was only an 8% increased enrollment of men in nursing programs.

Health professional ethnicity does not match the ethnic diversity in the United States, although 2004 graduate data suggest that diversity is improving in major health professions. In 2004, 74% of physicians and 82% of registered nurses were White (non-Hispanic) compared to 67% White (non-Hispanic) in the U.S. population

(U.S. Census Bureau, 2006). In contrast, 67% of graduating physicians and dentists and 64% of graduating pharmacists were non-Hispanic White in 2004, compared to 78% of graduating registered nurses (Health Resources and Services Administration, 2006a, 2006b). While 11.2% of graduating nurses and 9% of graduating pharmacists were Black, 5% of graduating dentists and 7% of physician graduates were Black (the U.S. population is 12.2% Black). The total Hispanic population in the United States is 14.1%, but only 4% to 6% of graduating dentists, physicians, nurses, and pharmacists were Hispanic in 2004. Asians are over-represented in medicine (20%), dentistry (22%), pharmacy (24%) graduates compared to 2004 population estimates of 4% Asians and Pacific Islanders. Graduating nurses were 4% Asian in 2004.

Health care occupations in the 21st century will have more women in them and will be slightly more ethnically diverse than they are today in terms of the number and proportion of women occupying jobs in the health labor force. Other implications of the changes (or lack of changes) in gender and ethnicity among the health work force will be explored further.

Occupational Roles for Women in Health Care

Occupational roles for women in health care reflect social conditions and values. Some examples of these social conditions that specifically impact women's roles in health care include changes in educational and social status of women along with population shifts, medical advances, and market-driven forces of the health care delivery system. The educational status of the population, particularly for women, has improved over the past several decades. The improved social and economic status of some women in Western societies has altered gender inequalities. The increasing numbers of women in medicine and other traditionally male health occupations have changed stereotypical ideas regarding roles. The numbers and types of health care workers have increased remarkably over the past decade, creating role overlap in an already fragmented system. Technological advances, rising health care costs, and increased consumer sophistication have raised societal expectations regarding the role of health professionals and the quality of care to be received. Shifts in disease patterns, lifestyle changes, and increased numbers of elderly individuals have altered the sites and settings where health care is provided. However, occupational roles and particular jobs in the health care field are likely to impact women more than men due to women's dual role obligations and socioeconomic status. First, some historical factors will be explored.

Historical Perspectives

The idea of formal education for women in the 19th century was not well accepted, let alone an occupation for women outside the home. Women in the 1800s were struggling to define a role for themselves in society through the women's suffrage movement of the 1840s as well as through the early women's health organizations of the time (Ehrenreich & English, 1973). Tremendous resistance was presented with "scientific reasons" for women to stay in what were their supposed physically and intellectually inferior positions in society. Hamilton (1885, in Ehrenreich & English, 1973) wrote that "the best education for girls, then, is that which best prepares them for the legitimate duties of womanhood" (p. 319; e.g., wife, mother, homemaker). He further asserted that attainment of high intellectual culture exacts too great a price and results in a "ruined or physically damaged constitution." Hamilton based his theory about education for women on a set of assumptions about physical and intellectual differences between the sexes. With respect to women, he described how "brain work" competes with the "vital forces of the body," and that such a diversion of "nerve power" to the mental labor involved in education could only lead to "greatly impaired or permanently ruined health, a life of sterility, general unhappiness, and uselessness" (p. 320). In the face of such heated (if erroneous) opposition as this, nursing was seen as at least a marginally respectable occupation for women given the close approximation of nursing work with the "legitimate duties of womanhood" (Hamilton, in Ehrenreich & English, 1973).

However, changes in societal attitudes toward patient care began to improve during this same time and women's talent for healing was widely acclaimed in the West for a short period during the mid- to late 19th century. Florence Nightingale, a member of British society, became a legend during the Crimean War and led the reform movement to improve conditions in hospitals and prisons (Jamieson & Sewall, 1944). Clara Barton received similar acclamation during the American Civil War when she organized nurses for the Union Army. However, health care was still considered largely a family matter. Women cared for their families, called on their friends and relatives, and traded advice through an oral tradition (Stevens, 1966). For a time, the United States became a leader in training women physicians during the late 1800s, when immigration increased demand for professional medical services. However, women's role in medicine declined during the first half of the 20th century, when medical colleges that admitted women closed for lack of funding and new antinepotism rules barred women from following their spouses into the expanding coeducational colleges and universities (Ehrenreich, 1975). It was at this time that physicians began to organize themselves in order to compete in a field of medical providers that was not dominated by any one provider regardless of gender. Contributing to the rise of a strong professional medical organization in the early 1900s was the rise of labor unions, corporations, and trusts that were dominated by men—and, in the case

| Percentage of Women in Selected Health Care Occupations

OCCUPATION	1970	1990	2000	2020	NUMBER OF WOMEN IN 2020
Registered nurses	97.3	94.2	94.5	89.0	2,259,000
Medical doctors	9.2	17.9	27.2	46.0	323,272
Dentists	3.4	8.6	16.0	36.0	59,400
Pharmacists	11.9	32.3	46.7	61.0	168,360

Note. Adapted from *Women as health care providers* by C. Leppa (1995), *in Women's Health Care* by C. Fogel and N. F. Woods (Eds.), Thousand Oaks, CA: Sage; *Statistical Abstract of the United States: 2000* (120th ed.), by U.S. Census Bureau, 2000, Washington, DC: Author; *Statistical Abstract of the United States: 2007* (126th ed.), by U.S. Census Bureau, 2007, Washington, DC: Author; "Occupational Employment Projections to 2014: Fastest Growing Occupations, 2004–2014," Table 2, *Monthly Labor Review*, by U.S. Department of Labor, Bureau of Labor Statistics, 2005, Washington, DC: Author; *Occupational outlook handbook* by U.S. Department of Labor, Bureau of Labor Statistics (2007). Washington, DC: Author; Career guide to industries, 2006–07 Edition, Health Care by U.S. Department of Labor, Bureau of Labor Statistics (2007), from http://www.bls.gov/oco/cg/cgs035.htm

United States Health Workforce Personnel Factbook, by Health Resources and Services Administration, Bureau of Health Professions, 1999, Washington, DC: Author; The National Sample Survey of Registered Nurses, March 2000: Preliminary Findings, by Health Resources and Services Administration, Bureau of Health Professions, 2000, Washington, DC: Author;.The United States Health Workforce Profile by Health Resources and Services Administration, Bureau of Health Professions, National Center for Health Workforce Information and Analysis, 2006, Washington, DC: Author, from http://bhpr.hrsa.gov/healthworkforce/ (found on HRSA grantee website, The NY Center for Health Workforce Studies, www.chws.albany.edu).

Projections are extrapolated from 2006 Department of Labor Statistics and 2006 Bureau of Health Professions statistics: RN work force to increase by 5% (2.6 million), physician work force to increase by 1% (788,000), dental work force to increase by 3% (165,000), and pharmacists to increase to 276,000 (approximately 15% increase).

of organized medicine, by wealthy White men. Medical education was restricted to universities that severely limited the number of students from low- and working-class backgrounds and deliberate policies of discrimination against Jewish people, women, and African Americans promoted even greater homogeneity (Starr, 1982).

After World War II, few women pursued careers in medicine, and a lower percentage of doctors were women in 1950 than in 1900. Fortunately, in the 1960s, new social forces shifted this history of women in medicine. The feminist movement, affirmative action programs, and women's own determination led women to seek higher education and particularly in the traditionally male medical careers. With expansion and rapid change in the health care system, new careers (not the traditional professions of nursing, medicine, pharmacy, or dentistry) are emerging in allied health occupations that now comprise 60% of all health-related jobs.

Nursing

Although nursing is the largest single health professional occupation, it continues to be subordinate to medicine and remains "women's work." While doctors have always been overwhelmingly men, nurses have been almost exclusively women. Historically, doctors were able to consolidate and homogenize their ranks by class, race, gender, and professional training; nursing has historically been much more stratified. This heterogeneity and size of nursing make it a mirror of women's experience in the U.S. work force for more than a century. The history of nursing parallels the history of women's work

and working conditions in the United States and worldwide. Further, the sexual and ethnic divisions that exist in health care provider roles are reflected in the history of nursing. However, the gendered nature of the nursing profession and the types of skills inherent in the healing capacity of nursing may in fact be critically important for the current and future health care system.

The History of Nursing Parallels the History of Women in Health Care

Little is written about nursing in ancient history, because the care of the sick was considered an ordinary event and did not warrant recording. In prehistoric ages, both men and women shared the activities of nursing and medicine—herbs and roots were gathered and dispensed to those who were ailing. However, records suggest that sexual divisions began even during these early times. Women tended to fulfill the caregiver role, and men tended to be medicine-givers (Dock & Stewart, 1938). Religion and medicine were united very early with medicine men and later physicians becoming priests while nuns provided nursing care.

Modern nursing is traditionally thought to begin with Florence Nightingale, who asserted that "every woman is a nurse" (Nightingale, 1860/1969). The development of nursing in the United States began during the mid 1800s and was strongly influenced by the programs established in England by Nightingale. The 19th century saw the organization of hospitals as centers for care for the sick as well as the organization of the education and profession of nursing. In the late 1850s, Elizabeth Blackwell, a friend of Florence Nightingale and the first American woman to become a physician, was instrumental in promoting Nightingale's methods for nursing education (e.g., practical experiential training in the hospital setting). Nursing had become a respectable occupation for women by the end of the 19th century due to the pioneering and collaborative efforts of Nightingale and Blackwell—along with other pioneers such as Dorothea Dix (who established nursing care in asylums for the mentally ill), Isabel Hampton Robb (who established the first school of nursing based on Nightingale's model), Lillian Wald and Mary Brewster (who established public health nursing), and Lavinia Dock and Adelaide Nutting (who published texts on the science and theory of nursing practice) (Jamieson & Sewall, 1944).

The 19th-century profession of nursing was created for women and by women—primarily middle- and upper-class women—and was molded by the restraints on women at that time (Ehrenreich & English, 1973). Historians have chronicled the developments of the nursing profession, nursing schools, nursing work in private duty and hospital environments, public health nursing, and war work; the recurrent cycles of nursing shortage; and the expanded roles of nurses. However, the close association between the status of women and the status of nursing and how this has affected the development of nurses and nursing has not received much attention from social and feminist scholars outside of nursing.

Jo Ann Ashley (1976) was one of the first to explore in depth the influence of gender on nursing and nurses. Her book, *Hospitals, Paternalism, and the Role of the Nurse,* is the first history of U.S. nursing from a feminist point of view. Ashley describes the discriminatory attitudes toward women that institutionalized their servitude in hospitals. By exploring and exposing the sexism within the hospital setting and its systematic oppression of the nursing profession, Ashley points out the far-reaching effects on the quality and delivery of health care in U.S. hospitals.

How sexism has affected nurses and nursing has been explored by others (Cleland, 1971; Darbyshire, 1987; Levitt, 1977; Weaver & Garrett, 1983). Of these, Cleland (1971) was the first to discuss how sexism is nursing's most pervasive problem. Roberts (1983) explored oppression and oppressed group behavior in nursing, discussing how oppression has fostered the horizontal violence of nurse against nurse. Muff and her colleagues (1988) identify the problems of nurses as the problems of women in the collection *Socialization, Sexism, and Stereotyping: Women's Issues in Nursing.* These authors explore the problems of rigid sex role socialization and the ways in which these stereotypes reflect societal values and prejudices. Feminism has brought both positives and negatives to nursing. On the positive side, feminists have encouraged women's participation and recognition in all work environments. On the negative

side, some feminists have identified nursing as an occupational ghetto that should be avoided by career-minded women.

The historical development of the nursing work culture, explored by Barbara Melosh in her 1982 book *The Physician's Hand,* complemented the history of nursing portrayed in nursing journals and texts (which promotes the ideal of professionalism). Melosh presents the history of nursing from the perspective of working nurses and the active and passive resistance that many nurses displayed toward professionalism in nursing. This is in contrast to the culture of professionalism created by academics and nursing leaders. Melosh explores the culture of nursing and "recasts nursing history from the viewpoint of working nurses and places it in the context of women's history, labor history, and medical history and sociology" (p. 6). In so doing, she illuminates the origins of some of the divisive issues within nursing that exist today—for example, the continued controversy over the required level of education for entry to practice. Melosh traces the labor history and the professional organizations that grew out of and supported the educational methods for licensed practical nurses (LPNs) and registered nurses (RNs). In addition, she describes the class differences between the educational elite (RNs) and the labor class workers (LPNs). The title of her work reflects the establishment and development of nursing as an extension of the physician—an image of handmaiden that nurses have long fought to eliminate. However, nurses were following the model of medicine that defined professional status on the basis of education.

The central work of nursing, caring, is the focus of Reverby's (1987a, 1987b) historical study of nursing. The history of nursing is inextricably intertwined with the development of medicine and political economy of the hospital as an institution. The "dilemma of caring" involves nurses being ordered to care (and to provide care) in a society that does not value caring. Taking the struggle that Nightingale faced in developing a respectable occupation for women one step further, Reverby examines how society has failed to value caring and caring activities. The profession of nursing has been demanding the right to care as opposed to obeying the order to care. This challenges the deeply held beliefs about the gender relations in and the structure of the health care hierarchy in that it opposes the traditional physician-male ordering the nurse-female to care for the patient-child. In contrast, with enactment of the ideal "right to care" process, the nurse and physician decide collaboratively, in consultation with the patient, on the methods and modes of care. The difficulty of finding a way to "care with autonomy" and the inability to separate caring from its societal (lack of) value leads many nurses to abandon the effort to care or to abandon nursing altogether. Reverby makes a strong argument to support the close connection between the social status of women and nurses and the problems that both face.

Unfortunately, by linking nursing's claim to professional status to caring, nursing both obscures the workings of the dominant culture (male and medical) and unintentionally maintains them (Fisher, 1995). Since caring is a gendered activity, if nurses (who are generally women) care, and doctors (who are still predominantly male) do not, then caring continues to be marginalized in both status and earning capacity. Arlie Hochschild (1983) linked the work of "caring" with occupational activities and economics. In a study of women service workers, she described how women are expected to sell their "emotional labor"—to pretend to have positive feelings they are not experiencing and to deny their negative responses in order to make others feel they are being cared for in a safe environment. This often results in "emotional dissonance"—core stress in which the task of managing an estrangement between self and feeling and between self and behavior. Although women in jobs with the greatest responsibility reported the most stress, it was those with the least say over their working lives who suffered the worst effects. Hochschild also reported that this experience leads to burnout and a loss of self as feelings and emotions became dulled as a defense against an intolerable situation. Subsequent studies have found that women workers with the least autonomy, job status, or control in their work suffered from physical and emotional disorders resulting in significant economic impact (Doyal, 1995). Pam Smith (1992) has transferred Hochschild's notion of emotional labor to nurses in an attempt to understand the nature of "caring" work. She documents the way in which some nurses have to suppress very powerful feelings of their own in order to care for and promote the well-being of those for whom they are caring. Two recent studies (Ishii, Iwata, Dakeishi, & Murata, 2004; Morikawa et al., 2005) demonstrate the physiologic effects of work stressors on nurses' well-being.

The relationship of gendered work to health outcomes has also been examined in the Nurses Health Study—a longitudinal cohort study that began in 1976 with 121,700 U.S. women registered nurses between the ages of 30 and 55 years (Colditz, 1995). In an analysis of 1992 cohort data from the Nurses Health Study, Amick and colleagues (1998) have shown that high-strain work was associated with lower vitality, poorer mental health, higher pain, and increased risks of physical and emotional role limitations among a sample of 33,689 nurses. Moreover, job insecurity was associated with poorer health status. Iso-strain (high job strain with low social support at work) was associated with functional declines over 4 years of follow-up of this cohort. In seven dimensions of healthy functioning (physical functioning, role limitations due to physical health problems, freedom from bodily pain, vitality, social functioning, role limitations due to emotional problems, and mental health), iso-strain predicted lower physical health and less improvement in mental health as seen in other women ($n = 21,290$).

These findings point to the hazards within service sector jobs, particularly for women. Notably, elements of the work women do, and the support they receive from their coworkers and supervisors, have important effects on their health and the health of their patients. Most studies of job strain in women have not included information on work-related social support or sex-specific occupational stressors, including sex discrimination as exemplified in inequitable treatment in hiring and promotion, salary differentials between men and women, limited career advancement opportunities, and sexual harassment. Alternatively, these findings suggest that women with high levels of support from peers and supervisors will have improved function and fewer role limitations despite high levels of job strain.

Other studies of nurses and physicians show that hazards and stressors such as workload and work environment factors also have an impact on patient outcomes. Riley (2004) found that demanding work, a subjective lack of control, and insufficient rewards were powerful sources of stress in doctors, resulting in burnout and physical or mental impairment. Research on patient safety and medical errors suggests a link between hospital staff workload and patient mortality as well as links between job satisfaction and the quality of patient care (Aiken, Clarke, & Sloane, 2001; Vahey, Aiken, Sloane, Clarke, & Vargas, 2004). Nurse burnout has been found to erode clinical decision making, and surveillance of patient safety and is negatively correlated with job satisfaction. Close to half of hospital nurses score in the high burnout and job dissatisfaction range on standardized tests (Aiken, Clarke, Sloane, Sochalski, & Silber, 2002). Essentially, more patients and fewer (or less-educated) staff combined with sicker patients and more complex responsibilities not only affects quality care but increases the risk of death. Essentially, the burden of dealing with hazards inherent in health care work—whether it is risks to self or risks to patients—become the burden of women.

Nursing's Roles in Providing Health Care

There are more than 2 million nurses in the United States practicing throughout the health care delivery system. The average nurse is a White, married, middle-aged mother working full-time in a hospital. Although most nurses are non-Hispanic White, the racial and ethnic diversity of student populations suggests that nursing is appealing to a more diverse population of individuals (28% of nursing students in baccalaureate programs were ethnic minorities in 2005). In 2004, the average age of nurses climbed to 46.8 years; just over 41% of RNs were 50 years and older, and 8% of nurses were under age 30. About half (52.2%) of these nurses have children or other adults living at home for whom they report caretaking responsibilities (Health Resources and Services Administration, 2006b).

While annual earnings of RNs ($59,963) are above average for all workers (approximately $45,650), they are markedly lower than physician, dentist, and pharmacy earnings (see Table 2.1) and below those for physical therapists and dental hygienists (Health Resources and Services Administration, 2006a, 2006b, 2006c). While the average earnings of RNs employed full-time in 2004 were estimated at $58,000 (U.S. Department of Labor, Bureau of Labor Statistics, 2006a, 2006b), when changes in the purchasing power of the dollar were taken into account utilizing the consumer price index, the "real" salary of an RN employed full-time in 2004 was $27,000. Real salaries remained relatively flat between 1992 and 2000, using the annual median salary for nurses estimated by the U.S. Department of Labor. However, between 2000 and 2004, real earning increased for the first time since 1992 (U.S. Bureau of Labor Statistics, 2006b, 2006c). In 1988, more than two-thirds of nurses worked in hospital settings; about 7% worked in nursing homes, community or public health settings, or ambulatory sites; and the remaining 11% worked in nursing education, student health, occupational, and private-duty nursing (O'Neil, 1993). Although hospitals remain the major employer of nurses, results from the 2004 National Sample Survey of Registered Nurses (Health Resources and Services Administration, 2006b) indicate a slight trend away from the hospital as the setting for the principal nursing position. In 2004, over half of RNs worked in hospitals (56.2%, approximately 4% less than in 2000), with about one-third (31.7%) employed in nursing homes, community or public health settings, or ambulatory settings (Health Resources and Services Administration, 2006b).

Although hospital census decreased during the 1980s, registered nurse employment in hospitals increased, reflecting the growing complexity of patient and expanded administrative roles for RN personnel. In the early 1990s, for cost-cutting reasons, unlicensed assistive personnel were hired in lieu of RNs. In addition, massive staff reduction occurred, leaving nurses feeling undervalued and overworked and resulting in a mass exodus of nurses from the profession. However, these market-driven models of health care management failed due to increasing patient acuities, concerns over medical errors, and declining numbers of ancillary personnel.

As many nurses have moved out of generic staff nurse roles in hospitals, some have gained new education and assumed new responsibilities in the delivery and management of care, particularly in primary care settings. Expanded roles for nurses, described as advanced practice nursing, include the more autonomous roles of clinical nurse specialist, nurse practitioner, nurse midwife, and nurse anesthetist. According to a 2004 survey, the number of nurses prepared to practice in at least one advanced practice role was estimated to be 240,460 (8.3% of the total RN population) compared to 161,712 (or 6.3%) in 1996 (Health Resources and Services Administration, 2006a, 2006b).

Most visible of the advanced practice roles for nurses are the approximately 141,209 licensed nurse practitioners (NPs) and the 10,340 licensed nurse midwives (28,855 dually certified as NPs and nurse midwives). Educated and licensed in many states to play a more collaborative leadership role in primary care with patients, their employment was split about 30% each in hospitals, community health, and ambulatory care settings, and about 5% were self-employed. Research findings consistently find that both NPs and midwives provide safe and effective care (Brown & Grimes, 1993; Rooks, 1997; Sox, 1979) and that collaborative physician/nurse practitioner care management of hospitalized medical patients results in improved outcomes (reduced length of stay and increased hospital profit) without altering readmissions or mortality (Cowan et al., 2006). A meta-analysis published in 1993 compared NP and Certified Nurse Midwife (CNM) care with physician care and found equivalent medical outcomes, along with greater patient adherence to treatment recommendations and less use of technology (Brown & Grimes, 1993). Another study reported that women with midwife attendants had 50% fewer cesarean sections than did those with physicians; their periods of labor were 25% shorter; they needed 40% less oxygen with 30% fewer painkillers during childbirth and suffered less postpartum depression (Rooks, 1997).

The majority of nurse practitioners provide primary health care—a combination of medical care and health promotion in the context of social and psychological caring, treating minor illnesses and chronic diseases and referring those with more complex medical conditions to specialists or hospitals. NPs devote more time than most physicians to whole patient care, focusing on psychological and social aspects of disease, such as stress, family issues, mental health, or neighborhood safety. But like most nurses, they also tend to recommend health-promoting regimens such as diet and exercise, rather than costly treatments more often prescribed by physicians (Avorn, Everitt & Baker, 1991; Baldwin, Hutchinson, & Rosenblatt, 1992; Lenz, Mundinger, Hopkins, Lin, & Smolowitz, 2002; Rosenblatt et al., 1997).

The expansion of the nursing role by these advanced practitioners has met with opposition from the medical practitioners who occupy the respective markets. Nurse midwives have had to fight obstetricians and gynecologists for practice privileges and reasonable insurance rates (Kendellen, 1987; Lubic, 1987). In addition, nurse midwives have struggled with the dilemma of lay midwives (whether or how to officially recognize and identify with these less formally educated practitioners), who have been making a comeback in the past 20 years (Kay, Butter, Chang, & Houlihan, 1988). The role of the nurse practitioner has required close collaboration with a physician due to restrictions on medication prescribing by NPs as well as limitations on direct reimbursement for NP services. While NPs (just like physicians) can bill patients directly, this has become the exception rather than the rule. While federal and state laws have been changed to allow NPs to bill their services under private and government health insurance programs (e.g., Medicaid and Medicare), patient access to NP care has been restricted due to a combination of factors—opposition from organized medicine and payment restrictions by managed care organizations (that are often controlled by physician groups).

Several studies conducted on the future of nursing point to a growing demand for nurses through the early years of the 21st century. The gap between the demand and supply of nurses is projected to increase significantly after 2005. While there will always be a need for traditional hospital nurses, a large number of new nurses will be needed in home health care (to perform complex procedures in patients homes), long-term care (for older, sicker patients and rehabilitation for stroke, head injury, or Alzheimer's disease patients), and ambulatory care (for patients having same-day surgery, rehabilitation, or chemotherapy).

As the nation's population ages, nurses are also growing older, but the rate of newcomers to the profession is slowing. Age isn't the only factor as fewer young people are taking up the profession and many nurses are increasingly finding opportunities in business, law, and other careers. However, many believe that nursing will not only survive into the next century, but that its values will prevail in the health care system of the future (Fagin, 1994; Fisher, 1999; Nursing Institute, 2001). The future of health care delivery is shifting some of its focus from cure to care. Nurses—especially nurse practitioners and midwives—link curing and caring with compassion, patience, people skills, an interest in healing as a team, a tendency to seek holistic cures, and a view of the patient as a whole person with social and psychological needs. With more NPs as primary care providers, health care costs could be reduced, primary care providers would be increased, and a change in the way medicine is practiced could occur. Although the nursing work force is aging, all women will be living and working longer. We have seen that middle-aged women become more assertive; thus, as educated, experienced, baby boomer women nurses age, they are likely to accelerate the historical trend toward economic and social equality between the sexes in health care. These nurses have the competence and the capacity to move from invisible and silent handmaidens to leaders in wellness and healing as well as caring.

Allied Health Care Providers

Allied and auxiliary health care workers[1] make up over 60% of the nation's 13.5 million people in the health care work force (Ruzek et al., 1999) and have been defined by the Committee on Allied Health Education and Accreditation as a "a large cluster of health care–related professions and personnel whose functions include assisting, facilitating, or complementing the work of physicians and other specialists in the health care system, and who choose to be identified as allied health personnel" (Lindeman & McAthie, 1999, p. 43). These workers, ranging from physical therapists and technicians at the allied level to unlicensed assistive personnel at the auxiliary level, play critical support roles in the health care system. Allied health care workers include more than 200 health professions and all personnel who provide therapeutic, diagnostic, informational, or environmental services in health care delivery settings. They may be licensed, certified, or registered and may provide either direct or indirect care and support services to patients. Not included in these categories are physicians, pharmacists, dentists, and nurses.

Auxiliary health care worker is a less well-defined group that can provide environmental and other support services. Typically, these workers are not licensed, certified, or registered (Tache & Chapman, 2006). These occupations have been predominantly hospital based. A range of extended practice roles for allied health professionals have been promoted and are being undertaken, but their health outcomes have rarely been evaluated. There is also little evidence as to how best to introduce such roles or how best to educate, support, and mentor these practitioners (McPherson et al., 2006).

Women make up a large proportion of the work force in many of these occupations. A 1998 study of allied health workers from California along with updated statistics from the Bureau of Health Statistics highlight the proportion of women in selected allied health occupations (Ruzek et al., 1999; U.S. Department of Labor, 2006b): Dental hygienists and dental assistants (97% women), speech and occupational therapists (90% women), health records technologists/technicians (87% women), nursing and home health aides (88% women), physical therapists (69% women), clinical laboratory technologists/technicians (74% women), radiology technicians (72% women), and respiratory therapists (51% women). Nursing aides represent the largest group of allied health workers (37%) followed by dental hygienists/assistants (21%). Men outnumber women in only one occupational category—emergency medical technicians and paramedics (U.S. Department of Labor, 2006b). Ethnic minority

---

1. Despite the linguistic confusion associated with the term *allied health worker*, it continues to be used by federal and state agencies to refer to supporting staff—therapists, technicians, clerks, aides, assistants, and a few other workers not classified as dentists, doctors, or nurses.

women (37%) are over-represented in the lowest paying allied health occupations such as nursing assistants and health aides.

The majority of technical allied health jobs are in hospitals—80% of nuclear medicine and clinical laboratory technologists and more than half of radiology technicians and respiratory therapists. Clinical laboratory workers are the largest group of hospital workers other than nurses. Dieticians, emergency medical technicians, and occupational and physical therapists are often employed by private contractors or state and local governments (public health departments). The majority of the lowest paid allied and auxiliary health workers are in nursing and personal care facilities and home health care. Two-thirds of the 250,000 medical assistants are employed in medical clinics or doctors' offices, and over half of the 1.5 million nursing and home health aides work in nursing homes. The service and support occupations attract many workers with little or no specialized education or training. In general, education and technical training is directly linked with earnings and wages for all health care workers, including allied health workers (see Table 2.1). Although a high school diploma and on-the-job training is the minimum for entry into most of the lowest-paid occupational categories, some college education or technical training is necessary for the technical and upper-level allied health occupations.

Allied health positions—in particular, medical assistants and home health aides—are expected to grow rapidly in the next 10 years, by approximately 55% (U.S. Department of Labor, 2005a; Tache & Chapman, 2006). Median annual earnings for these two groups ($20,000 to $22,000) was less than the average annual wage for all workers ($37,000) as well as the average wage for all health service workers ($24,000) in 2005 (U.S. Department of Labor, 2006b). Medical record and health information technicians are projected to be the fastest growing occupations due to rapid growth in the number of medical tests, treatments, and procedures that will be increasingly scrutinized by third-party payers, regulators, courts, and consumers. Although technical jobs often have higher wages, these occupations are often unstable for long-term employment. These technology-driven jobs (e.g., radiation imaging) have limited scopes of practice, and new technology will reduce the need for workers. In one of the higher paying allied health occupations, the demand for dental hygienists is increasing in response to increasing need for dental care and the greater substitution of hygienists for services previously performed by dentists. Overall within the allied and auxiliary health occupations, women's median earnings continue to be less than their male counterparts; women allied health workers earn 80% of men's salaries (U.S. Department of Labor, 2006b). While some authors have suggested that this disparity could reflect men's higher levels of responsibility rather

than unequal pay for the same work, others point to the fact that, in the occupations with the most women (e.g., dental assistants and dietitians), they earn less than similar categories of workers that have more men (Muller, 1994).

It has been widely believed that these jobs—because they tend to be thought of as women's jobs—are neither physically hazardous nor particularly stressful. Another myth is that women are working part-time to supplement a husband's salary. In a 1993 study (Himmelstein, Lewontin & Woolhandler, 1996), many poor and minority women, especially single African American mothers, were concentrated in the allied and auxiliary health occupations. Even more disturbing was that 12% did not have health insurance, and about 600,000 workers lived in poverty. Dietary workers report that they often prepare healthier foods professionally than they consume at home. Compared to other occupational sectors, there are more occupational injuries and illness in hospitals and nursing homes, and these affect the lower paid workers more frequently (Colligan, Smith & Hurrell, 1977; U.S. Department of Labor, 2005b). Work-related injuries and hazards include back strain; radiation or chemical exposure; and exposure to infectious diseases such as AIDS, tuberculosis, and hepatitis. In nursing facilities and home care, hazards are related to transportation accidents, overexertion, falls inside and outside the home, and injuries related to moving patients because mechanical lifting devices are usually not available.

The issues for nurses as health care providers are the same for many of the women-dominated allied health occupations, just more so. Waged work cannot be separated from women's lives. Nurses and women in the allied health occupations need employer support of regular and emergency care giving obligations. The lower paid allied health workers need family insurance for health care costs. Many of these women (as well as many minority men) need training, child care during training, entry jobs with career possibilities, and adequate wages in order to fill the future needs for a multiskilled health worker.

Women in Medicine, Pharmacy, and Dentistry

Three health care occupations—medicine, dentistry, and pharmacy—are identified as traditionally male in Table 2.1, which also identifies them as the highest paid health occupations. There is a considerable literature on women in medicine, less on women in dentistry and pharmacy. Women are changing the practice of these formerly male professions but in different ways. With an oversupply of physicians in some specialties and an undersupply in others (particularly in primary care), women physicians are helping to transform the practice of medicine by their dominance in primary care fields. However, shortages are looming for both dentistry and especially for pharmacy. Pharmacist shortages are most acute, with women pharmacists playing a role because few of them want to work full-time. Since almost half of the practicing pharmacists are women with 60% projected by 2010, the pharmacy work environment is drastically changing. The following section will focus on women in medicine as representative of the challenges facing women in these male-identified occupations. First, we will highlight some unique aspects of women in dental and pharmacy occupations.

Pharmacy

Pharmacists represent the third largest health professional group in the United States, with about 248,000 active pharmacists in 2005 (Health Resources and Services Administration, 2006c). Most pharmacists are employed and practice in pharmacies or drug stores, hospitals and medical centers, other retail stores with pharmacies (i.e., grocery stores and mass merchandising stores), and other institutional settings such as long-term care facilities. Smaller numbers of pharmacists are employed by pharmaceutical manufacturers, managed care and health insurance plans, consulting groups, home health care, and universities. Pharmacists practicing today provide a much broader range of services than pharmacists did in the past. In the 1990s, the pharmacy profession extended the educational requirements to a doctorate-level entry degree, requiring additional clinical training and expanded practice skills, thus preparing pharmacists to take on more complex clinical roles such as counseling patients, advising other health professionals on drug use issues, and participating in disease management programs.

While the overall supply of pharmacists has increased in the past decade, there has been an unprecedented demand for pharmacists and for pharmaceutical care services, which has not been met by the currently available supply. Some of the factors identified as contributing to the shortage include advances in new drug development and dispensing technology; changes in the organization of pharmaceutical distribution through pharmacy benefit management programs and growth of chain pharmacy stores; rapid expansion in the number of medications dispensed; increased numbers of pharmacy technicians; and a greater range of opportunities for clinical pharmacists (Knapp, 1999; U.S. Department of Health and Human Services, 2000a).

As with many professions—including medicine, law, and dentistry—pharmacy has seen increasing numbers of women enter the profession over the last three decades. In 1970, women pharmacists accounted for 13% of the pharmacy work force, progressing to 46% in 2004.

Many women pharmacists elect part-time work, which has become an important issue for the pharmacist shortage.

Dentistry

Dentists represent the nation's fourth largest health professional group. Dental care focuses on oral health and oral function provided by general dentists, dental specialists, and dental hygienists. Most practitioners in both dentistry and pharmacy practice as generalists, in sharp contrast with medicine, where the number of specialist physicians far exceeds generalists. Once focused on treatment, today the focus is on preventive aspects of oral health care. Like all other health professionals, technological advances, market evolution, and demographic changes have substantially altered types and quality of dental services. The U.S. public is increasingly interested in prevention of dental disease, good occlusion, pain-free joint and jaw function, good lip function for speech, and skeletal harmony in their faces for an attractive appearance. There also is a need for holistic dental providers with the capacity to consider overall health status. Concurrently, there has been a deterioration in oral health according to a recent U.S. Surgeon General Report that found over one-third of the U.S. population (100 million people) has no access to community water fluoridation and more than 108 million children and adults lack dental insurance (U.S.Department of Health and Human Services, 2000b).

The major practice mode of dentistry remains private practice, most commonly solo practice or groups with two or three dentists. There is no consensus on the optimal number of and ratio of health professionals to meet the population's health care needs. However, in the 1990s, dentist supply growth fell below overall population growth (Brown & Lazar, 1999). There is now concern that the supply of dentists will not be sufficient to meet the aggregate population dental care needs. As more Americans retain their teeth into older age, the demand for continued restorative care among older age groups will increase.

The rate of growth in the number of women in dentistry has been substantial, with almost a 50% increase in women dentists over the past 20 years. In 1980, women represented 14% of new graduates in dentistry; by 1996, they had increased to 36%. While women represented only 2% of practicing dentists in 1980, they represented almost 22% in 2005 (American Dental Association, 1999; U.S. Department of Labor, 2006b). In comparison to medicine and pharmacy, the number of women in dentistry lags, with only one out of six dentists being women, compared to a 1-to-2 ratio for pharmacy and a 1-to-4 ratio for medicine. Although earnings are high for dentists, the traditional solo practice model may be a deterrent for women entering the profession who want to balance work and family and prefer group or part-time practice.

Medicine

As described earlier in the history of the development of nursing, the history of women in medicine is clearly linked with women's social and political history. It is not surprising that women faced resistance in seeking entrance into the medical profession. In the 19th century, when women were organizing and fighting for their political (right to vote) and social (right to work outside the home and own property) rights and some women were fighting to establish nursing as a respectable career for women, others were arguing that women ought to be physicians "by virtue of their natural gifts as healers and nurturers" (Morantz-Sanchez, 1985). Although the feminist movement of the 19th century helped women gain access to medical education and careers, at the same time the feminist movement also incited a strong resistance to women in medicine (Shryock, 1966).

The early relative success in the 1850s in opening medicine to women was minimized or reversed in the late 19th and early 20th centuries. During this time, the Flexner Report was contracted by the Carnegie Corporation and published in 1910. The wealth of the industrial revolution had allowed the development of organized philanthropy, and medical reform was a high priority for these new foundations. In the name of standardizing (in accordance with the Johns Hopkins medical education model) and ensuring the quality of medical education, the majority of smaller, less well-endowed and -supported medical schools that trained women and minority physicians were effectively closed. Although this process did eliminate ineffective and dangerous small schools, it also eliminated those that were effective and successful but unable to finance the newly required facilities. Without access to training opportunities, the number of women physicians decreased markedly. Not until the 20th-century women's movement, which gained momentum in the 1960s, did women begin to increase significantly in numbers and proportion of medical school applicants, admissions, and graduates (Walsch, 1977).

As indicated in Table 2.2, the proportion of physicians who are women has been increasing significantly and is projected to continue to increase to more than 40% in 2020. Currently, there are almost 800,000 practicing physicians in the United States, with one woman for every 3 to 4 men physicians (U.S. Department of Labor, 2006b). There are no data about the proportion of minority women physicians, but ethnic diversity in medicine as been slow to improve. In 1989, 3% of all physicians were Black compared to the same proportion in 1910 (Hart-Brothers, 1994). While current medical school graduate data suggest that non-Hispanic White physicians are more representative of the national population, only 7% of graduates were Black and Hispanic in 2004 compared to 20% who were Asian (Health Resources and Services Administration, 2006a). However, in the past decade, the number of Black women physicians has increased more rapidly than the number of male physicians in the United States. These women have made it into a traditionally male work world, and, although they are at the top of the health care occupations hierarchy, they face problems similar to those faced by women in other occupations and in society as a whole.

First, making it into the world of medicine does not mean making it within the world of medicine—if *making it* means status and monetary success. More than 60% of all women physicians in 1992 were disproportionately concentrated in one of seven specialties (e.g., relatively lower-paying and lower-status medical specialties): internal medicine (22%), pediatrics (14%), family practice (10%), psychiatry (9%), obstetrics and gynecology (9.3%), anesthesiology (5%), and pathology (4%) (Frank & Lutz, 1999). Women have been underrepresented in all surgical specialties except gynecology and are particularly underrepresented in orthopedic and urologic surgery specialties (Ginzberg, 1994). The higher-paying (and therefore higher-status) specialties of diagnostic radiology (4% women) and surgery (4.4% women)—in particular, cardiothoracic surgery (less than 0.1% women)—have the lowest proportion of women (Council of Medical Specialty Society, 1990; U.S. Department of Labor, 2006b). Whether these specialty choices reflect women's preferences for practice type and environment or reflect a subtle pressure to choose "appropriate" specialties, it remains interesting that those specialties with a higher proportion of women are at the bottom of the medical hierarchy. In a 1998 survey of women physicians (Frank, McMurray, Linzer, & Elon, 2000), although most were satisfied with their medical career and choice of specialty, many would not become physicians if starting their careers again due to work stress, harassment, and poor control over their work environment.

The discrimination that women physicians have faced in medicine has been well documented (Kopriva, 1994; Lorber, 1984; Morantz-Sanchez, 1985; Walsch, 1977). The problems of combining a family with a demanding medical career have been explored with the not-surprising finding that women physicians feel the most strain in their personal lives, some strain in their family role, and minimal strain in their professional role (Bickel, 2000; Ducker, 1986; Frank, Harvey, & Elon, 2000). Women physicians, like women in general, sacrifice their own health and well-being for the sake of others. Women physicians struggle to combine a family life and a career (More & Greer, 2000; Woodward, Cohen,

& Ferrier, 1990). A female surgery resident who is married starts out "with a strike against her" because her attention is assumed to be divided between her career and her marriage/family responsibilities (Burnley & Burkett, 1986). The struggles that men physicians face in combining a family and career are not documented in the literature on physicians; therefore, comparisons are not currently possible. However, there is an indication among young physicians, both men and women, to reduce the traditionally long and rigorous training and practice schedules and to find ways to maintain a more healthy balance among their professional, family, and medical leadership responsibilities (Kopriva, 1994). There is also indication that the disparities in earnings between men and women physicians have begun to shrink. Although physician earnings are the highest of any occupation, women physicians earn about two-thirds of men physicians' mean annual income (U.S. Department of Labor, 2006b). With the growth of managed care and an increase of salaried physicians (for both men and women), gender differences in earnings are declining.

The increase in women in medicine may be related to a decline in men's applications to medical schools as well as more older men physicians leaving the practice. Medicine has been seen as a less attractive career choice for well-educated men (who have the greatest career options) due to constraints on professional fees and salaries, the expansion of managed care arrangements, and increasing government regulation of health care services (Ginzberg, 1994). Women may be in a more advantageous position, because their values tend to be more congruent with the shape of the new health care system. Many prefer salaried employment; many are attracted to primary care specialties; and many prefer the flexibility that medicine offers them to extend or contract their hours of work. And both men and women patients prefer women physicians (one and a half to three times more often), especially in the areas of obstetrics and gynecology, family practice, internal medicine, and psychiatry (Fenton, Robinowitz, & Leaf, 1987).

An unfortunate outcome of the increased number of women in medicine has been an increase in distancing behavior between women physicians and other women health care workers, especially nurses. Surveys in the past decade support the view that women physicians are no more collaborative in their relationships than men physicians (Fagin, 1994). Articles written by women physicians indicate that the problem may be worse when both professionals are women, because women physicians must demonstrate their differences from women nurses, thereby increasing their status while lowering nurses' status (National League for Nursing, 1990). Lorber (1987) and Wilson (1987) sum up the issues of women physicians by stating that women physicians face a choice—either they can align themselves with men physicians and perpetuate physician dominance of the health care system or they can align themselves with other women and work toward change of the health care system. Whether the increasing proportion of women physicians will result in women influencing the practice of medicine or whether the established medical profession will influence women physicians— or a combination of the two—the status of women physicians will continue to be linked with the status of women in society.

WOMEN AS PAID HEALTH CARE PROVIDERS IN THE 21ST CENTURY: A PREFERRED FUTURE

By the time you read this, the health care system will have taken another turn in its rapid fluctuations of market-driven change. Emerging trends and perceived and real threats on the horizon will impact all health professions (Fagin, 1994; O'Neil, 2003; O'Neil & The Pew Health Professions Commission, 1998). These include profound changes in the payment to and financing of doctors and hospitals, with increased competition among health care providers; a perceived surplus of physicians and concerns about the effects on the costs of health care generated by more physicians; a perceived shortage of other health workers with a long-lasting shortage of nurses; concerns about reduced interest of students in health professions, especially care giving occupations; new technologies in and outside hospitals; rapid growth of ambulatory and home care services, often in competition with hospitals; the growing problems in financing care for the uninsured and vulnerable populations (the working and nonworking poor, people with AIDS, the homeless, the chronically mentally ill, and frail elderly needing long-term care); and the changing patterns of disease created by changing demographics and social trends (e.g., the aging population, the drug epidemic, environmental diseases, or deaths from violence). An aging population will require more home health care services and new technologies; health networks will become larger and more complex, requiring more managerial and support workers. A shift from hospital care to less expensive ambulatory and home care is occurring because of a focus on disease prevention and health promotion as well as cost-containment and self-care practices by many Americans.

Unfortunately, little has been done to change health professions or to include them as change agents for education or health care delivery. Furthermore, little attention has focused on the dynamic between health care workers and the health care delivery system. In the current market-driven system, health care workers are treated as problems (liabilities and expenses) rather than as part of a solution (critical and participatory resources). The usual business approach of focusing on supply and demand fails to capture the fundamental problem that health care workers and professionals face today—the environment of care. With more than a decade of constant health system change and reorganization along with changes in reimbursement and funding mechanisms, the overall environment of care has deteriorated to such an extent that many health care workers, especially direct care providers, feel unable to care adequately for patients (Glazer, 1988; Ruzek et al., 1999; Smith, 1992; Taft, 2001). Stress of care giving is evidenced by the very high rates of turnover and dropout (Aiken et al., 2002; Vahey et al., 2004). And this problem is not new. Almost 25 years ago, the National Institute for Occupational Safety and Health ranked 130 occupations according to their incidence of mental health problems: women caregivers, nursing aides, and RNs were ranked 3, 10, and 27, respectively. Clearly, history informs us that we are experiencing not only massive changes in health care delivery but also an impending health-caring and care giving crisis.

Outside the health care delivery system, trends are affecting all work environments and provide a context in which the health-caring crisis is evolving. Many workers are choosing time over money with a priority on personal time instead of financial compensation. Employees want to balance their professional and personal roles rather than choosing one over the other. Young employees in their 20s and 30s view the work place differently than earlier generations, preferring greater autonomy and less bureaucracy. Their loyalty is to the work rather than to an employer. Subsequently, these younger workers are choosing independent work and freelancing, such as the temporary employment agencies in health care (Jovic, Wallace, & Lemaire, 2006). To attract workers, especially women, employers are offering services to reduce the stress of managing professional and personal lives (e.g., child or elder care, housecleaning, and on-site full-service banking). Outside of health care, management is increasingly collaborative, with flattened hierarchies and increased team structures. On the downside, however, as more employees opt for less stressful work or more personal time, a subgroup of workers are carrying extra workloads and long hours.

Women are also changing the work environment in the marketplace and creating a more humane work life. With more women in the workforce, industries outside of health care are recognizing the value of women's talent as well as temperament. Some research findings suggest that women take a more long-term, contextual view toward solving complex problems and often conduct business with fewer trappings of rank or hierarchy (Drucker, 1992; Fisher, 1999; Rosener, 1995). Women workers, managers, and professionals have demonstrated skills related to attention to detail, sensitive listening, and empathetic responses, as well as their ability to motivate, organize, and direct others. Many believe that, in the field of international development, women's grass-roots organizations will be the most significant economic catalysts and forces for social justice in the 21st century (Fisher, 1999). As traditional corporations are decentralizing and building staff networks based on teams of equals, they have found that women have been especially skilled at constructing and maintaining these networks. Women are also gravitating to companies that offer flexible work arrangements in order to balance work and family.

The health care industry can take lessons from other business sectors that value a diverse, productive, and healthy work force. Many people within health care have already recognized that the new health care system will require health professionals with different skills, attitudes, and values (O'Neil, 1993, 2003). As the boundaries of the health professions change, there is a growing demand for the skills of collaboration, effective communication, and teamwork. With women as the dominant work force in health care delivery, promoting and rewarding the skills and abilities of women will only improve health care delivery. Including women's experiences and concerns as a source of organizational vision can put the "care" back into health care.

Some successful hospitals have focused on improving the work environment, finding that shared governance and shared leadership creates a more satisfying work environment (Peterson, 2001; Cheung & Aiken, 2006). Other important attributes of health care services with effective administrative structures and quality patient care include participatory management, enhanced communication, adequate staffing, and investment in the development of nurses and staff. These organizations are involving staff—because they are closest to patients—in defining and developing the practice of care. Recognizing the link between cost and quality, some health care organizations are involving nurses in the financial management of their units.

Men have made and will continue to make enormous contributions to the practice of medicine, but women physicians bring new attitudes to the job of healing and health care leadership. Studies of women physicians find that they spend more time with patients, are more inclined to mix traditional allopathic medical practices with alternative or complementary cures, and they tend to work in teams with other professionals more regularly than men physicians (Braus, 1994; Mundinger et al., 2000). In a poll of medical students, they reported that women physicians were more sensitive and more altruistic than men doctors (Fisher, 1999).

Although future physicians will remain accountable for patients' medical care, the changing needs of patients suggest that medical care will be only one part of a person's health care needs. Rather than using medicine as the standard for all health care, the foundational model for care giving, healing, and health should be nursing. In the era of professional competition, nurses have been promoted as cheaper alternatives to physicians (e.g., nurse practitioners can provide equal or better care than primary care doctors). Unfortunately, what have been lost in this argument are the benefits, strengths, and contributions of nursing. Although not as well publicized compared to medical care, the characteristics and functions of nursing care have a long tradition of empirical support. In addition to direct patient care activities that restore or maintain health, nurses provide certain functions that are critically important to patient care and to the larger health care organization, such as coordination, advocacy, care management, and communication. Nurses have demonstrated the art and science of care management and advocacy extends beyond the patient to the community and public health problems. Research demonstrates that they have verbal and social skills combined with their empathy and holistic perspective; an ability to network; and a nurturing attitude toward people, society, and the environment (Lindeman & McAthie, 1999). The health care system is in need of these nursing care approaches not as an alternative to medicine—fully utilizing the strength of women's skills that they already have in the nursing work force—but as a partnership with medicine to expand the strengths of women physicians to improve medical care (Hoffman, Maraldo, Coons, & Johnson, 1997; Litaker et al., 2003; Taylor & Woods, 1996).

Women health care workers bring to the curing and caring arts a compassion, a patience, a precision touch, people skills, an interest in healing as a team, a tendency to seek holistic cures, and a view of the patient as a whole person with social and psychological needs. The challenge to women health care providers will be to work together across their multiple diversities. Just as women physicians must work with other women health care workers, nurses will be moving from a direct care role to a new role of organizing and coordinating teams of caregivers. Tensions currently exist about how to delegate, how to manage the workload and be accountable for outcomes, and how to provide for the growth and development of multiple caregivers and other support staff. Nursing and women physicians must consider delegation, along with shared governance, as another form of empowerment. Delegation must be learned, practiced, evaluated, and improved. The work environment must be created where delegation is supported and valued and positive outcomes are rewarded. A critical element of the redesign will be the evaluation of the effectiveness of health care provider roles. As we are making monumental changes in how we care for patients; we must also evaluate whether we are improving patient care or making it worse.

WOMEN AS UNPAID HEALTH CARE PROVIDERS

Clearly, health care is women's work, with the majority of health care providers being women. Turning the phrase around presents another truth—women's work is health care. Much of the work that women do in their unpaid, private lives is health care for themselves and their families. The "caring tricycle" of women is often a life time of responsibility that begins with care of children, continues into middle age with the care of an aging parent, and culminates in old age with responsibility for a frail partner (Doyal, 1995). Almost always a labor of love, it can also be a crushing burden for women who must balance work and other family responsibilities with constant care giving of a vulnerable, dependent human.

The arguments that used to gain women's access into the paid fields of health care were based on women's natural talents and interests in caring for their families. Chodorow (1996) argued that women's greater interest in and ability to care for family members is a socially constructed gender difference, not a biologically determined difference. The ancient socially proscribed roles of food gathering, cultivation, and preparation; keeping the home environment clean and safe; and the biological role of bearing and caring for children had singularly prepared women to care for the health and welfare of society.

Today, women do the majority of domestic work—housework, shopping, cooking, and care giving—regardless of whether they are employed outside of the home (Brody, 1995). The fact that more women are in the labor force and that the two-income family is fast becoming a necessity rather than a luxury has not altered women's socially proscribed roles and rarely has challenged responsibility for their care of the family.

One way of evaluating the socially recognized importance of women as health care providers for the family is an exploration of the marketing aimed at women as the health care decision maker for the family (e.g., the "ask Doctor Mom" commercial for cough medicine). Women provide health care and also decide from whom and where they will seek help for themselves and their families. To guide women consumers toward healthy choices in providing family health care, women are also targeted by food product advertisements that promote healthy children, heart health, low fat, low sugar, and smart buying as healthy buying, including all types of food products from soup to peanut butter. The importance of a clean house, clean clothes, healthy exercise—not to mention a beautiful body, preferably looking like a fashion model—are primarily advertised using women models and targeted to women who are responsible for the health and welfare of their families (Graham, 1985).

Beyond the standard of daily health care provided by women in families is the role of health care provider for the ill and infirm in the family (Finch & Groves, 1983; Robinson, 1998). Women as mothers and daughters have traditionally been the caregivers for family members in need, with one study finding that 75% of the caregivers of ill elders are women (Travelers Insurance Companies, 1988; U.S. Department of Labor, 2006b). While elderly spouses provide care to each other when one of them becomes ill or disabled, because of the discrepancy in life expectancy between men and women, most care giving spouses are women. Daughters outnumber sons by about four to one as primary caregivers to disabled parents and are the largest group of helpers for the disabled elderly (Brody, 1995; Robinson, 1998). Elaine Brody (1981) was the first to define the role of "women in the middle" as those women who have primary responsibility for dependent children as well as assuming care for their elderly parents and in-laws as the advances of medical science and public health have resulted in an extended life span. U.S. demographics are not encouraging for this group of women in the middle. Only 4% of the total U.S. population was aged 65 or older in 1900. In 1990, 12% of the population was 65 or older, which is projected to be 14% in 2010 and 20% by the year 2030 (Day, 1992). The oldest old (i.e., people over 85 years old) has also increased dramatically to almost 4 million, with a 27% rise since 1990 (U.S. Census Bureau, 2000). Not all people over the age of 65 are infirm; in fact, most are in good health. However, the increasing disability and episodic health needs of this age group rely primarily on daughters or daughters-in-law for assistance. The aging of the population has combined with a decrease in the birthrate (4 per family in 1900 to 1.2 per family in 1997). This means that there will be an increase in the number of needy elderly in the population corresponding to a decrease in the number of women (or men) available to provide health care assistance. Almost no data are available on the numbers of women providing care to children with serious ongoing health conditions, and most of this care is rendered without appearing on the ledgers of the nations' economy (Stein, Bauman, & Jessop, 1994). Advanced technology has improved the life span of many disabled children, allowing them to live at home but requiring significant caretaking. These caretakers, the women in the middle, will likely attend to the needs of their aging and young dependent family members to the detriment of their own health needs (Bull, 2001; Hoffman & Mitchell, 1998).

It is not only the increase in the numbers of elderly in the population that has placed additional burdens on women as family health care providers. The changes resulting from the implementation of diagnostic related groupings—which effectively limits the amount of time any particular patient stays in the hospital—have resulted in patients being discharged sooner and sicker than in the past. The majority of these patients are discharged home with the assumption that home care is cheaper than hospital care and just as safe, if not beneficial, after a certain stabilized point in recovery (Bull, 1990; Picot, 1995; Robinson, 1998). The majority of this at-home care—from assistance with daily living activities to complex cancer pain and treatment management to managing with the ever-changing demands of the Alzheimer's patient or the ventilator-assisted child—is provided by women, either an unpaid family member (80% to 90%) or a home health aide (Brody, 1995; Talley & Crews, 2007).

Beyond the family health care needs that women attend to, women are community activists in promoting health care. Whether it is campaigning for safe living environments in the inner city, combating toxic waste hazards, or working for clean water and proper sanitation in developing countries, women are leaders in identifying the problems and organizing the solutions (Doyal, 1995; Pizurki, Mejia, Butter, & Ewart, 1987). The World Health Organization has recognized the importance of women as health care providers in its emphasis on "Women, Health and Development" in the efforts for "Health for All by the Year 2000" through the mechanisms of primary, preventive health care (Pizurki et al., 1987). At local and state levels, women are organizing and advocating for new models of delivering health care (Taylor & Dower, 1997; Washington Women's Education Foundation, 1997).

But who cares for the caregivers? Little is known about the economic costs of physical and mental health care for care giving women whose health suffers. Nor do we know the costs to the system when family caregivers are deterred from entering the labor force, quit their jobs or work part-time, or are less efficient in their jobs due to care giving responsibilities. Since women's wages are generally lower than men's, women are more likely than men to leave paid employment to become unpaid family caregivers. Although there is evidence that more employers are providing incentives to women workers in the form of child and elder care services, the tension remains between changing values—new values about women's roles as paid workers and traditional values of women remaining the primary caregivers and health care providers for the family.

SUMMARY

Health care is women's work, and this work cannot be separated from women's lives. Although the increasing numbers of women doctors, dentists, and pharmacists receive a lot of attention and praise for "making it in a man's world," the vast majority of paid and unpaid health care providers are women, with unskilled, minority women at the bottom of the employment ladder. While the health care system is still controlled primarily by men, it is the skills and talents of women that are needed to provide the care. The challenge for women health care providers will be to participate in the evolving definitions of what their contributions should produce versus the historical traditions of professional authority. Women's talents for care giving, working in teams, and long-term problem solving provide the basis for real solutions to the current health-caring dilemmas.

REFERENCES

Aiken, L. H., Clarke, S. P., & Sloane, D. M. (2001). Hospital restructuring: Does it adversely affect care and outcomes? *Journal of the Health and Human Services Administration, 23*(4), 416–442.

Aiken, L. H., Clarke, S. P., Sloane, D. M., Sochalski, J., & Silber, J. H. (2002). Hospital nurse staffing and patient mortality, nurse burnout, and job dissatisfaction. *Journal of the American Medical Association, 288*(16), 1987–1993.

American Dental Association. (1999). *ADA Dental Workforce Model: 1997–2020.* Chicago: Author.

American Medical Association. (2004). *Physician characteristics and distribution in the U.S.* Chicago: Author.

Amick, B. C. 3rd, Kawachi, I., Coakley, E. H., Lerner, D., Levine, S., & Colditz, G. A. (1998). Relationship of job strain and isostrain to health status in a cohort of women in the United States. *Scandinavian Journal of Work Environment & Health, 24*(1), 54–61.

Ashley, J. (1976). *Hospitals, paternalism, and the role of the nurse.* New York: Teachers College Press.

Avorn, J., Everitt, D., & Baker, M. (1991). The neglected medical history and therapeutic choices for abdominal pain: A nationwide study of 799 physicians and nurses. *Archives of Internal Medicine, 151*(4), 694–698.

Baldwin, L. M., Hutchinson, H. L, & Rosenblatt, R. A. (1992). Professional relationships between midwives and physicians: Collaboration or conflict? *American Journal of Public Health, 82*(2), 262–264.

Berwick, D. M. (2003). Improvement, trust, and the healthcare workforce. *Quality and Safety in Health Care, 12*(6), 448–452.

Bickel, J. (2000). Women in academic medicine. *Journal of the American Medical Womens Association, 55*(1),10–20.

Braus, P. (1994). How women will change medicine. *American Demographics,* November, 40–47.

Brody, E. M. (1981). Women in the middle and family help to older people. *The Gerontologist, 21*(5), 471–480.

Brody, E. M. (1995). Women as unpaid caregivers: The price they pay. In E. Friedman (Ed.), *An unfinished revolution: Women and health care in America* (pp. 67–86). New York: United Hospital Fund.

Brown, C. (1982). Women workers in the heatlh service industry. In E. Fee (Ed.), *Women and health: The politicis of sex in medicine* (pp. 105–116). New York: Baywood.

Brown, L., & Lazar, V. (1999). Trends in the dental health work force. *Journal of the American Dental Association, 130,* 1743–1749.

Brown, S., & Grimes, D. (1993). *A meta-analysis of process of care, clinical outcomes and cost-effectiveness of nurses in primary care roles; nurse practitioners and certified nurse-midwives.* Washington, DC: American Nurses' Association.

Bull, M. J. (1990). Factors influencing family caregiver burden and health. *Western Journal of Nursing Research, 12*(6), 758–770, 771–776.

Bull, M. J. (2001). Interventions for women as family caregivers. In D. Taylor & N. F. Woods (Eds.), *Annual Review of Nursing Research: Women's Health Research, 19,* 125–143.

Bullough, B., & Bullough, V. (1975). Sex discrimination in health care. *Nursing Outlook, 23*(1), 40–45.

Burnley, C., & Burkett, G. (1986). Specialization: Are women in surgery different? *Journal of the American Medical Women's Assocaition, 41*(5), 144–147.

Butter, I., Carpenter, E., Kay, B., & Simmons, R. (1985). *Sex and status: Hierarchies in the health workforce.* Ann Arbor, MI: American Public Health Association.

Butter, I., Carpenter, E., Kay, B., & Simmons, R. (1987). Gender hierarchies in the health labor force. *International Journal of Health Services, 17*(1), 133–149.

Cheung, R., & Aiken, L. H. (2006). Hospital initiatives to support a better-educated workforce. *Journal of Nursing Administration, 36*(7–8), 357–362.

Chodorow, N. J. (1996). Theoretical gender and clinical gender: Epistemological reflections on the psychology of women. *Journal of the American Psychoanalytic Association, 44*(Suppl.), 215–238.

Cleland, V. (1971). Sex discrimination: Nursing's most pervasive problem. *American Journal of Nursing, 71*(8), 1542–1547.

Colditz, G. A. (1995). The nurses' health study: A cohort of US women followed since 1976. *Journal of the American Medical Women's Association, 50*(2), 40–44.

Colligan, M., Smith, M., & Hurrell, J. (1977). Occupational incidence rates of mental health disorders. *Journal of Human Stress, 3,* 34–39.

Council of Medical Specialty Society. (1990). *Choosing a medical specialty.* Lake Forest, IL: Author.

Cowan. M. J., Shapiro, M., Hays, R. D., Afifi, A., Vazirani, S., Ward, C. R., & Ettner, S. L. (2006). The effect of a multidisciplinary hospitalist/physician and advanced practice nurse collaboration on hospital costs. *Journal Nursing Administration, 36*(2), 79–85.

Darbyshire, P. (1987). Nurses and doctors: The burden of history. *Nursing Times, 83*(4), 32–34.

Day, J. (1992). Population projections of the United States, by age, sex, race and Hispanic origin: 1992–2050. Washington, DC: U.S. Government Printing Office.

Dock, L., & Stewart, I. (1938). *A short history of nursing.* New York: Putnam.

Doyal, L. (1995). *What makes women sick: Gender and the political economy of health.* New Brunswick, NJ: Rutgers University Press.

Drucker, P. (1992). *Managing for the future: The 1990s and beyond.* New York: Truman Talley Books/Plume.

Ducker, D. (1986). Role conflict in women physicians: A longitudinal study. *Journal of the American Medical Women's Association, 41*(1), 14–16.

Ehrenreich, B. (1975). The status of women as health providers in the United States. In *Proceedings of the International Conference on Wowen in Health, June 16–18* (DHEW Publication No. HRA 76-51, pp. 7–13). Washington, DC: Department of Health, Education and Welfare.

Ehrenreich, B., & English, D. (1973). *Witches, midwives, and nurses: A history of women healers.* New York: Feminist Press.

Fagin, C. (1994). Women and nursing: Today and tomorrow. In E. Friedman (Ed.), *An unfinished revolution: Women and health care in America* (pp. 159–176). New York: United Hospital Fund.

Fenton, W., Robinowitz, C., & Leaf, P. (1987). Male and female psychiatrists and their patients. *American Journal of Psychiatry, 144*(3), 358–361.

Finch, J., & Groves, D. (1983). *A labor of love: Women, work and caring.* Boston: Routledge and Kegan Paul.

Fisher, H. (1999). *The first sex.* New York: Random House.

Fisher, S. (1995). *Nursing wounds: Nurse practitioners, doctors, women patients, and the negotiation of meaning.* New Brunswick, NJ: Rutgers University Press.

Frank, E., Harvey, L., & Elon, L. (2000). Family responsibilities and domestic activities of US women physicians. *Archives of Family Medicine, 9*(2), 134–140.

Frank, E., & Lutz, L. (1999). Characteristics of women US family physicians. *Archives of Family Medicine, 8*(4), 313–318.

Ginzberg, E. (1994). The woman physician. In E. Friedman (Ed.), *An unfinished revolution: Women and health care in America* (pp. 135–142). New York: United Hospital Fund.

Glazer, N. (1988). Overlooked, overworked: Women's unpaid and paid work in the health services "cost crisis." *International Journal of Health Services, 18*(1), 119–137.

Graham, H. (1985). Providers, negotiators, and mediators: Women as the hidden carers. In E. Lewin and V. Olesen (Eds.), *Women, Health, and Healing: Toward a new perspective.* (pp. 25–52) London: Tavistock-Methuen.

Hart-Brothers, E. (1994). Contributions of women of color to the health care of America. In E. Friedman (Ed.), *An unfinished revolution: Women and health care in America* (pp. 205–222). New York: United Hospital Fund.

Health Resources and Services Administration, Bureau of Health Professions. (1999). *United States health workforce personnel factbook.* Washington, DC: Author.

Health Resources and Services Administration, Bureau of Health Professions. (2000). *The National Sample Survey of Registered Nurses, March 2000: Preliminary findings.* Washington, DC: Author.

Health Resources and Services Administration, Bureau of Health Professions, National Center for Health Workforce Information and Analysis. (2006a). *The United States Health Workforce Profile.* Rensselaer, NY: New York Center for Health Workforce Studies. http://chws.albany.edu

Health Resources and Services Administration, Bureau of Health Professions. (2006b). *The registered nurse population: Findings from the 2004 national sample survey of registered nurses, March 2006.* Washington, DC: Author. http://bhpr.hrsa.gov/healthworkforce/rnsurvey04

Health Resources and Services Administration, Bureau of Health Professions, National Center for Health Workforce Information and Analysis. (2006c). *The United States health workforce profile.* Washington, DC: Author. http://bhpr.hrsa.gov/health-workforce/ (found on HRSA grantee Web site, The New York Center for Health Workforce Studies, www.chws.albany.edu).

Himmelstein, D., Lewontin, J., & Woolhandler, S. (1996). Medical care employment in the United States, 1968 to 1993: The importance of health sector jobs for African Americans and women. *American Journal of Public Health, 86*(4), 525–528.

Hochschild, A. (1983). *The managed heart: Commercialization of human feeling.* San Francisco: University of California Press.

Hoffman, E., Maraldo, P., Coons, H., & Johnson, K. (1997). The woman-centered health care team: Integrating perspectives from managed care, women's health and the health professional workforce. *Women's Health Issues, 7,* 362–373.

Hoffman, R., & Mitchell, A. (1998). Caregiver burden: Historical development. *Nursing Forum, 33*(4), 5–11.

Ishii, N., Iwata, T., Dakeishi, M., & Murata, K. (2004). Effects of shift work on autonomic and neuromotor functions in female nurses. *Journal of Occupational Health, 46*(5), 352–358.

Jacox, A. (1997, December 30). Determinants of who does what in health care. *Online Journal of Issues in Nursing.* Retrieved December 2006, from http://www.nursingworld.org/Main MenuCategories/ANAMarketplace/ANAPeriodicals/OJIN/JournalTopics/Who DoesWhatinHealthCare.aspx

Jamieson, E., & Sewall, M. (1944). *Trends in nursing history* (2nd ed.). Philadelphia: Saunders.

Jovic, E., Wallace, J. E., & Lemaire, J. (2006). The generation and gender shifts in medicine: An exploratory survey of internal medicine physicians. *BioMed Central Health Services Research, 5*(6), 55–62.

Kay, B., Butter, I., Chang, D., & Houlihan, K. (1988). Women's health and social change: The case of lay midwives. *International Journal of Health Services, 18*(2), 223–236.

Kendellen, R. (1987). The medical malpractice insurance choice: An overview of the issues. *Journal of Nurse-midwifery, 32*(1), 4–10.

Knapp, K. (1999). Charting the demand for pharmacists in the managed care era. *American Journal of Health Systems Pharmacy, 56*(13),1309–1314.

Kopriva, P. (1994). Women in medicine. In E. Friedman (Ed.), *An unfinished revolution: Women and health care in America* (pp. 123–135). New York: United Hospital Fund.

Lenz, E. R., Mundinger, M. O., Hopkins, S. C., Lin, S. X., Smolowitz, J. L. (2002). Diabetes care processes and outcomes in patients treated by nurse practitioners or physicians. *Diabetes Education, 28,* 590–598.

Leppa, C. (1995). Women as health care providers. In C. Fogel & N. F. Woods (Eds.), *Women's Health Care* (2nd ed.). Thousand Oaks, CA: Sage.

Levinson, W., & Lurie, N. (2004). When most doctors are women: What lies ahead? *Annals of Internal Medicine, 141*(6), 471–474.

Levitt, J. (1977). Men and women as providers of health care. *Social Science and Medicine, 14,* 395–398.

Lindeman, C., & McAthie, M. (1999). *Fundamentals of contemporary nursing practice.* Philadelphia: Saunders.

Litaker, D., Mion, L., Planavsky, L., Kippes, C., Mehta, N., & Frolkis, J. (2003). Physician–nurse practitioner teams in chronic disease management: The impact on costs, clinical effectiveness, and patients' perception of care. *Journal of Interprofessional Care, 17*(3), 223–237.

Lorber, J. (1984). *Women physicians: Careers, status and power.* New York: Tavistock.

Lorber, J. (1987). Welcome to a crowded field: Where will the new women physicians fit in? *Journal of the American Medical Women's Association, 42*(5), 149–152.

Lubic, R. (1987). Nurse midwives and liability insurance. *Nursing Outlook, 35*(4), 174–177.

Marieskind, H. (1980) *Women in the health system: Patients, providers, and programs.* St. Louis, MO: Mosby.

McPherson, K., Kersten, P., George, S., Lattimer, V., Breton, A., Ellis, B., Kaur, D., & Frampton, G. (2006). A systematic review of evidence about extended roles for allied health professionals. *Journal of Health Services Research and Policy, 11*(4) 240–247.

Melosh, B. (1982). *The physician's hand: Work culture and conflict in American nursing.* Philadelphia: Temple University Press.

Morantz-Sanchez, R. M. (1985). *Sympathy and science.* New York: Oxford University Press.

More, E., & Greer, M. (2000). American women physicians in 2000: A history in progress. *Journal of the American Medical Women's Association, 55*(1), 6–9.

Morikawa, Y., Kitaoka-Higashiguchi, K., Tanimoto, C., Hayashi, M., Oketani, R., Miura, K., Nishijo, M., & Nakagawa, H. (2005). A cross-sectional study on the relationship of job stress with natural killer cell activity and natural killer cell subsets among healthy nurses. *Journal of Occupational Health, 47*(5), 378–383.

Muff, J. (Ed.). (1988). *Socialization, sexism, and stereotyping: Women's issues in nursing.* Prospect Heights, IL: Waveland.

Muller, C. (1994). Women in allied health professions. In E. Friedman (Ed.), *An unfinished revolution: Women and health care in America* (pp. 177–203). New York: United Hospital Fund.

Mundinger, M. O., Kane, R. L., Lenz, E. R., Totten, A. M., Tsai, W. Y., Cleary, P. D., Friedewald, W. T., Siu, A. L., & Shelanski, M. L. (2000). Primary care outcomes in patients treated by nurse practitioners or physicians: A randomized trial. *Journal of the American Medical Association, 283*(1), 59–68.

National League for Nursing. (1990). *Nurses of America Media Project.* New York: Author.

Navarro, V. (1975). Women in health care. *New England Journal of Medicine, 292*(8), 398–402.

Nevidjon, B., & Erickson, J. (2001, January 31). The nursing shortage: Solutions for the short and long term. *Online Journal of Issues in Nursing, 6*(1), manuscript 4. http://www.nursing world.org/MainMenuCategories/ANAMarketplace/ANA Periodicals/OJIN/TableofContents/Volume62001/Number1 January2001/NursingShortageSolutionsNightingale, F. (1969). *Notes on nursing: What it is and what it is not.* New York: Dover. (original work published 1860)

Nursing Institute, University of Illinois College of Nursing. (2001). *Who will care for each of us? America's coming health care labor crisis.* Chicago: Author. http://www.uic.edu/nursing/ nursinginstitute/policy/finalreports/finalreport.pdf

O'Neil, E. H. (1993). *Health professions education for the future: Schools in service to the nation.* San Francisco: Pew Health Professions Commission.

O'Neil, E. H. (2003). *Emerging workforce issues. Proceedings of the California Healthcare Foundation Leadership Program.* Sacramento, CA.

O'Neil, E. H., & the Pew Health Professions Commission. (1998). *Recreating health professional practice for a new century.* San Francisco: Pew Health Professions Commission.

Peterson, C. (2001). Nursing shortage: Not a simple problem—No easy answers. *Online Journal of Issues in Nursing, 6*(1), manuscript 5. http://www.nursingworld.org/MainMenuCategories/ ANAMarketplace/ANAPeriodicals/OJIN/TableofContents/Vol ume62001/Number1January2001/ShortageProblemAnswers. aspx

Picot, S. (1995). Rewards, costs, and coping of African American caregivers. *Nursing Research, 43,* 147–152.

Pizurki, H., Mejia, A., Butter, I., & Ewart, L. (1987). *Women as providers of health care.* Geneva, Switzerland: World Health Organization.

Reverby, S. (1987a). A caring dilemma: Womanhood and nursing in historical perspective. *Nursing Research, 36*(1), 5–11.

Reverby, S. (1987b). *Ordered to care: The dilemma of American nursing, 1850–1945.* New York: Cambridge University Press.

Riley, G. J. (2004). Understanding the stresses and strains of being a doctor. *Medical Journal of Australia, 181*(7), 350–353.

Roberts, S. J. (1983). Oppressed group behavior: Implications for nursing. *ANS Advances in Nursing Science, 5*(4), 21–30.

Robinson, K. (1998). Family caregiving: Who provides the care, and at what cost? *Nursing Economics, 15:* 243–247.

Rooks, J. (1997). *Midwifery and childbirth in America.* Philadelphia: Temple University Press.

Rosenblatt, R. A., Dobie, S. A., Hart, L. G., Schneeweiss, R., Gould, D., Raine, T. R., Benedetti, T. J., Pirani, M. J., & Perrin, E. B. (1997). Interspecialty differences in the obstetric care of low-risk women. *American Journal of Public Health, 87*(3), 344–351.

Rosener, J. (1995). *America's competitive secret: Women managers.* New York: Oxford University Press.

Ruzek, J. Y., Bloor, L. E., Anderson, J. L., Ngo, M., & the UCSF Center for the Health Professions. (1999). *The hidden health care workforce: Recognizing, understanding and improving the allied and auxiliary workforce.* San Francisco: UCSF Center for the Health Professions.

Shryock, R. H. (1966). *Medicine in America: Historical essays.* Baltimore: Johns Hopkins University Press.

Smith, P. (1992). *The emotional labor of nursing: How nurses care.* London: Macmillan.

Sox, H. (1979). Quality of patient care by NPs and PAs: A 10-year perspective. *Annals of Internal Medicine, 91,* 459–468.

Starr, P. (1982). *The social transformation of American medicine.* New York: Basic Books.

Stein, E., Bauman, L., & Jessop, D. (1994). Women as formal and informal caregivers of children. In E. Friedman (Ed.), *An unfinished revolution: Women and health care in America* (pp. 103–120). New York: United Hospital Fund.

Stevens, R. (1966). *American medicine in the public interest.* New Haven, CT: Yale University Press.

Tache, S., & Chapman, S. (2006). The expanding roles and occupational characteristics of medical assistants: Overview of an emerging field in allied health. *Journal of Allied Health, 35*(4), 233–237.

Taft, S. (2001, January 31). The nursing shortage: Introduction. *Online Journal of Issues in Nursing, 6*(1), manuscript 1. http://www.nursingworld.org/MainMenuCategories/ANA-Marketplace/ANAPeriodicals/OJIN/JournalTopics/Nursing Shortage.aspx

Talley, R. C., & Crews, J. E. (2007). Framing the public health of caregiving. *American Journal of Public Health, 97*(2), 224–228.

Taylor, D., & Dower, K. (1997). Toward a women-centered health care system: Women's experiences, women's voices, women's needs. *Health Care for Women International, 18*(4), 407–422.

Taylor, D., & Woods, N. F. (1996). Changing women's health, changing nursing practice. *Journal of Obstetrical, Gynecological & Neonatal Nurses, 25*(9), 791–802.

Travelers Insurance Companies and the American Association of Retired Persons. (1988). *National survey of caregivers: Summary of findings.* Hartford, CT: Author.

U.S. Census Bureau. (2000). S*tatistical abstract of the United States: 2000* (120th ed.). Washington, DC: Author.

U.S. Census Bureau. (2006). Resident population by sex race and Hispanic origin status: 2000–2004. In *Statistical abstract of the United States, 2006* (Table 13). Washington, DC: Author. http:// www.census.gov/compendia/statab/tables/08s0006.pdf

U.S. Census Bureau. (2007). *Statistical abstract of the United States: 2007* (126th ed.). Washington, DC: Author. http://www.census. gov/compendia/statab

U.S. Department of Health and Human Services, Health Resources and Services Administration, Bureau of Health Professions. (2000a). *The pharmacist workforce: A study of the supply and demand for pharmacists.* Washington, DC: Author.

U.S. Department of Health and Human Services, Public Health Service. (2000b). *Oral health in America: A report to the Surgeon General.* Washington, DC: Author.

U.S. Department of Labor, Bureau of Labor Statistics. (2005a). *Occupational employment projections to 2014: Fastest growing occupations, 2004–2014, Table 2, November 2005 Monthly Labor Review.* Washington, DC: Author.

U.S. Department of Labor, Bureau of Labor Statistics. (2005b). *Industry injury and illness data—2005.* Washington, DC: Author. http://www.bls.gov/iif/oshsum.htm

U.S. Department of Labor, Women's Bureau. (2006a). *20 leading occupations of employed women: 2006 annual averages.* Retrieved May 18, 2007, from http://www.dol.gov/wb/fact sheets/20lead2006.htm

U.S. Department of Labor, Bureau of Labor Statistics. (2006b). *Women in the labor force: A databook 2006,* Report 996. Washington, DC: Author. http://www.bls.gov/cps/wlf-databook2006.htm

U.S. Department of Labor, Bureau of Labor Statistics. (2006c). *Occupational employment statistics.* Washington, DC: Author. http://www.bls.gov/oes/home.htm

U.S. Department of Labor, Bureau of Labor Statistics. (2007a). *Occupational outlook handbook.* Washington, DC: Author.

U.S. Department of Labor, Bureau of Labor Statistics. (2007b). *Career guide to industries, 2006–07 Edition,* Health Care. Retrieved May 18, 2007, from http://www.bls.gov/oco/cg/cgs035.htm

Vahey, D. C., Aiken, L. H., Sloane, D. M., Clarke, S. P., & Vargas, D. (2004). Nurse burnout and patient satisfaction. *Medical Care, 42*(Suppl. 2), 57–66.

Walsch, M. R. (1977). *"Doctors wanted: No women need apply": Sexual barriers in the medical profession 1835–1975.* New Haven, CT: Yale University Press.

Washington Women's Education Foundation. (1997). *The health of Washington women.* Olympia, WA: Author.

Weaver, J., & Garrett, S. (1983). Sexism and racism in the American health care industry: A comparative analysis. In E. Fee (Ed.), *Women and health: The politics of sex in medicine* (pp. 79–104). New York: Baywood.

Wilson, M. (1987). Making a difference: Women, medicine and the twenty-first century. *Yale Journal of Biology and Medicine, 60*(3), 273–288.

Woodward, C., Cohen, M., & Ferrier, B. (1990). Career interruptions and hours practiced: Comparison between young men and women physicians. *Canadian Journal of Public Health, 81*(2), 16–20.

Yoon, J., Grumbach, K., & Bindman, A. B. (2004). Access to Spanish-speaking physicians in California: Supply, insurance, or both. *Journal of the American Board of Family Practice, 17*(3), 165–72.

Women and Health Care

Debbie Ward and
Nancy Fugate Woods

Women are redefining health. The many factors that contribute to personal and community well-being for women—economic and social status, work, public safety, community infrastructure, kin networks, interests, recreation, childbirth, menstruation, menopause, aging, sexuality, body size/shape and functionality—are all undergoing redefinition as women create their own health standards, rather than accept others' definitions. Women are also redefining health care systems and services. They have mounted a many-sided critique of U.S. health care, revealing aspects of personal and public health services, research, and health policies that do not address women's diverse views and needs. Women are working to create appropriate personal health services, conduct their own research on women's health, establish a women's public health agenda, and change U.S. health policy.

A focus on and by women is bringing about profound alterations in health care. As feminists analyze health care delivery systems, structural changes are being demanded that meet human needs—from secure parking for night-shift nurses to group support via conference call and chat room for women caring for housebound, chronically ill family members and friends. Community-wide work includes movements for environmental safety and against social and interpersonal violence.

THE ILLNESS CARE NONSYSTEM

But the hydra-headed U.S. illness care nonsystem (Ward, 1990) resists change and sometimes looms insurmountably in the paths of small and large schemes for improvement and rationalization. The United States pays more for less than any other country in its peer group of industrialized nations in regard to health care expenditures. The United States is first in spending among the 29 Organisation for Economic Co-operation and Development (OECD) countries, with 13% of its gross domestic product spent for health care in 2000. The second-, third-, and fourth-ranked countries are Switzerland (10.7%), Germany (10.6%), and France (9.5%) (OECD Health Data, 2002). Yet for all this cost, the United States is in the bottom quartile for life expectancy and infant mortality, and its relative ranking has declined since comparisons were first drawn in 1960 (Anderson, 1997).

The United States also does not begin to approach universal access to health care for all its inhabitants. The total number of uninsured Americans continues to rise, reaching some 41.2 million in 2001 data. The uninsured comprised 14.6% of the population under 65, an increase of 1.4 million over the previous year. Children, young adults age 18 to 39, Blacks, Hispanics, and low- and middle-income families are most likely to be uninsured (Carrasquillo, Himmelstein, Woolhandler, & Bor, 1999). Rates of uninsurance were found to be higher for men (17.1% for the period 1989 to 1996) than for women (14.2%) (Carrasquillo et al., 1999). Medicaid (state-administered health insurance for persons with low income and/or some categories of disability) costs currently threaten state budgets nationwide, both as a result of the national recession as well as from Medicaid costs that grew to an average of 20% of state spending (Levit et al., 2003). At the same time, the 1996 welfare reform law, which was intended to increase women's labor force participation as well as limit time on public aid, has led to higher rates of uninsurance for women and children and lower Medicaid participation (Mann, Hudman, Salganicoff, & Folsom, 2002).

Claims for reproductive care, especially childbirth costs, are believed to underlie reductions in the individual (as opposed to group and employer-based) insurance market. Medicaid has become the payer of last resort for reproductive care for many women; in contrast to women covered either by private insurance or Medicaid, uninsured women have significantly more difficulty obtaining care, and they receive fewer recommended services and report poorer quality care (Salganicoff & Wyn, 1999).

Cyclically, the unique U.S. approach to health insurance through the economically regressive link to employers is called into question. Some 69% of U.S. workers under age 65 are insured through an employer (Centers for Disease Control and Prevention [CDC], 1997). Fifty-two percent of U.S. businesses offered health insurance in 1993, the year of the national employer-sponsored health insurance study (CDC, 1997). Yet almost two-thirds of 1993's 41 million uninsured were in families headed by workers, and 56% of the uninsured were working adults (CDC, 1997). The growing number of uninsured Americans is due to the erosion of employment-based insurance: Fewer employers offer insurance, more employees are relegated to categories deemed ineligible for insurance (part-time, temporary), the growth in jobs has been in nonunionized, low-wage service-sector jobs without benefits, and employees opt out of job-based insurance due to their inability to meet co-pays and deductibles (Bodenheimer, 1998).

Another 31 million Americans are presumed to be underinsured, unable to access needed services without weighing their needs against the ability to meet excessive costs (Consumers' Union, 1998). They are either not covered for an existing illness or are compelled to spend at least 10% of their income on health care or insurance. The elderly—despite Medicare coverage—are particularly vulnerable to this condition, with the average 65-and-older couple spending 19% of its income on health costs (Consumers' Union, 1998).

Insurance premiums and pharmaceutical costs are the fastest growing segments of the rising costs for health care (Gruber & Levitt, 2000). From an increase of 4.7% in 1997, health care costs increased 5.6% in 1998 to a total of 1.1 trillion dollars, or $4,094 per capita, the largest increase since 1993 (Gruber & Levitt, 2000). Public costs are growing exponentially. Medicare spending rose from $3.3 billion in 1967 to almost $241 billion in 2001, or 19% of the overall total national spending for personal health care of $1.1 trillion. Once the first baby boomers reach Medicare eligibility age in 2010, costs are expected to jump even more sharply, placing the entire health care system at a new level of distress.

In addition to financial barriers, women experience additional hurdles to quality care, including rurality, culture, transportation, self-perception, and knowledge and attitudes about available services. For example, as Medicaid programs have expanded to include prenatal care, enrollment rates have nonetheless lagged. Studies of this population have shown that multiple factors are involved in initiating care, including difficulty in making an appointment, transportation, child care, and perceptions about the need for care and experience with previous pregnancies (Roberts et al., 1998).

Some changes in the U.S. health care *culture* can be recognized. Women no longer equate medical care with health. From unjustifiably high hysterectomy and cesarean birth rates to the Dalkon Shield, women have become acquainted with the detrimental potential of the *medical industrial complex* (the term comes from Relman, 1980). A report from the Institute of Medicine (2000) on medical errors has quantified the risks to the public's health from inadequate quality controls in medical care. Tens of thousands of unnecessary deaths are estimated to occur in hospitals and other regulated health settings. More unreported errors occur in nonhospital, unregulated sites such as private medical offices and clinics.

And women recognize that the health care industry relies on some of the worst aspects of commercialism—goods and services that serve to foster denial of death, pursuit of ageless beauty, individual success over community welfare—and continues to practice in patterns of sexism, elitism, and paternalism. Feminist analysts have long noted the focus on illness, not health, in the United States.

This chapter will survey women's health care. It explores problems women have historically faced in receiving personal health services, as well as the influence that professional education has had on the clinicians who care for women. Women's place in health research and health policy are considered. Attempts to predict some future trends conclude this survey.

DIAGNOSIS AND TREATMENT FOR WOMEN

The social and health sciences literature provides evidence of the complex role of gender in personal health services, in the education of health professionals, and in research on women's health. In the delivery of personal health services, investigators have found evidence of sexist bias in diagnosis, treatment, prescription of medications, and admission to hospital for psychiatric problems. Similarly, the diagnosis and treatment of women for a variety of medical and surgical conditions have also been gender-biased, with strong evidence that treatment practices and outcomes are affected.

Gender—a social category that includes changing definitions of appropriate roles, division of labor, economic power and political influence—and sex—a biological category—have different and multifaceted influences on health and health care. A new era of research with mandatory inclusion of women—since 1993, the National Institutes of Health (NIH), for example, have required the inclusion of women and minorities in all its funded research—has led to new understandings of these complexities. Community and public interest groups have dissected patterns of care and demanded new formulations. Analyses of the biases at work in the distribution of resources and the outcomes of health care interventions have moved from individual-level blame to more detailed, system-level probing at the structures that reinforce discrimination.

Diagnosis

Psychiatric

Classic studies (Aslin, 1977; Broverman et al., 1970) demonstrated that women judged to behave in gender-appropriate ways were also judged to be psychologically less healthy than men and that the gender of a therapist can influence expectations about women's mental health. Subsequent work has continued to delineate the demographic and epidemiological differences in women's mental disorders. Women have higher rates than men of many psychiatric disorders: mood, anxiety, eating, sleep, personality, somatoform, dissociative, obsessive-compulsive spectrum, and impulse control, as well as late-onset schizophrenia with prominent mood symptoms and dementia of the Alzheimers' type (Fankhauser, 1997). Studies of depression continue to critique early conclusions about the preponderance of women with the diagnosis, though current evidence indicates that women exhibit more depressive symptomatology than do men (Pajer, 1995). Psychiatric epidemiological studies, however, show that there is no significant difference in prevalence between men and women (Murphy, Laird, Monson, Sobol, & Leighton, 2000). Whether men and women fall into gender-neutral diagnostic categories as a result of gender-neutral evaluations or are guided into gender-biased diagnoses as a result of gender-biased evaluations are important questions that continue to be studied.

A new level of sophistication and detail is entering our understanding of women's mental health. Over their life times (years longer than men's), women suffer more frequently from acute and chronic psychiatric disorders, with higher comorbidity (Fankhauser, 1997). In a group of patients with affective disorders, for example, women were found to have more comorbid anxiety disorders, more family history of psychiatric illness, and more history of previous treatment than men (Rapaport et al., 1995). The effects of family relationships seem to be more significant for women than for men; women in methadone treatment, for example, were found to have more dysfunctional families of origin (as well as greater psychological and medical comorbidity) than men (Chatam, Hiller, Rowan-Szal, Joe, & Simpson, 1999).

Determining rates of women's alcohol and drug use remains difficult, but experts have moved from assuming women drink and drug less (because women are not as frequently observed in these behaviors) to illuminating the attitudes and stereotypes that stigmatize women substance abusers and make detection and treatment more difficult (Blum, Nielsen, & Riggs, 1998). Women—as compared to men—start drug use at a later age and move more quickly from early use to addiction (Grella & Joshi, 1999). Women are more likely than men to be introduced to drug use by their (men) partners; in a sample of cocaine users, women were more likely to have a drug-dependent partner than were men (Grella, & Joshi, 1999). This research group echoes others in speculating that gender has substantive and diverse effects on biological markers of psychiatric illness, treatment outcomes, and prognosis.

The intricate interweaving of socially constructed definitions of gender and their relation to diagnostic taxonomies is also illustrated by the continuing controversies surrounding various diagnoses in revisions of the *Diagnostic and Statistical Manual of Mental Disorders*, the standardized diagnostic manual that forms the basis for diagnosis and treatment, not to mention billing and data collection. Two diagnoses—late luteal phase dysphoric disorder, or premenstrual dysphoric disorder, and self-defeating personality disorder, or masochistic personality disorder—continue to be debated and their use unresolved (Frances, First, & Pincus, 1995).

Medical

The history of women's medical diagnosis is similarly rife with now-discredited categories such as hysteria (Leavitt, 1984). Many major national studies of women's health have been undertaken; they exemplify the much-needed, expanded understanding of women's diseases and concerns. In 1976, for example, 121,700 women registered nurses returned a mailed health questionnaire. This cohort of women was initially surveyed to examine the relation of oral contraceptive use and cigarette smoking to the risk of major illness, but the study has gone on to evaluate the health consequences of exercise, diet, vitamin supplement use, hormone replacement therapy, and other lifestyle practices (Colditz, Manson, & Hankinson, 1997). In addition, quality-of-life measures have been assessed, including work stress and care giving burden. Findings include a lack of association between dietary calcium intake and risk of osteoporotic fractures and multiple adverse effects from weight gain, including coronary heart disease, type 2 diabetes mellitus, and total mortality.

The Nurses' Health Study (Colditz et al., 1997) found support for a practice that had come into widespread acceptability: hormone replacement therapy (HRT) for menopausal women. The study supported a reduction in heart disease risk from HRT. This finding has subsequently been contradicted by results from another large trial, the Women's Health Initiative (Writing Group for the Women's Health Initiative Investigators, 2002). The latter study revealed that HRT increased heart disease risk (see chapter 6 for more detailed discussion of the results of the Women's Health Initiative Trial).

Another large study is the Study of Women's Health Across the Nation (Sowers et al., 2000). This work tracked 3,700 healthy premenopausal women over 5 years to measure, among other variables, differences in the transition to menopause for women of different ethnic groups. Functional limitations associated with menopause (including weight gain) varied among ethnicities, with only 2% to 3% of Asian women reporting limitations, compared to 12% to 14% of White and African American women (Sowers et al., 2006).

These studies exemplify the new dimensions that have been added to our understanding of women's health. Overall, the evidence about medical diagnosis suggests a complex segregation of men and women into different health care consumers. Men and women bring a variety of interdependent economic, cultural, social and gender-based expectations to the health care encounter, where they, in turn, are variably treated according to a complex mix of these same factors.

Treatment

Whatever our needs for health and illness care, we can only buy services that are available. Verbrugge and Patrick (1995) have suggested that care has been disproportionately shaped to deal with fatal conditions such as heart disease and cancer, while the impact of chronic, nonfatal conditions (arthritis and visual impairment, for example) is actually much greater. The additional roles of direct drug advertising, health care marketing, and other inducements to use health resources are extremely powerful shapers of our delivery system.

Quality-of-care studies are slowly moving from the rudimentary to the more sophisticated. The history of medical treatment is rife with discrimination against a variety of categories of people. The history of inpatient care for African Americans, for example, includes the era of outright denial of hospital admission, the separate-but-equal facilities legislation with the 1946 Hill-Burton Act, which brought about the stunning increase in hospitals, and the current era of subtle but telling discrimination

against Blacks in access, intensity of services, and quality of care in hospitals and nursing homes (Thomson, 1997).

Discriminatory disparities in hospital care are receiving closer examination: a large study of 2,200 Medicare patients admitted for pneumonia or heart failure to hospital in three large states found that Black patients received lower quality of care. Care by gender was found to be roughly equivalent; however, men were found to receive better care from doctors than did women, while women received better nursing care than men (Ayanian, Weissman, Chasen-Taber, & Epstein, 1999).

Comparisons drawn from cross-national studies of health care utilization demonstrate that, in populations with universal health insurance (the United Kingdom and Canada, for example) and after accounting for differences in reproductive biology and higher age-specific mortality rates among men, there is relatively little difference in utilization between genders (Mustard, Kaufert, Kozyrskyj, & Mayer, 1998). In other cross-national studies, women have been found to use more primary care, while men use more short inpatient stays and have more emergency room visits (Ruiz & Verbrugge, 1997). But the characterization of women as insatiable and inappropriate overusers of care is now demonstrated to be incorrect.

Included in these utilization analyses is discussion of the fact that women are primary care providers for children, and thus familiarize themselves with the medical waters on their families' behalf, whereas men tend to go to doctors only for their own treatment. Women as a group pay significant attention to health-promoting and illness-treating practices—their own and their families' (Taylor & Woods, 1996).

Admission and Referral for Psychiatric Treatment

Early studies of psychiatric treatment found evidence of gender differences and possible bias. In a study of hospitalization for psychosis, investigators suggested that men are more likely to be directed to psychiatric treatment at younger ages and stay institutionalized longer than women because social tolerance of mental illness in men is more limited than for women (Tudor, Tudor, & Gove, 1977). In a 1990 study of the psychiatric intake process, however, women outnumbered men at presentation. But men were again found to be more severely symptomatic and have more accompanying problems (comorbidity) at intake than women (Fabrega, Mezzich, Ulrich, & Benjamin, 1990). Instead of bearing out Tudor and colleagues' interpretation, the preponderance of women in the 1990 study may demonstrate society's unwillingness to tolerate even slight degrees of deviance in women. Women were found to enter treatment earlier than men, and men may not seek treatment until they are very ill. Women and men exhibited simple diagnostic conditions equally, but men exhibited higher degrees of social impairment associated with complex clinical conditions, including such accompanying disorders as substance abuse.

In studying social anxiety disorder (the most common anxiety disorder) from several national data sources, men were found to have lower lifetime prevalence than women, but men sought treatment more (Weinstock, 1999). Women who are not assertive and outgoing in school, work, and social settings are less likely to be sanctioned for their passivity than men, leading men more than women to seek treatment. These complex patterns of presentation undoubtedly reflect multiple factors, which include gender-based definitions of appropriate and desirable behavior.

Psychiatric Therapy

Women have been subject to discrimination in the provision of psychiatric services—for instance, when treatment is both qualitatively and quantitatively inadequate. Drug and alcohol treatment for women exhibits the changes in both public policy and research understanding that is slowly addressing women's needs for psychiatric treatment.

Surveying alcohol use disorders in women, Greenfield (2002) noted a significant lag before alcohol dependence research stopped using male study population findings to generalize to both sexes. We now know that women are increasing their rates of abusive drinking, have different physiologic responses from alcohol use than men, and tend to follow a shorter trajectory from problem drinking to adverse consequences. Critically for treatment policy, alcoholic women are more likely than alcoholic men to use primary care and mental health treatment, as opposed to targeted alcohol treatment (Greenfield, 2002). (See chapter 22 on substance abuse and women.)

In the 1980s and 1990s, federal and state set-asides were created to support women-only treatment units and program. Concerns with childbearing and child-rearing figured in this legislative mandate; Medicaid, model programs for drug-using pregnant and postpartum women through federal drug abuse agencies, and services for drug-dependent women and their children via the Child Abuse Prevention and Treatment Act are all examples of women-centered (albeit pronatalist) services. Women-centered programs tend to be less likely than mixed-gender programs to charge a fee; to use a more supportive and less confrontational approach; to focus on skill development in social, parental, and vocational arenas; and to use more women staff and role models (Grella, Polinsky, Hser, & Perry, 1999). Interestingly, this survey of treatment programs in Los Angeles county found that mixed-gender programs were more likely than women-only programs to provide group and family therapy, suggesting a model of family involvement that has been found to figure more for men than women addicts. Instead of family-focused approaches, these women-only programs used a social-model, peer-based approach, with peer support, 12-step meetings on site, and social outings.

In another study, husbands of women alcoholics in treatment were found to provide less support—qualitatively and quantitatively—than wives of men alcoholics (Brown, Kokin, Seraganian, & Shields, 1995). Among other implications of this study is the question raised for therapists about reflexively encouraging closer family involvement during treatment, without adequately assessing spousal capacities.

Noting the policy initiatives that underwrote expanded services for women, one review of services for drug-affected women and children in California found "wide gaps between the kinds of services that are appropriate for drug-affected families and the existing service system" (Soman, Brindis, & Dunn-Malhotra, 1996, p. 7). Gaps included variations in services offered, lack of comprehensiveness, onerous application procedures, and exclusionary medical or developmental criteria for eligibility (including exclusion of pregnant women from substance abuse treatment programs, exclusion of women with dual diagnoses, and exclusion of women with children). Funding was both uncoordinated (further segmenting services) and unpredictable. Engagement in comprehensive treatment has consistently been found to predict greater freedom from relapse; the search for and application of gender-appropriate mechanisms for fostering engagement continues (Fiorentine, Anglin, Gil-Rivas, & Taylor, 1997) just as does the struggle for policies and funding that ensure comprehensiveness and open access.

The therapeutic process itself has been the subject of a vigorous feminist critique. Mitchell's classic work (1974) presaged others who observed that Freudian theory and practice, which constitutes a major body of the psychotherapeutic canon, is anti-woman. In the growth of the psychoanalytic literature since the turn of the 20th century, a recurrent theme has been the association of neurosis with feminism: "Many twentieth-century psychiatrists and psychologists claimed that feminist aspirations either resulted from or led to neurosis" (Stage, 1979, p. 228).

Vigorous critiques have led to multiple changes, most of which can hardly be said to have resolved the continuing questions surrounding the role of gender in psychiatric therapy. Klinkenberg and Calsyn (1998) join a growing school of researchers who eschew gender reductionism and who treat gender not as a sole determinant of outcome but as only one variable among many and/or as a moderating variable—that is, one that affects the direction and/or strength of a relationship between independent and dependent variables. In their study of gender differences in aftercare and psychiatric hospitalization in severely ill adults who visited a psychiatric emergency room, they found that women were more affected by the responsiveness of the service system than men, who were more likely to come for follow-up care when they were accompanied to the emergency room by family or friends. This study, like others discussed previously, suggests that gender roles play a more complex role in treatment than stereotypes (women's greater connection to family, for example) dictated.

Medical Therapy

Coronary artery disease (CAD) is a well-studied example of differences in treatment related to gender. CAD is the leading cause of death in women. Men's risk is greater at younger ages, but at older ages, gender difference in risk disappears (Chandra et al., 1998). Women's risk factors (not all unique to their gender) include diabetes, hyperlipidemia, premature menopause, minority racial status, lower socioeconomic status, smoking, physical inactivity, and overweight (Wenger, 1999). Several factors may hold the key to discovering more about women's CAD risk, notably diabetes (which, more than any other risk factor, erases women's advantage over men in CAD risk at younger age) and central (upper-body/male-pattern) obesity (which appears to be related to androgen excess and higher risk for CAD in women with this pattern of body fat distribution) (Barrett-Connor, 1997). Targeted primary prevention is an obvious approach to the treatment of CAD in women, yet 80% of U.S. women and 33% of their primary care physicians were unaware that heart disease is the major cause of death in women, accounting for 22% of all women's deaths.

Another group of U.S. women—poor women of color at risk for HIV—is experiencing clear negative effects by gender; compared to men, U.S. women are not reaping the benefits of progress against HIV (Gollub, 1999). While men's infection rates dropped 8% in 1996, women's rose 1%. The drop in women's mortality for that year (12%) was less than half the decrease seen in men (26%). Arguing for interventions aimed at communities, Gollub laments the emphasis on individual, behavioral approaches instead of on approaches regarding welfare, drug treatment, and scientific research policies toward women.

Drug Therapy

Sexism also affects the prescription of medications. During office visits, physicians recommended over-the-counter medications to young women (and minority group patients) more than they did to men (Pradel, Hartzema, Mutran, & Hanson-Divers, 1999). In psychopharmacologic treatment, women have a 55% greater chance of receiving any psychotropic drug from an office visit than do men (Simoni-Wastila, 1998). Three-quarters of all psychotropic medications are prescribed for women (Fankhauser, 1997). Women are subsequently at higher risk than men for adverse drug reactions; women on antidepressants (two-thirds of all antidepressant prescriptions are for women) experience more—and more severe—side effects than do men. Complications from pharmaceutical use of all kinds disproportionately affect women; office visits for medication-related morbidity are greatest for women aged 65 to 74 (Aparasu, 1999).

As women appear to experience more medication-related adverse reactions, and, if they are the targets of over-the-counter drug advertising and physician recommendations for over-the-counter drugs, it could be speculated that clinicians' expectations and market forces might be powerful determinants of the care women receive. Might men physicians embrace certain expectations about women's behavior and adjustment and tend to determine that women are more in need of psychotropic drugs, for example, than their equally troubled but more reticent men patients? Do women request medication more than men and, if so, why? It is not known what the U.S. population of women has as a baseline standard of demand and need for care, apart from the products and services eagerly sold to them. As Ruiz and Verbrugge (1997) stated,

> We know little about how men and women voluntarily adopt some risk behaviours and risk exposures, their different perceptions of symptoms and expression of complaints, how their milieux of social support affect health and health behaviour, and their behavioural strategies for treating and adjusting to health problems. (p. 106)

The conditions that lead women more than men to use medicaments of all kinds await full explication. The historic development of women as herbalists clearly arose from their role as family nurse and healer (Ehrenreich & English, 1973). An argument can be made that faith in pharmaceutical therapy is a logical association with what has been called women's culture—a culture of connection and mutual aid rather than the individualism associated with male culture. Under this theoretical construct, women would be more likely to use drugs of all kinds—from diet pills to megavitamins—while men are more apt to be socialized to ignore or endure symptoms such as low energy, despondency, or overeating.

Women's physiology is increasingly thought to play a role in treatment. Differences in drug disposition and pharmacodynamics between men and women (Fankhauser, 1997), treatment in depression (Pajer, 1995), treatment in social anxiety disorder (Weinstock, 1999), and hospitalization for severe psychiatric disease (Klinkenberg & Calsyn, 1998) are only some of the arenas in which women are seen to be a distinct population with particular needs.

Surgery

The famous studies by Wennberg and others demonstrated a national pattern of extreme variability in physician practice patterns (Wennberg & Cooper, 1999). This variability is influenced by such factors as the practice patterns of regional peers, style and location of medical school training, and penetration by specialty practice. Patient gender has also been found to influence rates and types of surgery.

Gynecology was one of the first specialty areas to fall under the scrutiny of women's health care analysts. As of 1980, the hysterectomy had become the most frequently performed major operation for women of reproductive years. The American College of Obstetricians and Gynecologists estimated at that time that 15% of hysterectomies were performed to remove cancer, 30% to remove noncancerous fibroids, 35% for pelvic relaxation or prolapse, and 20% for sterilization (Scully, 1980). A hysterectomy should not be performed as an elective procedure or when more conservative treatment will suffice, and yet it was estimated that one-third of hysterectomies and half of cesarean sections performed in the United States were unnecessary (Seaman, 1972). Recent evidence continues to demonstrate that nonclinical factors (physician characteristics such as background, training, experience, and practice style) play a statistically significant role in this surgical decision (Geller, Burns, & Brailer, 1996). Although African American women have higher rates of fibroid tumors than Whites, other factors may contribute to this difference, including geographic variation in surgical rates.

Cardiology and cardiovascular surgery comprise another specialty practice arena studied for its utilization by gender. Although the risk of developing coronary artery disease has increased for women and decreased for men since 1950, women are less likely to be referred promptly for cardiac surgical consultation than men (Schwartz et al., 1997). In a survey of 720 physicians responding to a computerized survey instrument, women and Black patients were significantly less likely to be referred for cardiac catheterization than men and White patients (Schulman et al., 1999). Black women were least likely of all groups to be so referred. The authors concluded that, after careful controls were applied, race and patient gender independently influenced management of chest pain. When hospitalized for acute myocardial infarction, women undergo fewer diagnostic and therapeutic interventions than men (Chandra et al., 1998). These differences could mean that women are not receiving full benefit from the clinical advances in cardiology or that men are undergoing more coronary procedures than optimal. The researchers point out, however, that the differences in care included physicians' prescribing behavior and such common therapies as heparin, beta blockers, and aspirin, the administration of which was significantly lower in women than in men. What influences in the development of our illness care complex have led to the disproportionately high use of psychopharmacology by women and the low utilization of cardiovascular treatment?

At the same time as women need to be concerned that they are receiving all necessary interventions—surgical and otherwise—they also need to pay particular attention to the substantial cost—financial, personal, social—paid in health care errors (Institute of Medicine, 2000). The "wasteful overcapacity of the nation's hospital plant" (Ginzberg, 1998, p. 1539) is a force that continues to drive health care demand—by both providers and patients—and spending.

SEXISM AND THE EDUCATION OF HEALTH PROFESSIONALS

Analyses of professional education materials as well as influential advertising directed toward health professionals demonstrate continuing gender bias. Early work demonstrated inaccurate information in medical texts concerning such subjects as the strength of women's sexual drives, the roles of the vagina and clitoris in orgasm, and the incidence and prevalence of female sexual dysfunction (Scully & Bart, 1973). One text portrayed women as inherently sick and stated that the feminine core consists of masochism, passivity, and narcissism. At the same time, the text advised physicians to counsel their women patients to simulate orgasms if they were not orgasmic with their husbands.

Naomi Wolf, in her 1997 book *Promiscuities* on sexual coming-of-age, provides the lecture we never had on the clitoris. Identified and well-described in 1559 by the Venetian scientist Renaldus Columbus, the clitoris was described by midwives, anatomists, and physicians through the 18th century. But when sexual purity and ill health for women were popularized, and as the home and family were separated into their own private spheres in the 19th century, information on this sexual organ, along with cognizance of female sexual desire, was suppressed. Wolf argues that Freud was hardly the first authority to examine and misunderstand the clitoris, and she reminds readers that generations of social critics suggested that close attention to female anatomy and physiology could improve intimate relationships. The authors of *A New View of a Woman's Body* (Federation of Feminist Women's Health Centers, 1991) examined the basic research on the anatomy and physiology of the clitoris. They found it to be a vital sexual organ whose existence was omitted from medical texts. Textbook illustrations of women's genitals through the 1980s frequently excluded the clitoris.

Textbooks and advertisements aimed at gynecologists reinforced status and intellectual asymmetry between patients and doctors (Fisher, 1986). "By controlling women and their reproductive capacities," wrote Fisher, "medical domination functioned to sustain male domination" (p. 160). A newer generation of critic suggests that both texts and advertisements have moved away from portraying women as inferior and victim, and instead are portraying women as invincible to illness and especially age, so long as they make the right choices about their behavior and the medical goods and services they purchase (Kaufert & Lock, 1997). "Health is the new virtue for women as they age. . . . [I]f she allows her body to deteriorate, then she becomes unworthy, undeserving of support" (Kaufert & Lock, 1997, p. 86). Being characterized as invincible is not much of an improvement over being characterized as a victim, when both stereotypes prevent development of health care providers and systems that respond to women's complex and various needs.

As feminism and other critical social movements have encouraged both men and women to move beyond stereotype, the expressive capacities of those who provide personal health services are receiving more attention. This shift affects even the financing of health care: federally set physician fee schedules, revamped by the valuation system called resource-based relative value scales, provided increased payment for such cognitive services as taking a patient history, while payment for such technical procedures as sigmoidoscopy were lowered (Hsiao et al., 1988). The relative value units assigned to various interventions are multiplied by a dollar conversion factor to arrive at reimbursement levels for all procedures covered by Medicare, as well as for many private insurers. The use of this relative value scale figures in the setting of standards of provider productivity (Shackelford, 1999); such standard setting may benefit patients by reducing practice variability and may also aggravate patients uninterested in service delivery efficiency. The importance of gender-aware analysis figures here as well: in comparing pairs of gender-specific surgical procedures, work units were found to be similar or identical, while reimbursement for male-specific procedures were reimbursed at an amount 44% greater than female-specific procedures (Goff, Muntz, & Cain, 1997).

Women in physician practice are almost equal in numbers to men (Lorber, 2000). But Black women are only 2% of all practicing physicians, and when combined with Black men physicians, make up only 4% of the work group (Council on Graduate Medical Education, 1998)—a figure stable since 1910, when the Flexner report on medical education led to the abandonment of most medical education facilities for Blacks and for women (Starr, 1982). Medical practice—only one area affecting the use of health care resources but one of the most expensive—is characterized by a continuing excess of medical specialists practicing in affluent urban areas and a paucity of primary care physicians in rural and inner-city urban areas. Rural medicine, as one example,

is characterized by a ratio of men to women physicians of almost six to one (Council on Graduate Medical Education, 1998). Women physicians have been shown to practice more collaboratively with patients, spend more time with patients, and deal more often with feelings and emotions than their male counterparts (Elderkin-Thompson & Waitzkin, 1999). Woodward (1999) suggests cautious optimism about the decreasing sexism of medical students, as evidenced by reduced stereotyping of sex roles; willingness to collaborate rather than control the decision making of female patients; and similar conceptualizations of women, men, and adults. The professional and academic leadership of medicine is dominated by men: 15% of women medical school faculty in the United States hold the rank of full professor compared to 30% of men, and only 11% of all medical department chairs are women (Hamel, Ingelfinger, Phimister, & Solomon, 2006; Tesch, Wood, Helwig, & Nattinger, 1995).

Some improvements in care for women have been brought about by national initiatives, such as the establishment of offices for women's health in various federal agencies (the Food and Drug Administration, for example) and women's health services at the Veterans Administration. In addition, the Public Health Service has considered adding women's health courses to health professional school curricula (Schatzberg, 1997).

SEXISM AND RESEARCH ON WOMEN AND HEALTH

Like health care practice, health research also has been affected by gender-based bias and stereotype. All aspects of the research process may be influenced, including the conceptual frameworks that form the theoretical basis for research, the selection of problems for study, funding, the logistics of research methodology, and the conclusions drawn from the results. Just as there is a gender difference in the academic rank held by women in medical schools, so also is there a discrepancy in authorship of research. Although there has been an increase of first authorship by women from 5.9% in 1970 to 29.3% in 2004, and the percent of senior authors of articles in leading medical journals has increased from 3.7% to 19.3%, women's influence on published research remains clearly in the minority (Jagsi et al., 2006).

Conceptual Frameworks

The conceptual frameworks guiding research about women have their own historical context—the times in which the studies were conducted as well as the contemporaneous academic orientations. Social science research, for example, has been predicated upon certain beliefs about the social structure (Gouldner, 1970) and the family, such as the perception that children should be raised in families in which men perform the active, doing, instrumental roles while women perform the feeling, "expressive" roles (Parsons & Bales, 1955). The effects of such a normative conceptual framework was evident in psychoanalytic research, where illness in women was equated with rejection of culturally defined roles, such as loosing interest in housework. It can also be seen in the family care literature, in which women are automatically assigned nurturing roles in situations as different as family therapy or cardiac rehabilitation. While women's interest in the care giving aspects of family life is assumed, their interest in other family issues—economic health, for example—is ignored. Studies on the stress of chronic illness care, for example, routinely ask for women's responses on expressive items, while instrumental aspects of family life such as finances are left unstudied.

Women's health research remains illness oriented and concerns itself disproportionately with pathology rather than health. Such normal events as lactation, childbirth, menstruation, menopause, and sexual response have frequently been approached in the context of dysfunction or pathology. Although nurses and other researchers have focused on these nonpathologic points of view, their numbers and institutional support remains disproportionately small. The commercial marketplace for health-promoting products has apparently outstripped the research marketplace in its focus on disease and disability prevention, leaving consumers unsure of the context for and efficacy of a wide variety of approaches and regimens. The massive self-help and self-improvement industry is largely aimed at women, often without the benefit of confirmatory research as a resource. But alternative therapies, also long aimed at women, are increasingly the subject of research, including by the National Center for Complementary and Alternative Medicine, a part of the National Institutes of Health, established in 1992.

Topics for Study

The problems chosen for research also reflect widely held assumptions about women. Central among society's assumptions regarding women is the inherent otherness of women; in this context, normal, positive physiological functions are seen as pathologic. For example, many menstrual cycle studies conducted prior to the 1980s were designed to detect the problems women experience because they menstruate—for example, a hypothesized propensity for illness, violent crimes, or accidents.

Diseases primarily affecting men have traditionally received a large share of researchers' attention. Serious and costly conditions that affect women, such as osteoporosis, have been neglected. Osteoporosis was not studied until recently, despite clear evidence that hip fracture—only one of the consequences of increased bone fragility—is a leading cause of hospitalization, surgery, and nursing home placement among older women (McGowan & Pottern, 2000).

Although coronary artery disease is the leading cause of death in women, many years lapsed before it was targeted for study in women. Not until 1989 did the National Heart, Lung and Blood Institute (which has funded most of the clinical trials on heart disease) break tradition by funding its first women-only study, the Postmenopausal Estrogen Progestin Intervention, to study the effects of prescribed hormonal treatment on the risk of CAD in women (Stefanick, 1992).

The choice of study problems is obviously related to the research perspectives and tools available and popular at the moment. A biomedical orientation to research has emphasized specialization and an orientation to genetic and molecular events. Concentration on these aspects of illness ignores the final object of study: the total organism. Sophisticated instrumentation and specialization in research areas promote science that examines only a fragment of the patient, male or female, rather than the person as a whole. New methodologies (especially qualitative approaches), interdisciplinary research teams, and expanded venues for publication and discussion can encourage research directed at women as totalities. The recently updated *Agenda for Research on* Women's Health, now up to seven volumes, reflects important new efforts at promoting a new level of intellectual vigor in addressing women's health (see Office of Research on Women's Health at http://orwh.od.nih.gov and U.S. Public Health Service, 1999).

The 1999 women's health research agenda grew from an inclusive process in which women's health advocates as well as scientists participated in regional and national meetings and heard public testimony. Explicit consideration of various groups of women representing America's ethnic groups and those living with disabilities enriched the agenda-setting process. The final reports reflect the deliberations and recommendations from these hearings and assess the current status of research on women's health. Gaps in knowledge, sex and gender differences that may influence women's health, and factors that affect health of women from various populations were topics of discussion. Enhancing prevention, diagnosis, and treatment was an explicit focus of discussion, as was development of strategies to improve the health status of women regardless of race, ethnicity, age, or other characteristics. In addition, career issues for women scientists were addressed in the report.

Topics for research that are included in this agenda span a wide range of health issues. Among these are disorders and consequences of alcohol, tobacco, and other drug use; behavioral and social science aspects of women's health; bone and musculoskeletal disorders; cancer; cardiovascular diseases; digestive diseases; immunity and autoimmune idseases; infectious diseases and emerging infections; mental disorders; neuroscience; oral health; pharmacologic issues; reproductive health; and urologic and kidney conditions. Chapters also address the use of sex and gender to define and characterize differences between men and women. A special consideration was research design for studies of women, addressing consideration of special populations of women; racial, ethnic, and cultural diversity; and multidisciplinary perspectives. The creative ideas expressed in these chapters can have significant effects on the science of women's health if they are integrated with the disease-focused topics including the biomedical perspectives. The degree to which the ideas expressed in the research agenda are influential rests on how they are embraced by the senior scientists judging the scientific merit of research proposals and advisory councils who shape science policy for NIH (Woods, 2000).

Although the 1999 agenda promises to change the course of women's health research, several issues were not addressed. There is little emphasis on the health consequences of poverty in women, of the power differential between men and women that influences health, and the gendered allocation of work in U.S. society. A global perspective is needed to examine consequences of economic development and social policy on women's health (Woods, 2000).

Funding

To the extent to which such large funding sources as the National Institutes of Health allocate scarce resources for research programs, they define the nature of research about women. The NIH Revitalization Act of 1993 mandated that the NIH establish guidelines for including women and minorities in clinical research (NIH, 1994). All NIH-sponsored research from 1995 on had to comply with those guidelines, which mandated inclusion of women and minorities; that cost could not preclude such inclusion; and that outreach, recruitment, and retention efforts would be supported (NIH, 2002). The Food and Drug Administration (FDA) also instituted a 1993 policy change regarding women: to gain FDA approval of pharmaceuticals, drug companies were required to include women in clinical trials, study gender differences in phase 3 (safety and efficacy) trials, and study gonadal hormone interactions with new drugs (Herz, 1997).

The peer review process exerts at least an indirect influence as well. For example, the predominantly male composition of the study sections that reviewed proposals for scientific merit and allocation of funding certainly influenced the types of research funded. Were it not for the increasing visibility of women on these bodies, it is likely that the biomedical approach and the traditional orientations toward women's health would

have continued unchallenged. The Center for Scientific Review of the NIH, which sets guidelines and policy for research review, now explicitly includes gender, ethnicity, and geographic distribution among its principles for reviewer selection (Center for Scientific Review, 2000).

The research efforts of the largest single group of health care professionals—nurses—were not organizationally included in the NIH until 1986, when the National Center for Nursing Research was established. One of the smallest of the institutes, the nursing center received some $137 million in the 2007 budget, compared to much larger budgets for institutes focusing on prevalent diseases in the United States.

Funding for training new investigators in women's health has been established by NIH's Office of Research on Women's Health via the Building Interdisciplinary Research Careers in Women's Health program, as well as programs for nascent scientists among high school girls and for women already established in biomedical careers, but who are encountering barriers that limit their advancement. In addition, the Office of Research on Women's Health has funded specialized centers of research. The picture for funding health care research relevant to women has improved, but careful observers should keep in mind the continued disproportion and not forget the abysmal baseline from which we started and from which we still draw comparisons.

Sampling and Informed Consent

Women are not the only group who may be coerced and/or mistreated in research studies, but they deserve special attention from prospective researchers in regard to issues of power and information. Sechrest (1975) was an early reporter on the coercion and power that can be applied to foster women's participation in research projects. She noted that early research on oral contraceptives took advantage of relatively uniformed and low-resource Puerto Rican women who had few options for avoiding pregnancy. Financial incentives or provision of free medical care for women and their children may also be irresistible elements in recruiting.

In a review of federal standards for research involving human subjects and a policy-focused set of recommendations, the Human Research Ethics Group from the University of Pennsylvania (Moreno, Caplan, & Wolpe, 1998) took note of situations involving women. They recommended vigorous pursuit of the goal to include women, minorities, and children in biomedical and behavioral research. Noting the new federal policies and initiatives that are in place, the group nonetheless reported that the pace and scope of improvement with regard to fairness in subject selection are unclear. They noted that, while consensus exists about the importance of including reproductive aged women in research, debate continues about the inclusion of pregnant women as research subjects.

Mouton and colleagues (1997) from the University of Texas health science center studied the attitudes of Black women about participating in cancer research. Although death from malignant neoplasms among Blacks is about 20% higher than for Whites, and both Black women (56%) and White women (71%) had positive attitudes about cancer research in this telephone survey, 32% of Black women expressed distrust of scientists compared to only 4% of White women. These data are said to corroborate Harris poll findings that African Americans fear clinical trials and distrust the health care system.

African American women, in comparison to White and Hispanic women, also entered AIDS clinical trials at lower rates than their proportions in the HIV/AIDS population (Korvick et al., 1996). Women with a history of injection drug use participate at low rates as well. The importance of studying women is illustrated by the possibility that gender differences may play a role in toxicity and efficacy of HIV therapies; previous enrollment rates of women in drug trials did not allow for sufficient statistical power to evaluate these potential differences.

Data Analysis, Interpretation, and Conclusions

Woods (1992) has made clear that helpful research on women's health will not come about from old wine in new bottles. She advocated for a reformulation of science, clear views of women's experiences through lenses ground by women. This could include qualitative methods of analysis that are reaching new levels of rigor and reproducibility. It could include interpretation of biologic uniqueness as a sign of health rather than deviance or illness. And reformulated science could include designing research *for* rather than *on* women, with liberating rather than oppressive results.

> Simply adding a cohort of women to a study designed to illuminate issues grounded in thinking about men or increasing the proportion of women researchers in a male-dominated field will not solve the problem of advancing a more complete understanding of women's health. What is necessary is a reexamination of the nature of science that will foster a better understanding of the health of the many populations of women and serve emancipatory ends. (Woods, 1992, p. 1)

In their recommendations for the future protection of human subjects in biomedical and behavioral research, Moreno, Caplan, and Wolpe (1998) noted the important role of increased community understanding vis-à-vis the research process and the conclusions drawn.

Consumer demand for incompletely studied and sensationally portrayed technologies and cures have filled front pages and legislative hearing rooms. Even well-studied treatments have been found, on hindsight, to be less than foretold: high-dose chemotherapy followed by autologous bone marrow transplant was promoted as effective for late-stage breast cancer, and, without conclusive studies, insurers and governments were pressured to provide coverage. Randomized trial studies later revealed no significant advantage over conventional treatment. The picture was confused even further for consumers by a revelation of falsified data. Out of five studies of high-dose chemotherapy followed by transplant, only one held out the hope of effectiveness, and this South African study was subsequently discredited for apparently falsifying data (Neergaard, 2000).

One highly regarded expert in the field of clinical trials, David Eddy, has made a compelling case that insurers should continue to withhold routine payment for a new treatment until its effects are known. The reason, he argues, is not profits; it is quality of care (Eddy, 1997). This position is subject to continuing debate among women's and consumer groups, whose agitations demonstrate that a gold standard for scientific conclusion is not the same as a gold standard for patients' sense of satisfaction, deserving-ness, and adequacy of care. Personal health decisions continue to be made from a complex set of factors, but no woman can afford to be blind to the commercial and political decisions that guide the design, findings, and release of information from both private and publicly funded research.

HEALTH CARE ISSUES AND ARENAS FOR WOMEN
Personal Health Services

A notable shift in health care over the last few decades has been from a monopolistically physician-centered and traditionally authoritarian manner of delivering personal health services to a pluralistic array of clinicians, healers, and approaches to cure and care. Moving over time from word-of-mouth to the telephone book, services as diverse as acupuncture and music therapy are entering the everyday consumer vocabulary. Mainstream clinical groups have been surprised and even shocked to learn that more visits are paid to alternative than to mainstream clinicians (Eisenberg et al., 1998). More visits were paid to alternative providers (629 million in 1997) than to all U.S. primary care physicians, and more was spent out of pocket ($12.2 billion in 1997) than was spent out of pocket for all U.S. hospitalizations (Eisenberg et al., 1998). Women used alternative therapies more than men (49% versus 38%); higher-income persons and those with college education were more likely to use alternative therapies, but the national use of at least one alternative treatment was 42%, a significant increase from 34% in 1990 (Eisenberg et al., 1999). A survey of use of chiropractic services in the United States and Canada similarly showed that women patients predominate slightly more than men; the percentage of the population using chiropractic has doubled over the past 20 years, just as has the number of chiropractors (Hurwitz, Coulter, Adams, Genovese, & Shekelle, 1998).

The lure of 12-plus billion dollars in consumer buying power alone has been enough to bring window-dressing and even some fundamental change to health care service delivery. Although the evolution of some models of women's personal health care delivery has been the result of humanistic movements within some of the professions, women themselves have had a profound influence on the structure of personal health services. In some instances— such as the increasing use of midwives—traditional modes of health care, often culturally linked, have come into wider use (Paine, Dower, & O'Neil, 1999). In other instances, women have created new kinds of services, such as self-help clinics, caregiver support teams, and resource groups on the Internet. In some cases, professionals took over women's efforts, creating modified forms of personal health services that remain firmly under the control of professionals (e.g., the development and promotion of home-like birthing rooms in hospitals).

Health care settings such as self-help clinics arose from the women's health movement, which Marieskind (1975) described as a grass-roots organization dating from about 1970. Drawing parallels to the popular health movement of the mid-19th century, Marieskind saw modern interest in women's health linked to activism for political gains for women. Just as the popular health movement was associated with gaining the vote for women, the 20th century's women's health movement was linked to a progressive, feminist political and economic agenda (Leavitt, 1984). Ruzek (1978) and Marieskind reported some common features of women's health movement organizations: reduction in hierarchy, changes in the profit-making orientation, increased use of lay workers, involvement of clients in their own care, and a commitment to a feminist ideology.

Morgen and Julier (1991) revisited a sample of organizations arising from the women's health movement to document development and change over the decades since the late 1960s. They mailed questionnaires to 144 women's health clinics, advocacy, and education organizations. The authors reported that a significant number of questionnaires were returned, indicating that the organization was no longer in existence (the actual number was not reported). Three-quarters of the responding organizations described themselves as focused on prevention or self-care; two-thirds identified themselves as ideologically feminist. Commitment to low-income and minority women was high: most of the organizations served poor and minority women either in excess of or in direct proportion to the percentage of low-income and minority women in their communities. These characteristics conform to much of the original expressed intent of the women's health movement. In contrast to the organizational mission, the organizational structures have tended to change over the decades, from egalitarian staff models (for example, in some women's health clinics, pay was equal for all workers) to more traditional ranking of workers and from consensus decision making to hierarchical authority. Staff hiring, training, and development continue to reflect feminist principles such as diversity and group solidarity. This study suggests that the women's health movement continues to influence the delivery of health services and that, not without struggle, alternatives to the health business-as-usual continue their work. The Fair Haven Community Health Center in Haven, Connecticut, is one example of a community clinic dating from the early 1970s that still consciously asserts its community-focused, feminist roots in its management today. Salaries, scheduling, and organization-wide meetings with rotating chair responsibility all reflect its founding commitment to enacting alternatives to hierarchical, male-dominated medical models of health care delivery and system management. Consumer participation is also exemplified in organizations such as Group Health Cooperative, a health maintenance organization (HMO) in the Pacific Northwest dating from the 1940s, which is still governed by a consumer-elected board.

Managed Care

"Managed care, which, by default, became the instrument of health-care reform after the Clintons' failure, grates on the public when it fulfills its mission of restraining costs by restraining use of services" (Greenberg, 1999, p. 1799).

Some women may be surprised to consider that managed care organizations and their quality assurance activities may directly affect women's health issues. In contrast to the era in which no quality measures were available by which consumers could choose clinicians or clinical approaches, a variety of measures is now available: licensure and accreditation of clinicians and consumer ratings for health plans (through consumer assessment organizations, independent services such as Consumers Union's *Consumer Reports* magazine, and publications such as *Newsweek*). Many health plans support being accountable for quality and want consumers to have information.

In 1991, the nonprofit National Committee for Quality Assurance (NCQA) began accrediting health plans, using a standardized set of clinical performance measures called HEDIS (health plan employer data and information set). Health plans with NCQA accreditation and that publicly report their HEDIS data outperform those that are not NCQA accredited those that do not make their data public (measures include prenatal care, follow-up for mental illness, diabetic eye exams, immunization rates, breast cancer screening, and treatment with beta-blocker medication after heart attack). The HEDIS measures specific to women's health include breast and cervical cancer screening, prenatal care in the first trimester, post-delivery checkups, cesarean rates, vaginal birth after C-section, discharges and average length of stay for mothers and newborns. Additional HEDIS measures now include management of menopause and chlamydia screening and are being updated constantly (see http://www.ncqa.org and select HEDIS measures of interest). The NCQA is also studying for inclusion calcium intake, osteoporosis prevention and counseling, birth control counseling and coverage, postpartum depression screening, domestic violence screening, and benefits to people over a yet-to-be-determined percentage of body weight (Merrikin, 1999).

Among the challenges to women's health presented by managed care mechanisms are the inclusion of services that have often been marginalized. Drug and alcohol treatment is such an example. Child development services, early intervention, parental support, and care for children with special needs also risk marginalization or exclusion by health plans that focus only on illness care services. Plans that follow missions that truly emphasize health maintenance may find it easier (but not necessarily financially positive); the large staff model HMO Kaiser-Permanente screens pregnant women for risk of substance abuse and initiates early intervention services such as comprehensive assessment, counseling, case management, home visits, and targeted follow-up (Soman et al., 1996).

Long-Term Care

Women are the recipients of some and the providers of most long-term care. It is estimated that some 25 million Americans provide informal caregiving, at an average of 17.9 hours per week (Arno, Levine, & Memmott, 1999). Calculating a value for that work at even the minimum wage results in an annual figure well over $100 billion, far larger than an annual cost for formal home care ($32 billion) and nursing home care ($83 billion) (Arno et al., 1999).

Populations other than the elderly also need long-term care: those with chronic mental and physical illnesses, the developmentally delayed, and disabled persons of all ages. The AIDS epidemic has brought new populations into chronic care: HIV-positive children and adults. Grandmothers are a caregiving population with increasing responsibility for the care of their HIV-positive and drug- and alcohol-affected grandchildren.

Caregivers have been found to be burdened by multiple stressors associated with caregiving work. Caregiving stressors in one study were found to lead to depression; hours of care provided and caregiver perception of overload were found to be significant factors (Yates, Tennstedt, & Chang, 1999).

Two policy changes will bring about change in directions yet to be determined. One is the decline in the availability of home health care, in response to the 1997 Balanced Budget Act and its changes in Medicare funding. The second, longer-standing change has been in the availability of caregiving leave, albeit unpaid, under the 1993 Family and Medical Leave Act.

Nurse Practitioners

The nurse practitioner movement represents an important addition to the pluralistic U.S. health care labyrinth. Developed in the late 1960s, nurse practitioners are nurses with advanced training in the diagnosis and treatment of minor, acute, and chronic illness. They have evolved much as their original planners hoped they would (Lynaugh, 1986): nurse practitioners work with multiple communities, but have special representation among poor and underserved populations; they concentrate on patient education and advocacy as well as diagnosis and treatment, and they have gained a high level of consumer confidence. Their numbers have grown rapidly, from 55,000 to an estimated 106,000 in 2005 (Cooper, Laud, & Dietrich, 1998).

The question of nurse practitioners' effectiveness compared to physicians' has undergone decades of study. Brown and Grimes (1995) undertook a meta-analysis of nurse practitioners and nurse midwives in primary care. With careful discussion of methodological and analytic issues, they found nurse practitioner care equal to and sometimes better than physician care. Fewer than half of the studies randomized patients to provider; in these, patient compliance to treatment regimens was greater for nurse practitioners' patients. In studies that controlled for risk in ways other than randomization, patient satisfaction and resolution of pathologic conditions was greater with nurse practitioner patients; other care variables were found to be equivalent between nurse practitioner and physician patients. (In controlled studies, nurse midwives were similarly found to achieve neonatal outcomes equivalent to physicians', using less technology and less analgesia.)

Yet each study of nurse practitioner effectiveness is followed by refutation. In a recent round, Mundinger and colleagues' (2000) study of patients randomly assigned to nurse practitioners or primary care physicians with similar authority, responsibility, and administrative/productivity requirements demonstrated that health status and patient satisfaction did not differ. This study, praised for its randomization, sophisticated analysis, and internal validity has been faulted for its lack of external validity (applicability to a variety of other sites) (Sox, 2000). What continue to be at play are clinical outcome research and turf and income protection issues.

Brown and Grimes's (1995) important meta-analysis notes that cost-effectiveness has not been adequately evaluated from these data on nurse practitioner practice. And most importantly, studies in this vein have been designed around care provider, not process of care, as the independent variable. The whole range of clinician (and care system) activities that may lead to patient well-being awaits clear explication.

Popular Media Coverage on Health

Media coverage of health issues is inadequate in a variety of ways, including disproportionate emphasis on certain diseases (breast cancer over heart disease, for example), no acknowledgement of the limitations of research, no connections to other studies, and no discussion of confounding variables or multifactorial nature of the causes of disease. In reviewing the treatment of menopause in the popular press, nurse researchers found that unsubstantiated opinion played a large role, and that the biomedical approach to menopause predominated (Carlson, Li, & Holm, 1997).

Shuchman and Wilkes (1997) suggest that the dynamic relationship between scientists and journalists can be altered to improve public understanding of health news. The urge for dramatization, the push to publicize for increased funding potential, a bias in both the media and scientific communities against negative studies, jargon-filled technical writing, undisclosed links to profit-making health care enterprises, lack of follow-up and corroborative studies and their reporting all contribute to poor public service and can be alleviated.

Community Leadership

The Boston Women's Health Book Collective and the National Black Women's Health Project are two examples of groups arising from communities that are defining their own health concerns and seeking alternatives to paternalistic care.

Our Bodies, Our Selves is the Book Collective's most famous publication and represents a revolutionary and collective effort by women to answer questions about health issues for themselves. Starting as a mimeographed booklet in 1971, it has evolved into a regularly revised softcover book that has sold millions of copies and is now translated into multiple languages.

Billye Avery, founder of the National Black Women's Health Project, joined with women in southeastern communities to address their health problems through self-help chapters, educational presentations, a national newsletter, and national and local media productions and conferences. "We've worked on everyone else's issues; it's time to work on ours" was one of their slogans.

The late 20th century saw both the increased corporatization of care and a surge in community-based programs. Examples of community-based care include

- a nurse-run program in Detroit to link HIV-positive women with mental illness and substance abuse to care sources (Andersen, Smereck, Hockman, Ross, & Ground, 1999)
- the *de Madres a Madres* effort in Houston led by community mothers in forming a coalition with health clinics, social service agencies, local businesses, schools, churches, local officials, and the media to identify and redress their health needs (McFarland & Fehir, 1994)
- a home nurse-visiting program for high-risk, low-income primiparous women piloted in rural New York state and then replicated in Memphis, Tennessee, which reduced pregnancy-related hypertension, childhood injuries, and subsequent pregnancies (Kitzman et al., 1997)
- a 40-clinic system of breast and cervical cancer screening for Native American women that relied on community input and participation as well as highly planned system change, including data collection and a commitment to quality assurance (Kottke & Trapp, 1998).

A far-sighted group from East Carolina University in Greenville, North Carolina, has expanded thinking about the role of community structures in health in its study of "premature mortality," an age-adjusted measure of potential life-years lost before age 75, across U.S. counties (Mansfield, Wilson, Kobrinski, & Mitchell, 1999). They found that the proportions of women-headed households and Black populations were the strongest predictors, followed by low education, American Indian population, and chronic unemployment. The authors echo the thinking of many other observers in suggesting that strengthening community structure may be far more healthful than increasing the amounts of expensive medical care.

As federal and state policymakers seek to improve health, they should consider whether resources might not be better spent on programs to reduce social pathology instead of on more medical care. Social policy can diminish, cause, or exacerbate the social factors that underlie illness as we choose or choose not to encourage family integrity, improve education and economic equality, discourage teen pregnancy, and so forth.

A vital critique of U.S. health care practice has been added through the recent work of the Institute of Medicine (2002) in its report on health. David Williams, a member of the prestigious group assembled to study inequality in U.S. health care, has written on a number of factors that, resting on the bedrock of U.S. racism, continue to promote health disparities—for example, residential segregation (Williams & Collins, 2001). Minority women, in particular, suffer from health disparities largely on the basis of socioeconomic status, but also from geographic location, migration and acculturation, exposure to stress, resources, and the basic variability in quality of medical care (Williams, 2002).

Public Health Services

Although women are directly affected by personal health services, they are just as surely but less obviously affected by the public health system. The mission of public health services is the surveillance and promotion of the health of all people in the United States. Health care in the United States is private business; the government is less involved than in most other industrialized countries. But some elements of the health care system are government controlled: military health care, including the Veterans Administration hospital system, and the Indian Health Service are two examples of publicly run, personal health care delivery systems. Women's health issues confront these systems with problems as varied as domestic violence on military bases to fetal alcohol syndrome prevention on Native American reservations.

Two major divisions of the U.S. Department of Health and Human Services administer health programs: the Public Health Service and the Centers for Medicare & Medicaid Services (formerly the Health Care Financing Administration). The Public Health Service has five major agencies, including the National Institutes of Health and the Health Resources and Services Administration. The federal health programs are enormously complex and lack centralized, rational planning sustained over time. Although some analysts find beneficial the continuous creation of new programs in response to public demand in that it maintains the health system's link to reality, others fear the changing political tides that ebb and flow in funding and support.

A prime example of the variability of public funding and governmental support is the recent history of family planning, including access to contraception and abortion services. Despite a worldwide population explosion and a national explosion in the number of teen pregnancies over the past three decades, federal funding for international family planning has decreased and access to abortion services has been curtailed.

States and localities offer a highly variable range of public health services, from widely accepted traditional public health services such as vital statistics, communicable disease control, environmental sanitation, and public health education to providing personal health services of last resort to the poor and such special groups as the chronically mentally ill and persons with AIDS. These services too ebb and flow with unreliable funding, often affecting the services available to needy women such as county well-baby clinics and public health nurses.

Public health's ability to monitor community health should be a concern for women. As savvy community supervisors, women depend on the public health infrastructure to determine whether the multifaceted primary care resources of a state (for example) are meeting population needs (Starfield, 1996). The public health community's successes, on the other hand, should inspire hope: When the Public Health Service joined the Institute of Medicine to design Healthy People 2000, the goals set became an important benchmark for health status improvement. The creation of the goals for Healthy People 2010 has exerted the same, critical influence.

International Concerns

Criticism of the U.S. health system's shortchanging of women can be leveled on an international level as well. Habitual regard of women solely as reproductive organisms has pervaded the health policy of many nations. National and international health policies have often centered solely on this function—from outlawing abortion under pronatalist regimes to coercive sterilization and contraception in countries with exploding populations. At both extremes, the voices of the women are infrequently heard. Women's health advocates and activists have important responsibilities to foster public involvement and to monitor international health efforts in adult and child health, work place health and safety, contraception, and access to abortion. The focus on reproduction—to the exclusion of other important issues such as job creation, providing market access for women growers, and sponsoring credit and loan mechanisms to women—calls for continuing advocacy and the development of new priorities.

THE FUTURE

The personnel, institutions, research, and policies particular to women's health care will undoubtedly reflect the broad changes taking place in all of health care in the 21st century. If burgeoning health care costs are controlled, so profits in the health care business will be reduced, target incomes of clinicians may lower, and the pool of applicants for health care training will change. The numbers of women physicians will increase. Nurses may well come into their own with a scope of practice highly visible to the public. To meet the demand for primary care clinicians, workers such as nurse practitioners will see their numbers grow. The demand for nurses will continue, with increased pressure to place a variety of workers—some with shorter and less costly education—at the bedside. Professionals will be called on to balance their demands for the most highly trained colleagues with a clear-eyed look at the elitism that has kept the highest paid of the health professions from reflecting the population diversity of our country as a whole.

A variety of thinkers and prognosticators have worried about the composition of the primary care work force in the United States, most recently in a symposium reported in the *Annals of Internal Medicine,* which was predictably physician centered. However, calls for improved quality of care for all (Showstack, Lurie, Larson, Rothman, & Hassmiller, 2003) and new designs for chronic care (Rothman & Wagner, 2003) emphasize the need to involve multiple clinicians in true teams.

The demand for nursing aides and assistants will be influenced by the aging of the U.S. population; in-home assistance is an as-yet-underdeveloped segment of the health care industry. Training and supervision of in-home caregivers will pose new challenges for managers of public and private home care agencies. The movement of health care out of institutions and into the home may add additional pressure for change already underway in the nature of patient-provider relationships, a change from hierarchical to mutual. But this shift may also institutionalize women's role as family health provider—a role made even more demanding in the context of competing responsibilities from employment outside the home.

The first decade after the failed Clinton health care reform plan of 1994 showed not a steady movement toward a more rational health delivery system with reduced variability, but rather a ferocious competition among different varieties of health care businesses, often with competing values and missions (Gold, 1999). For-profit health plans fought for market share with long-established, not-for-profit health maintenance organizations. Alternative providers competed with physicians for access to patients through regulatory and financial routes. An era of extreme profit-taking seems to be past, but the health care industry is still in full-growth mode, with new horizons of technology and approaches to disease just ahead.

The anomaly of employer-based insurance continues to befuddle U.S. business as well as the health services industry. A shift can be seen as employers move from a *defined benefit* approach to health insurance (in which employers supply at least one, if not a choice of, health insurance plans) to *defined contribution* (an approach by which employers offer a subsidy to purchase insurance or care, the selection of which is no longer up to the employer, but the employee).

If much of the populace does move to insurance via defined contribution, even more importance will be attached to consumers' ability to evaluate health service delivery plans. Attention must be paid to issues such as the scope of services to be reimbursed. Benefits must not be limited to illness care; illness prevention and health promotion services are especially important for women—adult health screening, work site health and safety, contraceptive services, pelvic examinations, breast exams, pregnancy, childbirth care—and the children they tend. A health insurance plan that limits the number of providers would adversely affect women who tend to use more than one clinician—for example, a midwife and a family practitioner.

Current debates over employer-based insurance plans involve important issues for women. Women's employment patterns are different from men's, with more interruptions for family care—children, spouses, and parents all receive the majority of their care from their mothers, spouses, and daughters. Can employer-based insurance accommodate the employment interruptions women need? Women's health activists and advocates must be prepared to work at both the state and national levels to ensure that health care financing plans meet women's real needs.

Institutional changes now occurring will affect women's health care: the demise of small and rural hospitals; a move from private, independent physician practices to health maintenance organizations and other group practices; and the growth in home health care. Sentimental idealization of a past golden era of health care and demonization of the present will not serve women well; instead, women must carefully examine their needs and preferences to decide which modes of care will best serve them.

The role of public health departments in women's health is yet to be determined. Long the provider of specific services such as treatment for sexually transmitted disease, health departments may expand their personal health services, especially to women and children. Pilot projects in which public health and school nurses are the neighborhood primary care clinician may foretell a future community-based system of care, particularly in low-income neighborhoods. Nurses—the single largest group of health care professionals yet often the group least represented at policy and planning levels—could be an important group of women workers called upon to shape the health care systems for the future.

Although researchers and feminist authors have seriously addressed the problems women encounter in personal health service interactions, they only recently have begun to explore the connections between public policy and women's health. Labor and pension policy, the obligation to provide unpaid care to family members, child care and parental leave, welfare reform, and prison policies are women's health policy issues as well.

Improvements such as the federal requirement for women's participation in federally funded research may foster knowledge of women's health in the previously male-dominated world of biomedical research. Increased awareness of women's health issues has led to policy changes as diverse as funding for optimum supports to live with chronic disease and new programs that focus on the work place hazard of sexual harassment.

Many state governments have expanded their Medicaid programs to include women and children not otherwise insured for health care. Those same states are currently struggling with enormous budget deficits. In keeping with the incremental nature of social policy change in the United States and a history of distributing welfare resources group by group (rather than universally), women and children will continue to be a group readily identified as worthy of guaranteed health care. Recent national efforts to insure children through the Children's Health Insurance Plan reflect the patchwork of health policy to address access to health care for select population groups. Unfortunately, in budget crises, these same programs are at risk of service reductions and budget cuts. As states work on individual health insurance plans, the need to design dependable, basic, minimum sets of primary care services will include identification of appropriate primary care services specific to women. This could include a call for increased attention to preventive services for women, with the design and implementation of well-woman care that extends beyond its current class and economic boundaries to low-income women and women of color. Employment-based insurance continues to create many problems, including job lock and the dependence of middle-aged and older women on breadwinners' insurance. Long-term care will continue to be considered a financial black hole for public money; the private insurance industry's long-term care insurance products are now largely stagnant. What services and systems will meet the needs of women for some guarantee of long-term care in their senior years?

But the most fundamental questions about our health care system are only beginning to be asked: why do we pay more for less than any other country? Are the products and services that have been developed in our market economy actually the products and services most needed to promote health and treat illness? Does research support the development of approaches and treatments most needed by the public? Do we have the right personnel to provide care? And how much shall we spend for it all?

It remains to be seen whether the net outcome of a focus on women's health on women's terms will be the institutionalization of their values, the cooption of their health-related activities, or a useful if often strained dialectic between women's critique of the health care system and the traditional institutions. But the attitudinal changes brought about among patients and practitioners, the alterations wrought in modes of health care delivery, the continuing examination of sexism in illness care, and the movement of women's issues onto the nation's health agenda demonstrate a vital and enduring impact on U.S. health care.

REFERENCES

Anderson, G. F. (1997). In search of value: An international comparison of cost, access, and outcomes. *Health Affairs, 16*(6), 163–171.

Andersen, M. D., Smereck, G. A., Hockman, E. M., Ross, D. J., & Ground, K. J. (1999). Nurses ease barriers to health care by "hyperlinking" multiple-diagnosed women living with HIV/AIDS into care. *Journal of Nurses in AIDS Care, 10*(2), 55–65.

Aparasu, R. R. (1999). Visits to office-based physicians in the United States for medication-related morbidity. *Journal of the American Pharmaceutical Association, 39*(3), 332–337.

Arno, P. S., Levine, C., & Memmott, M. M. (1999). The economic value of informal caregiving. *Health Affairs, 18*(2), 182–188.

Aslin, A. L. (1977). Feminist and community mental health center psychotherapists' expectations of mental health for women. *Sex Roles, 3*(6), 537–544.

Ayanian, J. Z., Weissman, J. S., Chasen-Taber, S., & Epstein, A. M. (1999). Quality of care by race and gender for congestive heart failure and pneumonia. *Medical Care, 37*(12), 1260–1269.

Barrett-Connor, E. (1997). Sex differences in coronary heart disease: Why are women so superior? *Circulation, 95*(1), 252–264.

Blum, L. N., Nielsen, N. H., & Riggs, J. A. (1998). Alcoholism and alcohol abuse among women: Report of the council on scientific affairs. *Journal of Women's Health, 7*(7), 861–871.

Bodenheimer, T. (1998). How large employers are shaping the health care marketplace, part II. *New England Journal of Medicine, 388*(15), 1084–1087.

Broverman, I. K. et al. (1970). Sex role stereotypes and clinical judgments of mental health. *Journal of Consultative and Clinical Psychology, 34*(1), 1–7.

Brown, S. A., & Grimes, D. E. (1995). A meta-analysis of nurse practitioners and nurse midwives in primary care. *Nursing Research, 44*(6), 332–339.

Brown, T. G., Kokin, M., Seraganian, P., & Shields, N. (1995). The role of spouses of substance abusers in treatment: Gender differences. *Journal of Psychoactive Drugs, 27*(3), 223–229.

Carlson, E. S., Li, S., & Holm, K. (1997). An analysis of menopause in the popular press. *Health Care for Women International, 18*(6), 557–564.

Carrasquillo, O., Himmelstein, D. U., Woolhandler, S., & Bor, D. H. (1999). Going bare: Trends in health insurance coverage. *American Journal of Public Health, 89*(1), 36–42.

Center for Scientific Review. (2002). *How scientists are selected for study section service.* Retrieved May 17, 2003, from http://www.csr.nih.gov/events/studysectionservice.htm

Centers for Disease Control and Prevention. (1997). *Employer-sponsored health insurance: State and national estimates.* DHHS publication #98-1005. Retrieved January 18, 2003, from http://www.cdc.gov/nchs/data/misc/employer.pdf

Chandra, N. C., Zieglestein, R. C., Rogers, W. J., Tiefenbrunn, A. J., Gore, J. M., French, W. J., & Rubison, M. (1998). Observations of the treatment of women in the United States with myocardial infarction: A report from the national registry of myocardial infarction–I. *Archives of Internal Medicine, 158*(9), 981–988.

Chatham, L. R., Hiller, M. L., Rowan-Szal, G. A., Joe, G. W., & Simpson, D. D. (1999). Gender differences at admission and follow-up in a sample of methadone maintenance clients. *Substance Use and Misuse, 34*(8), 1137–1165.

Colditz, G. A., Manson, J. E., & Hankinson, S. E. (1997). The nurses' health study: 20-year contribution to the understanding of health among women. *Journal of Women's Health, 6*(1), 49–62.

Consumers Union. (1998). Medicare: New choices, new worries. *Consumer Reports, 63*(9), 27–38.

Cooper, R. A., Laud, P., & Dietrich, C. L. (1998). Current and projected workforce of nonphysician clinicians. *Journal of the American Medical Association, 280*(9), 788–794.

Council on Graduate Medical Education. (1998). *Physician distribution and health care challenges in rural and inner-city areas. Tenth report.* Rockville, MD: Department of Health and Human Services, Health Resoures and Services Administration.

Eddy, D. (1997). Investigational treatments: How strict should we be? *Journal of the American Medical Association, 278*(3), 179–185.

Ehrenreich, B., & English, D. (1973). *Witches, midwives, and nurses.* Old Westbury, NY: Feminist Press.

Eisenberg, D. M., Davis, R. B., Ettner, S. L., Appel, S., Wilkey, S., Van Rompay, M., & Kessler, R. C. (1998). Trends in alternative medicine use in the United States, 1990–1997: Results of a national follow-up survey. *Journal of the American Medical Association, 280*(18), 1569–1575.

Eisenberg, D. M., Davis, R. B., Ettner, S. L., Appel, S., Wilkey, S., Van Rompay, M., & Kessler, R. C. (1999). Trends in alternative medicine use in the United States, 1990–1997: Results of a national follow-up survey. *Obstetrical and Gynecological Survey, 54*(6), 370–371.

Elderkin-Thompson, V., & Waitzkin, H. (1999). Difference in clinical communication by gender. *Journal of General Internal Medicine, 14*(2), 112–121.

Fabrega, H., Mezzich, J., Ulrich, R., & Benjamin, L. (1990). Females and males in an intake psychiatric setting. *Psychiatry, 53*(1), 1–16.

Fankhauser, M. P. (1997). Psychiatric disorders in women: Psychopharmacologic treatments. *Journal of the American Pharmaceutical Association, 37*(6), 667–678.

Federation of Feminist Women's Health Centers. (1991). *A new view of a woman's body.* Los Angeles: Feminist Health Press.

Fiorentine, R., Anglin, M. D., Gil-Rivas, V., & Taylor, E. (1997). Drug treatment: Explaining the gender paradox. *Substance Use and Misuse, 32*(6), 653–678.

Fisher, S. (1986). *In the patient's best interest.* New Brunswick, NJ: Rutgers University Press.

Frances, A., First, M. B., & Pincus, H. A. (1995). *DSM-IV guidebook.* Washington, DC: American Psychiatric Press.

Geller, S. E., Burns, L. R., & Brailer, D. J. (1996). The impact of nonclinical factors on practice variations: The case of hysterectomies. *Health Services Research, 30*(6), 729–750.

Ginzberg, E. (1998). US health system reform in the early 21st century. *Journal of the American Medical Association, 280*(17), 1539.

Goff, B. A., Muntz, H. G., & Cain, J. M. (1997). Is Adam worth more than Eve? The financial impact of gender bias in the federal reimbursement of gynecologic procedures. *Gynecologic Oncology, 464*(3), 372–377.

Gold, M. (1999). The changing US health care system: Challenges for responsible public policy. *Milbank Quarterly, 77*(1), 3–37.

Gollub, E. L. (1999). Human rights is a US problem, too: The case of women and HIV. *American Journal of Public Health, 89*(10), 1479–1482.

Gouldner, A. (1970). *The coming crisis of Western sociology.* New York: Avon Books.

Greenberg, D. (1999). Health-care reform back on the US political agenda. *Lancet, 354*(9192), 1799.

Greenfield, S. (2002). Women and alcohol use disorders. *Harvard Review of Psychiatry, 10*(2), 76–85.

Grella, C. E., & Joshi, V. (1999). Gender differences in drug treatment careers among clients in the National Drug Abuse Treatment Outcome study. *American Journal of Drug and Alcohol Abuse, 25*(3), 385–406.

Grella, C. E., Polinsky, M. L., Hser, Y. I., & Perry, S. M. (1999). Characteristics of women-only and mixed-gender drug abuse treatment programs. *Journal of Substance Abuse Treatment, 17*(1–2), 37–44.

Gruber J., & Levitt, L. (2000). Tax subsidies for health insurance: Costs and benefits. *Health Affairs, 19*(1), 72–85.

Hamel, M. B., Ingelfinger, J. R., Phimister, E., & Solomon, C. G. (2006). Women in academic medicine: Progress and challenges. *New England Journal of Medicine, 355*(3), 310–312.

Herz, S. (1997). Don't test, do sell: Legal implications of inclusion and exclusion of women in clinical drug trials. *Epilepsia, 38*(Suppl. 4), S42–S49.

Hsiao, W. C., Braun, P., Becher, E., et al. (1988). *A national study of resource-based relative value scales for physician services: Final report.* Cambridge, MA: Harvard School of Public Health.

Hurwitz, E. L., Coulter, I. D., Adams, A. H., Genovese, B. J., & Shekelle, P. G. (1998). Use of chiropractic services from 1985 through 1991 in the United States and Canada. *American Journal of Public Health, 88*(5), 771–776.

Institute of Medicine, Committee on Quality of Health Care in America. (2000). In L. T. Kohn, J. M. Corrigan, & M. Donaldson (Eds.). *To err is human: Building a safer health system.* Washington, DC: National Academy Press.

Institute of Medicine, Committee on Understanding and Eliminating Racial and Ethnic Disparities in Health Care. (2002). In B. D. Smedly, A. Y. Stith, & A. R. Nelson (Eds.). *Unequal treatment: Confronting racial and ethnic disparities in health care.* Washington, DC: National Academy Press.

Jagsi, R., Guancial, E. A., Worobey, C. C., Henault, L. E., Chang, Y., Starr, R., Tarbell, N. J., & Hylek, E. M. (2006). The gender gap in authorship of academic medical literature: A 35-year perspective. *New England Journal of Medicine, 355*(3), 2.

Kaufert, P. A., & Lock, M. (1997). Medicalization of women's third age. *Journal of Psychosomatic Obstetrics and Gynecology, 18*(2), 81–86.

Kitzman, H., Olds, D. L., Henderson, C. R., Hanks, C., Cole, R., Tatelbaum, R., McConnochie, K. M., Sidora, K., Luckey, D.W., Shaver, D., Engelhardt, K., James, D., & Barnard, K. (1997). Effect of prenatal and infancy home visitation by nurses on pregnancy outcomes, childhood injuries, and repeated childbearing: A randomized controlled trial. *Journal of the American Medical Association, 278*(8), 644–652.

Klinkenberg, W. D., & Calsyn, R. J. (1998). Gender differences in the receipt of aftercare and psychiatric hospitalization among adults with severe mental illness. *Comprehensive Psychiatry, 39*(3), 137–142.

Korvick, J. A., Stratton, P., Spino, C., Huang, J., Bardequez, A. D., & Wofsy, C. (1997). Women's participation in AIDS clinical trials group (ACTG) trials in the USA: Enough or still too few? *Journal of Women's Health, 5*(2), 129–135.

Kottke, T. E. & Trapp, M. A. (1998). Implementing nurse-based systems to provide American Indian women with breast and cervical cancer screening. *Mayo Clinic Proceedings, 73*(9), 815–823.

Leavitt, J. W. (1984). *Women and health in America.* Madison: University of Wisconsin Press.

Levit, K., Smith, C., Cowan, C., Lazenby, H., Sensinig, A., & Catlin A. (2003). Trends in U.S. health care spending, 2001. *Health Affairs, 22*(1), 154–164.

Lorber, J. (2000). What impact have women physicians had on women's health? *Journal of the American Medical Women's Association, 55*(1), 13–15.

Lynaugh, J. (1986). The nurse practitioner: Issues in practice. In M. D. Mezy & D. O. McGivern (Eds.), *Nurses, nurse practitioners* (pp.137–145). Boston: Little, Brown.

Mann, C., Hudman, J., Salganicoff, A., & Folsom, A. (2002). Five years later: Poor women's health care coverage after welfare reform. *Journal of the American Medical Women's Association, 57*(1), 16–22.

Mansfield, C. J., Wilson, J. L., Kobrinski, E., & Mitchell, J. (1999). Premature mortality in the United States: The roles of geographic area, socioeconomic status, household type, and availability of medical care. *American Journal of Public Health, 89*(6), 893–898.

Marieskind, H. I. (1975). The women's health movement. *International Journal of Health Services, 5*(2), 217–223.

McFarland, J., & Fehir, J. (1994). De madres a madres: A community, primary health care program based on empowerment. *Health Education Quarterly, 21*(3), 381–394.

McGowan, J. A., & Pottern, L. (2000). Commentary on the women's health initiative. *Maturitas, 34*(2), 109–112.

Merrikin, K. (1999, November). *Improving women's health care: NCQA and HEDIS.* Address to Sun Mountain Women's Health Alliance/1999 Women's Health Legislative Summit, Leavenworth, WA.

Mitchell, J. (1974). *Psychoanalysis and feminism.* New York: Random House.

Moreno, J., Caplan, A. L., & Wolpe, P. R. (1998). Updating protections for human subjects involved in research. *Journal of the American Medical Association, 280*(22): 1951–1958.

Morgen, S., & Julier, A. (1991). *Women's health movement organizations: Two decades of struggle and change.* Eugene: Center for the Study of Women in Society, University of Oregon.

Mouton, C. P., Harris, S., Rovi, S., Solorzano, P., & Johnson, M. S. (1997). Barriers to Black women's participation in cancer clinical trials. *Journal of the National Medical Association, 89*(11), 721–727.

Mundinger, M. O., Kane, R. L., Lenz, E. R., Totten, A. M., Tsai, W. Y., Cleary, P. D., Friedewald, W. T., Siu, A. L., & Shelanski, M. L. (2000). Primary care outcomes in patients treated by nurse practitioners or physicians: A randomized trial. *Journal of the American Medical Association, 283*(1), 59–68.

Murphy, J. M., Laird, N. M., Monson, R. R., Sobol, A. M., & Leighton, A. H. (2000). A 40-year perspective on the prevalence of depression: The Stirling County study. *Archives of General Psychiatry, 57*(3), 209–215.

Mustard, C. A., Kaufert, P., Kozyrskyj, A., & Mayer, T. (1998). Sex differences in the use of health services. *New England Journal of Medicine, 338*(23), 1678–1683.

Neergaard, L. (2000, February 5). Scientist falsified data supporting cancer regimen. *Seattle Times.*

National Institutes of Health. (1994). NIH guidelines on the inclusion of women and minorities as subjects in clinical research. http://grants.nih.gov/grants/guide/notice-files/not94-100.html

NIH Tracking/Inclusion Committee. (2002, December). Monitoring adherence to the NIH policy on the inclusion of women and minorities as subjects in clinical research. Blue report. http://orwh.od.nih.gov/inclusion/updated 2002-2003.pdf

Paine, L. L., Dower, C. M., & O'Neil, E. H. (1999). Midwifery in the 21st century: Recommendations from the Pew Health Professions Commission/UCSF Center for the Health Professions 1998 Task Force on Midwifery. *Journal of Nurse-Midwifery, 44*(4), 341–348.

Pajer, K. (1995). New strategies in the treatment of depression in women. *Journal of Clinical Psychiatry, 56*(Suppl. 2), 30–37.

Parsons, T., & Bales, R. F. (1955). *Family socialization and interaction process.* Glencoe, IL: Free Press.

Pradel, F. G., Hartzema, A. G., Mutran, E. J., & Hanson-Divers, C. (1999). Physician over-the-counter drug prescribing patterns: An analysis of the National Ambulatory Medical Care Survey. *Annals of Pharmacotherapy, 33*(4), 400–405.

Rapaport, M. H., Thompson, P. M., Kelsoe, J. R., Golshan, S., Judd, L. L., & Gillin, J. C. (1995). Gender differences in outpatient research subjects with affective disorders: A comparison of descriptive variables. *Journal of Clinical Psychiatry, 56*(2), 62–72.

Relman, A. S. (1980). The new medical-industrial complex. *New England Journal of Medicine, 303*(17), 963–970.

Roberts, R. O., Yawn, B. P., Wickes, S. L., Field, C. S., Garretson, M., & Jacobsen, S. J. (1998). Barriers to prenatal care: Factors associated with late initiation of care in a middle-class midwestern community. *Journal of Family Practice, 47*(1), 53–61.

Rothman, A. A., & Wagner E. H. (2003). Chronic illness management: What is the role of primary care? *Annals of Internal Medicine, 138*(3), 256–261.

Ruiz, M. T., & Verbrugge, L. M. (1997). A two way view of gender bias in medicine. *Journal of Epidemiology and Community Health, 51*(2), 106–109.

Ruzek, S. B. (1978). *The women's health movement: Feminist alternatives to medical control.* New York: Praeger.

Salganicoff, A., & Wyn, R. (1999). Access to care for low-income women: The impact of Medicaid. *Journal of Health Care for the Poor and Uninsured, 10*(4), 453–467.

Schatzberg, A. (1997). The dynamics of sex: Gender differences in psychiatric disorders. *Journal of Clinical Psychiatry, 58*(Suppl. 15), 3–4.

Schulman, K. A., Berlin, J. A., Harless, W., Kerner, J. F., Sistrunk, S., Gersh, B. J., Dube, R., Taleghani, C. K., Burke, J. E., Williams, S., Eisenberg, J. M., Escarce, J. J., & Ayers,W. (1999). The effect of race and sex on physicians' recommendations for cardiac catheterization. *New England Journal of Medicine, 340*(8), 618–626.

Schwartz, L. M., Fisher, E. S., Tosteson, A. N., Woloshin, S., Chang, C. H., Virnig, B. A., Plohman, J., & Wright, B. (1997). Treatment and health outcomes of women and men in a cohort with coronary artery disease. *Archives of Internal Medicine, 157*(14), 1545–1551.

Scully, D. (1980). *Men who control women's health.* Boston: Houghton Mifflin.

Scully, D., & Bart, P. (1973). A funny thing happened on the way to the orifice: Women in gynecology textbooks. *American Journal of Sociology, 78*(4), 1045–1050.

Seaman, B. (1972). *Free and female.* Greenwich, CT: Fawcettc.

Sechrest, L. (1975). Ethical problems in medical experimentation involving women. In V. Olesen (Ed.), *Women and their health: Research implications for an era.* DHEW HRA 77-3138. Washington, DC: Department of Health, Education, and Welfare.

Shackelford, J. L. (1999). Measuring productivity using RBRVS cost accounting. *Healthcare Financial Management, 53*(1), 67–69.

Showstack, J., Lurie, N., Larson, E. B., Rothman, A. A., & Hassmiller S. (2003). Primary care: The next renaissance. *Annals of Internal Medicine, 138*(3), 268–272.

Shuchman, M., & Wilkes, M. S. (1997). Medical scientists and health news reporting: A case of miscommunication. *Annals of Internal Medicine, 126*(11), 976–982.

Simoni-Wastila, L. (1998). Gender and psychotropic drug use. *Medical Care, 36*(1), 88–94.

Soman, L. A., Brindis, C., & Dunn-Malhotra, E. (1996). The interplay of national state, and local policy in financing care for drug-affected women and children in California. *Journal of Psychoactive Drugs, 28*(1), 3–15.

Sowers, M., Crawford, S., Sternfeld, B., Morganstein, D., Gold, E., Greendale, G., Evans, D., Neer, R., Matthews, K., Sherman, S., Lo, A., Weiss, G., & Kelsye, J. (2000). SWAN: A multicenter, multiethnic community-based cohort study of women and the menopausal transition. In R. Lobo, J. Kelsey, & R. Marcus (Eds.), *Menopause: Biology and pathobiology* (pp. 175–188). San Diego: Academic Press.

Sowers, M., Jannausch, M. L., Gross, M., Karvonen-Gutierrez, C. A., Palmieri, R. M., Crutchfield, M., & Richards-McCullough, K. (2006). Performance-based physical functioning in African-American and Caucasian women at midlife: Considering body composition, quadriceps strength, and knee osteoarthritis. *American Journal of Epidemiology, 163*(10), 950–958.

Sox, H. C. (2000). Independent primary care practice by nurse practitioners. *Journal of the American Medical Association, 283*(1), 106–108.

Stage, S. (1979). *Female complaints: Lydia Pinkham and the business of women's medicine.* New York: Norton.

Starfield, B. (1996). Public health and primary care: A framework for proposed linkages. *American Journal of Public Health, 86*(10), 1365–1369.

Starr, P. (1982) *The social transformation of American medicine.* New York: Basic Books.

Stefanick, M. L. (1992). Post-menopausal hormone replacement and cardiovascular disease. *Stanford University Institute for Research on Women and Gender Newsletter, 16*(2), 2–3.

Taylor, D. L., & Woods, N. F. (1996). Changing women's health, changing nursing practice. *Journal of Obstetric, Gynecologic, and Neonatal Nursing, 25*(9), 791–802.

Tesch, B. J., Wood, H. M., Helwig, A. L., & Nattinger, A. B. (1995). Promotion of women physicians in academic medicine: Glass ceiling or sticky floor? *Journal of the American Medical Association, 273*(13), 1022–1025.

Thomson, G. E. (1997). Discrimination in health care. *Annals of Internal Medicine, 126*(11), 910–912.

Tudor, W., Tudor, J., & Gove, W. (1977). The effect of sex role differences on the social control of mental illness. *Journal Health Social Behavior, 18*(2), 98–112.

U.S. Public Health Service. (1999). A report of the Task Force on the NIH Women's Health Research Agenda for the Twenty-first Century. NIH Publication No. 99-4386. Bethesda, MD: National Institutes of Health.

Verbrugge, L., & Patrick, D. (1995). Seven chronic conditions: Their impact on US adults' activity levels and use of medical services. *American Journal of Public Health, 85*(2), 173–182.

Ward, D. (1990). National health insurance: Where do nurses fit? *Nursing Outlook, 38*(5), 206–207.

Weinstock, L. S. (1999). Gender differences in the presentation of management of social anxiety disorder. *Journal of Clinical Psychiatry, 6*(Suppl. 9), 9–13.

Wenger, N. K. (1999). Should women have a different risk assessment from men for primary prevention of coronary heart disease? *Journal of Women's Health and Gender-Based Medicine, 8*(4), 465–467.

Wennberg, J., & Cooper, M. M. (Eds.). (1999). *The Dartmouth atlas of health care.* Washington, DC: American Hospital Publishing.

Williams, D. R. (2002). Racial/ethnic variations in women's health: The social embeddedness of health. *American Journal of Public Health, 92*(4), 588–597.

Williams, D. R., & Collins, C. (2001). Racial residential segregation: A fundamental cause of racial disparities in health. *Public Health Reports, 116*(5), 404–416.

Wolf, N. (1997). *Promiscuities: The secret struggle for womanhood.* New York: Random House.

Woods, N. F. (1992). Future directions for women's health research. *NAACOG's Women's Health Nursing Scan, 6*(5), 1–2.

Woods, N. F. (2000). The U.S. women's health research agenda for the twenty-first century. *Signs: Journal of Women in Culture and Society, 25*(4), 1269–1274.

Woodward, C. A. (1999). Medical students' attitudes toward women: Are medical schools microcosms of society? *Canadian Medical Association Journal, 160*(3), 347–348.

Writing Group for the Women's Health Initiative Investigators. (2002). Risks and benefits of estrogen plus progestin in healthy postmenopausal women: Principal results from the Women's Health Initiative Randomized Controlled Trial. *Journal of the American Medical Association, 288*, 321–333.

Yates, M. E., Tennstedt, S., & Chang, B. H. (1999). Contributors to and mediators of psychological well-being for informal caregivers. *Journal of Gerontological and Psychological Science and Social Science, 54*(1), P12–P22.

Useful Web Sites

http://www.fda.gov/womens/informat.html; A gateway to information about the Food and Drug Administration and women's health issues.

http://www.ncqa.org; The work of the Measurement Advisory Panels to the National Committee on Quality Assurance (NCQA) is to establish standards to judge the quality of health care for women provided by health maintenance organizations and other health plans.

http://www.nwhn.org; The National Women's Health Network is a unique health site free of pharmaceutical advertising.

http://www4.od.nih.gov/orwh/index.html; This site for the Office of Research on Women's Health of the National Institutes of Health has information for both researchers and consumers.

Women's Bodies

Nancy Fugate Woods and Aileen MacLaren Loranger

Providing health care to women offers a special opportunity to educate women about their bodies and the intricacies of their female form and functions. Established as the major consumers of health care and the primary gatekeepers of their family's health, women are usually eager to learn about how their bodies work and how to keep them healthy (Hoffman & Johnson, 1995; Pinn, 2003). When given the chance, they often express curiosity about specifics related to their particular anatomy or physiology. Although a frequently neglected topic in routine health care, women also wonder about their sexuality and their body's ability to experience pleasure.

Discovering that there are unique biological differences about having a female body beyond solely the reproductive system interests many women, as well. Over the past decade, the advanced scientific study of cellular and molecular mechanisms of human biology have uncovered new, significant sex-based differences in physiological functions (Institute of Medicine Committee on Understanding the Biology of Sex and Gender Differences, 2001). Being familiar with these discoveries in biologic sex differences is important to anyone involved in health care in order to promote a better understanding of the implications for disease prevention and health maintenance of women.

The purpose of this chapter is to briefly highlight the key aspects of female anatomy and physiology so that this can be shared with women who seek nursing services, consultation, or education about their bodies. The chapter begins with a review of the structural and functional aspects of a woman's anatomy. The procreative and recreative functions of women's bodies will be compared and contrasted. Next, a brief discussion of the endocrine system and specifically, the physiologic influences of hormone secretion on women's bodies will set the stage for understanding the complexities of women's cyclic rhythms. As women's bodies mature across the life span, a description of initial sexual differentiation and development, pubertal development, and changes occurring during menarche and menopause are presented. Two important cyclic phenomena are women's menstrual cycles and sexual response cycles; how women's bodies participate in these cycles is described. The chapter concludes with some of the recently established biologic sex differences to appreciate how these affect the health and longevity of women's bodies.

WOMEN'S ANATOMY

Breasts

Although some Western societies socialize women to regard their breasts as symbols of their feminine attractiveness and nurturance while socializing men to regard women's breasts as sexual objects, women's breasts serve to provide both procreative powers and recreative pleasures. Indeed, the mammary gland is the distinguishing feature of an entire zoological class—mammals. Naturally round, protuberant breasts are exclusive to the human female and vary in their appearance more than most other parts of the female anatomy (Stoppard, 2002). These structures have a unique and complex anatomy.

Location

Considered organs of the integumentary system, breasts are highly specialized variants of sweat (or apocrine) glands, located between the second and sixth ribs and between the sternal and midaxillary line. About two-thirds of the breast lies superficial to the pectoralis major, the remainder to the serratus anterior.

Appearance

The breasts of healthy women are generally symmetrical in shape and amplitude, although they are often not absolutely equal in size. Breasts are typically measured by both chest circumference and their fullness. What are commonly defined as plural glands are actually two parts of a single, contiguous anatomic breast with a proliferation of a shared nerve, vascular, and lymphatic supply (Porth, 2007). The skin covering the breasts is similar to that of the abdomen. Hair follicles sometimes are noted around the darker pigmented area surrounding the nipple, called the areola. Often, women with fair complexions can note a vascular pattern in a horizontal or vertical dimension under the superficial skin of the breast tissue. When present, this pattern is usually symmetrical.

The areolar pigment varies in color from pink to brown, in position on the breast, and in size from woman to woman. The areola surrounds the nipple that is located at the tip of each breast. Several sebaceous glands can be seen on the areola as small elevations that are called Montgomery's tubercles to keep the nipple area soft and stretchy. The nipples are more darkly pigmented and usually protuberant because of erectile muscles. Nipple size and shape are highly variable from woman to woman, and the same woman may notice a great deal of variation in the size and shape of her nipples depending on the extent to which they are contracted. The erectile tissue of the nipple is responsive to emotional and tactile stimulation, thus promoting the recreative function of the breasts. Some women have inverted nipples, a condition in which the nipple is dimpled or its central portion flattened or depressed. A normal nipple that suddenly becomes inverted may indicate the presence of breast cancer.

Some women have supernumerary nipples, nipples and breasts, or breast tissue. This supernumerary tissue develops along the longitudinal ridges extending from the axilla to the groin, which existed during early embryonic development.

Visible changes in a woman's breast occur in conjunction with her development. Prior to the age of 10, there is little visible distinction between boys' and girls' breasts. At approximately the age of 10, the mammary buds appear in girls' breasts. The subareolar mammary tissue is not prominent at this point. The adult breast develops under the influence of estrogen and progesterone. During the transition to adulthood, the prominent subareolar tissue of adolescence recedes into the contour of the remainder of the breast and the nipple protrudes. (See the later section on puberty for a more complete description of breast changes that occur during puberty.)

Breast shape and texture are influenced by nutritional factors, heredity, endocrine factors, and hormonal sensitivity in addition to age, muscle tone, and pregnancy. Nodularity, tenderness, and size of the breasts may fluctuate with the menstrual cycle. Usually, women's breasts are smallest during days 4 to 7 of the menstrual cycle, shortly after menstruation. An increase in breast volume, tenderness, heaviness, fullness, and general or nipple tenderness may be experienced just before menstruation.

Short-lived changes of appearance are observed in many women during sexual response, including protuberance of the nipple, increase in breast size, and so forth. The breasts are highly erogenous organs for many women. They do not merely vary in shape and size with sexual excitement, but there is also a great deal of variation from woman to woman in those parts of the breasts perceived as erotic. For example, some women perceive erotic sensations in the areolae, others in the nipple, and still others in the breast tissue near the axilla.

A woman's breasts may also double or triple in size during pregnancy. Striae, engorgement of veins, and increased prominence and pigmentation of nipple and areolae are common during pregnancy. The glandular tissue of the breast gradually involutes after menopause and fat is deposited in the breasts. The breasts of postmenopausal women as they age, therefore, take on a more flattened contour and appear less firm than prior to menopause.

A convention useful in describing the appearance of women's breasts during physical examination is a division into four quadrants by vertical and horizontal lines crossing at the nipple (for example, upper, outer quadrant of left breast). Another landmark, the axillary tail (also called the tail of Spence) is a portion of breast tissue that extends into the axilla. A more precise description of breast landmarks is one that incorporates an analogy to the face of a clock: A lump could be described at 2 o'clock and include the appropriate number of centimeters from the nipple.

Although women are encouraged to wear brassieres to prevent a drooping of Cooper's ligaments, which makes breasts appear pendulous, there is no compelling evidence for the efficacy of the practice. Aside from fatigue or pain that some women with large breasts experience, there are no health consequences associated with not wearing a brassiere.

Components of Breast Tissue

There are three main components of tissue in women's breasts: glandular, fibrous, and fatty tissue. Most of the breast is composed of subcutaneous and retromammary (behind the breast) fat. Breast tissue is supported by fibrous tissue, including suspensory ligaments

(Cooper's ligaments), extending from the subcutaneous connective tissue to the muscle fascia (see Figure 4.1).

An important functional component of the breast is the glandular tissue, which consists of 12 to 25 lobes that terminate in ducts that open on the surface of the nipple. Each lobe is composed of 20 to 40 lobules, each of which contains 10 to 100 alveoli (sometimes called acini).

The alveolus is the basic component of the breast lobule. The hollow alveolus is lined by a single layer of milk-secreting columnar epithelial cells, which are derived prenatally from an ingrowth of epidermis into the mesenchyme between 10 and 12 weeks of gestation. These cells enlarge greatly and discharge their contents during lactation. The individual alveolus is encased in a network of myoepithelial strands and is surrounded by a rich capillary network. The lumen of the alveolus opens into a collecting intralobar (within the lobe) duct through a thin, nonmuscular duct. The intralobar ducts eventually end in the openings in the nipple and are surrounded by muscle cells.

Supporting Structures

The third and fourth branches of the cervical plexus provide the cutaneous nerve supply to the upper breast and the thoracic intercostal nerves to the lower breast. The perforating branches of the internal mammary artery constitute the chief external blood supply, although additional arterial blood supply emanates from several branches of the axillary artery. Superficial veins of the breast drain into the internal mammary veins and the superficial veins of the lower portion of the neck and from the latter into the jugular vein. Veins emptying into the internal mammary, axillary, and intercostal veins serve deep breast tissue.

The lymphatic drainage of the breast is of special interest and importance to women because of its role in dissemination of tumor cells as well as its ability to respond to infection. The lymphatic system of the breast is both abundant and complex. In general, the lymphatics drain both the axillary and internal mammary areas. Lymph from the skin of the breast, with the exception of areolar and nipple areas, flows into the axillary nodes on the same side of the body, whereas the lymph from the medial cutaneous breast area may flow into the opposite breast. The lymph from the areolar and nipple areas flows into the anterior axillary (mammary) nodes.

Lymph from deep within the mammary tissues flows into the anterior axillary nodes but may also flow into the apical, subclavian, infraclavicular, and supraclavicular nodes. Lymph from areas behind the areolae and the medial and lower glandular areas of breast tissue communicates with the lymphatic systems draining into the thorax and abdomen (see Figure 4.1).

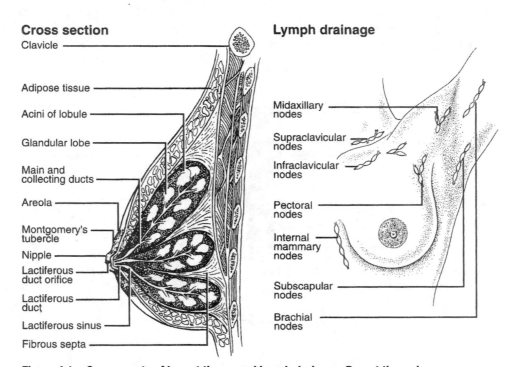

Cross section

Clavicle
Adipose tissue
Acini of lobule
Glandular lobe
Main and collecting ducts
Areola
Montgomery's tubercle
Nipple
Lactiferous duct orifice
Lactiferous duct
Lactiferous sinus
Fibrous septa

Lymph drainage

Midaxillary nodes
Supraclavicular nodes
Infraclavicular nodes
Pectoral nodes
Internal mammary nodes
Subscapular nodes
Brachial nodes

Figure 4.1   Components of breast tissue and lymph drainage. Breast tissue is composed of glandular, fibrous, and fatty tissue. Lymph from the skin of the breast flows to the axillary nodes and lymph from the medial cutaneous area of the breast flows to the opposite breast. Lymph from the areolae and the nipple flows into the mammary nodes.

Pelvic Organs

Like her breasts, many of a woman's pelvic structures serve both reproductive functions and recreative (or sexual) pleasures. Despite the unique functions served by their pelvic structures, women may be unaware of their appearance because they are located deep within the pelvic cavity or because women have not had an opportunity to visualize their external genitalia or they have been discouraged from examining themselves.

Many of a woman's genital structures can be visualized easily with a mirror (see Figure 4.2). The configuration of the genitals is strikingly unique to each woman and highly variable from woman to woman. For example, many paired structures, such as the labia, are not perfectly symmetrical.

Vulva

The external female genitalia are commonly referred to as the vulva. The older term for the vulva, the pudendum, derives from the Latin word meaning to be ashamed. For this reason, the term vulva is preferable.

The most obvious feature on an adult woman is her pubic hair, which is rather coarse, curly, and often darker than the hair on her head. Pubic hair not only covers parts of the vulvar area (mons pubis, labia majora) but may extend upward toward the abdomen and outward onto the inner thighs. The flattened area of pubic hair over the lower abdomen forms the base of an inverted triangle. The triangle is sometimes referred to as the female escutcheon. Although this is a somewhat

typical pattern, it is not uncommon for healthy women to exhibit variation in this pattern. For example, hair growth may extend up toward the umbilicus in a narrow diamond pattern or back toward the anus. Some women have little pubic hair or a well-delineated triangular area while others have a prolific hair pattern. Pubic hair eventually turns gray and thins with aging.

The mons veneris or mons pubis is composed of soft, fatty tissue and lies over the symphysis pubis. The labia majora consist of two larger, raised folds of adipose tissue. The inner surface of the labia majora consists of apocrine (scent), eccrine (sweat), and sebaceous (oil) glands that serve to lubricate as well as stimulate by releasing a classic, female musk scent during sexual arousal. The labia majora are heavily pigmented, and, in postpubertal women, their outer surfaces are covered with hair, whereas the inner surfaces are smooth and hairless. In postmenopausal women, the hair on the labia becomes thinner and the labia and mons appear less full as a result of the loss of fatty tissue.

The labia minora are two very thin folds of inner skin heavily endowed with blood vessels that lie within the labia majora and extend from the clitoris to the fourchette (vaginal outlet). Each of the labia minora divides into a medial and lateral part. The medial parts join anteriorly to the clitoris to form the clitoral hood (also called prepuce), and the lateral parts join posterior to the clitoris. There are more nerve endings in the labia minora than the outer labia majora. There are also more sebaceous glands to lubricate the opening into the vagina (the vestibule) to provide waterproof protection against urine, menstrual bleeding, and bacteria. In some women, the labia minora are completely hidden from view by the

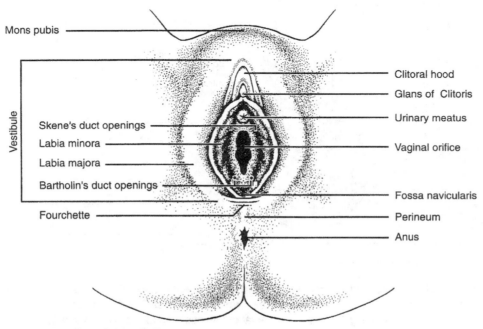

Figure 4.2   External genitalia.

labia majora, but in other women the labia minora protrude out from between the labia majora. Frequently, the labia minora are asymmetric.

The color and texture of the labia minora are highly individual, varying from pink to brown. The clitoral hood covers the clitoris and is believed to protect this extremely sensitive organ from irritation. In some women, the clitoral hood will adhere to the clitoris so that the hood cannot be pulled back very far to reveal the clitoris (see Figure 4.3).

The area between the labia minora is called the vestibule. It contains both the urethral and vaginal orifices. The hymen, a membranous covering at the vaginal opening, may be intact, but more frequently is seen as a ring of small, rounded skin fragments attached to the margins of the vaginal opening. This fluted or ruffled appearance is due to the natural erosion of the hymen from regular childhood activities such as running, jumping, and riding a bicycle. Some women have a more thick and rigid membrane that remains intact even after penile penetration. Approximately 1 out of every 2,000 women has a hymen that must be surgically removed (Stoppard, 2002).

Skene's glands are tiny, clustered paraurethral organs, the ducts of which open laterally and posteriorly to the urethral orifice. Bartholin's glands, located lateral and slightly posterior to the vaginal introitus, open into the groove between the labia minora and the hymen at the 5 and 7 o'clock positions in relation to the vaginal orifice. Both Skene's and Bartholin's glands are usually not visible, although they are located in tissues that can be visualized, and their openings on the vulva can be seen in some women. These racemose glands serve a lubricating function by secreting mucus. The perineum consists of the tissues between the vaginal orifice and the anus. Beneath the vestibule are two bundles of vascular tissue referred to as the bulbs of the vestibule or the perineal sponge. These tissues become congested during sexual response.

Clitoris

A woman's clitoris is an erectile organ unique to all of human anatomy. Its sole purpose is to serve as a receptor and transformer of sensual stimuli. This unique structure exists to initiate or elevate levels of sexual tension for women (Masters & Johnson, 1966). The various structural components of the clitoris are homologous to similar structures of the male penis (Federation of Feminist Women's Health Centers, 1981). The clitoris, from the Greek word meaning key, has the same number of nerve endings at its tips as the glans of the penis, making it extremely sensitive to tactile stimulation (Stoppard, 2002).

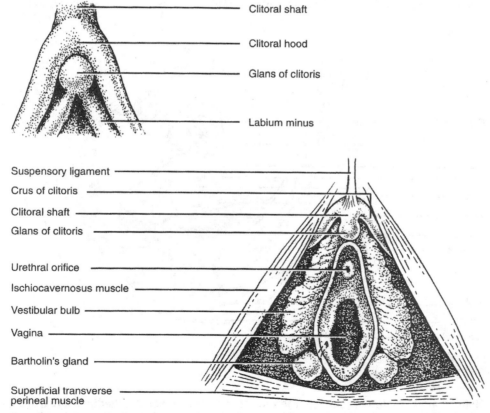

Clitoral shaft

Clitoral hood

Glans of clitoris

Labium minus

Suspensory ligament

Crus of clitoris

Clitoral shaft

Glans of clitoris

Urethral orifice

Ischiocavernosus muscle

Vestibular bulb

Vagina

Bartholin's gland

Superficial transverse perineal muscle

Figure 4.3   The clitoris. The sole purpose of the clitoris is reception and transformation of sexual stimuli.

The clitoris consists of two corpora cavernosa (cavernous bodies) enclosed in a dense fibrous membrane that is made up of elastic fibers and smooth muscle bundles. Each corpus is connected to the pubic ramus and the ischium. The clitoris is held in place by a suspensory ligament and two small ischiocavernosus muscles that insert into the crurae of the clitoris (Masters & Johnson, 1966).

Blood supply to the clitoris emanates from the deep and dorsal clitoral arteries that branch from the internal pudendal artery. The vasculature of the clitoris plays an important role in increasing its size during sexual response.

The length of the clitoral body (consisting of glans and shaft) varies markedly. The size of the clitoral glans may vary from 2 mm to 1 cm in healthy women and is usually estimated at 4 to 5 mm in both the transverse and longitudinal planes. There is also variation in the position of the clitoris, a function of variation in the points of origin of the suspensory and crural ligaments. The glans is capable of increasing in size with sexual stimulation, and marked vasocongestive increases in the diameter of the clitoral shaft have also been noted (Masters & Johnson, 1966).

The dorsal nerve of the clitoris is the deepest division of the pudendal nerve, and it terminates in the nerve endings of the glans and corpora cavernosa. Pacinian corpuscles, which respond to deep pressure, are distributed in both the glans and the corpora but have greater concentration in the glans. Their distribution is highly variable from woman to woman, which probably accounts for the rich variation in women's self-pleasuring techniques. For example, some women prefer very light touch whereas others prefer deep pressure. In some women, the anatomic arrangement of the labia minora that forms the clitoral hood makes it possible for mechanical traction on the labia to stimulate the clitoris indirectly. The clitoris is endowed with sensory nerve endings that respond to tactile stimuli as well as pressure. Although afferent stimuli can be received through afferent nerve endings in the clitoral glans and shaft, it is also possible that the clitoris serves as the subjective end point or transformer for efferent stimuli from higher neurogenic pathways (Masters & Johnson, 1966).

Vagina

Although the vagina can be considered an internal structure, it can be visualized easily with the assistance of a speculum, a light source, and a mirror. The vagina is a musculomembranous canal connecting the vulva with the uterus. It is lined with a reddish pink mucous membrane that is transversely rugated. Under the stratified squamous epithelial lining (much like the skin on the palm of the hand) is a muscular coat that has an inner circular layer and an outer fibrous layer (see Figure 4.4).

The vagina is typically a potential rather than a real space as it is ordinarily an empty, collapsed tube.

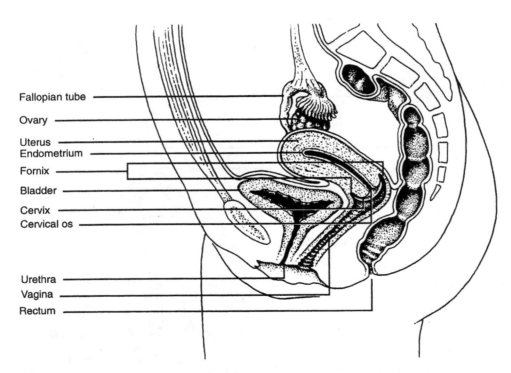

Fallopian tube

Ovary

Uterus
Endometrium

Fornix

Bladder

Cervix
Cervical os

Urethra
Vagina
Rectum

Figure 4.4   The internal genitalia. The vaginal canal is a potential rather than a real space and inclines posteriorly at a 45 degree angle. The cervix pierces the anterior superior wall of the vagina.

Although highly distensible, its unstimulated length is approximately 6 to 7 cm anteriorly and about 9 cm posteriorly. The vaginal canal inclines posteriorly at about a 45-degree angle. The cervix is the neck of the uterus and is encased in the vagina anteriorly and superiorly. There is a recessed portion of the vagina adjacent to the cervix, which, together with the cervix, is called the vaginal fornix. The fornix has anterior, posterior, and lateral portions.

Unlike the clitoris, the vagina has procreative as well as recreative functions. One of the important physiological functions of the vagina during sexual response is its ability to produce lubrication by means of transudation of mucoid material across its ruggated folds. In addition, vaginal lubrication occurs in a rhythmic 90-minute cycle throughout the day and night. The circulatory venous plexus (including the bulbus vestibuli, plexus pudendalis, plexus uterovaginalis, and possibly the plexus vesicalis and plexus rectalis) encircling the vaginal barrel probably provides the circulatory support for vaginal lubrication and a constant natural sloughing of dead epithelial cells. This vaginal discharge is normal and is called leukorrhea.

In addition to producing lubrication, the vagina demonstrates a remarkable distensive ability during both sexual response and childbirth. Both a lengthening of the vagina and a ballooning out of its inner portions have been observed during sexual response. The vascular changes occurring in conjunction with sexual response are profound. The reddish pink hue of the premenopausal woman's vagina changes to a darker purplish vasocongested appearance. In postmenopausal women, the color changes in the vagina and its expansion during sexual response are less pronounced. As the vagina distends, the rugae become flattened as a result of the thinning or stretching of the vaginal mucosa. The vagina, unlike the clitoris, is not well endowed with nerve endings; although there are deep pressure receptors in the innermost portion of the vagina, it is primarily in the outer third of the vagina that women report pleasurable sexual sensations (Masters & Johnson, 1966).

Cervix

Although the cervix might be regarded as an internal structure because it is a part of the uterus, it can be visualized for a clinician's exam with the aid of a speculum and a light source. The cervix extends from the isthmus of the uterus into the vagina, and it is through the small cervical opening (os) that the uterus and vagina communicate. The cervical os appears as a small closed circle in nulliparous women and may be enlarged or of an irregular shape in parous women. The cervix appears as an oval-shaped structure and is usually shiny and pale pink. In postmenopausal women, it may be smaller and less pigmented than in premenopausal

women. The stroma (connective tissue forming the supportive framework) of the cervix consists of connective tissue with unstriated muscle fibers as well as elastic tissue.

The stratified squamous epithelium of the outer cervix (the portio) is made up of several layers. The basal layer is a single row of cells resting on a thin basement membrane and is the layer where active mitosis (cell division) is seen. The parabasal and intermediate layers are next. In the intermediate layer are vacuoles containing glycogen. The superficial, keratinized layer varies in thickness in response to estrogen stimulation. The desquamation of this surface layer occurs constantly. The superficial layer contains a large amount of glycogen, as does the intermediate layer. It appears that glycogen plays an important role in maintaining the acid pH of the vagina. Glycogen released by cytolysis of the desquamated cells is acted on by the glycolytic bacterial flora in the vagina, forming lactic acid. In a healthy vaginal ecosystem with a basic pH, the vagina will typically smell salty and slightly musky. Each woman has a unique, characteristic odor that is more noticeable during the hormonal influences associated with ovulation, menstruation, and sexual stimulation (Stoppard, 2002).

Just as the endometrium is influenced by the hormonal fluctuations of the menstrual cycle, so is the mucus produced by the secretory cells of the glands in the endocervix (interior cervical canal). This is especially noticeable in premenopausal women. The fluctuations in cervical mucus during the course of the menstrual cycle will be discussed later in this chapter.

There is an abrupt transition from the stratified squamous epithelium covering the vagina and the outer surface of the cervix to the tall, glandular columnar cells rich in mucin (proteinaceous mucoid substance) located within the internal cervical canal. This junction between ectocervical cells and endocervical cells is designated as the transformation zone. This ever-changing squamocolumnar junction is actually a cellular dividing line where newly forming columnar epithelium in the cervix are merging with encroaching stratified epithelium lining. It is an area of increased susceptibility to infection and carcinogens. During a Pap smear to test for cervical cancer, desquamated (exfoliated) cells from the cervix are examined cytologically for cellular abnormalities. For an adequate test, endocervical cells at the squamocolumnar transformation zone as well as ectocervical squamous cells must be included.

Uterus

The uterus is a hollow, pear-shaped organ that is from 5.5 to 9 cm long, 3.5 to 6 cm wide, and 2 to 4 cm thick in nulliparous women. The uterus of a parous woman may be 2 to 3 cm larger in any of these three dimensions.

The uterus is usually inclined forward at a 45-degree angle from the longitudinal plane of the body. Usually, the uterus is anteverted or slightly anteflexed in position. However, it also may be retroflexed, retroverted, or in a midposition.

The portion of the uterus above the cervix is termed the corpus (body) and is constructed of a thick-walled musculature. It is covered with peritoneum on the exterior and lined interiorly with a mucoid surface called the endometrium. The body of the uterus is divided into three portions: the fundus, the corpus, and the isthmus. The fundus is the prominence above the insertion of the fallopian tubes, the corpus is the main portion, and the isthmus is the narrow lower portion of the uterus adjacent to the cervix. The uterus is not a fixed organ but can be moved about; for example, during the sexual response cycle, the entire uterus elevates from the true pelvis into the false pelvis.

Fallopian Tubes

Two fallopian tubes are laterally located at either horn of the uterine fundus, run laterally toward the ovaries, and are the site for ovum and sperm transport, sperm capacitation, ovum retrieval, fertilization, and embryo transport. Each tube is approximately 10 to 12 cm long. The distal portion of the oviduct is fimbriated; both the middle portion (the ampulla) and the portion of the tube closest to its insertion in the uterus (the isthmus) are extremely narrow. The wider funnel shaped end of the tubes is surrounded by irregular, fingerlike extensions called fimbriae. Although not actually attached to the ovary, the fimbriae come into contact with the ovary and are lined with ciliated epithelium that sweep uniformly toward the uterus, acting as a vaccuum for any newly released ovum. The outer, serous coat of the oviduct covers a muscular portion consisting of an inner circular layer and a thin, outer longitudinal layer. The mucosal layer, composed of a number of rugae that become more numerous approaching the fimbriated portion, lines the tubes.

Ovaries

The ovaries are paired, almond shaped, female gonads approximately 3 to 4 cm long, 2 cm wide, and 1 to 2 cm thick. They are located near the pelvic wall at the level of the anterior superior iliac spine. The external ovarian surface has a dull, whitish, opaque appearance. The ovary is composed of three major portions. First, there is an outer cortex lined by a single layer of cuboidal (cube-shaped) epithelium. Through this layer, blood vessels and nerves enter and leave the ovary. Follicles are embedded in the connective tissue of the outer cortex and are either growing or inactive. Second, the central medulla of the ovary is composed of loose connective tissue (stroma), lymphatics, and blood vessels. The ovarian stroma is comprised of contractile cells, connective tissue cells that provide structural support to the ovary, and interstitial cells that secrete sex steroid hormones (primarily androgens). In addition, the stroma contains the primordial follicles yet to be recruited. Not only do the ovaries release gametes, but they also produce sex steroid hormones—including estrogen, progesterone, and androgens—as well as a number of nonsteroidal factors that regulate endocrine regulation of ovarian function. The ovary has a rich lymphatic drainage, and an abundant supply of unmyelinated nerve fibers also enters the medulla through the rete ovarii (the hilum). The hilum is the point of ovarian attachment to the mesovarium, a peritoneal fold on the posterior surface of the broad ligament.

At birth, the ovary contains approximately 1 to 2 million germ cells after reaching the acme of follicular formation at 16 to 20 weeks gestation (6 to 7 million oocytes); no new germ cells are ever produced later in life. By the onset of puberty, the total content of germ mass is ultimately reduced through the process of atresia to 300,000 follicles and only 400 oogonia will achieve ovulation during a woman's reproductive life (Speroff & Fritz, 2005).

The follicle is the functional unit of the ovary, the source of both the gametes and the ovarian hormones. Each follicle is surrounded by a circular cellular wall called the theca folliculi. The theca contains an inner rim of secretory cells (the theca interna) and an outer rim of connective tissue (the theca externa). Within the theca—but separated from it by a layer of thin basement membrane—are the granulosa cells, which, in turn, surround the ovum. An acellular layer of protein and polysaccharide, the zona pellucida, separates the ovum from the granulosa cells. The theca interna is richly vascularized although neither the ovum nor the granulosa cells are in contact with any capillaries. The theca and granulosa cells are the primary sex steroid–secreting elements. These cells have receptors for gonadotropins and respond to those released by the anterior pituitary—follicle stimulating hormone (FSH) and lutenizing hormone (LH).

Development and maturation of the follicle is stimulated by FSH and consists of proliferation of the granulosa cells and the gradual elaboration of fluid within the follicle. Accumulation of the fluid increases rapidly with follicular maturation and causes the follicle to bulge into the peritoneal cavity. As the follicle swells, the ovum remains embedded in granulosa cells (cumulus oophorus), which remain in contact with the theca. As fluid accumulates, the cumulus thins until only a narrow thread of cells connects the ovum with the rim of the follicle. At ovulation, the ovum, surrounded by the corona of granulosa cells (sometimes called the corona radiata) while floating in the follicular fluid, ruptures.

The ovum and its corona extrude into the peritoneal cavity in a bolus of follicular fluid. This sometimes is perceptable as a crampy sensation, referred to as Mittel-schmerz. After ovulation, ingrowth and differentiation of the remaining granulosa cells fill the collapsed folli-cle to form a new endocrine structure called the corpus luteum. The corpus luteum continues to develop when a pregnancy occurs. When the ovum is not fertilized and dies, the corpus luteum no longer develops and leaves a remnant on the surface of the ovary called a corpus albicans (see Figure 4.5).

Pelvic Supporting Structures

Bones, muscles, ligaments, blood vessels, and nerves form supporting structures of the pelvic organs and are described below.

Bony Pelvis

The pelvis is composed of two innominate bones: the sacrum and coccyx. The innominate bones, in turn,

are composed of the ilium, ischium, and pubis. These constitute the hipbones. The pubic bones meet anteri-orly at the symphysis pubis, a fibrocartilaginous sym-physeal joint. The pubic arch is formed by the inferior borders of the pubic bones and symphysis. The ilium joins with the sacrum posteriorly to form the sacroiliac joint. A woman's pelvis is typically wider and more hol-low than a man's because of the flaring of the woman's iliac bones and a curved sacrum (see Figure 4.6).

Muscles

Several sets of pelvic muscles attach to the bony pelvis and can be divided into two main groups: the urogeni-tal triangle and the pelvic floor. These muscle groups both actively and passively support the pelvis and are involved in the voluntary contraction of the vagina and the anus. The layer of muscles that is closest to the skin is called the urogenital triangle. Two pairs of long, slender muscles (the ischiocavernosus) run alongside the pelvic outlet and form the two sides of the triangle, with the clitoris at its apex. The superficial transverse perineal muscle extends laterally and forms the base of this triangle. The bulbocavernosus muscles extend from the glans of the clitoris downward under the labia ma-jora, connecting at the perineum, and is shaped like a pair of parentheses. The deep transverse perineal mus-cle forms a solid triangular base of muscle immediately behind the open urogenital triangle and is bisected by the vagina and urethra. During orgasm, these muscles all contract simultaneously, compressing the engorged clitoral tissue between them, creating muscle tension and sexual pleasure. Behind the urogenital triangle is the pelvic floor, which is made up of the levator ani muscle (Frye, 1995). The pubococcygeus muscle, part of the levator ani group, has particular significance in women because it is important in sexual sensory function, blad-der control, and childbirth—by controlling relaxation and extension of the perineum and expulsion of the infant (see Figure 4.7).

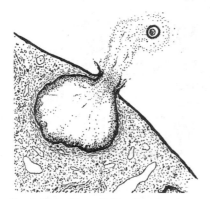

Figure 4.5 Ovulation. At ovulation the ovum, surrounded by the corona radiate and floating in the follicular fluid, ruptures into the peritoneal cavity.

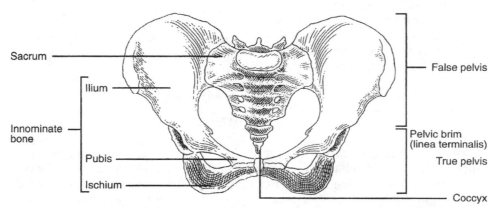

Figure 4.6 The bony pelvis. The pelvis is composed of two innominate bones, the sacrum and the coccyx. The innominates are composed of the ilium, the ischium, and the pubis.

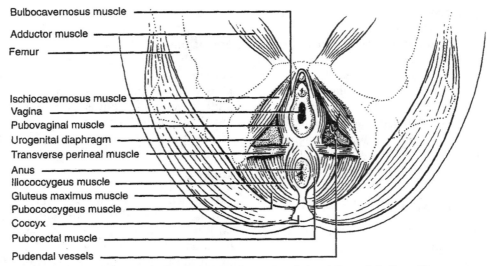

Bulbocavernosus muscle
Adductor muscle
Femur

Ischiocavernosus muscle
Vagina
Pubovaginal muscle
Urogenital diaphragm
Transverse perineal muscle
Anus
Iliococcygeus muscle
Gluteus maximus muscle
Pubococcygeus muscle
Coccyx
Puborectal muscle
Pudendal vessels

Figure 4.7   Pelvic muscles. Several sets of muscles support the pelvic floor. The bulbocavernosus and the puboccygeus have special significance for sexual function.

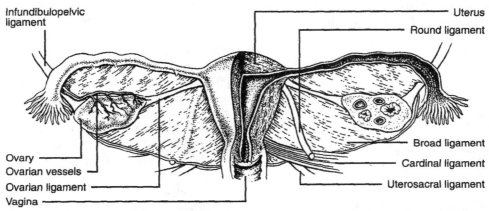

Infundibulopelvic ligament
Uterus
Round ligament
Ovary
Ovarian vessels
Ovarian ligament
Vagina
Broad ligament
Cardinal ligament
Uterosacral ligament

Figure 4.8   Ligaments. Four pairs of ligaments support the uterus, tubes, and ovaries. These are the cardinal, uterosacral, round, and broad ligaments.

Ligaments

Four pairs of ligaments—the cardinal, uterosacral, round, and broad ligaments—provide primary support for the uterus, and the ovarian ligaments and infundibulopelvic ligaments provide ancillary support (see Figure 4.8). Overstretching the ligaments is sometimes associated with minor discomfort during strenuous exercise or during pregnancy.

Vasculature

The ovarian arteries arise from the abdominal aorta, supply the fallopian tube and ovary, and ultimately anastamose with the uterine artery. The uterine artery arises from the anterior branch of the hypogastric artery and supplies the cervix and uterus. The vaginal artery arises similarly from the anterior branch of the hypogastric artery. The uterine veins run along the same channels as the uterine artery. The ovarian veins from the vena cava pass through the broad ligament en route to the ovarian hilus (neck of the ovary). On the right, the ovarian vein empties into the inferior vena cava; on the left, it empties into the renal vein.

Innervation

The internal genitalia are supplied by autonomic as well as spinal nerve pathways. The main autonomic supply to the uterus appears to consist of both sympathetic and parasympathetic fibers of the superior hypogastric plexus. The pudendal nerve is the main spinal nerve, providing the source of motor and sensory activation of the lower genital tract.

PHYSIOLOGIC INFLUENCES OF THE ENDOCRINE SYSTEM AND HORMONAL CONTROLS

Many of the unique functions of the female body are governed by hormonal influences resulting from the communication between the endocrine system and the central nervous system (CNS). Grasping the basic relationship between the hypothalamus, pituitary, and ovaries is important for understanding the rhythms of the menstrual cycle and specific biologic differences created by classic female steroid hormones, estradiol and progesterone.

The endocrine system is comprised of all the glands that secrete hormones (considered chemical messengers) that are carried by the blood from the glands to target cells elsewhere in the body to elicit systemic biologic responses. In addition to discrete organs such as the adrenal or thyroid glands, the definition of endocrine systems has been recently expanded to include single cells or clusters of cells that are not anatomically definable as a gland but that can also secrete or produce hormones. The effects of hormones can either be rapid or delayed, short or long term, depending on their structure and synthesis. A complex feedback system allows for the intricate balance between the hormones secreted and the responses elicited at the level of the target cells throughout the body.

On the target cell (the cell that responds to the presence of the hormone), receptors are the immediate recipients of the chemical messages or information units of hormones. These receptors are structurally organized so that they can specifically recognize and interact with their own cognate hormone, either inside the cell or, more frequently, on the plasma membrane of the cell. All receptors have two essential components: a ligand-binding region that binds the exact hormone for that receptor and an effector region that recognizes the presence of the hormone bound to the ligand region and then initiates the generation of the biological response. As a consequence of the specific receptor-hormone interaction (much like a specific lock and key), a cascade of events, or signal transduction pathways, occurs, and a specific biological response is generated in and, in some instances, around the target cell.

To maintain system precision, receptors have internal physiologic regulators to maintain a balance between the extracellular hormone messengers and the number of target cell receptor sites that elicit specific cellular responses. One of these mechanisms is called down regulation and has the effect of reducing the number of receptor sites (within target cells) in response to long periods of frequent or intense hormonal bombardment. The other mechanism—up regulation—increases the number of receptor sites on the target cell to increase the cell's response to prolonged periods of low concentrations of particular hormones. In other words, if a gland over- or undermanufactures a particular hormone, the master control gland in the brain notes this from the amount of hormones circulating in the blood stream and responds by modulating hormone secretion.

As key elements of the central nervous system, the hypothalamus and pituitary glands are located in the middle of the forebrain on its undersurface, inferior to the third ventricle. While these structures occupy a very small portion of the brain and account for less than one percent of the brain's weight, the hypothalamus and pituitary function as the master control center for the coordination of both neural and endocrine systems (Widmeier, Ruff, & Strong, 2004).

The hypothalamus is responsible for the homeostasis of the interior climate of the body such as temperature regulation, water balance, and emotional behaviors in addition to behaviors related to preservation of the species—hunger, thirst, and reproduction.

The pituitary gland sits in a hollow of the sphenoid bone, just below the hypothalamus. This endocrine gland is attached to the hypothalamus by a stalk that contains nerve filaments and small blood vessels. In adults, the pituitary is composed of two lobes—the anterior and posterior, each of which functions essentially as a distinct gland. The anterior pituitary releases hormones responsible for a wide variety of critical functions including growth, metabolism, steroid release, breast growth, and milk synthesis as well as gamete production and sex hormone secretions. These essential bodily capacities are produced by the release of growth hormone (GH), thyroid-stimulating hormone (TSH), adrenocorticotropic hormone (ACTH), prolactin, and two gonadotropic hormones—follicle stimulating hormone (FSH) and lutenizing hormone (LH). The posterior pituitary controls milk let-down and uterine contractility as well as water secretion by the kidneys and blood pressure through release of oxytocin or vasopressin.

The posterior pituitary is actually an extension of the hypothalamus and communicates through neural connections and electrical messages to release hormones. The anterior pituitary has a unique, localized circulatory connection to the hypothalamus that allows blood to transport special hormones secreted directly from the hypothalamus to the anterior pituitary (hypophysiotropic hormones) to stimulate the release of other, specific anterior pituitary hormones.

Of particular importance to the female body is the regulation of the menstrual cycle and the ovaries' ability to produce gametes. This signal transduction pathway is initially stimulated by gonadotropin releasing hormone (GnRH) secreted by the hypothalamus, which then stimulates the release of follicle stimulating hormone as well as lutenizing hormone from the anterior pituitary. FSH and LH are called gonadotropins because they stimulate the target cells—ovaries (gonads)—to release steroid hormones estradiol, progesterone, and androgens while a mature egg follicle develops and is subsequently released. The careful monthly orchestration of these various hormonal pathways in the interrelated CNS and endocrine communication system is referred to as the hypothalamic-pituitary-ovarian axis.

SEXUAL DIFFERENTIATION AND DEVELOPMENT

Sexual differentiation and development involves a complex series of events that ultimately transform an undifferentiated embryo into a human with a gender identity of female or male. As a result of the complexity of differentiation, one can be born with genotypic sex that is inconsistent with one's phenotypic sex. Phenotypic sex can be understood as the total perceptible characteristics displayed by an individual under specific environmental circumstances, regardless of the person's genotype. The developmental process of sexual differentiation begins at fertilization with establishment of genetic sex. Genetic sex refers to the chromosomal combination from the ovum and sperm, resulting in an XX (female), XY (male), or other combination. Gonadal sex refers to the structure and function of the gonads, whereas somatic sex involves the genital organs other than the gonads. Neuroendocrine sex refers to the cyclic or continuous production of gonadotropin releasing hormones. Although gonadal, somatic, and neuroendocrine sexual differentiation begins prior to birth, sexual differentiation continues after birth. Development of social, psychological, and cultural dimensions of sexuality as well as secondary sex characteristics occurs after birth (Blackburn, 2003).

Genetic Sex

Genetic sex is determined at the time of fertilization and is defined by the contribution of an X or Y chromosome from the father. Of interest is that, despite the genotype, sexual differentiation will produce a basic female phenotype unless testosterone is present and can be used by the cells of the developing human.

Gonadal Sex

At about 4 to 6 weeks of gestation, germ cells migrate to the site of the fetal gonad. At the 6th week, the gonads are sexually indistinguishable, containing a cortex and medulla layer. If the chromosomal sex is XX, the cortex will differentiate into the ovary, and the medulla will regress; if the chromosomal sex is XY, the medulla will differentiate into a testis and the cortex will regress under the influence of SRY, a gene from the sex-determining region of the Y chromosome.

Differentiation of the gonad occurs slightly earlier in male than in female fetuses. At 7 weeks, testicular differentiation begins under the influence of testosterone, which is stimulated by human chorionic gonadotropin (HCG). The ovary differentiates about 2 weeks after testicular differentiation and is identifiable by 10 weeks. By 16 weeks, the oogonia become surrounded by follicular cells, composing the primordial follicle. At 20 weeks' gestation, the fetal ovary contains mature compartmentalization with primordial follicles and oocytes, and there are 5 to 7 million germ cells present. Follicular maturation and atresia is already progressing. Approximately 1 million germ cells remain in the ovary at birth. The oocytes are surrounded by primordial follicles and are arrested in the prophase of the first meiotic (cellular division in which the diploid number of chromosomes is reduced to the haploid) division until the follicle is reactivated at the time of puberty.

Female differentiation is probably linked to a gene on the X chromosome that acts in the absence of androgen. Only one X chromosome is needed for primary ovarian differentiation, explaining why female differentiation may occur in fetuses with XY chromosomes who lack testosterone elaboration at a critical point in development or are unable to use testosterone.

Somatic Sex

The mesonephric (Wolffian duct) and the paramesonephric (Mullerian duct) coexist in all embryos regardless of chromosomal sex. During the third fetal month, one persists and the other disappears. The intrinsic tendency toward feminization produces differentiation of the paramesonephric (Mullerian) system. In the absence of Mullerian inhibiting factor, which inhibits the further development of the Mullerian ducts in male embryos, the paramesonephric system differentiates into the uterine tubes, uterus, and upper vagina.

At the 8th week of gestation, the embryo is bipotential—that is, it can differentiate into either a female or a male. Between 9 and 12 weeks of gestation, differentiation of external genitalia becomes evident. The urogenital sinus, labioscrotal swellings, and genital tubercle will differentiate into a female pattern in the absence of androgen stimulation and without a Y chromosome. In females, the urogenital folds remain open, developing into the labia minora. The labioscrotal folds differentiate into the labia majora, and the genital tubercle differentiates into the clitoris. The urogenital sinus becomes the vagina and the urethra. The lower vagina is formed as part of the external genitalia. The differentiation of these structures is illustrated in Figures 4.9a and 4.9b.

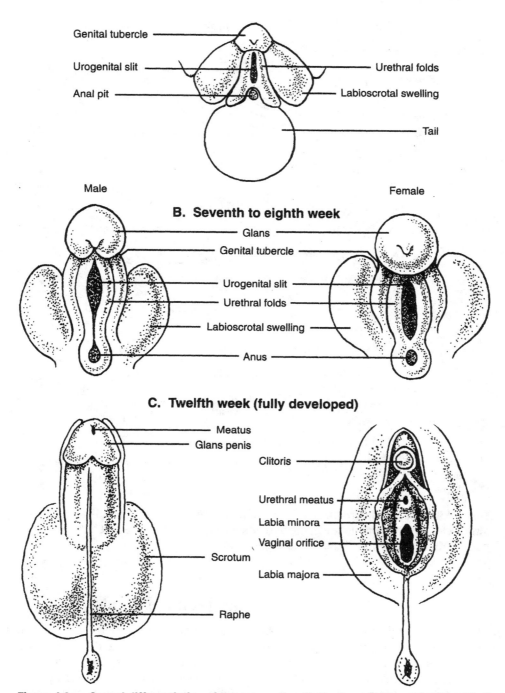

Genital tubercle

Urogenital slit

Anal pit

Urethral folds

Labioscrotal swelling

Tail

Male

Female

B. Seventh to eighth week

Glans

Genital tubercle

Urogenital slit

Urethral folds

Labioscrotal swelling

Anus

C. Twelfth week (fully developed)

Meatus

Glans penis

Clitoris

Urethral meatus

Labia minora

Vaginal orifice

Scrotum

Labia majora

Raphe

Figure 4.9a   Sexual differentiation of the external genitalia. As early as weeks 7 and 8 of fetal life, gender differentiation has begun. Before week 6, the embryo appears undifferentiated. By week 12, the external genitalia assume the differentiated appearance.

Fetal endocrine glands are supported by the placenta as well as the fetal gonads. By the 10th week of gestation, most of the pituitary hormones are apparent. They rise during the first 20 weeks of pregnancy, and then negative feedback mechanisms begin to limit their levels. Luteinizing hormone and follicle-stimulating hormone are apparent at 9 to 10 weeks and peak at about 20 to 22 weeks' gestation. FSH stimulates follicular development in females; LH stimulates steroid synthesis in the ovary and will later induce ovulation in FSH-primed follicles. Hypothalamic-releasing hormones stimulate adrenocorticotropin hormone production by about 8 weeks' gestation.

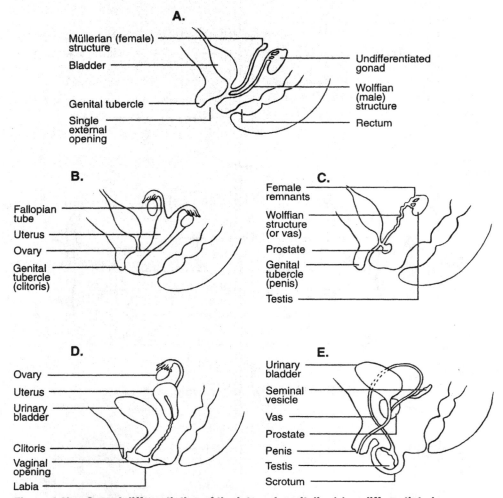

Figure 4.9b   Sexual differentiation of the internal genitalia. (a) undifferentiated structures, (b) female structure at the third month, (c) male structure at the third month, (d) female mature form, (e) male mature form.

PUBERTY

Puberty refers to the period of becoming capable of reproducing sexually and is indicated by the maturation of the genital organs, the development of secondary sex characteristics, and the first occurrence of menstruation in young women. Puberty and the menopausal transition share the characteristic of a transitional period during which a biological series of events culminating in a change in fertility occurs. During puberty, menarche occurs in girls; during the menopausal transition, the final menstrual period occurs in women.

A time interval of a decade or more separates birth and puberty. Puberty occurs during the later phases of human growth, long after the initial sexual differentiation. Both growth and differentiation continue during puberty, making it a distinctive part of the life span and requiring complex physiological mechanisms to initiate its occurrence (Plant, 1994; Venturoli, Flamigni, & Givens, 1985).

Initiation of Puberty

The initiation of puberty remains poorly understood, although it is recognized that a central nervous system program must be responsible for the onset of puberty. It appears that the HPO axis in girls develops in two definitive stages during puberty. First, early in puberty, gradually increasing gonadotropin secretion takes place because of a decrease in sensitivity of the hypothalamic centers to the negative inhibitory effects of low levels of circulating sex steroids. This can be viewed as a slowly rising set point of decreased sensitivity, resulting in increasing GnRH pulsatile secretions. This, in turn, leads to increasing gonadotropin production and ovarian stimulation. Second, later in puberty, there is a maturation of the positive feedback response from ovarian estrogen to the anterior pituitary, which stimulates the mid-cycle surge of LH with subsequent ovulation (Rebar, 2002). This explains why the first few menstrual cycles are annovulatory (for as long as 18 months), although there are frequent exceptions (Speroff & Fritz, 2005).

Current data suggest that the CNS inhibits the onset of puberty until the appropriate time. Thus, the neuroendocrine control of puberty is mediated by GnRH-secreting neurons in the hypothalamus, which act as an internal pulse generator. At puberty, the GnRH pulse generator is reactivated or disinhibited, leading to increasing amplitude, frequency, and regularity of GnRH pulses, especially at night (Speroff & Fritz, 2005). Consequently, the hormonal cascade of reproductive processes is triggered—hypothalamic GnRH pulsations stimulate the release of FSH and LH from the anterior pituitary, which then stimulates ovarian steroidal secretions. Just what causes the disinhibition of GnRH is still unknown (Rebar, 2002). It is important to understand that puberty is not merely turned on like a light switch but rather a functional convergence of all factors. It is more of a concept than an actual focal point of action (Speroff & Fritz, 2005).

Physiological Development and Puberty

Shortly after birth, neonatal FSH and LH levels are still elevated due to negative feedback provided by the maternal ovarian hormones during pregnancy. The gonadotropins remain high for approximately 3 months with resulting transient elevations of estradiol; FSH and LH then gradually decrease to reach a nadir at 1 to 2 years of age in females. Then, gonadotropin levels begin to rise slightly between 4 and 10 years. Low levels of gonadotropins in the pituitary and circulation during childhood yield little response of the pituitary to GnRH and maximal hypothalamic suppression. LH pulses appear during infancy although they are quite irregular. Thus, it appears that immaturity of the endocrine systems is not the factor that tempers the onset of puberty. Indeed, all components of the hypothalamic-pituitary-ovarian axis below the level of the hypothalamus can respond to GnRH from birth.

Prepubertal Phases

In girls, the first steroids to increase in the circulation from the adrenal cortex are androgens—dehydroepiandrosterone (DHEA), dehydroepiandrosterone sulfate (DHEAS), and androstenedione, which occurs from about 6 to 8 years of age, shortly before FSH begins to rise. Estrogen levels as well as LH do not begin to increase until 10 to 12 years of age.

During the prepubertal years, three phases are evident: adrenarche, decreasing the suppression of the gonadostat, and amplification of interactions leading to gonadarche. Adrenarche refers to the development of pubic and axillary hair and is a function of increased adrenal androgen production. An increase in the size of the inner zone of the adrenal cortex precedes a classic linear growth spurt by about 2 years. In addition, adrenarche precedes elevation of estrogens and gonadotropins seen during early puberty and menarche in midpuberty. However, the mechanisms governing adrenarche probably are not the same as those influencing GnRH-pituitary-ovarian axis maturation and gonadarche. Early adrenarche, occurring before 8 years, is not associated with early gonadarche. The mechanisms producing adrenarche remain obscure.

Decreasing repression of the gonadostat refers to the increased responsiveness of the anterior pituitary to GnRH and follicular activity to FSH and LH. Factors that are responsible for de-repressing the gonadostat, allowing the hypothalamus and pituitary to become less sensitive to the negative feedback of low levels of estrogens and permitting gonadotropin concentrations to rise, remain uncertain. Sustained elevation of growth hormone levels may play a role as the factor responsible for de-repressing the gonadostat.

Endogenous GnRH is important in establishing and maintaining puberty. An increasing amplitude and frequency of pulsatile GnRH probably enhances the responses of FSH and LH secretion. GnRH appears to induce cell surface receptors specific for itself and necessary for its action on the surface of gonadotrope cells of the anterior pituitary. Sleep-related pulsations of LH are seen during early puberty. By midpuberty, estrogen enhances LH secretory responses to GnRH (creating positive feedback) and maintains its negative feedback of FSH responses.

Puberty

A cascade of endocrine events initiated by release of pulsatile GnRH results in elevated gonadotropin levels and gonadal steroids, with subsequent appearance of secondary sexual characteristics and, later, menarche and ovulation. Between the ages of 10 and 16, the usual sequence includes the appearance of a pulsatile pattern of LH during sleep, followed by pulses of lesser amplitude throughout the day. Increasing levels of estradiol result in menarche, and, by the latter part of puberty, the positive feedback relationship exists between estradiol and LH that is necessary to stimulate ovulation.

Progression of puberty through a sequence of increased rate of linear growth, breast development, pubarche (onset of pubic hair growth), and menarche occurs over a period of approximately 4.5 years. Usually the first sign of puberty is acceleration of growth, which is followed by breast budding (thelarche). The growth peak (about 2 to 4 inches within 1 year) usually occurs about 2 years after breast budding. Pubarche usually appears following the appearance of breast budding; axillary hair growth occurs approximately 2 years later. In some girls, pubic hair growth is the first sign of puberty. The growth peak in height occurs about 1 year prior to menarche. Menarche occurs late in this sequence with a median age of about 12.8, after the growth peak has occurred. Growth hormone and gonadal estrogen are important factors in the increased growth velocity. In addition, increasing estrogen levels produce breast development, female fat distribution, vaginal and uterine growth, and skeletal growth.

Menarche

Menarche is a function of genetic and environmental influences and occurs between 9.1 and 17.7 years of age, with a mean age of 12.8 years. Improvements in the standard of living and nutrition have produced children who mature earlier than in the past. In cultures that are affluent, menarcheal age has become lower. After menarche, growth slows, with approximately 2.5 inches in height gained after menarche. Age of menarche is correlated for mothers and daughters and between sisters.

Although there has been discussion of a critical weight for menarche to occur (47.8 kg), it is likely that the shift in body composition from 16% to 23.5% fat is a more important factor. Recently, the peptide hormone leptin, secreted in adipose tissue, has revived the significance of a relationship between body fat and reproductive function. This hormone acts on the CNS to regulate eating behaviors and energy balance. Leptin levels increase during childhood until the onset of puberty, suggesting that there is a necessary threshold level of leptin (and, thus, a critical amount of adipose, the source of leptin) for puberty to occur (Garcia-Mayor et al., 1997). Earlier ages of menarche are associated with higher levels of leptin (Matkovic et al., 1997; Speroff & Fritz, 2005). What is also clear is that estrogen secretion, which produces endometrial proliferation, is essential for menarche to occur.

Fertility

Development of positive feedback effects of estrogen on the pituitary and hypothalamus that stimulates the midcycle LH surge necessary for ovulation is a late event in puberty. For this reason, menstrual cycles are often anovulatory for about 12 to 18 months after menarche. The frequency of ovulation becomes more regular with each menstruation and as girls progress through pubertal changes.

Development During Puberty

The five Tanner (1981) stages are a commonly used indicator of the stage of pubertal development. On the basis assessment of breast and pubic hair growth, it is possible to assess progression through puberty (see Figures 4.10a and 4.10b).

In Stage 1, a prepubertal stage, there is elevation of the papilla of the breast only. Although the feminine pelvic contour is evident, the breasts are flat. The labia majora

are smooth, and the labia minora are poorly developed. The hymenal opening is small, the mucous membranes are dry and red, and the vaginal cells lack glycogen.

In Stage 2, there is elevation of the nipple, with a small mound beneath the areola, which is enlarging and beginning to become pigmented. The labia majora become thickened, more prominent, and wrinkled. The labia minora are easily identified due to their increased size along with the enlarging clitoris. The urethral opening is more prominent, mucous membranes are moist and pink, and some glycogen is present in vaginal cells. Pubic hair first appears on the mons and then on the labia about the time of menarche. The pubic hair is scanty, soft, and straight. There is increased activity of the sebaceous and merocrine sweat glands and in the initial functions of the apocrine glands in the axilla and vulva.

In Stage 3, the rapid growth peak has occurred; menarche occurs most frequently during this stage following the acceleration of the growth peak. The areola and nipple enlarge, and pigmentation is more evident along with increased glandular size. The labia minora are well developed, and the vaginal cells have increased glycogen content. The mucous membranes are increasingly more pale. The pubic hair is thicker, coarser, and often more curly at this time. There is increased activity of the sebaceous and sweat glands, with the beginning of acne in some girls along with adult body odor.

In Stage 4, the areola project above the plane of the breast, and the areolar glands are apparent. Glandular tissue is easily palpable. Both the labia majora and minora assume the adult structure, and the glycogen content of the vaginal cells begins its cyclic pattern. Pubic hair is more abundant, and axillary hair is present.

In Stage 5, the breasts are more mature, with the nipples enlarged and protuberant and the areolar glands well developed. Pubic hair is more abundant and spreads to thighs in some women or may extend to the umbilicus. Facial hair may increase. Increased sebaceous gland activity of the skin and increased severity of acne may appear.

THE MENSTRUAL CYCLE

Coordination of the Menstrual Cycle

The menstrual cycle requires a complex sequence of physiological events coordinated by the hypothalamus in conjunction with the pituitary, ovary, and uterus and that adapts to environmental phenomena. Major components of the system coordinating the menstrual cycle include the GnRH pulse generator, GnRH released by the hypothalamus, the gonadotropins (FSH and LH) secreted by the pituitary, and estrogen and progesterone produced by the ovary and corpus luteum, respectively. GnRH is released from the hypothalamus in a

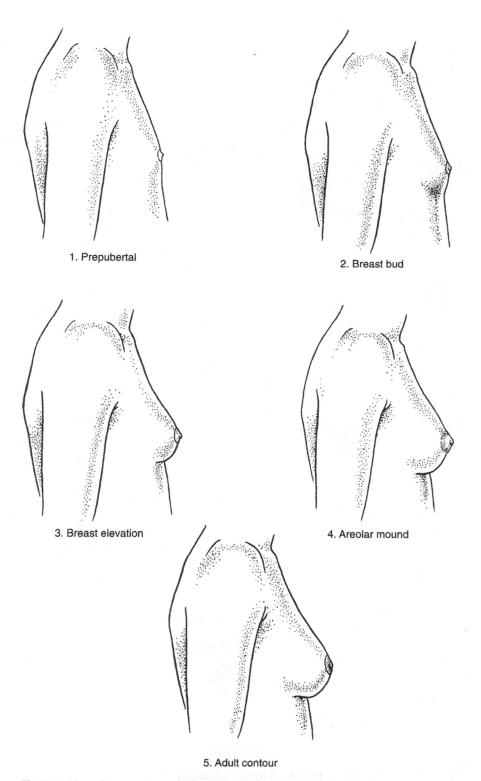

1. Prepubertal

2. Breast bud

3. Breast elevation

4. Areolar mound

5. Adult contour

Figure 4.10a   Tanner stages for breast development.

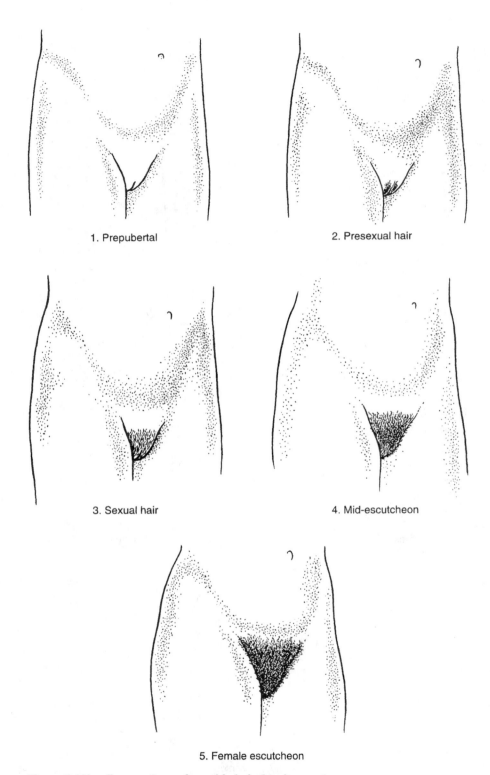

1. Prepubertal

2. Presexual hair

3. Sexual hair

4. Mid-escutcheon

5. Female escutcheon

Figure 4.10b   Tanner stages for pubic hair development.

pulsatile fashion into the pituitary portal circulation. The pituitary gonadotropins respond to the stimulus from GnRH with pulses of LH and FSH released into the peripheral circulation. In response to GnRH and the gonadotropic hormones, the follicles produce estradiol, and the corpus luteum produces progesterone in response to elevated LH.

This coordinating system can be modulated by many inputs from higher neural centers and peripheral factors influencing the GnRH pulse generator as well as other hormones. Norepinephrine seems to amplify GnRH secretion, whereas dopamine dampens GnRH secretion. Increased endorphin release inhibits gonadotropin secretion through suppression of the release of GnRH (Speroff & Fritz, 2005).

Ovarian Cycle: The Follicular Phase

The menstrual cycle consists of an ovarian and an endometrial component. The ovarian component is customarily divided into three phases to facilitate discussion: the follicular, ovulatory, and luteal (see Figure 4.11). The follicular phase consists of 10 to 14 days of hormonal influence that support the growth of the primordial

follicle through the preantral, antral, and preovulatory phases. The primordial follicle consists of the oocyte arrested in the diploid stage of development in which it still has 46 chromosomes. The initiation of follicular growth does not appear to be dependent on gonadotropins or estrogen. In fact, follicular growth may have begun during the days of the previous luteal phase, when the regressing corpus luteum secretes decreasing amounts of steroids. Indeed, follicles grow continuously, even during pregnancy, ovulation, and anovulation.

During the first few days of the cycle, the follicle that will ovulate is selected and recruited. The mechanism for determining which follicles or how many will grow appears to be the result of two estrogenic actions: a local interaction between estrogen and FSH with the follicle and the effect of estrogen on pituitary secretion of FSH (Speroff & Fritz, 2005).

Preantral Follicle

A rise in FSH stimulates a group of follicles to grow to the preantral phase (the phase before the antrum is identifiable). During this phase, the zona pellucida appears around the ovum and the thecal layer begins

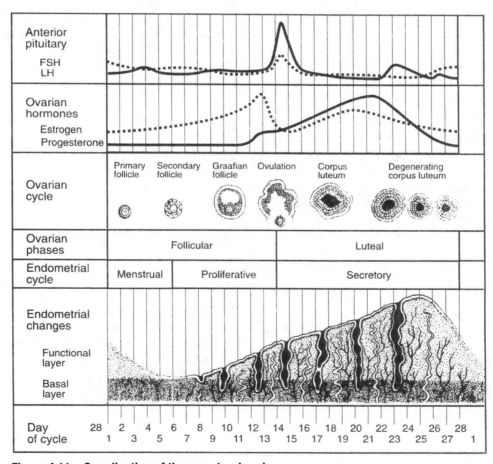

Figure 4.11 Coordination of the menstrual cycle.

to organize. The granulosa cells synthesize steroids, producing more estradiol than progestins or androgens. The follicle also can convert androgens to estrogens. Activated by FSH, the preantral follicle can generate its own estrogenic microenvironment. FSH can increase the concentration of its own receptors on the granulosa cells, thus inducing the production of estradiol. Moreover, at low concentrations, androgen enhances its transformation to estradiol. At higher levels, androgens cause the follicle to produce a more androgenic environment leading to atresia of the follicle. The follicle's development depends on its ability to convert androgen to estrogen.

Antral Follicle

Accumulation of follicular fluid in the antral follicle provides nurturance in an endocrine microenvironment. Influenced by FSH, estradiol becomes the dominant substance in follicular fluid. During the follicular phase, estrogen production occurs by a two-cell, two-gonadotropin mechanism. LH stimulates the theca cells to liberate androgens that are converted to estrogen, and FSH stimulates the granulosa cells to produce estradiol. Sensitivity to FSH determines the capacity for conversion of androgenic to an estrogenic environment in the follicle.

Selection of the follicle that will ovulate (often called dominant follicle) occurs during cycle days 5 through 7 and requires estrogenic action. By day 7, peripheral estradiol levels begin to rise significantly. Estradiol produces negative feedback that decreases gonadotropin support to other follicles. To survive, the selected follicle must increase its own FSH production. Because the dominant follicle has FSH receptors in the granulosa cells, it can enhance FSH action. These actions effectively allow the selected follicle to increase its own estradiol levels and suppress FSH release to other follicles. The theca doubles in vascularity by day 9, producing a siphon for gonadotropins for the selected follicle.

Although the midfollicular increase in estradiol levels produces negative feedback to suppress FSH, it exerts a positive feedback on LH. When estradiol levels reach a concentration necessary for positive feedback (more than 200 pg/ml sustained for at least 50 hours), the LH surge occurs (Speroff & Fritz, 2005).

Feedback systems involving the pituitary and hypothalamus also enable the selected follicle to control its own development. Estradiol exerts negative feedback effects at the hypothalamus and anterior pituitary. Progesterone exerts inhibitory feedback at the level of the hypothalamus and positive feedback at the level of the pituitary. FSH is particularly sensitive to estradiol, whereas LH is sensitive to negative feedback of estradiol at low levels and to positive feedback by estradiol at higher levels. Progesterone slows LH pulses.

GnRH is secreted in the hypothalamus in a pulsatile fashion that changes in amplitude and duration across the menstrual cycle. During the early follicular phase, GnRH is secreted at approximately 94-minute intervals; in the late luteal phase, it is secreted at 216-minute intervals with a decreased amplitude. In turn, the pituitary releases gonadotropic hormones in a pulsatile fashion.

Preovulatory Follicles

Initiated by the LH surge, the oocyte resumes meiosis, approaching completion of reduction division. Estradiol concentrations rise to maintain the peripheral threshold necessary for ovulation to occur. LH initiates luteinization of the granulosa cells and the production of progesterone in the granulosa. The preovulatory increase in progesterone facilitates positive feedback of estradiol and may be necessary for induction of the midcycle FSH peak. The midcycle increase in local and peripheral androgens deriving from the theca of the nonselected follicles may account for the increased libido some women report at midcycle.

Ovulation

Ovulation occurs about 10 to 12 hours after the LH peak, 24 to 36 hours after the estradiol peak. The onset of the LH surge is estimated to occur approximately 34 to 46 hours before the follicle ruptures. LH stimulates the completion of the reduction division in the oocyte (to 23 chromosomes), luteinization of granulosa cells, and synthesis of progesterone and prostaglandins. The continuing rise in progesterone in the follicle up to the time of ovulation may act to end the LH surge. Progesterone also enhances proteolytic enzymes and prostaglandins needed for digestion and rupture of the follicle. Progesterone influences the midcycle rise in FSH, which in turn frees the oocyte from the follicular attachments, converts plasminogen to plasmin (a proteolytic enzyme involved in follicular rupture), and ensures sufficient LH receptors for a normal luteal phase.

Ovarian Cycle: Luteal Phase

The luteal phase is named for the process of luteinization, which occurs following rupture of the follicle and release of the ovum. The granulosa cells increase in size and take on a yellowish pigment, lutein, from which they were named the corpus luteum or yellow body. Luteinization involves synthesis of androgens, estrogens, and progesterone. The process of luteinization requires the accumulation of LH receptors during the follicular phase of the cycle and continuing levels of LH secretion. Progesterone acts during this phase to suppress new follicular growth, rising sharply after ovulation with a peak at about 8 days after the LH surge. The length of the luteal phase tends to be more constant than the follicular phase and is consistently close to

14 days from LH midcycle surge to menses. Luteal phases ranging from 11 to 17 days are considered to be within normal limits. The corpus lutuem begins a rapid cessation of activity at about 9 to 11 days after ovulation, and the mechanism triggering this remains unknown. Some speculate that estrogen production and alteration in prostaglandin concentrations within the ovary are responsible. When pregnancy occurs, the corpus lutuem continues to function with the stimulus of HCG, which appears at the peak of corpus luteum function, 9 to 13 days after ovulation. HCG maintains corpus luteum function until approximately the 9th or 10th week of gestation.

The Endometrial Cycle

The first portion of the menstrual cycle is dominated by follicular development and follicular secretion and causes proliferation of the endometrium. The first portion of the menstrual cycle is named the follicular phase with respect to the ovary and the proliferative phase with respect to the endometrium. The second portion of the cycle is influenced by the corpus luteum, and the increasing levels of progesterone evoke secretory changes in the endometrium. The second portion of the menstrual cycle is named the luteal phase with respect to the ovary and the secretory phase with respect to the endometrium.

Immediately following menstruation, the endometrium is thin, only about 1 to 2 mm thick. Its surface endometrium is composed of low cuboidal cells, the stroma is dense and compact, and the glands appear straight and tubular.

Proliferative Phase

Under the influence of estrogen, the endometrium proliferates and thickens. The endometrium becomes somewhat taller and the surface epithelium becomes columnar. The epithelial lining becomes continuous with the stromal component containing spiral vessels immediately below the epithelial-binding membrane that form a loose capillary network. Although the stroma is still quite compact, the endometrial glands have become more tortuous. Mitotic activity is evident in both the surface epithelium and the basal nuclei of the epithelial cells lining the endometrial glands. Estrogenic effects are also seen in the secretions of the cervical glands and in the vaginal lining. The variability in length of this phase of the menstrual cycle is greater than that for the luteal phase. Indeed, the varying number of proliferative or follicular phase days accounts for the variation in total cycle length.

Secretory Phase

As a result of the developing corpus luteum, progesterone evokes and increases the secretory changes in the endometrium. The surface epithelium is now tall and columnar; the stroma is less compact than earlier in the cycle and somewhat edematous and vascular. The endometrial glands become increasingly tortuous and convoluted. In addition, by 7 days after ovulation, the spiral vessels are densely coiled. The confinement of the growing endometrium to a fixed structure produces the tortuosity of the glands and spiral vessels.

Implantation usually occurs within 7 to 13 days after ovulation. At this point, the midportion of the endometrium appears lacelike, a stratum spongiosum. The stratum compactum overlies the inner layers of the endometrium and is a sturdy structure.

Premenstrually, the surface epithelium is quite tall, about 8 to 9 mm. The stroma consists of large polyhedral cells. The endometrial glands are very convoluted and serrated, resembling a corkscrew. The lining epithelium of endometrial glands is less well demarcated and smaller because of loss of glycogen into the gland lumen. A large number of lymphocytes and leukocytes are seen, probably as a result of the beginning necrosis of the endometrium.

Menstruation

In the absence of fertilization, implantation, and sustaining HCG, estradiol and progesterone levels wane as the corpus luteum ceases to function.

Endometrial growth regresses a few days before the onset of menstruation; at the same time, there is stasis of blood flow to the coiled arteries, with intermittent vasoconstriction. Between 4 and 24 hours prior to the onset of menstrual bleeding, intense vasoconstriction occurs. The menstrual blood flows from coiled arteries that have been constricted for several hours. Prostaglandins, synthesized in the endometrium as result of progesterone stimulation, are released and produce more intense vasoconstriction. Dissolving of the endometrium liberates acid hydrolases from the cell lysosomes. The acid hydrolases further disrupt the endometrial cell membranes, completing the process of menstruation. White cells migrate through capillary walls, and red blood cells escape into the interstitial space along with thrombin-platelet plugs that appear in the superficial vessels. Leakage and interstitial hemorrhage occur. With increased ischemia, the continuous-binding membrane becomes fragmented and intercellular blood is extruded into the endometrial cavity. The loose, vascular stroma of the spongiosum desquamates. Menstrual flow stops due to prolonged vasoconstriction, desquamation of the spongy layer of the endometrium, vascular stasis, and estrogen-induced rebuilding. The lower layer of the endometrium (basalis) is retained, and the stumps of the basal glands and stroma for the ensuing cycle continue to grow from them. The surface epithelium regenerates rapidly and may begin even while other areas are being desquamated.

With menstruation, as much as two-thirds of the endometrium is lost. The menstrual flow may last from 2 to 8 days. Menstruation fluid consists of cervical and vaginal mucus as well as degenerated endometrial particles and blood. Sometimes clots may appear in the menstrual fluid. Usually from 2 to 3 ounces of fluid is lost with menses, but the amount of flow is highly variable. Women with more rapid loss experience a shorter duration of flow. Heavier flow and greater blood loss may indicate delayed or incomplete shedding of the endometrium.

Cyclic Changes in Other Organs

In addition to the uterus and ovary, other organs experience cyclic changes. The cervical canal contains about 100 crypts referred to as columnar glands; the secretory cells of these crypts secrete mucus into the endocervical canal. The mucus undergoes qualitative and quantitative changes during the menstrual cycle depending on the hormonal environment. Immediately after menstruation, the mucus is sparse, viscid, and sticky. When examined under a microscope, an abundance of vaginal and cervical cells and lymphocytes can be seen. From about the 8th day of the cycle until ovulation, the quantity and viscosity of the mucus increase. Sometimes an obvious plug of yellow, white, or cloudy mucus of a tacky consistency is present. At midcycle, the mucus is a thin hydrogel containing 2% solids and 98% water. The mucus resembles raw egg white, being clear, stretchy, and slippery. It will stretch without breaking or spin a thread (and is called spinnbarkheit). Ability of the mucus to stretch at least 5 to 6 cm has been established as a guideline for determining adequacy of the cervical mucus to support sperm transport. When the midcycle mucus is allowed to dry on a slide, it gives a fern or palm-leaf pattern. This pattern is absent after ovulation, during pregnancy, and after menopause. After ovulation, the mucus may again become cloudy, white, or yellow and tacky and may disappear altogether. Women can use the changes in cervical mucus as an indirect index of ovulation.

The cervix itself changes with the menstrual cycle. During the proliferative phase, the os progressively widens, reaching its maximum width just prior to or at ovulation. At the point of maximal widening, mucus can be seen extruding from the external os. After ovulation, the os returns to a smaller diameter, with the profuse and watery mucus becoming scanty and viscid. These changes are believed to be estrogen induced and are not seen in prepubertal or postmenopausal women nor in those whose ovaries have been removed.

The motility of the uterine tubes is greatest during the estrogen-dominant portion of the menstrual cycle. They demonstrate a decreased motility during the progesterone-dominant phase.

Estrogen stimulation leads to cornification of the vagina. Following progesterone stimulation, the vaginal epithelium shows an increase in the number of precornified cells, mucus shreds, and aggregates of cells.

MENOPAUSE

At between 38 and 42 years of age, ovulation becomes less frequent. Residual follicles have decreased in number from about 300,000 at puberty to a few thousand and are less sensitive to gonadotropin stimulation than earlier in life, are less likely to mature, and produce less estrogen. Menopause occurs when estrogen is insufficient to stimulate endometrial growth so that a woman no longer menstruates (Vom Saal & Finch, 1994; Wise, 1989; Wise, Weiland, Scarbrough, Larson, & Lloyd, 1990).

Menopause is said to have occurred when a woman has not menstruated for a period of 1 full year. Prior to menopause, women notice changes in their menstrual cycles, most likely due to a shortening of the follicular phase as a result of lower estradiol secretion. As a woman's cycles become more irregular, vaginal bleeding may occur at the end of a short luteal phase or after an estradiol peak without ovulation or corpus luteum formation.

Elevated FSH levels reflect an attempt to stimulate a follicle to produce estrogen. FSH levels of over 30–40 IU/L are used as an indicator that menopause is approaching, although women may still be bleeding. Elevated FSH levels probably reflect the decreased regulation by the negative feedback of inhibin produced by the granulosa cells. Recent studies have revealed that FSH is an unreliable predictor of the final menstrual period: thus, a single FSH level is not a useful clinical tool for predicting menopause (Randolph et al., 2006). Although FSH rises to 10 to 20 times its premenopausal level and LH rises to 3 times its premenopausal level within 1 to 3 years after menopause, there is a subsequent decrease in both gonadotropins to a new steady state. In postmenopausal women, the ovary continues to secrete testosterone from the stromal tissue, and androstenedione secretion decreases to approximately half the level seen premenopausally. As the follicles disappear and less estrogen is produced, the gonadotropins may stimulate secretion of testosterone. However, the total amount of testosterone produced is lower than premenopausally because peripheral conversion of androstenedione is reduced.

Circulating estradiol levels after menopause range from approximately 10 to 20 pg/ml. Most of this is derived from the conversion of estrone to estradiol in adipose tissue. Circulating levels of estrone are higher than estradiol with the mean levels of approximately 30 to 70 pg/ml. As women age, there are lower levels of DHEA and DHEAS, but estrone, testosterone, and androstenedione remain relatively constant. Although estrogen production by the ovaries does not persist beyond menopause, estrogen levels in postmenopausal women may be significant due to the conversion of androstenedione and testosterone to estrone. Because fat aromatizes androgen, women with more body fat have higher estrone levels than do those with less body fat. An increase in substrate for estrogen production, as occurs in stressful situations that increase adrenal androstenedione, may induce a menstrual flow in a woman who is postmenopausal. Estrogens from nonovarian sources sustain the breasts and other estrogen-stimulated surfaces such as the urethra.

Occasionally, ovulation occurs after months of amenorrhea and may result in an unplanned pregnancy during the menopausal transition. Elevation of both FSH and LH are thought to indicate that pregnancy cannot occur. Nonetheless, to prevent unwanted conception, women who are experiencing the menopausal transition need to be aware of their fertility status.

Physiological Aspects of Sexual Response

Masters and Johnson (1966) characterized physical phenomena that occur as humans responded to sexual stimulation as well as the psychosocial factors that influenced how people responded. Their observations during sexual response in 382 women and 312 men ranging from 18 to 89 years of age and representing a wide range of educational levels and ethnic groups contributed significantly to understanding sexual physiology.

Two principal physiological changes are responsible for events during the human sexual response cycle: vasocongestion and myotonia. Vasocongestion is congestion of blood vessels, usually venous vessels, and is the primary physiological response to sexual stimulation. Myotonia, increased muscular tension, is a secondary physiological response to sexual stimulation. These two changes are responsible for the phenomena observed during the sexual response cycle. Human sexual response is a total body response, not merely a pelvic phenomenon. Changes in cardiovascular and respiratory function as well as reactions involving skin, muscle, breasts, and the rectal sphincter occur during sexual response. The sexual response cycle originally included four phases: excitement, plateau, orgasm, and resolution (Masters & Johnson, 1966).

Research on sexual desire by Kaplan (1974) suggested that desire is another essential component of human sexual response. Desire initially supplies the catalyst or motivation for sexual receptivity. As with other aspects of sexuality, desire is influenced by health, physiology, past experiences, and cultural and environmental factors (MacLaren, 1995). Recent studies of women's sexual desire are discussed in greater detail in chapter 14.

Excitement Phase

Excitement develops from any source of bodily or psychic stimuli, and, if adequate stimulation occurs, the intensity of excitement increases rapidly. This phase may be interrupted, prolonged, or ended by other competing stimuli. During the excitement phase, the clitoral glans becomes tumescent or enlarged, and the clitoral shaft increases in diameter and length. The appearance of vaginal lubrication, caused by vasocongestion and transudation of fluid across the vaginal membrane, occurs within 10 to 30 seconds after initiation of sexual stimulation. The vaginal barrel expands about 4 cm in transcervical width and lengthens 2.5 to 3.5 cm. In addition, the vaginal wall develops a purplish hue due to vasocongestion. Partial elevation of the uterus may occur if it lies in the anterior position.

In nulliparous women, flattening and separating of the labia majora occur. In multiparous women, the labia majora move slightly away from the introitus due to a vasocongestive increase in their diameter. The vaginal barrel is lengthened approximately 1 cm as a result of the thickening of the labia minora.

During the excitement phase, changes also occur in women's extragenital organs. Nipples may protrude, breast size increases, the areolae become engorged, and the venous pattern on the breast becomes more obvious. The sex flush, a maculopapular rash, may appear over the epigastric area, spreading quickly over the breasts. Some involuntary muscle tensing may be evident, as in the tensing of intercostal and abdominal muscles. The heart rate and blood pressure also increase as sexual tension increases (see Figure 4.12a).

Plateau Phase

When stimulation is maintained, sexual tension becomes intensified to the level at which a person may experience orgasm. Like excitement, this phase also may be affected by competing stimuli. During the plateau phase, the clitoris retracts against the anterior body of the symphysis pubis, underneath the clitoral hood. Vasocongestion of the tissues of the outer third of the vagina and the labia minora causes an increase in size of this highly sensitive tissue, referred to as the orgasmic platform. Further increase in the depth and width of the vaginal barrel occurs. The uterus becomes fully elevated, and, as the cervix rises, it produces a tenting effect in the inner part of the vagina. Irritability of the corpus uteri continues to intensify.

In both nulliparous and multiparous women, the labia majora continue to become engorged, with the phenomenon being more pronounced in nulliparous women. The labia minora undergo a vivid color change from bright red to a deep wine-colored hue, considered a sign of impending orgasm. During the plateau phase,

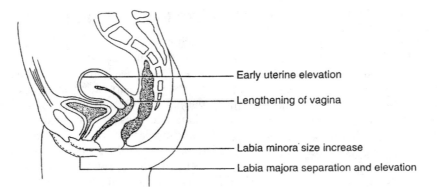

Early uterine elevation

Lengthening of vagina

Labia minora size increase

Labia majora separation and elevation

Figure 4.12a   Excitement phase of sexual response.

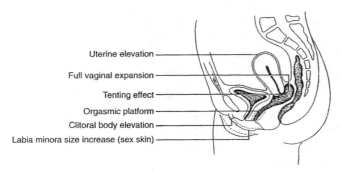

Uterine elevation

Full vaginal expansion

Tenting effect

Orgasmic platform

Clitoral body elevation

Labia minora size increase (sex skin)

Figure 4.12b   Plateau phase.

a drop or two of mucoid material is secreted from Bartholin's glands; this secretion probably assists slightly in vaginal lubrication.

Several extragenital responses occur in women during the plateau phase. Nipple stiffness continues to develop along with an increase in breast size and marked engorgement of the areolae. The sex flush, which began during excitement, may spread over the body. Facial, abdominal, and intercostal muscles contract; muscle tension is increased both voluntarily and involuntarily. Some women use voluntary rectal contractions to enhance stimulation during this phase. Hyperventilation occurs along with a heart rate of 120 to 175 beats per minute, elevation of the systolic blood pressure of 20 to 60 mm Hg, and diastolic elevation of 10 to 20 mm Hg (see Figure 4.12b).

Orgasmic Phase

Orgasm, the involuntary climax of sexual tension increment, involves only a few seconds of the cycle during which vasocongestion and muscle tension are released. During the orgasmic phase, the primary response occurs in women's orgasmic platform, as illustrated in Figure 4.12c. Approximately 5 to 12 contractions occur in the orgasmic platform at 0.8-second intervals. After the first three to six contractions, the interval between contractions increases and the intensity diminishes. The

pelvic floor muscles that surround the lower third of the vagina contract against the engorged vessels, thus forcing out the blood trapped in them. Contractions of the uterus begin at the fundus and progress to the lower segment of the uterus. The contractile excursion of the uterus parallels women's ratings of the intensity of the orgasmic experience.

Extragenital responses involve several organ systems during orgasm. The sex flush parallels the intensity of orgasmic experience and is present in about 75% of women. Involuntary contraction and spasm of muscle groups may be experienced, including contractions of the rectal sphincter, which occur at the same intervals as those of the orgasmic platform. Respiratory rates as high as 40 breaths per minute have been recorded, along with pulse rates from 110 to 180 beats per minute. Fluctuations in the pulse and respiratory rate tend to parallel the level of sexual tension. The systolic blood pressure may be elevated 30 to 80 mm Hg and the diastolic 20 to 40 mm Hg.

Resolution Phase

During the resolution phase, involutional changes restore the preexcitement state. With adequate stimulation, women may begin another sexual response cycle immediately before sexual excitement totally resolves. Usually the length of the resolution period parallels the length of the excitement phase. During the resolution phase, the clitoris returns to its usual position within 5 to 10 seconds after the contractions of the orgasmic platform cease. Vasocongestion and tumescence of the clitoris dissipate more slowly. There is rapid detumescence (loss of vasocongestion) of the orgasmic platform and relaxation of the walls of the vagina. The vaginal wall returns to its normal coloring in about 10 to 15 minutes. Gaping of the cervical os continues for 20 to 30 minutes. The uterus returns to its unstimulated position in the true pelvis, and the cervix descends into the dorsal area of the vagina. The nulliparous labia majora return to their preexcitement position, but in multiparas, the labial vasocongestion dissipates more slowly. The labia minora change from deep red to light pink, and they decrease in size as vasocongestion is lost.

Involution of nipple stiffness, a slow decrease in breast size, and rapid reversal of the sex flush are seen. Some myotonia may still be seen during resolution. The respiratory rate, pulse rate, and blood pressure return to usual levels. An involuntary widespread film of perspiration may appear (Figure 4.12d).

Although these physiological changes are common in women's sexual response, not every woman experiences each response. Indeed, the same woman may experience different aspects from cycle to cycle. Regardless of the difference in stimuli, some women will experience the same sexual responses whether the stimulus is self-pleasuring, pleasuring from another woman or from a man, or intercourse (Sherfey, 1972). Women also tend to be more whole-body oriented (versus genitally oriented) and thus more receptive to sexual touching and experiencing pleasurable, exciting sensations from their skin. Women tend to report a high degree of sensitivity from either mouth or finger contact (Masters & Johnson, 1966).

BIOLOGICAL SEX-BASED DIFFERENCES BEYOND REPRODUCTION

It is becoming more evident through recent scientific exploration that there are broader influences on a woman's health than solely her genetic assignment of two

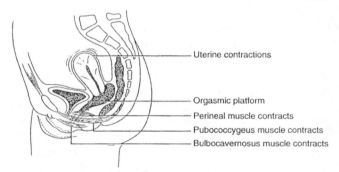

Figure 4.12c   Orgasmic phase.

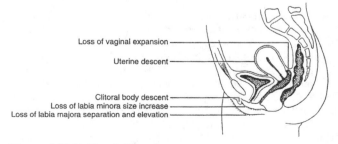

Figure 4.12d   Resolution phase.

X chromosomes. The interplay between genes, prenatal hormone exposure, natural hormone exposure throughout adulthood, female physiologic and biochemical responses, as well as behavioral and socioenvironmental factors all contribute to the way a woman's body responds to disease and illness (Bird & Rieker, 1999; Institute of Medicine Committee on Understanding the Biology of Sex and Gender Differences, 2001).

In 1999, the Institute of Medicine organized a large, interdisciplinary committee to evaluate and consider the current scientific evidence related to the determinants of sex differences at a biological level. What follows is the committee's summary of its identified key issues relevant to women's bodies (Institute of Medicine Committee on Understanding the Biology of Sex and Gender Differences, 2001, pp. 22–23).

Sex Chromosome

A special protective mechanism called X-chromosome inactivation allows females to possess a unique, mixed population of inherited X chromosomes—some from the mother and some from the father. Early in embryonic development, most female cells randomly inactivate one set of X chromosomes (within their normal XX chromosome genotypic assignment). This ability allows inactivation of potential X chromosome gene mutations that would cause disease or death. This ability is not seen in males (XY), who only have one X chromosome assigned and thus only one copy of the X chromosome gene that is thus vulnerable to any deleterious X chromosome gene mutation inherited from only one parent. Thus, if a male inherits a mutated X chromosome that is incompatible with life, death occurs. If a female inherits a mutated X chromosome, and random X chromosome inactivation occurs to this mutated chromosome, the other X chromosome is able to replace it and sustain life.

A good example of this protective effect is demonstrated in a skin disorder, incontinentia pigmenti, that is only seen in females because affected males die in utero or shortly after birth. When male fetuses inherit this X chromosome mutation, this gene alteration causes cell death and an inability to survive. When females inherit the mutated X chromosome from one copy of the gene, cells that contain the gene for the disease (on the active X chromosome) die, but the dead cells are replaced by cells expressing the functional gene from the other X chromosome. Survival results and most of the cells express the functional gene in females (Francis & Sybert, 1997; Goldsmith & Epstein, 1999).

Immune Function

Females have a more resilient immune system that protects them against infectious diseases. Yet this aggressive immune system also makes females more vulnerable to autoimmune diseases such as lupus or thyroiditis. Systemic lupus erythematosus is a predominantly female disease (9:1) in humans, though its severity is similar in females and males. Hashimoto thyroiditis is also clearly a female disease in humans (10:1).

Other examples of this distinction between female immune and inflammatory response differences are seen in vaccination responses of females. Higher antibody levels are induced in females from vaccinations than males. Yet a complication of vaccinations is arthritis, which occurs more frequently in females. Women are also more likely to experience multiple sclerosis and rheumatoid arthritis, which are other debiliatating and often painful autoimmune diseases.

Onset and Symptoms of Cardiovascular Disease

Heart disease has been identified as the most common cause of mortality in women (as in men). Women experience myocardial infarctions (MIs), on average, 10 years later than men and have poorer 1-year postattack survival rates. After an MI, women younger than 65 years of age are more than twice as likely to die as are men of the same age (Vaccarino, Parsons, Every, Barron, & Kurmbolz, 1999). Possible explanations include the increased prevalence of diabetes, heart failure, and stroke in younger women; the more frequent occurence of placque erosions in premenopausal women; less arterial narrowing and higher levels of reactive platelets are present in younger women.

Women have more "silent" heart attacks. Symptoms present differently for women than men in that women experience more shortness of breath and fatigue versus men, who have acute, crushing chest pain.

Response to Toxin

Recent studies suggest that women may be biologically predisposed to adverse responses to the toxins found in cigarettes. Women are at a 1.2- to 1.7-fold higher risk than men for all major types of lung cancer at every level of exposure to tobacco smoke, even after adjusting for smoking history and body size differences. Sex differences in metabolism or gene expression may be the underlying causes for these differences in cancer risk (Guinee et al., 1995; Manton, 2000; Shriver et al., 2000; Tseng et al., 1999).

Brain Organization

Women use both the left and the right inferior frontal gyri to carry out language tasks, while men use only the left inferior frontal gyrus when, for instance, they try to determine whether two nonsense words rhyme. Despite this, both women and men perform the task

equally accurately and rapidly. This sex difference may account for why women who experience a left-sided stroke do not experience a reduction in their language performance, and men do.

Response to Pain and Pain Therapies

Women have greater nociperception (a greater sensitivity by nerve centers to painful stimuli or injurious influences), particularly those that occur in internal organs. Coupled with this, women also have a higher prevalence of many painful disorders such as gallbladder disease, irritable bowel syndrome, carpal tunnel syndrome, and fibromyalgia. Recent data suggest that young adult women may be more responsive to kappa opioid drugs than young adult men (Berkely & Holdcroft, 1999; Gear et al., 1999).

As more women participate in ongoing research to determine sex-based differences in morbidity and mortality, it will be important to take into account *both* the biological factors and social factors that contribute to these health differences. Gender differences in social opportunities shape women's choices and expectations regarding role-related activities. This, in turn, can affect women's exposures to various risks (including stress, role overload, and occupational health problems such as carpal tunnel syndrome and exposure to toxic chemicals) and access to appropriate health resources (health insurance, income, social support) (Bird & Rieker, 1999).

SUMMARY

From this discussion, it is evident that certain structures and functions are unique to a woman's body. These are involved in the menstrual cycle and women's sexual response cycles. Several of the structures of a woman's body serve her reproductive powers as well as her recreative pleasures—with the exception of the clitoris, an organ whose sole raison d'être is to receive and transduce sexual pleasure. Women's bodies develop uniquely from the time of conception and early differentiation through pubertal and menopausal transitions.

REFERENCES

American Psychiatric Association. (2000). *Diagnostic and statistical manual of mental disorders, DSM-IV-TR* (4th ed., text revision). Washington, DC: Author.

Berkely, K. J., & Holdcroft, A. (1999). Sex and gender differences in pain. In P. D. Wall & R. Melzak (Eds.), *Textbook of pain* (4th ed., pp. 951–965). Edinburgh, Scotland: Churchill Livingstone.

Bird, C. E., & Rieker, P. P. (1999). Gender matters: An integrated model for understanding men's and women's health. *Social Sciences and Medicine, 48*(6), 745–755.

Blackburn, S. T. (2003). *Maternal, fetal, and neonatal physiology: A clinical perspective* (2nd ed.). St. Louis, MO: Saunders.

Federation of Feminist Women's Health Centers. (1981). *A new view of a woman's body.* New York: Simon & Schuster.

Francis, J. S., & Sybert, V. P. (1997). Incontinentia pigmenti. *Seminars in Cutaneous Medicine and Surgery, 16*(1), 54–60.

Frye, A. (1995). *Healing passage: A midwife's guide to the care and repair of the tissues involved in birth* (5th ed.). Portland, OR: Labrys Press.

Garcia-Mayor, R. V., Andrade, M. A., Rios, M., Lage, M., Dieguex, C., & Casanueva, F. F. (1997). Serum leptin levels in normal children: Relationship to age gender, body mass index, pituitary-gonadal hormones, and pubertal stage. *Journal of Clinical Endocrinology and Metabolism, 82*(9), 2849–2855.

Gear, R. W., Miaskowski, C., Gordon, N. C., Paul, S. M., Heller, P. H., & Levine, J. D. (1999). The kappa opioid nalbuphine produces gender- and dose-dependent analgesia and antianalgesia in patients with postoperative pain. *Pain, 83*(2), 339–345.

Goldsmith, L. A., & Epstein, E. H., Jr. (1999). Genetics in relation to the skin. In I. M. Feedberg, A. Z. Eisen, & K. Wolff (Eds.), *Fitzpatrick's dermatology in general medicine* (5th ed.). New York: McGraw-Hill.

Guinee, D. G. Jr., Travis, W. D., Trivers, G. E., DeBenedetti, V. M., Cawley, H., Welsh, J. A., et al. (1995). Gender comparisons in human lung cancer: Analysis of p53 mutations, anti-p53 mutation serum antibodies and C-erb-2 expression. *Carcinogenesis, 16*(5), 993–1002.

Hoffman, E., & Johnson, K. (1995). Women's health and managed care: Implications for the training of the primary care physician. *Journal of the American Medical Women's Association, 50*(1), 17–19.

Institute of Medicine Committee on Understanding the Biology of Sex and Gender Differences. (2001). T. M. Wizemann & M. L. Pardue (Eds.), *Exploring the biological contributions to human health: Does sex matter?* Washington, DC: National Academy Press.

Kaplan, H. S. (1974). *The new sex therapy: Vol. 1.* New York: Brunner-Mazel.

MacLaren, A. (1995). Primary care for women: Comprehensive sexual health assessment. *Journal of Nurse-Midwifery, 40*(2), 104–119.

Manton, K. (2000). Gender differences in cross-sectional and cohort age dependence of cause-specific mortality: The United States, 1962–1995. *Journal of Gender Specific Medicine, 3*(44), 47–54.

Masters, W., & Johnson, V. (1966). *Human sexual response.* Boston: Little, Brown.

Matkovic, V., Ilich, J. Z., Skugor, M., Badenhop, N. E., Goel, P., Clairmont, A., Klisovic, D., Nahhas, R. W., & Landoll, J. D. (1997). Leptin is inversely related to age at menarche in human females. *Journal of Clinical Endocrinology and Metabolism, 82*(10), 3239–3245.

Pinn, V. W. (2003). Sex and gender factors in medical studies: Implications for health and clinical practice. *Journal of the American Medical Association, 289*(4), 397–399.

Plant, T. (1994). Puberty in primates. In E. Knobil, J. O'Neill, et al. (Eds.), *The physiology of reproduction* (pp. 1763–1788). New York: Raven Press.

Porth, C. M. (2007). *Essentials of Pathophysiology: Concepts in altered health states.* Philadelphia: Lippincott.

Randolph, J. F., Crawford, S., Dennerstien, L., Cain, K., Harlow, S. D., Little, R., et al. (2006). The value of follicle-stimulating hormone concentration and clinical findings as markers of the late menopausal transition. *Journal of Clinical Endocrinology and Metabolism, 91*(8), 3034–3040.

Rebar, R. (2002). Puberty. In J. S. Berek (Ed.), *Novak's gynecology* (13th ed., pp. 805–841). Philadelphia: Lippincott, Williams & Wilkins.

Sherfey, M. (1972). *The nature and evolution of female sexuality.* New York: Random House.

Shriver, S. P., Bourdeau, A., Gubish, C. T., Tirpak, D. L., Davis, A. L., Luketich, J. D., et al. (2000). Sex-specific expression of gastrin-releasing peptide receptor: Relationship to smoking history and risk of lung cancer. *Journal of the National Cancer Institute, 92*(1), 24–33.

Speroff, L., & Fritz, M. (2005). Clinical gynecologic endocrinology and infertility (7th ed.). Baltimore: Lippincott, Williams & Wilkins.

Stoppard, M. (Ed.). (2002). *Woman's body: A manual for life.* New York: Dorling Kindersley.

Tanner, J. (1981). Growth and maturation during adolescence. *Nutrition Reviews, 39*(2), 43–55.

Tseng, J. E., Rodriguez, M., Roe, J., Liu, D., Hong, W. K., & Mao, L. (1999). Gender differences in p53 mutational status in small cell lung cancer. *Cancer Research, 59*(22), 5666–5670.

Vaccarino, V., Parsons, L., Every, N. R., Barron, H. V. & Krumbolz, H. M. (1999). Sex-based differences in early mortality after myocardial infarction. *New England Journal of Medicine, 341*(4), 217–225.

Venturoli, S., Flamigni, C., & Givens, J. (Eds.). (1985). *Adolescence in females.* Chicago: Medical Year Book.

Vom Saal, F., & Finch, C. (1994). Reproductive senescence: Phenomena and mechanisms in mammals and selected vertebrates. In E. Knobil, J. Neill, et al. (Eds.), *The physiology of reproduction* (pp. 2351–2413). New York: Raven Press.

Widmeier, E., Ruff, H., Strong, K. (Eds.). (2004). *Vander, Sherman, & Luciano's Human physiology: The mechanisms of body function* (9th ed.). Boston: McGraw-Hill.

Wise, P. (1989). Influence of estrogen on aging of the central nervous system: Its role in declining female reproductive function. In C. Hammond, F. Haseltine, & I. Schiff (Eds.), *Menopause: Evaluation, treatment, and health concerns* (pp. 53–70). New York: Alan Liss.

Wise, P., Weiland, N., Scarbrough, K., Larson, G., & Lloyd, J. (1990). Contribution of changing rhythmicity of hypothalamic neurotransmitter function to female reproductive aging. In M. Flint, F. Kronenberg, & W. Utian (Eds.), *Multidisciplinary perspectives on menopause* (pp. 31–43). New York: New York Academy of Sciences.

Young Women's Health

Janet Cady

The second decade of life is a time of rapid physical, emotional, social, and cognitive change. For young women, adolescence is a time to explore, learn, and grow in self-awareness as they form their own identities and prepare for their adult years. The state of a young woman's health and the decisions she makes during her adolescent and young adult years will impact her well-being for the rest of her life. It is essential, therefore, to focus on this unique period of change in a young woman's life and examine adolescent-specific research and clinical services.

This chapter contains an overview of young women's health, beginning with considerations of the demographic characteristics of adolescents in the U.S. population. Adolescent development occurs in stages as well as in several contexts, including the developing self in the context of family, peer, and community. Adolescents have typical and atypical experiences, and those who develop in the context of challenging circumstances require adaptations in their health care. Health services for adolescents are evolving in multiple settings, and the health services they need are driven by challenges in their development and the context in which they live their lives. Consideration of the special health challenges facing young women concludes the chapter.

AN OVERVIEW OF ADOLESCENCE IN THE UNITED STATES

Demographic Characteristics

Adolescents are a large and diverse part of U.S. society. Children ages 10 to 19 years old comprise approximately 14% of the U.S. population and total over 42 million (McKay, 2007). Geographically, adolescents are concentrated in urban and suburban communities, but their percentage of the overall population of the community is greatest in rural areas. They are more diverse than the general population, and that diversity will increase over the next decade due in large part to Hispanic, Asian, and Pacific Islander immigration (University of California, 2003). There has been a continued decrease in adolescents living in two-parent households over the last two decades. Overall, two-thirds of adolescents lived with two parents, yet the range is 77.8% for Asian adolescents to 38.4% for Black youth. Correspondingly, Black youth are most likely to live in poverty (32.3%), closely followed by Hispanic youth (28.6%), with a national average of 1 in 6 youth under 18 years of age living below the federal poverty line (University of California, 2003). This disparity is reflected in multiple health outcomes and has implications for health care policy and program design.

Each year, the Annie E. Casey Foundation publishes the *Kids Count Data Book*, intended to highlight key indicators of child well-being and assess trends at the state and national level. Ten key indicators are measured (see Table 5.1), and four of these specifically target adolescent health: teen death rate, teen birth rate, percent of teens who are high school dropouts, and the percent of teens not attending school and not working (Annie E. Casey Foundation, 2006). The trend for this decade in four key indicators focused on adolescent well-being has been positive.

The Centers for Disease Control and Prevention (CDC) have developed "21 Critical Objectives for Adolescent and Young Adults" as part of the *Healthy People 2010* initiatives (U.S. Department of Health and

Ten Key Indicators of Child Well-Being

KEY INDICATORS	2000	2004	% WORSE	% BETTER
Percent low–birth weight babies	7.6	8.1	7	
Infant mortality rate (deaths per 1,000 live births)	6.9	6.8		1
Child death rate (deaths per 100,000 children ages 1 to 14)	22	20		9
Teen death rate (deaths per 100,000 teens ages 15 to 19)	67	66		1
Teen birth rate (births per 1,000 females ages 15 to 19)	48	41		15
Percent of teens who are high school dropouts (ages 16 to 19)	11	7		34
Percent of teens not attending school and not working (ages 16 to 19)	9	8		11
Percent of children living in families where no parent has full-time, year-round employment	32	34	6	
Percent of children in poverty (income below $19,806 for a family of two adults and two children in 2005)	17	19	12	
Percent of children in single-parent families	31	32	3	

Note. From *2007 Kids Count Data Book,* by Annie E. Casey Foundation, 2007, Baltimore, MD: Annie E. Casey Foundation.

Human Services, 2000). These objectives prioritize the major morbidities and mortalities of 10- to 24-year-old youth and have set targets for measurable improvements. These initiatives are intended to focus public health interventions on adolescent and young adult death rate reductions, unintentional injury, violence, substance abuse, mental health, reproductive health, and chronic disease prevention.

Risk and Protective Factors

Although it is essential to develop interventions targeted at these health goals, the 21 Critical Objectives do not address the individual, family, or community's risk or protective factors, which have a direct link to health outcomes. Every two years, the CDC surveys 9th-through 12-grade youth in public and private schools with the Youth Risk Behavior Surveillance System

(YRBSS). The goals of the survey are to identify health problems in youth, identify trends in health risk-taking behaviors over time, and to focus the country on adolescent health problems. The YRBSS measures activities that contribute to unintended injuries; violence; tobacco, alcohol, and other drug use; sexual behavior; unhealthy eating patterns; and inadequate physical activity (Centers for Disease Control, 2006). The leading causes of death in adolescents are preventable. Motor vehicle accidents account for 31% of deaths in 10- to 24-year-olds followed by homicide (15%) and suicide (11%) (Derluyn & Broekaert, 2007). Although girls are less likely to die in adolescence than boys, they experience depressed moods, suicidal feelings, intimate partner violence, and bullying at alarming rates (Centers for Disease Control, 2006).

The negative consequences of adolescent risk taking, morbidity, and mortality have historically led to prevention and interventions focused on teen compliance, punishment, and shame. Over the last 20 years, examination of risk-taking adolescent behaviors and health outcomes revealed that both negative and positive factors contribute to health outcomes. Dahlberg and Potter (2001); Hawkins, Kosterman, Catalano, Hill, and Abbott (2005); and others have evaluated both risk and protective factors for violence and use of tobacco, alcohol, and other drugs. Their work has enhanced efforts of school-based and community intervention programs in building strengths and developing skills—in contrast to interventions that focus only on negative outcomes.

The Resiliency Model recognizes the ability of youth to buffer themselves from harm and remain healthy even when faced with multiple risk factors. Risk and protective factors are inversely related to each other as they affect health outcomes, and these factors can be identified in the individual, peers, family, school, and community. Youth with multiple risk factors and few protective factors have poorer health outcomes than youth with few risk factors and multiple protective factors. Examples of risk factors are individual lack of school commitment, friends who engage in drug use, family conflict, violence in the school, and community disorganization. Examples of protective factors include an individual's positive social orientation or resiliency, positive bonds with friends and within the family, a school's high expectation of youth, and opportunities for youth participation in the community. (Hawkins, Smith, & Catalano, 2002). Adelmann (2005) has linked protective factors with positive health behaviors in 6th-grade students: seat belt use, participation in exercise and recreation, quality nutrition intake, and academic achievement. Conversely, his findings reveal that individuals with multiple risk factors had significantly higher negative health behaviors. Because African American youth are disproportionately represented in every negative health measure (Centers for Disease Control, 2006), Barrow, Armstrong, Vargo, and Boothroyd (2007) examined the resiliency of African American adolescents and identified specific protective factors to be fostered: self-efficacy, positive ethnic and racial identity, and commitment to the family and community. In African American youth, the development of ethnic pride was linked with parental influence, self-esteem, and self-control and therefore had a protective impact on risk-taking behaviors (Wills et al., 2007). School environments and academic connectedness combine to create a strong protective factor for youth. Using social and school connectedness as predictors of future health outcomes, Bond and colleagues (2007) studied 8th-grade students and then measured them again in year 2 and year 4. They found that positive social and/or school connectedness was associated with positive outcomes (school achievement, mental health, and substance abuse) in the 10th and 12th grades. In addition, they found that having both social and school connectedness was associated with the best outcomes. Resiliency has a positive impact on youth development. Youngblade and colleagues (2007) studied a sample of over 42,000 adolescents, age 11 to 17, from the 2003 National Survey of Children's Health. They conclude that multiple family, school, and community protective factors have a positive influence on youth health behaviors. No single influence in an adolescent's life provides protection from violence, substance abuse, or poor health outcomes, but the individual, family, school, and community all contribute to a strong foundation for positive youth development.

Adolescent Stages of Development

In this context, throughout adolescence, young women are simultaneously individuating and in relationship with others. Development occurs in physical, social, spiritual, and emotional growth as well as in cognitive and moral development. Multiple theories have been developed to enhance our understanding of developmental stages. Each theory provides "an organized set of concepts and statements related to significant questions about a particular domain of knowledge" (Rew, 2005, p. 24). Throughout adolescence, young women are moving toward integration of the whole. Central to the discussion in this chapter is the notion that young women are simultaneously embodied selves and relational selves. The embodied self refers to the simultaneity of physical experiences with the self. The body is inseparable from the self, and yet a woman can contemplate her body. Although women's lives have historically been limited by others' assumptions that they are reducible to their bodily functions (for example, as reproductive machines), women also have unique bodily experiences, such as menstruation, that influence their life experiences and how they experience their bodies. Understanding embodiment means embracing the bodily being, not accepting the dualistic notions about the separateness of body and self.

The relational self refers to the self as one in which relationships are a central and positive aspect of development throughout the life span. Young women are confronted with the reaction in the self to a changing physical body at the same time they face complex reactions from others (Porter, 2002). Development occurs within the context of relationships (Cox & Brooks-Gunn, 1999). Self-in-relationship framework, a product of contemporary developmental theorists such as Jean Baker Miller and Carol Gilligan, defines a woman's orientation as it is influenced by socialization. In *Reviving Ophelia: Saving the Selves of Adolescent Girls,* Pipher (1994) acknowledges this female need for socialization and the conflicting messages young women receive from those connections. Young women, therefore, are challenged with internal reconciliation or discord from the personal and social worlds in which they exist.

Definitions of Adolescence: Stages

There are multiple ways to define the boundaries of adolescent development, and there is no consensus. Researchers, clinicians, parents, and youth themselves debate when adolescence begins and ends. For girls, thelarche marks the first physical sign of pubertal change and is often accompanied by some of the emotional changes of adolescence, but this may occur in girls as young as 7 or 8 years old. Another view of adolescence is to consider the academic periods of adolescence: middle school, high school, and post–high school. Considerations for extending adolescence up to 24 or 25 years of age reflect the emerging science on brain development and the tasks of emancipation that extend well into the 20s for some youth (Galvan, Hare, Voss, Glover, & Casey, 2007). Whatever marks the beginning and end of adolescence, there is wide acceptance of three distinct developmental periods (Neinstein, 2008).

Early adolescence: 10- to 13-year-olds, linked with middle school years

Middle adolescence: 14- to 17-year-olds, linked with high school

Late adolescence: 17- to 21-year olds, linked with later high school, college, military service, or employment

The essential goals of the adolescent years are to emerge with:

- Sound mind and body
- Basic life skills and abilities in critical thinking
- Responsible sexuality and ability to establish strong attachments
- Skills to avoid addiction to drugs and alcohol
- Intellectual and moral capability to participate in society (Carnegie Council on Adolescent Development, 1993)

Each phase of a young woman's development contributes to her overall health and well-being and will be the foundation for her successful emergence from adolescence and the transition to womanhood. Early, middle, and late adolescent young women are seeking independence, identity development, social skills and connections with peers, and body awareness. According to Erickson (1963, 1968), adolescents and young adults must develop their identity to avoid role confusion. In Piaget's (1973) cognitive theory, the focus is for the adolescent to proceed from concrete operational thinking to formal operational thoughts characterized by abstract thinking. This ability to think about thinking and seeing the future becoming a possibility is essential in identity formation. An extension of Piaget's work, Kohlberg's (1981) moral development theory discusses movement from conventional moral reasoning—making judgments based on what is right because of society's regulation—to postconventional morality—making judgments based on universal principles of justice. Carol Gilligan's work developed as a result of her affiliation with Kohlberg and examination of how gender variables challenged the moral development theory. Through further investigation, Gilligan (1982) identified how girls construct moral dilemmas in terms of caring, responsibility, and relationship and not in terms of right, wrong, and rule making. Rew (2005) points out that adolescent girls recognize a disparity between care and power and many choose to abandon the concern for attaining and maintaining power and adopt the concern for caring.

Early Adolescence

The hallmarks of early adolescence are accompanied by the rapid physical changes of puberty in most girls. She becomes less interested in family activities and more focused on peers and begins to critique parental influences. The struggle for independence while still being dependent frequently creates family discord and is accompanied by wide mood swings in the young adolescent. Young women make strong attachments to a peer group and explore the joys and emotion of that intensity. She becomes increasingly aware, and yet insecure about her body, frequently comparing herself to others. Often young women will experience confusion about their physical body's impact on others in their social network and in the community. She begins to have sexual feelings and begins to privately question her thoughts and emotions. At this stage in a young woman's development, she is expanding her knowledge, beginning to abstractly process information, fantasize about the future, and daydream about idealistic goals. There is an intense focus on the self, accompanied by an overwhelming self-consciousness that Elkind and Bowen (1979) termed the "imaginary audience."

Middle Adolescence

Middle adolescence is marked by continued withdrawal from the family with a heightened interest in peer connections and adopting peer group norms. This separation from the family increases conflict in the home, and, depending on the adopted norms, the girl also may experience school and community conflicts as well. Middle adolescence is the height of delinquency, gangs, sports, and clubs, as each young person tries to find the powerful connections of a peer group. The middle adolescent begins to accept the physical changes of puberty and focuses on developing a personal identity within the peer group norms in terms of clothing, make-up, and hairstyle. This creative self-expression enhances identity development and body image. During middle adolescence, a young woman often feels omnipotent and ignores risk with the false impression that, "it can't happen to me!"

Late Adolescence

The foundation established during the early and middle adolescent stages supports the last phase of adolescence. The late adolescent stage is a time for the young woman to begin the transition to adulthood. If her previous experience with independence, peer group support, and identity development have been empowering, the young woman is well equipped to trust this next phase of her life. If, on the other hand, her early and middle stages of adolescence were not completed because of addiction, mental illness, eating disorder, or other chronic problems, the young woman will not be optimally prepared to accept the responsibilities and challenges of adult life. The tasks during this phase are to have body acceptance, a clear self-identity, and the ability to critique both parents and peers to make independent choices. With these skills, the young woman transitions to adult life, having met the goals of adolescence and ready to actively participate in adult society.

Changing Bodies, Changing Selves

Prior to menarche, young women experience dramatic changes in their bodies during a relatively short period, including a deposition of adipose tissue (up to 11 kg of body fat) as well as an increase in height (up to 25 cm), called the growth spurt (Tanner, 1962). In addition, premenarcheal girls experience adrenarche (growth of pubic hair, stimulated by androgens), thelarche (breast development stimulated by estradiol), and, late in puberty, menarche. Nearly two-thirds of girls experience menarche during Tanner's (1981) Stage 4 (Brooks-Gunn & Warren, 1985; Brooks-Gunn, Warren, Rosso, & Gargiulo, 1987; Tanner, 1962). The physiological basis of puberty and menarche is discussed more fully in chapter 4, "Women's Bodies."

In addition to sexual maturation, bone mass or bone mineral density increases. Physical activity level, heredity, nutrition, endocrine function, and medications can positively or negatively impact bone mass in adolescents. Peak bone mass is acquired by early adulthood, so adolescence is a critical time in acquiring bone density necessary for lifelong bone health. Other physical changes of puberty include growth of the internal organs, including the liver, kidneys, and heart. Significant biochemical changes also occur, including changes in serum alkaline phosphatase concentrations, serum ferritin, and erythrocyte mass (Neinstein, 2008). Of all the physical changes associated with puberty, among the most dramatic, unexpected, and misunderstood is the change in adipose mass. On average, girls who mature earlier tend to have higher body mass index , and slightly shorter girls who mature later tend to be lighter, leaner, and slightly taller when puberty is complete.

In recent years, there has been increasing focus on the developing adolescent brain and its role in social, behavioral, and psychiatric disorders. This work has found that social skills, decision making, and impulsiveness are significantly linked to measurable physiological changes in the brain. Nelson, Leibenluft, McClure, and Pine (2005) describe the brain's social information processing network and identify three nodes based on function and developmental timing: detection node, affective node, and cognitive-regulatory node. The associations of the adolescent brain's maturation, social inhibition, and risk-taking impulsivity are individualized and remain an area of emerging science (Galvan, Hare, Voss, Glover, & Casey, 2007). A woman's relationship to her body evolves over the life span, and adolescence appears to be a critical period for changes in a young woman's self-concept, body image, physical strength, and emotional well-being (Patton & Viner, 2007). Body image, an individual's mental representation of one's body, is critical to the formation of an individual's sexual identity (Lauffer, 1991).

A growing body of literature (Haudek, Rorty, & Hender, 1999; Hayward et al., 1997; Hayward, Gotlib, Schraedley, & Litt, 1999; Siegel, Yancy, Aneshensel, & Schuler, 1999) indicates that early puberty can be especially challenging for White, Asian, and Hispanic girls. The earliest-maturing girls begin puberty when peers are not experiencing these events and thus are at risk for problems, perhaps because they are not prepared for the physical, psychological, and social changes that occur in puberty (Brooks-Gunn, Petersen, & Eichorn, 1985). Early pubertal status has been found to be a predictor of frequent problems seen among adolescent girls (Angold, Costello, & Worthman, 1998; Hayward et al., 1999).

Although few have investigated the implications of pubertal timing for adult functioning, Serepca (1996) examined whether women's objective pubertal timing (their menarcheal age) and subjective timing (perceived timing relative to peers of menarche and breast development) influenced their adult body image and self-esteem. Objective pubertal timing did not differ on any of the body image or self-esteem variables. However, adult women who perceived themselves as early in breast development as compared to their peers described themselves as heavier, and were more preoccupied with being or becoming overweight. They were also less satisfied with their physical appearance than late-maturing women. Late maturers on both subjective timing measures, reported more positive body image attitudes than on-time and early maturers. This suggests that girls' pubertal growth may have lasting implications for women.

The evolutionary model of individual differences in pubertal timing (Belsky, Steinberg, & Draper, 1991) and data (Graber, Brooks-Gunn, & Warren, 1995) suggest that an individual's experiences during childhood may influence the physiological mechanisms that initiate and control pubertal development. Based on this model, individuals who grow under conditions of family stress are predisposed to respond to the stress situation by maturing early and engaging in relatively indiscriminate sexual behavior, while children growing up in nonstressed families are not so predisposed. Population studies in Poland provide strong support for the evolutionary model of individual differences (Hulanicka, 1999). An 8-year prospective study of 173 girls and their families found that, consistent with the model, fathers' presence in the home, more time spent by fathers in child care, greater supportiveness in the parental dyad, more father-daughter affection, and more mother-daughter affection, as assessed prior to kindergarten, predicted later pubertal timing by daughters in 7th grade. The positive dimension of family relationships, rather than the negative dimension, accounted for these relations (Ellis, McFadyen-Ketchum, Dodge, Pettit, & Bates, 1999).

A large body of research suggests that early-maturing girls are more likely than other girls to exhibit depressive, eating, and delinquent symptoms, as well as general behavior problems (Attie & Brooks-Gunn, 1995; Caspi & Moffitt, 1991; Graber, Brooks-Gunn, Paikoff, & Warren, 1994; Graber, Lewinsohn, Seeley, & Brooks-Gunn, 1997; Hayward et al., 1997; Petersen, Sarigiani, & Kennedy, 1991). In a national probability sample of 5th- to 8th-grade girls, pubertal stage was the stronger predictor of panic attack occurrence and eating disorder symptoms. Frequency of panic attack and eating disorder symptoms increased dramatically with advanced pubertal development (Hayward et al., 1999). In these same studies, late-maturing girls demonstrated no consistent pattern of adjustment problems when compared with on-time maturers. Most of the research in this area has been conducted with a subject pool consisting of primarily White middle-class female adolescents. Not all studies have found an association between pubertal status and depression among predominantly White samples. Studies with small sample sizes, less than 110, with multiple predictors using multivariate methods and pubertal status as one variable, have not found pubertal status predictive of depression (Brooks-Gunn & Warren, 1989; Paikoff, Brooks-Gunn, & Warren, 1991; Warren & Brooks-Gunn, 1989).

Graber and colleagues (1997) found that the risk not only for internalizing, depression, and anxiety but also externalizing behaviors is conferred to girls by early maturation. In their epidemiological study of 1,709 students, early-maturing girls were most likely to have attempted suicide. Cultural pressures for thinness may be particularly strong for early-maturing girls because they gain weight when other girls are still thin.

Fewer Mexican American adolescent girls experience body image distortion than Whites (Guinn, Semper, Jorgensen, & Skaggs, 1997). In a growing body of research, African American girls have been found to have higher and more stable self-worth and greater satisfaction with physical appearance compared to White girls (Brown et al., 1998; Doswell, Millor, Thompson, & Braxter, 1998; Parker, Nichter, Nichter, & Vuckovic, 1995; Siegel et al., 1999). This was found despite a higher mean body mass index among African American girls (Striegel-Moore & Smolak, 1996). In the first longitudinal study of African American girls (ages 9 to 14 years) followed over 5 years, these girls had higher body image scores and greater tolerance for higher body mass index than White girls. The authors suggest that a reason may be cultural differences in attitude toward physical appearance and obesity among Blacks (Brown et al., 1998). However, Siegel et al. (1999) found that heavier African Americans felt more negatively about their bodies than those who were leaner, suggesting that taking pride in their bodies does not insulate them from dominant social norms. Exposure to a dominant culture that denigrates different physical features may impact body image among African American young women (Williamson, 1998). Black girls who reported peer pressure were as likely as White girls to be dissatisfied with their weight and try to lose weight by dieting (Schreiber et al., 1996).

Menarche

McDowell, Brody, and Hughes (2007) have analyzed the change in menarche timing over the last century. Data from the 1999–2004 National Health and Nutrition Examination Survey (NHANES) on 6,788 women reveals a significant (.9 year) decline in self-reported age at menarche in all racial and ethnic groups. For women born before 1920, the mean age of menarche was 13.6 years. For women born in 1980 to 1984, the mean age was 12.5 years. To account for this decrease, researchers have identified multiple variables, including nutrition status, obesity, race, socioeconomic class, genetic predisposition, as well as environmental and societal influences (Cesario & Hughes, 2007; Lee et al., 2007). Young women from large families, living at high altitude or in rural communities, tend to have a later onset of menarche (Neinstein 2008). Menarche occurs 2 to 2.5 years after breast buds emerge, after the peak height velocity is completed, and at a sexual maturity rating of 3 or 4 (see chapter 4).

In a study by Rapkin, Tsao, Turk, Anderson, and Zeltzer (2006), the ability of young women to self-identify pubertal status was compared with hormonal markers of pubertal development: estradiol and follicle-stimulating hormone concentrations. They examined 124 healthy girls ages 8 to 18 years old and found that self-report of sexual maturity/Tanner staging was as accurate as hormonal markers in evaluating pubertal stage of development.

FACTORS INFLUENCING ADOLESCENT DEVELOPMENT

Being Different

Being "different" during adolescence can impact all aspects of development, including identity formation, engagement with peers, and the transition to adulthood. As adolescents mature, there is a natural focus on the self and the self in relationship or comparison to others. All youth experience the feelings of not fitting in or questioning, "Am I normal?" Adolescents living outside the dominant norms of a society will have those feelings amplified in ways that impact their health, education, and social relationships. This section examines the impact on adolescents of disability; chronic illness; race and ethnicity; immigration and refugee status; socioeconomic and family status; and sexual orientation and identity.

Disability

Disabling conditions in adolescents have been recognized as having unique impacts on the progression of development. Children with special health care needs, as defined by the Maternal Child Health Bureau, include a broad array of disabilities: attention-deficit disorders, autism, cerebral palsy, developmental delay, and epilepsy, as examples (Sadof & Nazarian, 2007). For adolescents living with disabling conditions, there is a range of impact from each condition and some youth have multiple disabilities. Young women living with cerebral palsy, for example, may have mild to severe disability from the same diagnosis. It is, therefore, difficult to generalize the effect disability has on an individual adolescent.

It is essential to provide coordinated care by a health care team experienced in working with adolescents with special health care needs. This type of "Medical Home" provides services with a focus on transition to adulthood (for more information, consult the Web site MedicalHomeInfo.org). The coordination of health services for special needs children in rural areas can have a positive impact on reducing family stress, school absences, and utilization of ambulatory health care (Farmer, Clark, Sherman, Marien, & Selva, 2005). The Medical Home incorporates seven integral elements into the health care of young people and their families:

- Accessible
- Compassionate
- Comprehensive
- Continuous
- Coordinated
- Culturally Effective
- Family Centered (Medical Home Initiatives for Children With Special Needs Project Advisory Committee, 2004)

Transition services for youth with special health care needs are a requirement of the Individuals with Disabilities Education Act (Betz, 2007). These services assist in the preparation of youth to fully participate and be included in adult society by focusing on access to health care, educational and employment transition, social and recreation networks, community living skills, and quality of life (Betz, 2007; Sadof & Nazarian, 2007).

Chronic Conditions

Most adolescents are physically healthy when compared with the general population, amplifying the influence of chronic illness in this age group. It is estimated that 12% of adolescents live with a chronic health problem; the most common are diabetes mellitus, asthma, arthritis, epilepsy, and heart disease (Sawyer, Drew, Yeo, & Britto, 2007). Chronic health problems are defined as having three characteristics: (1) biological, psychological, or cognitive basis; (2) expected to last longer than 12 months; and (3) having limitations that require medication, diet, personal assistance, or medical technology, or limitations in function in activities or social roles, or the need for medical care or accommodating services that would be unique for the person's age (Sawyer et al., 2007). Youth with chronic conditions make decisions to take health risks at rates equal to or greater than their same-age peers, yet put themselves at greater risk for negative consequences; poor medication adherence, pregnancy, substance abuse, and so on can each compound chronic health conditions and influence the health status of young women (Sawyer et al., 2007). Women with disabilities experience up to 50% greater risk for violence and exploitation (Rosen, 2006). Women with disabilities and special health care needs are more likely to experience unemployment than are men, and Betz (2007) describes the long-term consequences of poverty, limited access to health care insurance, and barriers to community services as factors in the quality of life for disabled adults. Young women with disabilities and chronic health conditions need coordinated health services and reduced barriers to care to facilitate a safe transition to adulthood.

Race/Ethnicity

Adolescents and young adults from minority racial and ethnic groups experience inequities in health status and outcomes (Park, Paul Mulye, Adams, Brindis, & Irwin, 2006). Health disparities between African American and White women continue to exist when comparing reproductive health outcomes (infant and maternal mortality, unintended pregnancy, and access to preventive health care (Anachebe & Sutton, 2003). After age 18, many young adults have barriers to health insurance and experience low rates of coverage, but Black and Hispanic young adults are most likely to be uninsured (Adams, Newacheck, Park, Brindis, & Irwin, 2007). A study of adolescents in New York State with publicly funded health insurance demonstrated that youth utilized available health services and reduced unmet health needs (Klein et al., 2007). National, state, and community interventions to address racial and ethnic health disparities among youth must focus on improvements in access while also focusing on the quality of available care.

Immigrant/Refugee

The foreign-born population of the United States is increasing and the Center for Health and Health Care in Schools (2007) at George Washington University reports that most immigrants come from Mexico (39%), followed by Asia and Pacific Islands, Central America and the Caribbean, Europe, South America, and Africa. In the 2000 census, one in five children in the United States were born to immigrant parents, and it is projected that, by 2020, nearly one in four children will be of Hispanic origin (Center for Health and Health Care in Schools, 2007). Because they often lack health insurance and are more likely to live in poverty, immigrant and refugee youth are especially vulnerable in U.S. society. Yet those same youth often have protective factors that aid in their adjustment to a new country: two-parent families, strong commitment to the family unit, and a solid work ethic. In a survey of 5,801 youth in a California data sample, first-generation Asian and Latino youth, when compared with White youth, reported spending more time playing video games or viewing television and less time participating in physical activity. They also reported less use of seat belts, bike helmets, and sunscreen (Allen et al., 2007). In a study of parent refugee status and impact on adolescent risk taking, Spencer and Le (2006) found a strong link between parent refugee status and externalizing teen violence in Southeast Asian and Chinese youth. A review of mental health in child and adolescent refugees identified several mediating factors in their reaction to multiple stressors in their lives: coping strategies, belief systems, and social relations (Lustig et al., 2004). Immigration waves and refugee migration are linked with war and social unrest in the country of origin. Many of these families and youth have been exposed to violence and may have experienced or witnessed torture. A study of Somali and Oromo adolescents revealed a link between the amount of exposure to violent acts and resulting post-traumatic stress, as well as physical, psychological, and social problems (Halcon et al., 2004). The study also identified gender differences among the youth; girls were more likely to report feelings of aloneness, even though they were more likely to be partnered, married, or to be with their mothers. Silverman, Decker, and Raj (2007) examined YRBSS data from 1997 to 2003 in Massachusetts youth. They found immigrant girls reported less dating violence when compared with nonimmigrant peers, but this protective factor diminished once the girl became sexually active.

Sexual Orientation and Identity

Adolescence is a time for sexual identity development in all youth. Sexual orientation is a part of overall identity development, and the trajectory for this development varies among adolescents. Many youth experience same-sex attractions and romantic friendships, and, among girls, approximately 10% report sexual contact with another girl (Brown & Melchiono, 2006). There has been increasing study of gay, lesbian, bisexual, transgender, and questioning (GLBTQ) youth, their sexual identity development, and health risks (Saewyc et al., 2006). As a group, GLBTQ youth experience higher rates of family violence, homelessness, substance abuse, depression, and suicidality than their heterosexual peers. Kulkin (2006) has explored the impact of living in a heterosexist society on the coping skills and mental health of lesbian youth. The stress and stigma of homosexuality can account for many of the increased health risks associated with GLBTQ youth. Eisenburg and Resnick (2006) examined suicide ideation and suicide attempts among nearly 22,000 adolescents with same-sex experience in the 2004 Minnesota Student Survey and compared them to protective factors: family connectedness, teacher caring, other adult caring, and school safety. They concluded that lack of supportive and caring environments accounted for suicidality and that same-sex experience alone was not the predictive variable. Organizations such as the Safe Schools Coalition and Parents, Families, and Friends of Lesbians and Gays can provide education, support, and contribute to increasing protective factors for youth and their families. In one study, by Nerdahl et al. (1999), pediatric nurse practitioners were studied for their comfort level and knowledge in adolescent health care. The nurse practitioners identified their lowest skill level in areas of greatest risk to adolescent health, including GLBTQ issues. Nurses can enhance their communication skills, confront personal bias, and develop cultural competency by utilizing available resources, such as the Gay, Lesbian, Bisexual, Transgender Health Access Project.

Web Resources:

www.safeschoolscoalition.org

www.pflag.org

www.glbthealth.org

Out-of-Home Youth

Out-of-home youth are defined as adolescents not living in their immediate family's or a guardian's home. These can include youth experiencing homelessness with their family or those living with relatives, friends, in foster care, or in detention facilities, as well as runaway youth or unaccompanied minors. Youth leave home for a variety of reasons, but neglect and sexual abuse are often triggers and consequently put youth at extreme risk for additional victimization. Thrane, Hoyt, Whitbeck, and Yoder (2006) examined the precursors to youth leaving home and compared rural with urban youth. Their findings suggest that rural youth leaving homes with high levels of physical violence initially stayed at home longer, but once leaving home utilized more delinquent subsistence strategies for survival. In a sample of 84 GLBTQ youth matched with 84 heterosexual youth all experiencing homelessness, the GLBTQ youth were much more likely to have experienced higher rates of violence, substance abuse, and frequent runaway. In addition, they identified more sexual partners and more psychopathology (Cochran, Stewart, Ginzler, & Cauce, 2002).

Youth living in foster care may have multiple health and educational needs during adolescence that contribute to barriers to emancipation. Leathers and Testa (2006) surveyed Illinois foster care case workers in charge of 416 youth and found that one-third of the youth had barriers to transition: mental health problems, developmental disabilities, or other special needs. Urban youth were receiving less service than their rural counterparts, and the more disabled the child with regard to employment, education, or physical health barriers, the less likely he or she was to continue to receive child welfare benefits; the most vulnerable youth were the least likely to receive services beyond the age of 18. In an Oregon study of foster care youth in special education compared with other special education students, it was found that foster care youth had lower academic performance and were likely to be maintained in a more restrictive classroom (Geenen & Powers, 2006).

Runaway youth are a transient and ever-changing population. Sanchez, Waller, and Greene (2006) utilized the 1995 and 1996 National Longitudinal Study of Adolescent Health to identify a data sample of over 10,000 respondents, ages 12 to 17. They report that, during the study year, 6.4% of youth ran away. Girls (7.5%) were more likely than boys to leave home, as were older youth (6.8%) when compared to younger adolescents. Youth not living with either parent produced the highest rates of runaway in the previous year at 11.4%, and, yet, 99% of all runaway youth returned "home" within 12 months (Sanchez et al., 2006). Adolescents not living with a biological parent may be living with a grandparent. Grandmothers' experiences as caregivers and their perceived burdens were examined by Dowdell (2004), who found that parental drug abuse was reported as the reason for grandparent care giving in 80% of the cases. Grandmothers reported their personal health was strongly correlated with the health of their grandchildren; nurses must recognize the relationship between the health of the children and grandmother caregivers.

Social Contexts for Adolescent Development

Parents

Parental influence is linked to multiple health outcomes in adolescents (Youngblade et al., 2007). The National Adolescent Health Information Center and Child Trends have published a summary paper, "The Family Environment and Adolescent Well-Being: Exposure to Positive and Negative Family Influence," which cites the following findings from multiple studies:

- Over three-quarters of all parents report very close relationships with their adolescent children.
- Many 15-year-olds report difficulty talking with their mothers and fathers about things that really bother them.
- Adolescents who live with two parents are more likely to have parents who know their whereabouts after school.
- Hispanic parents are less likely than White and Black parents to know who most of their adolescent's friends are.
- Foreign-born adolescents are more likely than their native-born peers to eat meals with their family.
- Adolescents with better-educated parents are less likely to be exposed to smoking and heavy drinking by their parents.
- Adolescents whose parents exercise are less likely to be sedentary themselves (Aufausser, 2006).

Girls (53%) were more likely than boys (42%) to report it was difficult or very difficult to communicate with their fathers, and both girls and boys reported less difficulty with their mothers (32%) (Aufausser, 2006). Positive parental involvement (time together, monitoring whereabouts) has influence on an adolescent's health and behavior and is linked with stronger school performance, abstinence from sex and tobacco, and lower rates of delinquency. Negative parental involvement (abuse, alcohol addiction, domestic violence) has been linked with poor school performance, delinquency, sexual risk taking, and substance abuse (Aufausser, 2006; Pate, Dowda, O'Neill, & Ward, 2007; Power, Stewart, Hughes, & Arbona, 2005; Resnick, Ireland, & Borowsky, 2004; Spencer & Le, 2006). Girls may be more responsive to family involvement and support from parents. One study demonstrates that girls are more likely than boys to abstain or reduce alcohol use when there are high levels of family connectedness, family supervision, and clear messages from parents regarding alcohol use (Sale et al., 2005). In addition, sexually active girls who have mother involvement are more likely to choose more reliable birth control methods and have lower rates of high-risk behavior (Harper, Callegari, Raine, Blum, &Darney, 2004; for additional resources, see http://www.guttmacher.org). In a study of African American young women, the perception of a good quality parent-adolescent relationship and consistent parental attitudes regarding sex were predictive of higher levels of sexual abstinence in their adolescent daughters (Maguen & Armistead, 2006). There is evidence that parents overestimate and underestimate the risky behaviors (sex, substance abuse, and violence) in their adolescent children (Yang et al., 2006). It is clear that adolescence is a time for parents to remain engaged in their children's lives and to continue to provide guidance, support, and set reasonable boundaries. Other caring adults in young people's lives make vital contributions to the child's well-being as well. Teachers, coaches, religious leaders, neighbors, relatives, and mentors all have essential roles in the lives of youth; families and communities can support the role of nonparental adults and adolescents to foster necessary attachments (Grossman & Bulle, 2006).

School, Peer, and Community

School environments have an impact on the development of risk and protective factors in adolescents, and positive interventions are linked with positive outcomes into adulthood (Hawkins et al., 2005). The school context includes adult supervision, peer relationships, physical activity, dietary decision making, and problem solving. Early school connectedness and positive social relationships with peers are predictive of future academic achievement, reduced substance abuse, and improved mental health later in high school (Bond et al., 2007). From the same sample, low levels of school

connectedness and/or social connectedness in the 8th grade increased risk of school dropout. Feeling physically safe is necessary for optimal functioning, and one study demonstrated that the level of perceived safety at school is linked with social competence and lower levels of negative externalizing behaviors (Youngblade et al., 2007). Schools provide an opportunity for girls to be physically active. Studies that have examined the involvement of girls with attempts to increase overall physical exercise have demonstrated little impact; this remains an area for future evaluation and intervention (Robbins, Gretebeck, Kazanis, & Pender, 2006).

The CDC provides ongoing evaluation of the School Health Profiles, which include health education, physical education, health services, food services, school policy and environment, and family and community involvement. The Institute of Medicine recommends at least one semester of school health education classes in high schools (for useful tools, see www.cdc.gov/Healthy Youth/schoolhealth/tools/htm). The goals of health education are intended to contribute to the Healthy People 2010 goals. The content of sex education has been controversial. School district policies regarding sex education are guided by local, state, and federal rules and regulations. Evidence shows that comprehensive sex education programs that provide information about both abstinence and contraception can help delay the onset of sexual activity among teens, reduce their number of sexual partners, and increase contraceptive use when they become sexually active. These findings were underscored in "Call to Action to Promote Sexual Health and Responsible Sexual Behavior," issued by former Surgeon General David Satcher in June 2001 (Satcher, 2001).

Unsupervised time with peers is linked with substance abuse and aggressive behavior, and the more evenings out per week has been correlated with increased drug and alcohol abuse, as well as physical fights and carrying a weapon (Gage, Overpeck, Nansel, & Kogan, 2005). These findings held true for both boys and girls. Peer influences on adolescent risk taking can be positive or negative and have related consequences on young women's health.

School dropout for teens is recognized as one of the 10 key indicators for child well-being (Annie E. Casey Foundation, 2006). School dropout is linked with multiple risks to health and overall well-being during adolescence and extending into adulthood.

> According to the U.S. Department of Commerce, high school dropouts are more likely to be unemployed and, when they are employed, earn less than those who completed high school. According to the National Center for Health Statistics, those who did not complete high school report worse health than their peers who did complete high school, regardless of income. (U.S. Department of Health and Human Services, Health Resources and Services Administration, Maternal and Child Health Bureau, 2006)

Chen and Paterson (2006) investigated the role of neighborhood socioeconomic status (SES) with perceived family SES and individual physical and mental health characteristics—including blood pressure, basal cortisol levels, and body mass index (BMI)—of 315 adolescents. Neighborhood SES alone was more predictive of high BMI and low cortisol levels, and, when both neighborhood and family SES were low, there were significant impacts on psychological factors, including hostility. Neighborhoods can provide a community safety net, but some neighborhoods may be a danger zone for adolescents. An examination of the neighborhood by Lambert, Brown, Phillips, and Ialongo (2004) demonstrated the link between neighborhood safety and predicted substance abuse among African American youth. Seventh-graders who perceived their neighborhood to be more disorganized—particularly with drugs, violence, or concerns for safety—were more likely to use tobacco and other drugs in the 9th grade. It is interesting to note that, for young women, personal attitudes regarding drug use and drug harmfulness mediated the neighborhood influence.

Workplaces

The CDC reports that, in 2006, approximately 2.4 million youth 16 to 17 years old were employed. "Because of their biologic, social, and economic characteristics, young workers have unique and substantial risks for work-related injuries and illness" (Department of Health and Human Services [DHHS], 2004). The National Institute for Occupational Safety and Health reports that, in 2005, 54 youth under the age of 18 died from work-related injuries. Moreover, in 2003, an estimated 54,800 work-related injuries and illnesses among youth younger than 18 years of age were treated in hospital emergency departments. Because only one-third of work-related injuries are seen in emergency departments, it is likely that approximately 160,000 youth sustain work-related injuries and illnesses each year. The U.S. Public Health Service has a Healthy People 2010 objective to reduce youth emergency department injury rates to 3.4 injuries per 100 full-time equivalents by 2010; the rate in 2003 was 4.4 injuries per 100 full-time equivalents (DHHS, 2004).

Late adolescents and young adult women are participating in military service in record numbers since the institution of the all-volunteer force in the 1970s (Quester, 2005). Nursing care of women recruits, service members, and veterans require special skills and awareness of the demands of military service. The natural adolescent developmental tasks of individuation, experimentation, and emancipation are challenged in the hierarchical military structure, which values obedience (Hardoff & Halevy, 2006). One study conducted at a Veterans Administration facility examined the link between military sexual assault, civilian sexual assault, and childhood history of sexual assault with a diagnosis of post-traumatic stress disorder (PTSD) and health care utilization (Suris, Lind, Kashner, Borman, & Petty, 2004). PTSD was more likely to be associated with military sexual assault, but these same women were utilizing fewer health care services. The impact of war was reviewed in a recent study of over 100,000 veterans and their mental health after military service in the Afghanistan and Iraq wars between 2001 and 2005. One-quarter received mental health diagnoses, and 31% had either a mental health or a psychosocial diagnosis, with the youngest of the veterans (18 to 24 years old) being more likely to have a mental health diagnosis (Seal, Bertenthal, Miner, Sen, & Marmar, 2007). This study did not include currently deployed or hospitalized members of the military because they are not yet transitioned to veteran status. This study also did not explore the impact of military service on the mental health of spouses, partners, and children.

Communities

Adolescents respond to positive and negative pressure from peers, neighborhoods, families, and schools every day. In addition, young people are continually filtering the powerful media messages that surround them. Youth today have grown up with 24-hour-a-day access to the Internet, television, and other media. In a society where one-third of 3- to 6-year-old children have a television in their bedroom (Vandewater et al., 2007), the impact of the digital age cannot be understated in the world of adolescents. In the new millennia, the influence of media on adolescent health will require additional examination. A recent review of literature noted that much of the media research done in the past 20 years with adolescents is now outdated, and it is recommended that, as we look to the future for best-practice recommendations and advice for families, expanding on this work is essential (Escobar-Chaves et al., 2005). Fears abound regarding adolescent risk taking and the Internet, and a recent study revealed the practice of teens putting personal information on MySpace, a popular social networking site online (Hinduja & Patchin, 2007). Through a random sample of MySpace personal pages, the authors report 0.3% of youth included a phone number, 8.8% included their full names, and 57% included a photo of themselves. The authors suggest that adolescents are aware of Internet safety precautions and are attempting to use the Internet responsibly. One study of the influence of mass media—television, magazines, movies, and music—on adolescent sexual behavior and intentions (L'Engle, Brown, & Kenneavy, 2006) reports a dose effect, linking more sexual activity and intention to engage in sexual behavior with a greater exposure to mass media. Chow (2004) conducted research on focus groups with a small number of adolescent girls and their response to popular magazines' health-related messages. Young women reported magazine messages were equated with thinness and perfection, and the need for a male companion to provide protection. Adolescents are immersed in media: cell phones and text messages, the World Wide Web, television, music, magazines, and the list will continue to expand. The wise nurse will strive to understand the emerging media influences on young women and encourage the development of skills in media literacy.

HEALTH SERVICES FOR ADOLESCENTS

Utilization of Health Services

Adolescents have the lowest rates of utilization of health services among all age groups, and, when they do present for care, they receive poor-quality health counseling and promotion messages (Ma, Wang, & Stafford, 2005). Racial and ethnic minorities and boys were least likely to receive health care. Most frequent reasons cited for youth obtaining health care were respiratory illness, general physical examinations, and, for girls, prenatal care. Targeted interventions to promote quality in adolescent health services demonstrate effectiveness. Klein et al. (2001) examined the implementation of the Guidelines for Adolescent Preventive Services into five Community and Migrant Health Clinics. They report improvements in providers reporting having given and, most importantly, adolescents reporting having received positive health counseling messages, comprehensive age-appropriate health screening, and health education materials. Parent involvement can be hampered by language barriers and poor communication between health care workers (Clemans-Cope & Kenney, 2007), but parents have a vital role in the health care and promotion of their children. Most early adolescents have adequate health insurance, but with increasing age are more likely to be uninsured (Adams et al., 2007). The World Health Organization has created a framework for adolescent-friendly health care facilities. The main goals are to support adolescent health care that is equitable, accessible, acceptable, appropriate, and effective (Tylee, Haller, Graham, Churchill, & Sanci, 2007). State, national, and international efforts are underway to remove barriers to adolescent health care delivery, improve quality of the services provided, and focus on improving health outcomes.

School-Based Health Services

In response to adolescents' low utilization of traditional health services and high rates of preventable negative health outcomes, school-based health services are expanding across the country. The first school-based and school-linked health clinics (SBHCs) were established in the early 1970s with the main goals of reducing soaring teen pregnancy rates and rates of sexually transmitted diseases and infections; SBHCs have expanded into comprehensive health services in most clinic sites (Fothergill & Ballard, 1998). An excellent resource is the site for the National Assembly for School-Based Health Care at www.nasbhc.org. There have been multiple benefits demonstrated from SBHCs, including utilization increases in both mental health and physical health services, cost reductions, improved school attendance, and a reduction in emergency room utilization among regular users of the clinics (Key, Washington, & Hulsey, 2002). School-based health clinics are in addition to school nurse services provided in schools. The health clinics are often affiliated with a local health care facility—hospital, clinic, or public health department—and are funded by state general funds, maternal child health block grants, tobacco taxes, or tobacco settlement dollars (Center for Health and Health Care in Schools, 2002). The National Assembly for School-Based Health Care has advocated the following principles and goals for school-based health care: supports the school goals, responds to the community, focuses care on the student, provides comprehensive care, includes health promotion activities, implements high-quality systems, and provides leadership in adolescent and child health. Costello-Wells, McFarland, Reed, and Walton (2003) reviewed school-based mental health care provided to adolescents in four urban high schools and noted a reduction in barriers to care as well as opportunities for multidisciplinary teamwork on behalf of youth. Even with the advent of expanded services in some schools, gaps remain in linking the most high-risk students with appropriate care (Santor, Poulin, LeBlanc, & Kusumakar, 2006). SBHC complements community health care and is not intended to replace primary providers. SBHC provides increased access for all adolescents to both medical and mental health services. (Juszczak, Melinkovich, & Kaplan, 2003)

Consent and Confidentiality

In the United States, rules and regulations regarding adolescent rights to consent for health care vary by state. Consent defines the legal ability to obtain health services, and confidentiality is the ability to choose when to disclose the content of that care. Individual states govern the minor's rights to obtain reproductive health care, mental health services, and substance abuse assessment and treatment. Reproductive health care can include contraception, sexually transmitted diseases and infections assessment and treatment, pregnancy services, and termination of pregnancy care. Defining individual minor's rights in each state is outside the scope of this text, but updated information for each state and the District of Columbia can be found through the Center for Adolescent Health & the Law (www.cahl. org) and the Guttmacher Institute (www.guttmacher. org). Rights to confidentiality and the ability to consent change frequently, and each year there are new attempts by state legislatures to limit or expand rights of parents/ guardians and adolescents. A young woman must understand that there are legal and ethical situations when confidentiality will be broken. If she discloses intent to harm herself or someone else, it is the professional responsibility of the nurse to break confidentiality and obtain all necessary services to maintain safety for all involved. In addition, if the young woman is a minor and has been assaulted or abused, she is subject to state laws governing child protection (www.childwelfare. gov). It is the nurse's responsibility to understand and follow the rules in the state where she or he practices.

Health Care Visits for Adolescent Women

Young women may present for health care without their parents, or another caring adult, for the first time during their adolescence. If the parent or another adult is present, it is important to allow for a portion of the visit to be with the young woman alone. This can be accomplished by simply stating, "I am glad you are here for this visit together. Now that ___ is getting older, it is important for her to have part of this visit by herself. After we have talked together, I will ask you to leave, so she and I have a chance to talk in private." This is the optimal time to guide the young woman and her parent through her rights to confidentiality and consent. The parent or guardian may also have concerns to address without the adolescent present. It is essential to provide clear introductions, agree on the goals of the visit, and allow the young woman to express her health concerns. Preventive health care guidelines for adolescent girls have been developed by national health organizations: *Bright Futures: Guidelines for Health Supervision of Infants, Children, and Adolescents,* sponsored by a collaborative based in the Department of Health and Human Services and the American Academy for Pediatrics; Guidelines for Adolescent Preventive Services, developed by the American Medical Association; and Primary and Preventive Health Care for Female Adolescents, published by the American College of Obstetricians and Gynecologists. National guidelines are utilized to improve the quality of care and to emphasize comprehensive health services, including anticipatory guidance, targeted health screening, immunizations, and physical exam components. *Bright Futures: Guidelines for Health Supervision of Infants, Children, and Adolescents* (3rd ed.), recommend annual visits for health screening and anticipatory guidance (Hagen, Shaw, & Duncan, 2008).

Bright Futures incorporates a focus on the major morbidities and mortalities of adolescence and, therefore emphasizes the importance of risk reduction, injury prevention, pregnancy and sexually transmitted disease prevention, physical growth and development, social and school connectedness, and mental health. National guidelines are reviewed and updated regularly to reflect trends in health indicators and evidence-based research.

The first step in establishing care with adolescents is to create a foundation of a trusting relationship. Earlier in this chapter, we identified this concept as vital to the young woman. Making connections is time well spent and requires nursing skill and patience. The foundation is the clinician's introduction of herself or himself and her or his role, clarifying the goals of the visit and explaining consent and confidentiality. It is important to explain the transitions in the history so there are no surprises—for example, "Now I would like to talk with you about school." Offer the adolescent as many choices as are practical and provide justifications for clinical decision making. Based on the Imaginary Audience theory of Elkind and Bowen (1979), adolescents will be naturally self-conscious about personal discussions. It is useful to preface the discussion with, "I talk with all the young women I see about _____." The natural egocentrism of adolescents and the stages of psychosocial development necessitate careful use of feedback. Provide feedback that is direct, sincere, hopeful, and building on the young woman's protective factors and strengths. Barriers to effective communication with young women include generalizations and labeling, accusations, blaming, and threats; they have no role in harm reduction or health promotion.

Bright Futures (Hagen et al., 2008) recommends that components of a comprehensive adolescent health history include discussion of the following:

- Physical development
  - ☐ What changes have you noticed in your body since your last visit?
  - ☐ How do you feel about your body and how it is changing?
- Social and emotional development
  - ☐ What do you do for fun in your free time?
  - ☐ Do you have a best friend?
  - ☐ What are some of the things that make you sad? Angry?
  - ☐ What are four words you would use to describe yourself?
- Health habits
  - ☐ What do you do to stay healthy?
  - ☐ What do you do to get exercise and move your body?
  - ☐ When was the last time you saw a dentist?

- Nutrition and dietary habits
  - ☐ What and when do you usually eat?
  - ☐ How often does your family eat meals together?
  - ☐ Do you do things to gain, lose, or manage your weight?
- Safety—car, bike, personal, home, community
  - ☐ Do you wear a seatbelt? Sometimes, rarely, always, never?
  - ☐ Do you feel safe in your home?
  - ☐ Do you feel safe in your neighborhood?
  - ☐ Do you ever carry a weapon?
- Relationships and sexuality
  - ☐ Have you gone out with anyone or started dating?
  - ☐ Have you ever had sex before?
  - ☐ Do you have sex with males, females, or both?
  - ☐ Let's talk about birth control and sexually transmitted diseases.
- Family functioning
  - ☐ Every family is different—how do you get along with the people in your family?
  - ☐ Who lives in your home?
- School and/or vocational performance
  - ☐ Where do you go to school? What grade are you in?
  - ☐ How are you doing in school? Are you getting any special help in school?
  - ☐ Do you have a job?

An acronym is commonly used in adolescent health care to support a comprehensive focus of each visit, and Ginsburg (2007) has proposed one that includes protective factors in a young person's life and a review of the person's strengths. The new format is SSHADESS (see Table 5.2):

- **S**trengths
- **S**chool
- **H**ome
- **A**ctivities
- **D**rugs/substance abuse
- **E**motions/depression
- **S**exuality
- **S**afety

The Physical Examination and Laboratory Screening

The physical examination is a small component of the overall assessment of the adolescent patient. The new *Bright Futures* recommendations (Hagen et al., 2008) include a physical examination for each health supervision visit. The physical examination will include weight, height, body mass index, blood pressure,

 5.2 | The SSHADESS Dimensions: Protective Factors and Personal Strengths in Young Person's Lives

SSHADESS DIMENSIONS	SAMPLE QUESTIONS/COMMENTS
Strengths	Tell me some of the things you like best about yourself. Tell me what your friends would say are the best things about you.
School	How is it going for you in school? What are the best and hardest things about school?
Home	How is it going for you at home? What responsibilities or chores do you have in your home?
Activities	What do you like to do with your friends? If you had half a day and could do whatever you wanted, what would you do?
Drugs and substance abuse	At some point in growing up, everyone faces decisions about tobacco, alcohol, and drugs. Do you have friends that smoke or drink?
Emotions and depression	Being healthy is more than being able to run around the track or not having broken bones, but has a lot to do with how we feel about ourselves, how connected we are at home, school, and with our friends. How have you felt over the last couple of months? Do ever think about hurting yourself or dying?
Sexuality	What questions do you have about your body and how it works? If you were with someone you really liked and they wanted to have sex but you did not, what would you do?
Safety	When you are out with your friends, do you feel safe? Do you know how to swim? What would you do if your ride home was drunk or high?

a complete physical examination including dental screening, and sexual maturity rating/Tanner staging. Vision and hearing screening questions should be completed during each preventive care visit. Vision testing is recommended during each phase of adolescence—early, middle, and late (Hagen et al., 2008). Audiometry is performed based on risk assessment. The pelvic exam is no longer an essential part of every young woman's annual examination. With the advent of urine-based sexually transmitted disease and infection screening and consensus on national cervical screening guidelines, adolescents obtain pelvic examinations based on risk factors. The cervical screening guidelines for young women recommend initiating screening three years after coitarche and at least by age 21 (Saslow et al., 2002). The first pelvic examination is an excellent opportunity for health promotion and education about the female body. Providing a clear explanation about the equipment and the procedure, allowing time for the young woman to ask questions, and allowing a friend or family member to be present will reduce her anxiety and increase her cooperation. Creating a positive experience for the adolescent's first pelvic exam provides the foundation for future preventive gynecological care. It is also is an investment in developing a respectful partnership with the young woman. All young women who are sexually active, with males, females, or both must be screened for sexually transmitted infections. Screening recommendations are based on local incidence of infection, but generally any sexually active young woman is screened annually for chlamydia and gonorrhea (Branson et al., 2006). In September 2006, the CDC released revised recommendations for HIV testing of adults, adolescents, and pregnant women. The new recommendations advise routine HIV screening of all adolescents in health care settings in the United States. Implementation of these new guidelines and reducing the barriers to HIV testing are current challenges in ambulatory care settings. Syphilis screening is recommended for high-risk youth—which includes those who have multiple partners; do not use a condom or barrier method; exchange sex for drugs, money, or services; have spent time in jail or detention; are homeless; use intravenous drugs; and any adolescent with a sexually transmitted disease or infection. Other screening tests that may be performed as part of the young woman's preventive health visit, based on her history, include screening for anemia, tuberculosis, urinary tract infections, and dyslipidemia.

Immunizations

Immunizations are an essential and changing part of adolescent preventive health care services (Middleman et al., 2006). The CDC Advisory Committee on Immuni-

zation Practices (ACIP) currently recommends several vaccines for young adolescents ages 11 to 12:

■ Tetanus-diphtheria-acellular pertussis vaccine
■ Meningococcal conjugate vaccine
■ Human papillomavirus (HPV) vaccine for girls

In June 2006, the U.S. Food and Drug Administration approved Gardasil® for use among girls and young women aged 9 to 26. The vaccine prevents infection from the types of HPV most likely to lead to cervical cancer. Other vaccines for HPV are in development and will be available before the end of the decade.

It is recommended that all adolescents, if not previously immunized, receive the following vaccinations:

■ Hepatitis B series
■ Polio series
■ Measles-mumps-rubella series
■ Varicella (chickenpox) series—A second catch-up shot is recommended for adolescents who have previously received only one dose and have no history of chickenpox infection.

Additional vaccines are recommended for certain adolescents, either due to specific health conditions, exposure to household contacts, or employment that may increase their risk for transmission or infection:

■ Influenza
■ Pneumococcal polysaccharide
■ Hepatitis A

ACIP immunization recommendations are reviewed annually, and vaccine-preventable diseases or conditions are identified and vaccine schedules change. The CDC will maintain an up-to-date immunization schedule at www.cdc.gov/vaccines/recs/schedules/default.htm.

Sexual and Reproductive Health Concerns

Sexual and reproductive health is included in the care of all young women regardless of sexual behavior. As discussed in this chapter, sexual identity, sexual orientation, and sexual behavior are related but unique factors in adolescent development. In 2006, the Guttmacher Institute published Facts on American Teen's Sexual and Reproductive Health (Guttmacher Institute, 2006). This compilation of research on adolescent sexual behavior provides an overview of sexual activity, contraceptive use, access to contraceptive services, rates of sexually transmitted infections, pregnancy, childbearing, and abortion. The report states that nearly half of all 15- to 19-year-olds in the United States have had sex at least once. At age 15, approximately 13% of youth have had sex, but, by age 19, 7 in 10 teens have engaged in sexual intercourse. Most teenage girls (50%) report their first sexual partner was 1 to 3 years older than themselves. A striking number (10%) of young women aged 18 to 24 years old report their first sex was involuntary. Most teens (74% of girls and 82% of boys) report using some form of contraception during their first sexual experience. The most common method used by teens is condoms, and most youth (94%) report using them at least once. Teens are at risk for sexually transmitted infections; they represent one-quarter of the sexually active population yet account for nearly half of all new sexually transmitted infections.

The Guttmacher Institute reports that, each year, nearly 750,000 young women aged 15 to 19 become pregnant. This figure equates to 75 pregnancies per 1,000 young women aged 15 to 19 and represents a 36% decline from its peak in 1990. Delays in sexual activity and more consistent use of contraception in those who are sexually active have contributed to this decline. Pregnancy rates declined for all racial groups (36%), with the sharpest declines among Black teens (40%). Black young women continue to have the highest teen pregnancy rate (134 per 1,000 women aged 15 to 19), followed by Hispanics (131 per 1,000) and non-Hispanic Whites (48 per 1,000). Teen pregnancies are largely unplanned (82%). Two-thirds of teen pregnancies occur in older adolescents aged 18 to 19 years old. The birth rate to teens aged 15 to 19 dropped 31% from 1991 (62 births per 1,000) to 2002 (43 births per 1,000). Babies born to teens are at greater risk for health complications, including low birth weight. Teen mothers are also less likely to receive prenatal care or to engage in prenatal care late in their pregnancy. In 2002, 29% of 15- to 19-year-olds ended their pregnancies with abortion, compared to 21% for all women. Sixty percent of minors who had abortions involved at least one parent, and most of those parents supported their daughter's decision to terminate the pregnancy. The main reasons teens gave for having an abortion included concerns about how a baby would impact their lives, an inability to afford a child, and feeling insufficiently prepared to raise a child at that time in their lives.

Adolescent decision making regarding sexual behavior, contraceptive use, sexually transmitted diseases and infections, and pregnancy have lifelong impacts on young women's health, as well as that of their families and communities. Ginsburg (2007) emphasizes that providers of adolescent health services must balance the identification of risky behaviors while continuing to promote strengths. Providers and nurses can provide hope for the future and support risk reduction if there is an integration of health promotion, resiliency, and positive youth development into adolescent health care.

YOUNG WOMEN'S HEALTH PROBLEMS

Young women may experience other health problems that influence their quality of life and future health.

Breast health, contraceptive methods, and other topics related to adolescent health are covered in other chapters in this text. Multiple factors contribute to menstrual health. Primary amenorrhea is defined as no menarche by 14 years of age if there are no secondary sex characteristics, no menarche by 16 years old, no menses for 1 year after achieving sexual maturity stage (SMR) 5, or no menses in any female with the clinical features of Turner's syndrome (Neinstein, 2008). Primary amenorrhea requires an evaluation for potential congenital, hormonal, and genetic etiologies and is discussed in detail in other chapters. It is important to complete the medical evaluation while attending to the emotional and psychological needs of the adolescent.

Secondary amenorrhea occurs after menarche when a young woman has no subsequent menses for 6 months, or in a regularly menstruating female who has no menses for three cycles (Neinstein, 2008). By conducting a careful history, physical assessment, and standard laboratory tests, the etiology of amenorrhea can be determined. It is essential to rule out pregnancy as the first step in any evaluation. Menstrual health is a topic discussed in each health assessment for young women. The normal cycle is between 21 and 45 days, lasts 7 days or less, and is not excessively heavy (Adams Hillard, 2006). Dysmenorrhea is a common complaint in young women and usually is associated with normal ovulation in the absence of pelvic pathology. Ten percent of young women with dysmenorrhea, however, will experience severe symptoms and may have some pelvic abnormality (Harel, 2006). These women require further evaluation for underlying pathology that may contribute to their cyclic pain. Dysfunctional uterine bleeding is abnormal endometrial bleeding without structural pathology (Bravender & Emans, 1999). The most likely cause of dysfunctional uterine bleeding in adolescents is anovulatory cycles, yet there are a multitude of other possible etiologies, including pregnancy, pelvic inflammatory disease, hematologic disorders, endocrine disorders, systemic or chronic illnesses, trauma or abuse, medications, or previously undiagnosed gynecologic pathologies (Emans, Laufer, & Goldstein, 1998).

Polycystic ovarian syndrome (PCOS) is a complex progressive syndrome that can be observed in young adolescent girls and has future consequences on fertility and overall health. PCOS is caused by abnormalities in the hormonal feedback mechanisms of the hypothalamus-pituitary-ovary-adrenal axis and results in a constellation of possible signs and symptoms: hirsutism, chronic anovulation, weight gain or obesity, acne, and acanthosis nigricans (Jeffrey Chang & Coffler, 2007). These complications are the result of higher-than-normal levels of androgens and, if untreated, can cause damage to the ovaries, resulting in possible fertility problems and other health complications. Caught early in adolescence and with appropriate treatment, the clinical features of PCOS may be minimized. Ongoing investigation and clinical inquiry is necessary to know how future health may be impacted. Metabolic syndrome is linked to PCOS in some young women. This syndrome, with probable etiology in both genetic and environmental triggers, occurs in overweight and obese males and females resulting in hyperinsulinemia, hyperlipidemia, and hypertension (Harrell, Jessup, & Greene, 2006). The incidence of metabolic syndrome is correlated to the increasing rates of pediatric obesity and necessitates the involvement of the adolescent, family, school, and health care supports for successful intervention. Prevention of obesity, and early screening and identification of young women at risk, are paramount to preventing the development of heart disease, diabetes mellitus, and their sequelae. Helpful resources for young women with PCOS can be found at the Web site of the Center for Young Women's Health at Children's Hospital in Boston (http://www.youngwomenshealth.org/index. html). Identification of PCOS, treatment goals, and psychological supports must be developed in a partnership with the adolescent and parents, recognizing the complex emotional and identity development of adolescence.

Other topics of particular concern in young women's health are nutrition, dieting behaviors, eating disorders, mental health, and substance abuse.

Nutrition

Adolescence places new demands on nutritional status and emerging body image of growing young women. The body has increased demand for calories, protein, calcium, iron, zinc, vitamin C, and folic acid. Normal adolescent eating patterns are a challenge to evaluate, but, in contrast to childhood, teens have more meals independent of the family, frequently skip breakfast, eat frequent snacks, and increase their consumption of fast food or convenience foods. Ellyn Satter (1987), in her book, *How to Get Your Kid to Eat . . . But Not Too Much*, identifies "normal eating" as being able to choose foods that are enjoyable, becoming satisfied by them, and knowing when to stop. Satter also writes that normal eating is flexible and varies with emotions, schedules, hunger, and the availability of food. In a focus group study involving examination of the eating patterns and beliefs of 203 adolescent boys and girls, Croll, Neumark-Sztainer, and Story (2001) found a high level of knowledge about healthy eating recommendations, but identified multiple barriers in their daily routines: lack of time, limited availability of healthy food, and lack of concern about links to health consequences. Eating habits established during the new independence of adolescence are linked with lifelong eating behaviors and may contribute to future health status (Jenkins & Horner, 2005). Food availability and security, family socioeconomic status, and media advertising also play roles in determining food preferences and healthy eating (Taylor, Evers, & McKenna, 2005). Young women are at particular risk for establishing distorted eating patterns in early adolescence and during other periods of marked change, especially during the transitions of late adolescence. There is not one etiology for eating disorders, but rather a recognition of multiple contributing factors: biologic, familial, environmental, genetic, and social (Emans, 2000). Eating disorders are included in the *Diagnostic and Statistical Manual of Mental Disorders* (American Psychiatric Association, 2000) and include anorexia nervosa; bulimia nervosa; and eating disorder, not otherwise specified. The care of young women with disordered eating requires a team of professionals working in collaboration to support the adolescent, her family, and to manage the complex demands of her physical and emotional health.

Overweight and obesity are common concerns for young women and also have multifactor origins. Female awareness of weight, desire for thinness, and cyclic dieting patterns begin early in life and have been well documented to often start in grade school (Emans, 2000). As adolescent girls grow older, they are less likely to participate in vigorous physical activity or participate in school-based physical education. In a North Carolina study of 8th-grade girls, evaluated again in the 9th and 12th grades, a drop from 45% to 34% participation in vigorous exercise over the 4 years was identified. The results also note that 8th-grade participation in exercise was predictive of 12th-grade exercise patterns (Pate et al., 2007). Childhood and early adolescence must be the target of efforts to increase physical activity throughout adolescence and extending into adulthood.

Substance Abuse, Mental Health, and Suicidality

This chapter has addressed alcohol and substance abuse in the context of peer, family, and community influences on adolescents. Individual substance use is often best understood as a continuum: abstinence, experimental use, regular use, problem use, substance abuse, substance dependency, and secondary abstinence as part of recovery (Knight, Shrier, Bravender, Farrell, VenderBilt, et al., 1999). The CRAFFT questions developed by Knight and colleagues (1999) are suggested to review alcohol or other drug use and their impact in the adolescent's life (see Exhibit 5.1). The CRAFFT questions are intended for use in the development of a partnership with the adolescent and in forming an alliance for future health promotion. Two or more positive answers suggest a significant problem with alcohol or other drugs and necessitate further evaluation.

Tobacco use by teens in all age groups has been declining since the peak of the late 1990s. This may be the result of legislation to reduce access to tobacco, restrict smoking in public places, relatively high taxation

EXHIBIT 5.1 CRAFFT QUESTIONS

C Have you ever ridden in a **C**ar driven by someone (including yourself) who was high or had been using alcohol or drugs?

R Do you ever use alcohol or drugs to **R**elax, feel better about yourself, or fit in?

A Do you ever use alcohol or drugs while you are by yourself, **A**lone?

F Do you ever **F**orget things you did while using alcohol or drugs?

F Do your family or **F**riends ever tell you that you should cut down on your drinking or drug use?

T Have you ever gotten into **T**rouble while you were using alcohol or drugs?

of tobacco products, and social marketing campaigns aimed at youth (Evans et al., 2004). A positive note is the downward trend of tobacco use among 8th-, 10th-, and 12th-graders.

Mental health care is an integral component in the care of adolescent girls. In addition to eating disorders and substance abuse, young women are at risk for depression, anxiety, conduct and oppositional disorders, suicide, and the emergence of psychotic disorders. Women are more likely to experience depression across the life span and, during adolescence, are particularly vulnerable (Garber, 2006). In an examination of gender differences in coping styles by Li, DiGiuseppe, and Froh (2006), depressed young women were more likely to utilize ruminating and emotion-focused coping versus problem-focused and distractive coping skills.

Suicide is the third leading cause of death nationally, and in many states it is the second cause of death among adolescents. Suicide screening and prevention are recommended as part of health care for all adolescents. Young men are more at risk for dying by suicide, while young women report higher levels of depression and make more attempts at suicide (Centers for Disease Control, 2006). Young men typically choose more lethal methods in suicide—such as firearms, hanging, and motor vehicles—and consequently result in more deaths by suicide. Young women tend to choose medication or overdosing and self-cutting; these methods are usually not immediate and allow for help to arrive or be sought. There are questions regarding suicide ideations, planning, and attempts in the 2005 Youth Risk Behavior Surveillance System. By asking adolescents about their thoughts of sadness over the last year that occurred almost every day for 2 weeks or longer and that impacted their desire to participate in normal activities, 36.7% of girls and 20.4% of boys report feelings of depression. Hispanic girls report the highest levels of depression and have attempted suicide at higher rates than Black and White women. Suicidality is multifaceted and continues to be investigated to provide insights into adolescent mental health and suffering. In the United States in 2003, one-fifth of 12- to 17-year-olds received some counseling or mental health treatment and were most commonly seeking care for depressed feelings, breaking rules or

"acting out," disturbing feelings, or suicidal thoughts or attempts (U.S. Department of Health and Human Services, et al., 2006). There continue to be health disparities in access to quality mental health services, based on race/ethnicity, geography, socioeconomic status, and insurance coverage (Children's Defense Fund, 2003).

Adolescents are increasingly utilizing complementary and alternative medicine (CAM) to treat and manage their health concerns. In a study of a national sample of adolescents, 79% reported using CAM at some point in their lives and nearly 50% in the last month. Use of CAM was more common among girls and among middle and older adolescents (Wilson et al., 2006). In another focus group study, girls reported higher levels of use and knowledge of CAM, and adolescents with chronic health problems such as asthma, diabetes, and eating disorders were more likely to utilize alternatives to allopathic medicine. Examination of CAM use in youth with asthma revealed that nearly 80% of youth used some form of CAM and were most likely to use CAM if they had family exposure to CAM, a more severe illness, or had a past exposure to CAM (Reznik, Ozuah, Franco, Cohen, & Motlow, 2002). Commonly used CAM in this population were rubs, teas, supplements, prayer, and massage. In a national sample of parents of children and adolescents surveyed in 1996, only 2% of parents reported taking their child to a CAM practitioner, but those who did rarely reported this source of health care to their usual provider or clinic (Yussman, Ryan, Auinger, & Weitzman, 2004). It is important for nurses, families, and adolescents to work together to have a complete health history and shared goals for health promotion and healing.

With an understanding of adolescent development, health status, and health concerns, it is important to be skillful in health promotion and in establishing partnerships with youth. Traditional authoritarian methods have not been effective in changing behaviors or long-term health outcomes, but motivational interviewing (MI) has demonstrated promise in multiple fields (Gance-Cleveland, 2007). Motivational interviewing is a directive, client-centered counseling style for eliciting behavior change by helping clients to explore and resolve ambivalence (Rollnick & Miller, 1995). The purpose of MI is the establishment of a goal-oriented partnership that empowers the client to actively take responsibility for change. Rollnick and Miller (1995) describe MI as initiating from the client. MI does not utilize direct persuasion by a professional to resolve conflicts or ambivalence, but quietly and actively listens. MI recognizes that change is not absolute, but fluctuates over time.

In adolescent health promotion, these principles prove invaluable. Adolescents' developmental goals are to individuate, experiment, and begin to trust their ability to make health decisions independently. Utilization of MI aids the nurse in respectful care of the young woman, recognizing her current stage of development, and working with her to move toward responsible health care decisions. MI is being adapted to multiple settings other than the field of addiction and substance abuse treatment, where much of the research has been conducted (Resnicow, Davis, & Rollnick, 2006). One model that has been developed by Miller and Sanchez (1994) is FRAMES: *Feedback,* emphasis on *responsibility* for change, clear *advice* to change, *menu* of options, *empathetic* counseling style, and faith in *self-efficacy* to change.

Lifelong health patterns are established during adolescence and have profound consequences on individual development as well as the family's and community's health. Quality care of adolescents involves a comprehensive knowledge of the multiple factors that influence health and well-being, an ability to engage in effective communication with adolescents and their families, and advocacy in the community to promote access to quality care and reduce barriers to service. Nurses can participate in a dynamic partnership to enhance young women's health by recognizing risk and protective factors in the individual, family, peers, and community and working to build on the strengths and possibilities of adolescence.

REFERENCES

Adams Hillard, P. J. (2006). Adolescent menstrual health. *Pediatric Endocrinology Review, 3*(Suppl. 1), 138–145.

Adams, S. H., Newacheck, P. W., Park, M. J., Brindis, C. D., & Irwin, C. E., Jr. (2007). Health insurance across vulnerable ages: Patterns and disparities from adolescence to the early 30s. *Pediatrics, 119*(5), 1033–1039.

Adelmann, P. K. (2005). Social environmental factors and preteen health-related behaviors. *Journal of Adolescent Health, 36*(1), 36–47.

Allen, M. L., Elliott, M. N., Morales, L. S., Diamant, A. L., Hambarsoomian, K., & Schuster, M. A. (2007). Adolescent participation in preventive health behaviors, physical activity, and nutrition: Differences across immigrant generations for Asians and Latinos compared with Whites. *American Journal of Public Health, 97*(2), 337–343.

American Psychiatric Association. (2000). *Diagnostic and Statistical Manual of Mental Disorders* (4th ed.). Washington, DC: Author.

Anachebe, N. F., & Sutton, M. Y. (2003). Racial disparities in reproductive health outcomes. *American Journal of Obstetrics and Gynecology, 188*(4), S37–S42.

Angold, A., Costello, E. J., & Worthman, C. M. (1998). Puberty and depression: The roles of age, pubertal status and pubertal timing. *Psychological Medicine, 28*(1), 51–61.

Annie E. Casey Foundation. (2006). *Kids count databook.* Baltimore, MD: Annie Casey Foundation.

Attie, I., & Brooks-Gunn, J. (1995). The development of eating regulation across the life span. In D. Cicchetti & D. J. Cohen (Eds.), *Developmental psychopathology: Vol. 2. Risk, disorder, and adaptation.* New York: Wiley.

Aufausser, D., Jekielek, S., & Brown, B. (2006). The family environment and adolescent well-being: Exposure to positive and negative influences. Retrieved March 3, 2008, from http://nahic.ucsf.edu/downloads/FamEnvironBrief.pdf

Barrow, F. H., Armstrong, M. I., Vargo, A., & Boothroyd, R. A. (2007). Understanding the findings of resilience-related research for fostering the development of African American adolescents. *Child and Adolescent Psychiatric Clinics of North America, 16*(2), 393–413.

Belsky, J., Steinberg, L., & Draper, P. (1991). Childhood experience, interpersonal development, and reproductive strategy: An evolutionary theory of socialization. *Child Development, 62,* 647–670.

Betz, C. L. (2007). Facilitating the transition of adolescents with developmental disabilities: Nursing practice issues and care. *Journal of Pediatric Nursing, 22*(2), 103–115.

Bond, L., Butler, H., Thomas, L., Carlin, J., Glover, S., Bowes, G., et al. (2007). Social and school connectedness in early secondary school as predictors of late teenage substance use, mental health, and academic outcomes. *Journal of Adolescent Health, 40*(4), 357 359–318.

Branson, B. M., Handsfield, H. H., Lampe, M. A., Janssen, R. S., Taylor, A. W., Lyss, S. B., & Clark, J. E. (2006). Revised recommendations for HIV testing of adults, adolescents, and pregnant women in health-care settings. *Morbidity and Mortality Weekly Report, 55*(R-14), 1–17. Retrieved July 12, 2007, from http://www.cdc.gov/mmwr/preview/mmwrhtml/rr5514a1.htm

Bravender, T., & Emans, S. J. (1999). Menstrual disorders. Dysfunctional uterine bleeding. *Pediatr Clin North Am, 46*(3), 545–553.

Brooks-Gunn, J., Petersen, A., & Eichorn, D. (1985). The study of maturational timing effects in adolescence. *Journal of Youth and Adolescence, 14*(1), 149–161.

Brooks-Gunn, J., & Warren, M. (1985). Measuring physical status and timing in early adolescence: A development perspective. *Journal of Youth and Adolescence, 14*(3), 163–189.

Brooks-Gunn, J., & Warren, M. (1989). Biological and social contributions to negative affect in young adolescent girls. *Child Development, 60*(1), 40–55.

Brooks-Gunn, J., Warren, M., Rosso, J., & Gargiulo, J. (1987). Validity of self-report measures of girls' pubertal status. *Child Development, 58,* 829–841.

Brown, J. D., & Melchiono, M. W. (2006). Health concerns of sexual minority adolescent girls. *Curr Opin Pediatr, 18*(4), 359–364.

Brown, K. M., McMahon, R. P., Biro, F. M., Crawford, P., Schreiber, G. B., Similo, S. L., et al. (1998). Changes in self-esteem in Black and White girls between the ages of 9 and 14 years: The JHLBI Growth and Health Study. *Journal of Adolescent Health, 23*(1), 7–19.

Carnegie Council on Adolescent Development. (1993, June). *Promoting adolescent health: Third symposium on research opportunities in adolescence.* Retrieved July 11, 2007, from http://www.carnegie.org/sub/research/index.html#adol

Caspi, A., & Moffitt, T. E. (1991). Individual differences are accentuated during periods of social change: The sample case of girls at puberty. *J Pers Soc Psychol, 61,* 157–168.

Center for Health and Health Care in Schools. (2006.) Children of immigrant and refugees: What the research tells us. Retrieved August, 7, 2007, from http://www.healthinschools.org/%7E/media/Files/immigrantfs.ashx

Centers for Disease Control and Prevention. (2006). Youth risk behavior surveillance: United States, 2005. *Morbidity and Mortality Weekly Report, 55*(55-5).

Center for Health and Health Care in Schools. (2002). 2002 State survey of school-based health center initiatives. Retrieved August 7, 2007, from http://www.healthinschools.org/static/sbhcs/2002fs.pdf

Cesario, S. K., & Hughes, L. A. (2007). Precocious puberty: A comprehensive review of literature. *J Obstet Gynecol Neonatal Nurs, 36*(3), 263–274.

Chen, E., & Paterson, L. Q. (2006). Neighborhood, family, and subjective socioeconomic status: How do they relate to adolescent health? *Health Psychol, 25*(6), 704–714.

Children's Defense Fund. (2003, June). *Children's Mental Health Resource Kit.* Washington, DC: Children's Defense Fund.

Chow, J. (2004). Adolescents' perceptions of popular teen magazines. *J Adv Nurs, 48*(2), 132–139.

Clemans-Cope, L., & Kenney, G. (2007). Low income parents' reports of communication problems with health care providers: Effects of language and insurance. *Public Health Rep, 122*(2), 206–216.

Cochran, B. N., Stewart, A. J., Ginzler, J. A., & Cauce, A. M. (2002). Challenges faced by homeless sexual minorities: Comparison of gay, lesbian, bisexual, and transgender homeless adolescents with their heterosexual counterparts. *American Journal of Public Health, 92*(5), 773–777.

Costello-Wells, B., McFarland, L., Reed, J., & Walton, K. (2003). School-based mental health clinics. *Journal of Child and Adolescent Psychiatric Nursing, 16*(2), 60–70.

Cox, M., & Brooks-Gunn, J. (1999). *Conflict and cohesion in families: Causes and consequences.* Mahwah, NJ: Erlbaum.

Croll, J. K., Neumark-Sztainer, D., & Story, M. (2001). Healthy eating: What does it mean to adolescents? *J Nutr Educ, 33*(4), 193–198.

Dahlberg, L. L., & Potter, L. B. (2001). Youth violence: Developmental pathways and prevention challenges. *Am J Prev Med, 20*(Suppl. 1), 3–14.

Department of Health and Human Services (DHHS). (2004). *Worker health chartbook, 2004.* Retrieved March 3, 2008, from http://www2a.cdc.gov/NIOSH-Chartbook/ch5/ch5-2.asp

Derluyn, I., & Broekaert, E. (2007). Different perspectives on emotional and behavioural problems in unaccompanied refugee children and adolescents. *Ethnicity and Health, 12*(2), 141–162.

Doswell, W. M., Millor, G. K., Thompson, M. S., & Braxter, B. (1998). Self-image and self-esteem in African-American preteen girls: Implications for mental health. *Issues in Mental Health Nursing, 19,* 71–94.

Dowdell, E. B. (2004). Grandmother caregivers and caregiver burden. *MCN, The American Journal of Maternal Child Nursing, 29*(5), 299–304.

Eisenberg, M. E., & Resnick, M. D. (2006). Suicidality among gay, lesbian and bisexual youth: the role of protective factors. *Journal of Adolescent Health, 39*(5), 662–668.

Elkind, D., & Bowen, R. (1979). Imaginary audience behavior in children and adolescents. *Developmental Psychology, 15*(1), 38–44.

Ellis, B. J., McFadyen-Ketchum, S., Dodge, K. A., Pettit, G. S., & Bates, J. E. (1999). Quality of early family relationships and individual differences in the timing of pubertal maturation in girls: A longitudinal test of an evolutionary model. *Journal of Personality and Social Psychology, 77*(2), 387–401.

Emans, S. J. (2000). Eating disorders in adolescent girls. *Pediatrics International, 42*(1), 1–7.

Emans, S. J., Laufer, M. R., & Goldstein, D. P. (Eds.). (1998). *Pediatric and adolescent gynecology* (4th ed.). Philadephia: Lippincott Williams, and Wilkins.

Erickson, E. (1963). *Child and society* (2nd ed.). New York: Norton.

Erickson, E. (1968). *Identity, youth and crisis.* New York: Norton.

Escobar-Chaves, S. L., Tortolero, S. R., Markham, C. M., Low, B. J., Eitel, P., & Thickstun, P. (2005). Impact of the media on adolescent sexual attitudes and behaviors. *Pediatrics, 116*(1), 303–326.

Evans, W. D., Price, S., Blahut, S., Hersey, J., Niederdeppe, J., & Ray, S. (2004). Social imagery, tobacco independence, and the truthsm campaign. *Journal of Health Communications, 9*(5), 425–441.

Farmer, J. E., Clark, M. J., Sherman, A., Marien, W. E., & Selva, T. J. (2005). Comprehensive primary care for children with special health care needs in rural areas. *Pediatrics, 116*(3), 649–656.

Ford, C. A., English, A., & Sigman, G. (2004). Confidential health care for adolescents: Position paper. Society for Adolescent Medicine. *Journal of Adolescent Health, 35,* 160–167.

Fothergill, K., & Ballard, E. (1998). The school-linked health center: A promising model of community-based care for adolescents. *Journal of Adolescent Health, 23*(1), 29–38.

Gage, J. C., Overpeck, M. D., Nansel, T. R., & Kogan, M. D. (2005). Peer activity in the evenings and participation in aggressive and problem behaviors. *Journal of Adolescent Health, 37*(6), 517.

Galvan, A., Hare, T., Voss, H., Glover, G., & Casey, B. J. (2007). Risk-taking and the adolescent brain: Who is at risk? *Developmental Science, 10*(2), F8–F14.

Gance-Cleveland, B. (2007). Motivational interviewing: Improving patient education. *Journal of Pediatric Health Care, 21*(2), 81–88.

Garber, J. (2006). Depression in children and adolescents: Linking risk research and prevention. *American Journal of Preventive Medicine, 31*(6, Suppl. 1), S104–S125.

Geenen, S., & Powers, L. E. (2006). Are we ignoring youths with disabilities in foster care? An examination of their school performance. *Social Work, 51*(3), 233–241.

Gilligan, C. (1982). *In a different voice: Psychological theory and women's development.* Cambridge, MA: Harvard University Press.

Ginsburg, K. R. (2007). Viewing our adolescent patients through a positive lens. *Contemporary Pediatrics, 24*(1), 65, 67.

Gold, R. B. & Nash, E. (2001). State-level policies on sexuality, STD education. *4*(4). Retrieved March 3, 2008, from http://www.guttmacher.org/pubs/tgr/04/4/gr040404.htm

Graber, J. A., Brooks-Gunn, J., Paikoff, R. L., & Warren, M. (1994). Prediction of eating problems: An 8-year study of adolescent girls. *Developmental Psychology, 30,* 823–834.

Graber, J. A., Brooks-Gunn, J., & Warren, M. (1995). The antecedents of menarcheal age: Heredity, family environment, and stressful life events. *Child Development, 66,* 346–359.

Graber, J. A., Lewinsohn, P. M., Seeley, J. R., & Brooks-Gunn, J. (1997). Is psychopathology associated with the timing of pubertal development? *Journal of the American Academy of Child and Adolescent Psychiatry, 36*(12), 1768–1776.

Grossman, J. B., & Bulle, M. J. (2006). Review of what youth programs do to increase the connectedness of youth with adults. *Journal of Adolescent Health, 39*(6), 788–799.

Guinn, B., Semper, T., Jorgensen, L., & Skaggs, S. (1997). Body image perception in female Mexican-American adolescents. *Journal of School Health, 67*(3), 112–115.

Guttmacher Institute. (2006). *Facts on American teens' sexual and reproductive health.* Retrieved March 3, 2008, from http://www.guttmacher.org/pubs/fb_ATSRH.html

Hagen, J. F., Shaw, J. S., & Duncan, P. M. (Eds.). (2008). *Bright futures: Guidelines for health supervision of infants, children, and adolescents* (3rd ed.). Elk Grove Village, IL: American Academy of Pediatrics.

Halcon, L. L., Robertson, C. L., Savik, K., Johnson, D. R., Spring, M. A., Butcher, J. N., et al. (2004). Trauma and coping in Somali and Oromo refugee youth. *Journal of Adolescent Health, 35*(1), 17–25.

Hardoff, D., & Halevy, A. (2006). Health perspectives regarding adolescents in military service. *Current Opinion in Pediatrics, 18*(4), 371–375.

Harel, Z. (2006). Dysmenorrhea in adolescents and young adults: Etiology and management. *Journal of Pediatric and Adolescent Gynecology, 19*(6), 363–371.

Harper, C.,Callegari, L., Raine, T., Blum, M., & Darney, P. (2004). Adolescent clinic visits for contraception: Support from mothers, male partners and friends. *Perspectives on Sexual and Reproductive Health, 36*(1), 20–26.

Harrell, J. S., Jessup, A., & Greene, N. (2006). Changing our future: Obesity and the metabolic syndrome in children and adolescents. *Journal of Cardiovascular Nursing, 21*(4), 322–330.

Haudek, C., Rorty, M., & Hender, B. (1999). The role of ethnicity and parental bonding in the eating and weight concerns of Asian-American and Caucasian college women. *International Journal of Eating Disorders, 25*(4), 425–433.

Hawkins, J. D., Kosterman, R., Catalano, R. F., Hill, K. G., & Abbott, R. D. (2005). Promoting positive adult functioning through social development intervention in childhood: Long-term effects from the Seattle Social Development Project. *Archives of Pediatrics & Adolescent Medicine, 159*(1), 25–31.

Hawkins, J. D., Smith, B. H., & Catalano, R. F. (2002). Delinquent behavior. *Pediatrics in Review, 23*(11), 387–392.

Hayward, C., Gotlib, I. H., Schraedley, P. K., & Litt, I. F. (1999). Ethnic differences in the association between pubertal status and symptoms of depression in adolescent girls. *Journal of Adolescent Health, 25*(2), 143–149.

Hayward, C., Killen, J. D., Wilson, D. M., Hammer, L. D., Litt, I. F., Kraemer, H. C., et al. (1997). Psychiatric risk associated with early puberty in adolescent girls. *Journal of the American Academy of Child and Adolescent Psychiatry, 36*(2), 255–262.

Hinduja, S., & Patchin, J. W. (2008). Personal information of adolescents on the Internet: A quantitative content analysis of MySpace. *Journal of Adolescence, 31*(1), 125–146.

Hulanicka, B. (1999). Acceleration of menarcheal age of girls from dysfunctional families. *Journal of Reproductive and Infant Psychology, 17*(2), 119–132.

Jeffrey Chang, R., & Coffler, M. S. (2007). Polycystic ovary syndrome: Early detection in the adolescent. *Clinical Obstetrics and Gynecology, 50*(1), 178–187.

Jenkins, S., & Horner, S. D. (2005). Barriers that influence eating behaviors in adolescents. *Journal of Pediatric Nursing, 20*(4), 258–267.

Juszczak, L., Melinkovich, P., & Kaplan, D. (2003). Use of health and mental health services by adolescents across multiple delivery sites. *Journal of Adolescent Health, 32*(Suppl. 6), 108–118.

Key, J. D., Washington, E. C., & Hulsey, T. C. (2002). Reduced emergency department utilization associated with school-based clinic enrollment. *Journal of Adolescent Health, 30*(4), 273–278.

Klein, J. D., Allan, M. J., Elster, A. B., Stevens, D., Cox, C., Hedberg, V. A., et al. (2001). Improving adolescent preventive care in community health centers. *Pediatrics, 107*(2), 318–327.

Klein, J. D., Shone, L. P., Szilagyi, P. G., Bajorska, A., Wilson, K., & Dick, A. W. (2007). Impact of the state children's health insurance program on adolescents in New York. *Pediatrics, 119*(4), 885–892.

Knight, J. R., Shrier, L. A., Bravender, T. D., Farrell, M., VenderBilt, J., & Shaffer, H. J. (1999). CRAFFT: A new brief screen for adolescent substance abuse. *Archives of Pediatric and Adolescent Medicine, 153*(6), 591–596.

Kohlberg, L. (1981). *Essays on moral development.* New York: Harper & Row.

Kulkin, H. S. (2006). Factors enhancing adaptive coping and mental health in lesbian youth: A review of the literature. *Journal of Homosexuality, 50*(4), 97–111.

Lambert, S. F., Brown, T. L., Phillips, C. M., & Ialongo, N. S. (2004). The relationship between perceptions of neighborhood characteristics and substance use among urban African American adolescents. *American Journal of Community Psychology, 34*(3–4), 205–218.

Lauffer, M. (1991). Body image, sexuality and the psychotic core. *International Journal of Psycho-Analysis, 72,* 63–71.

Leathers, S. J., & Testa, M. F. (2006). Foster youth emancipating from care: Caseworkers' reports on needs and services. *Child Welfare, 85*(3), 463–498.

Lee, J. M., Appugliese, D., Kaciroti, N., Corwyn, R. F., Bradley, R. H., & Lumeng, J. C. (2007). Weight status in young girls and the onset of puberty. *Pediatrics, 119*(3), 624–630.

L'Engle, K. L., Brown, J. D., & Kenneavy, K. (2006). The mass media are an important context for adolescents' sexual behavior. *Journal of Adolescent Health, 38*(3), 186–192.

Li, C. E., DiGiuseppe, R., & Froh, J. (2006). The roles of sex, gender, and coping in adolescent depression. *Adolescence, 41*(163), 409–415.

Lustig, S. L., Kia-Keating, M., Knight, W. G., Geltman, P., Ellis, H., Kinzie, J. D., et al. (2004). Review of child and adolescent refugee mental health. *Journal of the American Academy of Child and Adolescent Psychiatry, 43*(1), 24–36.

Ma, J., Wang, Y., & Stafford, R. S. (2005). U.S. adolescents receive suboptimal preventive counseling during ambulatory care. *Journal of Adolescent Health, 36*(5), 441.

MacKay, A. P. & Duran, C. (2007). *Adolescent health in the United States, 2007.* National Center for Health Statistics.

Maguen, S., & Armistead, L. (2006). Abstinence among female adolescents: Do parents matter above and beyond the influence of peers? *American Journal of Orthopsychiatry, 76*(2), 260–264.

McDowell, M. A., Brody, D. J., & Hughes, J. P. (2007). Has age at menarche changed? Results from the National Health and Nutrition Examination Survey (NHANES) 1999–2004. *Journal of Adolescent Health, 40*(3), 227–231.

Medical Home Initiatives for Children With Special Needs Project Advisory Committee. (2004). Policy statement: Organizational principles to guide and define the child health care system and/or improve the health of all children. *Pediatrics, 113*, 1545–1547.

Middleman, A. B., Rosenthal, S. L., Rickert, V. I., Neinstein, L., Fishbein, D. B., & D'Angelo, L. (2006). Adolescent immunizations: A position paper of the Society for Adolescent Medicine. *Journal of Adolescent Health, 38*(3), 321–327.

Miller, W. R., & Sanchez, V. C. (1994). Motivating young adults for treatment and lifestyle change. In G. Howard (Ed.), *Issues in alcohol use and misuse by young adults* (pp. 55–82). Notre Dame, IN: University of Notre Dame Press.

National Institute for Occupational Safety and Health. (date). *Young worker safety and health.* Retrieved July 12, 2007, from www.cdc.gov/niosh/topics/youth

Neinstein, L. (2008). *Adolescent health care: A practical guide* (5th ed.). Philadelphia: Lippincott Williams & Wilkins.

Nelson, E. E., Leibenluft, E., McClure, E. B., & Pine, D. S. (2005). The social re-orientation of adolescence: A neuroscience perspective on the process and its relation to psychopathology. *Psychological Medicine, 35*(2), 163–174.

Nerdahl, P., Berglund, D., Bearinger, L. H., Saewyc, E., Ireland, M., & Evans, T. (1999). New challenges, new answers: Pediatric nurse practitioners and the care of adolescents. *Journal of Pediatric Health Care, 13*(4), 183–190.

Paikoff, R. L., Brooks-Gunn, J., & Warren, M. (1991). Effects of girls' hormonal status on depressive and aggressive symptoms over the course of one year. *Journal of Youth and Adolescence, 20*, 191–215.

Park, M. J., Paul Mulye, T., Adams, S. H., Brindis, C. D., & Irwin, C. E., Jr. (2006). The health status of young adults in the United States. *Journal of Adolescent Health, 39*(3), 305–317.

Parker, S., Nichter, M., Nichter, M., & Vuckovic, N. (1995). Body image and weight concerns among African-American and White adolescent females: Differences that make a difference. *Human Organizations, 54*, 103–114.

Pate, R. R., Dowda, M., O'Neill, J. R., & Ward, D. S. (2007). Change in physical activity participation among adolescent girls from 8th to 12th grade. *Journal of Physical Actvity & Health, 4*(1), 3–16.

Patton, G. C., & Viner, R. (2007). Pubertal transitions in health. *Lancet, 369*(9567), 1130–1139.

Petersen, C. C., Sarigiani, P. A., & Kennedy, R. E. (1991). Adolescent depression: Why more girls? *Journal of Youth and Adolescence, 20*, 247–271.

Piaget, J. (1973). *The child and reality.* New York: Grossman.

Pipher, M. (1994). *Reviving Ophelia: Saving the selves of adolescent girls.* New York: Ballantine.

Porter, C. P. (2002). Female "tweens" and sexual development. *Journal of Pediatric Nursing, 17*(6), 402–406.

Power, T. G., Stewart, C. D., Hughes, S. O., & Arbona, C. (2005). Predicting patterns of adolescent alcohol use: A longitudinal study. *Journal of Studies on Alcohol, 66*(1), 74–81.

Quester, G. H. (2005). Demographic trends and military recruitment: Surprising possibilities. *Parameters*, Spring, 27–40. Retrieved July 12, 2007, from http://carlisle-www.army.mil/usawc/Parameters/05spring/quester.pdf

Rapkin, A. J., Tsao, J. C., Turk, N., Anderson, M., & Zeltzer, L. K. (2006). Relationships among self-rated Tanner staging, hormones, and psychosocial factors in healthy female adolescents. *Journal of Pediatric and Adolescent Gynecology, 19*(3), 181–187.

Resnick, M. D., Ireland, M., & Borowsky, I. (2004). Youth violence perpetration: What protects? What predicts? Findings from the National Longitudinal Study of Adolescent Health. *Journal of Adolescent Health, 35*(5), 424.e1–424.e10.

Resnicow, K., Davis, R., & Rollnick, S. (2006). Motivational interviewing for pediatric obesity: Conceptual issues and evidence review. *Journal of the American Dietetic Association, 106*(12), 2024–2033.

Rew, L. (2005). *Adolescent health: A multidisciplinary approach to theory, research ,and intervention.* Thousand Oaks, CA: Sage.

Reznik, M., Ozuah, P. O., Franco, K., Cohen, R., & Motlow, F. (2002). Use of complementary therapy by adolescents with asthma. *Archives of Pediatrics and Adolescent Medicine, 156*(10), 1042–1044.

Robbins, L. B., Gretebeck, K. A., Kazanis, A. S., & Pender, N. J. (2007). Girls on the move program to increase physical activity participation. *Nursing Research, 55*(3), 206–216.

Rollnick, S., & Miller, W. (1995). What is motivational interviewing? *Behavioural and Cognitive Psychotherapy, 23*, 325–334. Retrieved July 2, 2007, from http://motivationalinterview.org/clinical/whatismi.html

Rosen, D. B. (2006). Violence and exploitation against women and girls with disability. *Annals of the New York Academy of Sciences, 1087*, 170–177.

Sadof, M. D., & Nazarian, B. L. (2007). Caring for children who have special health-care needs: A practical guide for the primary care practitioner. *Pediatrics in Review, 28*, e36–42. Retrieved July 11, 2007, from http://pedsinreview.aappublications.org/cgi/content/full/28/7/e36

Saewyc, E. M., Skay, C. L., Pettingell, S. L., Reis, E. A., Bearinger, L., Resnick, M., et al. (2006). Hazards of stigma: The sexual and physical abuse of gay, lesbian, and bisexual adolescents in the United States and Canada. *Child Welfare, 85*(2), 195–213.

Sale, E., Sambrano, S., Springer, J. F., Pena, C., Pan, W., & Kasim, R. (2005). Family protection and prevention of alcohol use among Hispanic youth at high risk. *American Journal of Community Psychology, 36*(3–4), 195–205.

Sanchez, R. P., Waller, M. W., & Greene, J. M. (2006). Who runs? A demographic profile of runaway youth in the United States. *Journal of Adolescent Health, 39*(5), 778–781.

Santor, D. A., Poulin, C., LeBlanc, J. C., & Kusumakar, V. (2006). Examining school health center utilization as a function of mood disturbance and mental health difficulties. *Journal of Adolescent Health, 39*(5), 729–735.

Saslow, D., Runowicz, C. D., Solomon, D., Moscicki, B.-A., Smith, R. A., Eyre, H. J., & Cohen, C. (2002). American Cancer Society guideline for the early detection of cervical neoplasia and cancer. *CA: A Cancer Journal for Clinicians, 52*, 342–362. Retrieved July 12, 2007, from http://caonline.amcancersoc.org/cgi/content/full/52/6/342

Satter, E. (1987). *How to get your kid to eat . . . But not too much.* Boulder, CO: Bull Publishing.

Sawyer, S. M., Drew, S., Yeo, M. S., & Britto, M. T. (2007). Adolescents with a chronic condition: Challenges living, challenges treating. *Lancet, 369*(9571), 1481–1489.

Schreiber, G. B., Robins, M., Striegel-Moore, R., Obarzanek, E., Morrison, J. A., & Wright, D. J. (1996). Weight modification efforts reported by black and white preadolescent girls. *Pediatrics, 98*, 63–70.

Seal, K. H., Bertenthal, D., Miner, C. R., Sen, S., & Marmar, C. (2007). Bringing the war back home: Mental health disorders among 103,788 US veterans returning from Iraq and Afghanistan seen at Department of Veterans Affairs facilities. *Arch Intern Med, 167*(5), 476–482.

Serepca, R. O. (1996). The implications of pubertal timing for women's body image and self-esteem. *Dissertation Abstracts International: Section B: The Sciences and Engineering, 57*(6-B), 4060.

Siegel, J. M., Yancy, A. K., Aneshensel, C. S., & Schuler, R. (1999). Body image, perceived pubertal timing, and adolescent mental health. *Journal of Adolescent Health, 25*(2), 155–165.

Silverman, J. G., Decker, M. R., & Raj, A. (2007). Immigration-based disparities in adolescent girls' vulnerability to dating violence. *Maternal Child Health Journal, 11*(1), 37–43.

Spencer, J. H., & Le, T. N. (2006). Parent refugee status, immigration stressors, and Southeast Asian youth violence. *Journal Immigrant and Minority Health, 8*(4), 359–368.

State Survey of School-Based Health Centers Initiative. (2002). Retrieved July 3, 2007, from http://www.healthinschools.org/home.asp

Striegel-Moore, R., & Smolak, L. (1996). The role of race in the development of eating disorders. In M. P. Smolak, R. Levine & R. Striegel-Moore (Eds.), *The developmental psychopathology of eating disorders: Implications for research prevention and treatment* (pp. 259–284), Hillsdale, NJ: Erlbaum.

Suris, A., Lind, L., Kashner, T. M., Borman, P. D., & Petty, F. (2004). Sexual assault in women veterans: An examination of PTSD risk, health care utilization, and cost of care. *Psychosomatic Medicine, 66*(5), 749–756.

Tanner, J. (1962). *Growth at adolescence* (2nd ed.). Springfield, IL: Charles C. Thomas.

Tanner, J. (1981). Growth and maturation during adolescence. *Nutrition Reviews, 39*(2), 43–55.

Taylor, J. P., Evers, S., & McKenna, M. (2005). Determinants of healthy eating in children and youth. *Canadian Journal of Public Health, 96*(Suppl. 3), S20–S26.

Thrane, L. E., Hoyt, D. R., Whitbeck, L. B., & Yoder, K. A. (2006). Impact of family abuse on running away, deviance, and street victimization among homeless rural and urban youth. *Child Abuse & Neglect, 30*(10), 1117–1128.

Tylee, A., Haller, D. M., Graham, T., Churchill, R., & Sanci, L. A. (2007). Youth-friendly primary-care services: How are we doing and what more needs to be done? *Lancet, 369*(9572), 1565–1573.

U.S. Department of Health and Human Services, Health Resources and Services Administration, Maternal and Child Health Bureau. (2006). *Child health USA 2006*. Rockville, MD: U.S. Department of Health and Human Services.

U.S. Department of Health and Human Services, Centers for Disease Control and Prevention. (2000, November). 21 critical health objectives for adolescents and young adults. *Healthy People 2010: Vols. 1 and 2*. Retrieved June 13, 2007, from http://www.cdc.gov/HealthyYouth/AdolescentHealth/NationalInitiative/pdf/21objectives.pdf

University of California, San Francisco (2003). *National Adolescent Health Information Center (2003) fact sheet on demographics: adolescents*. Retrieved March 3, 2008, from http://nahic.ucsf.edu//downloads/Demographics.pdf

Vandewater, E. A., Rideout, V. J., Wartella, E. A., Huang, X., Lee, J. H., & Shim, M. S. (2007). Digital childhood: Electronic media and technology use among infants, toddlers, and preschoolers. *Pediatrics, 119*(5), 1006–1015.

Warren, M., & Brooks-Gunn, J. (1989). Mood and behavior at adolescence: Evidence for hormonal factors. *Journal of Clinical Endocrinology and Metabolism, 69*(1), 77–83.

Williamson, L. (1998). Eating disorders and the cultural forces behind the drive for thinness: Are African American women really protected? *Social Work in Health Care, 28*(1), 61–73.

Wills, T. A., Murry, V. M., Brody, G. H., Gibbons, F. X., Gerrard, M., Walker, C., et al. (2007). Ethnic pride and self-control related to protective and risk factors: Test of the theoretical model for the strong African American families program. *Health Psychology, 26*(1), 50–59.

Wilson, K. M., Klein, J. D., Sesselberg, T. S., Yussman, S. M., Markow, D. B., Green, A. E., et al. (2006). Use of complementary medicine and dietary supplements among U.S. adolescents. *Journal of Adolescent Health, 38*(4), 385–394.

Yang, H., Stanton, B., Cottrel, L., Kaljee, L., Galbraith, J., Li, X., et al. (2006). Parental awareness of adolescent risk involvement: Implications of overestimates and underestimates. *Journal of Adolescent Health, 39*(3), 353–361.

Youngblade, L. M., Theokas, C., Schulenberg, J., Curry, L., Huang, I. C., & Novak, M. (2007). Risk and promotive factors in families, schools, and communities: A contextual model of positive youth development in adolescence. *Pediatrics, 119*(Suppl. 1), S47–S53.

Yussman, S. M., Ryan, S. A., Auinger, P., & Weitzman, M. (2004). Visits to complementary and alternative medicine providers by children and adolescents in the United States. *Ambulatory Pediatrics, 4*(5), 429–435.

Mid-Life Women's Health

Nancy Fugate Woods and
Ellen Sullivan Mitchell

Mid-life women account for a growing proportion of the U.S. population, but only recently have researchers and clinicians devoted much attention to mid-life women's health concerns. The purposes of this chapter are to: (1) define and summarize findings relating to women's perceptions of mid-life; (2) describe current understanding of the biological changes associated with mid-life, with a special emphasis on the menopausal transition; (3) propose approaches to health status assessment of mid-life women; (4) review current empirical work related to management of mid-life symptoms; and (5) propose a program of health promotion and prevention for mid-life women.

MID-LIFE: DEFINITIONS AND PERCEPTIONS

Mid-life can be defined using age boundaries, such as 35 to 65 years, to differentiate mid-life from young adulthood and old age. Alternatively, definitions can be based on reproductive aging stages using indicators of menstrual cycle changes or hormonal changes. Women's changing role patterns, using indicators such as a child leaving home or a woman's return to the work place to designate the beginning of mid-life, provides another option. Using women's own perceptions about whether they are in the middle of their lives provides yet another option. Brooks-Gunn and Kirsh (1984) stress the multidimensional and multidirectional nature of change in mid-life, describing the boundaries as fluid and constructed by the society and the individual rather than being determined by chronological age. Whatever the markers for mid-life might be, understanding the context in which women experience mid-life is extremely important. Anticipation of mid-life by each woman's age cohort (women born at the same time) as well as socialization by other women about what to expect during mid-life contribute to the framework with which women view and interpret the events of mid-life. Both anticipated and actual mid-life experiences can influence women's notions of health.

Meanings of Mid-Life

Mid-life women born during different eras, those from different birth cohorts, have lived in different worlds (Bernard, 1981); thus, it is important to locate women's mid-life experiences within the sociopolitical and historical context in which they occur. Contemporary mid-life women represent at least two birth cohorts who have had very different lives. Women born during the post–World War II era of the mid-1940s to mid-1950s experienced the gender revolution of the late 1960s and 1970s in the United States. Women born during the prior decade, from 1935 to 1945, lived their young adult years prior to the gender revolution and the subsequent changes (Coney, 1994). These different experiences are likely to have had an important effect on women who are part of the contemporary mid-life cohort, making it important to differentiate their experiences from those of cohorts of mid-life women born in prior decades.

Neugarten's (1968) work with both mid-life women and men studied prior to and during the 1960s indicated that, for women born prior to the end of World War II, mid-life meant being in control of a complex life. Those who participated in her interviews were socially privileged and recognized their roles as powerful norm-bearers and decision makers. They experienced mid-life as a time of heightened sensitivity to their power within a complex social environment. Reassessment of the self was a prevailing theme. Women, compared to men, estimated their age status in the timing of the family life cycle. Launching their children was an important marker of mid-life. Changing time perspectives were evident in the interviews with mid-life women and men: the time left was of concern. Another aspect of time, the time of one's life, was also a theme in Neugarten's interviews. Rubin's (1979) classic study *Women of a Certain Age* focused on 160 women who were 35 to 55 years of age when they were studied during the 1970s (born between the 1920s and 1940s). Rubin found that women "of a certain age" struggled with an uncertain identity she labeled the "elusive self." The women Rubin studied were part of a birth cohort that was beginning to be influenced by the women's movement of the 1960s and 1970s. Most had given up the job or careers of their youth for at least 10 years to devote themselves to full-time marriage and motherhood. Nearly 25% were unable to describe who they were. Few described themselves in relation to their work despite their employment. Many described themselves as having two selves, reflecting their difficulty integrating the achieving self with the emotional, intuitive self. Others made a distinction between who they were in relation to being and doing: their internal identity represented their being, whereas their work represented their doing. For these women, work was what they did, not who they were. Rubin found that these women were not devastated by the "empty nest," the time when their children left home.

The baby boomer cohort born after World War II differentiated itself from women of previous generations by fashioning their lives as individuals. Whereas past generations of women organized their life roles and goals around their family's objectives, baby boomer women now spend more of their lives as single, independent adults, organizing their lives to meet their personal and employment objectives. The baby boomer woman is better educated, lives alone longer than did her mother's generation, and participates in the labor force throughout her life regardless of her marital status and the age of her children. She experiences greater financial independence and fertility control than her mother. Marriage and family are no longer the single controlling institutions around which this generation of women organize their lives, but parenting, partnerships, and caregiving also remain significant components of women's work (McLaughlin, Melber, Billy, & Zimmerle, 1986).

The perceptions and experiences of baby boomer women during their middle years are likely to reflect this dramatic change in their life course. Gilligan (1982a) proposed restoring the missing text of women's development for this cohort rather than simply replacing it with work about men's development. She saw women's middle years as a risky time due to women's embeddedness in lives of relationship, their orientation to interdependence, their ability to subordinate achievement to care, and their conflicts over competitive success. Should mid-life bring an end to relationships and, with them, a sense of connection for women, then mid-life may be a time of despair. Gilligan stressed that the meaning of mid-life events for women is contextual, arising from the interaction between the structures of women's thought and the realities of their lives. Women approach mid-life with a different history than do men, and they face a different social reality with different possibilities for love and work (Gilligan, 1982a, 1982b).

A study of nearly 500 mid-life women (35 to 60 years in 1986) by the New Zealand Society for Research on Women (1988) indicated that 80% to 90% had positive attitudes about life, more than 80% had positive attitudes toward their physical appearance and health, and 80% were positive about their futures. Only 14% were unhappy with their daily lives. One-third of women reported some stress in their relationships with husbands or partners, such as unemployment, illness, work demands, or finances. Women's experiences with their children were a function of their ages: of the 35- to 40-year-olds, two-thirds found their children stressful, and of the 50- to 60-year-olds, two-thirds rated their children not at all stressful.

At the same time that women are experiencing the social transitions associated with parenting responsibilities, they are also experiencing the aging of their bodies. In a series of interviews with a convenience sample of mid-life women, Coney (1994) found that signs of aging, such as wrinkles and weight gain, produced grief in some women and no concern in others. Reflections of others' perceptions of aging that included sexist and ageist stereotypes about women, frequently reinforced by mass media, caused some women to be worried about their physical aging. Others were more worried about loss of physical abilities, such as hearing, eyesight, and mobility, and losing mental powers. Still others felt panicky and negative because they sensed that time was running out for them. The "empty nest" had both positive and negative associations for many of the women Coney studied. Despite negative attitudes toward menopause and aging women, inequities in employment and financial security, mid-life women had surprisingly high well-being. They expressed having made achievements, gained maturity, experience, and confidence that younger women do not have, and knowing what they are capable of doing. Having attained some seniority in employment and having launched their children, many women felt freer to concentrate on themselves and decide what they want for the next third of their lives. More secure in their own opinions and beliefs and less afraid of expressing them, mid-life women Coney studied emphasized increasing freedom.

Participants in the Seattle Midlife Women's Health Study—begun in 1990, when the women were 35 to 55 years of age—responded to these questions: What does "mid-life" mean? What events of mid-life do women believe are important? distressing? satisfying? A particular emphasis of this investigation was to determine whether menopause figured prominently in women's experiences of this part of the life span. Participants' most common image of mid-life was getting older (Woods & Mitchell, 1997). Their emphasis on defining mid-life as an age and aging process is consistent with findings from older cohorts of women (Rossi, 1985; Rubin, 1979) and is not surprising given the youthful value orientation of U.S. society. These women also associated changes of every kind with mid-life. They alluded to transitions with respect to their physical bodies, emotions, feelings about being older, outlook on life, relationships, and "change of life." A few referred to their changing health and vulnerability. The notion of mid-life as a time of transition is consistent with findings from older birth cohorts of women (Helsen & Wink, 1992; Neugarten, 1968). Given the prevalence of life changes among this cohort of mid-life women, their emphasis on transitions is not surprising. The centrality of personal achievements and employment in the Seattle women's lives stands in striking contrast to data from older birth cohorts of mid-life women. The distinction between images of mid-life described by the birth cohort of women Rubin interviewed and those of the women in this study reflect the dramatic changes in lifelong employment patterns women have experienced since the 1970s. The baby boomers did not seem to be trying to figure out what to do with the rest of their lives. They were still juggling the demands of integrating work and family responsibilities. Although emphasis on work-related events and personal goal attainment among this cohort resembled that in studies of men's development (Neugarten, 1968), emphasis on family and health-related events were among those considered most important. Children, spouses, and parents were mentioned frequently as women described the important events of mid-life.

Participants in the Seattle Midlife Women's Health Study ($N = 508$), with a median age of 41 years, reported a variety of stressful or distressing events, which included health problems, deaths, family problems, work-related problems, frustrated goal attainment, and financial problems (Woods & Mitchell, 1997). Women reported distressing health problems, including their own and those of their parents with similar frequency. Deaths were also commonly cited as the most distressing event and included the deaths of parents, in-laws, and husbands. Family problems included those with adolescent children, domestic violence, divorce or separation from a spouse, and the ending of relationships. Work problems were also mentioned frequently, including

inability to find work, work place conflicts, and downsizing of work places. Frustrated goal attainment included events such as being unable to finish an academic program on time or have personal time while working on an academic program. Women's financial events included financial problems such as inability to pay college tuition for a child or afford essentials.

Not surprisingly, the Seattle women's images of mid-life and the events they found most important and most stressful reflected their engagement in a broader, more complex world than that of their mothers. No longer focusing only on their roles as mothers and homemakers, contemporary mid-life women are attempting to balance the demands of work place and home, and this is reflected in how they characterized the best and worst of mid-life. Unlike Rubin's sample, this sample of mid-life women talked freely of their multidimensional selves and the social circumstances that necessitated their viewing themselves differently from their mothers' generation.

In sum, contemporary mid-life women described mid-life similarly to women from earlier birth cohorts with one important exception: the centrality of work and personal achievement in their lives. As women's roles have changed, so have the experiences that women count as important. Personal achievement and work-related events have assumed a central place, along with family events, in how women describe their lives. With a life course that is made more complex than their mothers' by lifelong employment, contemporary mid-life women are not wondering what to do with the rest of their lives as much as they are wondering how to juggle the demands of family and work-related responsibilities.

Perceptions of the Menopausal Transition

The years during which women make the transition to menopause (the menopausal transition) and the first few years after the final menstrual period (early post menopause) hold great fascination and sometimes frustration for the women experiencing them as well as their health care providers. When mid-life women were asked about what they anticipated menopause would be like, the most prevalent theme was uncertainty and mixed feelings (Woods & Mitchell, 1999). These sentiments suggested a need for knowledge about this part of the life span and changing biology.

As women anticipate mid-life, menopause is one focus of their concerns. Participants in the Seattle Midlife Women's Health Study voiced uncertainty about what to expect menopause would be like, and many had no expectations about the experience, revealing a need for information about this part of the lifespan (Woods & Mitchell, 1999). Indeed, women defined menopause as the cessation of menstrual periods, the end of reproductive capacity, a time of hormonal changes, a new or different life stage, a time of symptoms, changing emotions, changing bodies, part of the aging process. Of interest is that few defined this period of life as a time of disease risk or one necessitating medical care.

How various U.S. ethnic groups of women define menopause was unknown until the efforts of investigators for the Study of Women's Health Across the Nation (SWAN; Sowers et al., 2000). Results from the multisite study of multiple U.S. ethnic groups indicate widespread differences in women's expectations and experiences as well as areas of similarity across groups. Urban Latina women stressed the primacy of health and the importance of harmony and balance in their lives. They described menopause as *el cambio de vida*—something you have to go through. They also stressed that "this time is for me," referring to reorienting and restructuring their lives (Villaruel, Harlow, Lopez, & Sowers, 2002). Menopause conceptions among Japanese American and European American women differed. Change in self-focus, with self-satisfaction, ability to reprioritize their values accompanied menopause. Japanese American women described a metamorphosis from motherhood to nurturing, becoming a more complete human being (Kagawa-Singer et al., 2002). African American women's conceptions of menopause emphasized mid-life as a period of developmental changes. They recognized their personal mortality, changing family relationships, increasing authenticity, revaluing of life experiences, and setting new goals for personal growth and experiencing greater self-esteem. They emphasized increased self-acceptance and productivity (Sampselle, Harris, Harlow, & Sowers, 2002). Chinese American and Chinese women's conceptions of menopause were inextricably bound with meanings of mid-life. For this group, the borders and timing of the menopausal transition are ambiguous. The menopausal transition represents a natural progression through the life cycle.

Of interest is that expectations of women who have not yet experienced menopause did not match the experiences of postmenopausal women. Menopause was viewed as a marker for aging. Women believe that it is important to prepare for and manage the menopausal transition (Adler et al., 2000), but this belief exists in the context of a lack of access to information and uncertainty about the process. In contrast to women's perceptions of menopause is recent research focused on defining the menopausal transition.

CHANGING BIOLOGY: THE MENOPAUSAL TRANSITION AND BEYOND

During the past decade, efforts to predict the events of the menopausal transition have culminated in a model for staging reproductive aging. As part of this effort,

researchers and clinicians proposed and are beginning to test criteria that women and clinicians can use to anticipate the onset of the menopausal transition and postmenopause. Figure 6.1 includes a proposed model of reproductive aging from the Staging Reproductive Aging Workshop (STRAW) held in 2001 (Soules et al., 2001). The STRAW model is oriented around the final menstrual period (FMP), with the time period immediately preceding the FMP labeled the menopausal transition and the period immediately following the FMP postmenopause. The menopausal transition is divided into two stages: early and late. The STRAW participants suggested criteria for defining the onset of these stages and recommended they be tested with longitudinal data. STRAW recommended that the criterion for early menopausal transition was the beginning irregularity of menstrual cycles, with the length of one cycle varying by 7 or more days from the preceding or following cycle. The late menopausal transition is denoted by skipping periods, using the criterion that cycles be longer than 60 days. STRAW participants divided the reproductive stage into three parts—early, peak, and late—corresponding to women's experience of fertility. The late reproductive stage, just prior to the menopausal transition, was characterized by rising follicle stimulating hormone levels and regular menstrual cycle length. Figures 6.2 through 6.4 illustrate the late reproductive and early and late menopausal transition stages as indicated by women's menstrual calendars. STRAW participants divided postmenopause into early and late stages, with the early stage spanning the first 5 years after the FMP and the late stage spanning the remainder of a woman's life. The provisional STRAW criteria for staging the menopausal transition have been recently validated by the RESTAGE collaboration that compared results from several longitudinal studies of women's menstrual cycles as they approached the FMP (Harlow et al., 2006). Results supported the STRAW recommendations that 60 or more days of amenorrhea be used to define onset of late menopausal transition (Harlow et al., 2007) and that early menopausal transition onset be defined as a persistent 7 or more days difference in length of consecutive cycles (Harlow et al., 2008).

During the menopausal transition, women also frequently report spotting (bloody discharge that does not require use of a napkin or tampon) before, after, and in between episodes of menstrual bleeding and longer and heavier episodes of bleeding (menorrhagia or flooding) that cause them to worry and seek health care. They may define themselves as in menopause or menopausal based on their bleeding changes, but their definitions may not be consistent with those in the STRAW staging model. Menopause is defined as the end of menstruation as marked by the last menstrual period and is said to have occurred after women have not menstruated for 1 calendar year (Soules et al., 2001).

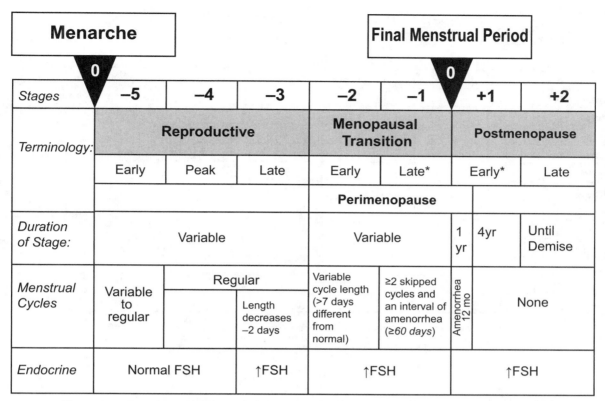

Figure 6.1 Proposed staging system for the menopausal transition (STRAW Conference).
Source: Soules, M. R., Sherman, S., Parrott, E., Rebar, R., Santoro, N., Utian, W., Woods N. (2001). Executive summary: Stages of reproductive aging workshop (STRAW). *Climacteric, 4*(4), 267–272.

Year *1998*   MENSTRUAL CYCLE RECORD   IDNO_____

Day	1	2	3	4	5	6	7	8	9	10	11	12	13	14	15	16	17	18	19	20	21	22	23	24	25	26	27	28	29	30	31
JAN									B_3	B_4	B_3	B_2	B_1	S^u																	
FEB			B_4	B_3	B_2	B_1	B_1	S^u																							
MAR	B_3	B_4	B_3	B_2	B_1	B_1^u	B_1																			B_3	B_3	B_2	B_2	B_1	B_1
APR	S																					B_3	B_3	B_2	B_2	B_1	B_1^u	B_1	S		
MAY															B_3	B_4	B_2	B_2	B_2	B_1^u	B_1										
JUN									B_3	B_4	B_3	B_2	B_2	B_1^u	B_1	B_1															
JUL				B_3	B_3	B_3	B_1	B_2	B_1^u	S																					B_2
AUG	B_4	B_3	B_1	B_2	B_1																					B_3	B_4	B_3	B_2	B_2	B_1
SEP	B_1																					B_2	B_4	B_3	B_2	B_2	B_1				
OCT																	B_2	B_4	B_3	B_1	B_2	B_1	B_1								
NOV									B_3	B_4	B_3	B_3	B_2	B_2	B_1	B_1															
DEC					B_3	B_4	B_2	B_2	B_1	B_1	S																				

For every day you spot or bleed enter an S or B in the appropriate square. Record a 1, 2, 3 or 4 next to every B day.
(1: light flow, 2: moderate, 3: heavy, 4: very heavy/flooding)
For any month no bleeding or spotting occurs write in NO BLEEDING.
If you forget to record for a month write in FORGOT TO RECORD.

Figure 6.2 Menstrual cycle calendar: Late reproductive stage (STRAW).

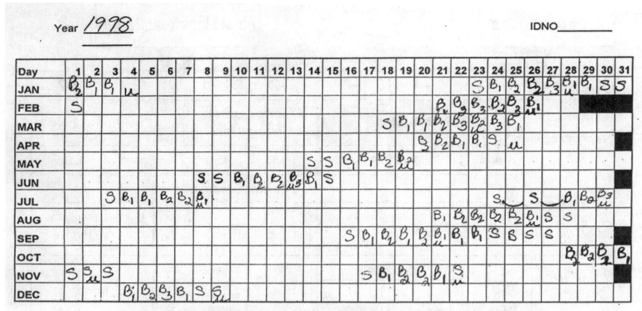

For every day you spot or bleed enter an S or B in the appropriate square. Record a 1, 2, 3 or 4 next to every B day.
(1: light flow, 2: moderate, 3: heavy, 4: very heavy/flooding)
For any month no bleeding or spotting occurs write in NO BLEEDING.
If you forget to record for a month write in FORGOT TO RECORD.

Figure 6.3   Menstrual cycle calendar: Early transition (STRAW).

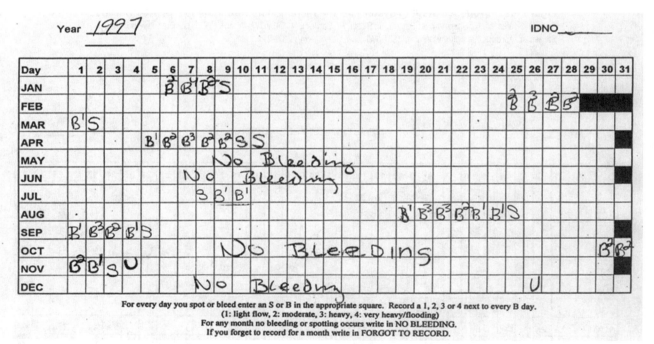

For every day you spot or bleed enter an S or B in the appropriate square. Record a 1, 2, 3 or 4 next to every B day.
(1: light flow, 2: moderate, 3: heavy, 4: very heavy/flooding)
For any month no bleeding or spotting occurs write in NO BLEEDING.
If you forget to record for a month write in FORGOT TO RECORD.

Figure 6.4   Menstrual cycle calendar: Late transition (STRAW).

Staging reproductive aging provides a useful framework for women to use in anticipating their progress through the menopausal transition. It is also useful to clinicians in organizing their understanding of the changing biology around the time of menopause (Santoro et al., 2007).

The Menopausal Transition: Part of Reproductive Aging

In the United States, most women experience their final menstrual period during their late 40s or early 50s, with the median age being 51 to 52 years (McKinlay,

| Duration and Age of Onset of Menopausal Transition Stages |

	MIDDLE STAGE				**LATE STAGE**				**POSTMENOPAUSE**			
	N	Mean	*SD*	Range	*N*	Mean	*SD*	Range	*N*	Mean	*SD*	Range
Age of onset	122	46.1	3.6	36.6–54.6	135	49.2	2.8	42.0–54.8	101	51.9	3.0	43.7–58.3
Duration (years)	80	2.8	1.5	0.2–6.5	73	2.6	1.4	0.4–8.1	n.a.	n.a.	n.a.	n.a.

Brambilla, & Posner, 1992; Mitchell & Woods, 2007). Although the final menstrual period occurs only once in a woman's life time, the natural menopausal transition is a biological process that usually occupies several years of a woman's life as opposed to being a single occasion (see Table 6.1 for information on ages at and duration of menopausal transition stages based on findings from the Seattle Midlife Women's Health Study). The early stage of the menopausal transition estimated from U.S. women's menstrual bleeding patterns recorded daily on menstrual calendars has been timed to start during the mid-40s and occurred at a median age of 45.5 years for a population of Midwestern White women (Treloar, 1981), at 47.5 years as reported in telephone interviews by participants in the Massachusetts Women's Health Study (MWHS) (McKinlay et al., 1992), and 46.1 years based on menstrual calendars obtained from participants in the Seattle Midlife Women's Health Study (Mitchell, Woods, & Mariella, 2000; Mitchell & Woods, 2007). The beginning of the late stage of menopausal transition occurred at 49.2 years in the Seattle Midlife Study. Duration of the menopausal transition is an average of 4 to 5 years across the studies but varies widely, with a range of 2 to 7 years and a median of 4.5 years in the Minnesota and 3.5 years in the Massachusetts Women's Health Study samples. Duration of the middle stage was 2.8 years and the late stage 2.5 years in the Seattle Midlife Women's Health Study sample (Mitchell & Woods, 2007).

Altered Hypothalamic-Pituitary-Ovarian Function During the Menopausal Transition

Irregularity of menstrual periods indicates progression through the menopausal transition and is associated with a logarithmic decrease in the number of ovarian follicles as women age. Comparing women aged 45 to 55 years who were menstruating regularly to women having irregular cycles and postmenopausal women, Richardson (1993) found that follicle counts decreased dramatically among women having irregular cycles and were nearly absent in the postmenopausal group.

In addition to changes in bleeding patterns and cycle regularity, elevated gonadotropins are commonly used indicators of changing ovarian function associated with the transition to menopause. Sustained increases of follicle stimulating hormone (FSH) occur on average 5 to 6 years and luteinizing hormone (LH) 3 to 4 years before the last period (Lenton, Sexton, Lee, & Cooke, 1988; Metcalf, 1988; Randolph et al., 2006). Elevated gonadotropins have been attributed to both ovarian aging (loss of follicles and therefore reduced estrogen and the reduction in inhibin levels that provide negative feedback to FSH) and central regulation of aging (decrease in sensitivity to feedback at the hypothalamus and/or pituitary). Wise and colleagues (2002) have proposed that central regulation of reproductive aging may play a role in the elevated LH and FSH levels occurring during the late reproductive stage and the menopausal transition. Klein and colleagues (1996) found that accelerated follicular development was associated with a monotropic rise in FSH in women between 40 and 45 years who were still cycling. As women near the end of regular ovulation, their estradiol levels obtained during the early follicular phases are higher and their estradiol levels rise earlier in the follicular phase than those measured among younger women. As reproductive age advances, progesterone levels diminish. Although increasing FSH levels are a useful indicator that the final menstrual period is approaching, they are not sufficiently specific to diagnose a menopausal transition stage, nor is there a clear-cut point distinguishing women in the menopausal transition within a specified time period compared to those not yet in the menopausal transition (Harlow et al., 2006; Randolph et al., 2006).

Data from the Melbourne Midlife Women's Health Project, a longitudinal study of Australian women during the menopause transition and postmenopause, revealed that estradiol levels drop between 1 and 2 years prior to the final menstrual period and continued to drop during the first years after the final menstrual period. In addition, FSH levels rose notably in the year prior to FMP, consistent with findings of other studies (Rannevik et al., 1995). Inhibin levels dropped in the 2 years prior to FMP as FSH levels rise, reflecting the diminishing size of the follicle pool (Burger et al.,1999; Burger, Dudley, Cui, Dennerstein, & Hopper, 2000; Burger, Dudley, Robertson, & Dennerstein, 2002). Dominant follicles continue to produce estradiol and inhibin A, probably as a result of the fall in inhibin B, which allows FSH to rise and stimulate the ovary. Thus, dramatic increases in FSH may be responsible for elevated levels of estrogens during the later phase of the menopausal transition, producing periods of hyperestrogenism in some women (Santoro, Brown, Adel, & Skurnick, 1996). As ovulation ceases, the levels of inhibin A fall, reflecting the inability of a dominant follicle to develop.

Androgens

Women produce androgens in the ovary and adrenal cortex, and studies have revealed that there is no difference in metabolic clearance for mid-life women regardless of whether they had completed the FMP. Although the conversion of estrone to estradiol decreased in middle-aged women who continued to menstruate, peripheral aromatization of androstenedione to estrone increased in all women regardless of their menopausal status (menstruating to menopausal, and menopausal at both occasions). Women begin producing increasing levels of estrone prior to FMP (Longcope & Johnson, 1990).

The adrenal gland secretes androgen precursors, including dehydroepiandrosterone sulfate, (DHEAS) dehydroepiandroterone (DHEA), androstenedione, and testosterone. Data from the Melbourne Midlife Women's Health Project revealed that testosterone levels remained unchanged during the transition to menopause (from 4 years before FMP to 2 years after), and DHEAS levels decreased as a function of age, not of the menopausal transition (Burger et al., 2000). In addition, sex hormone binding globulin (SHBG) decreased by 43% from 4 years before to 2 years after FMP, with the greatest drop 2 years before FMP. SHBG levels were associated with a drop in estradiol levels over the same period. Free androgen index (FAI), calculated as the ratio of testosterone to SHBG, rose by 80% during the same period, with the maximal change occurring 2 years before the FMP (Burger et al., 2000).

The Study of Women's Health Across the Nation (SWAN) is an ongoing multisite longitudinal study of a multiethnic population of U.S. women extending across the menopausal transition. Designed to characterize the physical and psychosocial changes that occur during the time of the menopausal transition and postmenopause and to observe their effects on later risk factors for age-related diseases and health, the SWAN study includes data from over 16,000 women between the ages of 40 and 55 years who were screened from 1995 to 1997. Of these women, 3,302 of them who were between 42 and 52 years of age were enrolled in a longitudinal cohort studied by annual visits and other data collection efforts for 6 years of follow-up, and 900 of these women are participating in a daily hormone study. The data being collected in SWAN include ovarian markers, lifestyle and behavior indicators, and markers of cardiovascular and bone health. Results of the SWAN study will make a significant contribution to the understanding of the natural history of the menopausal transition (Sowers et al., 2000).

The multiethnic nature of the SWAN cohort has allowed investigators to explore the variability of endocrine levels with women's ethnic/racial group as well as the stage of the menopausal transition. Although DHEAS has been found to decline as a function of age, there was a transient increase in DHEAS noted in some women during the transition to late perimenopause (the late stage of the menopausal transition using the STRAW terminology). Changes in testosterone (T) and estradiol were correlated with changes in DHEAS such that T rose with DHEAS. The correlation of DHEAS to estradiol was weaker than that to T. Because DHEAS can be metabolized to either a potent androgen or estrogen, it may play a role in testosterone production for women during the menopausal transition (Lasley et al., 2002). Serum FSH, SHBG, estradiol, testosterone, and DHEAS all are correlated with body mass. Estradiol levels adjusted for body mass do not differ across ethnic groups. Adjusted FSH levels were higher and adjusted T levels were lower in African American and Hispanic women. Thus, serum sex steroids, FSH, and SHBG levels vary by ethnicity, but this relationship is highly confounded by ethnic differences in body mass (Randolph et al., 2003).

The Menopausal Transition as a Time of Reregulation

Although some emphasize the dysregulation of the hypothalamic-pituitary-ovarian (HPO) axis functions occurring during the menopausal transition, this period in a woman's life may represent a time of reregulation of endocrine function. The ovary produces lower levels of estradiol as the ovarian follicles decrease in number, but the transition is punctuated by higher levels of estradiol in response to increasing levels of FSH. Ovulation ceases and progesterone levels become extremely low or unmeasurable. During the menopausal transition, a compensatory response with an increase in peripheral aromatization of the androgen androstenedione to estrone and a time-limited increase in DHEAS occur during the late transition stage. These events may signal a transition from ovarian to ovarian-adrenal metabolism of estrogens, thus supporting reregulation of the HPO axis to a new pattern not dependent on the ovarian production of higher levels of estrogen.

PHYSIOLOGIC CONSEQUENCES OF THE MENOPAUSAL TRANSITION

Widespread physiologic effects of estrogens, progesterone, and androgens would warrant compensatory changes in response to their production in order to re-regulate the HPO axis, and these alter physiologic functioning. Physiologic effects of estrogen and progesterone seen in menstruating women change over the course of the menopausal transition as estradiol production becomes more variable and eventually diminishes, progesterone production linked to ovulation ceases, testosterone and androstenedione levels may remain stable or fluctuate slightly, and the proportion of estrone to estradiol increases.

Physiologic effects of estrogens and progesterone influence an array of biological functions, including reproductive system tissues of the uterus, fallopian tubes, vagina, and breast. Gonadal steroids also influence bone, lipid, carbohydrate, and protein metabolism. Both alpha and beta receptors for estrogen and progesterone mediate hormonal effects. The cell types in which each type of receptor is functional have not yet been clearly demonstrated (McConnell, 2000). Some estrogenic effects are mediated by effects on hepatic protein secretion. In addition, there are widespread effects of estrogen and progesterone on bone, adipose tissue, and muscle; blood clotting, blood pressure, electrolytes, respiration, and nervous system and immune system functions.

Physiologic effects of estrogen on reproductive tissues include proliferation of the endometrium; contractile activities of the myometrium; up-regulation of uterine progesterone receptors; enhancement of the vascularity of the cervix and secretion of cervical mucus (clear, thin, spinbarkheit); contractile activity of the fallopian tubes; proliferation of the vaginal epithelium with glycogen deposition in superficial cells; promotion of breast development and maintenance, especially the ductal system, and increased breast mass. Progesterone effects include development of secretory endometrium; maintenance of placental implantation; relaxation of smooth muscle of the uterus; down-regulation of the progesterone receptor in the uterus; relaxation of the smooth muscle of the fallopian tubes; and stimulation of lobulo-alveolar growth of the breast tissue (in conjunction with estrogen) (Dyrenfurth 1982; Patton, Fuchs, Hille, Scher, & Steiner, 1989).

In addition to estrogen's and progesterone's effects on reproductive and sexual organs, both have important effects on metabolism, bone, muscle, adipose tissue, and functional effects on respiration, blood clotting, blood pressure, electrolytes, and immune response. Estrogenic effects on metabolism include increasing hepatic protein secretion, including lipoproteins, clotting factors, renin substrate, and binding proteins. In addition, estrogenic effects increase binding proteins, including sex hormone–binding globulin, corticosteroid-binding globulin, thyroxin-binding globulin, growth hormone–binding proteins, and ceruloplasmin. Estrogen also enhances the excretory capacity for bromosulphthalein (BSP), bilirubin, and bile salts and is responsible for changes in serum transaminase and alkaline phosphatase (Dyrenfurth, 1982; Patton et al., 1989).

Lipid effects of estrogen include increased secretion of lipoproteins, very low density lipoproteins (VLDL), low density lipoproteins (LDL), and high density lipoproteins (HDL) and decreased serum cholesterol and increased phospholipids. Progesterone is associated with diminished secretion of certain hepatic proteins—for example, VLDL and HDL.

Estrogen also influences carbohydrate metabolism, including increasing insulin secretion, decreasing blood sugar, and decreasing glucose tolerance. Progesterone diminishes insulin action, producing insulin resistance.

Protein metabolism effects of estrogen include increased hepatic protein secretion as outlined above, as well as increased binding proteins. Progesterone effects include enhanced nitrogen wasting.

Important tissue effects of estrogen include inhibition of bone resorption and increased adipose tissue mass. Progesterone is associated with enhanced fat breakdown and relaxation of the smooth muscle of the gut and arterioles.

Functional effects of estrogen on respiration include decreased metabolic rate, whereas progesterone enhances the hypothalamic respiratory center and stimulates respiration. Blood clotting effects of estrogen include increased clotting factors I, II, VI, VII, VIII, IX, and X and acceleration of platelet aggregation. Blood pressure and electrolyte balance are also influenced by estrogen with increased renin substrate (angiotensinogen) production and renin activity; increased aldosterone and sodium retention; and elevation of blood pressure. Progesterone increases sodium excretion by the kidney and decreases proximal tubular absorption. In addition, progesterone lowers blood pressure by relaxing the arterioles. Estrogen has an excitatory effect on neurons, whereas progesterone has a sedative effect. Estrogen also influences other endocrines: it stimulates pituitary secretion of prolactin and increases serum growth hormone secretion. Finally, estrogen has important effects on immune function. It modulates the immune response through estrogen receptors on T-lymphocyes and inhibits cell-mediated immunity in some lymphocytes—for example, low estrogen levels stimulate CD8 + suppressors, and high estrogen levels inhibit CD4 + helper cells. Estrogen also influences cytokines and growth factors: low estradiol stimulates interleukin-1, and higher estradiol levels inhibit interleukin 1 production and FNF-a (Dyrenfurth, 1982; Patton et al., 1989).

CONSEQUENCES OF REPRODUCTIVE AGING

Given the widespread and systemic effects of estrogen and progesterone, it is not surprising that their changing levels during the menopausal transition and postmenopause have been associated with changes in bone, adipose tissue, metabolism, and other aspects of integrative functioning. The ongoing SWAN study and other longitudinal studies of the menopausal transition have and will contribute much to understanding these longitudinal changes across the menopausal transition.

Changing Bone

Studies of the SWAN cohort revealed that, in 2,311 African American and White women followed for 4 years, bone density varied across ethnic groups of women, with highest bone mineral density levels among African American women and lowest in Whites (Finkelstein et al., 2002; Sowers et al., 2003). Dual-energy X-ray absorptiometry testing indicated that, over the 4-year period, women lost 5.6% of the lumbar spine mass as they experienced the menopausal transition and postmenopause. Women who experienced a surgical menopause lost 3.9% of their bone mass, and those who were in the late menopausal transition stage lost 3.2% over 4 years. Serum FSH predicted the 4-year bone loss, with women who had FSH levels of more than 35–45 mIU/ml losing the most bone. Estradiol levels of less than 35 pg/ml were associated with lower bone mineral density, but testosterone, free androgen index, and dehydroepiandrosterone sulfate were not (Sowers et al., 2006).

Body Composition: Fat and Muscle

In addition to bone, two other dimensions of body composition change with the menopausal transition: fat and muscle. Sowers and colleagues (2003, 2006, 2007) assessed body composition in 543 SWAN participants, following them over 7 years by measuring waist circumference and body composition (fat and muscle) using biological impedance measures. They found that women experienced an absolute cumulative 6-year increase in fat mass of 3.4 kg and a 6-year decrease in skeletal muscle mass of approximately 0.23 kg. The absolute 6-year increase in waist circumference was 5.7 cm. FSH changes were positively correlated with fat mass change. Waist circumference increased until 1 year following the FMP, when it slowed. Fat mass continued to increase after FMP with no change in rate (Sowers et al., 2006).

Metabolic Syndrome

The metabolic syndrome (in the past known as insulin resistance syndrome or syndrome X) is a clustering of metabolic abnormalities consisting of glucose intolerance, high blood pressure, high triglyceride levels, high LDL levels, hyperuricemia, adiposity, and insulin resistance.

Criteria for the metabolic syndrome (ATP III criteria discussed in chapters 12 and 26) include:

- Abdominal obesity (waist > 35 in)
- Atherogenic displidemia
  - □ Triglycerides > 150 md/dl
  - □ HDL-C < 50 mg/dl
  - □ > LDL-C levels
  - □ Small dense LDL
- Hypertension (BP > 130/85 mm Hg)
- Fasting blood glucose > 110 mg/dl (ATP III)

Metabolic syndrome is also associated with insulin resistance and glucose intolerance, a prothrombotic state, and a proinflammatory state.

During the menopausal transition, endocrine changes are associated with several characteristics of the metabolic syndrome. Studies of hemostatic and inflammatory factors and hormone levels during the menopausal transition revealed that both testosterone and estrogen play important roles. Androgens (testosterone and free androgen index) were positively associated with plasminogen activator inhibitor type I (PAI-1) and tissue plasminogen activator (t(PA)). FAI was positively associated with C-reactive protein (hs C-RP). Lower SHBG levels—which were associated with greater levels of bioavailable testosterone—were also associated with higher levels of PAI-1, hsC-RP, and factor VIIc. Androgens were strongly associated with fibrinolytic and inflammation markers, even when considering age, body size, smoking, and race/ethnicity in the SWAN cohort (Sowers et al., 2005a).

Estrogen was also significantly related to some hemostatic factors in the SWAN cohort: lower estradiol was associated with higher PAI-1 and t(PA) but not to fibrinogen, factor VIIc, or hs CRP. Elevated FSH was related to higher levels of PAI-1, factor VII levels and to lower fibrinogen and hs-CRP. Transitions to postmenopause were not associated with different levels of hemostatic factors. Endogenous estrogens may be associated with lower CVD risk via fibrinolytic but not coagulation or inflammatory mechanisms (Sowers et al., 2005b).

Data from the SWAN study also illuminate the relationship of hormone levels and lipids and insulin metabolism. FSH was associated with increased total cholesterol and LDL and lower insulin and homoeostasis model assessment for insulin resistance (HOMA-IR) measures. Estradiol was associated with increased triglycerides, lower LDL, higher HDL, lower PAI-1, and lower tPA levels. Testosterone was associated with greater BMI, higher triglyceride and glucose levels, and elevated diastolic blood pressure. Sex hormone binding globulin was associated with lower waist circumference, BMI, total cholesterol, LDL, and HDL as well as lower insulin, glucose, and HOMA insulin resistance measures. Free androgen index (a measure of bioavailable androgen) was associated with greater waist circumference, BMI, total cholesterol, triglycerides, insulin, glucose, and HOMA IR levels (Sutton-Tyrell et al., 2005). Taken together, there is mounting evidence that the endocrine changes during the menopausal transition have important effects on risk factors for heart disease—in particular, the metabolic syndrome. Higher free androgen and lower SHBG levels play an important role in cardiovascular risk factors for women during the menopausal transition.

Changes in blood pressure are of concern due to their relationship to stroke. There is little evidence supporting an effect of the menopausal transition on blood pressure. Prevalence of hypertension among the SWAN cohort varies significantly by ethnic/racial group, with Whites, Blacks, Hispanics, Chinese, and Japanese women having respective prevalences of hypertension of 14.5%, 381.%, 27.6%, 12.8%, and 11.0% (Lloyd-Jones et al., 2005).

Cognitive Function

Women worry about the effects of menopause on their cognitive function, particularly their memory functioning (Woods, Mitchell, & Adams, 2000; Mitchell & Woods, 2001). Recent attention to dementia has increased attention to the experiences of memory lapses. To date, only one longitudinal study has tracked changes in cognition across the menopausal transition. The SWAN study included measures of verbal memory, working memory, and cognitive processing speed. Results indicated that women did not experience significant declines in any of these areas, but measures improved for women in the late reproductive and early menopausal transition stages over a 2-year period. Significant decreases in Symbol Digit Modalities Test scores occurred only for postmenopausal women, a pattern consistent with expected age-related changes (Meyer et al., 2003).

Autonomic Nervous System Changes

Studies of autonomic nervous system responses across the menopausal transition have revealed differences in stress response when comparing premenopausal and postmenopausal women. Postmenopausal women exhibited greater increases in heart rate during all laboratory stressors when compared to premenopausal women, with a pronounced increase during a speech task stressor deemed to be socially relevant to middle-aged women. Postmenopausal women exhibited greater increases in systolic blood pressure and epinephrine during the speech task, but not in response to other stressors (Saab, Matthew, Stoney, & McDonald, 1989). Subsequent experiments confirmed this effect and demonstrated that women receiving estrogen therapy had attenuated stress response (Lindheim et al., 1992), but a more recent study with transdermal estrogen in postmenopausal women 52 to 56 years of age revealed that acute transdermal estrogen administration did not attenuate norepinphrine spillover or sympathetically mediate hemodynamic responses (Sofowora, Singh, He, Woods, & Stein, 2005). Recent studies also point out that muscle sympathetic nerve activity was not attributable to menopause, but that aging was accompanied by a greater increase in sympathetic traffic in women than in men (Narkiewicz et al., 2005).

Immune Response

The greater prevalence of autoimmune diseases—for example, thyroid disease, lupus erythematosus, scleroderma, and rheumatoid arthritis—among women compared to men makes the relationship of the MT to the immune response of interest. Estradiol can modulate immune response via estrogen receptors on T lymphocytes and by modulating cytokines and growth factors (Polan, Daniele, & Kuo, 1988). To date, no longitudinal studies document the effects of menopausal transition on immune function. Nonetheless, recent reports indicate that there are between-group differences among women who have not yet begun the menopausal transition, women in the transition, and women in early and late postmenopause. A study of 16 women not in the transition, 54 women in transition, and 32 women in early (first 5 years) postmenopause and 20 women who were between 5 and 10 years postmenopause revealed that: IL4 was higher in late postmenopausal women; IL 2 was higher in early postmenopause, as was granulocyte-macrophage colony-stimulating factor (GM-CSF) and granulocyte colony stimulating factor (G-CSF). Age was negatively related to IL-6, but MT was unrelated. Estradiol was negatively related to IL-6 levels and weakly negatively related to IL-2, IL-8, and GM-CSF (Yasui et al., 2007). Results from longitudinal studies are needed to clarify the relationship between the menopausal transition and these immune indicators.

ASSESSMENT OF MID-LIFE WOMEN'S HEALTH

Assessment of mid-life women negotiating the menopausal transition includes obtaining a thorough history, physical examination, laboratory testing, and differential diagnosis. Sometimes the differential diagnosis includes ongoing medical problems in addition to problems women associate with their transition from reproductive to postreproductive state (Hawkins, Roberto-Nichols, & Stanley-Haney, 2007). However, emphasis in this section is on menstrual cyclicity and symptoms women report during their transition to postmenopause.

History Related to Menstrual Cycling

When menstrual cycles dysregulate, a number of changes occur: Cycle lengths change, becoming shorter or longer or women may have alternating short and long cycles. As women approach the final menstrual period, they frequently experience very long cycles, which they often refer to as skipped periods. The number of bleeding days may increase or decrease, and the amount of menstrual flow may become more scanty or heavier, with some women experiencing extremely heavy bleeding referred to as flooding. A careful history of menstrual cycling would include the following items.

A. Presenting symptoms
1. Menstrual cycle changes (in comparison to women's menstrual regularity during the 20s and mid-30s). Asking women to keep a menstrual calendar and reviewing it at each appointment will provide the most accurate basis for the history.
   a. Menstrual periods more or less frequent or shorter or longer in duration
   b. Light menstrual flow
   c. Flooding
   d. Irregular periods
   e. Gradual or abrupt cessation of menses for 1 or more months
2. Changes women relate to the menopause transition or to aging
   a. Hot flashes or flushes
   b. Vaginal dryness
   c. Night sweats
   d. Dry skin and hair
   e. Skeletal pain or stiffness; joint pain
   f. Graying of hair; thinning of pubic hair
   g. Loss of skin turgor
   h. Sleep alterations
   i. Development issues: empty nest, caring for aging parents, role changes, retirement
3. Recent history of gynecologic surgery: hysterectomy, oophorectomy, salpingectomy, dilatation and curettage, cervical conization, cryosurgery, loop electrocautery (electrosurgery) excision procedure (LEEP) for abnormal Pap smear

B. Gather additional historical data
1. Menstrual history in past year and in previous year for comparison
2. Contraceptive use to present
3. Pregnancies, abortions, stillbirths
4. Gynecologic history: surgery, endometriosis, infertility, abnormalities, last Pap smear, any breast problems, sexually transmitted infection history, breast health promotion (such as self breast exam and last mammogram), symptoms of urinary incontinence
5. Sexual history: dysfunction, pain, recent changes
6. Life event changes: new or resumed career, retirement, care of older family members, adult children issues, divorce, separation, marriage, new sexual relationship, caring for grandchildren. These data enlighten about potential stressors in women's lives.
7. Health promotion behaviors: nutrition, exercise, stress reduction, recreation
8. Risk behaviors: smoking, stressors, alcohol use, recreational drugs
9. Medical history: chronic disease, prescription medications, over-the-counter medications, vitamins, herbal remedies
10. Use of alternative and complementary therapies: botanicals, homeopathy, acupuncture, traditional Chinese medicine, chiropractic, aromatherapy, Ayurvedic
11. Beliefs and expectations about the menopausal transition: Previous research reports suggest a relationship betwveen these and symptom perception and evaluation.

Physical Examination Elements

Physical examination elements for mid-life women negotiating the menopause transition do not differ from those for younger women. However, age-related changes as well as changes related to altered sex hormones require greater emphasis on certain elements of the speculum exam (evaluate for irritation, vaginal dryness, dyspareunia), bimanual (greater possibility of cystocele, rectocele, urethrocele, less palpable tubes or ovaries, and small uterine size), and rectal (greater risk of colorectal cancer) examinations.

A. Vital signs
B. General health examination
C. Gynecologic exam
1. External inspection and palpation for lesions, infection, atrophy, anomaly

2. Speculum examination
   a. Vaginal walls
   b. Discharge (wet mount, gonococcus [GC] culture, chlamydia culture, Pap smear if indicated)
   c. Lesions on vaginal walls or cervix
   d. Cervical inspection for inflammation, discharge
   e. Inspection of vaginal vault—note if posthysterectomy

D. Bimanual examination
   1. Adnexa: tenderness, masses, palpable tubes or ovaries, if present
   2. Uterus: position, size, mobility, tenderness, masses
   3. Evaluate for cystocele, rectocele, urethrocele

E. Rectal examination: masses, bleeding, test for fecal occult blood

Laboratory Testing

A. Appropriate cultures or smears if infection suspected

B. Papanicolaou (Pap) smear

C. Mammogram as directed by the American Cancer Society guidelines
   1. Baseline at age 35
   2. Annually at age 40 and beyond
   3. May be altered with significant family history or personal breast cancer risk factors

D. Testing serum FSH level is controversial for women in the early and late menopausal transition. It is commonly used to confirm menopause (12 consecutive months of amenorrhea); however, clinical history provides sufficient data. Results should be reviewed in conjunction with women's menstrual calendars

Differential Diagnosis for Menstrual Dysregulation

A. Genital tract abnormalities—for example, carcinoma

B. Endocrine disorders

C. Pregnancy

D. Poor nutritional state, obesity

E. Dramatic increase in exercise regimen resulting in lowered fat stores

Symptoms During the Menopausal Transition

During mid-life, women experience a variety of symptoms. Among these are hot flashes, sweats, depressed mood, sleep disturbances, sexual concerns or problems, memory symptoms, vaginal dryness, urinary incontinence, and somatic or bodily pain symptoms.

Hot flashes are sudden sensations of heat that usually arise on the chest and spread to the neck and face and sometimes to the arms. They may be accompanied by sweating in some women (Voda, 1981). Hot flashes and sweats increase in prevalence as women approach the final menstrual period, with an estimated 33% to 64% of women experiencing hot flashes during the late menopausal transition stage (Woods & Mitchell, 2005). Vasomotor symptoms have been associated with luteinizing hormone pulses (Casper, Yen, & Wilkes, 1979; Freedman, 2005), low estradiol (Guthrie, Dennerstein, Hopper, & Burger, 1996; Guthrie, Dennerstein, Taffe, Lehert, & Burger, 2004; Guthrie, Dennerstein, Taffe, Lehert, and Burger, 2005; Woods et al., 2007); low inhibin levels (Guthrie et al., 2005), and high levels of follicle-stimulating hormone (Freeman et al., 2001; Randolph et al., 2005; Woods et al., 2007). Sex hormone binding globulin and free estradiol levels were also associated with a lower prevalence of hot flashes (Randolph et al., 2005), and, in one study (Overlie, Moen, Holte, & Finset, 2002), androgen levels were associated with a decreased frequency of postmenopausal vasomotor symptoms. In acute studies of hot flashes where laboratory stimuli were used to provoke hot flashes, elevations in LH, adrenocorticotropic hormone, and cortisol all were closely associated in time with the experience of the hot flash, but no changes were reported in estradiol and FSH levels (Meldrum et al., 1980; Tataryn, Meldrum, Lu, Frumar, & Judd, 1979).

An estimated 30% to 45% of women experience disrupted sleep during the menopausal transition, with the prevalence of symptoms becoming higher during the late menopausal transition stage and early postmenopause (Dennerstein, Lehert, Burger, & Guthrie, 2005). Women believe that awakening during the night is due to hormonal changes and hot flashes (Woods & Mitchell, 1999) and that hot flashes are correlated with sleep disruption and estrogen levels (Woods et al., 2007), but evidence from a recent study indicates that women awaken, then have a hot flash (Freedman & Roehrs, 2004). Polysomnographic studies of sleep among women during the menopausal transition and postmenopause revelaed that there was both an increase in sleep disruption as women progressed to the postmenopause and that psychological distress was associated with subjectively experienced symptoms (Shaver et al., 1988, 1993). Sleep symptoms have been associated with higher FSH levels during the late reproductive stage and to lower estradiol levels in another study of women who were still cycling (Hollander et al., 2001), but these findings are not consistent across all studies (Woods et al., 2007). When women without hot flashes were monitored overnight, arousals that occurred were associated with sleep disordered breathing and age (Lukacs, Chilimigras, Cannon, Dormire, & Reame, 2004).

Depressed mood symptoms are prevalent among mid-life women, with 25% to 29% of women reporting depressed mood during the late menopausal transition stage and 23% to 34% during the early postmenopause (Woods & Mitchell, 2005). Higher FSH and LH levels and increased variability of estradiol, FSH, and LH (within women) were associated with depressed mood symptoms (Freeman, Samuel, Lin, & Nelson, 2004; Freeman et al., 2006), as were lower levels of estradiol (Avis et al., 2001a; Freeman et al., 2006) and dehydro-epiandrosterone sulfate (Morrison et al., 2001; Schmidt et al., 2002), but some studies show no relationship to endocrine levels (Woods et al., 2008). Evidence is beginning to suggest that the menopausal transition may be a period of vulnerability to depression, even for women who have no history of depression earlier in life (Bromberger et al., 2001, 2003, 2004, 2007; Freeman et al., 2006; Woods et al., 2008).

Women often notice cognitive symptoms such as forgetfulness or difficulty concentrating, but few rate them as serious and most attribute these symptoms to changing hormones as well as general aging and life stress (Mitchell & Woods, 2001; Woods, Mitchell, & Adams, 2000). The Study of Women Across the Nation reported stage-specific prevalence of forgetfulness ranging from 31% during the late reproductive stage to 42% in postmenopause (Gold et al., 2000). The single longitudinal assessment of cognitive functions indicated that the changes were related to aging and that women's cognitive function improved in some areas (Meyer et al., 2003). One study has demonstrated that women bothered by forgetfulness had higher FSH levels than those not so troubled; difficulty concentrating was associated with lower levels of testosterone (Woods et al., 2007).

Changes in sexual desire are troublesome to some women, and these changes become more pronounced in the late menopausal transition stage (Dennerstein et al., 2002, 2004; Avis, Stellato, Crawford, Johannes, & Longcope, 2000). Decreased sexual desire was negatively correlated with estradiol levels in one study (Woods et al., 2007), and lower sexual functioning scores in the Melbourne Midlife Women's Health Study were associated with higher FSH levels and lower estradiol levels (Dennerstein et al., 2002). Although there was no relationship with testosterone in the Melbourne study, participants in the Penn Ovarian Aging study who experienced fluctuation in testosterone levels experienced more problems with sexual desire (Gracia et al., 2004). Painful intercourse (dyspareunia) has been associated with low estradiol levels (Avis et al., 2000), and vaginal dryness has been associated with higher FSH levels and lower testosterone levels (Woods et al., 2007). Vaginal dryness increases in frequency as women progress from the menopausal transition to postmenopause; 21% of participants in the Melbourne study reported vaginal dryness during the late menopausal transition stage and 47% during early postmenopause (Dennerstein, Dudley, Hopper, Guthrie, & Burger, 2000).

Urinary incontinence symptoms are prevalent among women and appear to increase with age as well as over the menopausal transition. Approximately 47% of the Melbourne study participants reported being bothered by urinary leakage during the late menopausal transition and 53% during early postmenopause (Dennerstein et al., 2000).

Although musculoskeletal and joint aches and pains are a commonly experienced symptom in mid-life women (57% of the Melbourne study participants experienced them during the late menopausal transition and early postmenopause) (Dennerstein et al., 2000), they do not appear to be associated with the menopausal transition. As the ongoing longitudinal studies near completion, some of the associations between symptoms and aging and the menopausal transition will become clearer.

Finally, although the level of ovarian steroids or gonadotropins may not be directly related to symptoms, several studies point to the importance of variability or rate of change in hormones and symptoms. Rannevik and associates (1995) found no association between estradiol and depression symptoms but did find that women who experienced a greater drop in estradiol around the time of menopause were at greatest risk of having depressed mood. In addition, Freeman and colleagues' work (2006) suggests that variability in endocrine levels is important.

A Menopausal Syndrome?

Many assume that there is a "menopausal syndrome" that affects women universally, but there is not definitive evidence to support this assertion (Avis et al., 2001b). Findings from the SWAN study revealed that there is not a universal menopausal syndrome consisting of a variety of vasomotor and psychological symptoms. Instead, during the menopausal transition women who used hormones and women who had surgical menopause reported more vasomotor symptoms but no more psychological symptoms than do their counterparts. White women reported more psychosomatic symptoms than other ethnic groups, and African American women reported more vasomotor symptoms than other ethnic groups of women in the SWAN study (Avis, Brockwell, & Colvin, 2005).

The relationships among symptoms any one woman experiences may be important for clinicians to consider. Mitchell and Woods (1996) found that symptoms clustered together in vasomotor, dysphoric mood, sleep disturbance, and other groups. The vasomotor symptoms were least reliable across multiple occasions, indicating they were most likely to change across the menopausal transition. Avis and colleagues (2001a, 2001b) found that participants in the Massachusetts women's health study did not experience symptoms of depression as a result of changing estradiol levels. Instead, women who had hot flashes, night sweats, and trouble sleeping had more depressed mood. Avis suggested a "domino" hypothesis: depressed mood occurs among women who have vasomotor symptoms and sleep problems that are related to their changing hormone levels. When the vasomotor and sleep symptoms are taken into account, estradiol has no effect on depressed mood. Figure 6.5 shows the relationships among symptoms studied in a subset of participants in the Seattle Midlife Women's Health Study who had completed the transition to menopause. Of interest is that hot flashes were related to night-time awakening and to forgetfulness, but not related directly to depressed mood when patterns were examined within individual women over time (Woods et al., 2007). A careful history could elicit from women the symptoms they are experiencing and their impressions of which are related. Knowing the complement of symptoms may suggest a tailored therapy regimen—for example, one that is effective for both hot flashes and sleep disruption.

There is some evidence that symptoms women report during the menopausal transition and postmenopause are a culture-bound phenomenon because women from cultures not influenced by Western medicine report few symptoms or different symptoms than do Western women. For example, Lock, Kaufert, and Gilbert's (1988) work with Japanese women revealed that their most frequently reported symptom was shoulder pain, not hot flashes. Whether infrequent reporting of hot flashes by Japanese women may be attributable to the high phytoestrogen content in their diets or other features by which culture influences biology remains to be seen.

When considering the relationship of symptoms to the menopausal transition, it is important to consider the context in which they occur. Many women juggle multiple obligations for their families, such as parenting adolescent or young adult children, providing caregiving services for their elderly family members, grandparenting, and dealing with the challenges of material stress. The participants in the SWAN study who have trouble paying for basics are at greater risk for nearly every kind of symptom (Gold et al., 2000). Viewing symptoms in the broader context of women's lives may help tailor therapies likely to be most efficacious.

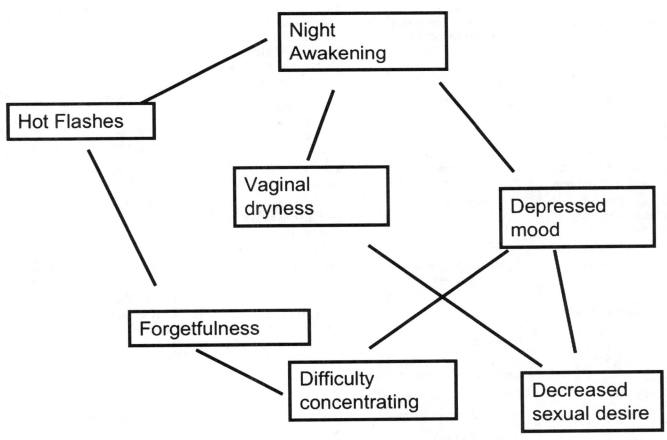

FIGURE 6.5   Relationships among symptoms: Intraindividual analyses.

SELF-MANAGEMENT AND COMPLEMENTARY AND ALLOPATHIC THERAPIES

Symptoms that women experience during the menopausal transition elicit an array of self-management attempts. Indeed, women often find that mid-life and symptoms they experience lead them to contemplate and implement changes in their health behavior patterns. A survey conducted by the North American Menopause Society revealed that women engaged in a wide variety of efforts to promote their health and often saw this time of life as an opportunity to appraise their health (Kaufert, 1986). Women reported trying exercise regimens, nutritional modification, vitamin supplementation, relaxation, and alteration of their mental attitudes as a means of managing their symptoms. In addition, contacts with health care providers during this time of life provide opportunities for health promotion and prevention counseling.

Women find that many symptoms such as hot flashes, blue mood, and sleep problems respond to self-management strategies, especially if the symptoms are mild. Some women may choose complementary and alternative therapies, although many have not been demonstrated to be efficacious. Finally, prescription therapies are indicated for some symptoms. Table 6.2 lists self-

 | Symptoms, Self-Management, Complementary, and Allopathic Therapies for Menopause

SYMPTOM	SELF-MANAGEMENT	COMPLEMENTARY THERAPIES	ALLOPATHIC THERAPIES
Hot flashes and night sweats	Identify triggers for symptoms and avoid or minimize exposure to them (e.g., avoid smoking, poorly ventilated rooms) Adjust ventilation or environmental temperature Avoid elevation of core temperature (e.g., drinking hot beverages)	Paced respiration and relaxation therapy[a] Isoflavone extracts[a] Phytoestrogen preparation Acupuncture Yoga Meditation Tai chi or qi gong Positive visualization Exercise regularly, avoiding exercise within a few hours of bedtime Black cohosh Chinese herbs Magnets Reflexology	Systemic estrogen therapy, estrogen/progestin, or progesterone[a] Nonhormonal drugs, including gabapentin,[a] clonidine,[a] and paroxetine[a]
Sleep disturbances and night-time awakening	Sleep hygiene measures	Valerian Melatonin	FDA-approved sleep medications
Mood symptoms, including depression and anxiety	Stress management Coping skills training	St. John's wort Omega 3 fatty acids Vitamin + Exercise + Light Exposure (LEVITY)	Antidepressants and talk therapy[a]
Vaginal dryness	Vaginal lubricants (water soluble) Vaginal moisturizers	Vitamin E oil[a]	Systemic or local estrogens such as the estradiol ring, estrogen creams[a]
Urinary incontinence	Bladder diary Kegel exercises Timed voiding	Biofeedback using vaginal cones	FDA approved medications Surgery
Sexual function	Available sexual stimulation Lubricants or moisturizers for comfort		None FDA approved
Cognitive	Memory aids (e.g., calendars)		
Somatic	None specific to menopause	None specific to menopause	None specific to menopause

[a]existing evidence for efficacy

management strategies that many women find useful for symptoms as well as complementary and allopathic therapeutic options.

Hot Flashes and Sweats

Few of the self-management strategies have been evaluated in randomized controlled clinical trials for efficacy. Voda's (1981) early studies of women's hot flash experiences identified several triggers that women may learn to identify and subsequently avoid or minimize exposure to them. Some of these include hot foods or beverages, spicy foods, poorly ventilated rooms, hot and humid environments, caffeine, certain alcoholic beverages, and other agents that could increase core body temperature or minimize heat loss. Dressing in natural fabrics that do not retain heat and in layers that can be removed also may be helpful.

Trials of complementary therapies have focused on the effects of biologically based agents such as phytoestrogens (plant-based estrogens); mind-body and behavioral therapies; manipulative, body-based, and energy therapies, and whole medical systems. Recent reviews find little evidence to warrant the use of many of these therapies, but in some cases sufficient evidence to encourage further study (Carpenter & Neal, 2005; Nedrow et al., 2006; Nelson et al., 2006).

Biologically based therapies include botanicals, animal-derived extracts, vitamins, amino acids, proteins, probiotics, whole diets, and functional foods (Nedrow et al., 2006). In the category of biologically based therapies, most trials for hot flashes have focused on phytoestrogens and soy extracts. Phytoestrogen preparations and dietary soy isoflavones have been studied most extensively. Isoflavones (50 to 70 mg per day for 4 to 6 weeks to 6 months) were associated with a reduction of one to two hot flashes per day (Nelson et al., 2006). The majority of evidence indicates that red clover isoflavones are not efficacious for managing hot flashes (Nelson et al., 2006). There is no evidence of the efficacy of phytoestrogen topical creams (Nedrow et al., 2006). Further research on soy therapies with varying doses and better methods may reveal helpful effects. To date, there are no known hazardous effects of these therapies.

Black cohosh (Remifemin®) has been evaluated with inconsistent results until recently. A large randomized controlled clinical trial of black cohosh 160 mg per day; multibotanical with black cohosh and nine other ingredients 200 mg per day; and mutibotanical plus dietary soy counseling versus conjugated equine estrogens 0.625 mg per day and/or medroxyprogesterone acetate 2.5 mg daily or placebo revealed that vasomotor symptoms did not differ between the herbal interventions and placebo at 3, 6, or 12 months. Results of this trial suggest that black cohosh used in isolation or with a multibotanical regimen had little effect on vasomotor symptoms (Newton et al., 2006).

Dong quai, ginseng extract, and evening primrose seed oil do not have demonstrated efficacy in well-conducted trials (Low Dog, 2005). To date, there is no evidence of effectiveness of DHEA or vitamin E. Kava is not recommended owing to the risk of liver failure. (Nedrow et al., 2006)

Mind-body therapies focus on the interactions among mind-body and behavior, with some including emotional, mental, social, spiritual, and behavioral dimensions related to health. Self-knowledge and self-care capacity are the focus of guided imagery and meditation and paced respiration (Nedrow et al., 2006). Exercise, relaxation therapy, progressive muscle relaxation, audiotaped relaxation training, stress management, and menopausal transition education and counseling have also been studied for hot flashes.

Of the mind-body therapies, paced respiration and relaxation (Freedman, 2005; Irvin, Domar, Clark, Zuttermeister, & Friedman,1996) have received the most attention. Paced respiration was effective in helping women reduce the number of hot flashes in two studies, although it is unclear what the mechanism is (Freedman, 2005). Women were randomized to six weekly sessions of progressive muscle relaxation and slow, deep breathing (paced respiration) or alpha wave biofeedback as a placebo. Relaxation and paced respiration reduced by 50% the number of hot flashes recorded in the laboratory and the hot flashes women experienced and recorded in a daily symptom diary. In a second study, paced respiration was compared with muscle relaxation and alpha EEG biofeedback control. Paced respiration resulted in 50% fewer hot flashes as demonstrated by ambulatory monitoring. Assessment of the effects of paced respiration on 3-methoxy-4-hydroxyphenylglycol (MHPG), epinephrine, norepinephrine, cortisol, and platelet alpha-2 receptors in blood samples did not indicate any change despite reduction of the hot flash frequency by 50%. Another investigator group (Irvin et al., 1996) tested the effects of relaxation therapy training using paced respiration and mental focusing compared with a reading control group and a no-treatment control group. They found that paced respiration reduced the severity of hot flashes but not the frequency. Taken together, these studies suggest that paced respiration is an effective and low-cost therapy that women can use for self-management of hot flashes. A comprehensive assessment of symptoms during the menopausal transition, education and counseling, and intervention with pharmaceutical and behavioral therapies was effective in reducing symptoms of hot flashes, vaginal dryness, and stress urinary incontinence among women with breast cancer (Ganz et al., 2000). These results suggest that bundling of interventions may be an optimal approach for symptom management.

Trials of exercise for reduction of hot flashes have not demonstrated efficacy. It is likely that exercise is ineffective because it has been shown to stimulate hot flashes in laboratory conditions, probably because it raises core temperature (Freedman, 2005). Nonetheless, the effects of exercise warrant encouraging women with hot flashes to exercise for other health benefits.

Energy therapies include those manipulating energy fields through the use of electromagnetic and sound waves as well as human energy fields (therapeutic touch, Reiki). To date, there is no evidence of efficacy with magnet therapy and hot flashes (Carpenter & Neal, 2005).

Manipulative therapies such as chiropractic or osteopathic manipulation include massage, the Feldenkrais, and Rolfing approaches. There is no evidence of efficacy of these therapies for hot flashes (Carpenter & Neal, 2005). Low-force osteopathic manipulation of the spine, pelvis, and cranium versus sham treatment has been shown effective for reducing hot flashes and several other symptoms (Cleary & Fox, 1994).

Whole medical systems include the Eastern approaches, such as Chinese medicine and Ayurvedic schools from India. Western approaches, including homoeopathy and naturopathy, also are in this category. Acupuncture has been studied using randomized controlled trials with demonstrable improvement in hot flashes over time in the treatment group in some studies and no improvement of hot flashes in others (Nedrow et al., 2006).

Acupuncture and yoga trials are in process, and their efficacy awaits further evidence (Carpenter & Neal, 2005 Nedrow et al., 2006). Use of these interventions requires an understanding of their effectiveness within the context of the whole medical system, but Western studies tend to focus on a single component. Thus, it is unclear what the efficacy of these treatments would be if tested as they are typically delivered—for example, within a Chinese medicine treatment framework.

Trials of allopathic therapies emphasized hormone therapy until the publication of the results of the Women's Health Initiative (La Croix, 2005). Hormone therapy trial results provided evidence of efficacy for symptom relief for transdermal estradiol, oral estrogens, including estrogen and progestins/progesterone and estrogen alone (Nelson et al., 2006).

Recent trials of the anticonvulsant gabapentin (900 mg per day) showed efficacy, as have trials of the antidepressant SNRI paroxetine (12 to 25 mg per day) and the alpha-adrenergic agonist antihypertensive drug clonidine (Nelson et al., 2006). None of these drugs is without risk, and there tend to be fewer side effects at lower doses of these drugs.

Sleep Disturbances

Sleep hygiene interventions include avoiding heavy meals in the evening; modifying environment factors such as ventilation, lighting, noise, and temperature; avoiding stimulants such as caffeine and nicotine; avoiding alcohol; and exercising several hours before bedtime. Lifestyle changes may not alleviate sleep symptoms. When night-time awakening, inability to go to sleep, and early morning awakening persist, clinical exams should rule out other potential causes, including sleep disorders, sleep disordered breathing, thyroid anomalies, allergy, restless leg syndrome, and clinical depression.

Valerian trials have not demonstrated efficacy. Although kava has been studied for anxiety and sleep problems, its association with severe liver damage makes it dangerous. Estrogen therapies for hot flashes may alleviate sleep symptoms, but estrogen therapy is not indicated for treatment of sleep problems by the U.S. Food and Drug Administration (FDA). Primary therapies for sleep symptoms should be explored.

Mood Symptoms

Tearfulness, mood swings, and feeling blue, irritable, or anxious are symptoms that women experience throughout the lifespan and some women may experience them during the menopausal transition. Recent studies that suggest an increase in depressed mood and clinical depression during the menopausal transition link these mood changes to past history of depression, premenstrual syndrome, postpartum depression, having a longer menopausal transition, and experiencing more severe hot flashes (Freeman et al., 2006; Woods et al., 2008; Avis et al., 2001a). Some women may be vulnerable to depression during the time when they experience hormonal change; this would account for the link between premenstrual syndrome and postpartum depression history and depression during the menopausal transition. It is also important for clinicians to explore other causes for mood symptoms, such as thyroid imbalance, medication side effects, and concurrent life stresses.

Self-management for mood symptoms has included strategies effective in other parts of the life span: coping skills training, social support, and an integrated treatment approach with vitamin therapies, exercise or physical activity, and exposure to light (Brown & Robinson, 2002). Sometimes effective treatment of hot flashes will improve both sleep patterns and mood. However, depression that persists for longer than 2 weeks should be assessed by a clinician and treated with both talk therapy as well as antidepressants. A recent head-to-head trial of the antidepressant escitalopram (a selective serotonin reuptake inhibitor, or SSRI) and ethinyl estradiol and norethindrone acetate revealed that the SSRI was three times as effective as estrogen in relieving depressive symptoms. In addition, 56% of women using the SSRI experienced relief of their hot flashes (Soares et al., 2006).

Anxiety symptoms have been correlated with hot flashes in some studies (Freeman, 2005). Whether the symptoms of anxiety are related to hormonal changes remains unclear. As with depression, anxiety disorders should be treated with appropriate talk therapy and psychotropic medication (Frank et al., 2000).

Vaginal Symptoms

Women experience vaginal symptoms that include dryness, discharge, irritation, burning, dryness, itching, and pain at many points in their lives. It is important for clinicians to rule out infections, bacterial vaginosis, sexually transmitted infections, skin conditions, pelvic radiation history, Crohn's disease, pelvic nerve injury and vulvodynia, allergy, and irritation as underlying causes. Thinning of the vaginal tissue, reduction in vaginal lubrication, and increase in vaginal pH occur during the later parts of the menopausal transition and postmenopause. Self-management strategies may include the use of lubricants such as K-Y® personal jelly or vaginal moisturizers such as Replens®. Some women find vitamin E oil effective. Local estrogen therapy can be delivered in creams, tablets, or rings impregnated with hormone. Women with a uterus who use local estrogen therapy should also take a progestin preparation to protect themselves from endometrial cancer.

Sexual Functioning Symptoms

Sexual functioning symptoms that women experience during the menopausal transition resemble those they may experience at other points in their lives. Recent attention has been devoted to symptoms of sexual desire as well as dyspareunia during the menopausal transition. The relationship among vaginal dryness and night-time awakening to decreased sexual desire was noted in a longitudinal study of women as they made the transition to menopause (Woods et al., 2007). Hormonal and other changes such as fatigue, dissatisfaction with body image, low self-esteem, dissatisfaction with a partner, or sexual dysfunction in a partner may play a role in influencing sexual desire. Although some recommend the use of testosterone systemically or in creams, there is no evidence for its efficacy, and the use of testosterone for women for enhancing sexual desire is not approved by the FDA. The menopausal transition is an important time to reinforce safe sexual practices for women and for many women to enjoy their sexuality without the risk of pregnancy.

Urinary Incontinence

Urinary incontinence symptoms may be related to stress incontinence or urge incontinence. Careful assessment is important in developing a treatment plan. Women can take the initial steps by keeping a bladder diary that tracks their fluid intake (amount, type, and time) and urinary output (amount and time). In addition, keeping rack of urge symptoms and leaking (amount and time) are important as a foundation for diagnosis and further treatment. Self-management strategies such as timed voiding are strategies that women can try prior to seeking treatment. The Women's Health Initiative study revelaed that women treated with hormone therapy had a greater incidence of incontinence than women in a control group (Hendrix et al., 2005).

Cognitive Symptoms

Cognitive symptoms women experience during the menopausal transition cause worry about developing dementia. Worries may be particularly profound for women who have a family history of dementia. Use of memory aids such as calendars and lists may help. In addition, because many women associate these symptoms with role overload, assessment of life stress and use of stress management strategies may help. The Women's Health Initiative study revealed that women randomized to hormone therapy had no beneficial effects with respect to mild cognitive impairment or dementia (Rapp et al., 2003; Shumaker et al., 2003).

Somatic Symptoms

Somatic symptoms women experience during the menopausal transition include musculoskeletal and joint aches and pains. Although these symptoms are not specific to menopausal transition, their occurrence may be noticeable and bothersome. Persistent painful symptoms should be evaluated to determine whether they are linked to underlying disease processes such as osteoarthritis or osteoporosis.

Although it is important to focus symptom management on the symptoms women find most troublesome, some symptoms may improve as others are managed. For example, when women are treated with an antidepressant such as paroxetine for depression, they may notice their hot flashes improve. When some women achieve management of their hot flashes, their sleep improves.

Hormone Therapy for Symptom Management and Disease Prevention

Prevention of diseases associated with aging, promoting women's health during mid-life, and focusing on symptom management are important. Often women's consultation of health professionals for symptom management affords the opportunity for offering counsel related to health promotion.

Hormone therapy has been the primary therapy used for management of hot flashes and vaginal dryness, with established efficacy as described earlier. Estrogen was first approved for use by postmenopausal women during the 1940s, but the prevalence of estrogen use did not increase substantially until the 1960s, when clinicians prescribed it for relief of menopausal hot flashes and urogenital symptoms. During the early 1970s, evidence of an increased incidence of endometrial cancer associated with estrogen therapy and worries about possible associations with increased risk of vascular disease (as had occurred with the use of oral contraceptives) led to a decrease in prescription of estrogen therapy (Bush, 1991). In the 1980s, clinicians added a progestin to prescriptions of estrogen therapy to reduce the risk of endometrial cancer (Hemminki, Kennedy, Baum, & McKinlay, 1988). In 1986, the FDA approved the use of postmenopausal estrogen for the prevention and management of osteoporosis based on evidence supporting effectiveness of estrogen reducing hip and vertebral fractures (Weiss, Ure, Ballard, Williams, & Daling, 1980). Retrospective studies linked use of estrogen therapy to reduced incidence of cardiovascular disease, generating enthusiasm for using hormone therapy for preventive purposes (Bush et al., 1987).

Despite enthusiasm for using hormone therapies for prevention, the American College of Physicians (1992) advocated separate consideration of hormone therapy for symptom management and disease prevention. They advised a limited course of therapy, ranging from 1 to 5 years for symptoms, and recommended careful consideration of using hormones for disease prevention. The U.S. Preventive Services Task Force (1996) concluded that there was insufficient evidence to recommend for or against use of hormone therapy by women.

Although hormone therapy had been shown to be efficacious for managing symptoms of hot flashes and vaginal dryness, evidence was lacking for disease prevention. Three large clinical trials sponsored by the National Institutes of Health—the Postmenopausal Estrogen and Progestin Intervention (PEPI) study, the Heart and Estrogen/Progestin Replacement Study (HERS) study, and the Women's Health Initiative (WHI) trial—contributed important information about the relative benefits and risks of hormone therapy for preventing diseases of advanced age. The PEPI study examined the effects of estrogen and progestin on LDL and HDL cholesterol levels and other risk factors. The trial included 875 healthy postmenopausal women aged 45 to 64 years who had no known contraindication to hormone therapy. The women were randomized into five groups: placebo; conjugated equine estrogen (CEE) 0.625 mg; CEE 0.625 mg plus cyclic medroxyprogesterone acetate (MPA) 10 mg per day for 12 days per month; CEE 0.625 mg plus consecutive MPA 2.5 mg per day; or CEE 0.625 mg plus cyclic micronized progesterone (MP) 200 mg per day for 12 days per month. Results indicated that estrogen alone or with a progestin had positive effects on cardiovascular risk factors, including improved lipoproteins and lowered fibrinogen levels, without adverse effects on post-challenge insulin or blood pressure. Although unopposed estrogen provided optimal elevation of HDL-C, there was a high rate of endometrial hyperplasia among women who used unopposed estrogen, restricting recommendations for its use to women without a uterus (Writing Group for the PEPI Trial, 1995). Women treated with estrogens or estrogen and progestin gained bone mass at the hip and spine (from 3.5% to 5%) over a 3-year period (Writing Group for the PEPI Trial, 1996). Women who had a uterus responded most favorably to CEE with cyclic micronized progesterone with respect to HDL-C and had no excess increased risk of endometrial hyperplasia. MPA had no detrimental effects on lipids compared with the risk for those not taking hormones.

Two later clinical trials revealed different disease outcomes that contrasted with the positive effects seen on risk factors. The HERS study, a randomized, blinded, placebo-controlled trial of estrogen plus progestin therapy in postmenopausal women with documented heart disease ($N = 2,763$), included women from 55 to 79 years of age with a mean of 67 years. After 4 years of follow-up, researchers noted a higher risk of coronary events during the first year with unclear benefit after years 3 to 5 (Hulley et al., 1998). Follow-up studies revealed confusing results about evidence for efficacious reduction of cardiovascular disease and other health outcomes after nearly 7 years of tracking (Grady et al., 2002; Hulley et al., 2002).

The Women's Health Initiative, begun in 1993, includes a set of three interrelated clinical trials and an observational study in an apparently healthy postmenopausal sample. At entry to the study, 7.7% of women had prior cardiovascular disease. The randomized, blinded, controlled hormone therapy study included two treatment arms, one using estrogen alone for women without a uterus ($n = 10,739$) and one using combined conjugated estrogen and progestogen therapy for women with a uterus ($n = 16,608$). Postmenopausal women between 50 and 79 years were enrolled (mean age 63.2 years). The combined conjugated estrogen and progestogen therapy arm was terminated in July 2002 after an average of 5 years of follow-up because the overall risks exceeded benefits, including increased risk of breast cancer (Writing Group for the Women's Health Initiative Investigators, 2002). The estrogen-only arm was terminated in 2004 after 6.6 years of intervention based on an observed increased risk of stroke, low probability of establishing heart disease benefit, and low probability of demonstrating an increased risk of breast cancer (Anderson et al., 2004). In summary, women treated with estrogen plus progestogen experienced increased risk of breast cancer, coronary heart disease (including heart attacks, strokes, and blood clots in the legs and lungs), and dementia and mild cognitive impairment but decreased risk of colon cancer and hip and other fractures (Writing Group, 2002). Women treated with estrogen alone had increased risk of stroke, blood clots in the legs, mild cognitive impairment, and dementia, reduced incidence of hip fractures, and no change in coronary heart disease (CHD), colorectal, or breast cancer (Anderson et al., 2004).

Because women in both treatment arms of the study were instructed to stop therapy abruptly, it was possible to assess the return of symptoms after stopping hormone therapy. Vasomotor symptoms, pain and stiffness, fatigue, sleep problems, bloating or gas, and depressed mood were more prevalent among those who had been treated with estrogen plus progestogen than those who had received the placebo (Ockene et al., 2005).

Results of the WHI ancillary studies, the WHI Memory Study, and the WHI Study of Cognitive Aging revealed that the incidence of probable dementia in postmenopausal women was twice as high among women treated with estrogen plus progestogen versus those taking a placebo. In addition, treatment effects of estrogen plus progestogen versus placebo on mild cognitive impairment were not significantly different (Shumaker et al., 2003). In addition, women who used estrogen plus progestogen treatment versus a placebo had a substantial and clinically important decline in the indicators of global cognitive function measured annually with the modified Mini-Mental Status Examination (Rapp et al., 2003). Results were similar for the estrogen-alone treatment group (Shumaker et al., 2004).

Based on data from the WHI trial, the HERS studies, and other clinical trials, the North American Menopause Society (2004, 2007a, 2007b) Advisory Panel on Postmenopausal Hormone Therapy recommended that:

■ Treatment of menopausal transition-related symptoms (vasomotor symptoms and urogenital symptoms such as vaginal dryness) remains the primary indication for estrogen therapy.
■ Treatment of vulvar and vaginal symptoms in women without vasomotor symptoms with local estrogen therapy is indicated.
■ The only menopausal transition-related indication for progestogen treatment appears to be protection from endometrial hyperplasia induced by estrogen therapy (women without a uterus who use estrogen do not need to use a progestogen); use of a progestogen may not be indicated when low-dose local estrogen therapy is used.
■ No estrogen or estrogen plus progestogen therapy regimen should be used for primary or secondary prevention of heart disease; instead, proven heart disease prevention regimens should be considered. Further study of the timing of administration of hormone therapy (around the time of the FMP versus later) and effects on cardiovascular disease is recommended.
■ Use of hormone therapy for treatment of depression or prevention of dementia is not warranted.
■ Although estrogen and estrogen plus progestogens are FDA approved for the prevention of postmenopausal osteoporosis, other alternatives should be considered.
■ Use of estrogen or estrogen plus progestogen should be considered only for the shortest possible duration consistent with the treatment goals, risks, and benefits of individual women; indications for extended use might include treatment of osteoporosis when other treatments are contraindicated.
■ Lower than standard doses should be considered and effects on disease end points studied.
■ For women who have severe symptoms, such as hot flashes, or are nonresponsive to alternative treatments, estrogen or estrogen plus progestogen can be considered carefully by the woman and her health care provider.
■ Alternate routes of administration of estrogen and progestogen administration (patches, creams) carry unknown risks and need further study related to disease end points.
■ Individual risk profiles for each woman contemplating estrogen or estrogen plus progestogen should be considered, and women should be informed about possible risks.

In January 2003, the FDA recommended that a warning be included on all products containing estrogen, advising that extended use could lead to increased risk of heart attacks, stroke, breast cancer, and life-threatening blood clots with either estrogen alone or estrogen plus progestogen. In May 2005, the U.S. Preventive Services Task Force (2005) recommended against the routine use of combined estrogen and progestin for the prevention of chronic conditions in postmenopausal women and against the routine use of unopposed estrogen for the prevention of chronic conditions in postmenopausal women who have had a hysterectomy.

Many questions remain to be answered. Among these are the definition of short-term versus long-term treatment, the length of treatment for symptom management for vasomotor symptoms, justification for any long-term use of estrogen or estrogen plus progestogen, use of continuous combined therapy versus sequential combined therapy, use of hormones for women with premature menopause, methods for weaning women from hormone therapy, which agents other than those tested in the recently reported large clinical trials are likely to have the same outcomes, optimum timing for treatment with hormone therapy, and gene-environment interactions influencing the effects of hormones.

Bioidentical Hormones

In the wake of the publication of the WHI results, there has been a surge of interest in bioidentical hormones. Bioidentical hormones refer to hormones that are structurally identical to those produced by the ovary (North American Menopause Society, 2007a). Most bioidentical estrogens are derived from soy, whereas bioidentical progesterone is derived from the wild Mexican yam. These hormones are manufactured in laboratories as are synthetic hormones. Some popular literature encourages women to use these "natural" hormones instead of synthetics. There are two types of bioidentical hormone preparations: those approved by the FDA and those made at compounding pharmacies. The production process, purity, and safety of the latter group is unknown, and health insurance reimbursement is usually not available for these. Estrogen preparations don't always include an indication for need to use progesterone to protect the uterus, but it should be assumed that the same safety issues exist with bioidentical hormones as with synthetic hormones.

Bioidentical hormones with FDA approval include estradiol delivered by oral, percutaneous gel, percutaneous lotions, transdermal patches, vaginal cream, vaginal rings, and vaginal tablets. Progesterone is delivered orally and by gel (North American Menopause Society, 2007a, 2007b). Gels are the newest type of preparation and are absorbed to the stratum corneum as a reservoir from which they diffuse through other skin layers to the circulations. This route avoids the pass through the liver and demonstrates stable serum concentrations.

Contraindications are the same as for all estrogens: undiagnosed genital bleeding, breast cancer history, estrogen-dependent neoplasia, history of or active deep vein thrombosis (DVT) or pulmonary embolism (PE), thrombotic disease, liver dysfunction or disease, hypersensitivy to the gels, and known or suspected pregnancy. Progesterone should be used by women with a uterus (North American Menopause Society, 2007a, 2007b). The Endocrine Society's (2006) position statement on bioidentical hormones supports FDA regulation and oversight of all hormones regardless of their chemical structure or method of manufacture.

Health Promotion and Disease Prevention Strategies: Beyond Hormone Therapy

In addition to studying the preventive effects of hormone therapy, the Women's Health Initiative study examined the effects of dietary modification and supplementation with calcium and vitamin D on multiple health outcomes. The WHI Dietary Modification Trial enrolled 48,835 women, randomizing them to a dietary change or a comparison group, making this the largest diet trial ever conducted. The goals of the trial were to reduce fat consumption and to increase servings of fruits and vegetables and grains to five per day. Women began the trial with an average of 35% of energy derived from fat and completed it with about 29%. After 8.1 years of follow-up, women in the diet change group had a 9% lower incidence of breast cancer than the comparison group, but this was not a statistically significant change. Women in the dietary change group who started the trial with a higher fat intake and who reduced their fat intake had a lower incidence of breast cancer than women with a lower fat intake. The low-fat diet also reduced blood estrogen levels by about 15%. Women who were in the diet change group did not reduce the incidence of colorectal cancer but did reduce the incidence of colorectal polyps. This finding may portend a reduction in colorectal cancer incidence if the diet were modified for a longer period of time. Cardiovascular disease rates were not reduced by following the dietary modifications, but this is likely to be attributable to the focus on all fats versus only trans fats and saturated fats (Howard et al., 2006). Because a low-fat dietary pattern is consistent with the dietary Guidelines for Americans 2005 (U.S. Department of Health and Human Services and U.S. Department of Agriculture, 2005), it is likely to be a health pattern for mid-life women to follow, with specific emphasis on reducing saturated and trans fats (Prentice et al., 2006).

Calcium and vitamin D supplementation (CAD) was studied in 36,282 women randomized to the CAD and a comparison group. All participants were instructed to take 1,000 mg calcium and 400 IU of vitamin D daily. Participants were followed for 7 years. Overall, women taking CAD had 12% fewer hip fractures than those taking the placebo, which was not a significant difference. When women who adhered to the study pills regularly were compared, they had 29% fewer hip fractures than those taking the placebo (Jackson et al., 2006). In addition, women over 60 years of age experienced a 21% lower incidence of hip fractures when compared to the placebo group. Women taking CAD also had a 17% increase in kidney stones, but no other side effects differed. CAD also improved bone density by 1% more than the control group, but this was not a statistically significant difference (Jackson et al., 2006). There were no differences between the treatment and comparison groups in incidence of colorectal cancer (Beresford et al., 2006; Wactawski-Wende et al., 2006). Current recommendations for women over 50 years of age are for 1,000 to 1,200 mg of calcium and 400 to 600 IU of vitamin D daily. For women who have completed their final menstrual period (postmenopause), 1,200 mg of calcium is the minimum dose with 400–600 IU of Vitamin D daily. Osteoporosis prevention, as well as fracture prevention, relies on adequate intake of calcium and Vitamin D. Dietary intake of calcium-rich foods or beverages, especially dairy products, is discussed in greater detail in chapter 12. Calcium and Vitamin D are essential to reduce bone loss and prevent fractures. Vitamin D is essential for calcium intake to be beneficial. Because calcium is absorbed leses efficiently after menopause, an increased intake of calcium is essential as previously outlined (North American Menopause Society, 2006a, 2006b).

In addition to dietary modification and use of nutritional supplements, mid-life women are often motivated to change their activity patterns as a means to lose weight and enhance their fitness. Activity regimens such as those discussed in chapter 11, focusing on exercise, are appropriate prescriptions for health promotion. Also, attention to other nutrients, aside from CAD and dietary fat reduction should be contemplated.

Based on data on hip fracture experience among postmenopausal women between the ages of 50 and 79 who participated in the Women's Health Initiative study, a hip fracture risk calculator has been published for women and clinicians to use in assessing their risk. The fracture risk estimates are intended to be used by healthy women in conjunction with their health care providers. Factors included in the risk assessment are:

General health
Ethnicity
Physical activity
Smoking
Fracture history after 55 years of age
Hip fracture history of parents
Use of corticosteroids
Insulin-dependent diabetes
Age
Weight and height.

The origin of the risk estimates are given by Robbins and colleagues (2007). The risk is estimated and women are given the likelihood of hip fracture in the next five years, for example, the probability of hip fracture in the next five years is less than 5% (see http://hipcalculator.fhcc.org). The date provide a useful basis for dialog with a health care provider about ways to reduce fracture risk. It is possible to see what change in risk would occur if behavior were changed, for example, if physical activity increased or smoking ceased.

REFERENCES

Adler, S., Fosket, J., Kagawa-Singer, M., McGraw, S., Wong-Kim, E., Gold, E., et al. (2000) Conceptualizing menopause and midlife: Chinese American and Chinese women in the U. S. *Maturitas, 35,* 11–23.

American College of Physicians. (1992). Guidelines for counseling postmenopausal women about preventive hormone therapy. *Annals of Internal Medicine, 117*(12), 1038–1041.

Anderson, G., Limacher, M., Assaf, A., et al. (2004). Effects of conjugated equine estrogen in postmenopausal women with hysterectomy: The Women's Health Initiative randomized controlled trial. *Journal of the American Medical Association, 291,* 1701–1712.

Avis, N., Brockwell, S., & Colvin, A. (2005). A universal menopausal syndrome? *American Journal of Medicine, 19*(118 Suppl 12B), 37–46.

Avis, N. E., Crawford, S., Stellato, R., et al. (2001a). Longitudinal study of hormone levels and depression among women transitioning through menopause. *Climacteric, 4*(3), 243–249.

Avis, N., Stellato, R., Crawford, S., Bromberger, J., Ganz, P., Cain V., & Kagawa-Singer, M. (2001b). Is there a menopause syndrome? Menopause status and symptoms across ethnic groups. *Social Science and Medicine, 52*(3), 345–356.

Avis, N. E., Stellato, R., Crawford, S., Johannes, C., & Longcope, C. (2000). Is there an association between menopause status and sexual functioning? *Menopause, 7*(5), 297–309.

Beresford, S. A., Johnson, K. C., Ritenbaugh, C., Lasser, N. L., et al. (2006). Low-fat dietary pattern and risk of colorectal cancer: The Women's Health Initiative Randomized Controlled Dietary Modification Trial. *Journal of the American Medical Association, 295*(6), 643–654.

Bernard, J. (1981). *The female world.* New York: Free Press.

Bromberger J. T., Assmann, S. F., Avis, N. E., et al. (2003). Persistent mood symptoms in a multiethnic community cohort of pre- and perimenopausal women. *American Journal of Epidemiology, 158*(4), 347–356.

Bromberger, J., Harlow, S., Avis, N., et al. (2004). Racial/ethnic differences in the prevalence of depressive symptoms among middle-aged women: The Study of Women's Health Across the Nation (SWAN). *American Journal of Public Health, 94*(8), 1378–1385.

Bromberger, J., Matthews, K., Brockwell, S., Schott, L., Gold, E., Avis, N., et al. (2007). Do depressive symptoms increase during the menopause transition? The Study of Women's Health Across the Nation (SWAN). *Journal of Affective Disorders, 103*(1–3), 267–272.

Bromberger, J., Meyer, P., Kravitz, H., Sommer, B., Cordal, A., Powell, L., et al. (2001). Psychological distress and natural menopause: A multi-ethnic community study. *American Journal of Public Health, 91*(9), 1435–1442.

Brooks-Gunn, J., & Kirsh, B. (1984). Life events and the boundaries of midlife for women. In G. Baruch & J. Brooks-Gunn (Eds.), *Women in midlife* (pp. 11–30). New York: Plenum.

Brown, M., & Robinson, J. (2002). *When your body gets the blues.* New York: Berkley Trade.

Burger, H., Dudley, E., Cui, J., Dennerstein, L., & Hopper, J. (2000). A prospective longitudinal study of serum testosterone dehydroepianderosterone sulfate and sex hormone binding globulin levels through the menopause transition. *Journal of Clinical Endocrinology and Metabolism, 85*(8), 2832–2838.

Burger, H., Dudley, E., Hopper, J., Groome, N., Guthrie, J., Green, A., & Dennerstein, L. (1999). Prospectively measured levels of serum FSH, estradiol and the dimeric inhibins during the menopausal transition in a population-based cohort of women. *Journal of Clinical Endocrinology and Metabolism, 84*(11), 4025–4030.

Burger, H., Dudley, E., Robertson, D., & Dennerstein, L. (2002). Hormonal changes in the menopause transition. *Recent Progress in Hormone Research, 57,* 257–275.

Bush, T. (1991). Feminine forever revisited: Menopausal hormone therapy in the 1990's. *Journal of Women's Health, 1,* 1–4.

Bush, T., Barrett-Connor, E., Cowan, L., et al. (1987). Cardiovascular mortality and noncontraceptive use of estrogen in women: Results from the Lipid Research Clinics Program Follow-up Study. *Circulation, 75*(6), 1102–1109.

Carpenter, J., & Neal, J. (2005). Other complementary and alternative medicine modalities: Acupuncture, magnets, reflexology, and homeopathy. *American Journal of Medicine, 118*(12B), 109–117.

Casper, R., Yen, S., & Wilkes, M. (1979). Menopausal flushes: A neuroendocrine link with pulsatile luteinizing hormone secretion. *Science, 205*(4408), 823–825.

Cleary, C., & Fox, J. (1994). Menopausal symptoms: An osteopathic investigation. *Complementary Therapies in Medicine, 2*(4), 181–186.

Coney, S. (1994). *The menopause industry: How the medical establishment exploits women.* Alameda, CA: Hunter House.

Dennerstein, L., Dudley, E., Hopper, J., Guthrie, J., & Burger, H. (2000). A prospective population-based study of menopausal symptoms. *Obstetrics and Gynecology, 96*(3), 351–358.

Dennerstein, L., & Lehert, P. (2004). Modeling mid-aged women's sexual functioning: A prospective, population-based study. *Journal of Sex and Marital Therapy, 30*(3), 173–183.

Dennerstein, L., Lehert, P., Burger, H., & Guthrie, J. (2005). Sexuality. *American Journal of Medicine, 118*(12B), 59–63.

Dennerstein, L., Randolph, J., Taffe, J., Dudley, E., & Burger, H. (2002). Hormones, mood, sexuality, and the menopausal transition. *Fertility and Sterility, 77*(Suppl. 4), S42–S48.

Dyrenfurth, I. (1982). Endocrine function in women's second half of life. In A. Voda, M. Dennerstein, & S. O'Donnell (Eds.), *Changing perspective on menopause* (pp. 307–334). Austin: University of Texas Press.

Endocrine Society. (2006, October). *Position statement on bioidentical hormones.* Chevy Chase, MD: Endocrine Society. Retrieved February 17, 2008, from www.endo-society.org/publicpolicy/insider/2006/positionstatement-onBHArt1cfm

Finkelstein, J., Lee, M., Sowers, M., Ettinger, B., Neer, R., Kelsey, J., Cauley, J., Huang, M., & Greendale, G. (2002). Ethnic variation in bone density in premenopausal and early perimenopausal women: Effects of anthropometric and lifestyle factors. *Journal of Clinical Endocrinology and Metabolism, 87*(7), 3057–3067.

Frank, E., Grochocinski, V. J., Spanier, C. A., Buysse, D. J., Cherry, C. R., Houck, P. R, Stapf, D. M., & Kupfer, D. J. (2000). Interpersonal psychotherapy and antidepressant medication: Evaluation of a sequential treatment strategy in women with recurrent major depression. *Journal of Clinical Psychiatry, 61*(1), 51–57.

Freedman, R. (2005). Hot flashes: Behavioral treatments, mechanisms, and relation to sleep. *American Journal of Medicine, 118*(12B), 124–130.

Freedman, R., & Roehrs, T. (2004). Lack of sleep disturbance from menopausal hot flashes. *Fertility and Sterility, 82*(1), 138–144.

Freeman, E., Sammel, M., Grisso, J., Battistini, M., Garcia-Espagna, B., & Hollander, L. (2001). Hot flashes in the late reproductive years: Risk factors for African American and Caucasian women. *Journal of Women's Health & Gender-Based Medicine, 10*(1), 67–76.

Freeman, E., Sammel, M., Lin, H., & Nelson, D. (2006). Associations of hormones and menopausal status with depressed mood in women with no history of depression. *Archives of General Psychiatry, 63*(4), 375–382.

Freeman, E. W., Sammel, M. D., Liu, L., et al. (2004). Hormones and menopausal status as predictors of depression in women in transition to menopause. *Archives of General Psychiatry, 61*(1), 62–70.

Ganz, P., Greendale, G., Petersen, L., Zibecchi, L., Kahn, B., & Belin, T. (2000). Managing menopausal symptoms in breast cancer survivors: Results of a randomized controlled trial. *Journal of the National Cancer Institute, 92*(13), 1054–1064.

Gilligan, C. (1982a). Adult development and women's development: Arrangements for a marriage. In J. Giele (Ed.), *Women in the middle years: Current knowledge and directions for research and policy* (pp. 89–114). New York: Wiley.

Gilligan, C. (1982b). *In a different voice: Psychological theory and women's development.* Cambridge, MA: Harvard University Press.

Gold, E. B., Sternfeld, B., Kelsey, J. L., et. al. (2000). Relation of demographic and lifestyle factors to symptoms in a multi-racial/ethnic population of women 40–55 years of age. *American Journal of Epidemiology, 152*(5), 463–473.

Gracia, C., Sammel, M., Freeman, E., et al. (2004). Predictors of decreased libido in women during the late reproductive years. *Menopause, 11*(2), 144–150.

Grady, D., Herington, D., Bittner, V., et al. (2002). Cardiovascular disease outcomes during 6.8 years of hormone therapy: Heart and Estrogen/Progestin Replacement Study follow-up (HERS II). *Journal of the American Medical Association, 288*(1), 49–57.

Guthrie, J., Dennerstein, L., Hopper, J., & Burger, H. (1996). Hot flushes, menstrual status, and hormone levels in a population-based sample of midlife women. *Obstetrics and Gynecology, 88*(3), 437–442.

Guthrie, J., Dennerstein, L., Taffe, J., Lehert, P., & Burger, H. (2004). The menopausal transition: A 9-year prospective population-based study. The Melbourne Women's Midlife Health Project. *Climacteric, 7*(4), 375–389.

Guthrie, J., Dennerstein, L., Taffe, J., Lehert, P., & Burger, H. (2005). Hot flushes during the menopause transition: A longitudinal study in Australian-born women. *Menopause, 12*(4),460–467.

Harlow, S. D., Crawford, S., Dennerstein, L., Burger, H. G., Mitchell, E. S., et al. (2007). Recommendations from a multistudy evaluation of proposed criteria for Staging Reproductive Aging. *Climacteric, 10*(2), 112–119.

Harlow, S., Cain, K., Crawford, S., Dennerstein, L., Little, R., Mitchell, E., Nan, B., Randolph, J., Taffe, J., & Yosef, M. (2006). Evaluation of four proposed bleeding criteria for the onset of late menopausal transition. *Journal of Clinical Endocrinology and Metabolism, 91*(9), 3432–3438.

Harlow, S., Mitchell, E., Crawford, S., Nan, B., Little, R., Taffe, J., et al. (2008). The ReSTAGE Collaboration: Defining optimal bleeding criteria for onset of early menopausal transition. *Fertility and Sterility, 89*(1), 129–140.

Hawkins, J., Roberto-Nichols, D., & Stanley-Haney, J. (2007). *Peri- and postmenopause: Guidelines for nurse practitioners in gynecologic settings* (9th ed., pp. 250–255). New York: Springer Publishing.

Helson, R., & Wink, P. (1992). Personality change in women from the early 40's to the early 50's. *Psychology and Aging, 7*(1), 46–55.

Hemminki, E., Kennedy, D., Baum, C., & McKinlay, M. (1988). Prescribing of noncontraceptive estrogens and progestins in the United States, 1974–1986. *American Journal of Public Health, 78*(11), 1479–1481.

Hendrix, S., Cochrane, B., Nygaard, I., Handa, V., et al. (2005). Effets of estrogen with and without progestin on urinary incontinence. *Journal of the American Medical Association, 293*(8), 935–948.

Hollander, L., Freeman, E., Sammel, M., Berlin, J., Grisso, J., & Battistini, M. (2001). Sleep quality, estradiol levels and behavioral factors in late reproductive age women. *Obstetrics and Gynecology, 98*(3), 391–397.

Howard, B. V., Van Horn, L., Hsia, J., Manson, J. E., et al. (2006). Low-fat dietary pattern and risk of cardiovascular disease: The Women's Health Initiative Randomized Controlled Dietary Modification Trial. *Journal of the American Medical Association, 295*(6): 655–666.

Hulley, S., Furberg, C., Barrett-Connor, E., et al. (2002). Noncardiovascular disease outcomes during 6.8 years of hormone therapy: Heart and Estrogen/Progestin Replacement Study follow-up (HERS II). *Journal of the American Medical Association, 288*(1), 58–66.

Hulley, S., Grady, D., Bush, T., et al, for the HERS Research Group. (1998). Randomized trial of estrogen plus progestin for secondary prevention of coronary heart disease in postmenopausal women. *Journal of the American Medical Association, 280*(7), 605–613.

Irvin, J., Domar, A., Clark, C., Zuttermeister, P., & Friedman, R. (1996). The effects of relaxation response training on menopausal symptoms. *Journal of Psychosomatic Obstetrics and Gynecology, 17*(4), 202–218.

Jackson, R. D., LaCroix, A. Z., Gass, M., Wallace, R. B., et al. (2006). Calcium plus vitamin D supplementation and the risk of fractures. *New England Journal of Medicine, 354*(10), 1102.

Kagawa-Singer, M., et al. (2002). Comparison of the menopause and midlife transition between Japanese-American and Euro-American women. *Medical Anthropology Quarterly, 16*(1), 64–91.

Kaufert, P. (1986). Menstruation and menstrual change: Women in midlife. *Health Care for Women International, 7*(1–2), 63–76.

Klein, N., Battaglia, D., Fujimoto, V., Davis, G., Bremner, W., & Soules, M. (1996). Reproductive aging: Accelerated follicular development associated with a monotropic follicle-stimulating hormone rise in normal older women. *Journal of Clinical Endocrinology and Metabolism, 81*(3), 1038–1045.

La Croix, A. (2005). Estrogen with and without progestin: Benefits and risks of short-term use. *American Journal of Medicine, 118*(12B), 79–87.

Lasley, B., Santoro, N., Gold, E., Sowers, M., Crawford, S., Weiss, G., McConnell, D., & Randolph, J. (2002). The relationship of circulating dehydroepiandrosterone, testosterone, and estradiol to stages of the menopausal transition and ethnicity. *Journal of Clinical Endocrinology and Metabolism, 87*(8), 3760–3767.

Lenton, E. A., Sexton, L., Lee, S., & Cooke, I. D. (1988). Progressive changes in LH and FSH and LH: FSH ratio in women throughout reproductive life. *Maturitas, 10*(1), 35–43.

Lindheim, S. R., Legro, R. S., Bernstein, L., Stanczyk, F. Z., Vijod, M. A., Presser, S. C., & Lobo, R. A. (1992). Behavioral stress responses in premenopausal and postmenopausal women and the effects of estrogen. *American Journal of Obstetrics and Gynecology, 167*(6), 1831–1836.

Lloyd-Jones, D., Sutton-Tyrrell, K., Patel, A., Matthews, K., Pasternak, R., Everson-Rose, S., Cuteri, A., & Chae, C. (2005). Ethnic variation in hypertension among premenopausal and perimenopausual women: Study of Women's Health Across the Nation. *Hypertension, 46*(4), 689–695.

Lock, M., Kaufert, P., & Gilbert, P. (1988). Cultural construction of the menopausal syndrome: The Japanese's case. *Maturitas, 10*(4), 317–322.

Longcope, C., & Johnston, C. C., Jr. (1990). Androgen and estrogen dynamics: Stability over a two year interval in perimenopausal women. *Journal of Steroid Biochemistry, 35*(1), 91–95.

Low Dog, T. (2005) Menopause: A review of botanical dietary supplements. *American Journal of Medicine, 118*(12B), 98–108.

Lukacs, J., Chilimigras, J., Cannon, J., Dormire, S., & Reame, N. (2004). Midlife women's responses to a hospital sleep challenge: Aging and menopause effects on sleep architecture. *Journal of Women's Health, 13*(3), 333–340.

McConnell, D. (2000). Molecular pharmacology of estrogen and progesterone receptors. In R. Lobo, J. Kelse, & R. Marcus (Eds.), *Menopause biology and pathobiology* (pp. 3–11). New York: Academic Press.

McKinlay, S., Brambilla, D., & Posner, J. (1992). The normal menopause transition. *Maturitas, 14*(2), 103–115.

McLaughlin, S., Melber, B., Billy, J., & Zimmerle, D. (1986). *The changing lives of American women.* Chapel Hill: University of North Carolina Press.

Meldrum, D., Tataryn, I., Frumar, A., Erlik, Y., Lu, K., & Judd, H. (1980). Gonadotropins, estrogens, and adrenal steroids during the menopausal hot flash. *Journal of Clinical Endocrinology and Metabolism, 50*(4), 685–689.

Metcalf, M. G. (1988). The approach of menopause: A New Zealand study. *New Zealand Medical Journal, 101*(841), 103–106.

Meyer, P. M., Powell, L. H., Wilson, R. S., et al. (2003). A population-based longitudinal study of cognitive functioning in the menopausal transition. *Neurology, 61*(6), 801–806.

Mitchell, E., & Woods, N. (2007). Duration and age of onset of menopausal transition stages. Unpublished data from the Seattle Midlife Women's Health Study.

Mitchell, E. S., & Woods, N. F. (1996). Symptom experiences of midlife women: Observations from the Seattle Midlife Women's Health Study. *Maturitas, 25*(1), 1–10.

Mitchell, E. S., & Woods, N. F. (2001). Midlife women's attributions about perceived memory changes: Observations from the Seattle Midlife Women's Health Study. *Journal of Women's Health and Gender Based Medicine, 10*(4), 351–362.

Mitchell, E. S., Woods, N. F., & Mariella, A. (2000). Three stages of menopausal transition from the Seattle Midlife Women's Health Study: Toward a more precise definition. *Menopause, 7*(5), 334–349.

Morrison, M., Have, T., Freeman, E., et al. (2001). DHEA-S levels and depressive symptoms in a cohort of African American and Caucasian women in the late reproductive years. *Biological Psychiatry, 50*(9), 705–711.

Narkiewicz, K., Phillips, B., Kato, M., Hering, D., Bieniaszewski, L., & Somers, V. (2005). Gender-selective interaction between aging, blood pressure, and sympathetic nerve activity. *Hypertension, 45*(4), 522–525.

Nedrow, A., Miller, J., Walker, M., Nygren, P., Huffman, L., & Nelson, H. (2006). Complementary and alternative therapies for the management of menopause-related symptoms: A systematic evidence review. *Archives of Internal Medicine, 166*(14), 1453–1465.

Nelson, H., Vesco, K., Haney, E., Fu, R., Nedrow, A., Miller, J., Nicolaidis, C., Walker, M., & Humphrey, L. (2006). Nonhormonal therapies for menopausal hot flashes: Systematic review and meta-analysis. *Journal of the American Medical Association, 295*(17), 2057–2071.

Neugarten, B. (1968). The awareness of middle age. In B. Neugarten (Ed.), *Middle age and aging* (pp. 93–98). Chicago: University of Chicago Press.

North American Menopause Society. (2004). Recommendations for estrogen and progestin use in peri- and postmenopausal women: October 2004 position statement of the North American Menopause Society. *Menopause, 11*, 589–600.

North American Menopause Society. (2006a). The role of calcium in peri- and postmenopausal women: 2006 position statement of the North American Menopause Society. *Menopause, 13*(6), 862–877.

North American Menopause Society. (2006b). Management of osteoporosis in postmenopausal women: 2006 position statement of the North American Menopause Society. *Menopause, 13*(3), 340–367.

North American Menopause Society. (2007a). Position statement: Estrogen and progestogen use in peri and postmenopausal women: March 2007 position statement of the North American Menopause Society. *Menopause, 14*(2), 168–182.

North American Menopause Society. (2007b). The role of local vaginal estrogen for treatment of vaginal atrophy in postmenopausal women: 2007 position statement of the North American Menopause Society. *Menopause, 14*(3, Pt 1), 355–369.

Ockene, J., Barad, D., Cochrane, B., Larson, J., Gass, M., Wassertheil-Smoller, S., et al. (2005). Symptom experience after discontinuing use of estrogen plus progestin. *Journal of the American Medical Association, 294*(2), 183–193.

Overlie, I., Moen, M., Holte, A., & Finset, A. (2002). Androgens and estrogens in relation to hot flushes during the menopausal transition. *Maturitas, 41*(1), 69–77.

Patton, H., Fuchs, A., Hille, B., Scher, A., & Steiner, R. (1989). *Textbook of physiology: Vol. 2.* Philadelphia: Saunders.

Polan, M. L., Daniele, A., & Kuo, A. (1988). Gonadal steroids modulate human monocyte interleukin-1 (IL-1) activity. *Fertility and Sterility, 49*(6), 964–968.

Prentice, R., Caan, B., Chlebowski, R., et al. (2006). Low-fat dietary pattern and risk of invasive breast cancer: The Women's Health Initiative Randomized Controlled Dietary Modification Trial. *Journal of the American Medical Association, 285*(6), 643–654.

Randolph, J. F., Crawford, S., Dennerstien, L., Cain, K., et al. (2006). The value of follicle-stimulating hormone concentration and clinical findings as markers of the late menopausal transition. *Journal of Clinical Endocrinology and Metabolism, 91*(8), 3034–3040.

Randolph, J., Sowers, M., Bondarenko, I., et al. (2005). The relationship of longitudinal change in reproductive hormones and vasomotor symptoms during the menopausal transition. *Journal of Clinical Endocrinology and Metabolism, 90*(11), 6106–6112.

Randolph, J., Sowers, M., Gold, E., Mohr, B., et al. (2003). Reproductive hormones in the early menopausal transition: Relationship to ethnicity, body size, and menopausal status. *Journal of Clinical Endocrinology and Metabolism, 88*(4), 1516–1522.

Rannevik, G., Jeppsson, S., Johnell, O., Bjerre, Y., Laurell-Borulf, B., & Svanberg, L. (1995). A longitudinal study of the perimenopausal transition: Altered profiles of steroid and pituitary hormones, SHBG and bone mineral density. *Maturitas, 21*(2), 103–113.

Rapp, S., et al. (2003). Effect of estrogen plus progestin on global cognitive function in postmenopausal women: The Women's Health Initiative Memory Study: A randomized controlled trial. *Journal of the American Medication Association, 289*(20), 2663–2672.

Richardson, S. J. (1993). The biological basis of the menopause. *Balliere's clinical endocrinology and metabolism, 7*(1), 1–16.

Robbins, J., Aragaki, A. K., Kooperberg, C., Watts, N., et al. (2007). Factors associated with 5-year risk of hip fracture in postmenopausal women. *Journal of the American Medical Association, 298*(20), 2389–2398.

Rossi, A. (1985). *Gender and the life course.* New York: Aldine.

Rubin, L. (1979). *Women of a certain age.* New York: Harper

Saab, P. G., Matthews, K. A., Stoney, C. M., & McDonald, R. H. (1989). Premenopausal and postmenopausal women differ in their cardiovascular and neuroendocrine responses to behavioral stressors. *Psychophysiology, 26*(3), 270–280.

Sampselle, C., Harris, V., Harlow, S., & Sowers, M. (2002). Midlife development and menopause in African American and Caucasian Women. *Health Care for Women International, 23*(4), 351–363.

Santoro, N., Brockwell, S., Johnston, J., Crawford, S. L., Gold, E. B., Harlow, S. D., Matthews, K. A., & Sutton-Tyrrell, K. (2007). Helping midlife women predict the onset of the final menses: SWAN, the Study of Women's Health Across the Nation. *Menopause, 14*(3), 1–9.

Santoro, N., Brown, J., Adel, T., & Skurnick, J. H. (1996). Characterization of reproductive hormonal dynamics in the perimenopause. *Journal of Clinical Endocrinology and Metabolism, 81*(4), 1495–1501.

Schmidt, P., Murphy, J., Haq, N., Danaceau, M., Simpson, & St. Clair L. (2002). Basal plasma hormone levels in depressed perimenopausal women. *Psychoneuroendocrinology, 27*(8), 907–920.

Shaver, J., Giblin, E., Lentz, M., & Lee, K. (1988). Sleep patterns and sleep stability in perimenopausal women. *Sleep, 11*(6), 556–561.

Shaver, J., & Paulsen, V. (1993). Sleep, psychological distress, and somatic symptoms in perimenopausal women. *Family Practice Research Journal, 13*(4), 373–384.

Shumaker, S. A., Legault, C., Kuller, L., et al. for the Women's Health Initiative Memory Study Investigators. (2004). Conjugated equine estrogens and incidence of probable dementia and mild cognitive impairment in postmenopausal women: Women's Health Initiative Memory Study. *Journal of the American Medical Association, 291*(24), 2947–2958.

Shumaker, S. A., Legault, C., Thal, L., et al. for the Women's Health Initiative Memory Study Investigators. (2003). Estrogen plus progestin and the incidence of dementia and mild cognitive impairment in postmenopausal women: The Women's Health Initiative Memory Study: A randomized controlled trial. *Journal of the American Medical Association, 289*(20), 2651–2662.

Soares, C., Joffe, H., Bankier, B., Cassano, P., Petrillo, L., & Cohen, L. (2006). Escitalopram versus ethniyl estradiol and norethindrone acetate for symptomatic peri- and postmenopausal women: Impact on depression, vasomotor symptoms, sleep, and quality of life. *Menopause, 13*(5), 780–786.

Society for Research on Women in New Zealand. (1988). *The time of our lives: A study of mid-life women.* Christchurch, New Zealand: Christchurch Branch of SRWO.

Sofowora, G., Singh, I., He, H., Woods, A., & Stein, C. (2005). Effect of acute transdermal estrogen administration on basal, mental stress and cold pressor-induced sympathetic responses in postmenopausal women. *Clinical Autonomic Research, 15*(3), 193–199.

Soules, M. R., Sherman, S., Parrott, E., Rebar, R., Santoro, N., Utian, W., Woods N. (2001). Executive summary: Stages of reproductive aging workshop (STRAW). *Climacteric, 4*(4), 267–272.

Sowers, M., Crawford, S., Sternfeld, B., Morganstein, D., Gold, E., Greendale, G., Evans, D., Neer, R., Matthews, K., Sherman, S., Lo, A., Weiss, G., & Kelsye, J. (2000). SWAN: A multicenter, multiethnic community-based cohort study of women and the menopausal transition. In R. Lobo, J. Kelsey, & R. Marcus, *Menopause: Biology and pathobiology* (pp. 175–188). San Diego, CA: Academic Press.

Sowers, M., Finkelstein, J., Geendale, G., Donbarenko, I., Cauley, J., Ettinger, B., Sherman, S., & Neer, R. (2003). The association of endogenous hormone concentrations in bone mineral density (BMD) and bone mineral apparent density (BMAD) in pre- and perimenopausal women. *Osteoporosis International, 14*(1), 44–52.

Sowers, M., Jannausch, M., McConnell, D., Little, R., Greendale, G. A., Finkelstein, J. S., Neer, R. M., Johnston, J., & Ettinger, B. (2006). Hormone predictors of bone mineral density changes during the menopausal transition. *Journal of Clinical Endocrinology and Metabolism, 91*(4), 1261–1267.

Sowers, M., Jannausch, M., Randolph, J., McConnell, D., et al. (2005a). Androgens are associated with hemostatic and inflammatory factors among women at the mid-life. *Journal of Clinical Endocrinology and Metabolism, 90*(11), 6064–6071.

Sowers, M., Matthews, K., Jannausch, M., Randolph, J., McConnell, D., Sutton-Tyrrell, Little, R., Lasley, B., & Pasternak, R. (2005b). Hemostatic factors and estrogen during the menopausal transition. *Journal of Clinical Endocrinology and Metabolism, 90*(11), 5942–5948.

Sowers, M., Zheng, H., Tomey, K., Karvonen-Gutierrez, C., Jannausch, M., Li, X., Yosef, M., & Symons, J. (2007). Changes in body composition in women over six years at midlife: Ovarian and chronological aging. *Journal of Clinical Endocrinology and Metabolism, 92*(3), 895–901.

Sutton-Tyrell, K., Wildman, R., Matthews, K., Chae, C., Lasley, B., Brockwell, S., Pasternak, R., Lloyd-Jones, D., Sowers, M., & Torrens, J. (2005). Sex-hormone-binding globulin and the free androgen index are related to cardiovascular risk factors in multiethnic premenopausal and perimenopausal women enrolled in the Study of Women Across the Nation (SWAN). *Circulation, 111*(10), 1242–1249.

Tataryn, I., Meldrum, D., Lu, K., Frumar, A., & Judd, H. (1979). LH, FSH, and skin temperature during menopausal hot flash. *Journal of Endocrinology and Metabolism, 49*(1), 152–154.

Treloar, A. E. (1981). Menstrual cyclicity and the pre-menopause. *Maturitas, 3*(3–4), 249–264.

U.S. Department of Health and Human Services and U.S. Department of Agriculture. (2005). *Dietary guidelines for Americans, 2005* (6th ed.). Washington, DC: U.S. Government Printing Office.

U.S. Preventive Services Task Force. (1996). Postmenopausal hormone prophylaxis. In *Guide to clinical preventive services* (2nd ed.). Baltimore: Williams & Wilkins.

U.S. Preventive Services Task Force. (2005). Hormone replacement therapy for the prevention of chronic conditions in postmenopausal women. http://www.ahrq.gov/clinic/uspstf/uspspmho.htm

Villaruel, A., Harlow, S., Lopez, M., & Sowers, M. (2002). El cambio de vida: Conceptualizations of menopause and midlife among urban Latina women. *Research and Theory for Nursing Practice, 16*(2), 91–102.

Voda, A. (1981). Climacteric hot flash. *Maturitas, 3*(1), 73–79.

Wactawski-Wende, J., Kotchen, J. M., Anderson, G. L., Assaf, A. R., et al. (2006). Calcium plus vitamin D supplementation and the risk of colorectal cancer. *New England Journal of Medicine, 354*(7), 684–696.

Weiss, N., Ure, C., Ballard, J., Williams, A., & Daling J. (1980). Decreased risk of fractures of the hip and lower forearm with postmenopausal use of estrogen. *New England Journal of Medicine, 303*(21), 1195–1198.

Wise, P., Smith, M., Dubal, D., Wilson, M., Rau, S., Cashion, A., Bottner, M., & Rosewell, K. (2002). Neuroendocrine modulation and repercussions of female reproductive aging. *Recent Progress in Hormone Research, 57*, 235–256.

Women's Health Initiative Steering Committee. (2004). Effects of conjugated equine estrogen in postmenopausal women with hysterectomy: The Women's Health Initiative randomized controlled trial. *Journal of the American Medical Association, 291*(14), 1701–1712.

Woods, N. F., Mariella, A., & Mitchell, E. S. (2006). Depressed mood symptoms during the menopausal transition: Observations from the Seattle Midlife Women's Health Study. *Climacteric, 9*(3), 195–203.

Woods, N. F., & Mitchell, E. S. (1997). Women's images of midlife: Observations from the Seattle Midlife Women's Health Study. *Health Care for Women International, 18*(5), 439–453.

Woods, N. F., & Mitchell, E. S. (1999). Anticipating menopause: Observations from the Seattle Midlife Women's Health Study. *Menopause, 6*(2), 167–173.

Woods, N. F., & Mitchell, E. S. (2005). Symptoms during perimenopause: Prevalence, severity, trajectory, and significance in women's lives. *American Journal of Medicine, 118*(12B), 14S–24S.

Woods, N. F., Mitchell, E. S., & Adams, C. (2000). Memory functioning among midlife women: Observations from the Seattle Midlife Women's Health Study. *Menopause, 7*(4), 257–265.

Woods, N. F., Smith-DiJulio, K., Percival, D. B., Tao, E. Y., Mariella, A., & Mitchell, E. S. (2008). Depressed mood during the menopausal transition and early postmenopause: Observations from the Seattle Midlife Women's Health Study. *Menopause, 15*, 223–232.

Woods, N. F., Smith-DiJulio, K., Percival, D. B., Tao, E. Y., Taylor, H. J., & Mitchell, E. S. (2007). Symptoms during the menopausal transition and early postmenopause and their relation to endocrine levels over time: Observations from the Seattle Midlife Women's Health Study. *Journal of Women's Health, 16*(5), 667–677.

Writing Group for the PEPI Trial. (1995). Effects of estrogen or estrogen/progestin regimens on heart disease risk factors in postmenopausal women. The Postmenopausal Estrogen/Progestin Interventions (PEPI) trial. *Journal of the American Medical Association, 273*(3), 199–208.

Writing Group for the PEPI Trial. (1996). Effects of hormone therapy on bone mineral density: Results from the Postmenopausal Estrogen/Progestin Interventions (PEPI) trial. *Journal of the American Medical Association, 276*, 1389–1396.

Writing Group for the Women's Health Initiative Investigators. (2002). Risks and benefits of estrogen plus progestin in healthy postmenopausal women: Principal results from the Women's Health Initiative Randomized Controlled Trial. *Journal of the American Medical Association, 288*, 321–333.

Yasui, T., Maegawa, M., Tomita, J., Myatani, Y., Yamada, M., Uemura, H., Matsuzaki, T., Kuwahara, A., Kamada, M., Tuschiya, N., Yuzurihara, M., Takeda, S., & Irahara, M. (2007). Changes in serum cytokine concentrations during the menopausal transition. *Maturitas, 56*, 396–403.

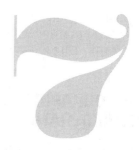

Older Women's Health

Barbara B. Cochrane and
Heather M. Young

Our beliefs and assumptions about older women—their capabilities, interests, and goals—influence how we behave toward them. Likewise, our behavior and the care we provide to older women affect their images of themselves. Just as sexism and racism are associated with stereotyping and discrimination simply because of one's gender or skin color, ageism can lead to systematic stereotyping of and discrimination against people because they are old (Butler & Lewis, 1975). Getting old is an inevitable and universal process, but personal fears and denial about our own aging can negatively influence our attitudes toward older women. Societal attitudes are not easily changed, but an understanding of aging and older adults' strengths and challenges can increase the effectiveness of the care we provide to this population.

The goal of this chapter is to increase understanding of the multifaceted nature of being an older woman in the United States today and serve as a knowledge base for providing appropriate health care. The population of older adults in the United States is composed mostly of women, many of whom are poor and have chronic illnesses, so most issues of aging and older adults' health can be thought of as women's issues. Although many of the solutions to the problems facing older women today are gender based, the context within which these issues arise can be more broadly described as a sociocultural phenomenon in which youth is valued over the age of either gender.

The term *older women*, as used in this chapter, refers to women 65 years and older. Women's health issues have often focused on reproductive health and the changes associated with menopause, but until recently, women's postmenopausal years have been largely neglected. The lives of older women may span three or four decades (e.g., young old, middle old, oldest old, centenarians), such that this age group encompasses three or more birth cohorts of women who have led diverse lives and experienced a wide variety of challenges and opportunities. As young girls, some experienced the Great Depression, whereas others were born just before the attack on Pearl Harbor and the beginning of World War II. The sociocultural contexts of these older women's lives have been influenced by history and personal experience, current norms and expectations, and visions and possibilities for the future. Topics included in this chapter are the demographic patterns and contexts that shape older women's lives, age-related changes, key health concerns experienced by older women, and considerations for healthy aging and health promotion.

The U.S. Census has provided important information about the population, including older adults, for over two centuries. Over the last two decades, there has been a dramatic increase in research on older women's health and factors that influence their health and quality of life. Much of what we know about older women's health comes from long-term, observational studies of men and women, such as the Baltimore Longitudinal Study of Aging, Cardiovascular Health Study, Framingham Heart Study, and Seattle Longitudinal Study. All of these studies have followed participants for a decade or more. Longitudinal studies of women's health have included the Nurses' Health Study and Women's Health Initiative. Some of these studies followed only older adults; others followed young or mid-life adults (and, in some, their children) through their older adult years. Many of these studies are still ongoing, and analyses of their data will contribute to our understanding of older women's health for many years to come.

DEMOGRAPHIC AND ECONOMIC CONSIDERATIONS

Population Trends

The older population in the United States, those 65 years and older, has grown rapidly throughout the 20th century, from 3.1 million in 1900 to 35 million in 2000, with projections that these numbers will double to 72 million by 2030 (Federal Interagency Forum on Aging-Related Statistics, 2006). Why this rapid increase over only 30 years? It is a combination of improvements in infant mortality and treatment of infectious diseases and a function of a large cohort—the baby boom generation. This large segment of the U.S. population was born between 1946 and 1964 and will start turning 65 in 2011. As of the most recent census year in 2000, the percentage of adults 65 and older made up approximately 12% of the total U.S. population, but they will represent nearly 20% of the total U.S. population by 2030 (He, Sengupta, Velkoff, & DeBarros, 2005). The relative impact of this rapid growth on U.S. population patterns can be represented graphically in "population pyramids," which show how different age groups, as a percentage of the population, change over time (see Figure 7.1). The shape of the 2030 pyramid is becoming wider at the top, where the oldest age groups are represented. Similar population trends and projections are being charted globally.

In the United States, as in most countries of the world, adult women outnumber adult men (He et al.,

2005). Although male births outnumber female births, men generally have higher mortality rates at every age (National Center for Health Statistics, 2006), so the higher percentage of women compared to men is most pronounced at older ages, reflecting their increased life expectancy. These differences can be visualized on population pyramids (Figure 7.1) and are highlighted when one examines sex ratios, the number of men per 100 women. Based on the year 2000 census data, the sex ratio for adults 65 and over was 70 (70 men per 100 women), but the ratio ranged from 86 for those aged 65 to 69 to 41 for those aged 85 and over (He et al., 2005). Sex differences in life expectancy, however, are declining; they stood at 7.6 years in 1970 and at 5.4 years in 2000 (He et al., 2005).

Economics

The economic status of older women is an important factor in their health status and is influenced not just by current income and poverty rates, but by their social security and retirement benefits, relative health care costs, and health care insurance coverage. Although economic trends for older women are rapidly changing, particularly as more women enter and remain in the work force full-time, women still experience profound economic disadvantages compared to men, in part because of historical differences in life trajectories. For example, men and women in younger cohorts are earning college degrees at about the same rate, but the economic status of the current cohort of older women has been influenced by previous gender gaps in educational opportunity. In 2003, 23% of older men, compared with 13% of older women had attained a bachelor's degree (He et al., 2005).

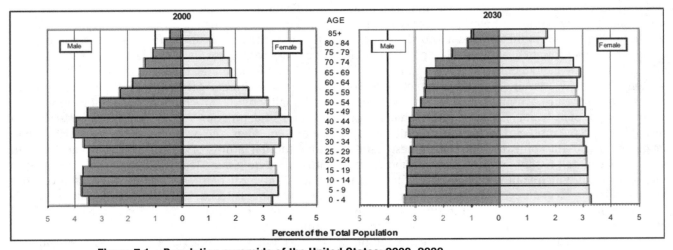

Figure 7.1   Population pyramids of the United States: 2000–2030.
Source: U.S. Census Bureau. (2005, April 21, 2005). Population pyramids and demographic summary indicators for U.S. regions and divisions. Retrieved August 15, 2007, from http://www.census.gov/population/www/projections/regdivpyramid.html

Income and Poverty

In each age group of working adults, women earn less than men for comparable work, such that older men who work full-time and year-round have higher median earnings than older women (Gist & Hetzel, 2004). To this day, then, more older women than older men will live lives of poverty—regardless of race or ethnicity, urban or rural residence, and age or labor force participation—and they are more likely than men to be poor (Dimond, 1989; Gist & Hetzel, 2004; Perales, 1988). Although poverty rates of older adults in the United States have decreased over the last half-century (from 35% in 1959 to 10% in 2003), age and sex disparities still exist (He et al., 2005). Women still earn less than men for comparable work and have lower total lifetime earnings (Weitz & Estes, 2001). This disparity is even more pronounced for racial/ethnic minority women. Latina and Pacific Islander women in the work force more commonly receive lower wages, fewer benefits, and no retirement plan (Hayes-Bautista, Hsu, Perez, & Gamboa, 2002). Among adults 65 years and older, 40.6% of all African American women and 47.1% of Hispanic women who lived alone in 2002 had incomes below the poverty level, compared to 17.4% of White women and 12.1% of White men (Federal Interagency Forum on Aging-Related Statistics, 2004). Being older, female, a member of a minority group, and living alone constitutes the greatest risk for poverty.

Social Security and Retirement Benefits

Initially planned in 1935, Social Security benefits were designed for dependents following the wage earner's retirement, disability, or death. Under the current regulations, Social Security is biased against some older adults and nearly all older women because benefits are still calculated based on pre-1950s family and work structures and more continuous career trajectories (Weitz & Estes, 2001). Many older women have grown old functioning in the dual role of homemaker and head of household while employed in low- or minimum-wage jobs with much lower lifetime earnings than men. Older women, therefore, are far more likely than older men to be poor on the basis of Social Security and other retirement benefits earned in the work place. Older women are penalized because they have a career trajectory that has been interrupted by childbearing, child rearing, and caring for other family members. Despite the economic value of this caregiving, spousal Social Security benefits may be limited if the woman's earned income is above a certain minimum level. The disparity in benefits is further widened by women's lower wages for work comparable to their male counterparts, and fewer working women than working men have pensions or

save for retirement (69% compared to 74%, respectively) (He et al., 2005).

Health Care Costs

Older adults use more health care services than any other age group, make up a significant percentage of the acute care population, and have had increasing needs for services in the nursing home setting (Federal Interagency Forum on Aging-Related Statistics, 2006). These trends are expected to increase as the baby boomers age. There are various national and state health programs to which older women may turn, but significant barriers still exist to good health care. In many situations, the criteria for medical insurance coverage are more easily met by men than by women.

The two major sources of reimbursement for health care used by older women are Medicare and Medicaid. Although most older women have health insurance through Medicare, they still spend the same proportion of their income (15% or more) on health care as they did before the passage of Medicare in 1965 (Prospective Payment Assessment Commission, 1989). Medicare covers only about half of the health care costs of older Americans (Federal Interagency Forum on Aging-Related Statistics, 2006), and the current reimbursement system discriminates against women because of its heavy emphasis on acute illness and high-technology medical care. Men submit claims primarily for acute care, whereas women have more chronic illness and disability and are over-represented in nursing homes (Weitz & Estes, 2001). Increased out-of-pocket costs for health care, therefore, become a considerable worry for many older women and may, in fact, limit or prevent their access to care. Each of the potentially reimbursable services has exceptions, co-payments, deductibles, and other requirements that place considerable limitations on the coverage overall and cause considerable confusion for older adults. In addition to these restrictions, Medicare does not cover, or covers in extremely limited ways, many important health care services, such as extended long-term care in nursing homes, hearing aids, eyeglasses, dentures, foot care, and outpatient psychotherapy.

Medicare Part D was instituted in 2006 to provide Medicare recipients with coverage for prescription drugs, regardless of income, health status, or prescription drugs used. Although many issues and concerns associated with the implementation of this coverage have been addressed, including a low-income subsidy, there remains a great deal of confusion and concern about having appropriate coverage, given enrollment periods and the wide variety of plans and associated formularies and costs. The Centers for Medicare & Medicaid Services (www.medicare.gov/pdphome.asp), AARP (www.aarp.org/health/medicare), and other groups offer helpful online information about the new coverage, as well as searchable databases to identify plans from which to chose, given an individual's current prescription drug needs.

The feminization of poverty among older women, particularly women who live alone and for women of color, makes out-of-pocket costs for older women a critical issue that becomes untenable for some women (Sofaer & Abel, 1990; Stone, 1989). The average out-of-pocket expenditure for older adults is approximately $90,000 for uncovered medical expenses in late life: $12,000 for prescription drugs, $16,000 for medical care not paid by Medicare or private insurance, $18,000 for private insurance (e.g., Medigap policies), and $44,000 for long-term care (Knickman & Snell, 2002). These costs are disproportionately borne by women who are less likely to have private insurance and available family caregivers, and who have a higher burden of chronic illness (Weitz & Estes, 2001). As the primary source of health care coverage for the poor in the United States, Medicaid becomes an important health care support for older women. Among older men and women (over 65 years), women represent 62% of those eligible for Medicaid. Therefore, Medicaid coverage is both a class and gender issue, because more older women than men are likely to be poor (Muller, 1988).

CONTEXTS OF OLDER WOMEN'S LIVES
Relationships With Family and Friends

Demographic trends for older adults, particularly sex ratios of men to women, help explain why older women are much less likely to be married than older men (41% of women 65 and older compared to 71% of men) (He et al., 2005). Predictably, widowhood is more common among older women than older men, with 35% of men 85 and older being widowed compared to 78% of women in the same age range (He et al., 2005). Even though older women live alone, their connectedness to other family members and friends is substantial (Brody, 1985) and reflects the importance with which women view their relationships and themselves in relation to others (Jack, 1987; Surrey, 1991). With the higher likelihood of being unpartnered with age, close and intimate relationships for older women, many of which are long-term friendships, take on even more importance in older women's daily lives.

Older women have many roles in the lives of their families. One of the most important roles is that of caregiver. Informal caregivers in the home are 72% women and 28% men. Mid-life and older women are the most frequent caregivers of aging parents and spouses and can expect to spend up to 18 years providing this care. This fact is quite extraordinary when compared with the

17 years spent, on average, caring for their own dependent children (Estes, 1991) and the fact that some older women are the primary caregivers for their grandchildren (Weitz & Estes, 2001). Although mid-life women are sometimes described as being in the "sandwich" generation (caring for both their children and their parents), some older adult women provide care for three or more generations of family members.

An extensive literature on caregiving has established both the rewards and strains of this experience, including a sense of meaning, meeting interpersonal obligations, pleasure in providing care to a loved one, satisfaction, as well as feelings of burden and emotional stress. The impact of caregiving on older women is a function of many factors, including vulnerabilities and strengths, the demands of the care situation, social support, characteristics of the care recipient, the type and quality of the dyad's relationship, and health (Cartwright, Archbold, Stewart, & Limandri, 1994; Chappell & Reid, 2002; Young, 2003). The physical and emotional demands over a long period of time, can result in negative health outcomes, including increased morbidity and mortality, for caregivers (Vitaliano et al., 2002).

Many older women will be the primary providers of end-of-life care for their spouses, and their release from caregiving responsibilities comes with the death of the spouse. Death of a spouse is one of the most significant losses for older women, often requiring great changes in lifestyle. Along with the death of friends, family, and other relatives, most aging women will eventually cope with widowhood. By age 75 or older, 65% of women are widows, whereas, at the same age, 37% of men are widowed. Given the mean age of widowhood for women at 56 years and their life expectancy of 80 years, many women can expect more than 20 years of widowhood (U.S. Senate Special Committee on Aging, 1986). Thus, spousal bereavement and widowhood have become almost natural components of aging women's lives. Most studies do not support major gender distinctions with respect to coping with this loss (Lund, 1989). Older bereaved spouses demonstrate an extraordinary degree of resiliency, resourcefulness, and adaptability. Loneliness is the single greatest difficulty experienced by older bereaved spouses, and it persists at least for 2 years and possibly longer.

Living Arrangements

Older women, because of their increased longevity and fewer available potential partners, are more likely than men to live alone (40% of women compared to 19% of men) (He et al., 2005). By 2020, women will account for close to 85% of those who live alone, and, of these, approximately 50% will be 75 years or older. In every ethnic and racial group, as well as in each age group, women are more likely than men to live alone. However, non-Hispanic White women and African American women are more likely to live alone than Hispanic and Asian women, who are more likely to live with relatives (He et al., 2005). Marital history and number of children may influence these findings, as may cultural variations in beliefs about the care of older relatives or more available extended family members and thus more resources for care (Choi, 1991). Relatives are the main source of assistance for older adults who live alone, but approximately 20% of those who live alone have no one to help them even for a few days. Among African American elders living alone, 37% have no living children, compared with 26% of older White persons who live alone (Commonwealth Fund Commission, 1988). In other words, older women often provide care to others at no economic cost, but most must pay for their own care when their health care needs change (Weitz & Estes, 2001).

Nursing homes are the most common institutional setting for older adults, but most women (95%) live in the community, not in nursing homes (Federal Interagency Forum on Aging-Related Statistics, 2006). Relocation to a long-term care facility increases as older adults age; approximately 1% of older adults ages 65 to 74 are in long-term care facilities, whereas 17% of those 85 years and older are in such facilities (Federal Interagency Forum on Aging-Related Statistics, 2006). Older women from racial/ethnic minority are more likely than Whites to postpone entering a nursing home, and, when they do enter such facilities, they are more likely to have greater functional and cognitive impairments (Engle & Graney, 1995). However, it is possible that biases and prejudices within the long-term care system impede access for single women from racial and ethnic minority groups (Young, 2003). Rates of nursing home residence also have declined in recent years (Federal Interagency Forum on Aging-Related Statistics, 2006), reflecting the wider variety of long-term care living arrangements available for older adults.

A variety of new living arrangements for older adults are emerging on the national scene—for example, continuing care retirement communities, life care communities, assisted-living residences, and adult day care. Many older adults are looking for living arrangements that provide access to high-quality health services but closely resemble ordinary home life, and a culture change (e.g., person-centered care, Eden Alternative, Green House) is taking place in long-term care (Baker, 2007; Thomas, 2004; Weiner & Ronch, 2003). Assisted living is the fastest growing sector in long-term care and is increasingly admitting more frail older adults with complex health needs (Gelhaus, 2001; Mollica, 1998). With an emphasis on independence and choice, assisted living offers a less institutional option and is appealing to many consumers. However, at this time, the assisted living industry is predominately private pay. These trends in housing offer a wider array of service options for older women, but research regarding the health and well-being outcomes of older adults who live in these settings remains limited. There are concerns about both the affordability of these living arrangements and the extent of coordination required to assure optimal care for older women taking advantage of community-based options.

Rural and Urban Contexts

Three out of four people 65 and older lived in urban areas in 2000; those 85 and older were also more likely to live in urban areas (He et al., 2005). However, economic security and access to health care are significant problems for rural residents, many of whom are older adults with chronic illness and disability. Rural residents have lower average incomes and higher poverty rates than urban residents. They are less likely to have a regular source of health care or sufficient health insurance (National Institute on Aging, 1991; Rosenblatt & Moscovice, 1982). Rural older adults living alone are more dependent on Medicaid than their urban-dwelling counterparts, are unlikely to have private insurance, and rely heavily on Medicare (Coward, Lee, Dwyer, & Seccombe, 1993). At the same time, they are more likely to have higher rates of chronic illness (little of which is covered by Medicare) and to have limitations in activity as a result of chronic conditions (National Center for Health Statistics, 1986; Young, 2003). In rural settings, community-based resources for managing chronic illness are limited, such that more rural older adults, per capita, reside in nursing homes (Penrod, 2001).

Retirement

Women are less prepared and less likely to retire when they reach retirement age, in large part because of the economic disadvantages related to their work and work-related benefits (He et al., 2005). However, participation in the labor force is changing and the gap between men's participation and women's is narrowing considerably. These trends mandate a closer examination of women's adjustment to retirement and the changes in social and personal resources as well as psychological and physical well-being following retirement. To date, most retirement research has focused primarily on men, and studies that have included women do not always examine gender differences. Most studies of women and retirement focus on timing of retirement and retirement planning. In a review of retirement research on women, Simmons and Betschild (2001) conclude that, because of different life paths and career trajectories, women do not prepare for retirement in the same way that men do, in terms of their decision making or their consideration of risk.

For women, their choices about retirement may be based on being able to contribute to social life more than their productivity. Research has shown that women report less retirement satisfaction than men (Quick & Moen, 1998), although this difference is small. Factors that contribute to the quality of and satisfaction with women's retirement include good health, fewer years spent in part-time employment, an early retirement, and a good postretirement income, as well as more frequent and a greater variety of social contact (Quick & Moen, 1998). Additional research is needed to clarify the contemporary relationships between retirement and measures of women's health. As a culture, we lack the societal map for ongoing engagement and meaning following retirement (Friedan, 1993). One of the developmental challenges of late life is determining how one remains involved in connections and activities that are meaningful, despite changes in social network (Erikson, Erikson, & Kivnick, 1986).

Racial/Ethnic Contexts

Population projections indicate that, by the year 2030, the older population will be much more diverse. In 2003, non-Hispanic Whites accounted for nearly 83% of the older population, whereas African Americans, Asians, and Hispanics accounted for 8%, 3%, and 6%, respectively (He et al., 2005). These percentages are projected to change by 2030, such that 72% of the older population will be non-Hispanic Whites, and African Americans, Asians, and Hispanics will account for 10%, 11%, and 5%, respectively. Currently, nearly 10% of older adults were foreign-born (Gist & Hetzel, 2004). Immigrant older adults of Hispanic or Asian/Pacific Islander heritage represent considerable diversity in their countries of origin, with wide-ranging languages and cultural traditions (Hayes-Bautista et al., 2002). Women from under-represented racial/ethnic groups will face the greatest problems with poverty and disease, and it is this segment of the older female population that is growing the fastest. Among older women living alone in 2003, poverty rates were 17% for non-Hispanic White women and about 40% for African American and Hispanic women (He et al., 2005).

Any consideration of the status of older women of color must be tempered by the fact that accurate information on the demographics of this population has been lacking until recently (Angel & Hogan, 2004). Zambrana (1988) notes that the undercount of African American and Hispanic populations in the 1970 census led to a political advocacy movement by these groups to obtain more accurate national data. Documentation of the increasing diversity of older adults now challenges the health care system to incorporate greater flexibility in its programs and services to meet the varying needs of this changing population.

Lesbian Older Women

With the aging of the population, there is a growing number of older gay, lesbian, and bisexual adults. Although older lesbians may not have revealed their sexual identity publicly during their lives, they have unique health concerns and often remain relatively invisible and underserved within the health care system (Brotman, Ryan, & Cormier, 2003; Claes & Moore, 2000). In the context of societal intolerance for same-sex relationships, older lesbians can face particular challenges in advocating for and participating in decision making for their partners during acute and chronic illness episodes, as well as accessing partner health benefits for their own health care.

AGE-RELATED PHYSICAL CHANGES

Is the end of life built into its beginning? Several theories of aging focus on aging at a cellular level. For example, the free radical theory of aging suggests that aging is due in part to by-products of oxidative metabolism that attack cellular DNA and result in mutations (Martin, 1992); the thesis of genetic instability refers to faulty copying in dividing cells or the accumulation of errors in information-containing molecules (Kane, Ouslander, & Abrass, 2003). The Baltimore Longitudinal Study of Aging investigators (U.S. Department of Health and Human Services, 1984) identified six patterns of age-related physical changes: (1) stability or the absence of significant change with age (e.g., personality); (2) declines with age due to age-related illnesses (e.g., arthritis); (3) steady declines in physical function even in the context of general good health (e.g., muscle strength); (4) more precipitous change in function, often associated with disease (e.g., dementia); (5) compensatory change to maintain function (e.g., aerobic capacity); and (6) changes over time that are unrelated to aging but instead reflect more secular trends (e.g., changes in diet due to increased processing of foods). Most physical changes of aging are not gender specific, but age-related changes do occur at different rates between individuals, and systems age at different rates within an individual, resulting in great heterogeneity of the process of primary aging among older women (Masoro & Austad, 2005).

Cardiovascular

Age-related structural and functional changes in the heart are similar for both older men and women. Increasing vascular thickening and resultant stiffness, which correlates with the onset of hypertension in advancing age, is found in both sexes. While not strictly a normal change of aging, the effects of lifestyle and heredity on atherosclerotic changes begin fairly early in life and accumulate over time such that most older women and men have some degree of subclinical or clinical coronary heart disease. (See chapter 6, on mid-life women's health, for a discussion of the effect of menopause on heart health.)

Immune Function

Age-related changes in the immune system, sometimes described as biological immunosenescence, are often accompanied by an increased incidence of cancer, auto-immune diseases, and infections in older adults (Chatta & Dale, 1991). For example, the reactivation of the herpes zoster virus in older adults is linked to a decline in the immune system with age (Chatta & Dale, 1991). In addition, age is a risk factor for many of the cancers that affect older women, such as breast cancer, colorectal cancer, and ovarian cancer (Jemal et al., 2007).

Cognition

Cognition refers to the various thinking processes through which knowledge is gained, stored, manipulated, and expressed (Rabins, 1992). Changes in cognition associated with old age involve a range of capacities, such as motivation, short- and long-term memory, intelligence, learning and retention of tasks, as well as other factors that facilitate or impede these capacities. Some memory impairment may occur as women get older, but dementia, even mild cognitive impairment, is not considered a part of normal aging (National Institute on Aging, 2005).

Sensory

Presbyopia, a gradual loss of the eyes' focusing ability, resulting in increased far-sightedness, is a normal visual change of aging, whereas glaucoma and cataracts, which commonly occur in older adults, are more age-related changes but do not occur in all older adults. Likewise, presbycusis (gradual, slight impairment, primarily for higher-pitched tones), is a condition that is seen in many, but not all, older adults. Hearing and visual impairments affect one in three women age 65 and older (Lichtenstein, 1992), but the purchase of appropriate corrective devices, such as eyeglasses and hearing aids, is a challenge for many older women, who have less supplemental insurance and reduced income to cover out-of-pocket expenses that are not covered by Medicare.

SELECTED HEALTH ISSUES FOR OLDER WOMEN

Given the diversity of older women's experiences and daily lives, older women's health issues vary widely. Older women report higher levels of hypertension,

asthma, chronic bronchitis and arthritis than men, and their lives are impacted by high risks of heart disease, cancer, and diabetes (see Figure 7.2) (Federal Interagency Forum on Aging-Related Statistics, 2006). These chronic illnesses cause much of the morbidity older women experience, and their increasing longevity places them at high risk for multiple, concurrent chronic conditions.

Cardiovascular Disease

Cardiovascular disease—including hypertension, coronary heart disease (CHD), and stroke—is known to develop at a later age in women than in men (Manolio, Kronmal, Burke, O'Leary, & Price, 1996; Rosamond et al., 2007). Unlike men, women are also more likely to be diagnosed with CHD based on clinical signs and symptoms of angina, rather than myocardial infarction. In addition, women more frequently experience atypical myocardial infarction symptoms (e.g., jaw ache, arm pain without chest discomfort), rather than the more typical substernal chest pain (McSweeney et al., 2003; Rosenfeld, 2004). These findings suggest there are important differences in the mechanisms of cardiovascular disease development in women compared to men, such as the influence of hormone receptors (Cochrane, 1992), a hypothesis that has been supported by animal research (Clarkson, Adams, Kaplan, & Shively, 1989).

Cancer

Over 75% of all cancers are diagnosed at 55 years or older (Jemal et al., 2007). Although breast cancer is diagnosed more frequently in women than any other cancer, lung cancer is the leading cause of cancer death in women (Jemal et al., 2007). Mortality due to lung cancer has declined among older men, but it has increased among older women, a finding that may reflect the fact that cigarette smoking has not declined in women to the extent that it has in men (He et al., 2005). Other leading causes of cancer death in women, besides lung cancer and breast cancer, include colorectal cancer, pancreatic cancer, and ovarian cancer (Jemal et al., 2007). Strategies for preventing cancer focus primarily on lifestyle modification, including healthy eating, physical activity, and weight control.

Diabetes

Adult-onset or type 2 diabetes mellitus, characterized by a decreased sensitivity to insulin, confers a greater risk for CHD in women than in men (Mosca et al., 2007; Rosamond et al., 2007). Obese and overweight older women are at an even greater risk for developing diabetes. However, lifestyle factors such as healthy eating, physical activity, and weight loss may improve or even resolve

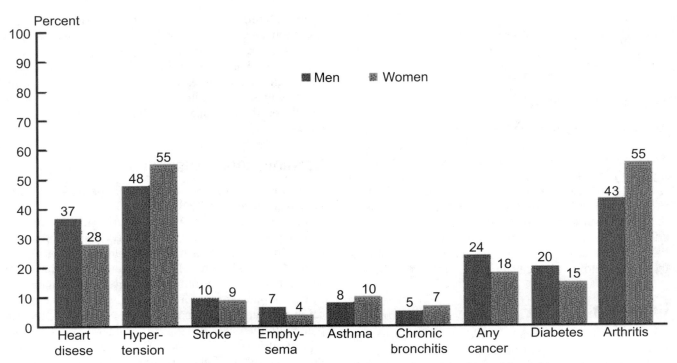

Figure 7.2   Percentage of people age 65 and older with selected health problems, by sex, 2003–2004.
Adapted from Federal Interagency Forum on Aging-Related Statistics (2006). *Older Americans update 2006: Key indicators of well-being.* Washington, DC: U.S. Government Printing Office.
Source: Centers for Disease Control and Prevention, National Center for Health Statistics, National Health Interview Survey.

problems with glucose control and obviate the need for medication (Paterson, Thorne, & Dewis, 1998).

Arthritis

Approximately 55% of older women report arthritic conditions (Federal Interagency Forum on Aging-Related Statistics, 2004), which may be classified as degenerative or osteoarthritis, with changes in the cartilage of the joint and associated pain, and inflammatory or rheumatoid arthritis, with joint inflammation and stiffness. Medications or surgery can address some of the functional difficulties and pain associated with arthritis, but weight loss and judicious physical activity remain important interventions for arthritis-associated symptoms.

Hip Fractures

Hip fractures, usually related to low bone density or osteoporosis, is a major cause of morbidity and mortality in older women, with only 40% of women regaining their functional status and independence following diagnosis and treatment of hip fracture (National Osteoporosis Foundation, 2003) and up to 25% dying within 1 year of the fracture (U.S. Congress Office of Technology Assessment, 1994). Vertebral fractures may be even

more common than hip fractures and can have a marked impact on women's functional health, particularly activities that involve bending and reaching, because of debilitating back pain, loss of height, and kyphosis. (See the chapter 6, on mid-life women's health, for a discussion of the effects of menopause on bone health.)

Alzheimer's Disease

Alzheimer's disease (AD) is an age-related, brain disorder that is characterized by memory loss, confusion, behavior and personality changes, and progressive decline in other cognitive abilities, such that the individual eventually experiences a severe loss of mental function (National Institute on Aging, 2005). Approximately 4.5 million people are currently estimated to have AD, and its prevalence rates nearly double for every 5-year age group beyond 65 years (National Institute on Aging, 2005). Low cognitive functioning is a major risk factor for entering a skilled nursing facility or nursing home (Mehta, Yaffe, & Covinsky, 2002), and dementia is a primary diagnosis in 60% of residents in nursing homes, 70% of whom are older women. Although AD and dementia are more commonly seen in older women, this increased prevalence may simply be due to older women's increased life expectancy compared to men, rather than any true gender differences (Siegler, Bastian, Steffens, Bosworth, & Costa, 2002).

AD is irreversible, but medical treatment options have been developed that slow its progression, enhance memory, improve functioning, and minimize problem behaviors, such as agitation, sleep disturbances, and wandering. Medications approved to treat AD generally act by cholinesterase inhibition or lowering glutamate levels in the brain and, therefore, improving certain cognitive skills and behavioral symptoms (National Institute on Aging, 2005). The long period of time between diagnosis and death, coupled with generally poor medical insurance coverage, makes the economic and psychological burdens on families of AD victims enormous. Interventions have been developed for families and caregivers of AD patients to enhance caregivers' coping skills and better manage behavioral disturbances (Teri, 1999; Teri, McCurry, Logsdon, & Gibbons, 2005; Zarit, Gaugler, & Jarrott, 1999).

Depression

Depression is an important mental health indicator that may represent a recurrent, chronic condition in older adults. Clinically relevant depression affects a higher percentage of older women than men, but it often goes under-diagnosed or under-treated. Women with depressive symptoms often experience high rates of physical illness, functional disability, and greater utilization of health services (Mehta et al., 2002). Medication, counseling, and physical activity, ideally in combination, have been effective in treating depression in older adults (Blumenthal et al., 1999), but insurance coverage restrictions on its treatment can create economic barriers to care for older women who are on fixed incomes.

Urinary Incontinence

Although not a disease, urinary incontinence (UI) accounts for significant functional disability in older women. UI is prevalent in 15% to 65% of older adults (depending on the study population, with a higher prevalence in frail, nursing home residents) (Wilson, 2006). Compared to men, UI is twice as likely in women, who may experience stress (leakage brought on by coughing, sneezing, laughing, or straining), urge (associated with overactive bladder syndrome or not being able to get to the toilet in time), nocturnal, or a combination of types (Hendrix et al., 2005). Decreased quality of life, depression, diminished social involvement, restricted sexual activity, and falls are frequent consequences of UI. Transient UI may be an outcome of urinary tract infections, which are frequent among older women. Drugs commonly prescribed for women, such as antihypertensives and antidepressants, also can result in transient UI (Agency for Health Care Policy and Research, 1992).

In the past, menopausal hormone therapy was recommended as a treatment for UI, but it has been shown to increase risk and worsen symptoms of UI in postmenopausal women (Hendrix et al., 2005). Pharmacological treatment with antimuscarinic agents or more invasive treatments, such as surgery, are used for women with severe UI symptoms (Wilson, 2006).

Functional Changes and Frailty

Older women's daily functioning may be impaired by acute or chronic illness, injury, or mental health problems. These changes can have a profound impact on women's instrumental activities of daily living (e.g., light housework, laundry, meal preparation, grocery shopping, getting around outside, managing money, taking medications, telephoning) as well as their basic activities of daily living (e.g., bathing, dressing, getting into or out of bed, getting around inside, toileting, and eating) (Federal Interagency Forum on Aging-Related Statistics, 2006). Although disability and functional limitations among the older population is declining, about 14 million noninstitutionalized older adults, 43% of older women, were identified as having some type of disability in 2000 (He et al., 2005).

Older women with severe functional limitations, disability, or multiple comorbid disease conditions may be described as frail, but more recently the term *frailty* has been used to describe a phenotype that may be distinct from disability or comorbidity but predictive of profound functional decline or mortality (Fried et al., 2001; Woods et al., 2005). Fried and colleagues (2001) have defined frailty as three or more of the following indicators: shrinking (unintentional weight loss or sarcopenia), poor endurance or self-reported exhaustion, weakness, slow walking speed, and low physical activity. Research on frailty—including measurement issues, biomarkers, other risk factors, and outcomes—is expanding rapidly. Our understanding of this phenomenon may one day help prevent its development and minimize its effects on older women's health.

Elder Mistreatment

Elder mistreatment is a growing, but often hidden, problem in the United States (Baker & Heitkemper, 2005; Fulmer, 2002). It includes acts of commission (abuse) or omission (neglect) that results in harm or threatened harm to the health or welfare of an older adult. These acts may be intentional or unintentional, may occur in the community or institutions, and occur across socioeconomic groups. Although research and advocacy has focused on domestic violence of women and there has been an increased awareness of elder abuse, the special problems of mistreatment of older women are sometimes ignored, particularly long-standing, unreported wife abuse, abuse of aging caregivers, and exploitation and neglect of older women (Fulmer, 2002; Phillips, 2000; Straka & Montminy, 2006). Elder mistreatment is sometimes difficult to identify with certainty, but health care professionals have a responsibility to ensure that it does not go unrecognized or untreated. Management of this complex phenomenon is best accomplished through interprofessional collaboration (Baker & Heit-kemper, 2005).

HEALTHY AGING AND HEALTH PROMOTION

Healthy aging for older women can involve negotiating a wide variety of challenges and transitions, as well as recognizing and building on various opportunities for growth. It does not necessarily represent a life that is free of chronic illness or functional impairment (Young & Cochrane, 2004). Although some older women live for several decades with excellent health and high function, others with chronic conditions still view themselves as healthy and functional. Therefore, health promotion and maintenance of function are key goals for many older women, regardless of their current health condition. Lifestyle modifications, an active role in one's health care management, physical activity, nutrition, enhancing safety, and minimizing risk are important components of a healthy lifestyle program for older women.

Self-Management of Health

To promote personal growth and optimal aging, women must secure adequate information about their bodies as well as behavioral strategies that ensure a healthy lifestyle. Meeting these goals requires skills in information processing, decision making, and action. Older women have been described as health conscious and resilient, and they are more likely than older men to have a regular physician, to have seen their physician in the last year, and to seek immediate care if symptomatic (Haber, 2003). With adequate information and skills and an environment that promotes physical, mental, economic, and social health, older women are in a position to maintain independence and achieve late-life health goals.

Regular health screening is an important component of self-management of one's health. Rates of breast cancer increase with age, and mammogram screening can aid in early detection while breast cancer is at a treatable stage. Mammograms with or without clinical breast exams are recommended every 1 to 2 years for women 40 years and older (Humphrey, Helfand, & Chan, 2002), a guideline followed by 60% to 70% of women ages 65 and older (Federal Interagency Forum on Aging-Related Statistics, 2006). Reminders from health care providers have been one of the most effective strategies for promoting mammogram screening in women, regardless of age or ethnicity (Levy-Storms, Bastani, & Reuben, 2004; Lukwago et al., 2003; Tu et al., 2003).

Physical Activity

Fewer than 20% of men or women 65 years of age or older engage in leisure-time physical activity on a regular basis (Federal Interagency Forum on Aging-Related Statistics, 2006). Yet there is growing evidence that, with appropriate cautions, the benefits of physical activity, particularly weight-bearing aerobic exercise such as walking, far outweigh possible risks in older adults. Cardiovascular fitness, mobility, muscle strength and gait, body fat, quality of life, depressive symptoms, pain, and cognition have shown improvement in older women who engage in physical activity, even those with chronic health conditions or who are very frail (Manson et al., 2002; Oh & Seo, 2003; Reynolds & Garrett, 1992; Rogers, Sherwood, Rogers, & Bohlken, 2002; Schwartz, Mori, & Jao, 2001; Villareal, Banks, Sinacore, Siener, & Klein, 2006; Wolin, Glynn, Colditz, Lee, & Kawachi, 2007). Despite these benefits, participation in physical activity and exercise adherence among older women remain low (LaCroix, Newton, Leveille, & Wallace, 1997). (See chapter 12, on exercise.)

Healthy Eating

Healthy eating can play an important role in preventing or delaying the onset of or morbidity associated with many chronic diseases, such as coronary heart disease, cancer, stroke, and diabetes (Federal Interagency Forum on Aging-Related Statistics, 2006). In addition, dietary quality can reduce controllable risk factors for chronic disease, such as obesity, hypertension, and hypercholesterolemia (Artinian, Jen, Shreve, & Templin, 2000). For many older women, who tend to gain weight as they age, healthy eating can be synonymous with good weight control (Burke & Raskind, 1991).

Although caloric needs decrease with age, the need for variety and quality of nutritional intake remains. Older women's diets may be deficient in certain vitamins and minerals, such as vitamin B-12, vitamin A, vitamin C, vitamin D, calcium, iron, zinc, and other trace minerals (Chernoff, 2005). Factors that influence older women's eating habits include living alone (and not focusing on one's own nutrition or regular meals), lower income (and trying to conserve money by purchasing less expensive processed and fast foods), and chronic disease (with complicated treatment regimens and effects on appetite). Some older women who live alone can meet their social and nutritional needs by taking advantage of their friendships with other older women and dining together regularly. (See chapter 11, on nutrition.)

Weight Control

Obesity and overweight has been described as an epidemic in the United States today, yet it is one of the key preventable risk factors for disease, morbidity from chronic disease, and death. Obesity is associated with increased risk of coronary heart disease, hypertension, diabetes, some cancers, asthma and other respiratory problems, osteoarthritis, and disability (Manson et al., 1990). Older women have slightly higher rates of obesity than older men (Federal Interagency Forum on Aging-Related Statistics, 2006).

Prevention of Falls

Hip fractures and most other nonvertebral fractures in older women occur because of a fall (North American Menopause Society, 2006), making fall prevention a key safety concern for older women that can have a major impact on morbidity and mortality. A Cochrane Review of fall prevention interventions showed that programs likely to be beneficial included multidisciplinary and multifactorial programs with both health and environmental risk factor screening and modification in the community and residential facilities; home hazard assessment and modification; muscle strengthening and balance retraining programs; and withdrawal of psychotropic medications (Gillespie et al., 2003). However, the effectiveness of these programs in preventing fall-related injuries has yet to be determined.

Medication Management

Prescription drug use has increased dramatically over the years as more and more new medications are introduced. Polypharmacy, or the use of multiple medications, can be a significant safety issue for older adults, particularly older women who consume the majority of prescription medications. With the higher number of chronic illnesses with age, the drug burden increases, along with the potential for drug interactions. Community-dwelling older adults use an average of 2.7 to 3.9 daily medications, while those in skilled nursing facilities consume an average of 8.9 medications daily (Hanlon, Ruby, Shelton, & Pulliam, 1999). In addition to prescribed medications, older adults regularly use 1 to 3.4 nonprescribed medications (Stewart & Cooper, 1994). Certain drugs are generally recognized as being inappropriate for older adults (Fick et al., 2003), yet these continue to be prescribed.

While polypharmacy has long been a topic of concern in geriatrics, there is increasing evidence of undertreatment of older adults according to evidence-based guidelines (Rochon & Gurwitz, 1999; Simon et al., 2005). The coexistence of multiple diseases (McCormick & Boling, 2005), with sometimes conflicting treatment guidelines, presents challenges for medication management. Increasingly, the focus in health care is on appropriate prescribing rather than simple polypharmacy reduction, assuring that prescriptions take into consideration age-related changes, evidence-based guidelines, and potential drug interactions, while attempting to minimize the total medication burden.

Older adults are at particular risk for adverse drug reactions due to age-related changes in pharmacokinetics and pharmacodynamics, resulting in slower excretion and differences in drug metabolism. Adverse drug reactions are the most preventable form of iatrogenic illness, resulting in considerable disability for older adults (Kane et al., 2003). The likelihood of an adverse drug reaction is heightened by inappropriate prescribing, multiple prescribers, or inadequate understanding of the drug indications, administration guidelines, and side effects. Confusion about medication management is greater among older adults who are experiencing mild to moderate memory impairment (which may or may not be a side effect of one or more medication). Psychotropic medications (e.g., antidepressants, anxiolytics, sedatives), for example, are commonly prescribed by health care providers to treat symptoms of mood or sleep disturbances in older adults but carry greater risks for adverse drug reactions, such as risk for falling, changes in cognition, and other neurological side effects. Innovative solutions to promote adherence, such as compliance devices and reminders (Fulmer et al., 1999; Stewart & Cooper, 1994), as well as strategies to ensure appropriate prescribing and coordination of care are essential for addressing this important health care concern.

Social Relationships

Most older persons seek active engagement in society, particularly when they have the support of others to meet the challenges of aging. Women often form an identity of themselves in relation to others, and this focus on relationships throughout life offers them some advantages in terms of social networking compared with older men (Surrey, 1991). With changing sociodemographic trends—such as increased population mobility, diminishing fertility, and increasing divorce rates—changing patterns of support by family are also seen. In response to these changes, older women's friendships can serve as a source of support that enhances and promotes health (Aday, Kehoe, & Farney, 2006; Armstrong, 2000; Siu & Phillips, 2002).

Sexuality

Older women are sexual beings who are capable of meaningful sexual relationships. Although they may experience some changes in sexual function, decreased sexual desire is not a normal change of aging (Addis et al., 2006). A number of factors influence sexual function for older women: normal physiological changes of aging, established behavioral patterns, illness, and societal values. Loss of a partner has been reported to be the main reason older women are no longer sexually active (Ginsberg, Pomerantz, & Kramer-Feeley, 2005). If a healthy older woman has remained sexually active, is not inhibited by societal stereotypes and myths against sex with advanced age, and has a partner who has maintained sexual interests, it is likely that she will have continued satisfactory sexual relationships. (See chapter 14, on sexuality in women's lives, for a comprehensive life span discussion of sexuality.)

SUMMARY

This chapter focused on women in the later years of their lives. The experience of aging is shaped by the social-political context of women's lives and the disparities in access to health care and services that are related to gender, race, and class. The economic lives of older women are improving, but economic disadvantages compared to older men are expected to continue; this is particularly true for women of color, who experience the triple effects of gender, age, and ethnicity. The diversity of the older population is growing, and the coming wave of baby boomers represents a challenge for policymakers, private enterprises, families, and health care providers (Young, 2003). We are already seeing an increased focus on aging in our debates about Social Security, Medicare, retirement and disability benefits, and health care allocations, and this debate will heighten as the number and proportion of older adults expands.

A woman's experience of aging depends on her individual characteristics, access to resources that promote health, and ability to develop strategies for coping with loss and change. Coping with the changes that accompany aging involves some losses that may not be anticipated, but many of the normal psychological and physiological changes that affect older women may be predicted. Improving outcomes for older women starts with primary prevention to improve general health, delay the onset of disability, and increase productivity and well-being. If women are educated about age-related changes and given time to assimilate and plan for the process of transition from one phase of life to the next, the potential for optimal aging will be enhanced. Sensitivity to the needs and issues of older women and advocacy for appropriate access and service are essential to promote the health and well-being of this significant population.

REFERENCES

Aday, R. H., Kehoe, G. C., & Farney, L. A. (2006). Impact of senior center friendships on aging women who live alone. *Journal of Women and Aging, 18*(1), 57–73.

Addis, I. B., Van Den Eeden, S. K., Wassel-Fyr, C. L., Vittinghoff, E., Brown, J. S., Thom, D. H., et al. (2006). Sexual activity and function in middle-aged and older women. *Obstetrics & Gynecology, 107*(4), 755–764.

Agency for Health Care Policy and Research. (1992). *Urinary incontinence in adults: Clinical practice guideline* (No. 92-0038). Washington, DC: U.S. Government Printing Office.

Angel, J. L., & Hogan, D. P. (2004). Population aging and diversity in a new era. In K. E. Whitfield (Ed.), *Closing the gap: Improving the health of minority elders in the new millenium* (pp. 1–12). Washington, DC: Gerontological Society of America.

Armstrong, M. J. (2000). Older women's organization of friendship support networks: An African American–White American comparison. *Journal of Women & Aging, 12*(1/2), 93–108.

Artinian, N. T., Jen, K.-L. C., Shreve, W., & Templin, T. (2000). Dietary problem-solving skills among older adults with coronary heart disease. *Journal of Gerontological Nursing, 26*(5), 21–29.

Baker, B. (2007). *Old age in a new age: The promise of transformative nursing homes.* Nashville, TN: Vanderbilt University Press.

Baker, M. W., & Heitkemper, M. M. (2005). The roles of nurses on interprofessional teams to combat elder mistreatment. *Nursing Outlook, 53*(5), 253–259.

Blumenthal, J. A., Babyak, M. A., Moore, K. A., Craighead, E., Herman, S., Khatri, P., et al. (1999). Effects of exercise training on older patients with major depression. *Archives of Internal Medicine, 159*, 2349–2356.

Brody, E. (1985). Parent care as a normative family stress. *The Gerontologist, 25*(1), 19–29.

Brotman, S., Ryan, B., & Cormier, R. (2003). The health and social service needs of gay and lesbian elders and their families in Canada. *The Gerontologist, 43*(2), 192–202.

Burke, W., & Raskind, W. H. (1991). Preventive health care of the older woman. In M. A. Stenchever & G. Aagaard (Eds.), *Caring for the older woman* (pp. 65–120). New York: Elsevier.

Butler, R., & Lewis, M. (1975). *Why survive? Being old in America.* New York: Harper & Row.

Cartwright, J., Archbold, P. G., Stewart, B. J., & Limandri, B. (1994). Enrichment processes in family caregiving to frail elders. *Advances in Nursing Science, 17*(1), 31–43.

Chappell, N. L., & Reid, R. C. (2002). Burden and well-being among caregivers: Examining the distinction. *The Gerontologist, 42*(6), 772–780.

Chatta, G., & Dale, D. (1991). Alterations of host-defense mechanisms and the susceptibility to infections. In M. Stenchever & G. Aagaard (Eds.), *Caring for the older woman* (pp. 37–55). New York: Elsevier.

Chernoff, R. (2005). Micronutrient requirements in older women. *American Journal of Clinical Nutrition, 81*(5), 1240S–1245S.

Choi, N. G. (1991). Racial differences in the determinants of living arrangements of widowed and divorced elderly women. *The Gerontologist, 31*, 496–504.

Claes, J. A., & Moore, W. (2000). Issues confronting lesbian and gay elders: The challenge for health and human services providers. *Journal of Health and Human Services Administration, 23*(2), 181–202.

Clarkson, T. B., Adams, M. R., Kaplan, J. R., & Shively, C. A. (1989). Pathophysiology of coronary artery atherosclerosis: Animal studies of gender differences. In P. S. Douglas (Ed.), *Heart disease in women* (pp. 147–158). Philadelphia: F. A. Davis.

Cochrane, B. L. (1992). Acute myocardial infarction in women. *Critical Care Nursing Clinics of North America, 4*(2), 279–289.

Commonwealth Fund Commission. (1988). *Aging alone: Profiles and projections.* Baltimore: Author.

Coward, R., Lee, G., Dwyer, J., & Seccombe, K. (1993). *Old and alone in rural America.* Washington, DC: American Association of Retired Persons.

Dimond, M. (1989). Health care and the aging population. *Nursing Outlook, 37*(2), 76–77.

Engle, V. F., & Graney, M. J. (1995). Black and White female nursing home residents: Does health status differ? *Journal of Gerontology, 50A,* M190–M195.

Erikson, E. H., Erikson, J. M., & Kivnick, H. Q. (1986). *Vital involvement in old age: The experience of old age in our time.* New York: Norton.

Estes, C. L. (1991). The Reagan legacy: Privatization, the welfare state, and aging. In J. Myles & J. Quadagno (Eds.), *States, labor markets, and the future of old age* (pp. 54–83). Philadelphia: Temple University Press.

Federal Interagency Forum on Aging-Related Statistics. (2004). *Older Americans 2004: Key indicators of well-being.* Washington, DC: U.S. Government Printing Office.

Federal Interagency Forum on Aging-Related Statistics. (2006). *Older Americans update 2006: Key indicators of well-being.* Washington, DC: U.S. Government Printing Office.

Fick, D., Cooper, J. W., Wade, W., Waller, J., Maclean, J., & Beers, M. (2003). Updating the Beers criteria for potentially inappropriate medication use in older adults: Results of a U.S. consensus panel of experts. *Archives of Internal Medicine, 163*(22), 2716–2724.

Fried, L. P., Tangen, C. M., Walston, J., Newman, A. B., Hirsch, C. H., Gottdiener, J. S., et al. (2001). Frailty in older adults: Evidence for a phenotype. *Journal of Gerontology: Medical Sciences, 56A*(3), M146–M156.

Friedan, B. (1993). *The fountain of age.* New York: Simon & Schuster.

Fulmer, T. (2002). Elder mistreatment. *Annual Review of Nursing Research, 20,* 369–395.

Fulmer, T. T., Feldman, P. H., Kim, T. S., Carty, B., Beers, M., Molina, M., et al. (1999). An intervention study to enhance medication compliance in community-dwelling elderly individuals. *Journal of Gerontological Nursing, 25*(8), 6–14.

Gelhaus, L. (2001). More reasons to stay: Increasing services such as medication management and extra assistance with ADLs leads assisted living providers into uncharted territory. *Provider, 27*(8), 18–20, 23, 26–28.

Gillespie, L. D., Gillespie, W. J., Roberston, M. C., Lamb, S. E., Cumming, R. G., & Rowe, B. H. (2003). Interventions for preventing falls in elderly people. *Cochrane database of systematic reviews* (4; Art. No. CD000340. DOI: 10.1002/14651858.CD000340).

Ginsberg, T. B., Pomerantz, S. C., & Kramer-Feeley, V. (2005). Sexuality in older adults: Behaviours and preferences. *Age and Ageing, 34,* 475–480.

Gist, Y. J., & Hetzel, L. I. (2004). *U.S. Census Bureau, Census 2000 special reports, CENSR-19, We the people: Aging in the United States.* Washington, DC: U.S. Government Printing Office.

Haber, D. (2003). *Health promotion and aging: Practical applications for health professionals* (3rd ed.). New York: Springer Publishing.

Hanlon, J., Ruby, C., Shelton, P., & Pulliam, C. (1999). Geriatrics. In J. DiPiro, R. Talbert, G. C. Yee, G. Matzke, B. Wells, & L. Posy (Eds.), *Pharmacotherapy: A pathophysiological approach.* Stamford, CT: Appleton & Lange.

Hayes-Bautista, D. E., Hsu, P., Perez, A., & Gamboa, C. (2002). The "browning" of the graying of America: Diversity in the elderly population and policy implications. *Generations, 26*(3), 15–24.

He, W., Sengupta, M., Velkoff, V. A., & DeBarros, K. A. (2005). *U.S. Census Bureau, current population reports, P23-209, 65+ in the United States: 2005.* Washington, DC: U.S. Government Printing Office.

Hendrix, S. L., Cochrane, B. B., Nygaard, I. I., Handa, V. L., Barnabei, V. M., Iglesia, C., et al. (2005). Effects of postmenopausal hormone therapy on urinary incontinence in the Women's Health Initiative. *Journal of the American Medical Association, 293*(8), 935–948.

Humphrey, L. L., Helfand, M., & Chan, B.K.S. (2002). Breast cancer screening: A summary of the evidence for the U.S. Preventive Services Task Force. *Annals of Internal Medicine, 137* (5, Part 1), 347–360.

Jack, D. (1987). Self-in-relation theory. In R. Formanek & A. Gurian (Eds.), *Women and depression: A lifespan perspective* (pp. 41–45). New York: Springer Publishing.

Jemal, A., Siegel, R., Ward, E., Murray, T., Xu, J., & Thun, M. J. (2007). Cancer statistics, 2007. *CA: A Cancer Journal for Clinicians, 57*(1), 43–66.

Kane, R., Ouslander, J., & Abrass, I. (2003). *Essentials of clinical geriatrics* (5th ed.). New York: McGraw-Hill.

Knickman, J., & Snell, E. (2002). The 2030 problem: Caring for the aging baby boomers. *Health Services Research, 37*(4), 849–884.

LaCroix, A. Z., Newton, K. M., Leveille, S. G., & Wallace, J. (1997). Healthy aging: A women's issue. *Western Journal of Medicine, 167*(4), 220–232.

Levy-Storms, L., Bastani, R., & Reuben, D. B. (2004). Predictors of varying levels of nonadherence to mammography screening in older women. *Journal of the American Geriatrics Society, 52,* 768–773.

Lichtenstein, M. J. (1992). Hearing and visual impairments. *Clinics in Geriatric Medicine, 8*(1), 173–182.

Lukwago, S. N., Kreuter, M. W., Holt, C. L., Steger-May, K., Bucholtz, D. C., & Skinner, C. S. (2003). Sociocultural correlates of breast cancer knowledge and screening in urban African American women. *American Journal of Public Health, 93*(8), 1271–1274.

Lund, D. (1989). *Older bereaved spouses: Research with practical applications.* New York: Hemisphere.

Manolio, T. A., Kronmal, R. A., Burke, G. L., O'Leary, D. H., & Price, T. R. (1996). Short-term predictors of incident stroke in older adults: The Cardiovascular Health Study. *Stroke, 27*(9), 1479–1486.

Manson, J. E., Colditz, G. A., Stampfer, M. J., Willett, W. C., Rosner, B., Monson, R. R., et al. (1990). A prospective study of obesity and risk of coronary heart disease in women. *New England Journal of Medicine, 322*(13), 882–889.

Manson, J. E., Greenland, P., LaCroix, A. Z., Stefanick, M. L., Mouton, C. P., Oberman, A., et al. (2002). Walking compared with vigorous exercise for the prevention of cardiovascular events in women. *New England Journal of Medicine, 347,* 716–725.

Martin, G. (1992). Biological mechanisms of aging. In J. G. Evans & T. F. Williams (Eds.), *Oxford textbook of geriatric medicine* (pp. 41–48). Oxford, England: Oxford University Press.

Masoro, E. J., & Austad, S. N. (Eds.). (2005). *Handbook of the biology of aging* (6th ed.). London: Academic Press.

McCormick, W. C., & Boling, P. (2005). Multi-morbidity and a comprehensive Medicare care-coordination benefit. *Journal of the American Geriatrics Society, 53,* 2227–2228.

McSweeney, J. C., Cody, M., O'Sullivan, P., Elberson, K., Moser, D. K., & Garvin, B. J. (2003). Women's early warning symptoms of acute myocardial infarction. *Circulation, 108,* 2619–2623.

Mehta, K. M., Yaffe, K., & Covinsky, K. E. (2002). Cognitive impairment, depressive smptoms, and functional decline in older people. *Journal of the American Geriatrics Society, 50*(6), 1045–1050.

Mollica, R. L. (1998). *State assisted living policy: 1998.* Washington, DC: Office of the Assistant Secretary for Planning and Evaluation, U.S. Department of Health and Human Services.

Mosca, L., Banka, C. L., Benjamin, E. J., Berra, K., Bushnell, C. D., Dolor, R. J., et al. (2007). Evidence-based guidelines for cardiovascular disease prevention in women: 2007 update. *Circulation, 115*(11), 1481–1501.

Muller, C. (1988). Medicaid: The lower tier of healthcare for women. *Women and Health, 14*(2), 81–102.

National Center for Health Statistics. (1986). *Vital and health statistics* (Series 10, No. 160). Washington, DC: U.S. Government Printing Office.

National Center for Health Statistics. (2006). *Health, United States, 2006 with chartbook on trends in the health of Americans.* Washington, DC: U.S. Government Printing Office.

National Institute on Aging. (2005). *Progress report on Alzheimer's disease, 2004–2005: New discoveries, new insights* (NIH Publication No. 05-5724). Washington, DC: U.S. Government Printing Office.

National Institute on Aging (Ed.). (1991). *Research on older women: Highlights from the Baltimore Longitudinal Study of Aging.* Washington, DC: U.S. Government Printing Office.

National Osteoporosis Foundation. (2003). *Physician's guide to prevention and treatment of osteoporosis.* Washington, DC: Author.

North American Menopause Society. (2006). Management of osteoporosis in postmenopausal women: 2006 position statement of the North American Menopause Society. *Menopause, 13*(3), 340–367.

Oh, H., & Seo, W. (2003). Decreasing pain and depression in a health promotion program for people with rheumatoid arthritis. *Journal of Nursing Scholarship, 35*(2), 127–132.

Paterson, B. L., Thorne, S., & Dewis, M. (1998). Adapting to and managing diabetes. *Journal of Nursing Scholarship, 30*(1), 57–62.

Penrod, J. (2001). Functional disability at nursing home admission: A comparison of urban and rural admission cohorts. *Journal of Rural Health, 17*(3), 229–238.

Perales, C. (1988). Introduction. *Women and Health, 14*(2), 1–20.

Phillips, L. R. (2000). Domestic violence and aging women. *Geriatric Nursing, 21*(4), 188–193.

Prospective Payment Assessment Commission. (1989). *Medicare prospective payment and the American health care system: Report to the Congress.* Washington, DC: U.S. Government Printing Office.

Quick, H. E., & Moen, P. (1998). Gender, employment, and retirement quality: A life course approach to the differential experiences of men and women. *Journal of Occupational Health Psychology, 3*(1), 44–64.

Rabins, P. (1992). Cognition. In J. G. Evans & T. F. Williams (Eds.), *Oxford textbook of geriatric medicine* (pp. 463–479). Oxford, England: Oxford University Press.

Reynolds, B. J., & Garrett, C. J. (1992). Elderly exercise: Relationship to ambulatory function, fall behavior, and well being. In S. G. Funk, E. M. Tornquist, M. T. Champagne, & R. A. Wiese (Eds.), *Key aspects of elder care: Managing falls, incontinence, and cognitive impairment* (pp. 104–109). New York: Springer Publishing.

Rochon, P., & Gurwitz, J. H. (1999). Prescribing for seniors: Neither too much nor too little. *Journal of the American Medical Association, 282*(2), 113–115.

Rogers, M. E., Sherwood, H. S., Rogers, N. L., & Bohlken, R. M. (2002). Effects of dumbbell and elastic band training on physical function in older inner-city African-American women. *Women & Health, 36*(4), 33–41.

Rosamond, W., Flegal, K., Friday, G., Furie, K., Go, A., Greenlund, K., et al. (2007). Heart disease and stroke statistics—2007 update. *Circulation, 115,* e69–e171.

Rosenblatt, R., & Moscovice, I. (1982). *Rural health care.* New York: Wiley.

Rosenfeld, A. G. (2004). Treatment-seeking delay among women with acute myocardial infarction: Decision trajectories and their predictors. *Nursing Research, 53,* 225–236.

Schwartz, A., Mori, M., & Jao, R. (2001). Exercise reduces chemotherapy fatigue in breast cancer patients. *Physician & Sports Medicine, 29,* 5–6.

Siegler, I. C., Bastian, L. A., Steffens, D. C., Bosworth, H. B., & Costa, P. T. (2002). Behavioral medicine and aging. *Journal of Consulting and Clinical Psychology, 70*(3), 843–851.

Simmons, B. A., & Betschild, M. J. (2001). Women's retirement, work and life paths: Changes, disruptions and discontinuities. *Journal of Women & Aging, 13*(4), 53–70.

Simon, S. R., Chan, K. A., Soumerai, S. B., Wagner, A. K., Andrade, S. E., Feldstein, A. C., et al. (2005). Potentially inappropriate medication use by elderly persons in the U.S. health maintenance organizations. *Journal of the American Geriatrics Society, 53*(2), 227–232.

Siu, O. L., & Phillips, D. R. (2002). A study of family support, friendship, and psychological well-being among older women in Hong Kong. *International Journal of Aging and Human Development, 55*(4), 299–319.

Sofaer, S., & Abel, E. (1990). Older women's health and financial vulnerability: Implications of the Medicare benefit structure. *Women and Health, 16*(3/4), 47–67.

Stewart, R. B., & Cooper, J. W. (1994). Polypharmacy in the aged. Practical solutions. *Drugs & Aging, 4*(6), 449–461.

Stone, R. A. (1989). The feminization of poverty among the elderly. *Women's Studies Quarterly, 17*(1/2), 20–34.

Straka, S. M., & Montminy, L. (2006). Responding to the needs of older women experiencing domestic violence. *Violence Against Women, 12*(3), 251–267.

Surrey, J. L. (1991). The "self-in-relation": A theory of women's development. In J. V. Jordan, A. G. Kaplan, J. B. Miller, I. P. Stiver, & J. L. Surrey (Eds.), *Women's growth in connection: Writings from the Stone Center* (pp. 51–66). New York: Guilford Press.

Teri, L. (1999). Training families to provide care: Effects on people with dementia. *International Journal of Geriatric Psychiatry, 14,* 110–119.

Teri, L., McCurry, S. M., Logsdon, R., & Gibbons, L. E. (2005). Training community consultants to help family members improve dementia care: A randomized controlled trial. *The Gerontologist, 45*(6), 802–811.

Thomas, W. H. (2004). *What are old people for? How elders will save the world.* Acton, MA: VanderWyk & Burnham.

Tu, S. P., Yasui, Y., Kunihuki, A. A., Schwartz, S. M., Jackson, J. C., Hislop, T. G., et al. (2003). Mammography screening among Chinese-American women. *Cancer, 97,* 1293–1302.

U.S. Census Bureau. (2005, April 21, 2005). Population pyramids and demographic summary indicators for U.S. regions and divisions. Retrieved August 15, 2007, from http://www.census.gov/population/www/projections/regdivpyramid.html

U.S. Congress Office of Technology Assessment. (1994). *Hip fracture outcomes in people age 50 and over: Background paper* (Publication OTA-BP-H-120). Washington, DC: U.S. Government Printing Office.

U.S. Department of Health and Human Services. (1984). *Normal human aging: The Baltimore Longitudinal Study of Aging.* Washington, DC: U.S. Government Printing Office.

U.S. Senate Special Committee on Aging. (1986). *Aging America: Trends and projections, 1985–1986.* Washington, DC: U.S. Government Printing Office.

Villareal, D. T., Banks, M., Sinacore, D. R., Siener, C., & Klein, S. (2006). Effect of weight loss and exercise on frailty in obese older adults. *Archives of Internal Medicine, 166,* 860–866.

Vitaliano, P. P., Scanlan, J. M., Zhang, J., Savage, M. V., Hirsch, I. B., & Siegler, I. C. (2002). A path model of chronic stress, the metabolic syndrome, and coronary heart disease. *Psychosomatic Medicine, 64,* 418–435.

Weiner, A. S., & Ronch, J. L. (Eds.). (2003). *Culture change in long-term care.* New York: Haworth Press.

Weitz, T., & Estes, C. L. (2001). Adding aging and gender to the women's health agenda. *Journal of Women & Aging, 13*(2), 3–20.

Wilson, M.-M. G. (2006). Urinary incontinence: Selected current concepts. *Medical Clinics of North America, 90,* 825–836.

Wolin, K. Y., Glynn, R. J., Colditz, G. A., Lee, I.-M., & Kawachi, I. (2007). Long-term physical activity patterns and health-related quality of life in U.S. women. *American Journal of Preventive Medicine, 32*(6), 490–499.

Woods, N. F., LaCroix, A. Z., Gray, S. L., Aragaki, A., Cochrane, B. B., Brunner, R. L., et al. (2005). Frailty: Emergence and consequences in women ages 65 and older in the Women's Health Initiative Observational Study. *Journal of the American Geriatrics Society, 53*(8), 1321–1330.

Young, H. (2003). Challenges and solutions for care of frail older adults. *Online Journal of Issues in Nursing, 8*(2), Manuscript 4.

Young, H. M., & Cochrane, B. B. (2004). Healthy aging for older women. *Nursing Clinics of North America, 39*(1), 131–143.

Zambrana, R. (1988). A research agenda on issues affecting poor and minority women: A model for understanding their needs. *Women and Health, 14*(2), 137–160.

Zarit, S. H., Gaugler, J. E., & Jarrott, S. E. (1999). Useful services for families: Research findings and directions. *International Journal of Geriatric Psychiatry, 14*(3), 165–178.

PART II

Frameworks for Practice

Feminist Frameworks for Nursing Practice With Women

Cheryl L. Cooke

The frame of reference used in delivering health care, if not in everyday living, influences how clinicians think and what they do. Over the past 35 years, clinicians have been steadily encouraged to specify the frame of reference that guides their delivery of health care services, the ways they conduct inquiry, and how they expose students to theoretical orientations. Nursing has an identifiable metaparadigm that undergirds much of its theoretical writings. In this chapter, we will explore how that metaparadigm guides our thinking about women and the notions we have about their health care needs. We will begin with a discussion of feminism, including feminist theory and inquiry, as background against which to consider concepts central to nursing practice: the person, environment, health, and nursing. We will conclude by considering new models for health care for and with women that are informed by feminist perspectives.

FEMINISM

The word *feminism* stimulates a variety of responses reflecting confusion and lack of awareness of the large body of feminist theory. It is not uncommon to find women and men who insist they are not feminists, yet who advocate feminist agendas. For some, feminism conveys threatening images of a social order in which everything is different from the status quo. For others, feminism conveys promising images of a social order in which women and men would have political, economic, and social rights that are equal. Definitions of feminism are multiple, but most consider the role of women in political and social life. Many definitions include not only equality for women with men, but changes in our social reality that some argue are linked to the possibility that earthly life can go on in the future. Indeed, Dinnerstein (1989) says that the question for women is "what kind of public power we want to share: the kind that is killing the world or the kind that is focused on keeping the world alive" (p. 16). In linking feminism not only to change in our uses of gender but also to our reversal of our involvement in nuclear and ecological disaster, Dinnerstein points out the need for feminist survival activists who are concerned with more than equality with men.

However, it remains difficult to limit feminism to a single definition as Elam (1994) suggests; feminism is not "in any simple way, one thing" (p. 4). Feminists are interested with a wide range of concerns influenced by the particular philosophical, cultural, political, and economic perspectives from which we view, interact within, interpret, and represent our worlds. Feminists are concerned with rapid change: changes in which women (and men) are responsible for both our self-creation and the preservation of the ecosphere—focusing our energy on protection of the life web for future generations.

In the few years prior to and in the several years following the events of September 11, 2001, the role of feminism has been challenged in ways that seem focused on dismantling the forward movement in many areas of women's issues, gender identity, and democratic equality. Language that was once used to support the ideals of inclusion and achievement for women and other traditionally marginalized groups is now being appropriated and used to fragment and dismantle groups that have traditionally promoted human rights for one another. Losses based on both racial and gender group are ongoing struggles in pay equity and health disparities (Correa-de-Marajo et al., 2006; Dey & Hill, 2007). Fear-based reactions to women's struggle for equality must be met head-on, making it essential to continue to explore how gender is experienced and enacted.

FEMINIST THEORY

Just as there is a range of definitions of feminism, there are many feminist theories or perspectives. Each attempts to describe women's oppression, explain its causes and consequences, and prescribe strategies for the development of a liberator or transformative politics for women and men. Feminist thought has emerged from a variety of philosophical traditions, including liberal Marxist, psychoanalytic, socialist, existentialist, postmodern, and postcolonial philosophies. In this chapter, we will consider a specific and frequently changing category called feminist theory. We provide an overview of several traditions of feminist philosophical thought. It must be noted that the philosophical traditions upon which much of feminist thought are based have disciplinary uses in other areas. For example, Marxist thought is a philosophical tradition that is often used in understanding economic theory, but it is also useful in understanding the history and subjugation of women in society.

Feminist theory also is described as occurring in waves, with our current time thought of as the third wave (sometimes referred to as postfeminism). The first wave of feminism is classically thought of as the events surrounding women's suffrage. The second wave of feminism centered on organizing women and using feminism as a resource for seeking equality in social organizations. The emerging third wave of feminism is committed to increasing the understanding and integration of feminist perspectives from the perspective of gendered identities, developing countries, and within the post- and neo-colonial worlds. This chapter contains historical citations and material from the late 1700s through current times in order to represent the breath and depth of thought in feminist theory.

The use of feminist theory is a relatively new addition to the discipline of nursing, most strongly emerging since the mid-1980s. The lines between certain types of feminism are not always clearly defined. The borders between different types of feminist theory are fluid, debated, and change across time. Feminism is concerned with the relations of women in society, but men are included as participants in constituting these relations.

Because most nursing students are unfamiliar with feminist theories, we consider feminism from what

appears to be a series of clearly marked out categories of thought—a rhetorical move that would be critiqued by many feminist scholars for its attempt to develop some clear taxonomy of feminism. For example, many scholars consider much of feminist theory as emerging from and existing within the liberal humanist tradition, rather than liberal feminism being a single feminist theory. Another example is the use of psychoanalytic feminist theory. Psychoanalytic feminist theories of desire presented from a poststructuralist perspective can be useful in understanding mothering and attachment, a theoretical positioning that requires more than one form of feminism to present its case (see Heriques, Hollway, Urwin, Venn, & Walkerdine, 1998). In these examples, categories of feminism overlap into one another. For these reasons, the categories below should be considered as a broad guide that underscores the differences in feminist theory, which in many ways reflects the differences in individuals and groups.

TRADITIONAL PERSPECTIVES IN FEMINIST THEORY

Liberal Feminism

Liberal feminists advocate gender justice, with gender equity replacing the politics of exclusion (Tong, 1998). Liberal feminism is exemplified in works such as Mary Wollstonecraft's *A Vindication of the Rights of Woman* (1796) and John Stuart Mills's *On the Subjection of Women* (1869). Liberal feminism often draws on and works within the framework of liberal political theory. The work of the National Organization of Women, in support of equal rights for women, reflects contemporary liberal feminism. Central to the beliefs of liberal feminists is the assumption that women's subordination is rooted in customary and legal constraints blocking women's entrance to and or success in the public world. Because society has viewed women as less than men, women have been excluded from many arenas of public life. Liberal feminism seeks to expose these injustices and to develop strategies for enhancing the position of women in society.

Marxist and Socialist Feminism

Marxist feminists, exemplified in some of Angela Davis's (1981, 1989), Catharine MacKinnon's (1989), and Iris Young's (1990) writings, believe it is impossible for anyone, especially a woman, to obtain genuine equal opportunity in a class society where wealth is produced by many powerless for a powerful few. Marx and Engels were influential voices whose work explored the capitalist economic philosophy that underwrites most of Western political and economic thought and action.

Marxist philosophy is also a factor influencing feminist responses to the subjugation of women worldwide. Tracing their works to Engels, Marxist feminists assert that women's oppression originates in the introduction of private property. Beasley (1999) concurs, suggesting that sexual oppression is a form of class oppression. To eradicate sexual oppression, Marxist feminists advocate replacing capitalism with a socialist system. In this new system, the means of production would belong to everyone, and women would no longer be economically dependent on men (Beasley, 1999; Tong, 1998).

Radical Feminism

Radical feminists, as exemplified by Mary Daly (1978), Andrea Dworkin, Gena Corea, and Shulamith Firestone, believe the patriarchal system oppresses women. They advocate that a system characterized by power, dominance, hierarchy, and competition cannot be reformed, but must be eradicated. Radical feminist thought suggests that institutions that produce and reproduce hierarchy and dominance—especially the family, the church, and the academy (academic institutions)—need to be replaced to achieve equality. Some radical feminists question the concept of "natural order," in which men are "manly" and women are "womanly," with a goal of overcoming whatever negative effects this thinking about biology as destiny has had on women and men. Radical feminists assert that biology, gender (masculinity, femininity), and sexuality (heterosexuality and homosexuality are some forms) are sources of women's oppression (Weedon, 1997). Many radical feminists focus on ways in which gender and sexuality have been used to subordinate women to men. They support reproductive rights as a means of enhancing women's choices. Some advocate escaping the confines of heterosexuality through celibacy, autoeroticism, or lesbianism, emphasizing acceptance of women's own desires (Rich, 1981).

In the 1980s, a political backlash against feminist theory and activism was initiated by conservative forces in the U.S. political landscape, most notably occurring during the Reagan-Bush era of the mid-1980s to the early 1990s. The backlash consisted of the reinsurgence of discourses that criticized the women's movement for its support of women's rights, abortion rights, and the movement of women out of the home and into the work place. Much of the backlash against feminism is centered on what is perceived to be the radical aspects of feminist theory, including gender difference and women's sexuality, and serves to undermine the progress of women in society (Rich, 1977, 1981). The results of this backlash against feminism are still being felt through continued challenges to the 1973 *Roe v. Wade* court case over abortion rights and in challenges to affirmative rights and other civil rights legislation that benefited women and other marginalized groups. In recent years, these arguments have been appropriated by neoconservatives in the United States and used as a politically centered fear tactic to limit equality and self-determination for women in public and private life.

Psychoanalytic Feminism

Psychoanalytic feminist theorists believe that the centrality of sexuality arises out of Freudian theory and concepts, such as the Oedipus complex. Chodorow (1978, 1989, 1994) and Dinnerstein (1976, 1989) exemplify early psychoanalytic, primarily Freudian, feminist thought. Central to their work is the assumption that the root of women's oppression is embedded deeply within her psyche. These theorists recommend dual parenting and dual participation in the work force as means to solve women's oppression. A prominent group of French feminist theorists includes Hélène Cixous, Luce Irigaray, and Julia Kristeva, whose work is conducted in critique of Freudian psychoanalysis. These French feminists challenge the theoretical perspectives of Jacques Lacan, a psychoanalyst whose work furthered that of Freud. Theory presented by the French feminists is often conceptualized from both a psychoanalytic and poststructuralist position (discussed below) and focuses on explorations of subjectivity and agency, abjection, and psychosexual identity formation (Weedon, 1997).

Existentialist Feminism

Work in this tradition is exemplified by Simone de Beauvoir's work, *The Second Sex* (1949). A central assumption is that women are oppressed by "otherness." In other words, women are oppressed because they are not men, but the "other." From an existentialist framework, women's meaning is from and by a male perspective. These theorists assert that, if woman is to become a self, she must transcend the definitions, labels, and essences that limit her existence (Tong, 1998). The work historically conducted under the umbrella of existentialist feminism is currently explored across many areas of feminist thought.

Socialist Feminism

Socialist feminist theory is exemplified in works like Juliet Mitchell's *Woman's Estate* (1971) and Nancy Hartsock's *Money, Sex, and Power* (1983). Tong (1998) suggests that this group has woven together several strands of feminist theory. Socialist feminist theory premises that human nature does not have essential characteristics; instead, it is socially constructed and, therefore, open to change (Weedon, 1997). Socialist feminists assert that women's conditions are overdetermined by structures of production (from Marxist feminism), socialization of children (from liberal feminism), and reproduction and sexuality (from radical feminism). They believe that women's status and functions must be changed in all these structures. In addition, a woman's interior world must be transformed (from psychoanalytic feminism) to be liberated from patriarchal thought that undermines her confidence (as emphasized by the existential feminists). Allison Jaggar pointed out the interrelationship of forms of women's oppression, emphasizing the concept of alienation: under capitalism, everything (sex, work, and play) and everyone (family and friends) that could be a source of integration becomes a source of disintegration (Jaggar & Rothenberg, 1984). Most socialist feminists maintain that only complex explanations can account for women's subordination and emphasize integration of women's lives and the usefulness of a unified feminist theory.

EMERGING PERSPECTIVES IN FEMINIST THEORY

Postmodernism and Feminist Theory

Postmodernism is expressed in feminist theory as a series of theoretical perspectives that view language as constructing our understanding and uses of gender. Much of what is known as postmodern work is conducted from a poststructuralist perspective, a philosophical perspective that relies heavily on the work of Michel Foucault, a French philosopher whose work heavily critiqued how power and knowledge are constructed and reified. Feminist writing from a poststructuralist perspective critiques the ideas of essentialism, the use of power in social relations, and how, through the use of language and power, knowledge about the world is produced and legitimated (Butler, 2000; Weedon, 1997). These orientations involve no single standpoint, but several perspectives that can account for the experiences of difference, an aspect of feminist theory that has been recently approached from postmodern and poststructuralist perspectives.

Women of Color and Feminist Theory

The voices and experiences of women of color are increasingly finding a place in feminist theory. Writers using postmodern, poststructuralist, and critical race theories enable this by calling out the use of metanarratives to describe the lives of women of color as essentially similar to those of White women. For example, the experiences of African American women are not interchangeable with those of White women. Works by and about African American women challenge us to think about their life experiences and consequences for their well-being (Collins, 1989a, 1989b, 2000;

Crenshaw, 1995; Davis, 1981, 1989, 1991; Dill, 1983, 1987; Gillispie, 1984; Gorden-Brashaw, 1987; Herman, 1984; hooks, 1984, 1997, 1999; Lorde, 1984a, 1984b, 1988a, 1988b; Smith, 1982).

Another example of feminist theory is authors writing from the womanist traditions. Womanist traditions offer a feminist theoretical perspective that seeks to encompass the uniqueness of African American women's experiences, accentuating the similarities and differences between African American women and women of other groups (Banks-Wallace, 2000; Taylor, 1998, 2002, 2005).

In the United States, Latinos are a rapidly growing demographic, representing one-seventh of the population. This change in national demographics presents an opportunity for the voices of Latina feminists to emerge and advocate for improvement in health care resource allocation. Works about Latina or Chicana women provide insight into the challenges for women within an emerging ethnic group (Anzaldua, 1987; Apodaca, 1977; Chavez, Cornelius, & Jones, 1986; del Portillo, 1987; Ginorio & Reno, 1985; Hurtado, 1989, 1996; Kelly, Bobo, MacLachlan, Avery, & Burge, 2006; Moraga, 1983, 1997; Moraga & Anzaldua, 1983; Sanchez, 1984; Sanchez-Ayendez, 1989; Segura, 1989). Writing about and by Asian American (Chow, 1987; Im, 2000; Im, Meleis, & Park, 1999; Johnson et al., 2004; Neufeld, Harrison, Hughes, Spitzer, & Stewart, 2001; Tsutakawa, 1988, Visweswaran, 1994; Woods, Lentz, Mitchell, & Oakley, 1994) and Native American/First Nations scholars (Browne & Fiske, 2001; Hale, 1985; Pirner, 2005; Witt, 1984) provide powerful accounts of issues central to different women's lives, illustrating points of difference that may help account for health experiences.

Queer Theory

Queer theory was brought about by a resistance movement that describes feminism from gay, lesbian, bisexual, and transgendered (GLBT) perspectives with an emphasis of "affinity and solidarity over identity" (Marcus, 2005). Queer theory provides an opportunity for understanding gender, offering a lens through which lesbian, gay, and transgendered people understand and interpret their lives in a heterosexually focused world (Butler, 1993, 2000; Jagose, 1996). As nurses, we want to shrink from language that is disparaging of individuals or groups, but the use of the term *queer* is taken up as an umbrella term "for a coalition of culturally marginal sexual self-identification" GLBT studies and theory (Jagose, 1996, p. 1). Queer theory calls on us to question how our discomfort with difference can be directed to work for the good of an often marginalized group. Using queer theory as a framework for understanding the health challenges of GLBT groups, we begin to understand how social identity operates in ways that amplify health issues. As the current research exploring the lives and health of the GLBT community focuses on lesbian health issues, additional research focusing on the health of gay, bisexual, and transgendered individuals is necessary (Clear & Carryer, 2001; Ensign, 2001; Glass, 2002; Spinks, Andrews, & Boyle, 2000).

Less prominent but equally important are feminist theoretical traditions from ecofeminism and feminist liberation theology. Ecofeminism provides a space for feminists to consider the conditions of women in the context of the environment and nature (Griffin, 1978; Haraway, 1989; Sturgeon, 1997). Feminist liberation theologies (Christian, mujerista, and some womanist traditions) provide a theoretical framework for women to use religious and spiritual traditions to enhance their understandings of women's subjugation and oppression (Fulkerson, 1994; Harrison, 1985; Isasi-Diaz, 1993; Isasi-Diaz & Tarango, 1992; Tigert, 2001). With the emergence of ecofeminism, feminist liberation theologies, and queer theory, issues of the ecological, racialized, and gendered experiences of women, communities of color, and GLBT communities are gaining theoretical prominence and becoming increasingly legitimized.

Postcolonial and Transnational Feminist Theories

Postcolonial theory calls into question the history of colonial dominance of the West over other geographical regions and people. As the overarching framework for feminist theory, transnational feminist theory adds support to the notion of the need for multiple forms of feminism in a postcolonial world (Scott, Kaplan, & Keates, 1997). Postcolonial theory has initiated discussions about how Western ideas are transmitted into non-Westernized regions and the effects of this transmission, including loss of native languages and traditions and the Westernization of social structures and institutions. Postcolonial theory offers an opportunity to think and develop strategies that resist contemporary forms of Western colonialism that "undermine and sabotage the self-determining aspirations" of citizens in independent states (Yeatman, 1994, p. 9). In the post–September 11 environment, the ideals of postcolonialism and transnational feminist theories and movements have become increasingly important.

Postcolonial theory questions the transfer of Western economic strategies and knowledge into more traditional economic systems, often to the economic benefit of the West (sometimes referred to as the North in opposition to countries in the Southern hemisphere). While Western technologies and economic strategies have been useful in some ways to some populations, the effects of these technologies have been detrimental

to the social structures, environments, and health of many populations. Another use for postcolonial theory is its provision of a theoretical frame for feminists to critique the effects of transnationalism on the lives of women and children. Anderson (2000, 2004a, 2004b) and Mohammed (2006) use postcolonial theory to describe both issues of racial and social marginalization in their research describing the lives and health of South Asian and Native Americans.

Issues for nurses to consider include the use of child labor and its effects on the family structure, the health effects of transnationalism, and the transfer of health technologies to populations that may not have the infrastructure to support their effective use. Understanding a country's political economy and how it affects the availability of health and social services is another important topic that drives improvement or deterioration of a population's health outcomes. Postcolonial theories and transnational feminism allow nurses to move between local and global ideas, placing the individual within a more globally oriented response to women's health. In doing so, nurses can work beside women in non-Western countries to deal with the effects of transnationalism such as inadequate infrastructure and the subsequent health effects that are accentuated in its wake.

PERSPECTIVES FOR INQUIRY

Awareness of the multiple feminist theories provides a useful analytic schema for those interested in understanding women's lives and promoting women's health. What is a feminist research perspective? What are the consequences of a feminist perspective for health research and for knowledge about women's health? Feminist theoretical orientations have influenced the process of inquiry about women and women's health. Some have asked: What are the consequences to these theories for inquiry? Is there a feminist method? If so, what is it? If not, is it sufficient to simply add women to research in order to answer feminist criticisms? Answers to these questions can influence development of research agendas for nursing and other health-related sciences, knowledge about women's health, policies regarding women's health care, and models for the delivery of nursing and other types of health care.

Just as there is no single feminist theory, there is no single feminist method. As a basis for considering what feminist science is, Harding (1987) emphasized the interrelationship of method, methodology, and epistemology. Method refers to techniques for gathering evidence, such as by listening, observing, and examining historical traces. In contrast, methodology refers to the theory and analysis of how research should proceed. Epistemology refers to issues about what is adequate theory of knowledge and strategies that are acceptable for justification of a theory. Epistemological issues concern who can be a knower, what tests must be passed in order to legitimize knowledge, and what kinds of things can be known. Epistemological concerns are exemplified in the concern about whether subjective truth counts as knowledge (Berman, Ford-Gilboe, & Campbell, 1998).

Feminists claim that mainstream science has its origins in a masculine voice, that the history of science emerges from dominant gender, class, and racial groups, and that women have not been regarded as legitimate knowers. Most feminists would assert that adding women—as scientists, as participants in studies, and as contributors to knowledge—is not enough. Instead, contemporary feminist theorists have recommended new directions for the conduct of research.

MacPherson's (1983) recommendations and McBride and McBride's (1982) consideration of new paradigms for nursing research initiated early discussion of a topic that has persisted in the literature. Duffy (1985), Duffy and Hedin (1988), Campbell and Bunting (1991), Hall and Stevens (1991), Allen, Allman, and Powers (1991), and Parker and McFarlane (1991), among others, have contributed to a growing understanding of feminist research and its possibilities in nursing.

Origin of the Questions for Feminist Researchers

Contemporary feminists advocate finding new empirical and theoretical resources in women's reports of their (lived) experiences. They emphasize the importance of the origins of scientific problems or research questions. They believe the questions asked are at least as important as the answers to those questions. In a context of discovery (theory development) versus justification (theory testing), concern for the origin of the question is particularly important. Questions grounded in men's experiences as the norm are not likely to illuminate the nature of women's experiences. Moreover, questions not grounded in women's experiences are not likely to generate knowledge for women, and probably do not generate valid knowledge about women (Duffy & Hedin, 1988; Klein, 1983).

Feminist researchers identify problems from the perspective of women's experiences, recognizing that there is no single woman's experience. That is, class, race, and culture must be considered as intersecting with gender (Crenshaw, 1995). Women's fragmented identities, such as African American feminist or Japanese American feminist give rise to partial perspectives that allow researchers to see phenomena from a viewpoint that is limited by their own particular racial, gendered, and class-based perspectives (Campbell & Bunting, 1991; Code, 1995; Haraway, 1988; Taylor, 1998).

In addition, feminist researchers are concerned with ways to transform conditions rather than with merely uncovering a series of truths about women's lives. It is not enough to describe women's oppression; it is as important to change the conditions that create and sustain it. This concern gives legitimacy to an action component as part of the research process, a concern for praxis as part of the research process. It follows that researchers should concern themselves with questions that women want answered (Lather, 1991).

Purposes of Feminist Science

The purposes of feminist science are to provide information for women rather than merely about women. The goal is seeking explanations for women that are liberating, that have the capacity to be used by women for women's good. Moreover, feminist researchers are explicit about their purpose: enhancing the well-being of women through providing information that has the possibility to be helpful to women. They are also explicit about their politics, asserting the value systems that undergird their science rather than maintain the pretense of objectivity.

Nature of the Subject Matter

The nature of the subject matter for feminist researchers may not differ dramatically from that concerning researchers with nonfeminist perspectives. Studying women is not new. Studying women from the perspective of their own experiences so that women can understand themselves and their world is a novel aspect of feminist research. For example, studying gender as a social construction rather than studying gender as a biological absolute illustrates an important distinction in feminist and nonfeminist research perspectives (Allen, Allman, & Powers, 1991; Campbell & Bunting, 1991).

The act of questioning the category known as *woman* is part of an ongoing debate in feminism that evolved following the so-called second wave of feminism, in the late 1960s to the early 1980s. The writings and discussions of this period made calls for *all* women to challenge the patriarchal stance of men in society and move toward a more equitable social order, with little regard to the social situations of many women. Called into question was the notion of woman as an essence, where differences between women are seen as negligible and/or without meaning. Poor women, lesbians, and women of color found themselves and their experiences as women outside the experience of those women most prominent in feminism's second wave— namely, White, middle-class women whose work place was in the home. These "other" women did not see the mandate against patriarchy and for work as feminism's most important goals, because, for many, work and/or patriarchy were, rather than a choice, necessary factors in their lives.

Feminism's late second wave and current writers and thinkers have challenged monolithic notions of *woman* by complicating ideas of who can be known as a woman, differences between women and the lives they lead, and the use of gender as a meaningful concept within which to understand multiple experiences of women and men (Beasley, 1999; Weedon, 1997). In the second and third waves of feminism, the movement has largely concentrated on an interrogation of difference rather than forging a shared identity for women. The movement toward marking difference and critiquing woman as a subject of inquiry are ways of exploring and identifying social and political forces that seek to unify women at the loss of individual differences in women's economic, social, sexual, and racial conditions. Critiques of a single category called *woman* have provided a way to analyze when using the category is meaningful for describing the lives of women with disparate histories and experiences (Spivak, 1990).

A related issue in feminist research is *how* women are studied. Although a nonhierarchical relationship would be ideal, it is impossible to completely equalize social, political, and historical experiences between women. Historically, most researchers "study up," meaning that the women who are the subjects of inquiry generally have less education and/or are in a different (usually lower) economic class than that of the researcher. Studying up as well as studying down are both legitimate and necessary. For example, nurses cannot merely study the behavior of their women clients; it is also important for women to study nurses' behavior to have more than a partial perspective of a phenomenon.

The racialization of both the researcher and study participant is another potential concern. How does the racialization of the research process influence researcher and participant and the types of questions that are asked, how they are answered, and how the study findings are interpreted and disseminated (Anderson, 2006; Kirkham & Anderson, 2002)? A researcher is a situated knower—that is, an individual who can have only a partial perspective of a problem. Only through multiple perspectives can multiple truths inform a topic. A woman seeking health care, a nurse, and a biostatistician are each able to contribute a different, but partial, perspective on the problem. Together, these individual and partial perspectives do not constitute a whole, but contribute a more complete understanding of the topic (Haraway, 1988).

Methods and Methodology

Harding (1987) suggested that it is the purpose of the inquiry, the alternative hypotheses being considered, and the relationship between the researcher and the person participating in the research that make feminist research distinctive. Because the frame of reference for women is relational and contextual, qualitative research methods often have been identified with feminist research (see MacPherson, 1983; McBride & McBride, 1982). Yet methods such as observation or listening are not bound to a certain philosophical stance; methods do not drive the assumptions grounding the research. While debates over appropriating feminist methods are likely to continue in nursing and other sciences, there are some common dimensions underlying the search for an appropriate methodology for feminist research. These grow from an understanding of epistemology in feminist theory (Campbell & Bunting, 1991; Code, 1995).

Feminist researchers recognize the validity of women's perceptions as truth for them (Campbell & Bunting, 1991). Women are regarded as a legitimate source of knowledge, capable of telling about and reflecting on their own experiences. Women themselves, then, are the appropriate participants in research about and for women. Research participants are experts on their own lived experiences. Methods of inquiry that involve eliciting women's perceptions about their experiences and their health yield appropriate information for feminist inquiry (Campbell & Bunting, 1991; Code, 1995).

Because knowledge is relational and contextual, research methods that acknowledge and reflect the importance of the interrelationship between history and contemporary observations are essential. Moreover, both historical and concurrent events should be considered in designing, conducting, and interpreting research endeavors (Campbell & Bunting, 1991). Boundaries between the personal and public or political spheres are artificial. Sharp dichotomies and boundaries should be carefully scrutinized in research involving women (and all humans). What is regarded as a personal problem may also be understood as a social or political problem (Campbell & Bunting, 1991).

Researchers should be attentive to the power relations between researcher and participant. These differences between researcher and study participant are situations in which the exercise of power can be inequitable, and the research relationship can become potentially exploitive (Bloom, 1998; Wolf, 1996). Nurses conducting research with women from a feminist perspective are mindful of the ways power relations function and are managed in the research process. *Participants* is an appropriate term to describe individuals who are actively engaged in studies. Indeed, the researchers can think of themselves as participants in a cooperative effort in which the researcher's role is helping produce knowledge that will be useful to the participants (Bloom, 1998; Campbell & Bunting, 1991). Interpretations of the data and conclusions by the researcher are validated by the participants and shared with them for their own use. Because the goal of the research is producing knowledge that will benefit the participants, they have a stake in interpreting the results (Campbell & Bunting, 1991).

Analyses

Cultural beliefs and behaviors shape the results of analyses and interpretations. Paradoxically, introducing the subjective element into the analyses enhances the objectivity of the research by revealing to the public the point of view of the investigator. Reflexivity as a methodological feature involves looking at oneself as the researcher, examining one's own position and values relative to the participants in a study. Some recommend that researchers identify their age, ethnicity, and feminist stance in publishing their works (Reinharz, 1983).

Feminist researchers have suggested the use of specific criteria for judging the adequacy of the analysis. We can ask:

1. Are women's experiences used as the test of adequacy of problems, concepts, hypotheses, research design, data collection, and interpretation?

2. Is the research project for women versus men and institutions men control?

3. Does the researcher or theorist place herself in the same class, race, culture, and gender-sensitive critical plane as the people being studied?

4. How does the process of racialization (e.g., how we categorize individuals and groups into social constructed categories [Anderson, 2006]) influence who and what is studied; how research questions are asked, answered, and interpreted; and how interventions are developed and carried out?

FEMINIST PERSPECTIVES FOR NURSING PRACTICE

Feminist perspectives for nursing practice mirror some of the major assumptions underlying the group of feminist theories. Moreover, feminist perspectives point to the need to redefine the concepts central to nursing's conceptual models for practice. The metaparadigm reflected in most of nursing's theoretical works includes the concepts of the person/client, environment, health, and nursing. In the following discussion, we will explore each of these concepts as the basis for proposing a feminist model for nursing practice.

PERSON/CLIENT

In most theoretical formulations, the person who receives nursing care is central. Usually the person is conceived of as an individual; however, groups of persons, families, or communities are also nursing's "client." The most consistent view of the person/client emphasizes wholeness. Some conceive of wholeness or holism as meaning that the person is a bio-psycho-social-spiritual organism whose environment can be manipulated to maintain or promote health. The person is more than and different from the sum of her or his parts. Still others assert that the person and environment are inseparable: considering the individual in isolation from the context is not possible (Chinn & Jacobs, 1987; Parse, 1987).

Feminist writings about women mirror many dimensions of contemporary nursing theorists' concepts of person. In fact, many revisionist accounts of women's development emphasize the importance of understanding women as products of their social, political, and historical experiences. Thus, the person/client becomes a less generalizable entity. Drevdahl (1999) reminds us that nursing must begin to contrast notions of "holism and uniqueness" with difference in conceptions of person/client in order to fully represent the complexities of individuals' lives and experiences (p. 1). Concepts of self, role, and body (corporeality) frequently appear in feminist writings about women's health. Consideration of these concepts as they inform nursing practice with women follows.

Self and Role

Self-in-relation theory, a product of thinkers such as Jean Baker Miller (1986), Nancy Chodorow (1987), and Carol Gilligan (1982), defines a woman's orientation to her relationships as a central, positive aspect of development beyond childhood. This body of theory emphasizes the differences between women and men in the strengths and vulnerabilities that develop out of their relational contexts and the norms that regulate their lives. A woman's concept of self is a relational self, one that exists in a web of relationships with others. Social intimacy organizes her experiences. Most women experience interdependence, not autonomy and separation, as is emphasized in theories about men's development.

Differentiation for women occurs in these ongoing relationships throughout life. Creativity, autonomy, competence, and self-esteem develop in a relational context. Indeed, relationships are essential for well-being and healthy development (Miller, 1986; Surrey, 1991). Development of a more complex sense of self in an increasingly complex web of relationships to others is the result (Miller, 1986). Developmental failure occurs not as a result of a failure to separate, but as the result of a failure to remain connected while asserting a distinct sense of self (Gilligan, 1977). Indeed, Gilligan suggests that the relational self is foundational to a morality grounded in an ethic of care (Gilligan, 1982).

A dilemma for women arises from their social contexts. Women are simultaneously pushed to define themselves through relationships in a society that views orientation to relationships as a sign of dependence or immaturity and that values achievement over affiliation (Jack, 1987).

Body

At the same time that feminist theorists have constructed new visions of the self, they have considered the body. Women have lived with the consequences of "biology as destiny" ideology. Our possibilities as humans have been defined by society's beliefs about what women can and should do—often based on reproductive capacities. Biological essentialism refers to the assumption that the essence of a woman is her body and its bodily functions. Although feminists reject the assumptions of biological essentialism, some feminist theorists have focused on biological difference and women's reproductive roles without reducing women to an identity with their bodies. By insisting that gender differences are socially constructed, some have pointed out that women's perceptions of their bodies are culturally controlled. Throughout history, women have been considered to be ruled by their bodies—bodies that are seen as inherently unstable and weak. Biological difference has been and still is used to justify the subjugation of women.

Scheper-Hughes and Lock (1987) consider three bodies: the individual body, referring to the lived experience of the body-self; the social body, referring to the representational uses of the body as a symbol with which to think about nature, society, and culture; and the body politic, referring to the regulation, surveillance, and control of bodies (individual and collective) in reproduction, sexuality, work and leisure, sickness, and other forms of human difference. The Cartesian legacy of separateness of the body and mind persists in health sciences literature about women. Separation of the self and the body, if not alienation of the body from the self, appears in women's descriptions of menstruation, menopause, labor, and birthing. Women describe these experiences as "something that happens to you," not as "something you do" (Martin, 1987). Women's conversations about their bodies revealed their beliefs that "your body needs to be controlled by your self" and that "your body sends you signals." This fragmentation and alienation in women's concepts of body and self link the notions women have of their bodies to the social body and the body politic: women's bodies have come to symbolize something that is separate from their person. The body politic has constructed ideas about women's bodies that allow them to be regulated in ways that disregard their attachment to personhood. Restricting attention to the nature of women's bodies, for example, by locating women's problems in their bodies, has served to deflect attention from the broader sociopolitical environments influencing women's health.

ENVIRONMENTS AND CONTEXTS

The contexts of women's lives and environments are multidimensional, despite the fact that many nurse theorists restrict their concepts of environment to the immediate surroundings of the hospitalized individual (Chinn & Jacobs, 1987). Beginning with Nightingale's conception of the environment as the origin of health and health problems, nurse theorists focused on dimensions of the physical environment such as air and water quality, cleanliness, and light. Over time, these concerns gave way to concern with the social environment and how it required adaptation, if not accommodation, of the individual. The ideas of environment also encompass context or how women experience the social, cultural, political, and environmental aspects of their lives.

Chooporian (1986) pointed out that focusing almost exclusively on the adaptation of individuals to their environments has excluded concern for persons or groups who refuse to accommodate to their environments that present intolerable or unacceptable social, political, or economic circumstances. She encouraged analysis of the environment as a social, political, and economic world that influences both well-being of clients and nursing practice. She urged stretching beyond a concept of environments as client relationships to a conception of environments along dimensions of social, political, and economic structures producing class relationships, economic policies, and ideologies such as sexism, ageism, racism, and classism, all with the power to influence health.

One consequence of nursing's limited view of environments is that persons must adjust, assimilate, or accommodate, and nurses support them in the process. Persons, not societal structures or institutions, are seen as the focus for change or adaptation. As an example, when women are considered as members of a family, from a family systems perspective, emphasis is often on what is adaptive for the family system, rather than the individual woman (Allen, 1986). Works such as those on women's friendships by Raymond (1986) and women's relationships in prison by Maeve (1999) provide evidence of women's ability to create socially supportive environments. Works of ecofeminists, encouraging women to renew their ties to the Earth, link women to the life of the planet (Schuster, 1990; Sturgeon, 1997).

Chooporian urged nurses to assume activist roles, diagnosing and treating the root of health problems rather than human responses to them. Beginning by reconceptualizing the environment as social, political, and economic structures, social relationships, and everyday life, nurses would extend their arenas for intervention beyond the boundaries of health care institutions.

Chooporian's urging to consider multiple dimensions of environments for human health is consistent with many feminist theories that link women's lives to social, political, and economic structures as context. Moreover, the emphasis on social relationships, including domination, power, and authority within organizations and families, leads one to examine exploitation of women and other forms of sexism and their relationships to women's health. Finally, emphasis on understanding everyday life for women and its meaning is consistent with feminist conceptions of the importance of women's experience.

HEALTH

Health is another concept central to nursing's metaparadigm, a concept with many meanings. Judith Smith (1981) identified four models of health from published literature: the eudaimonistic, adaptive, role performance, and clinical. The eudaimonistic model connotes exuberant well-being and wellness and the ability to actualize the self, whereas the adaptive model connotes health as flexible adjustment to the environment, the ability to cope with stressful events. The role performance model emphasizes health as performance of one's socially defined roles, the ability to engage in activities of daily living at an expected level. The clinical model emphasizes health as the absence of disease, symptoms, or bad feelings as well as the absence of need for medical care.

Despite decades of work about women's health, there is not consensus on a definition of women's health to guide scientists and clinicians in their work. The U.S. Public Health Service Task Force on Women's Health Issues (1985) defined women's health issues from a statistical standpoint, including those "areas where circumstances for women are unique, the noted condition is more prevalent, the interventions are different for women than for men, or the health risks are greater for a woman than for a man" (p. 6). McBride and McBride (1982) examined the concept of women's health as it was used during the 1970s. They found a growing emphasis on women's health as more than reproductive health. Beyond concern about the physical and psychological well-being of women, they found emphasis in health literature on inclusion of women as participants in studies about health, investigation of sociocultural factors leading to health problems, analysis of unnecessary surgery for women, examination of exclusion of women from decision making and treatment choices, recognition that men were not the norm,

identification of sexist bias in therapy, and recognition that women were worthy of serious scientific consideration. They found that a common theme in defining the focus of work about women's health was an emphasis on women's overall health concerns, not just reproduction. In addition, emphasis on the health consequences of changing sex roles for women was common in the 1970s and early 1980s. In short, they found evidence of interest in more than sex differences, but no well-articulated frameworks for studying women's health. They concluded that the growing emphasis on women's health, as opposed to the diagnosis and treatment of women's diseases, implied a rejection of the traditional patriarchal medical model in favor of one generally concerned with attaining, retaining, and regaining health. They cautioned that women's health, at the core, meant taking women's experiences as the starting point for all health efforts.

When over 500 women participating in a women's health survey responded to the question "What does being healthy mean to you?" their statements reflected the four models of health Smith proposed. Moreover, women identified several dimensions of the eudaimonistic model of health as seen in Table 8.1. These dimensions span a wide range of being and doing, supporting the assumption that women themselves articulate the meaning of health for them. Conversely, while women's literacy of health meanings is increasing, current research with women is exposing disparities in services and treatments between men and women and across racial and economic groups (Anderson, 2006; Williams, 2005; Williams et al., 2007; Williams & Jackson, 2005).

NURSING

The final concept in nursing's metaparadigm is nursing. Variously described in nursing's theoretical literature, nursing is conceived of as health promotion, care and cure of the sick, and prevention of illness. Some theorists conceive of the goal of nursing care as helping people adapt to their health-related situations. Other theorists have focused on the goal of nursing as promoting optimal quality of life from the patient's perspective. In this paradigm, the nurse focuses on guiding a person who determines the activities for changing health patterns. Outcomes of nursing practice are determined by the person who develops a plan for changing health patterns as they relate to the quality of her or his life (Parse, 1987).

The concept of caring has become part of nursing's ideology, if not an ethic. Works by Leininger, Watson, Swanson, and others have elucidated definitions and dimensions of caring as nurses practice it. Swanson (1990) defines caring as "acting in a way that preserves human dignity, restores humanity, and avoids reducing

8.1 | Women's Images and Health Definitions

IMAGE	DEFINITION
Clinical	Health as absence of illness, infrequency or absence of symptoms; freedom from addiction; ability to recover quickly from illness; absence of need for medical care or medication
	Role performance health as ability to perform one's activities of daily living as expected
Adaptive	Health as ability to adjust flexibly to the environment, cope with stressful events
Eudaemonistic	Health as exuberant well-being, including the following dimensions:
	Actualizing the self—reaching one's optimum, achieving one's goals
	Practicing healthy life ways—taking action to promote health or to prevent disease
	Positive self-concept—feeling good about oneself, having a positive sense of one's worth
	Social involvement—ability to interact, love, care, enjoy relationships; give and receive pleasure in relationships
	Fitness—feelings of stamina, strength, energy, in good shape
	Cognitive function—thinking rationally; being creative; having many interests, being alert and inquisitive
	Positive mood—feeling positive affect, such as happiness, joy, affection, excitement, exhilaration
	Harmony—feeling spiritually whole, centered, in balance, contentment

Note. From "Being Healthy: Women's Images," by N. F. Woods, S. Laffrey, M. Duffy, M. J. Lentz, E. S. Mitchell, D. Taylor, and K. Cowan, 1988, *Advances in Nursing Science, 11*(1), 36–46.

persons to the moral status of object" (p. 64). Grounded in her studies of women, she has identified several dimensions of caring:

- Knowing: striving to understand an event as it has meaning in the life of the person being cared for.
- Being with: being emotionally present to the person.
- Doing for: doing for the person as she would do for herself if it were possible.
- Enabling: facilitating the person's passage through life transitions and unfamiliar events.

- Maintaining belief: sustaining faith in the person's capacity to get through an event or transition and to face a future of fulfillment (Swanson, 1990).

Caring, as central to nursing practice, has been the object of feminist analysis. MacPherson (1988) pointed out that a radical feminist analysis has yet to be integrated in thinking about caring and nursing. The concept of caring does not incorporate the concepts of patriarchy and misogyny to explicate common women's health problems such as depression; nor does it inform nurses of uncaring roles such as that of "token torturers," the witnessing of and participation in unnecessary or harmful treatment of women (Daly, 1978). Moreover, socialist feminist critique has not led to incorporation of a focus beyond the individual to the social collective and an emphasis on the importance of caring as a societal responsibility, not an individual one. Visions of feminist nursing practice attempt to integrate these critical dimensions.

FEMINIST MODELS OF NURSING PRACTICE

Feminist nursing practice refers to nursing care that is informed by feminist theory. Within this perspective, women's health is more than reproductive health. Women's health care focuses on women's overall well-being and quality of life as women themselves define it. For example, women's experiences of role strain and anxiety about balancing child care, care for an elderly parent, and work roles are not diagnosed as a problem to be located within the woman, but are seen as arising within a nonsupportive social context (Sampselle, 1990).

Feminist practice values women as women. Men are not the norm, although historically they have been used as such. Within feminist practice, concern is about more than whether women are equal to men. A feminist perspective presupposes definitions of health and health care that are grounded in the woman's own perspective. Feminist practice rejects patriarchy that values men more than women and biological essentialism that restricts a woman's possibilities to her reproductive functions. The use of inclusive language and demonstration of respect for women and their information about their health reflect feminist values. A woman's basis for value to her society is not limited to her reproductive capacity. Moreover, feminist practitioners recognize that a woman's body belongs to her and is not owned by someone else or regarded only as a sexual object (Sampselle, 1990).

Western women have demonstrated their desire for health care that encompasses their total person, not simply their reproductive functions. Women consumers of health care expressed a preference for a pluralism of health services and health care providers. The range of services they desired included:

- Care for menstrual cycle problems and menopausal problems
- General health promotion, including prevention, nutrition, sexual, and exercise counseling
- Counseling for eating disorders
- Care for women experiencing substance use/abuse issues
- Mental health services, especially for depression
- Occupational health and career counseling
- Stress management services
- Reproductive services, including infertility, contraception, and genetic counseling
- Family and marital counseling
- Problems of aging, including caretaker stress, transitions, loss, osteoporosis, and care for chronic illness
- Pregnancy and childbirth services, child care counseling
- Services for abused women, including women who had been sexually abused, battered, and raped and women with same-sex partners who are experiencing abuse or violence
- Care for sexually transmitted diseases
- Aesthetic services, including cosmetic procedures
- Services for adolescent women
- Environmental risks affecting women's health

These services span women's lives, and few would be encompassed within the traditional domain of obstetrics/gynecology (Woods, 1985). Although some of these services reflect women's concerns about reproductive issues, such as pregnancy or infertility care, many reflect a broader range of concerns regarding health, such as child care counseling and services for sexual abuse. Still others reflect social pressures for women to adapt to their environments, such as cosmetic surgery and stress management. These services do not adequately reflect the desires of women who are often invisible to the health care system: those who are poor, from under-represented ethnic groups, lesbians and transgendered people, women who are part of a diaspora (emigrating populations, leaving and coming to countries due to the effects of war, economic hardship, threat of marital violence, or religious persecution), and aging populations.

Goals of Feminist Practice

One of the goals of feminist nursing practice is to improve the lot of all women. Emancipatory feminist paradigms orient practice to praxis, active engagement and participation in the larger society—another goal of feminist practice. The notion of praxis reflects awareness that women are in the world and that their actions affect the world. Being actively engaged and participating in the larger society unites their individual concerns with the concerns for all women. The goals of feminist practice thus transcend the boundaries of traditional practice in which the client is an individual and instead encompasses the well-being of all women.

Bermosk and Porter (1979) advocate a balanced complementarity in the relationships between nurses and women clients. In a symmetrical partnership, nursing care reflects these goals: increasing women's awareness of their human wholeness; promoting opportunities for women for expansion of their mind-body-spirit-environment interactions; fostering women's willingness to take responsibility for and make decisions about their health; and promoting women's effective participation with health care providers as facilitators of health. In their model, the woman client is seen as ever-evolving, ever-changing, and repatterning. Feminism is an integrative process that helps women expand their consciousness about health and identity. Promotion of health, in this model, is a function of transforming one's life through the expansion of one's consciousness rather than merely engaging in periodic medical checkups (Bermosk & Porter, 1979). Women's subjectivity and agency are prominent within a feminist practice. Women have awareness of themselves and others and the ability to appreciate the complexity of many diverse situations while acting in their own best interest (Beasley, 1999).

Linking Theory and Feminist Practice

Theory and practice are inextricably linked, each constituting the other. Theory is used to create practice, and practices change as a result of emerging theories. Feminist theory is a fairly new application for nursing research and care. With all new experiences, one first has to learn the tenets of the theory, begin to identify and uncover situations where the theory is applicable, and, ultimately, use the theory to create practice. Feminist theory has spent many years at the margins of theory in nursing, slowing moving toward central positions in research and practice. Nurse researchers and practitioners currently use feminist theory primarily as a framework to conceptualize issues or as a form of feminist critique of research and practice (Anderson, 2006; Bunting, 1997; Im, 2000; Im et al., 2001; Johnson et al., 2004; Maxwell-Young, Olshansky, & Steele, 1998; Richman, Jason, Taylor, & Jahn, 2000; Schroeder & Ward, 1998). The future will see nurses advancing feminist theories in ways that consistently inform nursing practice (Andrist, 1997; Liaschenko, 1999; Tang & Anderson, 1999). The use of feminist theory can be taken up as a form of consciousness that directs nurses' interactions with clients, peers, and the world-community.

An Ethical Feminist Practice

A feminist practice in nursing understands the category of woman as multiple, shifting, and constantly changing. Nursing practice that understands the complexities of women, the contexts of their lives, and the multiple and shifting landscape of their health is desirable and attainable. Educating nursing students about how women's health needs vary and how knowledge of the context of women's lives is essential to their developing an ethical feminist practice. Nurses' knowledge about women's health problems and the differences in how their health is experienced should be offered through work sites, college, and community educational offerings that are timely and economically accessible to a wide variety of nursing professionals. Encouraging nurses to further their education in master and doctoral programs translates into improved health opportunities for the development of an ethical nursing practice using feminist theory as a central feature of this education, using feminist theory to advance research agendas and programs. Research from a feminist perspective then informs the ethics that govern a nursing practice that is woman centered. An ethical practice demands attention to intersectionality, reflexive thinking, and self-reflection while avoiding a narcissistic perseveration and self-awareness. It also values local action as a way to influence women's health on a global level.

A Feminist Model for Nursing Practice for Women

Wilma Scott Heide (1982), a nurse and past president of the National Organization of Women, characterized nursing as nurturance and nourishment of the whole person. She advocated a vision of health care in which power enabled the "self to be and become," not to control others. In her book, *Feminism for the Health of It,* she asserted that "feminist values provide the experiential reality whereby health care encounters are affectively positive, conducive to healing and nurturing of positive self-images for both clients and practitioners" (p. 34–35). Like the self-health movement that provided women assertive nurturance based on discovery and sharing of knowledge and skills, nursing care can empower women through demystification, consciousness raising, and recognition of the constitutive nature of power relations. Like the self-help model, a feminist nursing model can reflect valuing scientific knowledge as well as intuitive and experiential knowledge, can focus on the whole person in context, and is cognizant of women's power to produce and experience wellness.

An end to patriarchy implies that the practitioner attempts to demystify health care in a way that values women's perspectives in the context of a partnership for health. This includes uncovering the ideological underpinning of practices that unintentionally promote disparities in health care provision. Attempting to create interpersonal and social relations that protect and preserve the types of principles diverse women value will lead to recognition of the need for a "fundamentally transformed, nonexploitive social order" (p. 11). The dimensions of this order will emerge through the exploration of women's experiences when they are no longer devalued (Bricker-Jenkins & Hooyman, 1989).

Empowerment implies an enabling, nonviolent, problem-solving orientation to practice that occurs in an egalitarian relationship between a woman and a health professional. Empowerment involves liberating the energy of women and others in a way that uses the energy in a noncoercive fashion (Bricker-Jenkins & Hooyman, 1989). However, the use of and ability to enable power is not a one-sided venture, but a description of a relationship between two entities (Foucault, 1977; Weedon, 1997). Both health care providers and clients are able to exercise power in their relationships, but the effects of this exercise of power have different outcomes. For the practitioner, unawareness of the authority that her or his advice carries is a form of exploitation within the power relationship may be damaging to clients, particularly women. Conversely, clients are able to exercise power in the provider-client relationship through an ability to express their needs and choices, in how and when they make their bodies available for health service, and through active participation in the provider-client relationship. Process as product reflects concern for the ends that are part of the means. The process of care itself is a product. Being "in process" means that conditions and consciousness are in constant flux. Caring involves mutually educating, democratizing, and enabling responsibility (Bricker-Jenkins & Hooyman, 1989).

The ideology that the personal is political implies that personal problems women experience have historical, material, and cultural origins and dimensions. The way women feel about themselves has political origins. In addition, this principle implies that we change our world as we change ourselves as we change the world. This awareness confirms that failure to act is one type of an action, it *is* acting. Moreover, our interconnections with others make us responsible to others for our acts (Bricker-Jenkins & Hooyman, 1989).

Another dimension of feminist practice ideology is the notion of unity-diversity. This implies that diversity is a source of strength and growth. Although conflict in human relations is inevitable, peace is achievable. Sisterhood reflects the concern that none is free until all are free. Racism, classism, heterosexism, ableism, anti-Semitism, and other forms of oppression affect all. Awareness of and value for difference is a beginning to creating conditions for peace (Bricker-Jenkins & Hooyman, 1989).

Validation of the nonrational is another dimension of feminist practice. This orientation allows for multiple competing definitions of problems, many "truths." It emphasizes women's ability to reconstruct their own experiences, to find a meaning of events that they alone can determine. For example, a woman may perceive that her mastectomy is not a sexual phenomenon, but raises existential issues for her. The process of problem definition is recognized as subjective. Nonlinear, multidimensional thinking is encouraged (Bricker-Jenkins & Hooyman, 1989; Weedon, 1997).

Finally, consciousness raising and praxis are central to a feminist model. The intended outcome of consciousness raising is a new set of values, assumptions, and expectations. It is part of an evolving process of social change. Praxis references the component of feminist consciousness that leads to social transformation. An awareness of the reality that shapes women's lives becomes infused into public values. Reality is renamed according to women's experiences. Recognition of the small group as a unit of social change is explicit. Self-help is one means of change but does not substitute for the provision of adequate services from the state. Struggles to implement values such as egalitarianism, consensus democracy, nonexploitation, cooperation, collectivism, diversity, and nonjudgmental spirituality are central to feminist practice (Andrist, 1997; Bricker-Jenkins & Hooyman, 1989; Sampselle, 1990). However, consciousness raising is an ongoing process, often undertaken at some risk to many women. Facilitating consciousness raising with women cannot be abandoned mid-process, because this risks leaving women more vulnerable than before the process began (Wolf, 1996).

STRUCTURE AND PROCESS OF THE RELATIONSHIP

Caring for women occurs in the context of an open and collaborative relationship. This implies that the relationship is structured so the professional power of the nurse is balanced with the power of the woman seeking health care. Mutual recognition of one another's expertise, sharing of information, and defining goals in collaboration are central elements of the process. Women are regarded as experts about their own bodies and self-care, and nurses are regarded as experts in the health problems that populations of women experience and the processes that can be used to facilitate health. Information is shared freely between the nurse and woman seeking care so that the woman can have as much of the necessary data possible to make informed choices about her health. The woman seeking care is an active participant in her own self–health care, not a passive recipient. At times, she alone makes decisions about her own self-care. The nurse as a consultant provides information to women about the full range of alternatives for health. The woman makes prescriptions for her own health based on information about self-care options. She is part of a relationship in which she strives for health as she defines it.

The focus of the relationship is on the woman as a person, her self as she defines herself, in the context of her lived experience. A woman seeking care is not defined simply in terms of her biology, her diagnosis, or her role. She is not seen as a mother simply because she seeks pregnancy care. She may define herself in terms of her roles as a care provider for an aging parent, a worker, a wife, or a mother, or perhaps all of these. She may not define herself in terms of any role, but as feeling overwhelmed by obligation or challenged by her environment. She may be unable to define herself, unable to voice who she is.

Data to be collected relate to the woman herself, not only to her reproductive system structure and function. Data include potential or emergent health problems as defined by changing health patterns of populations of women and by the woman's own individual concerns. The woman provides the nurse with her own data regarding her health. She is invited to share the data she believes to be relevant. Nurses may point to other useful data to consider. This is in contrast to systems in which the nurse decides what data are relevant, and the woman's only contribution is responding to nurse-initiated questions.

The goals are set by the woman, with the nurse as a consultant. Nurses share their own impressions about possibilities and facilitate women's ability to perform processes important for self-care. This may involve helping women alter their environments to support them rather than helping women adapt to their environments.

Evaluation of care is process oriented. The woman compares the goals she has set for herself with her own self-care agency, using process-oriented criteria. It is important for women to have an improved understanding of their health and self-care abilities as a result of their encounters with health care providers. Women should have an improved ability to collect data about their own health and make appropriate judgments based on the data. Another goal of the encounter is to expand a woman's ability to perform processes important to her self-care. Finally, women will have an improved capacity for making decisions about their health. This system of care rests on the assumption that women's values will be respected during encounters with health care professionals, and their health problems or concerns will be managed in a way that is congruent with their values.

Requirements for the Practitioner

Requirements for feminist practice include identifying implications of the issues that arise for women; recognizing patterns of institutionalized sexism and other oppressive ideologies (racism, classism, heterosexism, ableism) and behaviors that create problems for all but for women in particular; developing strategies to remove material and ideological barriers to the fullest development of individuals and groups; and recognizing that feminist nursing practice is political practice if it enables women to control the conditions of their lives by encouraging equity in power relationships (Bricker-Jenkins & Hooyman, 1989; Wolf, 1996).

Some feminists would insist that any specialized skills for assisting women with menstruation, orgasm, childbirth, and early abortion should be practiced by women only. While this might ensure the representation of a greater number of women in some of the male-dominated health fields, one cannot assume that gender confers on the health practitioner freedom from sexism and sex-role stereotyping. On the other hand, a woman should have access to a woman health care provider if that is her preference. Moreover, men who practice women's health care will benefit from studying with and about women in order to gain a more complete perspective of women's lives.

REFERENCES

Allen, D. (1986). Nursing and oppression: "The family" in nursing texts. *Feminist Teacher, 2*(1), 15–20.

Allen, D., Allman, K., & Powers, P. (1991). Feminist nursing research without gender. *Advances in Nursing Science, 13*(3), 49–58.

Anderson, J. M. (2000). Gender, "race," poverty, health and discourses of health reform in the context of globalization: A postcolonial feminist perspective in policy research. *Nursing Inquiry, 7*(4), 220–229.

Anderson, J. M. (2004a). Discourse. The conundrums of binary categories: Critical inquiry through the lens of postcolonial feminist humanism. *Canadian Journal of Nursing Research, 36*(4), 11–16.

Anderson, J. M. (2004b). Lessons from a postcolonial-feminist perspective: Suffering and a path to healing. *Nursing Inquiry, 11*(4), 238–246.

Anderson, J. M. (2006). Reflections on the social determinants of women's health: Exploring intersections: Does racialization matter? *Canadian Journal of Nursing Research, 38*(1), 7–14.

Andrist, L. (1997). A feminist framework for graduate education in women's health. *Nursing Inquiry, 4*(4), 268–274.

Anzaldua, G. (1987). *Borderlands = La Frontera: The New Mestiza.* San Francisco: Aunt Lute Books.

Apodaca, M. L. (1977). The Chicana woman: An historical materialist perspective. *Latin American Perspectives, 4*(1/2), 70–89.

Banks-Wallace, J. (2000). Womanist ways of knowing: Theoretical considerations for research with African American women. *Advances in Nursing Science, 22*(3), 33–45.

Beasley, C. (1999). *What is feminism? An introduction to feminist theory.* London: Sage.

Berman, H., Ford-Gilboe, M., & Campbell, J. (1998). Combining stories and numbers: A methodological approach for a critical nursing science. *Advances in Nursing Science, 21*(1), 1–15.

Bermosk, L., & Porter, S. (1979). *Women's health and human wholeness.* New York: Appleton Century Crofts.

Bloom, L. (1998). *Under the sign of hope: Feminist methodology and narrative interpretation.* New York: State University of New York Press.

Bricker-Jenkins, M., & Hooyman, N. (1989). *Not for women only: Social work practice for a feminist future.* Silver Spring, MD: National Association of Social Workers.

Browne, A., & Fiske, J. (2001). First nations women's encounters with mainstream health care services. *Western Journal of Nursing Research, 23*(2), 126–147.

Bunting, S. M. (1997). Applying a feminist analysis model to selected nursing studies of women with HIV. *Issues in Mental Health Nursing, 18*(5), 523–537.

Butler, J. (1993). *Bodies that matter: On the discursive limits of sex.* London: Routledge.

Butler, J. (2000). *Gender trouble: Feminism and the subversion of identity.* London: Routledge.

Campbell, J., & Bunting, S. (1991). Voices and paradigms: Perspectives on critical and feminist theory in nursing. *Advances in Nursing Science, 13*(3), 1–15.

Chavez, L. R., Cornelius, W. A., & Jones, O. W. (1986). Utilization of health services by Mexican immigrant women in San Diego. *Women & Health, 11*(2), 3–20.

Chinn, P., & Jacobs, M. (1987). *Theory and nursing: A systematic approach.* St. Louis, MO: Mosby.

Chodorow, N. (1978). *The reproduction of mothering: Psychoanalysis and the sociology of gender.* Berkeley: University of California Press.

Chodorow, N. (1989). *Feminism and psychoanalytic theory.* New Haven, CT: Yale University Press.

Chodorow, N. (1994). *Feminisms, masculinities, sexualities: Freud and beyond.* Lexington: University of Kentucky Press.

Chopoorian, T. (1986). Reconceptualizing the environment. In P. Moccia (Ed.), *New approaches to theory development* (pp. 39–54). New York: National League for Nursing.

Chow, E. N. (1987). The development of feminist consciousness among Asian American women. *Gender & Society, 1*(3), 284–299.

Clear, G. M., & Carryer, J. (2001). Shadow dancing in the wings: Lesbian women talk about health care. *Nursing Praxis in New Zealand, 17*(3), 27–39.

Code, L. (1995). How do we know: Questions of method in feminist practice. In S. Burt & L. Code (Eds.), *Changing methods: Feminists transforming practice.* Peterborough, Ontario, Canada: Broadview Press.

Collins, P. H. (1989a). The social construction of black feminist thought. *Signs, 14,* 745–773.

Collins, P. H. (1989b). A comparison of two works on Black family life. *Signs, 14,* 875–884.

Collins, P. H. (2000). *Black feminist thought* (2nd ed.). New York: Routledge.

Correa-de-Marajo, R., Stevens, B., Moy, E., Nilasena, D., Chesney, F., & McDermott, K. (2006). Gender differences across racial and ethnic groups in the quality of care for acute myocardial infarction and heart failure associated with comorbidities. *Women's Health Issues, 16*(2), 44–55.

Crenshaw, K. (1995). Mapping the margins: Intersectionality, identity, politics, and violence against women of color. In K. Crenshaw, N. Gotanda, G. Peller, & K. Thomas (Eds.), *Critical race theory: The key writings that formed the movement.* New York: New Press.

Daly, M. (1978). *Gyn/ecology: The metaethics of radical feminism.* Boston: Beacon Press.

Davis, A. Y. (1981). *Women, race and class.* New York: Vintage Books.

Davis, A. Y. (1989). *Women, culture, and politics.* New York: Random House.

Davis, A. Y. (1991). *A Place of Rage* (Videorecording). Channel Four Television. New York: Women Making Movies.

De Beauvoir, S. (1949). *The second sex.* New York: Bantam.

Del Portillo, C. T. (1987). Poverty, self-concept, and health: Experience of Latinas. *Women & Health, 12*(3/4), 229–242.

Dey, J. G., & Hill, C. (2007). *Beyond the pay gap.* Washington, DC: American Association of University Women Educational Foundation.

Dill, B. T. (1983). Race, class, and gender: Prospects for an all-inclusive sisterhood. *Feminist Studies, 9*(1), 131–149.

Dill, B. T. (1987). The dialectics of black womanhood. In S. Harding (Ed.), *Feminism and methodology: Social science issues* (pp. 97–108). Bloomington: Indiana University Press.

Dinnerstein, D. (1976). *The mermaid and the minotaur: Sexual arrangements and human malaise.* New York: Harper & Row.

Dinnerstein, D. (1989). What does feminism mean. In A. Harris & Y. King (Eds.), *Rocking the ship of state: Toward a feminist peace politics* (pp. 13–23). Boulder, CO: Westview Press.

Drevdahl, D. (1999). Sailing beyond: Nursing theory and the person. *Advances in Nursing Science, 21*(4), 1–13.

Duffy, M. E. (1985). A critique of research: A feminist perspective. *Health Care for Women International, 6,* 341–352.

Duffy, M., & Hedin, B. (1988). New directions for nursing research. In N. Woods & M. Catanzaro (Eds.), *Nursing research: Theory and practice* (pp. 530–539). St Louis, MO: Mosby.

Elam, D. (1994). *Feminism and deconstruction: Ms. en Abyme.* London: Routledge.

Ensign, J. (2001). "Shut up and listen": Feminist health care with out-of-the-mainstream adolescent females. *Issues in Comprehensive Pediatric Nursing, 24*(2), 71–84.

Foucault, M. (1977). *The history of sexuality, an introduction: Vol. 1.* New York: Vintage Books.

Fulkerson, M. (1994). *Changing the subject: Women's discourses and feminist theology.* Minneapolis, MN: Fortress Press.

Gillespie, M. A. (1984). The myth of the strong black woman. In A. M. Jaggar & P. S. Rothenberg (Eds.), *Feminist frameworks: Alternative theoretical accounts of the relations between women and men* (2nd ed., pp. 32–35). New York: McGraw-Hill.

Gilligan, C. (1977). In a different voice: Women's conception of the self and of morality. *Harvard Educational Review, 47,* 481–517.

Gilligan, C. (1982). *In a different voice: Psychological theory and women's development.* Cambridge, MA: Harvard University Press.

Ginorio, A., & Reno, J. (1985). Violence in the lives of Latina women. *Working Together, 5*(5), 7–9.

Glass, N. (2002). Difference still troubles university environments: Emotional health issues associated with lesbian visibility in nursing schools. *Contemporary Nurse, 12*(3), 284–293.

Gordon-Bradshaw, R. H. (1987). A social essay on special issues facing poor women of color. *Women & Health, 12*(3/4), 243–259.

Griffin, S. (1978). *Woman and nature: The roaring inside her.* New York: Harper & Row.

Hale, J. C. (1985). Return to the bear paw. In J. W. Cochran, D. Langston, & C. Woodward (Eds.), *Changing our power: An introduction to women's studies* (pp. 55–60). Dubuque, IA: Kendall/Hunt.

Hall, J., & Stevens, P. (1991). Rigor in feminist research. *Advances in Nursing Science, 13*(3), 16–30.

Haraway, D. (1988). Situated knowledges: The science question in feminism and the privilege of partial perspective. *Feminist Studies, 14,* 575–599.

Haraway, D. (1989). *Primate visions: Gender, race, and nature in the world of modern science.* London: Routledge.

Harding, S. (Ed.). (1987). *Feminism and methodology: Social science issues.* Bloomington: Indiana University Press.

Harrison, B. (1985). *Making the connections: Essays in feminist social ethics.* Boston: Beacon Press.

Heide, W. S. (1982). *Feminism for the health of it.* Buffalo, NY: Margaret Daughters Press.

Heriques, J., Hollway, W., Urwin, C., Venn, C., & Walkerdine, V. (1998). *Changing the subject: Psychology, social regulations, and subjectivity.* London: Routledge.

Herman, A. M. (1984): Still . . . Small change for black women. In A. M. Jaggar & P. S. Rothenberg (Eds.), *Feminist frameworks: Alternative theoretical accounts of the relations between women and men* (2nd ed., pp. 36–39). New York: McGraw-Hill.

hooks, b. (1984). The myth of black matriarchy. In A. M. Jaggar & P. S. Rothenberg (Eds.), *Feminist frameworks: Alternative theoretical accounts of the relations between women and men* (2nd ed., pp. 369–373). New York: McGraw-Hill.

hooks, b. (1997). *Wounds of passion.* New York: Holt.

hooks, b. (1999). *Feminism is for everybody: Passionate politics.* Cambridge, MA: South End Press.

Hurtado, A. (1989). Relating to privilege: Seduction and rejection in the subordination of White women and women of color. *Signs, 14*(4), 883–856.

Hurtado, A. (1996). *The color of privilege: Three blasphemies on race and feminism.* Ann Arbor: University of Michigan Press.

Im, E. (2000). A feminist critique of breast cancer research among **Korean women** . . . **including** commentary by M. A. Hautman and B. Keddy with author response. *Western Journal of Nursing Research, 22*(5), 551–570.

Im, E., Meleis, A. I., & Park, Y. S. (1999). A feminist critique of research on menopausal experience of Korean women. *Research in Nursing & Health, 22*(5), 410–420.

Isasi-Diaz, A. (1993). En la lucha/In the struggle: Elaborating a mujerista theology. Minneapolis, MN: Fortress Press.

Isasi-Diaz, A., & Tarango, Y. (1992). Hispanic women: Prophetic voices in the church. Minneapolis, MN: Fortress Press.

Jack, D. (1987). Self-in-relation theory. In R. Formanek & A. Gurian (Eds.), *Women and depression: A lifespan perspective* (pp. 41–45). New York: Springer Publishing.

Jaggar, A. M., & Rothenberg, P. S. (1984). *Feminist frameworks: Alternative theoretical accounts of the relations between men and women* (2nd ed.). New York: McGraw-Hill.

Jagose, A. (1996). *Queer theory: An introduction.* New York: New York University Press.

Johnson, J. L, Bottorff, J. L., Browne, A. J., Grewal, S., Hilton, B. A., & Clarke, H. (2004). Othering and being othered in the context of health care services. *Health Communication, 16,* 255–271.

Kelly, P., Bobo, T., McLachlan, S., Avery, S., & Burge, S. (2006). Girl World: A primary prevention program for Mexican-American girls. *Health Promotion Practice, 7*(2), 174.

Kirkham, S. R., & Anderson, J. M. (2002). Postcolonial nursing scholarship: From epistemology to method. *Advances in Nursing Science, 25*(1), 1–17.

Klein, G. (1983). How to do what we want to do: Thoughts about feminist methodology. In G. Bowles & R. D. Klein (Eds.),

Theories of women's studies (pp. 88–104). London: Routledge & Kegan Paul.

Lather, P. (1991) *Getting smart: Feminist research and pedagogy with/in the postmodern.* New York: Routledge.

Liaschenko, J. (1999). Can justice coexist with the supremacy of personal values in nursing practice? *Western Journal of Nursing Research, 21*(1), 35–50.

Lorde, A. (1984a). Scratching the surface: Some notes on barriers to women and loving. In A. M. Jaggar & P. S. Rothenberg (Eds.), *Feminist frameworks: Alternative theoretical accounts of the relations between women and men* (2nd ed., pp. 432–436). New York: McGraw-Hill.

Lorde, A. (1984b). *Sister outsider: Essays and speeches.* Trumansburg, NY: Crossing Press.

Lorde, A. (1988a). *A burst of light: Essays.* Ithaca, NY: Firebrand Books.

Lorde, A. (1988b). Age, race, class and sex: Women redefining difference. In C. McEwen & S. O'Sullivan (Eds.), *Out the other side* (pp. 269–276). London: Virago Press.

MacKinnon, C. (1989). *Toward a feminist theory of the state.* Cambridge, MA: Harvard University Press.

MacPherson K. I. (1983). Feminist methods: A new paradigm for nursing research. *Advances in Nursing Science, 5*(2), 17–25.

MacPherson, K. (1988). Looking at caring and nursing through a feminist lens. In *Caring and nursing: Explorations in the feminist perspectives.* Conference Proceedings. Denver: University of Colorado School of Nursing.

Maeve, M. K. (1999). The social construction of love and sexuality in a woman's prison. *Advances in Nursing Science, 21*(3), 46–65.

Marcus, S. (2005). Queer theory for everyone: A review essay. *Signs, 31*(1), 191–219.

Martin, E. (1987). *The woman in the body: A cultural analysis of reproduction.* Boston: Beacon Press.

Maxwell-Young, L., Olshansky, E., & Steele, R. (1998). Conducting feminist research in nursing: Personal and political challenges. *Health Care for Women International, 19*(6), 505–513.

McBride, A. B., & McBride, W. L. (1982). Theoretical underpinnings for women's health. *Women and Health, 6*(1/2), 37–53.

Miller, J. B. (1986). *Toward a new psychology of women* (2nd ed.). Boston: Beacon Press.

Mohammed, S. A. (2006). Moving beyond the "exotic": Applying postcolonial theory in health research. *Advances in Nursing Science, 29*(2), 98–109.

Moraga, C. (1983). A long line of vendidas. In C. Moraga (Ed.), *Loving in the war years: Lo que nunca paso por sus labios* (pp. 90–144). Boston: South End Press.

Moraga, C. (1997). *Waiting in the wings: Portrait of a queer motherhood.* Ithaca, NY: Firebrand Books.

Moraga, C., & Anzaldua, C. (Eds.). (1983). *This bridge called my back: Writings by radical women of color.* New York: Kitchen Table: Women of Color Press.

Neufeld, A., Harrison, M. J., Hughes, K. D., Spitzer, D., & Stewart, M. J. (2001). Participation of immigrant women family caregivers in qualitative research. *Western Journal of Nursing Research, 23*(6), 575–591.

Parker, B., & McFarlane, J. (1991). Feminist theory and nursing: An empowerment model for research. *Advances in Nursing Science, 13*(3), 59–67.

Parse, R. (1987). *Nursing science: Major paradigms, theories, and critiques.* Philadelphia: Saunders.

Pirner, D. (2005). "Multiple margins" (being older, a woman, or a visible minority) constrained older women's access to Canadian health care. *Evidence-Based Nursing, 8*(4), 128.

Raymond, J. G. (1986). *A passion for friends: Toward a philosophy of female affection.* Boston: Beacon Press.

Reinharz, S. (1983). Experiential analysis: A contribution to feminist research. In G. Bowles & R. Klein (Eds.), *Theories of women's studies.* Boston: Routledge & Kegan Paul.

Rich, A. (1977). *Of women born: Motherhood as experience and institution.* London: Virago.

Rich, A. (1981). *Compulsory heterosexuality and lesbian experience.* London: Onlywomen Press.

Richman, J. A., Jason, L. A., Taylor, R. R., & Jahn, S. C. (2000). Feminist perspectives on the social construction of chronic fatigue syndrome. *Healthcare for Women International, 21*(3), 173–185.

Sampselle, C. (1990). The influence of feminist philosophy on nursing practice. *Image, 22*(4), 243–247.

Sanchez, C. L. (1984). Sex, class and race intersections: Visions of women of color. In B. Brant (Ed.), *A gathering of spirit* (pp. 150–155). New York: Sinister Wisdom.

Sanchez-Ayendez, M. (1989). Puerto Rican elderly women: The cultural dimension of social support networks. *Women & Health, 14*(3/4), 239–252.

Scheper-Hughes, N., & Lock, M. (1987). The mindful body: A prolegomenon to future work in medical anthropology. *Medical Anthropology Quarterly, 1*(1), 6–39.

Schroeder, C., & Ward, D. (1998). Women, welfare, and work: One view of the debate. *Nursing Outlook, 46*(5), 226–232.

Schuster, E. (1990). Earth caring. *Advances in Nursing Science, 13*(1), 25–30.

Scott, J., Kaplan, C., & Keates, D. (1997). *Transitions, environments, translations: Feminisms in international politics.* London: Routledge.

Segura, D. A. (1989). Chicana and Mexican immigrant women at work: The impact of class, race, and gender on occupational mobility. *Gender & Society, 3*(1), 37–52.

Smith, B. (1982). Black women's health: Notes for a course. In R. Hubbard, M. S. Henifin, & B. Fried (Eds.), *Biological woman—The convenient myth* (pp. 227–239). Rochester, VT: Schenkman Books.

Smith, J. (1981). The idea of health: A philosophical inquiry. *Advances in Nursing Science, 3,* 43–50.

Spinks, V., Andrews, J., & Boyle, J. (2000). Providing health care for lesbian clients. *Journal of Transcultural Nursing, 11*(2), 137–143.

Spivak, G. (1990). *The post colonial critic: Interviews, strategies, dialogues.* New York: Routledge.

Sturgeon, N. (1997). *Ecofeminist natures: Race, gender, feminist theory and political action.* London: Routledge.

Surrey, J. L. (1991). The "self-in-relation": A theory of women's development. In J. V. Jordan, A. G. Kaplan, J. B. Miller, I. P. Stiver, & J. L. Surrey (Eds.), *Women's growth in connection* (pp. 51–66). New York: Guilford Press.

Swanson, K. (1990). Providing care in the NICU: Sometimes an act of love. *Advances in Nursing Science, 13*(1), 60–73.

Tang, S.Y.S., & Anderson, J. M. (1999). Human agency and the process of healing: Lessons learned from women living with a chronic illness—"Re-writing the expert." *Nursing Inquiry, 6*(2), 83–93.

Taylor, J. (1998). Womanism: A methodological framework for African American women. *Advances in Nursing Science, 21*(1), 53–64.

Taylor, J. Y. (2002). The straw that broke the camel's back: African American women's strategies for disengaging from abusive relationships. *Women & Therapy, 25*(3/4), 79–93.

Taylor, J. Y. (2005). No resting place: African American women at the crossroads of violence. *Violence Against Women, 11*(12), 1473–1489.

Tigert, L. M. (2001). The power of shame: Lesbian battering as a manifestation of homophobia. *Women & Therapy, 23*(3), 73–85.

Tong, R. (1998). *Feminist thought: A more comprehensive introduction.* Boulder, CO: Westview Press.

Tsutakawa, M. (1988). Chest of kimonos—A female family history. In J. W. Cochran, D. Langston, & C. Woodward (Eds.), *Changing our power: An introduction to women's studies* (pp. 76–83). Dubuque, IA: Kendall/Hunt.

U.S. Public Heath Service Task Force on Women's Health Issues. (1985). *Women's health: Report of the Public Health Services: Vol. 2.* No. PHS-85-50206. Washington, DC: U.S. Department of Health and Human Services.

Visweswaran, K. (1994). *Fictions of feminist ethnography.* Minneapolis: University of Minnesota Press.

Weedon, C. (1997). *Feminist practice and poststructuralist theory.* Cambridge, MA: Blackwell.

Williams, D. R. (2005). The health of U.S. racial and ethnic populations. *Journals of Gerontology, Series B: Psychological Sciences and Social Sciences, 60*(2), 53–62.

Williams, D. R., Gonzalez, H. M., Neighbors, H., Nesse, R., Abelson, J. M., Sweetman, J., et al. (2007). Prevalence and distribution of major depressive disorder in African Americans, Caribbean Blacks, and non-Hispanic Whites: Results from the national survey of American life. *Archives of General Psychiatry, 64*(3), 305–315.

Williams, D. R., & Jackson, P. B. (2005). Social sources of racial disparities in health. *Health Affairs (Project Hope), 24*(2), 325–334.

Witt, S. H. (1984). Native women today: Sexism and the Indian woman. In A. M. Jaggar & P. S. Rothenberg (Eds.), *Feminist frameworks: Alternative theoretical accounts of the relations between women and men* (2nd ed., pp. 23–31). New York: McGraw-Hill.

Wolf, D. (1996). *Feminist dilemmas in fieldwork.* Boulder, CO: Westview Press.

Woods, N. F. (1985). New models of women's health care. *Health Care for Women International, 6,* 193–208.

Woods, N. F., Laffrey, S., Duffy, M., Lentz, M. J., Mitchell, E. S., Taylor, D., & Cowan, K. (1988). Being healthy: Women's images. *Advances in Nursing Science, 11*(1), 36–46.

Woods, N., Lentz, M., Mitchell, E., & Oakley, L. (1994). Depressed mood and self-esteem in young Asian, black, and white women in America. *Health Care for Women International, 15,* 243–262.

Yeatman, A. (1994). *Postmodern revisions of the political.* London: Routledge.

Young, I. M. (1990). *Justice and the politics of difference.* Princeton, NJ: Princeton University Press.

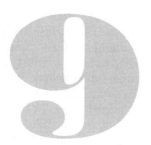

Well-Woman Assessment

Donna W. Roberson and
Catherine Ingram Fogel

At the beginning of the 20th century, women were most likely to die from childbirth or infectious disease. Today, women rank close to men in mortality from cardiovascular disease, stroke, and cancer (Agency for Healthcare Quality and Research, 2006). Rather than a homogeneous group of women, most providers find their patients come from varied cultural and socioeconomic backgrounds with a host of personal beliefs regarding health care (Nunez, 2000). Women may use alternative and complementary health care practices, research information on health questions using the Internet, or rely entirely on family or cultural values and knowledge for their health care needs. The well-woman examination is a priceless opportunity to educate women about their bodies and their health risks and support women in meeting what they desires for their own health. The well-woman examination entails obtaining a careful health history, providing a thorough physical examination, assessing an array of screenings based on age, and educating women in health promotion and preventative care as needed and desired. This chapter offers suggestions for conducting a health history, special considerations for adolescents and older women, and a review of the physical examination unique for women, including laboratory testing.

HEALTH HISTORY

Women are recommended to have routine well-woman care at 1- to 3-year intervals (Agency for Healthcare Quality and Research, 2007). Many women forgo their own health care needs while caring for others (Tharpe, 2006). For women in their childbearing years, an annual reproductive care visit for birth control or pregnancy planning may be the only opportunity to provide well-woman care. Adolescents and older women may be seen only for episodic care and need encouragement to obtain well-woman health care. The collection of the health history may be the best time to begin establishing a relationship that permits the advanced practice nurse to provide information on well-woman care.

A new patient requires a comprehensive health history; however, with subsequent visits, updates may be sufficient. Those updates should review the same elements in the original, comprehensive report. The health history is much more than soliciting answers to common health questions. It is an opportunity to discover what health care needs the woman has and how she views her health. The health history allows time for assessing risk, education needs, and values and identifying need for referral. This section discusses the health history in detail, including helpful hints for asking difficult or potentially sensitive questions.

Initiating the Interview

Few nurses would argue that nursing is both an art and a science. Advanced practice nurses must employ both art and science in conducting an interview. Helping a patient to feel comfortable improves the likelihood that difficult questions will be answered truthfully. Use of active listening skills such as leaning forward, nodding, encouraging further description by saying "tell me more" or "go on" indicates interest and instills a sense of trust in the clinician. Once the patient feels the nurse has concern for her as a person, rapport builds rapidly and both nurse and patient benefit from a more holistic encounter. Many nurses find certain elements of the health history difficult to address, including drug use, sexual history, and assessing for abuse. The nurse may experience discomfort from fear the question implies a judgment. However, if the nurse avoids asking the sensitive question, the patient may suffer consequences of incomplete health care. Suggested interview techniques follow that may help hone nurses' interviewing skills—even for hard-to-ask questions.

Whenever possible, observe the patient entering the examination room. If language is a barrier for your patient, a translator may be necessary. Use of family members as translators can be an uncomfortable practice. Family may alter the patient's answers to fit what they perceive is the "right" answer. Furthermore, the patient may not answer all questions as truthfully through the family as she would for a more neutral translator. In areas with a concentrated population with similar language issues, it is worth the expense to have quality translation available.

Consider collecting the patient's health history while she is clothed, before she disrobes for an examination. Sit at eye level and face the woman. Begin your health history with consideration for her cultural background. Some cultures may find it offensive to start with the common question: What brings you in today? Benign social conversation generally puts the patient at ease and is a nonthreatening way to begin the interview. Ask how the patient would like to be addressed, and include family or significant others if the patient desires. At some point in the interview, you will need to attempt to speak with the patient alone. Explaining that you typically like to speak with each patient alone for a few moments is usually accepted. Occasionally, for various reasons, the companion will not leave. Asking sensitive questions in front of family or friends may result in incomplete answers. Attempt to contact the patient later to fill in the important information.

Watch the patient as she talks. Pay attention to wording and emphasis, body language, and appearance as you listen to her answers. Allow ample time for the woman to tell her story. The woman should not be interrupted as she explains her concerns or reason for the visit. Beginning advanced practice nurses may feel the need to jot down notes as the patient is speaking. Keep note-taking to a minimum and consider explaining the purpose of your actions. With many practices utilizing electronic medical records, avoid the temptation to talk to the computer screen rather than address the patient directly.

Components of the History

Reason for Seeking Care (Chief Complaint)
> Description of the problem
> Precipitating/alleviating factors

Duration
Patient's perception of the problem and desired treatment

Social History
> Stress
>> Family, school, work, or other-related
> Support
>> Who is the person you turn to for support?
>> Who is important to you in your life?
> Relationships
>> Satisfaction with relationships

Marital status, number of marriages
Who lives with the patient
> Living arrangements
>> Primary residence
>> Length of time at current residence
>> Resources if no permanent residence
>> Safety of residence
> Work
>> Main source of income
>> Length of time on the job/working
>> Concerns about work/job
> Education
>> Highest grade completed
>> Future plans for schooling
>> Reasons for discontinuing education (as appropriate)

Racial/Cultural/Ethnic History
> Birthplace
> First language
> Length of time in United States (when appropriate)
> Special cultural practices

Religious History
> Importance of religion/spirituality
> Religious preference

Reproductive History
> Age at menarche
> Age of menopause (when appropriate) or age of mother's menopause if known
> Last menstrual period
> Menstrual patterns, frequency of cycles
> Length and amount of menstrual flow
> Pain associated with menses
> Perimenopausal or menopausal symptoms
>> Mood swings, crying, depression, irritability
>> Weight gain

Painful breasts, headache, cramps

Hot flashes

Management of menses or menopause

Breast self-examination practices

Last Pap smear

> ### HELPFUL HINTS
>
> ■ Younger patients may have difficulty recalling their last menstrual period, so have a calendar handy. Try to help jog the woman's memory by asking if she remembers an event or somewhere she went when she was menstruating.
> ■ Knowing the approximate age a woman's mother experienced menopause may be helpful in predicting perimenopause.
> ■ For categorization of flow, ask what size tampon or pad the woman uses and how often she has to change during her menses.
> ■ If pain is a complaint, you can ask what remedies the woman uses at this time, or ask during the medication review later.

Sexual History

Sexual orientation

New or change in partners

Exposure to Sexually Transmitted Infections—Include HIV Screening History

Abnormal Pap smear history

Pelvic infection

Endometriosis

Urinary incontinence

Method of birth control (if appropriate) and previous birth control methods

Concerns

Painful intercourse, bleeding, or discharge

Sex when intoxicated or high

Satisfaction with sex life

Obstetrical History

Gravity, parity

Infertility or miscarriages

Concerns

Plans for future pregnancies

Medical/Surgical History

Allergies

Medications—include prescription, over-the-counter, and supplements

> ### HELPFUL HINTS
>
> ■ Use open-ended questions to elicit sexual history.
> ■ Use of checklists with sexual history information may be less embarrassing for patients, but requires a certain level of literacy.
> ■ Ask what type of treatment the patient received for common conditions such as an abnormal Pap smear
> ■ Ask what causes urinary incontinence to determine type—for example, "does laughing or coughing cause you to leak urine?"
> ■ When the patient is an older woman, do not omit sexual activity questions. Using the words *love life* might be less embarrassing for the older patient versus using the word *sex*. If an older woman is returning to the dating world after the death of a spouse, it is important to assess her risk of sexually transmitted infection.

> ### HELPFUL HINTS
>
> ■ Asking about abortions, infertility, or pregnancy losses can be difficult. Practice a matter-of-fact tone in a nonjudgmental manner.
>   □ Good practice: "Tell me about your history of pregnancies."
>   □ Poor practice: "You haven't had an abortion, right?"

Immunization status

Tetanus

Meningococcal vaccine

Human papillomavirus vaccine

Hepatitis B vaccine

Measles, mumps, and rubella; chicken pox; polio

Pneumococcal vaccine

Influenza vaccine

Chronic disease—some common chronic diseases and problems to assess for may include:

Seizures	Urinary tract infection
Anemia	Hypertension
Cancer	Clotting disorder
Headaches/migraines	Heart disease
Thyroid disease	Lung disease
Stroke	Diabetes
Lupus	Irritable bowel/gastrointestinal disorders

Renal disease

Past surgical procedures

Foreign travel

Blood transfusions

Injuries

Last cholesterol check

HELPFUL HINTS

- Allergies should include food, medications, and environmental sources with reaction. Some patients say they have an allergy, but they relate a side effect rather than a true allergic response. For example, a common reaction to morphine is itching, but this does not indicate allergy.
- Attempt to obtain either dates or age at diagnosis, injury, or surgery.
- Document family history, indicating whether the disease is found on the mother's side, the father's side, or both.
- Always ask if there are any other problems that the patient has on a chronic basis.

Mental Health History

Common mental health disorders

Depression

Bipolar disorder

Anxiety

Eating disorders

Other

Counseling

HELPFUL HINTS

- Mental illness continues to have stigma, so use care when asking about mental health issues.
- If patient's history is positive for mental health disorders, ask if there is a family history.
- Document types of therapy and outcomes, including medications, psychotherapy, support groups, and so on.

Abuse/Violence Assessment

Emotional abuse

Physical abuse

Domestic violence

Rape

Substance abuse

HELPFUL HINTS

- Ask about past and present abuse.
  - ☐ Has anyone ever called you names or put you down? Does anyone do that now?
  - ☐ Has anyone ever shoved you, pulled your hair, or thrown things at you? Does anyone now?
  - ☐ Have you ever been forced to have sex when you did not want to?
  - ☐ Do you feel safe in your home/living situation?
  - ☐ Have you ever used alcohol or drugs to feel better about a bad situation or to reduce stress? Do you sometimes do that now?
- Rather than asking if the patient uses alcohol or drugs, ask "How much alcohol do you drink on a daily basis?" "How often do you get high?" "What drug do you most commonly use to get high?"

Lifestyle

Nutrition

Typical diet

Thoughts about current weight

Change in weight or dieting

Amount of caffeine consumed per day and its source

Amount of water consumed per day

Dietary restrictions—religious, personal preference, disease related

Vitamins

Calcium intake and sources

Sleep

Hours per night

Naps

Insomnia

Satisfaction with sleep patterns

Exercise

Type

Amount

Frequency

Tobacco

Age started using tobacco

Amount used daily

Attempts to quit or desire to quit

Exposure to smoke from others

Alcohol

How much alcohol used daily/weekly/monthly

Alcohol of choice

Age first started drinking

Ever been criticized for drinking

Problems with drinking

Binge drinking

Passing out from drinking

Driving while intoxicated

Arrested, lost job, or harmed relationship because of drinking

Drugs

What type of recreational drugs do you use?

How have you taken drugs—smoked, injected, snorted?

Blackouts

Age started using

Drug treatment program

Desire to stop using drugs

Current Trends

Tattoos

Piercings

Tanning

Skin popping

Previous Health Care Visits

Reason

Dates

Treatments or medications

HELPFUL HINTS

- In addition to cigarettes, some patients may use snuff ("dip") or other tobacco products.
- Record methods used to quit smoking, lose weight, or stop drug use and the outcomes of each method.
- It may be necessary to remind the patient you are asking about drug use not to report to the police, but to have a better understanding of how her body will respond to potential medications or treatments.
- Reassure adolescents that the information is confidential and will not be shared with their parents unless they want to share, except when they pose a safety risk to themselves or others. In such cases, the nurse must legally report pertinent information to the authorities.
- If the patient has tattoos or piercings, discuss where they were obtained and ask about any problems with infection, poor healing, and so on.
- Discuss the dangers of sun exposure and increased risk when using sun tanning machines.

Medication History

Prescribed medications

Daily use

Episodic use

Use of another person's prescription

Over-the-counter medications

Type, amount and reason for use

Supplements or herb use

The health history can appear quite intimidating on paper to the new clinician, but with practice, a health history can be obtained with little obvious effort. It is not necessary to follow any particular format; in fact, allowing the interview to flow naturally tends to elicit more information in a less threatening manner. Follow-up questions, when warranted, should follow the topic of conversation. Close the health history with the question, "Is there anything else I should know about you before we move on?"

After a thorough health history has been taken, a separate review of systems may not be necessary. The nurse should briefly review the history and determine whether further questions are required based on body system.

SPECIAL ADOLESCENT CONSIDERATIONS

Adolescents can be quite uneasy about having a well-woman examination. They may fear the pelvic examination or being undressed with a stranger. Adolescents are often body-conscious and wonder if they look like other adolescents. Adolescent may have questions about their body and sexuality that they are embarrassed to ask (Alexander, LaRosa, Bader, & Garfield, 2007; Fogel & Woods, 1998; Youngkin & Davis, 1998). Adolescents should be asked about unwanted physical contact (who, what, where, and when), contraceptive use (what and how), risk for suicide, substance abuse, and body image. Ask about school and after-school activities, friends, relationship with parents or older people, and sibling relationships. A simple question like "are you happy?" can yield tremendous insight into the world of the adolescent patient.

Interviewing adolescents requires great skill on the part of the nurse to put the patient at ease. Many teens will be accompanied by a parent, who will also need to feel comfortable with you. Establishing rapport with the parent greatly assists the clinician when it comes time to ask that parent to leave while you continue examining their child. Most adolescents will not disclose information about alcohol and drug use, sexual history, or reproductive concerns with a parent present. When talking about sensitive topics with a teen, it is imperative that the nurse remains open and nonjudgmental. Moreover, the nurse must inform the adolescent that her information will be kept confidential unless she is at risk for harming herself or someone else or if abuse is suspected. It may be necessary to give the adolescent permission to admit a behavior using statements such as, "Some girls your age have used drugs like marijuana or pot. Has this been something you've tried?" You can build on the assessment based on her answer.

SPECIAL OLDER WOMAN CONSIDERATIONS

As women age, questions related to cardiovascular health, breast changes, thyroid function, menses/menopause, and musculoskeletal status change focus to include effects of aging. Vaginal bleeding for the postmenopausal woman is important to identify. Depression may be present but not acknowledged due to stigma or a belief a person can "be strong" and overcome feelings of sadness. Elder abuse is becoming more apparent and should be assessed carefully for. Older patients may use several clinicians and pharmacies. Asking where prescriptions are filled and having the patient bring all current medications can shed light on a potential polypharmacy problem. Ask about risk factors for breast, colon, and lung cancers; cardiovascular disease; osteoporosis; and diabetes. Many older women may be on a fixed income and have difficulty affording medications or buying nutritious foods. A careful interview includes questions about purchasing medications and groceries. If the woman is perimenopausal, assessment of contraception is imperative.

PHYSICAL EXAMINATION

Most physical assessment textbooks contain excellent descriptions of the physical examination. To ensure all elements of a physical examination are assessed, the nurse should develop a systematic method for conducting the physical examination. Most find a head-to-toe approach is easy to follow and often puts the patient at ease by saving the more personal aspects of the exam for last.

The Breast Examination

Begin the breast examination by asking the woman whether she performs breast self-examination (BSE) and how she does the procedure. If she does not do BSE, ask if she knows how to perform BSE and explore reasons for not using BSE. Encouraging a woman to be familiar with how her breasts look and feel can help her detect changes in her breasts as she ages or as her health changes. Many Web sites have free BSE cards in a variety of languages that you can give to patients.

The clinical breast examination (CBE) should begin with inspection of the woman's breasts. Look for symmetry; however, many women have one breast slightly larger than the other. Note position of the nipple and look for discolorations, puckering, or unusual vascular patterns. Have the patient place her hands on her hips and flex her pectoral muscles as you observe for changes in the breast appearance. Explain what you are looking for as you conduct your survey. Next, with the patient in a supine position, place a small towel or pillow behind the patient's scapula on the side you are preparing to examine. Have the patient raise her arm above her head. This positioning should distribute the breast tissue more evenly over the rib cage. Discuss your examination as you proceed and demonstrate how to methodically examine the breast. Several acceptable methods are possible, including the wagon-wheel method, the vertical strip, or spiral method. The important feature to emphasize is regular BSE and including all breast tissue from mid-chest to clavicle to mid-axillary areas and the tail of Spence. Patients who have never performed BSE or who have questions about the technique should be encouraged to palpate normal breast structures with your guidance as well as cystic changes or other common variations.

The Pelvic Examination

The first pelvic examination is a source of fear for many women. Use of a caring, even humorous, approach can allay many fears. The pelvic exam is a unique opportunity to teach a woman about her body and remove myths or misconceptions about the female reproductive system. Keep a mirror handy to show the woman her anatomy, naming each part with the proper term as well as the common terminology as appropriate. Discuss how the pelvic exam will be conducted, and prepare the woman for physical sensations during the exam. For example, show the speculum and explain how it is used. The open speculum presses upward on the bladder and downward on the rectum causing a sensation of needing to void or pass flatus. Reassure the woman that these sensations are common and that she most likely will do neither (especially if she is encouraged to void prior to the exam).

With a first pelvic examination, discuss with the patient the steps in the exam, and show the speculum to those women who indicate an interest in seeing the equipment used. Some women will not want to see the speculum and prefer the exam to commence with little fanfare. Gloves are worn throughout the examination, and all equipment, testing supplies (Pap smear kits, swabs for wet mount or sexually transmitted infection testing), and trash receptacle should be within easy reach for the nurse seated at the foot of the examination table. The patient should be draped and assisted to insert one foot in each stirrup and slide down to the foot of the table. If the patient is positioned so her buttocks are almost off the edge of the table, the pelvic floor muscles will be more relaxed and the examination will be more comfortable for the patient. Be sure your light source is within easy reach and is in working order before positioning the patient in the lithotomy position.

1. Inspection: To avoid startling the patient, inform her of your motion before touching her. Most nurses will start by touching the inner thigh and move up to the perineum after warning the patient of the impending touch. Inspect the external genitalia by looking for lesions, discharge, erythema, or edema. Visually examine the external anal area for hemorrhoids, lesions, or masses. If you touch the anus, change gloves before touching the labia or vagina to avoid cross-contamination from the gastrointestinal tract to the vagina. Gently palpate the labia, and ensure you examine between labial folds for variances. Tell the patient you will next place one finger in the vagina slightly. Insert the index finger of your dominant hand in the vaginal opening about 1.5 to 2 inches, rotate so the base of the finger is pressed toward the urethra and milk the urethra and Skene's glands. Culture any discharge. Rotate the finger downward toward the 5 o'clock and 7 o'clock position and palpate the Bartholin's glands between the internal index finger and the external thumb of the dominant hand. There should be no tenderness or masses with palpation. Finally, place two fingers of the dominant hand on the base of the vagina and assess vaginal tone by having the patient bear down and then tighten the vaginal muscles. Bulging of tissue anteriorly may be a cystocele and posteriorly may be a rectocele.

2. Speculum exam: Select a speculum based on the size of the vaginal opening. For the first pelvic examination on a woman who has never delivered vaginally, select the Pederson speculum. Select the Graves speculum for other women. The speculum should be warmed. Stainless steel speculums can be warmed in the examination table drawer on a warming pad or by running warm water over the blades of the device. Plastic speculums should be warmed under warm water. Never use lubricants for insertion—water should be sufficient and is rarely necessary for premenopausal women. Lubricants alter the results of diagnostic tests. Use two fingers of the dominant hand to widen the opening of the vagina while inserting the closed speculum with the nondominant hand. The speculum is usually inserted diagonally then rotated once introduced into the vaginal canal. Most vaginal canals run downward toward the base of the woman's spine. Remove the dominant hand fingers and fully insert the speculum. Slightly open the speculum and look for the cervix. The cervix can be anywhere at the back of the vaginal canal. Occasionally, you may have to remove the speculum and find the cervix digitally and then reinsert the speculum toward the cervix. For heavy patients, have the woman, with or without assistance, pull her knees toward her chest. This maneuver will cause the cervix to pop up and can be captured with the speculum blades. Then the woman's feet can be returned to the stirrups for the remainder of the exam. Lock the speculum blades in position.

3. Completing the speculum examination: Note the color and appearance of the cervix. The cervix should be moist, pink, and rounded. Nulliparous women tend to have a closed cervical os, while those who have had cervical dilation (such as during vaginal delivery) may have a "fish mouth" or open os. Common cervical variations include pale (anemia or postmenopause), bluish (pregnancy), or protrusions (polyps). Assess for discharge, odor, and lesions along the vaginal canal and on the cervix.

   In the United States, most annual pelvic examinations include screening for chlamydia and gonorrhea. Insert the appropriate swab into the cervical os. Warn the patient she may feel a bumping sensation. There should not be pain with this specimen collection. Follow the manufacturer's directions for collection of this specimen. Next, use the Pap smear specimens by rotating the spatula over the entire 360 degrees of the surface of the cervix. Insert the endocervical brush into the os and rotate about one-quarter turn. Both specimens should be treated according to the Pap smear kit directions. If the patient has no cervix, use the spatula over the vaginal cuff and swab the vaginal pool for the Pap smear. If there is unusual drainage, odor, or complaints of itching by the patient, a wet mount is obtained by swabbing the vaginal wall or directly in the drainage. Loosen the locked speculum blades, withdraw the speculum from the cervix, and close the blades for removal from the vagina.

4. Bimanual examination: A bimanual examination is done to palpate the uterus and adenexa and evaluate pelvic floor support. Keeping the woman in the lithotomy position, stand and lubricate the first two fingers of the nondominant hand. Gently insert the fingers into the vaginal canal after explaining your actions to the patient. Take care that your thumb does not brush or compress the clitoris or urethra during the bimanual exam. Palpate the interior vaginal canal, locate the cervix, and palpate around the cervix to assess for masses or irregularities. The exam of the cervix should not be painful. Cervical motion tenderness is an abnormal finding and may indicate ectopic pregnancy, pelvic inflammatory disease, or infections of the cervix. A cervix positioned toward the anterior canal indicates a retroflexed uterus. A

posteriorly positioned cervix indicates an anteverted uterus. If the uterus and cervix are shifted left or right, this may indicate a pelvic mass.

Place the dominant hand over the symphysis pubis on the patient's abdomen and press inward toward the internally placed nondominant fingers to palpate the uterus. The uterus should be firm, smooth, and nontender. Note the position of the uterus. An enlarged uterus may indicate pregnancy, fibroid tumors, endometriosis, or carcinoma. Estimate the size of the enlarged uterus by weeks of gestation (for example, 12 weeks). The uterus should be pear shaped, but variations are possible, including bicornate or horned, which feel heart-shaped on palpation. The uterus should be slightly mobile; an immobile uterus may indicate infection, carcinoma, or adhesions.

Assessment of the ovaries is accomplished by shifting the internal fingers to the examiner's left (for the right ovary) and to the right (for the left ovary). The external hand presses downward toward the internal to capture the ovary. On prepubescent and postmenopausal women, the ovaries should not be palpable. Otherwise, the ovaries should be firm, oval in shape, and mobile. The ovaries should not be tender. An ovary that is over approximately 5 cm in diameter requires further evaluation. Fallopian tubes are not usually palpable unless in the presence of ectopic pregnancy, in which case they should not be firmly palpated to avoid rupture.

5. Rectovaginal examination: Some providers choose to perform a rectovaginal examination with each pelvic exam. Some sources suggest a rectal examination is not necessary unless medically indicated until age 40. The rectovaginal examination should be performed quickly, because it is uncomfortable for the patient. After explaining this last part of the exam to the patient, lubricate the middle finger and insert in the rectum, noting sphincter tone. Having the patient bear down as if having a bowel movement eases the insertion. Insert the index finger into the vagina and ask the patient to stop bearing down. Use the dominant hand placed externally on the lower abdomen to assess the posterior of the uterus and palpate for masses in the lower rectum. Remove your internal hand and examine the gloved finger for stool. Note color and presence of blood. For women over the age of 50, a test for occult blood should be performed from the stool on the gloved hand. If the stool appears bright red or dark and tarry, test for occult blood regardless of age.

With the pelvic examination complete, wipe the perineum from front to back and assist the patient to a sitting position. Remove gloves and wash hands.

Offer the patient cleansing wipes to remove excess lubricant and allow her to dress privately.

Routine Health Screening

- Pap smear
  - ☐ Should be completed by age 21 or when a younger woman is sexually active. Pap smears may be repeated annually for birth control maintenance, if sexual partners change, or as risk indicates. Women with normal Pap smears and no change in their sexual partner may opt to have Pap smears every 3 years.
- Sexually transmitted infection (STI) screening
  - ☐ every well-woman visit with the Pap smear.
  - ☐ Human Immunodeficiency Virus (HIV) at routine visits, not based on risk.
  - ☐ Women over the age of 64 should be offered STI and HIV screening if there has been a change in their risk factors.
- Mammography
  - ☐ every one to two years starting at age 40 or sooner as indicated.
- Cholesterol
  - ☐ baseline cholesterol panel age 45 and re-assessed based on findings/risk factors or every 5 years.
  - ☐ baseline panel checked by age 20 if family history of heart disease, the patient smokes or has diabetes.
- Colorectal cancer screen
  - ☐ stool for occult blood with well-woman visits starting at age 40.
  - ☐ sigmoidoscopy or colonoscopy recommend at age 50 or if family history, 10 years before relative was diagnosed with colon cancer.
  - ☐ Low risk, repeat screening every 5 years.
- Annual blood pressure evaluation after age 45 or with risk.
- Assessment for overweight/obesity or underweight with each well-woman visit.
- Bone density/osteoporosis screening for women at risk beginning with menopause.
  - ☐ Prevention of osteoporosis education begins with adolescent visit.
- For women over age 65, consider need for thyroid function studies, hearing and vision screen every 3 to 5 years. (adapted from Alexander et al., 2007)

Immunizations

The general immunization schedule is shown in Tables 9.1 and 9.2 for teens and college students and by age for adult women. This is a general overview, and nurses should review current guidelines, because the

9.1 Immunization Recommendations for Teens and College Students

VACCINE	RECOMMENDATION
Tetanus-diptheria-pertussis vaccine	Repeat every 10 years
Meningococcal vaccine	Recommended for high school freshmen or previously unvaccinated college freshmen living in dormitories
HPV vaccine series	Three-injection series for women younger than age 26
Hepatitis B vaccine series	If not previously vaccinated as an infant or in 6th grade
Polio vaccine series	No recommendation
Measles-mumps-rubella (MMR) vaccine series	Two doses, separated by a minimum of one month
Varicella (chickenpox) vaccine series	Second vaccine recommended for those who received one dose as an infant or child
Influenza vaccine	Annually, especially with high-risk patients
Pneumococcal polysaccharid (PPV) vaccine	More for high-risk patients
Hepatitis A vaccine series	Assess for need

Note. Adapted from "Recommended Adult Immunization Schedule—United States, October 2006–September 2007," by Centers for Disease Control and Prevention, 2006, *MMWR QuickGuide, 55*(40). Retrieved October 2, 2007, from http://www.cdc.gov/mmwr/pdf/wk/mm5540-Immunization.pdf

9.2 Female Immunization Recommendations by Age

	RECOMMENDATIONS		
VACCINE	**AGES 19 TO 49 YEARS**	**AGES 50 TO 64 YEARS**	**AGES 65 YEARS AND OLDER**
Tetanus	Every 10 years	Every 10 years	Every 10 years
HPV	Three doses if younger than 26 years		
MMR	One or two doses	One dose if indicated	One dose if indicated
Varicella	Two doses	One dose if no immunity	One dose if no immunity
Influenza	Annually, if indicated	Annually	Annually
Pneumonia	One to two doses, if indicated	One to two doses, if indicated	One dose
Hepatitis A	Three-injection series offered based on history, occupational, or lifestyle risks		
Hepatitis B	Three-injection series offered based on history, occupational, or lifestyle risks		
Meningitis	One dose based on risk	One dose based on risk	One dose based on risk

Note. Adapted from "Recommended Adult Immunization Schedule—United States, October 2006–September 2007," by Centers for Disease Control and Prevention, 2006, *MMWR QuickGuide, 55*(40). Retrieved October 2, 2007, from http://www.cdc.gov/mmwr/pdf/wk/mm5540-Immunization.pdf

recommendations change as new information and vaccines are made available.

A new vaccine of special interest is the human papillomavirus vaccine (HPV), now available to prevent infection with strands of HPV found to cause cervical cancer. The Advisory Committee on Immunization Practices recommends the three-dose injection series (at 0, 2, and 6 months) for women under age 26 and offered to girls age 11 to 12, but may be started in girls as young as age 9. It is recommended that women receive the series before becoming sexually active but is not contraindicated if the woman has had sexual intercourse. For women who have been infected with HPV, the vaccine will only protect them from infection with strands they have not yet acquired (Centers for Disease Control and Prevention, 2007).

REFERENCES

Agency for Healthcare Quality and Research. (2006). *Women's health highlights: Recent findings.* Rockville, MD: Author. Retrieved September 4, 2007, from http://www.ahrq.gov/research/womenh1.htm#intro

Agency for Healthcare Quality and Research. (2007). *Women: Stay healthy at any age—Your checklist for health.* Rockville, MD: Author. Retrieved September 18, 2007, from http://www.ahrq.gov/ppip/healthywom.htm

Alexander, L., LaRosa, J., Bader, H., & Garfield, S. (2007). *New dimensions in women's health* (4th ed.). Sudbury, MA: Jones and Bartlett.

Centers for Disease Control and Prevention. (2006). Recommended adult immunization schedule—United States, October 2006–September 2007. *MMWR QuickGuide, 55*(40). Retrieved October 2, 2007, from http://www.cdc.gov/mmwr/pdf/wk/mm5540-Immunization.pdf

Centers for Disease Control and Prevention. (2007). *Human papillomavirus: HPV information for clinicians.* Atlanta, GA: Author. Retrieved October 2, 2007, from http://www.cdc.gov/std/hpv/common-clinicians/ClinicianBro.txt

Fogel, E., & Woods, N. (1998). *Women's health dare: A comprehensive handbook.* Thousand Oaks, CA: Sage.

Nunez, A. (2000). Transforming cultural competence into cross-cultural efficacy in women's health education. *Academic Medicine, 75,* 1071–1080.

Tharpe, N. (2006). *Clinical practice guidelines for midwifery & women's health.* Sudbury, MA: Jones and Bartlett.

Youngkin, E., & Davis, M. (1998). *Women's health: A primary care clinical guide.* Stamford, CT: Appleton & Lange.

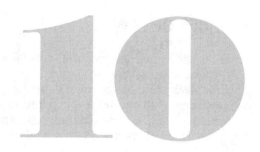

Legal Issues in the Care of Women

Diane K. Kjervik

You've got to rattle your cage door. You've got to let them know that you're in there, and that you want out. Make noise. Cause trouble. You may not win right away, but you'll sure have a lot more fun.

—*Florynce Kennedy (Warner, 1992)*

The historical, political disempowerment and disenfranchisement of women in the United States fueled a legal debate that resulted in the improvement of women's legal status. Although the health of women is a more invisible form of disempowerment, the political upheaval from the suffrage movement in the early 1900s and the struggle for the Equal Rights Amendment in the 1970s led to legal changes directly related to the health of women. This chapter addresses some areas of law that affect women's health, such as domestic violence, reproductive rights, and women's participation as human subjects in research. The analytical framework used to examine these changes will incorporate both feminist and therapeutic forms of jurisprudence. Therapeutic jurisprudence (TJ) is the study of whether legal systems actually result in improvement of emotional life and psychological well-being of individuals and communities (La Fond, 1999; Wexler, 2000; Wexler & Winick, 1996). Feminist jurisprudence (FJ) also examines the harms and benefits of legal decisions, particularly those relating to women, and theorizes a remedial structure to eliminate the negative results of patriarchal law (Scales, 1986; Sheldon & Thomson, 1998; Wishik, 1985). The chapter begins with a review of the areas of law that affect health of women and describes how law is a source of power. Several areas of law affecting women's health will be addressed followed by a discussion of strategies used to empower women legally.

AREAS OF LAW AFFECTING WOMEN

Both civil and criminal law influence women's health. The civil area of law addresses relationships among people and allows lawsuits for such concerns as disputed contractual relationships, employer-employee relationships (agency law and labor law), negligent or intentional harm to another (tort law), family law (divorce, child custody), and discriminatory practices. Through its system of criminal law, state and federal governments mandate behavior and practices that strive to provide an organized approach to human relationships—for example, business, health, and social relationships. Law also seeks justice (even-handed application of rules, regulations, and court decisions), but whether these goals are achieved for women is worth careful examination.

The critical analyses of TJ and FJ allow scholars to consider whether the law is truly neutral in terms of gender. The blindfold on the eyes of the depiction of justice (who is a woman) represents the neutrality the law is to embody. Some policies appear neutral in words, but in application thrust a heavier burden on women than men. For instance, policies that assume, but do not explicitly recognize, that women are the at-home caregivers of dependents, the sick, older persons, and the disabled institutionalizes the oppression of women (Wuest, 1993). Even in countries where women hold high government positions (e.g., Scandinavia), the assumption that women will care for elderly persons at home without pay exists (Covan, 1997). All areas of law should be examined to identify assumptions about women's health and work that underlie articulated policy and the effects that these assumptions have on women's lives.

SOURCES OF LAW

Legal decisions are derived from several sources. The U.S. Constitution is the primary source of law federally, and each state has its own constitution that must be consistent with the federal constitution. The equal protection, due process, free speech, and interstate commerce provisions are examples of areas governed by the U.S. Constitution. The state and federal constitutions also establish the three branches of government—legislative, judicial, and executive—that make, interpret, and execute the law, respectively. All states except Louisiana draw upon the common law of England. Common law is based on judicial precedent rather than statutes. Louisiana follows a civil code that is based on the Napoleonic Code from Roman, Spanish, and French systems (Aiken, 1994).

Law must be studied prior to and while practicing it because of the complexity of the relationships among the branches and levels of government, the common law, and constitutional law. As issues related to women's health become visible internationally, such as those examined by the International Council on Women's Health Issues, legal analysis must cross numerous legal systems and address substance and process of international law. Internationally, a pervasive neglect of women's health across the life span has reduced their physical, mental, and social well-being (Cook, 1994). The United Nation's Women Convention is considered the leading statement on women's legal rights and has been widely accepted by countries around the world (Cook, 1994). The Convention pledges countries to eliminate discrimination against women and, in terms of women's health specifically, to promote and protect women's health and enhance their dignity and self-determination (Cook, 1994).

The legal system in the United States espouses a goal of justice, and equality is the crucial component of justice in both legal and ethical contexts (Veatch, 1986). Women must prove they are *like* men before they are treated equally, and, as a result, areas in which obvious differences exist—for example, reproductive capacity—women's struggle for fair treatment is hampered (Scales, 1996).

LAW AS A SOURCE OF EMPOWERMENT

Whether law assists or blocks women in exercising their voice relates to the role played by women in legal proceedings. Women serve, for instance, as lobbyists, plaintiffs, or defendants in lawsuits and as lawyers, judges, and legislators. The percent of women in these roles, however, is not representative of the entire population, and, by virtue of this, the power exercised by women is not as extensive as it could be. The media play a key role in making women involved with law visible. However, images developed by the media have not created positive role models for women. For instance, recent media images of women lawyers conveyed negative messages (showing them making serious mistakes, having serious mental problems, or displaying unprofessional sexual conduct) despite the fact that the numbers of women in law had increased exponentially during the 1970s and 1980s (Caplow, 1999).

WOMEN AS RESEARCH SUBJECTS

Although women were excluded from many research studies in the 1970s and 1980s because risks to women were considered too great, these barriers were removed in 1993 by the Food and Drug Administration (Weijer & Crouch, 1999). The Institute of Medicine found evidence that women had been excluded or not adequately sampled in studies of AIDS and heart disease (Mastroianni, Faden, & Federman, 1994). Studies of cardiovascular disease funded by the National Institutes of Health (NIH) during the 1970s and 1980s did not include women subjects, although women die from these diseases in equal numbers to men in the United States (Dickersin & Schnaper, 1996). Women subjects were also excluded from initial research on HIV/AIDS (Teare & English, 1996). In 1994, the NIH issued guidelines that required representative numbers of women to be included in research funded by NIH and mandated that randomized controlled trials (RCTs) result in effective treatment for women (National Institutes of Health, 1994). In RCTs, uncertainty about the outcomes of the two treatments must exist, and clinical equipoise (professional disagreement about the preferable treatment) can be used as ethical justification for subgroup analysis directed at gender effects (Weijer & Crouch, 1999). Whether the federal approach will be adopted by other funding agencies remains unclear, but Weijer and Crouch (1999) recommend that the concerted effort by NIH to include women be adopted by other funding agencies and researchers.

DOMESTIC VIOLENCE AND RAPE

The problem of violence directed against women is well documented. The law can be used to empower women as they seek to protect themselves from the violence directed against them and their children. Using the law by calling police for help is considered "fighting back," part of the process women experience as they leave abusive partners (Merritt-Gray & Wuest, 1995). However, the law can also create barriers to the help women need to exit abusive situations. For instance, legal approaches to child custody when mothers are battered by spouses or partners have resulted in children being moved into foster care and the battered woman being charged with failure to protect under child abuse statutes. One feminist legal scholar recommends an approach that preserves the relationship between mother and child rather than punishing the woman by removing her child from her care (Daigle, 1998). This author recommends that courts examine the reasonableness of the mother's conduct during the time that precedes, accompanies, and succeeds the battering (Daigle, 1998).

Research has shown that battered women delay prenatal care whether they are White, Hispanic, or African American (Taggert & Mattson, 1996). The reasons for this delay are unclear, and the authors suggest further research to elucidate the process. Violence against ex-wives continues to be a problem, possibly because men feel a sense of ownership of women that entitles them to strike back when their "possession" leaves them (McMurray, 1997). An attitudinal/educational campaign to eliminate this belief is highly recommended by the author. Directing this campaign to legal officials may affect the choice of policy enacted or decided by them. Judges are, for instance, often surprised by the number of domestic violence cases that come before them and the number of "thick jackets" that occur (in which women return time after to time to either retract or reinitiate a request for a restraining order) (Almeida, Gujavarty, Scott, & Williams, 1999, p. 78).

The importance of good communication and interviewing skills cannot be over-emphasized. Women's health and legal concerns will often be revealed during routine physical examinations. As Siegel, Hill, Henderson, Ernst, and Boat (1999) found, many women will discuss domestic violence during pediatric office visits. Likewise, legal authorities who use good interviewing skills will learn of abuse directed at women or their children and are in a position to advise women of their legal options—for example, restraining orders to keep the abusive partner at a distance.

The Violence Against Women Act (VAWA) (1994) is a federal statute that allows women who have been assaulted to sue their attackers for damages. In addition, VAWA funds direct services for women who are victims of violence and funds research and training related to the problem (Almeida et al., 1999). A challenge to this statute was heard in the U.S. Supreme Court in January 2000 (*U.S. v. Morrison*), and the portion of the statute providing a civil remedy for a violent act against women was found unconstitutional. In this case, the plaintiff, Christy Brzonkala, alleged that she was raped in her college dorm by two men shortly after she met them. Under the VAWA, she brought a suit against the alleged perpetrators for monetary damages. The Na-

tional Organization for Women's Legal Defense and Education Fund (NOW LDEF, 1999–2000) appeared in court to defend the constitutionality of the VAWA. However, the court held that the act's provision to provide a civil remedy for acts of violence was not supported by the commerce clause or the 14th amendment of the U.S. Constitution.

NOW LDEF is an example of a consumer-driven legal action group that changes law to help women. This organization has produced a videotape to train judges about rape myths, sex offender treatment, and the impact of rape on victims (NOW LDEF, 1999–2000). Women often appear *pro se* (representing themselves) in legal proceedings, and thus jeopardize the success of their cases by, for example, not knowing the rules of evidence (Almeida et al., 1999). Effective advocacy groups such as NOW LDEF give women effective legal voice.

MENTAL HEALTH

As with HIV/AIDS, stigmatization by virtue of mental illness occurs in society at large, but feminist groups rarely identify mental illness as an issue in need of attention (Stefan, 1996). The invisibility of the concerns of mentally ill women even among women's groups probably relates to the mystification of diagnosis and treatment of mental illness. Legally, women can be forced into a hospital if they are considered dangerous to themselves or someone else, and then can be treated by force. While the same is true for men, women are more vulnerable to powerful decisions by those in authority because they are considered to be less authoritative than men. Rarely addressed by mental health experts are differing needs among men and women patients, including contraception or reproductive matters (Stefan, 1996). A feminist approach to reform of the mental health system would include participation rather than hierarchy, control rather than dependency, connection rather than isolation, recovery models rather than a pathology focus, and attention to context instead of objectification (Stefan, 1996). She suggests that organizations that fund mental health services for women keep these philosophical shifts in mind. This feminist approach would build incentives to a model of care that would preserve rather than destroy or disrupt strong family relationships and would give greater voice to women.

ABORTION

Since 1972, the law has considered family planning to fall within a "zone of privacy" protected by the U.S. Constitution (Charo, 1997, p. 74). This followed over 100 years of efforts to control fertility treatment and birth control by the medical community (Charo, 1997). Policy debates that pit the mother's interests against those of children or fetuses create tremendous problems in the law. Deference to children or fetuses has been considered a form of social control of women exercised by medical authorities (Hagell, 1993). Legal challenges to abortion have not succeeded in eliminating the basic right to abortion delineated by the U.S. Supreme Court in *Roe v. Wade* (1973), but state requirements that mandate disclosure of certain types of information to the woman prior to abortion (e.g., risks of abortion, age of and details about the fetus, alternatives to abortion) have been allowed by the U.S. Supreme Court (Rozovsky, 1999). Fertility control is, in essence, a matter of gender equality whereby community demographic goals cannot be served by coerced pregnancy (Charo, 1997). Because of continuing legal challenges to abortion, women and health care providers are not entirely clear about what is expected of them. Therefore, hospitals and clinics need to make clear what policies and procedures they will follow to obtain the woman's consent to abortion (Rozovsky, 1999).

DRUG ABUSE DURING PREGNANCY

Women who take drugs or drink alcohol during pregnancy are considered at risk to the fetus, and thus the law may choose to intervene to protect the fetus by exercising its *parens patriae* power. The extent of the state's right to intervene and how to intervene is not clear at this point. There are several ways in which jurisdictions have attempted to handle the growing problem of drug exposure to the fetus, none of which have been very successful.

Child endangerment statutes have been enacted to impose criminal sanctions on women for ingesting illegal substances while they are pregnant (*Whitner v. State*, 1997). Prosecutions under these statutes have not been successful in eliminating or preventing prenatal drug use because courts traditionally have been unwilling to stretch child endangerment and child support statutes beyond their most obvious purpose—to protect already-born children. Women have been charged with the "delivery" of a controlled substance to a "child" via the umbilical cord while in the womb or a few moments after birth. These prosecutions have also met with little success (*Johnson v. State*, 1992). Both of the above approaches usually come down to whether the fetus or newborn was a child within the legislative intent and protection of the statute. Charging the mother with involuntary manslaughter or using child custody statutes that provide for the temporary and permanent removal of children abused or neglected by their parents have been tried. The civil approach has met with some success in a few states, but the greater weight of legal authority supports not allowing intervention to protect a fetus from maternal drug abuse during pregnancy (*Unborn Child of Starks v. Oklahoma*, 2001). Several states have enacted statutes specifically addressing the use of illegal drugs during pregnancy in the context of child abuse and neglect, all of which can support the termination of parental rights to the child.

In 1998, Wisconsin legislators (followed immediately by South Dakota) enacted an amendment to child protection statutes that allows judges to confine these women for the remainder of the pregnancy (De Ville & Kopelman, 1999). Whether this legislation will withstand constitutional scrutiny in light of its burden on the woman's right to be secure in her person remains to be seen. The legislation reduces her rights to move around, to freely associate, and to her individual liberty (all constitutionally protected rights) (De Ville & Kopelman, 1999). Marshall (1999) points out that the weight of policy such as the Wisconsin and South Dakota legislation will fall disproportionately on minority and poor women, because evidence exists that minority and poor women are most often prosecuted for substance abuse while pregnant. Also worth considering, according to Marshall (1999), is the impact of the policy on the woman's willingness to seek treatment if she knows that her freedom may be infringed. Indeed, this policy may have a chilling effect on the woman and exacerbate the problem it is hoping to resolve—that is, ways to get the woman into treatment.

Numerous difficult legal issues arise such as whether existing statutes give proper notice to a pregnant woman that she can be prosecuted for harming her fetus, whether prosecuting a pregnant woman violates her right to privacy or endangers her abortion rights, whether such action violates the 8th or 14th Amendment to the U.S. Constitution, concerns about the discriminatory application of the law, and whether criminal sanctions actually promote the interests of the unborn or, in fact, create more harm than is justified.

CHILD CARE AND BREAST-FEEDING

Breast-feeding in public is an evolving focus in legal forums. While numerous states have passed legislation allowing women to breast-feed in public, very few have included provisions to enforce the right to breast-feed (Cruver-Smith, 1998). A law without enforcement provisions is worth little to women who are harassed for breast-feeding in public. Cruver-Smith (1998) recommends that states consider provisions such as those passed in New Jersey, New York, and Connecticut that impose fines or the right to sue the person who violates the statute. Slippery slope arguments are used by opponents of this legislation—for example, the fear articulated by one legislator that women will use breast-feeding as an excuse to make public displays of breast feeding (Warren, 1995). Negative attitudes toward breast-feeding are premised upon the breast as an object of sexual pleasure and thus "indecent" to expose. Covering femaleness in this way is another example of invisibility of women and women's needs. Although federal regulations support the value of breast-feeding, the federal judiciary has not clarified the scope of the right in case law (Cruver-Smith, 1998). Thus, women must work within their own states to obtain legislation that protects breast-feeding in public by drafting the protection explicitly and delineating the means to enforce the state policy.

Because women are often the primary child care providers in the family, day care for working mothers is a continuing problem that rises to the level of a legal concern. NOW LDEF (1999–2000) has initiated an Adopt a Politician program in which persons or companies who participate contact a given politician on a regular basis to let them know about the needs for child care in their communities. In this way, bills proposed by legislators are based on information from the voting public and, as such, make visible women's needs as caregivers of children.

BREAST IMPLANTS

Numerous lawsuits about faulty breast implants have been brought and won by women, and the Food and Drug Administration (FDA) has placed restrictions on their future use (Rozovsky, 1999). Although the choice of breast implants or other forms of alteration of one's appearance is a question of female self-esteem and self-acceptance, the law doesn't question the motives of the woman who seeks a medical procedure. Rather, tort law examines the standard of care that should have been used, whether the standard was breached, and whether injury was caused by the breach. As with abortions, clear policies and procedures related to consent obtained from women prior to implantation are necessary to adequate risk management (Rozovsky, 1999).

HIV

Several legal problems arise for women with HIV. Exclusions of HIV and inclusion only of AIDS cases by the Centers for Disease Control and the Social Security Administration meant that women who died of HIV without AIDS were excluded from policy considerations, including financial benefits (Teare & English, 1996). This policy was revised in 1992 to include HIV cases, and invasive cervical cancer was added to the list of complicating conditions of AIDS (Teare & English, 1996).

Legal issues around consent to HIV testing also exist. Because of the stigma associated with HIV, most women wish to maintain their HIV status as a private concern. However, public health officials seek this information for public health reasons. Approximately one-third of women have been tested for HIV either during blood donation or physical examination (Teare & English, 1996). The most frequently cited reason offered for testing women is that they may transmit HIV to others, particularly fetuses or infants (Teare & English, 1996). Many state laws require that informed consent be required prior to testing, but the voluntariness of women's choice to be tested has been questioned (Teare & English, 1996). Women may feel pressured into testing by relatives, health care providers, or friends who are worried about their own health or that of others.

Federal and state finance policy affects women's ability to be treated for HIV or other disease. Since most women and girls with HIV are poor or from minority populations, their access to care is directly affected by federal and state Medicaid provisions (Teare & English, 1996).

STRATEGIES TO IMPROVE THE LEGAL STATUS OF WOMEN

Since many policies contribute to the invisibility of women or are harmful to women's health, strategies to examine and change these effects are required.

Tort Law Reforms

Efforts to reform tort law by placing ceilings on malpractice awards or to limit certain types of awards (e.g., pain and suffering) exemplify proposed policy that, on its face, appears to be gender neutral. However, tort reform targets primarily products liability and medical malpractice, areas in which defective products such as the Dalkon Shield and diethylstilbestrol or negligent gynecological or obstetrical care fall (McConnell, 1996). Legislative changes have become critical to giving women access to hospitals after delivery of a child and to their ability to sue negligent managed care organizations. Women's needs should be brought into these debates so that generalizations about motives of injured plaintiffs are understood and the realities of the injuries suffered by women are considered.

Knowledge Generation

Action based on knowledge and information is necessary to the political process. Information and action (theory and practice) interact continuously over time to produce the most effective results. As Malterud (1993, p. 365) points out, "knowledge is constructed by voice." Knowledge, of course, is a form of power, and, thus, to achieve power, women must find their own voice. Malterud suggests the use of a "feminine medical epistemology" (p. 365) that records women's reality and translates it into medical knowledge. This necessitates a research methodology that reflects the reality of women's experiences. This should include research designs, for example, that examine subgroups in which women are disproportionately represented, such as the elderly (Weijer & Crouch, 1999).

The medical profession believes that its approaches are gender neutral (Malterud, 1993). For example, chronic illness and disability analyses are rarely approached from a gender perspective (Thorne, McCormick, & Carty, 1997). Similarly, the mainstream legal profession assumes that laws are gender neutral (Cook, 1994), and so FJ has evolved as a legal research approach that uses critical analysis of policy and practice. Sometimes the best approach to a woman's health problem is a caring confirmation of the existence of the problem and a respect for the woman's view of it (Malterud, 1993). Sexist policies are, at times, as pointed out recently by President Vest of the Massachusetts Institute of Technology, a matter of perception (Leo, 1999). Confirmation of the woman's perception results in giving the woman's viewpoint and voice expression.

FJ scholars also track and challenge esoteric legal battles—for example, the standard of scrutiny for cases involved the Equal Protection Clause of the U.S. Constitution (Matthews, 1998). A stricter scrutiny of legislation means that the court will take a very close look at the reasons for the differential treatment. A case involving a nursing school raised the question of which scrutiny standard to use and settled on the current intermediate level rather than strict scrutiny used for race discrimination cases (*Mississippi University for Women v. Hogan*, 1982). At issue in this case was a policy denying men academic credit for courses at a women-only nursing school. The court allowed the policy to be used by applying the intermediate rather than strict scrutiny test.

Community Advocacy

The legal system historically is not well equipped to engineer large social change, and rather is called into play when someone is injured (Moss, 1996). The proactivity, thus, will need to be generated from women who experience problems. Even if a sympathetic legislator or bureaucrat proposes a legal change, it will fail without broad-based support and a basis upon a sense of community obligation (Moss, 1996). The media can play a pivotal role in sending the message of women's health needs to the public. NOW LDEF planned its Women, Policy and Media Program to examine ways women are affected by policy issues such as budget surplus, taxes, and international policy changes (NOW LDEF, 1999–2000).

In June 2000, Legal Momentum (then known as NOW LDEF) launched Women's Enews, the first, and only, major initiative of the Women, Policy, and Media Program (Legal Momentum, 2000). This news source provides coverage of women's issues on the Internet in daily news updates to media outlets and its own subscribers. According to Altagracia Dilone Levat, Vice President for Communications and Marketing of Legal Momentum, Women's Enews is alive and well today (A. D. Levat, personal communication, March 3, 2008).

Policies considered must recognize differences between individuals and among groups of women. Social class and racial differences must be accounted for in whatever policy is proposed (Krieger & Fee, 1996). But as Minow (1990) cautions, differences among persons should not stereotype those within groups, but rather examine the relationships between the persons and the systems in which they find themselves disenfranchised. Thus, the best legal analysis examines the person and the system, with individual response the key to understanding the problem and its resolution.

While individuality is an important value in the United States, other countries may not share this value as a foundation to law and public health policy (Charo, 1997). Legal rights won here, therefore, will not necessarily follow in other countries in which a more communitarian view exists.

The National Women's Health Network established in 1976 is an example of an effective advocacy group for concerns of women (Norsigian, 1996). The Network continues to work in Congress and federal agencies such as the FDA to represent the needs of women. Successes the Network claims include the Patient Package Insert program of the FDA, the increase in the number of nurse practitioners who provide primary care to women, regulations to reduce the use of sterilizations, less invasive breast cancer treatment, and the Women's Health Initiative at NIH (Norsigian, 1996). *De Madres a Madres* is a Houston-based women's political action group that works for early prenatal care for Hispanic women (McFarlane, Kelly, Rodriguez, & Fehir, 1994). The coalition built partnerships with business, health, social service, religious, and school organizations to use feminist theory and principles to increase the voice of all women in the community. In New Jersey, the Manavi organization advocates on behalf of South Asian women (those from the Indian subcontinent) who are victims of violence, provides a rent-free Ashiana (transitional home) where women can stay for up to 18 months, brochures in three languages, and other bibliographic resources (Almeida et al., 1999). In New Zealand, women and consumers worked together to successfully pass an act of Parliament to create independent practice for midwives in 1990 after midwifery had nearly disappeared from the practice arena (Fleming, 1996).

Conflict Resolution

The traditional legal way to resolve conflict is for two parties to challenge each other in court as adversaries, to elect leaders to governmental bodies in a win-lose framework, or to lobby for changes sought with the strongest lobbyist winning the contest. FJ seeks the solution to problems by considering the relationship among people and things, rather than opposition between them, and, like TJ, seeks an adequate psychology for human behavior and motivation (Scales, 1986). This means that the subjective component (unconscious processes) is examined in FJ and TJ more than in traditional legal methods. For example, FJ examines the inherent biases of judges or legislators and the policies created by them and then makes these biases visible. With TJ, "legal rules, legal procedures, and the roles of legal actors (such as lawyers and judges) constitute social forces that, *whether intended or not*, often produce therapeutic or anti-therapeutic consequences" (Winick, 1996, p. 646, emphasis added). A relevant point of analysis, therefore, is whether the policy in reality maintains the power imbalance between men and women despite intentions to the contrary.

Alternative dispute resolution has been used as an alternative to an adversarial system that considers itself objective and blind to gender. Mediation and arbitration are forms of alternative dispute resolution that have been recommended to promote flexible solutions to problems that affect parties and nonparties who are involved in the dispute (Menkel-Meadow, 1997). Rather than the acrimonious battles in court or in legislative committee hearing rooms, agreement is reached by consensus of the parties without public spectacle and with face-to-face discussion in the presence of a neutral third party who helps the parties create collaborative solutions. Menkel-Meadow (1998), who served as an arbitrator in some of the Dalkon Shield cases, says that face-to-face discussion with the decision maker and the ability to express one's own version of the claims creates a sense of fairness among the participants. New forms of conflict resolution that address needs of women will improve the confidence women feel in the legal system and provide the voice they need to improve their influence on the law. In this sense, women are empowered to see their values become policy for themselves, their families, and society.

CONCLUSION

Ideals of the law guided by ethical principles do not always appear in practice. As Stern (1993) so eloquently points out, the law may be followed to the letter without considering that certain behaviors (breaking parole rules) are evidence of illness. The tension between "oughts" and "shalls" drives policy development and

provides balance between conservative and extremist views. However, the law as written is only as strong as the law as practiced. Strategies directed at the individual level such as lawsuits against rapists or those directed by organizations against a group or a government cause ripple effects in a sexist society. Changes toward equality are evolving slowly. Documentation of the effects of these policy changes will give birth to the next generation of laws that hopefully will be more supportive of women than has been true in the past.

Jurisprudential scholarship questions the assumptions behind seemingly gender-neutral policies. For instance, as Stefan (1993, p. 814) points out, "competence doctrine assumes unconstrained autonomy on the part of atomized individuals acting in a social vacuum." Competency is a key requirement for consent to treatment, sexual relationships, divorce, adoption of a child, and other matters affecting women's health. FJ, therefore, provides the theory to change practice by challenging law that thwarts women's voices. Research approaches must be adequate to capture women's experiences. Examination of the effects of law on the health of women using the TJ and FJ models has and will continue to inform women and lawmakers of paths that can be taken to improve health and achieve justice.

REFERENCES

Aiken, T. (1994). *Legal, ethical, and political issues in nursing.* Philadelphia: F. A. Davis.

Almeida, R., Gujavarty, S., Scott, S., & Williams, A. (1999). Advocating for victims of domestic violence. *Women's Rights Law Reporter, 20*(2/3), 73–84.

Caplow, S. (1999). Still in the dark: Disappointing images of women lawyers in the movies. *Women's Rights Law Reporter, 20*(2/3), 55–71.

Charo, R. A. (1997). The interaction between family planning policies and the introduction of new reproductive technologies. In K. Petersen (Ed.), *Intersections: Women on law, medicine and technology* (pp. 73–97). Hants, England: Ashgate.

Cook, R. J. (1994). *Women's health and human rights.* Geneva, Switzerland: World Health Organization.

Covan, E. K. (1997). Cultural priorities and elder care: The impact on women. *Health Care for Women International, 18*(4), 329–342.

Cruver-Smith, D. (1998). Protecting public breast-feeding in theory but not in practice. *Women's Rights Law Reporter, 19*, 167–180.

Daigle, L. E. (1998). Empowering women to protect: Improving intervention with victims of domestic violence in cases of child abuse and neglect: A study of Travis County, Texas. *Texas Journal of Women and Law, 7*, 278–317.

De Ville, K. A., & Kopelman, L. M. (1999). Fetal protection in Wisconsin's revised child abuse law: Right goal, wrong remedy. *Journal of Law, Medicine & Ethics, 27*(4), 332–342.

Dickersin, K., & Schnaper, L. (1996). Reinventing medical research. In K. L. Moss (Ed.), *Man-made medicine: Women's health, public policy, and reform* (pp. 57–76). Durham, NC: Duke University Press.

Fleming, V.E.M. (1996). Midwifery in New Zealand: Responding to changing times. *Health Care for Women International, 17*(4), 343–359.

Hagell, E. I. (1993). Reproductive technologies and court-ordered obstetrical interventions: The need for a feminist voice in nursing. *Health Care for Women International, 14*(1), 77–86.

Johnson v. State, 602 So. 2d 1288 (Fla. 1992). Florida was the first state to successfully prosecute a woman for drug use during pregnancy, but the Florida Supreme Court ultimately reversed the conviction of Jennifer Johnson for delivering a controlled substance to her child via the umbilical cord.

Krieger, N., & Fee, E. (1996). Man-made medicine and women's health: The biopolitics of sex/gender and race/ethnicity. In K. L. Moss (Ed.), *Man-made medicine: Women's health, public policy, and reform* (pp. 15–35). Durham, NC: Duke University Press.

LaFond, J. Q. (1999). Can therapeutic jurisprudence be normatively neutral? Sexual predator laws: Their impact on participants and policy. *Arizona Law Review, 41,* 375–415.

Legal Momentum. (2000). Women's enews up, live and online. *In Brief,* p. 7.

Leo, J. (1999). Gender test at MIT. *U.S. News & World Report, 127*(24), 14.

Malterud, K. M. (1993). Strategies for empowering women's voices in the medical culture. *Health Care for Women International, 14*(4), 365–373.

Marshall, M. F. (1999). Commentary: Mal-intentioned illiteracy, willful ignorance, and fetal protection laws: Is there a lexicologist in the house? *Journal of Law, Medicine & Ethics, 27*(4), 343–346.

Mastroianni, A. C., Faden, R., & Federman, D. (Eds.). (1994). *Women and health research: Ethical and legal issues of including women in clinical studies: Vol. 1.* Washington, DC: National Academy Press.

Matthews, D. M. (1998). Avoiding gender equality. *Women's Rights Law Reporter, 19,* 127–154.

McConnell, J. E. (1996). For women's health: Uncoupling health care reform from tort reform. In K. L. Moss (Ed.), *Man-made medicine: Women's health, public policy, and reform* (pp. 99–121). Durham, NC: Duke University Press.

McFarlane, J., Kelly, E., Rodriguez, R., & Fehir, J. (1994). *De Madres a Madres:* Women building community coalitions for health. *Health Care for Women International, 15*(5), 465–476.

McMurray, A. (1997). Violence against ex-wives: Anger and advocacy. *Health Care for Women International, 18*(6), 543–556.

Menkel-Meadow, C. (1997). When dispute resolution begets disputes of it own: Conflicts among dispute professionals. *UCLA Law Review, 44*(6), 1871–1933.

Menkel-Meadow, C. (1998). Taking the mass out of mass torts: Reflections of a Dalkon Shield arbitrator on alternative dispute resolution, judging, neutrality, gender, and process. *Loyola Law Review, 31,* 513–548.

Merritt-Gray, M., & Wuest, J. (1995). Counteracting abuse and breaking free: The process of leaving revealed through women's voices. *Health Care for Women International, 16*(5), 399–412.

Minow, M. (1990). *Making all the difference: Inclusion, exclusion, and American law.* Ithaca, NY: Cornell University Press.

Mississippi University for Women v. Hogan, 458 U.S. 718 (1982).

Moss, K. L. (Ed.). (1996). *Man-made medicine: Women's health, public policy, and reform.* Durham, NC: Duke University Press.

National Institutes of Health. (1994). NIH guidelines on the inclusion of women and minorities as subjects in clinical research. *Federal Register, 59,* 14508–14513.

National Organization for Women Legal Defense and Education Fund (NOWLDEF). (1999–2000). Women, policy and media: News that women want and need. *In Brief,* 1–8.

Norsigian, J. (1996). The women's health movement in the United States. In K. L. Moss (Ed.), *Man-made medicine: Women's*

health, public policy, and reform (pp. 79–97). Durham, NC: Duke University Press.

Roe v. Wade, 410 U.S. 113, 93 S.Ct. 756, 35 L.Ed.2d 147 (1973).

Rozovsky, F. A. (1999). *Consent to treatment: A practical guide* (2nd ed., cumulative supplement). Gaithersburg, MD: Aspen.

Scales, A. C. (1986). The emergence of feminist jurisprudence: An essay. *Yale Law Journal, 95*(7), 1373–1403.

Scales, A. (1996). Abortion, law, and public health. In K. L. Moss (Ed.), *Man-made medicine: Women's health, public policy, and reform* (pp. 219–248). Durham, NC: Duke University Press.

Sheldon, S., & Thomson, M. (Eds.). (1998). *Feminist perspectives on health care law.* London: Cavendish.

Siegel, R. M., Hill, T. D., Henderson, V. A., Ernst, H. M., & Boat, B. W. (1999). Screening for domestic violence in the community pediatric setting. *Pediatrics, 140,* 874–877.

Stefan, S. (1993). Silencing the different voice: Competence, feminist theory and law. *University of Miami Law Review, 47,* 763–815.

Stefan, S. (1996). Reforming the provision of mental health treatment. In K. L. Moss (Ed.), *Man-made medicine: Women's health, public policy, and reform* (pp. 195–218). Durham, NC: Duke University Press.

Stern, P. N. (1993). It's the law. *Health Care for Women International, 14*(2), v–vii.

Taggert, L., & Mattson, S. (1996). Delay in prenatal care as a result of battering in pregnancy: Cross-cultural implications. *Health Care for Women International, 17*(1), 25–34.

Teare, C., & English, A. (1996). Women, girls, and the HIV epidemic. In K. L. Moss, (Ed.), *Man-made medicine: Women's health, public policy, and reform* (pp. 123–160). Durham, NC: Duke University Press.

Thorne, S., McCormick, J., & Carty, E. (1997). Deconstructing the gender neutrality of chronic illness and disability. *Health Care for Women International, 18*(1), 1–16.

Unborn Child of Starks v. Oklahoma, 18 P. 3d. 342, 2001 OK 6 (2001).

U.S. v. Morrison, 29 U.S. 598, 120 S.Ct. 1740 (2000).

Veatch, R. M. (1986). *The foundations of justice: Why the retarded and the rest of us have claims to equality.* New York: Oxford University Press.

Violence Against Women Act. (1994). 42 U.S.C. Sec. 13931.

Warner, C. (1992). *Treasury of women's quotations.* Englewood Cliffs, NJ: Prentice-Hall.

Warren, J. (1995, May 11). Panel kills bill on breast-feeding assembly: Republicans block effort to grant women the explicit right to nurse in public. *Los Angeles Times,* A3, A30.

Weijer, C., & Crouch, R. A. (1999). Why should we include women and minorities in randomized controlled trials? *Journal of Clinical Ethics, 10*(2), 100–106.

Wexler, D. B. (2000). *International network on therapeutic jurisprudence.* http://www.law.arizona.edu/upr-intj-welcome.html

Wexler, D. B., & Winick, B. J. (Eds.). (1996). *Law in a therapeutic key.* Durham, NC: Carolina Academic Press.

Whitner v. State, 492 S.E.2d 777 (S.C. 1997), cert. denied, 118 S. Ct. 1857 (1998). South Carolina is the only state to uphold a criminal conviction of a substance-abusing mother.

Winick, B. J. (1996). The jurisprudence of therapeutic jurisprudence. In D. B. Wexler & B. J. Winick (Eds.), *Law in a therapeutic key* (pp. 645–668). Durham, NC: Carolina Academic Press.

Wishik, H. (1985). To question everything: The inquiries of feminist jurisprudence. *Berkeley Women's Law Journal, 1*(1), 64–77.

Wuest, J. (1993). Institutionalizing women's oppression: The inherent risk in health policy that fosters community participation. *Health Care for Women International, 14*(5), 407–417.

PART III

Health
Promotion

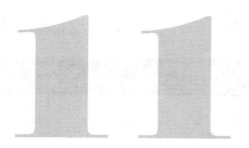

Healthy Practices: Nutrition

Betty Lucas

Until recently, women's health and subsequent nutrition implications revolved around the reproductive system. Now more research and clinical efforts address a broad spectrum of women's health concerns, especially those unique to or more prevalent in women. With increased life expectancy, women in the United States can have 35 to 40 additional years after childbearing years cease. Those later years can be productive, healthy, and mobile if acute or chronic diseases are prevented or well managed. Although genetic phenotypes are now more widely described relative to disease susceptibility, environment and lifestyle choices can have a significant role in controlling or modifying the course of diseases. Of the 10 leading causes of death in women, nutrition is involved in the etiology or treatment of 5 of them—heart disease, cancer, stroke, diabetes, and kidney disease (Centers for Disease Control and Prevention, 2002). This chapter focuses on the contributions of diet and nutrition to the developmental and reproductive process and to the prevention and management of selected diseases and conditions in women.

THE NUTRIENTS—A BRIEF REVIEW

Survival requires not only oxygen and water but food as well. Food provides the energy needed for life-sustaining processes, and it also contains the materials to build and maintain all body cells. These materials are referred to as nutrients; each plays a role in ensuring that the biochemical machinery of the human body runs smoothly.

Nutrients are classified into six categories: carbohydrates, lipids, proteins, vitamins, minerals, and water (see Table 11.1). Carbohydrates, lipids, and protein all produce energy and are called macronutrients; vitamins and minerals are micronutrients. Their basic features include:

Carbohydrates—contain carbon, hydrogen, and oxygen combined in small molecules called sugars and large molecules represented mainly by starch.

Lipids (fats and oils)—contain carbon, hydrogen, and oxygen-like carbohydrates, but the amount of oxygen is much less. Triglyceride is the main form of food fat.

Proteins—contain carbon, hydrogen, nitrogen, oxygen, and sometimes sulfur atoms, arranged in small compounds called amino acids. Chains of amino acids make up dietary proteins.

Vitamins—organic compounds that serve to catalyze or support a number of biochemical reactions in the body.

Minerals—inorganic compounds that play important roles in metabolic reactions and serve as structural compounds of body tissue, such as bone.

Water—vital to the body as a solvent and lubricant and as a medium for transporting nutrients and waste.

To determine standards for dietary adequacy for individuals of various age and sex, the Food and Nutrition Board of the Institute of Medicine regularly publishes updates of the recommended dietary allowances (RDAs) based on current research. Although the RDAs were designed for population groups with

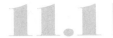

| Essential Nutrients in the Human Diet | | | | | | |

CARBOHY-DRATE	FAT (LIPID)	PROTEIN (AMINO ACIDS)	VITAMINS	MINERALS		WATER
Glucose (or a carbohydrate that yields glucose)	Linoleic acid (omega-6) Linolenic acid (omega-3)	Histidine Isoleucine Leucine Lysine Methionine Phenylalanine Threonine Tryptophan Valine	A C D E K Thiamin Riboflavin Niacin Pantothenic acid Biotin B-6 B-12 Folate	Arsenic Boron Calcium Chloride Chromium Copper Cobalt Fluoride Iron Magnesium	Manganese Molybdenum Nickel Phosphorus Potassium Selenium Silicon Sodium Sulfur Zinc	Water

the goal of preventing nutritional deficiencies, more recent concern has focused on preventing chronic diseases. The newer dietary reference intakes (DRIs) include both RDAs and adequate intakes (AIs) as guides for determining dietary adequacy, as well as tolerable upper intake levels (ULs) (Barr, Murphy, & Poos, 2002; Otten, Hellwig, & Meyers, 2006). See Table 11.2 for the RDAs and AIs of nutrients for females

Supplements

Almost three-quarters of U.S. noninstitutionalized adults take a dietary supplement regularly, about 85% being a multivitamin/multimineral supplement (Timbo, Ross, McCarthy, & Lin, 2006). Older persons and women tend to use more supplements than younger people and men. There has also been a dramatic increase in the use of herbs, botanicals, and single-ingredient vitamin/mineral supplements, particularly among those with chronic conditions. These supplements commonly are used with allopathic therapy and/or prescription medications. There can be negative interactions between supplements and some medications. Supplements plus dietary sources of nutrients can provide levels that exceed the UL and have risk of negative consequences. Nurses and other health care professionals should screen women for use of dietary supplements and other complementary and alternative therapies, assess any risks, and provide appropriate counseling regarding supplement safety and effectiveness. The National Institutes of Health Office

of Dietary Supplements (2007) provides resources for professionals and consumers.

NUTRITIONAL NEEDS THROUGHOUT THE LIFE CYCLE

Infancy and Childhood

The quality and quantity of children's diets are the most constant environmental factors affecting growth and development. Food, feeding, and the satiation of hunger are also important contributors to parent-infant bonding, parent-child interactions, and the child's ability to attend to her environment and learn. Feeding progresses from the newborn's total dependence on breast milk or formula to the preschool girl, who can feed herself, use utensils, make food choices, and communicate clearly regarding hunger and satiety. Food habits developed in childhood may have far-reaching effects on adult nutritional status and eating patterns. Excess weight gain in childhood or adolescence will increase the risk of adult obesity and its related diseases; inadequate calcium intake in the growing years will result in reduced bone density in adulthood. Malnutrition in the prenatal period or in the early years can negatively impact developmental and reproductive abilities later, even in subsequent generations.

Although small body composition differences are seen in boys and girls from about age 6, the nutritional needs do not differ by sex until puberty. The national

11.2 | Dietary Reference Intakes: Recommended Dietary Allowances and Adequate Intakes for Women

	AGES 14–18	AGES 19–30	AGES 31–50	AGES 51–69	AGES 70 AND OLDER	PREGNANT	LACTATING
Energy (kcal)	2,368	2,403[a]	2,326[a]	2,193[a]	2,060[a]	(14–18 years) (19 years and older) 2,368 (lst trimester) 2,403[a] 2,708 (2nd trimester) 2,743[a] 2,820 (3rd trimester) 2,855[a]	(14–18 years) (19 years) 2,698 (lst 6 months) 2,733[a] 2,768 (2nd 6 months) 2,803[a]
Protein (g)	46	46	46	46	46	71	71
Vitamin A (ug RE)	700	700	700	700	700	770 750 (<18 yrs)	1,300 1,200 (<18 yrs)
Vitamin D (ug)	5	5	5	10	15	5	5
Vitamin E (mg a-TE)	15	15	15	15	15	15	19
Vitamin K (ug)	75	90	90	90	90	90 75 (<18 yrs)	90 75 (<18 yrs)
Vitamin C (mg)	65	75	75	75	75	85 80 (<18 yrs)	120 115 (<18 yrs)
Thiamin (mg)	1.0	1.1	1.1	1.1	1.1	1.4	1.4
Riboflavin (mg)	1.0	1.1	1.1	1.1	1.1	1.4	1.6
Niacin (mg NE)	14	14	14	14	14	18	17
Vitamin B_6 (ug)	1.2	1.3	1.3	1.5	1.5	1.9	2.0
Folate (ug)	400	400	400	400	400	600	500
Vitamin B_{12} (ug)	2.4	2.4	2.4	2.4	2.4	2.6	2.8
Biotin (ug)	25	30	30	30	30	30	35
Pantothenic acid (mg)	5	5	5	5	5	6	7
Choline (mg)	400	425	425	425	425	450	550
Chromium (ug)	24	25	25	20	20	30 29 (18 years and younger)	45 44 (18 years and younger)
Calcium (mg)	1,300	1,000	1,000	1,200	1,200	1,000 1,300 (18 years and younger)	1,000 1,300 (18 years and younger)
Copper (ug)	890	900	900	900	900	1,000	1,300
Phosphorus (mg)	1,250	700	700	700	700	700 1,250 (18 years and younger)	700 1,250 (<18 yrs.)
Magnesium (mg)	360	310	320	320	320	400 (18 years and younger) 350 (19–30 years) 360 (31–50 years)	360 (18 years and younger) 310 (19–30 years) 320 (31–50 years)
Manganese (mg)	1.6	1.8	1.8	1.8	1.8	2	2.6

(continued)

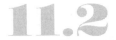

11.2 | Dietary Reference Intakes: Recommended Dietary Allowances and Adequate Intakes for Women (*continued*)

	AGES 14–18	AGES 19–30	AGES 31–50	AGES 51–69	AGES 70 AND OLDER	PREGNANT	LACTATING
Molybdenum (ug)	43	45	45	45	45	50	50
Fluoride (mg)	3	3	3	3	3	3	3
Iron (mg)	15	18	18	8	8	27	9 10 (18 years and younger)
Zinc (mg)	9	8	8	8	8	11 12 (18 years and younger)	12 13 (18 years and younger)
Iodine (ug)	150	150	150	150	150	220	290
Selenium (ug)	55	55	55	55	55	60	70
Fiber (g)	26	25	25	21	21	28	29

Note. From *Dietary Reference Intakes: The Essential Guide to Nutrient Requirements,* by J. Otten, J. Hellwig, and L. Meyers (Eds.), 2006, Washington, DC: Institute of Medicine, National Academies Press.
ª Subtract 7 kcal per day for women for each year of age above 19 years.

DRIs are delineated by sex from 9 years of age (Otten et al., 2006).

Adolescence

Adolescence is one of the most dynamic periods in human development, with pubertal changes beginning between ages 9 to 11 in girls. The rapid velocity of physical growth and the development of secondary sexual characteristics increase the demand for energy and other nutrients. At the same time, tremendous social, cognitive, and emotional growth occurs. There is increased nutritional vulnerability in the teenage years due to the high nutrient demand, which is impacted by lifestyle and food habits, possible use of alcohol and drugs, and special situations such as pregnancy, sports, and excessive dieting or eating disorders.

Changes in body composition are likely a trigger for the initiation of puberty and menarche. Girls have about 19% body fat prepubertally, and 22% to 26% body fat as young adults. Because these changes can occur at different ages in girls, using age as an indicator of nutrient needs is limiting. The use of sexual maturity ratings, often called Tanner stages, is more appropriate in determining energy and nutrient needs. These ratings are based on the assessment of secondary sexual characteristics from 1 (prepubertal) to 5 (adult) (Spear, 2004).

Developing an adult body image is an emotional and cognitive task of adolescent girls that has nutritional implications. Their appropriately maturing bodies with increased body fat are in direct contrast to today's culture of excessive thinness, reinforced by the popular media, fashion, and emphasis on dieting. It is no wonder that teenage girls are very dissatisfied with their bodies, frequently attempt weight loss diets, and are vulnerable for developing eating disorders (Spear, 2004). Those who diet to lose weight are more likely to have poorer nutrient intake than those who don't (Story, Neumark-Sztainer, Sherwood, Stang, & Murray, 1998).

Nutritional Needs

Energy needs in adolescent girls are determined by rate of growth, stage of maturation, and physical activity. This individual variability is shown in the DRIs for energy for healthy, moderately active girls: 2,071 kcal/day (11 years old); 2,368 kcal/day (16 years old), and 2,403 kcal/day (19 years old). Protein needs parallel the growth rate; the typical diet in the United States provides more protein than needed. Protein intake becomes a concern only when the energy intake is so low that dietary protein is used for energy needs instead of synthesis of new tissue and tissue repair.

Some of the micronutrients (vitamins and minerals) are more marginal in the diets of teenage girls. Because inadequate consumption of fruits and vegetables is linked with certain cancers and other diseases, national recommendations are to eat five or more servings of fruits and vegetables daily. A recent national survey, however, revealed that fruit and vegetable intake is the most insufficient, with about 25% of girls age 9 to 18 years eating the recommended five servings per day (Guenther, Dodd, Reedy, & Krebs-Smith, 2006).

Calcium needs are highest during puberty and adolescence than any other time, with 45% of the adult skeletal mass added during this time. Since the greatest retention of calcium as bone mass occurs in the early to middle period of adolescence, the recommended adequate intake is 1,300 mg for all adolescents age 9 to 18 years. By comparison, less than 20% of adolescent girls consume that amount (Larson, Story, Wall, & Neumark-Sztainer, 2006). Increasing soft drink consumption also has a negative effect on calcium status for this age group, because sodas frequently replace milk. Because sodas have a high phosphorus content, a low calcium-to-phosphorus ratio can be an added impact on bone by causing bone mineral loss. Thus, the stage is set early in life for bone health and risk for osteoporosis in later years.

Iron requirements are high in adolescent girls because of the increased muscle mass and blood volume, as well as the iron losses that occur with menses. National studies have noted that iron consumption is often less than the RDA in this population (Lytle et al., 2002). Although the incidence of iron deficiency anemia is low, the problem of low iron stores is common.

The needs for vitamins and other minerals increase in adolescence, but can be met by a well-chosen diet. Risk for marginal or inadequate intakes increases with omission of fruits and vegetables, cigarette use, eating disorders, chronic diseases, and fad diets.

Teenagers tend to have irregular and somewhat chaotic eating patterns, in part because of school and work schedules, sports and activities, and peer relationships. Breakfast and lunch are skipped frequently by girls, but snacking may contribute substantial energy (and variable nutrients) to their intake. Fast food restaurants are a common eating place because they are quick, inexpensive, a place to meet friends, and frequent employers of teenagers.

Young Adulthood

The young adult or childbearing years are a time when women create and establish careers, have babies and nurture families, actively participate in their communities, and attempt to balance it all. Nutrient needs are less than in the growing years, yet a variety of factors make achievement of optimal nutrition a challenge for many. These factors include delay in marriage and children and the continuance of the single lifestyle with frequent eating irregularities and poor intake; stressful work and family schedules that leave little time and energy for food shopping and meal preparation; single motherhood (which constitutes the majority of women on welfare, who have limited food resources); and the increasing lack of basic food knowledge and cooking skills among many young women.

Diet and nutrition theories and interventions have been proposed over the years for women with premenstrual syndrome (PMS), even though there is no evidence that poor diet or nutrient deficiencies are linked to the disorder. A variety of dietary, medication, and herbal treatments are popular despite lack of research to support these interventions. There is a high placebo response rate to many of these treatments. Some evidence exists that high dietary intakes of calcium and vitamin D are correlated with lower incidence of PMS (Bertone-Johnson et al., 2005). A Cochrane Library evidence-based review found no support for many common therapeutic treatments for PMS, including vitamin B_6 (Douglas, 2002). High doses of vitamin B_6 taken over a long period of time can cause neurological symptoms. Some women who experience PMS symptoms report higher intakes (i.e., cravings) of sugar, refined carbohydrates, and sodium than those without PMS (Cross, Marley, Miles, & Willson, 2001). Management of the symptoms certainly should include a healthy diet with complex carbohydrates, regular exercise, and stress reduction techniques.

Although routine vitamin/mineral supplementation has not been indicated in healthy young adult women, this has recently changed regarding folic acid. Randomized trials have demonstrated the role of folic acid in the prevention of neural tube defects, such as spina bifida and anencephaly. Studies have shown that the optimal red cell folate levels for preventing neural tube defects (906 mmol/L) are achieved from folic acid supplementation, not from diet alone (Shabert, 2004). Because the neural tube closes by 28 days of gestation (before most women realize they are pregnant), the folic acid is needed preconceptually. Therefore, the Centers for Disease Control and Prevention (1992) have recommended that all women of childbearing years increase their intake of folic acid. One public health measure to address this was the implementation in 1998 of the addition of folic acid to products made with enriched flour or grain products, such as bread, rice, and pasta. In addition to good dietary sources of folic acid (dark green leafy vegetables, legumes, enriched cereals and grains, orange juice, soy, wheat germ, and almonds and peanuts), women planning a pregnancy should begin folic acid supplementation of 400 mcg per day (Centers for Disease Control and Prevention, 1992).

Perimenopause/Menopause

The decrease of estrogen production in the natural process of menopause results not only in physical symptoms, but also in physiological changes that affect nutritional needs. Bone health is altered as less estrogen is available to trigger bone remodeling in response to bone resorption. As bone mass decreases, the risk of osteoporosis increases. However, optimal prevention in the early decades (adequate calcium intake, weight-bearing activity) will ensure optimal bone density at menopause. Reduced estrogen levels also affect blood lipids, resulting in higher total cholesterol and low-density lipoprotein (LDL) cholesterol levels, and lower high-density lipoprotein (HDL) levels—all negatively impacting cardiovascular health.

Recent interest and research has centered on phytochemicals found in plant-based foods such as fruits, vegetables, whole grains, legumes, nuts, seeds, and herbs. Phytochemicals are not micronutrients such as vitamins and minerals, but are naturally occurring, biologically active, chemical components of plant foods. They are being studied for the prevention or treatment of chronic diseases, such as cardiovascular disease and cancers. Phytochemicals include carotenoids, lycopene, flavonoids, isoflavones, thiols, and lignans. Phytoestrogens, such as isoflavones and genistein (found in soy), are phytochemicals that have weak, nonsteroidal estrogen effects when bound to estrogen receptor sites.

Isoflavones in soy have been suggested to decrease the frequency of hot flashes in menopausal women. A review and meta-analysis of randomized, controlled studies, however, showed that isoflavones had a modest or inconsistent impact on hot flashes (Nelson et al., 2006). With reduced use of hormone replacement in postmenopausal women, there has been increased interest and studies on soy isoflavones and bone health, including bone density, risk of fractures, and bone for-

mation. The studies have had inconsistent results, but federally funded, long-term intervention trials are underway. The quantity of soy needed to show results is more than typically consumed in the United States. To make an impact on the general population, education efforts would be necessary to increase the familiarity and intake of soybeans and their products.

The Older Woman

As the numbers of people 65 years and older continues to increase, there is more interest in the health and nutritional needs of this population. With the natural aging process, however, many physiological and psychosocial changes can alter appetite, digestion, absorption, nutrient requirements, and functional skills needed for food acquisition and preparation (see Table 11.3). As women get older, there is increased prevalence of chronic diseases such as heart disease, hypertension, diabetes, and cancer. These conditions may require an additional modified diet or changes in eating patterns that can be particularly challenging to this population.

Energy requirements decrease with age due to reduced basal metabolic rate and physical activity. Weight gain and increase in body fat can occur with a decreasing dietary intake. Despite a lower energy intake, requirements for protein, vitamins, and minerals do not decline,

11.3 | Factors Affecting Nutritional Status in Elderly Women

ALTERED STATUS	POSSIBLE CONSEQUENCES
Decreased lean body mass	Decreased basal metabolic rate, strength, activity
Increased body fat (especially abdominal)	Cardiovascular disease
Gastric hypochlorhydria	Decreased nutrient absorption
Xerostomia (dry mouth)	Chewing and swallowing problems, food avoidance
Reduced production of provitamin D by skin	Osteoporosis, vitamin D deficiency
Decreased glucose tolerance	Non–insulin-dependent diabetes
Diminished lactase secretion	Gastrointestinal distress, lactose intolerance
Increase in total and LDL cholesterol	Cardiovascular disease
Increased blood pressure	Cardiovascular disease, stroke
Reduced sense of taste (dysgeusia)	Reduced appetite and sensory stimulation
Reduced sense of smell (hyposmia)	Reduced appetite and sensory stimulation
Constipation	Inadequate intake of food and fluids
Depression	Poor appetite and intake
Social isolation or loss	Poor appetite, limited intake
Loss of independence and mobility	Limited food access and ability to prepare food
Reduced finances	Decreased food choices; limited intake

and some increase. Anorexia secondary to physiological and psychosocial changes can result in underweight (and higher mortality risk), dehydration, and likelihood of protein-energy malnutrition (American Dietetic Association, 2005a). Dietary protein needs may increase in the elderly as a result of diminished protein stores in the declining muscle mass, as well as altered gastrointestinal function and the presence of acute and chronic diseases. Low serum albumin levels have been correlated with the onset of pressure ulcers in nursing home residents (American Dietetic Association, 2005a). Although the RDA for protein for all adults is 0.8 gm/kg body weight, some evidence indicates that 1.0–1.3 gm/kg may better maintain positive nitrogen balance in the elderly (Morais, Chevalier, & Gougeon, 2006).

National surveys of food consumption and nutritional status indicate that elderly in the United States are at nutritional risk. With decreased mean energy intakes, nutrients at greatest risk are calcium, riboflavin, folate, vitamin B_{12}, vitamin B_6, iron, and zinc (American Dietetic Association, 2005a). One nutrient with an increased recommended intake for those over 70 years of age is vitamin D (see Table 11.2). Vitamin D is needed for absorption of calcium and

phosphorus into bone. In addition to possible limited dietary intake, active vitamin D may be reduced in elderly women due to decreased sunlight exposure (especially for the homebound and those in institutions), and diminished conversion of precursors in the liver and kidney. Older adults produce about one-fourth the vitamin D in the skin compared to young adults. Supplementation of vitamin D should be considered for those at risk—for example, women in long-term care facilities. Although providing moderate calcium and vitamin D supplements to healthy elderly has been common practice, other nutrients are also important to improve bone health, including protein, vitamins A and K, magnesium, and phytoestrogens (Kitchin & Morgan, 2003).

Because the nutritional status of otherwise healthy older adults can deteriorate without much notice, the American Dietetic Association, the American Academy of Family Physicians, and the National Council on Aging developed the Nutrition Screening Initiative for older adults who live independently. The simple screening tool evaluates risk factors such as body weight, living environment, eating habits, and functional status (see Exhibit 11.1). Based on the National Screening

EXHIBIT 11.1 CHECKLIST TO DETERMINE YOUR NUTRITIONAL HEALTH

The warning signs of poor nutritional health are often overlooked. To see whether you (or people you know) are at nutritional risk, take this simple quiz. Read the statement below and circle the number in the yes column for those that apply. To find your total nutritional score, add up all the numbers you circled.

	Yes
I have an illness or condition that made me change the kind and/or amount of food I eat.	2
I eat fewer than two meals per day.	3
I eat few fruits, vegetables, or milk products.	2
I have three or more drinks of beer, liquor, or wine almost every day.	2
I have tooth or mouth problems that make it hard for me to eat.	2
I don't always have enough money to buy the food I need.	4
I eat alone most of the time.	1
I take three or more different prescribed or over-the-counter drugs a day.	1
Without wanting to, I have lost or gained 10 pounds in the past 6 months.	2
I am not always physically able to shop, cook, and/or feed myself.	2

Total nutritional score: _____

If your total nutritional score is

0 to 2: Good! Recheck your nutritional score in 6 months.

3 to 5: You are at moderate nutritional risk. See what can be done to improve your eating habits and lifestyle. A local office on aging, senior nutrition program, senior citizens center, or health department can help. Recheck your nutritional score in 3 months.

6 or more: You are at high nutritional risk. Bring this checklist next time you see your doctor, dietitian, or other qualified health or social service professional. Talk with them about any problems you have experienced. Ask for nutritional counseling.

Note. Reprinted with permission of the Nutrition Screening Initiative, a project of the American Academy of Family Physicians, the American Dietetic Association, and the National Council on the Aging, Inc., and funded in part by a grant from Ross Products Division, Abbott Laboratories Inc.

Initiative, a more thorough nutritional assessment can be completed, followed by appropriate intervention. This kind of early detection and prevention can help keep elderly women healthy and avoid hospitalizations and disease.

PREGNANCY

Although numerous factors influence the progress and outcome of pregnancy, the nutritional status of the pregnant woman is certainly a key contributor. The historical studies of food deprivation in Russia and the Netherlands during World War II showed significant decrease in fertility and increase in stillbirths, neonatal deaths, and low–birth weight infants (Shabert, 2004). Some low–birth weight infants are the result of intrauterine growth retardation—that is, the infant in utero experiences malnutrition due to a reduction in maternal nutrient supply or placental transport. Maternal malnutrition is a crucial factor in fetal growth.

The timing and duration of nutritional restriction are significant. During the embryonic stage of fetal development, cells differentiate into three germinal layers. Growth during this time occurs only by an increase in the number of cells. The fetal stage is the time of most rapid growth. During this time, growth is almost continuous and is accompanied by increase in cell size. Most organ cells continue to proliferate after birth. It is thought that growth in cell size begins at around 7 months' gestation and can continue for 3 years after birth. Given this sequence of growth, it is possible to suggest the effects malnutrition might have at different stages of gestation. During the embryonic phase, a severe limitation in nutrients could have teratogenic effects, causing malformation or death. Although malnutrition occurring after the third month of gestation would not generally have teratogenic effects, it could cause fetal growth retardation. During the last trimester, nutritional needs are at a peak as cells increase in both size and number. Poor nutrition in the latter stages of pregnancy affects fetal growth, whereas malnutrition in the early months affects embryonic development and survival.

The outcome of pregnancy is also influenced by the pregnant woman's own nutritional and growth history. Bigger women tend to have bigger babies who have less morbidity and mortality. Maternal size is believed to be a controlling factor on the ultimate size of the placenta, which in turn determines the amount of nutrition available to the fetus. Women who have lower prepregnant weights tend to have much lighter-weight placentas than women with higher prepregnant weights (Shabert, 2004). Preconceptional and periconceptional health care providers should assess the weight status of women who eventually plan to get pregnant.

Weight Gain During Pregnancy

The optimal weight gain in pregnancy follows a pattern of little gain in the first trimester, a rapid increase in the second, and slow gain in the third trimester. Most of the weight gain associated with the products of conception takes place in the second half of pregnancy, while maternal stores are laid down very rapidly before mid-pregnancy, then slow down and appear to stop before term. By the time of delivery, the weight gain can be accounted for in the fetus, placenta, amniotic fluid, maternal blood, maternal extracellular fluid, maternal breast and uterus, and maternal fat (see Table 11.4). The fat stores represent an emergency energy reserve to be drawn on in case of food deprivation during either pregnancy or lactation.

Monitoring weight gain during pregnancy serves to estimate the adequacy of pregnancy progress, including dietary sufficiency. Although historically weight gain in pregnancy was restricted even through the 1960s, the current recommendation for women of normal body weight for height is to gain 25 to 35 pounds. The Institute of Medicine in 1990 recommended guidelines for pregnancy weight gain for subgroups of American women (see Table 11.5). These groups include women who are underweight, overweight, short, and very young. The weight gain goals are based on prepregnancy body mass index (BMI), which is weight (in kilograms) divided by height (in meters squared). Weight gain charts based on these guidelines have been developed for clinical use so that patterns of weight gain can be monitored, but they are not based on longitudinal evaluation of a large group of women.

Women who enter pregnancy significantly under- or overweight are at risk for poor outcome. Deviations

11.4 | Estimated Components of Weight Gain During Pregnancy

WEIGHT COMPONENT	WEIGHT GAIN (IN POUNDS)
Infant at birth	7¾
Placenta	1½
Increased maternal blood volume	6
Increased maternal tissue fluid	3
Increased size of maternal uterus	2
Increased size of maternal breasts	3
Fluid to surround fetus in amniotic sac	2
Mother's fat stores	4¾
Total	30

11.5 | Recommended Total Weight Gain Ranges for Pregnant Women, by Prepregnancy Body Mass Index

WEIGHT-FOR-HEIGHT CATEGORY	RECOMMENDED TOTAL GAIN	
	Kilograms	Pounds
Low (BMI < 19.8)	12.5–18.0	28–40
Normal (BMI 19.8–26.0)	11.5–16.0	25–35
High (BMI 26–29)	7.0–11.5	15–25
BMI > 29	at least 7.0	15
Other		
Twin pregnancy	15.9–20.4	34–45
Triplet pregnancy	22.7 overall	50

Note. Body mass index is weight in kilograms divided by height in meters squared. From *Nutrition During Pregnancy: Weight Gain and Nutrient Supplements,* by Institute of Medicine, 1990, Washington, DC: National Academy Press; and "Position of the American Dietetic Association: Nutrition and Lifestyle for a Healthy Pregnancy Outcome," by the American Dietetic Association, 2002, *Journal of the American Dietetic Association, 102*(10), pp. 1479–1490.

in weight gain are common problems in obstetric practice. The following definitions have been suggested:

Underweight—prepregnant weight of 10% or more below standard weight for height and age.

Overweight—prepregnant weight of 20% or more above standard weight for height and age.

Extreme overweight (obese)—prepregnant weight of 35% or more above standard weight for height and age.

Inadequate gain—less than 2.2 pounds per month in second and/or third trimester,

Excessive gain—more than 7 pounds gained in 1 month,

Total weight gain of 15 to 25 pounds is recommended for overweight women (BMI of 26 to 29) to account for the weight of the fetus and the maternal support tissues. Obese women (BMI of 29 or greater) who become pregnant are at risk for hypertension, preeclampsia, gestational diabetes, and neural tube defects regardless of folic acid intake (American Dietetic Association, 2002a; Shabert, 2004). In a study of women with two consecutive pregnancies, those whose BMI increased at least three units between the first and second pregnancies were more likely to experience gestational diabetes, preeclampsia, hypertension, cesarean delivery, and large-for-gestational newborns (Villamor & Cnattiquis, 2006). The recommended target weight for obese women is at least 15 pounds. Energy restriction, even if adequate protein is provided, may result in use of protein for energy, making it unavailable for tissue growth and repair, and for fetal needs. In addition,

when maternal intake is severely restricted, maternal fat stores are catabolized to meet energy requirements, resulting in ketosis and ketonuria, which can cause neurological damage to the fetus. Pregnancy weight gain in overweight women should be monitored carefully and referral made to a nutrition professional for appropriate dietary management.

Underweight women who become pregnant may have inadequate stores to meet the increased nutritional demands. The additional metabolic needs of pregnancy, nausea and vomiting in early pregnancy, and the psychological adjustments to pregnancy may all compound the problem. The principal hazard is delivery of a low–birth weight infant. The underweight category also includes women who are disinterested in food and those who do not appreciate the link between food and health. Underweight women should be encouraged to gain to the recommended goals and referred to a nutritionist for nutrition education and diet recommendations.

There appears to be a relationship between excessive weight gain in pregnancy and subsequent obesity (Suitor, 1997). This is serious, given the increasing prevalence of obesity in the United States. Although many factors are involved in adult obesity, women who gain excessive weight in pregnancy and do not lose it afterward are likely contributing to the problem, especially in successive pregnancies. Misinterpreting "eating for two" as permission to overconsume is as misguided as restricting weight gain or following fad diets. Rather, a sound diet based on the food guide pyramid and limited in nutrient-poor calories is needed.

Energy

Since growth requires energy, additional energy above that required for maintenance is needed for pregnancy. Table 11.2 gives the recommended dietary allowances for energy that provide optimal weight gain at various stages; meet growth needs of the fetus, placenta, and other maternal tissues; and take care of the increased maternal basal metabolism. The DRI for pregnancy is an additional 340 kcal/day for the second trimester and an additional 452 kcal/day for the third trimester, but this will vary with the woman's level of physical activity during her pregnancy. As long as the rate and amount of weight gain is within acceptable limits, the range of energy intakes can be quite variable. More energy expenditure for movement is required with increasing body weight, but most pregnant women slow or decrease their activity as pregnancy progresses. Enough energy is needed to protect protein to be used for growth rather than energy expenditure. Caloric restrictions in animals and humans have demonstrated profound negative effects on maternal physiological adjustments and fetal growth and development.

Protein

Protein needs increase during pregnancy. Protein is essential for synthesis of hemoglobin and provides the nitrogen and amino acids essential for forming body tissue. The RDA for protein during pregnancy is 71 gm per day, higher than in previous recommendations. This level is 25 gm more than the RDA for nonpregnant women.

Vitamins

Folic Acid

Folic acid requirements increase during pregnancy because of augmented maternal erythropoiesis and fetal and placental growth. It is also an essential coenzyme in metabolism and in DNA synthesis. Folic acid deficiency results in megaloblastic anemia. Although it is not as common as iron deficiency anemia, megaloblastic anemia can occur in high-risk women, such as those of low socioeconomic status and those with a multiple pregnancy or chronic hemolytic anemia. It may not be diagnosed until the third trimester, but biochemical and morphological signs may be seen earlier. Maternal folic acid deficiency in animals is associated with congenital malformations; some evidence in humans suggests an association with pregnancy complications, but well-done studies have not been conducted (Tsunenobu & Picciano, 2006).

The current RDA for folate is 600 mcg for pregnancy, 200 mcg more than the recommendation for nonpregnant women (see Table 11.2). The Institute of Medicine also recommends that 400 mcg of folic acid per day be provided from fortified foods or supplements (Centers for Disease Control and Prevention, 1992) in addition to the folate from a healthy diet. The DRI established a tolerable upper intake level of 800 to 1,000 mcg per day from fortified foods and supplements.

The most significant influence of folic acid in pregnancy is its role in preventing neural tube defects. Randomized clinical trials of several thousand women in Europe in the late 1980s and early 1990s resulted in unequivocal results (Tsunenobu & Picciano, 2006). However, because the neural tube closes by day 28 of gestation, most women do not know they are pregnant, much less are taking prenatal supplements. Therefore, good dietary sources of folic acid and supplements are needed before and between conceptions.

Vitamin A

The RDA for vitamin A for pregnant women, 770 retinol equivalents, is slightly more than the nonpregnant level. The concern is that excessive intake of vitamin A can be teratogenic. Cases of adverse pregnancy outcome such as malformations have been associated with a daily ingestion of 25,000 IU (7,500 retinol equivalents) or more of vitamin A (Rosa, Wilk, & Kelsey, 1986). In addition, epidemiological evidence indicates that the drug isotretinoin (a vitamin A analogue used to treat cystic acne) causes major malformations involving craniofacial, central nervous system, cardiac, and thymic changes (Lammer et al., 1985). Some findings indicate that pregnant women who take vitamin A supplements at levels as low as 2.5 times the RDA increase the risk of delivering a baby with a cranial neural crest defect (Rothman et al., 1995). The Teratology Society (1987) urges that women in their reproductive years be informed that the excessive use of vitamin A shortly before and during pregnancy could be harmful to their babies. It also suggests that manufacturers of vitamin A–containing supplements should lower the maximum amount of vitamin A per unit dosage to 5,000 to 8,000 IU and identify the source of vitamin A. Beta-carotene, a precursor of vitamin A, is not associated with these pregnancy risks.

Minerals

Iron

Pregnancy imposes a severe burden on the maternal hematopoietic system. With the natural increase in maternal blood supply in pregnancy, total erythrocyte volume increases by 20% to 30%. Normal hematopoiesis requires a nutritionally adequate diet. To produce hemoglobin, there must be protein to provide essential amino acids and sufficient additional iron. Other vitamins and minerals—such as copper, zinc, folic acid, and vitamin B_{12}—are needed to serve as cofactors in synthesis of heme and globin. The limiting factor in this synthesis is usually the availability of iron.

The requirement for iron during pregnancy is less than 1 gm. Fetal needs are approximately 300 mg at term, and the iron in the placenta, umbilical cord, and maternal blood lost at delivery account for another 100 to 500 mg. The average healthy young American woman has approximately 300 mg of iron stores. A significant number of women, however, enter pregnancy with minimal iron stores due to menstrual blood loss, previous pregnancy, and/or poor dietary intake. Because of these factors plus the sizable demand for iron during pregnancy, it is currently recommended that all pregnant women take a low-level iron supplement, especially during the latter half of pregnancy. The Centers for Disease Control recommends a well-balanced diet plus a 30-mg supplement of ferrous iron, beginning with the first prenatal visit (Centers for Disease Control, 1998; American Dietetic Association, 2002a). For optimal absorption, the supplement should be taken between meals and not with milk, tea, or coffee.

Anemia is a relatively common complication of pregnancy, because the small amounts of usable dietary iron ingested combined with low iron storage cannot meet the increased need for iron. Anemia is defined as hemoglobin lower than 11 gm/100 ml during the first and third trimesters and less than 10.5 gm/100 ml during the second trimester. When anemia is diagnosed, supplemental iron should be given in therapeutic doses of a total of 60 to 120 mg per day, in divided doses, along with 300 ug folate daily (American Dietetic Association, 2002a). If anemia persists after treatment, inquiries should be made about compliance with the iron supplementation, and further laboratory evaluation should be done. If anemia is reversed, iron at the lower dose of 30 mg daily can be resumed. Excessive iron supplementation should be avoided due to associated gastrointestinal discomfort in some women, and the possibility that iron taken in high doses might inhibit zinc absorption.

Calcium

Calcium metabolism is altered in pregnancy due to the effect of maternal hormones, which result in increasing calcium retention. Calcium deposition in fetal bones and teeth occurs primarily in the third trimester; the newborn has accumulated approximately 25 grams of calcium. The current adequate intake for calcium during pregnancy (1,000 mg/day for adults and 1,300 mg/day for those younger than 19 years of age) is not an increase over the nonpregnant state because of the increased efficiency of absorption and utilization.

Although available data are insufficient to support routine calcium supplementation for the prevention of osteoporosis in younger women, prenatal nutrition counseling should address dietary strategies to meet calcium needs. Dairy products are an obvious major source of dietary calcium, but other food sources contribute, including calcium-fortified products such as juice and soy milk. In situations where dairy products are omitted or restricted in the diet (allergy, lactose intolerance, vegan), or where calcium intake is chronically low, calcium supplementation should be considered.

Calcium deficiency has been suggested as an etiology of pregnancy-induced hypertension for some time. Although evidence is inconclusive, those at risk for pregnancy-induced hypertension, including pregnant adolescents, might benefit from increased calcium intakes (Ritchie & King, 2000).

Sodium

Sodium restriction in the diet of pregnant women was standard practice for decades. It is now recognized, however, that healthy pregnant women retain salt normally, and moderate edema appears to be a normal consequence of pregnancy. The normal increased fluid retention increases the body's need for sodium.

A positive sodium balance occurs in normal pregnancy, resulting from significant changes in renal and hormonal function. The glomerular filtration rate increases by 50% in early pregnancy and remains elevated until late in the third trimester, filtering sodium into the renal tubules. Simultaneously, progesterone produces a salt-losing action in the kidneys, slowing absorption of filtered sodium through the tubules.

To prevent an electrolyte imbalance, the renin-angiotensin-aldosterone system acts as a compensatory mechanism in normal pregnancy. This counterbalances the salt-losing tendencies of progesterone and decreases urinary sodium excretion. The result is that sodium is conserved to meet the needs of the expanded tissue and fluid. Severe sodium restriction can stress the physiological mechanism of sodium conservation, resulting in hyponatremia. Moderation in sodium intake is appropriate for everyone, and during pregnancy should not be less than 2 to 3 g per day.

Zinc

Animal studies have shown that maternal zinc deficiency is associated with abnormal fetal development and prolonged labor. Clinical and epidemiological studies in pregnant women have been less clear. A study of zinc supplementation in women with low prepregnant weights and low plasma zinc levels produced infants with higher birth weights (Goldenberg et al., 1995).

The RDA for zinc in pregnancy is 11 mg per day (12 mg for those younger than 18 years old). Because iron inhibits zinc absorption, high levels of prenatal iron supplementation may negatively impact maternal zinc status. For women taking more than 30 mg of iron daily, supplements of 15 mg zinc and 2 mg of copper are recommended (American Dietetic Association, 2002a). Good sources of zinc include meat, fish, poultry, dairy products, nuts, whole grains, and legumes.

Other Vitamins and Minerals

The DRIs of most other vitamins and minerals increase moderately, or not at all, during pregnancy. The RDA for vitamin B$_6$ during pregnancy is 1.9 mg per day, with an upper intake level of 80–100 mg per day. High doses of vitamin B$_6$ (as much as 75 mg/day) have been used to treat severe nausea and vomiting in pregnant women. Data on this treatment is only anecdotal; such high levels of supplementation should be closely monitored by a medical provider.

It is common practice to recommend a prenatal vitamin-mineral supplement to all pregnant women, even though not all are at risk based on dietary restrictions and practices, and most supplementation doesn't begin until well into the first trimester. There is some suggestion that periconceptional vitamin supplementation might decrease incidence of preeclampsia, but more research is needed (Bodnar, Tang, Ness, Harger, & Roberts, 2006). Women who are pregnant with two or more fetuses should take a multivitamin and mineral supplement (American Dietetic Association, 2002a).

Alcohol, Artificial Sweeteners, and Caffeine

The teratogenic effects of excessive alcohol consumption are well accepted. In addition to the outcomes of fetal alcohol syndrome and fetal alcohol effects, alcohol use in pregnancy has been associated with spontaneous abortion, low birth weight, and abruptio placentae. Since no safe level of alcohol intake in pregnancy can be guaranteed, promoting abstinence before and during pregnancy is recommended. Inquiring about alcohol intake can sometimes be less threatening when done within the context of a dietary history and usual patterns of food and beverage intake.

Artificial sweeteners used in the U.S. food supply include saccharin, aspartame, and acesulfame-K. Saccharin has been shown to be a weak carcinogen in animals, but not teratogenic. Acesulfame-K is considered safe, but is relatively new in food use and no long-term studies during pregnancy have been conducted. A product of aspartame metabolism is the amino acid phenylalanine, which can cause brain damage in persons with phenylketonuria. Moderate intake of aspartame in women without phenylketonuria, however, does not increase serum phenylalanine levels high enough to affect the fetal brain. Dietary assessment of pregnant women should include the use of artificial sweeteners, found primarily in soft drinks but also in flavored yogurt, baked goods, and as a substitute for added sugar. Counseling should encourage the use of nutrient-containing milk and juice instead of soft drinks.

Extensive research has been conducted on caffeine's effect on pregnancy outcome, with mixed results depending on study design and population. A meta-analysis found increased risk of low birth weight and spontaneous abortion in women who consumed more than 150 mg per day of caffeine, but the effect of alcohol and smoking on pregnancy outcomes could not be determined (Fernandes et al., 1998). Although no direct effect of caffeine has been demonstrated consistently in humans, massive doses of the substance are teratogenic in mice. Caffeine likely interacts with a variety of socioeconomic and lifestyle factors such as alcohol consumption, smoking, and drug use, resulting in an adverse pregnancy outcome. Although there is no evidence to recommend elimination of caffeine during pregnancy, women should limit their intake to no more than 300 mg per day, and others can be supported for omitting caffeine totally during pregnancy (American Dietetic Association, 2002a). In addition to coffee and tea, soft drinks are a major source of caffeine in the United States. Average caffeine content of common beverages are 85 mg in a 5-ounce cup of regular coffee, 40 mg in a 1-ounce espresso, 30 mg in a 5-ounce cup of tea, and 36 mg in 12 ounces of cola.

Diet-Related Problems in Pregnancy

Nausea and Vomiting

Morning sickness is common in the early months of pregnancy but typically disappears by the second trimester. The standard dietary recommendations include frequent, small, relatively dry meals of easily digested foods, with liquids taken between meals. Foods containing carbohydrates are usually well tolerated, and fats are often reported as hard to digest. Many women report odors as primary triggers of nausea. Rather than a specific diet for managing nausea, pregnant women should be encouraged to eat whatever they tolerate and avoid odors that result in nausea (American Dietetic Association, 2002a).

For a small percentage of pregnant women, the vomiting can be frequent and severe enough (hyperemesis gravidarum) to impact their nutritional status, resulting in weight loss, decreased nutrient intake, and electrolyte imbalance. These women need medical management and frequently require hospitalization for fluid and electrolyte replacement as well as nutrition support (Broussard & Richter, 1998).

Pregnancy-Induced Hypertension

The cardinal symptoms of pregnancy-induced hypertension (PIH) are hypertension, proteinuria, and edema, usually occurring after the 20th week of gestation. This condition is unique to pregnancy and resolves only by the termination of the pregnancy. Sometimes referred to as preeclampsia and eclampsia, the latter is an extension of preeclampsia, with more severity—that is, grand mal seizures and high risk of maternal and infant mortality. PIH, a more appropriate description of this disorder, is most often seen in first pregnancies, young women, obese women, and those from low socioeconomic status. Criteria for diagnosing PIH include:

Hypertension: 140/90 or an increase of 20 to 30 mm Hg systolic or 10 to 15 mm Hg diastolic above the woman's usual baseline; at least two observations at 6 or more hours apart.

Proteinuria: 500 mg or more in 24-hour urine collection or random 2+ protein; develops late in the course of PIH.

Edema: significant; usually in hands and face; if left unattended, seizures may occur; can be fatal to either mother or infant.

The etiology of PIH has been a mystery for many years. Although a number of theories have been proposed and studied, the precise cause of this disorder of pregnancy is unknown. Nutritional deficiency is suspected, however, because of the association of PIH with poverty, lack of prenatal care, and poor nutritional status. Protein deficiency has been proposed as a causative factor, but evidence has not been conclusive. A meta-analysis study found that calcium supplementation lowered systolic and diastolic blood pressure but did not have a significant effect on maternal and infant morbidity and mortality (Bucher et al., 1996). Providing supplements of magnesium, zinc, and fish oils has not been demonstrated to be effective treatments for PIH (American Dietetic Association, 2002a; Dekker & Sibai, 2001). A healthy diet—including good potassium sources (fruits and vegetables), low-fat dairy products, and high fiber—is associated with a reduced risk of preeclampsia (Frederick et al., 2005).

Sodium restriction, a previous treatment strategy for PIH, is not effective and should not be implemented. The use of diuretics is also contraindicated and can have negative effects on intravascular volume and kidney function. Women at risk for PIH should receive early prenatal care and a balanced diet providing adequate energy and protein.

Diabetes

With increasing overweight and type 2 diabetes on the rise in the general population, more women are entering pregnancy with diabetes, insulin resistance, or they will develop diabetes during their pregnancies. This increases the risk for pregnancy complications and poor birth outcomes.

Pregnancy is a diabetogenic event in which energy needs and fuel requirements are increased. Glucose is the primary fuel, particularly for the growing fetus, who has an uptake rate of glucose at least twice that of an adult. To meet fetal needs, glucose is transferred rapidly from mother to fetus through simple diffusion and active transport. Although glucose crosses the placental barrier, insulin does not, and the fetus is dependent on its own supply for development. Maternal fasting blood glucose levels drop as a result of rapid fetal uptake, which decreases her fasting insulin levels. Even brief fasting can result in the production of ketones, which is an alternative fuel source, but carries the risk of fetal brain damage. Normal glucose tolerance is maintained, however, by increased maternal secretion of insulin.

The normal energy metabolism of pregnancy and the maternal-fetal relationship have implications for women with insulin-dependent diabetes mellitus. During the first half of pregnancy, the increased transfer of maternal glucose to the fetus, along with the usual lower food intake because of nausea, may result in reduced insulin requirements. In the second half of pregnancy, the diabetogenic effects of the placental hormones override the continuous fetal drain of glucose so that insulin requirements are increased by as much 70% to 100% over prepregnant requirements. Risk of ketoacidosis is also increased; pregnant women with diabetes mellitus need frequent monitoring. Because of frequent changes in diet and insulin, these women are best served by a team of professionals including a skilled registered dietitian.

Diet is critical in the management of pregnant women with diabetes (American Diabetes Association, 2003a). Increased energy intake is dependent on prepregnancy weight, physical activity level, and adequacy of weight gain. It is important to maintain regular meals and snacks, including a bedtime snack to avoid overnight ketonemia. More structured eating schedules and balanced distribution of food in the pregnant state is usually needed to achieve a normoglycemic state. More frequent follow-up visits are need for women with diabetes for the team to monitor weight gain, blood glucose control, energy and nutrient intake, and then make needed adjustments in meal and snack plans or insulin doses.

Maintenance of satisfactory control of blood glucose levels during pregnancy is associated with a marked improvement in pregnancy course and outcome. Rates of congenital malformations, spontaneous abortion, and macrosomia are much reduced; these improvements are directly related to reduced perinatal mortality.

Gestational Diabetes

Pregnant women should be screened for gestational diabetes between the 24th and 28th week of gestation. This involves a nonfasting 50-gm oral glucose challenge followed by a glucose determination 1 hour later. Low-risk women who do not need to be screened include those who are under 25 years of age, have a normal prepregnancy weight, have no family history of diabetes, and are not a member of an ethnic or racial group with a high prevalence of diabetes (American Diabetes Association, 2003b). If the 1-hour plasma glucose level is greater than 140 mg per dL, a 100-gm oral glucose tolerance test is scheduled.

Following diagnosis of gestational diabetes, the nutritional recommendations are similar to those with pre-existing diabetes mellitus. Management goals include providing adequate energy and nutrients to support optimal weight gain without episodes of hyperglycemia or ketonemia. Frequent monitoring of blood glucose, weight gain, dietary intake and meal/snack timing, and urinary ketones by a health care team is essential, followed by appropriate adjustments in food intake and meal plans (American Diabetes Association, 2003b). It is generally recommended to limit carbohydrate intake at the morning meal, usually to no more than 30 gm, with larger amounts of carbohydrate later in the day.

For obese women with gestational diabetes (body mass index greater than 30), a moderate restriction of 30% to 33% in energy intake (25 kcal/kg actual weight per day) has reduced hyperglycemia without increasing ketonuria (American Diabetes Association, 2003b).

Pica

Pica is the behavior of eating nonfood substances. Although occurring in the broad population, it is most common in pregnant women. Usual substances consumed are clay, starch (laundry starch, chalk), and ice. Pica is associated with a higher incidence of malnutrition, because it displaces foods providing needed nutrients. There is a strong link between pica and iron deficiency; it is thought that some of those substances may bind to iron, preventing absorption (Rainville, 1998). Other negative consequences from pica can include intestinal obstruction and toxic levels of heavy metals such as lead.

The reasons for pica have not been clearly identified. Culture and tradition passed from generation to generation is certainly an important factor. Some reports indicate that women believe these substances relieve nausea, prevent vomiting, relieve dizziness, cure swelling, and stop headaches. Pica behavior is not easy to discourage, but the potentially dangerous consequences should be avoided.

For the practitioner, the immediate need is to identify the pica behavior, which is rarely revealed spontaneously. A dietary intake assessment can address this by asking about cravings or eating unusual substances while obtaining an overall diet pattern. If pica behavior is acknowledged, the practitioner should identify the extent of the amount and frequency, followed by a more thorough dietary and biochemical assessment. The client then can be offered nutrition education regarding the potential harm of the pica behavior, as well as nutritional guidance for strategies to improve her diet for pregnancy.

Food Safety

Pregnant women should take cautions to avoid food-borne illnesses, including salmonella, helicobacter, shigella, and Escherichia coli. Listeriosis, caused by listeria monocytegenes, can cause premature delivery, stillbirth, or newborn infection. During pregnancy, women should avoid unpasteurized juices; raw sprouts; unpasteurized dairy products; raw or undercooked meat, fish, and poultry; and soft or homemade cheeses (American Dietetic Association, 2002a). The U.S. Food and Drug Administration (2004) also recommends that pregnant women avoid eating large fish, such as shark, swordfish, king mackerel, and tilefish, since they may accumulate high levels of methylmercury. However, since fish contains healthy omega-3 fatty acids, it should be included in their diets. Up to 12 ounces per week is considered safe, and no more than 6 ounces per week of albacore tuna. Women are also advised to contact their state or local health departments regarding methylmercury or other contaminants in local fish and seafood.

Food Taboos

Superstitions and taboos about food are as old as human life. Pregnancy seems to be a time of great concern about food taboos, with strong connotation as to what is beneficial or harmful. When these taboos are grounded in ignorance, they can have a deleterious effect on the pregnant woman's diet. Many superstitions have been associated with protein and protein-rich foods, which can be particularly harmful. Some food beliefs in pregnancy center on limiting weight gain in order to have a smaller baby who is easier to deliver. Many food avoidances are rooted in religious or cultural practices that are believed to impart positive qualities in the offspring.

Health care practitioners should remember that a belief doesn't necessarily imply practice. In our rapidly changing multicultural society, assumptions cannot be made about dietary beliefs and practices based on ethnicity or culture. In working with pregnant women who have unhealthy dietary practices based on beliefs or taboos, it is essential to understand and listen to the woman's view, provide explanation and information, and then negotiate.

Adolescent Pregnancy

Pregnancy in adolescence poses potential physical and psychological risks because adolescence is a period of rapid growth and development with increased nutrient requirements. Teenage girls who become pregnant at a young gynecologic age (the number of years between onset of menses and date of conception) or who are undernourished at conception have the highest nutritional needs.

It has long been accepted that adolescent girls who are more physiologically mature have no more pregnancy complications than adult women, but a longitudinal study demonstrated that both the young women and their infants are at increased risk (Scholl, Hediger, & Schall, 1997). With increasing maternal weight gains, infant birth weights remained low. Explanations for this disparity include (1) disruption in fetal-placental blood flow associated with the physiology of maternal growth and (2) increases of insulin and growth hormone that enhance maternal fat and weight gain but diminish circulating nutrients available to the fetus. The same longitudinal study of adolescent pregnancies revealed an increased risk of later overweight and obesity. There was deposition of excess subcutaneous fat in central body sites during gestation, which can increase risk for later cardiovascular disease, noninsulin diabetes mellitus, and hypertension (Hediger, Scholl, & Schall, 1997).

Weight gain recommendations for pregnant teenagers are at the higher end of the recommendations for adult women—that is, 30 to 35 pounds. For those who are underweight before pregnancy, 35 to 40 pounds may be desirable (Institute of Medicine, 1990). Many young women who are concerned about body image and weight have difficulty accepting the appropriate pregnancy weight gain. And some of them may not benefit from the Institute of Medicine recommendations for weight gain, especially the older adolescents with high BMIs (Groth, 2006). They need education and counseling regarding the weight gain needed for the various products of conception in order to produce a healthy, full-term infant.

Requirements for energy and most other nutrients are the same as those for pregnant adults, individualized according to activity and weight gain. Calcium, phosphorus, and magnesium recommendations are higher than the pregnant adult recommendations (see Table 11.2). Given teenage girls' typical patterns of dieting, habitual poor food selection, and meal skipping, it can be a challenge to get pregnant adolescents to consume the nutrient-rich diet needed for a healthy pregnancy. For some young women, limited financial resources and food access create additional barriers. Pregnant adolescents are best served by a team that includes social services, nutritional counseling, and other health and community resources. A review of enhanced prenatal care interventions for adolescents showed positive pregnancy outcomes, but more research is needed to develop effective behavior change strategies (Nielsen, Gittelsohn, Anliker, & O'Brien, 2006).

Prenatal Nutrition Assessment and Counseling

Nutrition assessment of pregnant women includes a thorough history, physical examination, and laboratory tests. Many factors may place pregnant women at increased nutritional risk (see Table 11.6). The presence of one or more of these factors indicates the need for a more intensive nutritional assessment.

Obtaining dietary data is an essential component of the assessment, although it is rarely done as part of routine clinical practice. This may result from lack of training and experience, time constraints, or lack of recognition of its value. Several tools for collecting dietary information exist, each with strengths and limitations (Hammond, 2004). The 24-hour recall is commonly used in clinical practice but does not reflect intake over time and depends on accurate memory. Food records (3 to 7 days) require literacy and commitment to recording, but are representative when reviewed by a health professional for completeness. An in-depth diet history requires a trained nutritionist who obtains food intake and frequency over time, as well as food practices and resources; this is not often practical in clinical settings except for high-risk clients. A food frequency questionnaire, which can be self-administered, includes lists of foods and food groups and a scale for checking frequency of use—for example, servings per day, week, month. It can identify missing nutrient sources, but does not include eating practices and habits, or quantity consumed.

A modified diet history, combined with a food frequency questionnaire, can be used as a baseline for assessment and counseling in early prenatal care. This should include cultural food beliefs, living and cooking facilities, finances or other resources for food, food allergies or intolerances, use of supplements and medications, and unusual food practices. Follow-up visits can monitor diet by use of a 24-hour recall or repeat food frequency questionnaire. If specific diet information is

11.6 | Nutritional Risk Factors in Pregnancy

FACTOR	SIGNIFICANCE
Age	The adolescent whose reproductive biological age (chronological age minus menarche age) is less than 3. Adolescent pregnancy can be associated with emotional, financial, and educational risks. Advanced age may be associated with high parities. Age of menarche is significant in that it can be delayed by poor nutrition.
Reproductive performance	Short interconceptual periods, particularly when coupled with high parity. Past obstetric history of abortions, poor weight gain, anemia, generalized edema, stillbirth, toxemia, low–birth weight infants, and premature labor.
Chronic systemic illness	Anemia, thyroid dysfunction, diabetes, chronic infection, malabsorption syndromes, severe psychosocial problems, drugs used to treat these illness that may interfere with nutrition.
Weight	Low pregnant weight or low weight (less than 85%) for height, inadequate weight gain during pregnancy, obesity above 120% of standard weight for height.
Atypical eating patterns	Food fads, constant dieting, pica, dietary restrictions based on ethnic or cultural factors.
Substance abuse	Use of tobacco, drugs, or alcohol.
Economic deprivation	Inability to purchase adequate amounts of food to provide needed nutrients; chronic low level nutritional inadequacy.

available, nutrient intake can be estimated using food-nutrient tables and compared to recommendations for pregnancy. Less specific food intake data can be compared to recommended servings of food groups. By combining the evaluation of diet with history, laboratory results, and weight gain, the goals for nutrition counseling can be developed.

Most pregnant women are motivated and receptive to make positive changes in their diets. Nutrition counseling should be individualized, beginning with determining the woman's level of nutrition knowledge and reinforcing already established good food habits. The goals for changes in diet should be clearly identified, including an understandable rationale related to a healthy outcome of pregnancy—for example, more protein is needed not only for the baby's growth but also for mother's placenta, uterus, and increased blood. Positive results are more likely when the professional collaborates with the woman (and her partner, if possible) to identify strategies to reach these goals, an example of which might be a vegetarian mother who offers to increase her intake of cheese, tofu, nuts, and milk to get more protein.

Cultural and ethnic food patterns are important for many women, and need to be appreciated by health care practitioners. Positive aspects can be reinforced and alternative nutrient sources identified by the client or a nutritionist. The exception is atypical food taboos or beliefs that might have negative nutritional consequences.

Many non-White women are lactose intolerant, meaning they have diminished lactase enzyme needed to hydrolyze the lactose in milk to glucose and galactose. Undigested lactose in the intestine results in symptoms of lactose intolerance: abdominal cramps, bloating, diarrhea, and flatulence. Most individuals with lactose intolerance, however, can take in small quantities of dairy products without symptoms, especially when in combination with other foods. Cheese and yogurt are also well tolerated since most of the lactose has already been broken down in the cooking and fermentation process. In addition, lactase-treated milk is now available in grocery stores, and commercial enzyme products can be purchased to add to milk or eat with lactose-containing foods. If necessary, additional calcium supplements may be indicated for some pregnant women.

Despite a good diet, pregnant women are more likely to experience constipation due to the pressure of the enlarging uterus on the intestine and a decrease in physical activity. The components of an optimal prenatal diet, however, will help prevent constipation. This includes whole-grain breads and cereals, plenty of fruits and vegetables (raw, cooked, and dried), legumes, nuts, and seeds. In addition, adequate fluids (at least six to eight glasses of milk, water, or juice) are needed for water resorption in the large intestine. Regular physical activity also supports normal bowel function. Despite the best efforts, some women may occasionally need a fiber supplement.

LACTATION

Each year, more evidence accumulates to show that breast-feeding is the preferred method for infant feeding, with many benefits for both the infant and mother (see Table 11.7). The American Academy of Pediatrics (2004) and the American Dietetic Association (2005b) have developed position statements to encourage breast-feeding until the first birthday. There was an increase in breast-feeding rates in the 1970s and 1980s, followed by a decline in the 1990s and a recent increase, with more than 70% of women breast-feeding their babies when leaving the hospital in 2002 (American Dietetic Association, 2005b). After initiating breast-feeding, rates then decrease by 3 to 6 months of age. Barriers to continue breast-feeding include mother's work hours, lack of support (family and professional), changes in health care service delivery, sociocultural factors, inadequate information, and fatigue. Nurses and other professionals who provide prenatal and perinatal care are in a prime position to assist pregnant women with information and counseling regarding the breast-feeding decision and to provide resources and support for those who choose to nurse their infants.

From a nutrition perspective, lactation places a greater nutritional demand on a woman than pregnancy does. The DRI of most nutrients are increased (see Table 11.2). Milk volume is not affected by the mother's diet; rather, the infant's regular sucking triggers the hormones prolactin (for milk production) and oxytocin (for milk ejection and let-down). The composition of breast milk does reflect the maternal diet, however, such as in fatty acid content, the levels of some B vitamins, and alcohol and caffeine. For other nutrients, such as calcium, the level in the breast milk will be maintained at the expense of the maternal reserves if her diet is inadequate.

In addition to the host of anti-infective and immune properties of breast milk, there is now interest in certain long-chain polyunsaturated fatty acids and their role in early human development. Breast milk is fairly rich in docosahexaenoic acid (DHA) and arachidonic acid (AA), which are major components of brain and nervous tissue lipids early in life. In utero, the placenta appears to supply these fatty acids to the developing fetus. Studies of preterm infants who received human milk rather than formula showed a significantly higher IQ at 7½ to 8 years of age (Lucas, Morley, Cole, Lister, & Leeson-Payne, 1992). Trials of feeding formula supplemented with DHA and AA to term infants have produced mixed results (Hoffman et al., 2003; Scott et al., 1998) and rely on visual acuity tests in the infants. More controlled long-term studies are warranted. Most European countries have been supplementing infant formula with

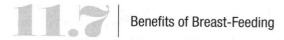

11.7 | Benefits of Breast-Feeding

Nutritionally superior for infants
Contains antibodies and immune cells
Contains omega-3 fatty acids
Nonallergenic
Difficult to overfeed
Promotes mother-infant bonding
Safe and hygienic
Usually less expensive than formula
Convenient

these fatty acids for some time, and U.S. infant formula manufacturers are following that lead.

The recommended energy increase for breast-feeding reflects the average production of approximately 750 ml per day, but varies with each woman. This assumes exclusive breast-feeding; mothers of infants who receive supplemental infant formula will produce less milk and require less energy. Energy needs are higher if the postpartum woman is also very active or nursing more than one infant. The amount of milk produced usually decreases after 6 months of age as solids are added to the infant's diet. Women who are obese before pregnancy or gain excessive weight during pregnancy may not need much more energy intake. The maternal fat stores accumulated during pregnancy are expected to provide some of the energy for breast milk production in the early months of life.

The postpartum pattern of weight loss during lactation varies greatly from woman to woman. Many will gradually lose 1 to 2 pounds per month while nursing, while others do not. Food intake and physical activity are likely factors in these differing weight patterns. One study of lactating women who were significantly overweight used a diet and exercise program in the first 14 weeks postpartum. Results showed that the women lost about 0.5 kg per week and that the growth of their infants was the same as those in the control group (Lovelady, Garner, Moreno, & Williams, 2000). These women had an average of 34% body fat, and the diet was reduced by 500 kcal per day. This type of intervention would not be indicated for women who were not significantly overweight. Lean women who attempt restrictive dieting may be at risk for reduced milk production, as is the case of malnourished women in developing countries. It is generally recommended that breast-feeding women take in at least 1,800 kcals daily (Shabert, 2004).

Early in lactation, the primary issues include dealing with sore nipples, engorgement, infection, and leaking. Nurses who counsel lactating women should reinforce a varied and healthy diet, urge avoidance of restrictive dieting attempts, and recommend 2 to 3 quarts of liquid daily for adequate milk production. Since women may not automatically feel thirsty to consume that amount, practitioners suggest that the nursing mother drink something while she is nursing or sitting down.

Breast-fed infants as a group tend to grow somewhat slower than do bottle-fed infants. On occasion, a nursing infant may fail to thrive while appearing to nurse adequately. Rather than providing a supplemental bottle right away, possible contributing factors should be thoroughly explored. These include maternal factors (stress, fatigue, use of oral contraceptives or other drugs, smoking, illness, poor diet, excessive caffeine) and infant factors (poor suck, infrequent feeding, increased energy needs, infection, malabsorption, vomiting, diarrhea). The nurse can be critical in identifying the contributing factors and working with the mother and infant to find the best strategies to solve the problem.

Nursing mothers are likely to bring up other concerns about diet and breast-feeding issues. These include:

1. Vitamin and mineral supplementation for the infant: Vitamin D and fluoride are recommended.
2. Allergic reaction of the baby to a compound in the breast milk: Most babies tolerate breast milk very well. A minority, however, may demonstrate an adverse reaction to a diet-derived component in breast milk. This is more often seen in highly allergic families. Cow's milk protein is reported to be the major culprit. If this occurs, lactating women should be advised to avoid the potentially problematic food and assess the infant's behavior in the next few days. If the dietary change is beneficial for the baby, the mother should make sure her own diet is adequate.
3. Contaminants in breast milk: Lactating women are often exposed to a variety of non-nutritional substances that may be transferred to their milk. These substances include drugs, environmental pollutants, viruses, caffeine, and alcohol. Although moderate amounts of many of these agents are believed to pose no risk to nursing infants, some substances provoke concern because of known or suspected adverse reactions (Lawrence & Lawrence, 2005)
4. HIV/AIDS and breast milk: Evidence suggests that the AIDS virus can be transmitted through breast milk. In developed countries, it is recommended that HIV-positive mothers be discouraged from breast-feeding their infants (American Dietetic Association,

2005b). The World Health Organization, however, supports the concept that infants in many developing countries have a greater risk of dying from diarrheal disease if they are not breast-fed than of developing AIDS from breast milk exposure.

Promotion of Breast-Feeding

The decision to breast-feed or not is usually made during pregnancy. Therefore, information and counseling about nursing should be provided to the mother and her partner during prenatal visits, in childbirth classes, and through community programs. Nurses working in a variety of settings can play an important role in providing this education and counseling (American Dietetic Association, 2005b). Additional knowledge (the specific how-to) and supportive counseling are key to later successful and sustained nursing. The hospital nurse or lactation specialist can provide practical tips and demonstration before the mother and baby go home. Hospitals that adopt the guidelines of the Baby Friendly Hospital Initiative provide trained staff that initiate nursing in the first half hour of life, offer 24-hour rooming-in, do not give bottles or pacifiers, and provide discharge support or referral for breast-feeding help (American Dietetic Association, 2005b; Ebrahim, 1993).

The La Leche League International, an educational and support group founded by nursing mothers, is found in most communities. Hospitals that have a lot of deliveries often have lactation specialists or other trained nurses available for phone consultation to new mothers. Those with the credentials IBCLC have completed the International Board of Lactation Consultant Examiners certification process. The national Healthy Mothers–Healthy Babies programs include breast-feeding promotion, as does the Special Supplemental Nutrition Program for Women, Infant, and Children program. Trained peer counselors are available in some community programs; they frequently work with groups who have low rates of breast-feeding, such as low-income women, teens, and minority women.

NUTRITION-RELATED CONCERNS OF WOMEN

Obesity and Weight Management

Obesity is a serious public health problem in North America, particularly because the prevalence continues to increase. Based on body mass index of 30 or more, 32.2% of Americans were obese in 2003–2004 (Ogden et al., 2006). Between 1999 and 2004, there was a significant increase in overweight prevalence of men, while women showed no increase during that 6-year period. African Americans have the highest rate of obesity at

45%. Women are more overweight than men, and Black women are more overweight than White women.

Definition of Overweight and Obesity

Although tables of desirable weight for height have been used for many decades to determine overweight and obesity, the use of body mass index is preferred today. BMI is calculated by dividing a person's weight in kilograms by his or her height in meters squared. For instance, a woman who is 64 inches (1.63 m) tall and weighs 130 pounds (59 kg) has a BMI of 22.3. The use of BMI eliminates the dependence on body frame size. Health risks from excess weight begin when BMI exceeds 25, and this is determined overweight. Obesity is defined by a BMI of 30 or greater (see Table 11.8).

Abdominal obesity may be a better predictor than overall obesity for disease risks and causes of mortality. Waist circumference is another measure of overweight that is associated with abdominal obesity. More than half of all adults in the United States in 2003–2004 had abdominal obesity, and some with BMIs between 25 and 29 (Li, Ford, McGuire, & Mokdad, 2007). From 1988 to 2004, the mean waist circumference and the prevalence of abdominal obesity in adults have increased continuously. Obesity, especially when combined with elevated waist circumference and high BMI, can lead to metabolic syndrome, which is a risk factor for diabetes and coronary heart disease (Haffner, 2006).

Consequences of Obesity

Higher BMIs are associated with increased mortality in both men and women, more so in White than in Black individuals (Ogden, Carroll, & Flegal, 2003). It is well known that obesity increases the risk of many chronic diseases such as hypertension, coronary heart disease, diabetes mellitus, stroke, gallbladder disease, osteoarthritis, asthma, sleep apnea, and certain cancers (ovarian, endometrial, colon) (Mokdad et al., 2003; Ogden et al., 2003). Menstrual abnormalities and ovarian dysfunction are more common in obese women, as is a greater risk of adverse pregnancy course and outcome. Excess weight gain in women contributes to decreased physical functioning, more bodily pain, and less vitality (Fine et al., 1999). More difficult to measure are the emotional consequences of obesity, such as discrimination, low self-esteem, depression, social rejection, and the use of food for consolation and as a coping mechanism. Many women try a variety of dieting regimens to lose weight, which frequently has short-term success, followed by weight gain and no real change in eating and activity patterns. As a result, it is not unusual for overweight and obese women to develop disordered eating patterns and cycles of weight loss and gain early in life, which often continues until older adulthood (Allaz, Bernstein, Rouget, Archinard, & Morabia, 1998).

Etiology of Obesity

Nature versus nurture as the cause of obesity has been debated for decades. Much of normal weight regulation is genetically determined, and with increased human gene mapping, knowledge of specific genes and other markers linked with obesity has increased (Laquatra, 2004). Although weight status is heritable to a degree, the dramatic increase in obesity in the past 30 years is associated primarily with environment.

Two hormones have been studied relative to obesity: leptin, which induces satiety, and ghrelin, which promotes feeding. Obese individuals have high levels of plasma leptin but exhibit leptin resistance (Monti, Carlson, Hunt, & Adams, 2006). Ghrelin is the only known circulating appetite stimulant and is involved in the deposition of adipose tissue. It induces weight gain and the appetite control system, working in balance with leptin (Wren et al., 2001).

It must be remembered that genes provide the susceptibility for obesity but do not actually cause it. Weight gain occurs when more energy is consumed than expended. Therefore, dietary and activity patterns are key factors in weight changes. It is easy to overconsume with ready food access at home, school, and work; large portions served in eating establishments; and food tied to many social situations. Decreased physical activity plays an even greater role in excess weight gain, as Americans spend more time in sedentary activities such as watching sports instead of doing them, in front of the computer, and in their cars.

11.8 | Definition of Overweight and Obesity by Body Mass Index

CLASSIFICATION	BODY MASS INDEX
Underweight	Less than 18.5
Normal	18.5–24.9
Overweight	25.0–29.9
Obesity, class I	30.0–34.9
Obesity, class II	35.0–39.9
Obesity, class III	More than 40

Note. Body mass index is weight in kilograms divided by height in meters squared. *From:* National Institutes of Health, National Heart, Lung, and Blood Institute. (1998). Clinical guidelines on the identification, evaluation, and treatment of overweight and obesity in adults—The evidence report. NIH Publication No. 98-4083.

Weight Management

Americans spend billions of dollars each year on a multitude of weight loss efforts, including diet books, commercial weight-loss programs (some providing food), weight-loss and healthy lifestyles classes, exercise programs and equipment, liquid and powdered meal replacements, drugs, herbal products and supplements, acupuncture, hypnosis, and surgery. Despite the high level of resources spent on various weight-loss efforts, the percentage of Americans who are overweight or obese has never been higher. Many weight-loss efforts are not successful over time because they have a single narrow treatment focus, appeal to individuals as a new diet but are too restrictive, do not address needed changes in eating and activity behaviors, and do not provide information and support.

Most long-term successful weight-management efforts are neither fast nor flashy. They work over time because they include modifications in food choices, activity, and lifestyle. A chronic disease prevention model that incorporates professionals from medicine, nutrition, exercise physiology, and behavior psychology will provide the best intervention program (American Dietetic Association, 2002b). Dieting alone rarely addresses the weight problem on a permanent basis. Many women trying to lose weight set ideal goals for themselves that are frequently hard to achieve, thus resulting in disappointment and a sense of failure, which colors future attempts. Weight cycling (losing and gaining weight several times over years) is particularly common in overweight women. Although it is not clear whether weight variability has negative long-term health effects, it certainly has negative psychological effects. Many health professionals recommend a gradual reduction in weight, to a level of better overall health if not slimness (American Dietetic Association, 2002b). Obese individuals, who lose as little as 5% to 10% of their body weight, have demonstrated improved blood glucose control, blood pressure, and lipid levels (*Clinical Guidelines*, 1998). There is a growing movement for size acceptance that emphasizes healthy eating and activity to be more fit, rather than focusing on fatness and BMI.

A moderate restricted-energy diet as part of a weight management program should contain 50% to 55% of energy as carbohydrate, 15% to 20% as protein, and no more than 30% as fat. A daily energy deficit of 500 to 1,000 kcalories is expected to result in a weight loss of 1 to 2 pounds per week, assuming moderate physical activity (American Dietetic Association, 2002b). Since fat is the most energy-dense macronutrient (9 kcal per gram versus 4 kcal per gram for protein and carbohydrate), reducing the fat content allows for a greater variety and volume of nutrient-rich food. For most women, a diet providing less than 1,200 to 1,300 kcal per day can result in fatigue and hunger and usually requires vitamin and mineral supplements. Overall, a sound weight loss diet should:

Meet nutritional needs—except for energy.

Allow adaptation to individual habits and tastes.

Emphasize slow and steady weight loss.

Minimize hunger and fatigue.

Contain common, readily available foods.

Be socially acceptable and incorporated into family meals.

Help promote regular and healthy eating habits.

Provide enough energy for regular physical activity.

Exercise is a key component in any successful weight loss program, as well as to maintain weight. A combination of aerobic and resistance training is optimal. The aerobic exercise helps use fat stores for fuel and has positive cardiovascular effects. Strength training increases resting metabolic rate and lean body mass, as well as improves bone density. Exercise alone, without changing diet, can result in slow weight loss. Other benefits of physical activity include stress reduction, a sense of accomplishment, relief of boredom, increased self-control, and improved sense of well-being. Consistency with the exercise program is important in weight management; the activity should be convenient, affordable, pleasant, and relatively easy to do. Many women find classes and group activities to be supportive and reinforcing, but any activity that a woman enjoys should be encouraged—for example, walking the dog or gardening.

Lifestyle modification in successful weight-management efforts includes analyzing and modifying behaviors relating to weight gain. The use of self-monitoring, problem-solving, stimulus control, and cognitive restructuring help implement these changes (Laquatra, 2004). Examples include:

Self-monitoring—recording the what, where, and when of food intake, as well as feelings and actions affecting eating helps identify the settings where eating occurs and the antecedents.

Problem-solving—defining the eating or weight problem, considering possible solutions, and choosing one to implement, evaluating the outcome, reimplementing that one or trying another, and reevaluating.

Stimulus control—altering the environment to minimize the stimuli for eating (for example, storing food out of sight in the kitchen, slowing the pace of eating by putting down the utensils between bites, avoiding the purchase of "problem" foods).

Cognitive restructuring—helping identify and correct the negative thoughts that undermine weight-management efforts. For example, instead of overeating when angry, call a friend or go for a walk; rather than considering a dietary lapse as "blowing my diet," use positive self-talk to continue healthy eating.

Many Americans use commercial weight-loss programs, including Internet-based programs. Some include meal replacement formulas instead of, or with, food. The diets used are generally well balanced, but each program has different components, such as behavior modification and group sessions. In addition, there are always new popular diets in the media—the dietary approach may vary from appropriate to unhealthy. Diets promising fast results with little effort are appealing to those who are overweight but usually have unrealistic expectations and result in feelings of failure. Consumers should be helped to evaluate these popular diets (Laquatra, 2004).

Osteoporosis

Osteoporosis is a bone disease characterized by decreasing bone mineral density (BMD) with the aging process, resulting in increased likelihood of fractures. Women are four times as likely as men to develop the condition, but this is changing as men live longer. Osteoporosis is defined as BMD greater than 2.5 standard deviations below the mean peak bone mass in young women. Osteopenia is BMD between 1 and 2.5 standard deviations below the mean peak value in young women (Anderson, 2004). So, although osteoporosis is a disease of the aging, its origins develop during the early years of skeletal development and peak bone mass accumulation in childhood and puberty. National surveys indicate that almost 44 million Americans are affected by osteoporosis or osteopenia, mostly women (National Osteoporosis Foundation, 2007). The subsequent fractures costs billions in health care dollars and can result in long-term care, decreased mobility and independence, and death.

There are two types of osteoporotic processes in women. Postmenopausal osteoporosis (type 1) is the loss in trabecular bone in postmenopausal women secondary to decreased estrogen. Lumbar vertebrae and wrist fractures are more frequent at this stage. Age-related osteoporosis (type 2) is the loss of trabecular and corticol bone seen in those over 70 years of age, most likely resulting in hip and other bone fractures (Anderson, 2004).

Osteoporosis can be prevented or delayed by maximizing peak bone mass in the first three decades of life and establishing positive dietary and exercise habits that can sustain the natural bone changes of menopause and aging (American Dietetic Association, 2004). Many nutrients or food components are linked to bone health, especially calcium and vitamin D, but also protein, phosphorus, magnesium, fluoride, and sodium. High levels of sodium, protein, or caffeine in the diet increase urinary calcium losses (Anderson, 2004). Excessive alcohol intake also increases the risk of osteoporosis. This shifts the calcium balance in a negative direction, especially if there is a low calcium dietary intake.

Optimal calcium intake is essential for bone health in postmenopausal women. Since hormone therapy is currently not indicated for most postmenopausal women, diet becomes more critical. The DRI for calcium increases from 1,000 to 1,200 mg per day for those over 50 years of age (see Table 11.2). For many women, this level of calcium intake cannot be achieved with diet alone, and supplements are needed. Although calcium supplementation does not have much effect on BMD in the first few years of menopause, it does slow bone loss in the late postmenopausal period (Heaney & Weaver, 2005). Food sources to emphasize include low-fat dairy products, which are the most well absorbed. Other products fortified with additional calcium include some orange juice, soy milk, rice milk, and breads.

Adequate vitamin D is required for normal bone metabolism because it is integral to calcium absorption. Older persons are more at risk for vitamin D deficiency due to their skin being less able to convert sunshine exposure to vitamin D, plus less exposure for those confined indoors or living in northern climates. Most studies show positive benefits from vitamin D. The recommended amounts of this nutrient are increased for older women (see Table 11.2). An adequate vitamin D intake of at least the DRI from food and supplements has been shown to significantly reduce hip fractures in postmenopausal women (Feskanich, Willet, & Colditz, 2003).

Isoflavones found in soybeans function as phytoestrogens, which may result in the inhibition of bone resorption similar to the action of selective estrogen receptor modulators. Some populations with low dietary calcium intakes, such as Japanese women, may be protected from osteoporosis by high intakes of soy foods. Although the potential for phytoestrogens in bone health is promising, further long-term trials will define the role more clearly.

Phosphorus intake becomes a problem when it is excessive relative to calcium intake, leading to decreased bone formation. Phosphates are widely available in the food supply, particularly in carbonated beverages. Intake of cola beverages has been associated with decreased bone mineral density (Tucker et al., 2006).

Cardiovascular Disease

Nearly half a million women die yearly from coronary heart disease (CHD) and stroke in the United States, which is more than the next four causes of death combined (Thom et al., 2006). To emphasize causes of mortality, 1 in 30 female deaths is from breast cancer, while 1 in 2.6 is from cardiovascular disease. Almost twice as many women as men die within a year of having a heart attack. These gender differences are believed to be due, in part, to "too little and too late" medical intervention. Increasing obesity and high rates of hypertension and obesity in women over 45 years of age mean more women are at risk for cardiovascular disease.

The risk factors for CHD in women are listed in Table 11.9. Many of these are diet-related; all are modifiable by changes in lifestyle. A consensus statement provides guidelines for preventing CHD in women, including lifestyle factors such as smoking cessation, increased physical activity, and stress management (Mosca et al., 1999). The recommendations include striving for a BMI no greater than 25 and avoiding excess weight gain during pregnancy. Optimal management of diabetes to reduce concomitant risk factors is strongly supported.

The revised National Cholesterol Education Program (NCEP, 2002) provides both community and clinical goals. The therapeutic lifestyle changes approach includes less than 7% of fat as saturated fat, less than 200 mg/d cholesterol, 10–25 g of soluble dietary fiber, 2 g plant stanols/sterols (added to commercial margarines), physical activity, and avoidance of overweight. Compared to previous recommendations, total fat can be 25% to 35% of total calories, with up to 10% as polyunsaturated fat and up to 20% as monounsaturated fat. For every reduction of 1% of saturated fatty acid as energy intake, there is a 2% decrease in cholesterol and additional decrease in LDL (NCEP, 2002).

The monounsaturated oleic acid, found in large amounts in olive and canola oils, lowers LDL cholesterol. On the other hand, trans-fatty acids (polyunsaturated fatty acids that are hydrogenated—solid vegetable fats such as margarine and shortening) are known to have a negative impact on total cholesterol, LDL, and high-density lipoprotein (Willett, 2006). Because fish and shellfish are rich in omega-3 fatty acids, eating these foods two to three times per week is encouraged. These short-chain fatty acids assist in clearing very low-density lipoproteins and chylomicrons and have antithrombotic effects. In addition, both soluble dietary fiber and soy protein appear to have positive, but moderate, impacts on blood lipids.

Recent research has explored the relationship between homocysteinemia and CHD. A high level of homocysteine appears to be a risk factor independent of other CHD risks. Plasma homocysteine is inversely associated with serum levels of folate, vitamin B_6, and vitamin B_{12} (Selhub, 2006). Although some data have suggested that high folate and vitamin B_6 are associated with low risk of CHD, an analysis of 43 studies on the topic revealed that, in prospective studies, there was no (or very small) association between homocysteine levels and cardiovascular risk (Christen, Ajani, Glynn, & Hennekens, 2000). Although there seem to be associations between elevated plasma homocysteine and increased mortality from heart disease, stroke, and Alzheimer's disease, more controlled prospective studies are needed on this issue (Selhub, 2006).

The role of antioxidants such as vitamin E, beta-carotene, and vitamin C in reducing heart disease has been studied for some time, with the promise of a protective effect. However, large human studies were based on diet questionnaires, and controlled intervention trials have been inconclusive. There is not enough evidence at this point to recommend antioxidant supplements to prevent heart disease, but women should consume a diet that meets the DRI levels for those nutrients, including fruits, vegetables, nuts, and oils.

Eating Disorders

Eating disorders such as anorexia nervosa (AN) and bulimia nervosa (BN) are psychiatric and medical conditions seen primarily in young females. Most eating disorder onsets occur during adolescence and are more frequently reported in athletes (American Dietetic Association, 2006a). Weight preoccupation, food control, and psychological vulnerability are hallmarks of eating disorders. Although AN and BN have been identified and treated for many decades, the range of eating

11.9 | Risk Factors for Coronary Heart Disease in Women

RISK FACTOR	RISK CRITERIA
Hypertension	Systolic blood pressure 140 mm Hg or higher; disastolic blood pressure 90 mm Hg or higher
Dyslipidemia	Total cholesterol 200 mg/dL or higher HDL cholesterol 40 mg/dL or lower LDL cholesterol 130 mg/dL or higher Triglycerides 150 mg/dL or higher
Diabetes mellitus	
Smoking	
Obesity	Body mass index 27 or higher
Poor diet	More than 30% of calories from fat More than 10% from saturated fats Fewer than 5 servings of fruits and vegetables daily Less than 25 g of fiber daily

disorders to include recurrent binge eating indicates a wider spectrum. See Exhibit 11.2 for diagnostic criteria for eating disorders. AN is characterized by low body weight, amenorrhea, distorted body image, and obsessive-compulsive features. Key characteristics of BN include binge eating, inappropriate compensatory behaviors, and symptoms of depression and mood disorders. Eating disorders not otherwise specified have partial symptoms of either AN or BN and are believed to be more common than either AN or BN. Binge eating disorder is similar to bulimia nervosa but without all the components; many of those with binge eating

EXHIBIT 11.2 DIAGNOSTIC CRITERIA FOR EATING DISORDERS

Anorexia Nervosa (AN)

- Refusal to maintain body weight at or above a minimally normal weight for age and height (i.e., weight loss leading to maintenance of body weight < 85% of that expected; or failure to make expected weight gain during period of growth, leading to body weight < 85% of that expected)
- Intense fear of gaining weight or becoming fat, even though underweight
- Disturbance in the way in which one's body weight or shape is experienced, undue influence of body weight or shape on self-evaluation; or denial of the seriousness of the current low body weight
- Amenorrhea in postmenarchal females, i.e., the absence of at least three consecutive menstrual cycles

Types of AN:

1. Restricting—during the current episode of AN, the person has not regularly engaged in binge eating or purging behavior
2. Binge eating/purging—during the current episode of AN, the person has regularly engaged in binge eating and purging behavior

Bulimia Nervosa (BN)

- Recurrent episodes of binge eating, characterized by both of the following:
  1. Eating, in a discrete period of time (e.g., within any 2-hour period), an amount of food that is definitely larger than most people would eat during a similar period of time and under similar circumstances
  2. A sense of lack of control over eating during the episode (e.g., a feeling that one cannot stop eating or control what or how much one is eating)
- Recurrent inappropriate compensatory behavior in order to prevent weight gain, such as self-induced vomiting, misuse of laxatives, diuretics, enemas, or other medications, fasting, or excessive exercise
- The binge eating and inappropriate compensatory behaviors both occur, on average, at least twice a week for 3 months
- Self-evaluation is unduly influenced by body shape and weight
- The disturbance does not occur exclusively during episodes of AN

Types of BN:

1. Purging—during the current episode of BN, the person has regularly engaged in self-induced vomiting or the misuse of laxatives, diuretics, or enemas
2. Nonpurging—during the current episode of BN, the person has used other inappropriate compensatory behaviors, such as fasting or excessive exercise, but has not regularly used purging behaviors

Eating Disorders Not Otherwise Specified (do not meet criteria for specific eating disorders); examples:

- All of the criteria for AN are met except that the person has regular menses
- All of the criteria for AN are met except that, despite significant weight loss, the individual's current weight is in the normal range

(continued)

EXHIBIT 11.2 DIAGNOSTIC CRITERIA FOR EATING DISORDERS (*CONTINUED*)

- All of the criteria for BN are met except that the binge eating and inappropriate compensatory mechanisms occurs at a frequency of less than twice a week or for a duration of less than 3 months
- The regular use of inappropriate compensatory behavior by an individual of normal body weight after eating small amounts of food
- Repeatedly chewing and spitting out, but not swallowing, large amounts of food

Binge Eating Disorder

- Recurrent episodes of binge eating (as above)
- A sense of lack of control over eating during the episode
- Binge eating associated with at least three of the following:
  1. eating more rapidly than normal
  2. eating until feeling uncomfortable full
  3. eating large amounts of food when not feeling physically hungry
  4. eating alone because of being embarrassed by how much one is eating
  5. feeling disgusted with oneself, depressed, or feeling very guilty after overeating
- Marked distress regarding binge eating
- Binge eating occurs, on average, at least 2 days per week for 6 months
- The binge eating is not associated with the regular use of inappropriate compensatory behaviors (e.g., purging, fasting, excessive exercise) and does not occur exclusively during the course of AN or BN

Note. From *Diagnostic and Statistical Manual of Mental Disorders* (4th ed., text revision), by American Psychiatric Association, 2000, Washington, DC: Author.

---

disorder are, or have been, overweight, and they suffer significant emotional distress related to eating control (American Dietetic Association, 2006a). A continuum of disordered eating, with more or less severity and complexity, is seen in the U.S. population due to dieting behavior and focus on weight loss.

Etiology and Medical Complications

Anorexia Nervosa. The etiology of AN is unknown but most evidence suggests an interaction of biological and psychosocial factors (Schebendach & Reichert-Anderson, 2004). A genetic component is indicated by the observation that the disorder is much more common in pairs of identical twins than in pairs of fraternal twins. It is well documented that there is a disturbance in the hypothalamic-anterior pituitary-gonadal axis, but this is likely secondary to malnutrition. The chronic dieting appears to trigger a continuous weight loss and hypometabolic adaptation in vulnerable individuals, leading to a vicious cycle that becomes self-perpetuating.

The typical girl who develops AN is conscientious, achievement oriented, and a perfectionist. Family interactional patterns characterized by enmeshment, overinvolvement, overprotectiveness, rigidity, and poor conflict resolution have been implicated; however, a variety of other family dynamics have been described.

The cultural obsession with thinness can be a powerful influence on vulnerable individuals. Concern about dieting may lead to gradual self-starvation, leading to significant weight loss that is denied.

The medical complications relate primarily to the progressive starvation. These include protein-energy malnutrition, hypoproteinemia, hypokalemia, decreased gastric motility, hypotension, arrested growth, and prolonged reduction of estrogen, which leads to osteopenia and osteoporosis (American Dietetic Association, 2006a). In children and adolescents, normal growth and development may be compromised by pubertal delay, reduction in peak bone mass, and brain abnormalities (American Dietetic Association, 2006a). Serious electrolyte imbalances can occur when vomiting, laxative, or diuretic abuse is present. Muscular weakness, cardiac arrhythmias, and renal impairment may occur. These complications can lead to cardiac and renal damage or to sudden death.

Bulimia Nervosa. The etiology theories for BN include addiction, family dysfunction, cognitive-behavioral, sociocultural, and psychodynamic (Schebendach & Reichert-Anderson, 2004). Depending on the model, different treatment strategies are emphasized. Onset of this disorder is most often seen in the late teens or early 20s, when young women leave home to attend college or to join the work force. This transitional time in life appears to be a high-risk period for the development of problematic eating behaviors. Since persons with BN are usually in a normal weight range and they are also very secretive, symptoms are more difficult to detect (see Table 11.10 for signs and symptoms). Most of the medical complications are a result of the inappropriate compensatory behaviors used to counter the binge eating—self-induced vomiting and excessive use of laxatives, diuretics, and enemas.

Intervention for Eating Disorders

Persons with eating disorders are best served by interdisciplinary teams, which include primary care providers, nutritionists, and psychotherapists. These teams should be trained and experienced in working with this population. Settings may include outpatient, day treatment, or psychiatric units; for some patients with anorexia nervosa, a crisis medical state may warrant hospitalization and nutritional rehabilitation, including tube feeding.

Nutrition Assessment and Intervention

In addition to the standard diet history, anthropometric (height, weight, BMI) indices, and biochemical data, the nutrition assessment by a trained dietitian should include eating attitudes and behaviors and some determination of metabolic rate (Schebendach & Reichert-Anderson, 2004). Reported energy intakes may be less than 1,000 kcal per day in young women with AN and low or as high as several thousand kcal per day in patients with BN. Because of the often limited quantity

| 11.10 | Signs and Symptoms of Bulimia Nervosa |

Abdominal distention

Anal tear and fissures (laxative abuse)

Binge eating

Diuretic abuse

Dehydration

Hypokalemia

Erosion of dental enamel, dental caries

Parotid gland enlargement

Esophagitis, esophageal tears

Cardiac arrhythmias

Scarring of the dorsum of one hand (used to stimulate gag reflex)

Vomiting

Weight fluctuating by 10 or more pounds in a month

and variety of food consumed, attention must be given to nutrient adequacy (macronutrients and micronutrients) and fluid and electrolyte balance. Taking the time to determine the woman's attitudes, beliefs, and behaviors regarding food and eating is essential to later developing appropriate nutrition education and therapy objectives. Some red flags to look for include:

Avoidance of certain foods or food groups—for example, animal foods, all fats, sweets.

Preoccupation with food and calorie content.

Strictly grouping foods as "good" or "bad."

Ritualistic eating schedules, preparation, and timing.

Misconceptions regarding usual portion sizes.

Certain foods that can trigger a binge episode.

Nutrition therapy for AN initially focuses on refeeding to promote a positive energy balance and eventual weight gain. Increments of the caloric prescription are increased slowly, and weight gain goals may be as modest as 1 to 2 pounds per week. The dietary plan needs to address the level of physical activity, food aversions, and subtle efforts of noncompliance. Diets that provide 25% to 30% of energy as fat are usually better accepted by patients who fear fat. Detailed guidance for the nutrition practitioner is available in other sources (Schebendach & Reichert-Anderson, 2004).

For patients with BN, nutrition therapy will depend on current weight status. For someone trying to lose weight, a diet plan that does not promote weight gain yet stimulates increased metabolic rate is appropriate. A balanced diet providing adequate intake of vitamins and minerals eaten at regular meals and snacks will begin to address the cycling periods of restrained eating and bingeing. Use of self-monitoring techniques, such as keeping a food diary, can sometimes provide a sense of control over eating and help avoid bingeing. A counseling approach incorporating cognitive behavioral therapy, interpersonal psychotherapy, or dialectical behavior therapy, can be helpful in challenging the erroneous beliefs and thought processes of the person with eating disorders (American Dietetic Association, 2006a).

Nutrition education, combined with psychotherapy, is key in addressing the long-term outcomes of eating disorders. The specific nutrition therapy will work best when there is a collaborative relationship between the patient and the nutritionist. Helping the patient separate the food and weight issues from the psychological issues will help ensure more cooperation and progress. Although many of these young women appear to be knowledgeable about nutrition, they have many misconceptions and concrete thinking processes. Nutrition education sessions can include metabolism, energy expenditure, nutrient and energy values of foods, and other topics, but using abstract thinking and a problem-solving process.

Monitoring and Outcome

Because eating disorders tend to be chronic conditions, regular and ongoing monitoring by appropriate team members is important. Outcome criteria include appropriate weight for height; adequate and balanced food intake; regular menses; realistic understanding of food, weight, and shape; and improved psychological adjustment. Therapy can last for years. Follow-up studies indicate that one-third of persons with AN recover fully, and the remaining demonstrate lifelong problems with disordered eating (American Psychiatric Association, 2000b). Although early identification and treatment have significantly reduced mortality from eating disorders, this population is vulnerable to relapse.

NUTRITION AND HEALTH PROMOTION

Because nutrition and dietary factors are associated with the major causes of morbidity and mortality in U.S. women, it makes sense that nutrition is a key component of health promotion and disease prevention efforts. The role of nutrition and diet in promoting health and reducing chronic diseases has been documented for many conditions, including diabetes mellitus, cardiovascular disease, and cancer and for preventing low birth weight (American Dietetic Association, 2006b; Centers for Disease Control and Prevention, 2000). The national prevention agenda, Healthy People (originally published in 1979) is updated each decade with specific health objectives based on priority areas. The Healthy People 2010 includes 18 specific nutrition objectives to achieve between 2000 and 2010 (Centers for Disease Control and Prevention, 2000). An example of one objective is: Reduce anemia among low-income pregnant women in their third trimester by 20%.

Nutrition can be included in the three levels of disease prevention: primary prevention (broad health promotion in communities), secondary prevention (screening to detect risk followed by early intervention), and tertiary prevention (treatment and rehabilitation for identified health conditions) (American Dietetic Association, 2006b). An example of primary nutrition prevention is the 5-a-Day Program, an education program to encourage people to eat a minimum of five servings of fruits and vegetables a day. The Dietary Approaches to Stop Hypertension (DASH) is an example of a secondary prevention program for individuals at risk for hypertension. Studies have shown that a diet high in fruits and vegetables (8 to 10 servings per day), low in saturated and total fat, and including nonfat dairy foods can decrease systolic blood pressure significantly (Champagne, 2006). The DASH diet can also be considered a primary prevention for the broad population as well as part of a medical management program for those with identified hypertension.

The Dietary Guidelines for Americans are the current national recommendations for dietary guidance that have evolved over the past 30 years. Reviewed and updated every 5 years, the Dietary Guidelines target the common nutrition-related chronic diseases (U.S. Department of Health and Human Services and U.S. Department of Agriculture, 2005) (see Exhibit 11.3). To assist in implementing these broad guidelines into food choices and planning nutritious meals, the most recent MyPyramid was developed (U.S. Department of Agriculture, 2007). It is meant to be used by consumers in selecting a healthy eating pattern and by health professionals who counsel clients. Based on color-coded food groups, the online version is interactive and can be individualized by age, gender, and activity level. The amounts and servings of protein and dairy foods are less (emphasizing low fat), followed by more minimal use of fats and sugars.

Several federal food and nutrition programs, primarily from the U.S. Department of Agriculture and the U.S. Department of Health and Human Services, serve the most vulnerable—infants and children, pregnant women, and those with low income. These nutrition programs include the National School Lunch and Breakfast Program (where all children can obtain school meals; low-income children receive free or reduced-price meals); Summer Food Service Program (free meals for low-income children at day camps and summer programs); Special Supplementary Nutrition Program for Women, Infants, and Children (for low-income pregnant women and children up to 5 years of age who have nutritional risk); Head Start (includes meals and nutrition services); the Title III Elderly Nutrition Program for Older Americans (congregate and home-delivered meals for seniors), and the Food Stamp Program (Dodd & Bayerl, 2004).

Many national health organizations also provide community-based nutrition prevention programs, including the American Heart Association, American Cancer Society, March of Dimes, American Diabetes Association, and others. Nutrition efforts in health promotion and disease prevention for women are most likely to succeed if they address lifestyle factors, environment, economics (personal and public), and the social and political climates that impact individuals and communities. Partnerships and coalitions among a variety of agencies and organizations can utilize limited resources, even though they take time and energy to develop. Possible partners for promoting good nutrition include public health agencies, primary care providers, schools (early childhood through college), supermarkets, the food industry, agricultural growers and farmers' markets, and print and electronic media.

EXHIBIT 11.3 DIETARY GUIDELINES FOR AMERICANS, 2005

Key Recommendations for the General Population
Adequate Nutrients Within Calorie Needs

- Consume a variety of nutrient-dense foods and beverages within and among the basic food groups while choosing foods that limit the intake of saturated and trans fats, cholesterol, added sugars, salt, and alcohol.
- Meet recommended intakes within energy needs by adopting a balanced eating pattern, such as the U.S. Department of Agriculture (USDA) Food Guide or the Dietary Approaches to Stop Hypertension (DASH) Eating Plan.

Weight Management

- To maintain body weight in a healthy range, balance calories from foods and beverages with calories expended.
- To prevent gradual weight gain over time, make small decreases in food and beverage calories and increase physical activity.

Physical Activity

- Engage in regular physical activity and reduce sedentary activities to promote health, psychological well-being, and a healthy body weight.
  - □ To reduce the risk of chronic disease in adulthood: Engage in at least 30 minutes of moderate-intensity physical activity, above usual activity, at work or home on most days of the week.
  - □ For most people, greater health benefits can be obtained by engaging in physical activity of more vigorous intensity or longer duration.
  - □ To help manage body weight and prevent gradual, unhealthy body weight gain in adulthood, engage in approximately 60 minutes of moderate- to vigorous-intensity activity on most days of the week while not exceeding caloric intake requirements.
  - □ To sustain weight loss in adulthood, participate in at least 60 to 90 minutes of daily moderate-intensity physical activity while not exceeding caloric intake requirements. Some people may need to consult with a health care provider before participating in this level of activity.
- Achieve physical fitness by including cardiovascular conditioning, stretching exercises for flexibility, and resistance exercises or calisthenics for muscle strength and endurance.

Food Groups to Encourage

- Consume a sufficient amount of fruits and vegetables while staying within energy needs. Two cups of fruit and 2½ cups of vegetables per day are recommended for a reference 2,000-calorie intake, with higher or lower amounts depending on the calorie level.
- Choose a variety of fruits and vegetables each day. In particular, select from all five vegetable subgroups (dark green, orange, legumes, starchy vegetables, and other vegetables) several times a week.
- Consume 3 or more ounce-equivalents of whole-grain products per day, with the rest of the recommended grains coming from enriched or whole-grain products. In general, at least half the grains should come from whole grains.
- Consume 3 cups per day of fat-free or low-fat milk or equivalent milk products.

Fats

- Consume less than 10% of calories from saturated fatty acids and less than 300 mg per day of cholesterol, and keep trans fatty acid consumption as low as possible.
- Keep total fat intake between 20% and 35% percent of calories, with most fats coming from sources of polyunsaturated and monounsaturated fatty acids, such as fish, nuts, and vegetable oils.
- When selecting and preparing meat, poultry, dry beans, and milk or milk products, make choices that are lean, low-fat, or fat-free.
- Limit intake of fats and oils high in saturated and/or trans fatty acids, and choose products low in such fats and oils.

(continued)

EXHIBIT 11.3 DIETARY GUIDELINES FOR AMERICANS, 2005 (*CONTINUED*)

Carbohydrates

■ Choose fiber-rich fruits, vegetables, and whole grains often.
■ Choose and prepare foods and beverages with little added sugars or caloric sweeteners, such as amounts suggested by the USDA Food Guide and the DASH Eating Plan.
■ Reduce the incidence of dental caries by practicing good oral hygiene and consuming sugar- and starch-containing foods and beverages less frequently.

Sodium and Potassium

■ Consume less than 2,300 mg (approximately 1 teaspoon of salt) of sodium per day.
■ Choose and prepare foods with little salt. At the same time, consume potassium-rich foods, such as fruits and vegetables.

Alcoholic Beverages

■ Those who choose to drink alcoholic beverages should do so sensibly and in moderation—defined as the consumption of up to one drink per day for women and up to two drinks per day for men.
■ Alcoholic beverages should not be consumed by some individuals, including those who cannot restrict their alcohol intake, women of childbearing age who may become pregnant, pregnant and lactating women, children and adolescents, individuals taking medications that can interact with alcohol, and those with specific medical conditions.
■ Alcoholic beverages should be avoided by individuals engaging in activities that require attention, skill, or coordination, such as driving or operating machinery.

Food Safety

■ To avoid microbial foodborne illness:
  □ Clean hands, food contact surfaces, and fruits and vegetables. Meat and poultry should not be washed or rinsed.
  □ Separate raw, cooked, and ready-to-eat foods while shopping, preparing, or storing foods.
  □ Cook foods to a safe temperature to kill microorganisms.
  □ Chill (refrigerate) perishable food promptly and defrost foods properly.
  □ Avoid raw (unpasteurized) milk or any products made from unpasteurized milk, raw or partially cooked eggs or foods containing raw eggs, raw or undercooked meat and poultry, unpasteurized juices, and raw sprouts.

Note. From U.S. Department of Health and Human Services and U.S. Department of Agriculture, 2005.

Nurses working in a variety of settings—public health, primary care, ambulatory care, school health, and teaching—can have a positive impact on preventive nutrition in the female populations they serve. They are also key team members in providing nutrition intervention and counseling for those at risk for diet-related diseases, as well as those with acute and chronic conditions.

REFERENCES

Allaz, A. F., Bernstein, M., Rouget, P., Archinard, M., & Morabia, A. (1998). Body weight preoccupation in middle-age and ageing women: A general population survey. *International Journal of Eating Disorders, 23*(3), 287–294.

American Academy of Pediatrics. Committee on Nutrition. (2004). *Pediatric nutrition handbook* (5th ed.). Elk Grove, IL: Author.

American Diabetes Association. (2003a). Evidence-based nutrition principles and recommendations for the treatment and prevention of diabetes and related complications. *Diabetes Care, 26*(Suppl.), S51–S61.

American Diabetes Association. (2003b). Gestational diabetes mellitus. *Diabetes Care, 26*(Suppl.), S103–S105.

American Dietetic Association. (2002a). Position of the American Dietetic Association: Nutrition and lifestyle for a healthy pregnancy outcome. *Journal of the American Dietetic Association, 102*(10), 1479–1490.

American Dietetic Association. (2002b). Position of the American Dietetic Association: Weight management. *Journal of the American Dietetic Association, 102*(8), 1145–1155.

American Dietetic Association. (2004). Position of the American Dietetic Association and dietitians of Canada: Nutrition and women's health. *Journal of the American Dietetic Association, 104*(6), 984–1001.

American Dietetic Association. (2005a). Position of the American Dietetic Association: Nutrition across the spectrum of aging. *Journal of the American Dietetic Association, 105*(4), 616–633.

American Dietetic Association. (2005b). Position of the American Dietetic Association: Promoting and supporting breastfeeding. *Journal of the American Dietetic Association, 105*(5), 810–818.

American Dietetic Association. (2006a). Position of the American Dietetic Association: Nutrition intervention in the treatment of anorexia nervosa, bulimia nervosa, and other eating disorders. *Journal of the American Dietetic Association, 106*(12), 2073–2082.

American Dietetic Association. (2006b). Position of the American Dietetic Association: The role of registered dietitians and dietetic technicians, registered, in health promotion and disease prevention. *Journal of the American Dietetic Association, 106,* 1875–1884.

American Psychiatric Association. (2000a). *Diagnostic and statistical manual of mental disorders* (4th ed., text revision). Washington, DC: Author.

American Psychiatric Association. (2000b). *Practice guidelines for the treatment of patients with eating disorders.* Washington, DC: Author.

Anderson, J. (2004). Nutrition for bone health. In L. Mahan & S. Escott-Stump (Eds.), *Krause's food, nutrition and diet therapy* (11th ed., pp. 642–666). Philadelphia: Saunders.

Barr, S. I., Murphy, S. P., & Poos, M. I. (2002). Interpreting and using the dietary reference intakes in dietary assessment of individuals and groups. *Journal of the American Dietetic Association, 102*(6), 780–788.

Bertone-Johnson, E. R., Hankinson, S. E., Bendich, A., Johnson, S. R., Willet, W. C., & Manson, J. E. (2005). Calcium and vitamin D intake and risk of incident premenstrual syndrome. *Archives of Internal Medicine, 165*(11), 1246–1252.

Bodnar, L. M., Tang, G., Ness, R. B., Harger, G., & Roberts, J. M. (2006). Periconceptional multivitamin use reduces the risk of preeclampsia. *American Journal of Epidemiology, 164*(5), 470–477.

Broussard, C. N., & Richter, J. E. (1998). Nausea and vomiting of pregnancy. *Gastroenterology Clinics of North America, 27*(1), 123–151.

Bucher, H. C., Guyatt, G. H., Cook, R. J., Hatala, R., Cook, D. J., Lang, J. D., & Hunt, D. (1996). Effect of calcium supplementation on pregnancy-induced hypertension and preeclampsia: A meta-analysis of randomized controlled trials. *Journal of the American Medical Association, 275*(14), 1113–1117.

Centers for Disease Control. (1992). Recommendations for use of folic acid to reduce the number of cases of spina bifida and other neural tube defects. *Morbidity and Mortality Weekly Report, 41,* 1.

Centers for Disease Control. (1998). Recommendations to prevent and control iron deficiency in the United States. *Morbidity and Mortality Weekly Report, 47,* 1–36.

Centers for Disease Control and Prevention. (2000). *Healthy People 2010.* Retrieved January 25, 2007, from http://www.healthypeople.gov/default.htm

Centers for Disease Control and Prevention Office of Women's Health. (2006). Leading causes of death in females—United States, 2002. Retrieved December 18, 2006, from http://www.cdc.gov/women/lcod.htm

Champagne, C. C. (2006). Dietary interventions on blood pressure: The dietary approaches to stop hypertension (DASH) trials. *Nutrition Reviews, 64*(Suppl. 1), 53–56.

Christen, W. G., Ajani, U. A., Glynn, R. J., & Hennekens, C. H. (2000). Blood levels of homocysteine and increased risks of cardiovascular disease: Causal or casual? *Archives of Internal Medicine, 160*(4), 422–434.

Clinical guidelines on the identification, evaluation, and treatment of overweight and obesity in adults—The evidence report. (1998). National Institutes of Health [published erratum appears in *Obesity Research, 6*(6), 464.] *Obesity Research, 6*(Suppl. 2), 51S–209S.

Cross, G. B., Marley, J., Miles, H., & Willson, K. (2001). Changes in nutrient intake during the menstrual cycle of overweight women with premenstrual syndrome. *British Journal of Nutrition, 85*(4), 475–482.

Dekker, G., & Sibai, B. (2001). Primary, secondary, and tertiary prevention of pre-eclampsia. *Lancet, 357*(9251), 209–215.

Dodd, J. L., & Bayerl, C. T. (2004). Nutrition in the community. In L. Mahan & S. Escott-Stump (Eds.), *Krause's food, nutrition and diet therapy* (11th ed., pp. 340–362). Philadelphia: Saunders.

Douglas, S. (2002). Premenstrual syndrome. Evidence-based treatment in family practice. *Canadian Family Physician, 48,* 1789–1797.

Ebrahim, G. J. (1993). The Baby Friendly Hospital Initiative [Editorial]. *Journal of Tropical Pediatrics, 39*(1), 2–3.

Fernandes, O., Sabharwal, M., Smiley, T., Pastuszak, A., Koren, G., & Einarson T. (1998). Moderate to heavy caffeine consumption during pregnancy and relationship to spontaneous abortion and abnormal fetal growth: A meta-analysis. *Reproductive Toxicology, 12*(4), 435–444.

Feskanich, D., Willet, W. C., & Colditz, G. A. (2003). Calcium, vitamin D, milk consumption, and hip fractures: A prospective study among postmenopausal women. *American Journal of Clinical Nutrition, 77*(2), 504–511.

Fine, J. T., Colditz, G. A., Coakley, E. H., Moseley, G., Manson, J. E., Willett, W. C., & Kawachi, I. (1999). A prospective study of weight change and health-related quality of life in women. *Journal of the American Medical Association, 282*(22), 2136–2142.

Frederick, I. O, Williams, M. A., Dashow, E., Kestin, M., Zhang, C., & Leisenring, W. M. (2005). Dietary fiber, potassium, magnesium and calcium in relation to the risk of preeclampsia. *Journal of Reproductive Medicine, 50*(5), 332–344.

Goldenberg, R. L., Tamura, T., Neggers, Y., Copper, R. L., Johnston, K. E., DuBard, M. B., & Hauth, J. C. (1995). The effect of zinc supplementation on pregnancy outcome. *Journal of the American Medical Association, 274*(6), 463–468.

Groth, S. (2006). Adolescent gestational weight gain: Does it contribute to obesity? *American Journal of Maternal Child Nursing, 31*(2), 101–105.

Guenther, P., Dodd, K., Reedy, J., & Krebs-Smith, S. (2006). Most Americans eat much less than recommended amounts of fruits and vegetables. *Journal of the American Dietetic Association, 106*(9), 1371–1379.

Haffner, S. M. (2006). Relationship of metabolic risk factors and development of cardiovascular disease and diabetes. *Obesity (Silver Spring), 14*(Suppl. 3), 121S–127S.

Hammond, K. A. (2004). Dietary and clinical assessment. In L. Mahan & S. Escott-Stump (Eds.), *Krause's food, nutrition, and diet therapy* (11th ed., pp. 407–435). Philadelphia: Saunders.

Heaney, R. P., & Weaver, C. M. (2005). New perspectives on calcium nutrition and bone quality. *J Am Coll Nutr, 24*(Suppl. 6), 574S–581S.

Hediger, M. L., Scholl, T. O., & Schall, J. I. (1997). Implications of the Camden Study of adolescent pregnancy: Interactions among maternal growth, nutritional status, and body composition. *Annals of the New York Academy of Science, 817,* 281–291.

Hoffman, D. R., Birch, E. E., Castaneda, Y. S., Fawcett, S. L., Wheaton, D. H., Birch, D. G., & Uauy, R. (2003). Visual function in breast-fed term infants weaned to formula with or without long-chain polyunsaturates at 4 to 6 months: A randomized clinical trial. *Journal of Pediatrics, 142*(6), 669–677.

Institute of Medicine. (1990). *Nutrition during pregnancy: Weight gain and nutrient supplements.* Washington, DC: National Academy Press.

Kitchin, B., & Morgan, S. (2003). Nutritional considerations in osteoporosis. *Current Opinions in Rheumatology, 15,* 476–480.

Lammer, E. J., Chen, D. T., Hoar, R. M., Agnish, N. D., Benke, P. J., Braun, J. T., Curry, C. J., Fernhoff, P. M., Grix, A. W., Jr., Lott, I. T., et al. (1985). Retinoic acid embryopathy. *New England Journal of Medicine, 313*(14), 837–841.

Laquatra, I. (2004). Nutrition for weight management. In L. Mahan & S. Escott-Stump (Eds.), *Krause's food, nutrition, and diet therapy* (11th ed., pp. 558–593). Philadelphia: Saunders.

Larson, N. I., Story, M., Wall, M., & Neumark-Sztainer, D. (2006). Calcium and dairy intakes of adolescents are associated with their home environment, taste preferences, personal health beliefs, and meal patterns. *Journal of the American Dietetic Association, 106*(11), 1816–1824.

Lawrence, R., & Lawrence, R. (2005). *Breastfeeding: A guide for the medical profession* (6th ed.). Philadelphia, PA: Elsevier Saunders.

Li, C., Ford, E. S., McGuire, L. C., & Mokdad, A. H. (2007). Increasing trends in waist circumference and abdominal obesity among U.S. adults. *Obesity (Silver Spring), 15*(1), 216–224.

Lovelady, C. A., Garner, K. E., Moreno, K. L., & Williams, J. P. (2000). The effect of weight loss in overweight, lactating women on the growth of their infants. *New England Journal of Medicine, 342*(7), 449–453.

Lucas, A., Morley, R., Cole, T. J., Lister, G., & Leeson-Payne, C. (1992). Breast milk and subsequent intelligence quotient in children born preterm. *Lancet, 339*(8788), 261–264.

Lytle, L. A., Himes, J. H., Feldman, H., Zive, M., Dwyer, J., Hoeschler, D., Webber, L., & Yang, M. (2002). Nutrient intake over time in a multi-ethnic sample of youth. *Public Health Nutr, 5*(2), 319–328.

Mokdad, A. H., Ford, E. S., Bowman, B. A., Dietz, W. H., Vinicor, F., Bales, V. S., & Marks, J. S. (2003). Prevalence of obesity, diabetes, and obesity-related health risk factors, 2001. *Journal of the American Medical Association, 289*(1), 76–79.

Monti, V., Carlson, J. J., Hunt, S. C., & Adams, T. D. (2006). Relationship of ghrelin and leptin hormones with body mass index and waist circumference in a random sample of adults. *Journal of the American Dietetic Association, 106*(6), 822–828.

Morais, J. A., Chevalier, S., & Gougeon. R. (2006). Protein turnover and requirements in the healthy and frail elderly. *Journal of Nutrition, Health and Aging, 10*(4), 272–283.

Mosca, L., Grundy, S. M., Judelson, D., King, K., Limacher, M., Oparil, S., Pasternak, R., Pearson, T. A., Redberg, R. F., Smith, S. C., Jr., Winston, M., & Zinberg, S. (1999). AHA/ACC scientific statement: Consensus panel statement. Guide to preventive cardiology for women. American Heart Association/ American College of Cardiology. *Journal of the American College of Cardiology, 33*(6), 1751–1755.

National Cholesterol Education Program (NCEP) Expert Panel on Detection, Evaluation, and Treatment of High Blood Cholesterol in Adults (Adult Treatment Panel III). (2002). Third Report of the National Cholesterol Education Program (NCEP) Expert Panel on Detection, Evaluation, and Treatment of High Blood Cholesterol in Adults (Adult Treatment Panel III) final report. *Circulation, 106*(25), 3143–3421.

National Institutes of Health, Office of Dietary Supplements. Retrieved January 29, 2007, from http://dietary-supplements. info.nih.gov

National Institutes of Health, National Heart, Lung, and Blood Institute. (1998). Clinical guidelines on the identification, evaluation, and treatment of overweight and obesity in adults—The evidence report. NIH Publication No. 98-4083.

National Osteoporosis Foundation. (2007). America's bone health: The state of osteoporosis and low bone mass in our nation. Washington, DC: Author. Retrieved January 25, 2007, from http://www.nof.org/advocacy/prevalence

Nelson, H. D., Vesco, K. K., Haney, E., Fu, R., et al. (2006). Non-hormonal therapies for menopausal hot flashes: Systematic review and meta-analysis. *Journal of the American Medical Association, 295*(17), 2057–2071.

Nielsen, J. N., Gittelsohn, J., Anliker, J., & O'Brien, K. (2006). Intervention to improve diet and weight gain among pregnant adolescents and recommendations for future research. *Journal of the American Dietetic Association, 106*(11), 1825–1840.

Ogden, C. L., Carroll, M. D., Curtin, L. R., McDowell, M. A., Tabak, C. J., & Flegal, K. M. (2006). Prevalence of overweight and obesity in the United States, 1999–2004. *Journal of the American Medical Association, 295*(13), 1549–1555.

Ogden, C. L., Carroll, M. D., & Flegal, K. M. (2003). Epidemiologic trends in overweight and obesity. *Endocrinol Metab Clin North Am, 32*(4), 741–760, vii.

Otten, J., Hellwig, J., Meyers, L. (Eds.). (2006). *Dietary reference intakes: The essential guide to nutrient requirements.* Washington, DC: Institute of Medicine, National Academies Press.

Rainville, A. J. (1998). Pica practices of pregnant women are associated with lower maternal hemoglobin level at delivery. *Journal of the American Dietetic Association, 98*(3), 293–296.

Ritchie, L. D., & King, J. C. (2000). Dietary calcium and pregnancy-induced hypertension: Is there a relationship? *American Journal of Clinical Nutrition, 71,* 1371S–1374S.

Rosa, F. W., Wilk, A. L., & Kelsey, F. O. (1986). Teratogen update: Vitamin A congeners. *Teratology, 33*(3), 355–364.

Rothman, K. J., Moore, L. L., Singer, M. R., Nguyen, U. S., Mannino, S., & Milunsky, A. (1995). Teratogenicity of high vitamin A intake. *New England Journal of Medicine, 333*(21), 1369–1373.

Schebendach, M., & Reichert-Anderson, P. (2004). Nutrition in eating disorders. In L. Mahan & S. Escott-Stump (Eds.), *Krause's food, nutrition and diet therapy* (11th ed., pp. 594–615). Philadelphia: Saunders.

Scholl, T. O., Hediger, M. L., & Schall, J. I. (1997). Maternal growth and fetal growth: Pregnancy course and outcome in the Camden Study. *Annals of the New York Academy of Science, 817,* 292–301.

Scott, D. T., Janowsky, J. S., Carroll, R. E., Taylor, J. A., Auestad, N., & Montalto, M. B. (1998). Formula supplementation with long-chain polyunsaturated fatty acids: Are there developmental benefits? *Pediatrics, 102*(5), E59.

Selhub, J. (2006). The many facets of hyperhomocysteinemia: Studies from the Framingham cohorts. *Journal of Nutrition, 136*(Suppl. 6), 1726S–1730S.

Shabert, J. K. (2004). Nutrition during pregnancy and lactation. In L. Mahan & S. Escott-Stump (Eds.), *Krause's food, nutrition, and diet therapy* (11th ed., pp. 182–213). Philadelphia: Saunders.

Spear, B. (2004). Nutrition in adolescence. In L. Mahan & S. Escott-Stump (Eds.), *Krause's food, nutrition, and diet therapy* (11th ed., pp. 284–301). Philadelphia: Saunders.

Story, M., Neumark-Sztainer, D., Sherwood, N., Stang, J., & Murray, D. (1998). Dieting status and its relationship to eating and physical activity behaviors in a representative sample of US adolescents. *Journal of the American Dietetic Association, 98*(10), 1127–1135, 1255.

Suitor, C. W. (1997). *Maternal weight gain: A report of an expert work group.* Arlington, VA: National Center for Education in Maternal and Child Health.

Teratology Society. (1987). Teratology Society position paper: Recommendations for vitamin A use during pregnancy. *Teratology, 35*(2), 269–275.

Thom, T., Haase, N., Rosamond, W., Howard, V. J., et al. (2006). Heart disease and stroke statistics—2006 update: A report from the American Heart Association Statistics Committee and Stroke Statistics Subcommittee. *Circulation, 113*(6), 85–151.

Timbo, B. B., Ross, M. P., McCarthy, P. V., & Lin, C. (2006). Dietary supplements in a national survey: Prevalence of use and reports of adverse events. *Journal of the American Dietetic Association, 106*(12), 1966–1974.

Tsunenobu, T., & Picciano, M. F. (2006). Folate and human reproduction. *American Journal of Clinical Nutrition, 83*(5), 993–1016.

Tucker, K. L., Morita, K., Qiao, N., Hannan, M. T., Cupples, L. A., & Kiel, D. P. (2006). Colas, but not other carbonated beverages, are associated with low bone mineral density in older women: The Framingham Osteoporosis Study. *Am J Clin Nutr, 84*(4), 936–942.

U.S. Department of Agriculture. *MyPyramid.* Retrieved January 26, 2007, from http://www.mypyramid.gov

U.S. Department of Health and Human Services and U.S. Department of Agriculture. (2005). *Dietary guidelines for Americans* (6th ed.). Washington, DC: U.S. Government Printing Office. Retrieved January 29, 2007, from http://www.health.gov/dietaryguidelines

U.S. Food and Drug Administration. (2004). *What you need to know about mercury in fish and shellfish.* Retrieved January 18, 2007, from http://www.cfsan.fda.gov/~dms/admehg3.html

Villamor, E., & Cnattiquis, S. (2006). Interpregnancy weight change and risk of adverse pregnancy outcomes: A population-based study. *Lancet, I*(9542), 1164–1170.

Willett, W. C. (2006). Trans fatty acids and cardiovascular disease—Epidemiological data. *Atherosclerosis Supplements, 7*(2), 5–8.

Wren, A. M., Seal, L. J., Cohen, M. A., et al (2001). Ghrelin enhances appetite and increases food intake in humans. *Journal of Clinical Endocrinology and Metabolism, 86,* 5992–5995.

12

Healthy Practices: Exercise Interventions

Cheryl A. Cahill Lawrence

Regular physical exercise is an essential component of a healthy lifestyle (*Physical Activity and Health,* 1999). In 1999, a report submitted by the Surgeon General of the United States stated that significant health benefits were derived by daily moderate exercise. Benefits include reduced risk of premature mortality, coronary heart disease, hypertension, colon cancer, diabetes, and enhanced psychological well-being. Evaluation of the exercise habits of women should be a part of any health assessment, and interventions to maximize exercise benefits should be included in health care plans.

EXERCISE AND CARDIOVASCULAR RISK FACTORS

In the United States, cardiovascular disease is the leading cause of death (Rosamond et al., 2007). Causes for the high incidence of cardiovascular disease have been laid at the feet of the U.S. lifestyle that is sedentary, includes diets that are high in saturated fat, and obesity. Lack of physical activity and an increase in obesity is epidemic even among U.S. children (Kirk, Scott, & Daniels, 2005; Warburton, Nicol, & Bredin, 2006; Wormald, Waters, Sleap, & Ingle, 2006). Many argue that altering the lifestyles of Americans could reduce deaths due cardiovascular disease. Increasing physical activity is one change in the U.S. lifestyle that could make a profound difference in this statistic.

Several investigators have examined the relationship between activity levels and cardiovascular risk factors in apparently healthy individuals. Cardiovascular risk factors include elevated serum total cholesterol (TC) and LDL-C (low-density lipoprotein) cholesterol, low HDL-C (high-density lipoprotein) cholesterol, elevated blood pressure, cigarette smoking, diabetes mellitus, and age. Contributing risk factors include family history of early onset coronary heart disease, physical inactivity, obesity, abdominal obesity, and psychosocial factors. Several other biological markers associated with possible increased risk for cardiovascular disease include elevated serum triglycerides, small LDL particles, elevated homocysteine, elevated lipoprotein (a), thrombotic factors, and inflammatory markers (Pearson, 2002). Endurance exercise improves the vasculature of the heart and skeletal muscles, lowers blood pressure, and alters lipid levels in the blood. Genetic and gender differences, intensity and frequency of exercise, and patterns of physical activity over time influence the extent of these changes (D'Eon & Braun, 2002; Shaw et al., 2006; Zehnder et al., 2005).

Assessment of Cardiovascular Risk in Women

Several assessment tools are available to clinicians to compute risk severity. Most clinicians base estimates of risk assessment on algorithms derived from the Framingham Heart study (U.S. Department of Health and Human Services, 2001). Instruments based on the Framingham Study permit clinicians to quantify the risk of future cardiovascular events for individuals. That score can then be compared with stratified risk of an event occurring within 5 years. Several calculators are available on the Internet (National Cholesterol Education Program, 2007b). The indices used to calculate risk of a cardiovascular event occurring within 5 years are: age, gender, total cholesterol levels, high density cholesterol levels, tobacco smoking, systolic blood pressure, and current use of antihypertensive drugs. Tables specifying risk are available (National Cholesterol Education Program, 2007a). Risk is reported in percent probability of experiencing an event and ranges from a low-risk score of 1% to more than 30%. Separate tables are available for men and women (National Cholesterol Education Program, 2007a).

Several investigators have reported that risk assessment using the Framingham norms are not accurate for women, those in lower socioeconomic brackets, and some international populations (Brindle et al., 2005; Lloyd-Jones, Liu, Tian, & Greenland, 2006; Matthews et al., 2005). For women, an alternative clinical tool has recently been validated by Ridker and colleagues (2007) that is purported to give a more accurate assessment of cardiovascular risk. The Reynolds Risk Score is calculated using a brief interactive instrument and bases the computed 10-year risk based on age, smoking, C-reactive protein levels, cholesterol levels, and family history (*Reynolds Risk Score,* 2007). The normative data were generated through the Woman's Health Study. Data from 24,558 women over 45 years of age who were followed for a median time of 10.2 years were used to calculate risk and to stratify it into risk categories. The authors argue that the criteria used to assign risk by the Reynolds Risk Score algorithm are superior to Framingham-based risk scores because application of the Reynolds score resulted in 40% of the participants' reassignment to either greater or lower risk categories. The Reynolds Risk Score is a new clinical instrument that has not been widely used, but the simplicity of use and apparent validity may prove it to be useful.

Biological Markers of Cardiovascular Disease

Recent reports suggest that biologic markers of inflammation and exercise testing increase the accuracy of estimates of cardiovascular risk. Novel biological markers that seem to have some prognostic value for women are C-reactive protein (CRP) and interleulin-6 (IL-6). Both are markers of inflammation.

Inflammation of the vascular wall has been associated with atherosclerotic changes in arteries. C-reactive protein (CRP) is a component of acute inflammation (Bruce, 2005; Koh, Han, & Quon, 2005; Libby, 2006; Napoli et al., 2006; Paffen & DeMaat, 2006). Several studies have examined the relationship between high-sensitivity C-reactive protein (hsCRP) and cardiovascular events including myocardial infarction and stroke (Boekholdt et al., 2006; Koenig et al., 2006). Recent review articles and reports of meta-analyses of published data suggest that hsCRP levels are of minimal or no predictive value (Lloyd-Jones et al., 2006; Paffen & DeMaat, 2006). Boekholdt and colleagues (2006) completed a prospective population study of the relationship

between hsCRP and cardiovascular risk for 25,663 men and women between 45 and 79 years of age. HsCRP levels were among the strongest predictors of a coronary artery event (coronary thrombosis or stroke) or mortality. Furthermore, the Shaw group has reported that hsCRP improved the accuracy of predictions related to risk for cardiovascular events within 5 years. Both the American Heart association and the Centers for Disease Control recommend obtaining hsCRP for those individuals with one or more reported risk factor. While the data are inconsistent regarding the usefulness of hsCRP in predicting cardiovascular risk, it is clear that diagnosis and management of cardiovascular disease in perimenopausal women is clinically difficult. Thus, risk assessment in women may require more testing than that needed to diagnose men.

Resting electrocardiogram (ECG) is a common measure used to identify cardiac pathology even in individuals who are asymptomatic. Resting ECG is rarely diagnostic of cardiovascular risk. In men, exercise ECG or stress testing reveals cardiovascular disease, but may provide an imprecise picture of the amount of ischemic heart disease (IHD) present in women. Data from the National Heart, Lung, and Blood Institute–sponsored Women's Ischemic Syndrome Evaluation study suggest that exercise duration is the best predictor of IHD in women (Shaw et al., 2006). Exercise testing is expensive and is not a recommended component of general cardiovascular risk assessment for individuals who report no symptoms of coronary disease. Alternative measures have been proposed to assess women who are asymptomatic but who are at risk for cardiovascular disease. They include exercise tolerance or endurance and assessment of the woman's ability to perform activities of daily living (D'Amore & Mora, 2006; Shaw et al., 2006). Because risk of cardiovascular disease increases in women after menopause, age is an important risk factor to assess. Other factors that contribute to increased risk of cardiovascular disease include obesity (especially abdominal obesity), insulin-resistance, and diabetes. Furthermore, women who experience medically induced menopause at a young age or early menopause may be at risk at a younger age. Most normative tables take age into consideration, but not age of menopause. A detailed discussion of tools and clinical interventions beyond exercise is outside the scope of this work. More information about the accuracy of the Framingham-based instruments is available in articles by Brindle, Boswick, Fahey, and Ebrahim (2006) and Brindle and colleagues (2005).

Comprehensive assessment of cardiovascular risk is a key element of a health care strategy of disease prevention. Several of the risk factors associated with cardiovascular disease are modifiable by lifestyle changes. They include dietary modifications to reduce total cholesterol levels, weight, and triglyceride levels.

Increased physical activity and diet combine to manage weight, and exercise has a direct effect on lipid metabolism, blood pressure regulation, and glycemic control. However, lifestyle modification therapies are difficult to maintain. Current clinical practices urge early, aggressive treatment of plasma lipid levels with medications, increased physical activity, weight reduction, and diet in individuals at high risk of a cardiovascular event. For those in lower risk categories, diet, weight reduction, and exercise are the usual treatments. Increased endurance exercise is a key element of interventions to reduce cardiovascular risk.

Endurance exercise involves the repetitive use of large muscles over time. Intensity and duration of the exercise modifies the physiologic effect of the activity, but, overall, the expected outcome is greater endurance for activity. Cardiovascular and skeletal muscle adaptations to increased demand are responsible for increased endurance. Cardiovascular adaptations are associated with increased capacity to deliver oxygen and nutrients to the working muscles and removal of waste products of metabolism (Campos et al., 2002; DiPietro, Dziura, Yeckel, & Neufer, 2006; Motohiro et al., 2005; Stisen et al., 2006). As muscle activity increases, the demand for oxygen increases and the amount of carbon dioxide to be excreted increases. To meet these increased demands, blood flow to the lung increases. Respiratory rate increases to increase ventilation of the alveoli. At the same time, the oxygen diffusion rate increases. Training—frequent sessions of repetitive endurance exercises—confers greater capacity to exercise because of increased efficiency in these mechanisms.

Measures of Cardiopulmonary Fitness

Cardiopulmonary fitness is a measure of exercise endurance. The most precise measure of an individual's cardiopulmonary fitness is the determination of maximal oxygen uptake (VO_2max). VO_2max is measured during strenuous exercise, contraindicated in some clinical populations, using sophisticated equipment that may not be available in clinical settings. Yet the direct measurement of oxygen uptake remains the most accurate and precise measure of cardiopulmonary capacity. The measured value may be compared to normative values based on age, gender, and usual level of activity, yielding an estimate of the individual's cardiopulmonary fitness level (Sports, 2007). Through a program of regular aerobic exercise, people can improve their VO_2max to equal or exceed predicted VO_2max.

To better understand the conceptual basis of this measure, consider the usual procedure used to capture the needed breath samples. The procedure is similar to the treadmill stress test used to identify cardiac pathology. Therefore, individual participants should first be assessed to rule out any obvious pathology that would interfere with performance of maximal exercise. Exercise testing of patients, those individuals with known or suspected coronary artery disease, must be done under the direct supervision of a cardiologist in a setting where emergent care is readily available. Discussion of diagnostic stress testing is beyond the scope of this chapter. The remainder of this discussion will relate to measurement of cardiopulmonary fitness for research purposes or as an assessment of a healthy individual's capacity to perform physical exercise.

Testing of apparently healthy individuals for research purposes may not require physician supervision; however, all research involving humans must be approved by human studies institutional review boards. Most institutional review boards have established guidelines to assure the safety of humans participating in exercise testing. A general rule would be that young individuals with no obvious sign of cardiovascular or pulmonary disease may be tested without physician supervision, but a plan for management of acute cardiopulmonary difficulties should be in place. All members of the research team should be certified in cardiopulmonary resuscitation methods. Research facilities within some institutions may include a human performance laboratory specifically designed to safely perform exercise tests as well. If available, these facilities should be used.

The primary investigator retains primary responsibility for participant safety and so is required to the best of his or her ability to rule out pathologies that could interfere with testing. The assessment should include resting heart rate and rhythms, respiratory rates, and systolic and diastolic blood pressure. If the exercise modality includes a treadmill or a bicycle, the individual should be free of neurological, bone, and joint pathology that could interfere with movements required to operate the instrument safely. Further, the person should be free of syncope or other balance issues that could result in falls.

The first step in the procedure once participant eligibility has been established is to estimate a measurable target for maximal exertion. The participant's age is used to estimate maximal heart rate. The formula used is 220 minus the individual's age. In the case of a 25-year-old woman, maximal heart rate would be 220 minus 25 or 195 beats per minute. An individual's ability to achieve and maintain maximal heart rate depends on his or her fitness level. Less fit individuals may not be able to achieve the calculated maximal heart rate.

Generally, electrodes to monitor heart rate are applied to provide feedback to the participant and to monitor cardiac activity. Participants hold a mouthpiece in their mouth or wear a mask that is attached to a gas analyzer. During the exercise session, the participant breathes through the gas analyzer. Several standardized exercise protocols are commonly used to achieve maximal exertion. Details of them are beyond the scope of this chapter. For more information, refer to handbooks and standards endorsed by the American College of Sports Medicine (Dwyer & Shala, 2005; Kaminsky & Kimberly, 2006). Differences in the methods relate to the speed at which the participant accelerates toward maximal achievable exertion, and so techniques may be selected based on the population under study.

Modern equipment permits breath-by-breath measurement of the rate of oxygen uptake or oxygen consumption (VO_2). As the individual reaches the point of exhaustion, the demand for oxygen exceeds the capacity to provide it. VO_2 reaches a plateau called maximal oxygen consumption (VO_2max) (Hawkins, Raven, Snell, Stray-Gundersen, & Levine, 2007). Because individuals with greater muscle mass have added capacity for oxygen consumption, VO_2 is normalized by dividing it by weight in kilograms. Therefore, VO_2max is expressed as milliliters of oxygen per minute per kilogram of body weight (ml/m/kg). Less fit individuals become fatigued and stop exercising before they reach that plateau. This point is called the VO_2 peak. Therefore, VO_2 peak is often used equivalently with VO_2max to indicate the oxygen consumption at the maximum workload *achievable*.

A number of protocols have been validated that estimate VO_2max values rather than directly respired gases. The procedures utilize direct measures of heart rate over time while following a prescribed exercise protocol. The VO_2max value is computed using standardized equations for the particular exercise protocol. The advantage of these tests is that they do not require costly gas analyzers (Noonan & Dean, 2000) and may be done in field settings.

In conducting research in populations unable to engage in vigorous maximal exercise, several less strenuous measures have been used to measure exercise capacity. These submaximal exercise tests include the Six-Minute and Twelve-Minute Walk Tests, the Self-Paced Walking Test, the Modified Shuttle Walking Test, the Bag and Carry Test, Time Up, and Go Test (Noonan & Dean, 2000). Each of these tests is designed to provide a measure of functional capacity that reflects exercise capacity. If one is unable to exercise or has limited capacity to work, she or he will perform less well on the functional tasks. For clinicians interested in an individual's abilities to carry out activities of daily living in the face of loss of fitness, these tests may be useful in the clinical assessment and monitoring. Researchers interested in evaluating interventions that enhance abilities to perform activities of daily living have used these measures.

The Six-Minute Walk Test and the Twelve-Minute Walk Test are methods to quantify exercise tolerance (Camarri, Eastwood, Cecins, Thompson, & Jenkins, 2006; Grindrod, Paton, Knez, & O'Brien, 2006; Jonsdottir, Andersen, Sigurosson, & Sigurosson, 2006).

Individuals are asked to walk on a premeasured circuit for 6 or 12 minutes. The total distance covered is used as an indicator of capacity to exercise. The method has been used in clinical populations with known cardiopulmonary limitations (Jonsdottir et al., 2006; Reardon, Lareau, & ZuWallack, 2006), aged individuals (Camarri et al., 2006), and individuals with neurological impairments (Courbon et al., 2006; Patterson et al., 2007). The Modified Shuttle Test is similar to timed walk tests except that the investigator or tester controls the pace of the walk. Participants are told to walk at a comfortable pace over a premeasured course and instructed to turn around and walk back toward the beginning when signaled. The required speed to complete one lap is increased over repeated trials. The test continues until the individual experiences breathlessness. The more fit an individual, the more trials they will complete and the faster they will walk. A similar test is the Self-Paced Walking Test, in which participants are asked to walk at three speeds: slow, moderate, and quick. Presumably, those who are more fit will choose a higher rate at all levels than those who are not and will cover longer distances during each trial. The Bag and Carry Test requires the individual to carry a package across a specified course and up and down a four-step set of stairs. After successful completion of each trial, the weight of the package is increased. The test ends when the participant is unable to carry the package over the course. The final maximum weight is recorded as the result of the test. None of these tests provides an empirical estimate of cardiovascular fitness as indicated by oxygen consumption, but they do reflect limitations in function associated with reduced aerobic capacity.

Although all of the aforementioned tests are useful for research purposes, clinicians may use them to evaluate the effectiveness of a program of exercise intended to improve cardiovascular fitness. Evidence is emerging that moderate exercise improves cardiopulmonary fitness and that the time spent in moderate activity per session is not as critical as the total time spent per day. Furthermore, incidental walking and other sorts of exercise that a person does in the course of the day contribute to fitness. Therefore, simply asking an individual how much they exercise may not provide the full picture. Clinicians may use one of the functional capacity methods to evaluate cardiopulmonary capacity to establish a baseline of performance and subsequently to detect improvements or diminishing capacity.

Exercise and Cardiovascular Disease Risk Reduction

Exercise is an effective intervention to prevent cardiovascular disease and as a therapy to restore and enhance function when cardiovascular disease is present.

Fewer cardiovascular risk factors have been observed in women and in men who exercise regularly (Murphy, Murtagh, Boreham, Hare, & Nevill, 2006; Palaniappan et al., 2002; Zahner et al., 2006). Fewer cardiovascular risk factors associated with regular exercise are due to the direct effects on the heart and vascular bed as well as the effects on lipid metabolism, glucose metabolism, and body composition (Belza & Warms, 2004; Stewart, Ouyang, Bacher, Lima, & Shapiro, 2006; Tune, Richmond, Gorman, & Feigl, 2002).

Epidemiological studies demonstrate a strong association between regular physical exercise and lower risk of cardiovascular illness (Belza & Warms, 2004; Boreham et al., 2004; Franco, Oparil, & Carretero, 2004; Reynolds & He, 2005). Cohort and longitudinal studies have been undertaken to validate the relationship (Belza & Warms, 2004; Boreham et al., 2004; Franco et al., 2004; Reynolds & He, 2005; Shaw et al., 2006). The evidence is incomplete regarding the amount, type, and intensity of exercise required to reduce cardiovascular risk, but some studies provide guidance for clinicians. However, effective interventions have not been reported that sustain increased physical activity for long-term effects on cardiovascular risk. Adherence to interventions requiring lifestyle modifications remains a challenge.

Regular exercise contributes to lower weight and has a direct effect on resting blood pressure and heart rate. Other risk factors are not amenable to intervention. Family history and the genetic consequences of that cannot be changed. While absolute chronological age cannot be changed, some of the consequences of aging may be delayed or mitigated by exercise. Therefore, simply increasing physical activity levels could have a potent effect on cardiovascular risk.

The effect of age on cardiovascular risk is different in men and women. Prior to menopause, the prevalence of coronary artery disease is rare among women; however, by age 70 the prevalence is the same for men and women (Shaw et al., 2006). The effects of estrogen prior to menopause seem to confer some cardiovascular protection, although cigarette smoking appears to reduce that effect. Women are less likely to engage in endurance exercise as they age. Thus, as they approach menopause and become more vulnerable to cardiovascular disease, they are less physically active, perhaps contributing to the rapid development of cardiovascular disease. Interventions to support healthy diets, weight management, and physical exercise in younger women and in girls, therefore, are important for long-term health. Fortunately, cultural attitudes have changed over the past 20 years, and more girls are involved in sports. But participation in organized sports does not guarantee lifelong exercise patterns that are required to prevent cardiovascular disease.

Gender differences in the cardiovascular system result in differences in vulnerability to disease, symptoms experienced associated with disease states, and responses to exercise. Women have smaller hearts and major blood vessels (Huxley, 2007). Consequently, there are differences in homeostatic responses between men and women. Because women have smaller hearts, the amount of blood expelled during each contraction of the heart is smaller, resulting in lower cardiac output. To compensate for lower cardiac output, women tend to have a higher resting heart rate than men. Homeostatic mechanisms expressed during exercise and in response to other cardiovascular stresses differ between men and women. In response to acute demands for greater blood flow, the autonomic nervous system is activated. The sympathetic nervous system activation causes the heart rate to increase and cardiac muscle contractility to increase, resulting in increased stroke volume. In the peripheral vasculature, autonomic arousal causes vasoconstriction, resulting in increased total peripheral resistance or increased blood pressure. The parasympathetic nervous system helps to slow the heart, allowing for more adequate filling of the ventricles with blood and thus maintaining adequate stroke volume. Women exhibit less robust sympathetic nervous system responses than men and rely more heavily on parasympathetic mechanisms to maintain homeostasis (Huxley, 2007). Differences in these compensatory mechanisms influence disease development and vulnerabilities. For example, women are more prone to orthostatic hypotension after vigorous exercise, prolonged standing, and return to gravity from outer space. Men are more likely to develop hypertension in response to vascular remodeling related to increased peripheral resistance. Furthermore, the effects of exercise on cardiovascular risk are different.

Cardiopulmonary fitness is associated with lower resting heart rate and blood pressure. A program of regular exercise has direct effects on cardiac muscle stamina and on the vasculature of the heart muscle. During exercise, the heart muscle as well as skeletal muscle require increased blood flow to meet the demands for oxygen and nutrients and for elimination of waste products. Blood flow is increased in two ways. Immediately, blood vessels expand to carry a larger volume of blood. Over the long term, regular exercise stimulates the expansion of the capillary bed to increase tissue perfusion (Prior, Lloyd, Yang, & Terjung, 2003; Prior, Yang, & Terjung, 2004).

Repeated and regular cardiopulmonary training induces remodeling of the vasculature of the heart and other blood vessels. Structural changes in blood vessels involve a number of complex mechanisms that result in enlargement of existing arteries and generation of new capillaries. Arteriogenesis is the term used to describe enlargement of existing arterial vessels. Enlargement is not the simple dilation of the vessel but rather remodeling of the endothelium, resulting in a larger lumen.

Angiogenesis is the formation of new capillaries from existing ones. Two distinct processes are involved in development of new capillaries. Capillary intussusception is the process by which one capillary splits to form two capillaries. Sprouting angiogenesis entails activated endothelial cells within existing capillaries extending through the existing structure to form a cord-like structure that develops into a new capillary. Adaptation to exercise includes increased capillarity in large muscles (Prior et al., 2004).

Furthermore, exercise training contributes to the maintenance of arterial compliance or elasticity. The aging process includes stiffening of the walls of the arteries, resulting in increased peripheral resistance to blood flow (Jani & Rajkumar, 2006). Increased resistance to blood flow is manifested as higher blood pressure. Elevated peripheral resistance increases the work of the heart and contributes to cardiovascular risk. Thus, regular endurance exercise is an important intervention to maintain cardiovascular health. Exercise enhances the health of the myocardium, improves blood flow, and maintains the elasticity of the blood vessels—resulting in lower resting heart rate, more rapid return to resting heart rate after stress and exercise, and keeping blood pressure low by maintaining vascular elasticity.

Clearly, prevention of cardiovascular disease in individuals with little or no existing risk is the easiest and most effective approach to overall reduction in morbidity and mortality due to heart disease. Programs of exercise have been shown to reduce risk factors, including hypertension, hyperlipidemia, and obesity for people with known risk of cardiovascular disease.

Exercise and Blood Pressure

The relationship between cardiovascular fitness and blood pressure has been investigated in a number of ways. Barlow et al. (2006) reported that level of fitness as measured by maximal stress test was predictive of the development of hypertension in a group of 4,884 women followed for 28 years. Similar findings were reported by Kokkinos and colleagues (2006). In this study, blood pressure was monitored for 24 hours in men and women with systolic blood pressures between 120 mmHg and 139 mmHg and diastolic blood pressures between 80 mmHg and 89 mmHg. The cardiovascular fitness level was measured and the group stratified into three fitness categories (low, medium, and high). A strong inverse relationship between 24-hour blood pressure and fitness levels was observed for both men and women. The investigators concluded that moderate physical exercise would be sufficient to prevent progression to hypertension in this vulnerable population.

In addition to gender differences, practitioners should consider ethnicity in evaluating blood pressure

and exercise treatments (Bond et al., 2005). A group of African Americans who demonstrated exaggerated blood pressure response to exercise were studied. Exaggerated blood pressure responses are thought to be predictive of the development of hypertension. Seven African American women between 18 and 26 years of age were studied. Participants were selected because they demonstrated at least a 50 mmHg difference in systolic blood pressure at rest and during exercise at 50% peak oxygen uptake (VO_2peak). Participants completed an 8-week bicycle ergometer training program. At the end of the treatment program, blood pressure increases associated with exercise were diminished, and the group demonstrated increased exercise capacity. The results suggest that increased fitness is associated with better arterial compliance. Again, the intervention studied is intensive and requires commitment to be sustained. Persons at risk for hypertension are usually sedentary and do not choose to exercise. Staffileno and colleagues (2007) have investigated a more acceptable strategy and one that has a greater chance of being effective over the long term. The intervention in this study consisted of an individualized home-based program. The participants were 24 African American women between the ages of 18 and 45 years. Participants had blood pressures that were considered prehypertensive or stage 1 hypertension. They were randomized to either the exercise group or the no exercise group. The exercise intervention consisted of instructions to walk or climb stairs or other lifestyle compatible exercise that was sufficient to increase heart rate prescribed level for 10 minutes three times per day for 5 days per week. The no exercise group was instructed to continue with their usual level of activity. After 8 weeks, the exercise group had significant reductions in systolic and diastolic blood pressure. Although the sample size is small, the effectiveness of multiple, short bouts of exercise suggest a promising approach to increasing exercise levels in sedentary individuals.

A meta-analysis of clinical trial research designed to explore the effects of exercise on blood pressure indicated that a program of aerobic exercise resulted in lowered systolic and diastolic blood pressure in both normotensive and hypertensive individuals (Whelton, Chin, Xin, & He, 2002). Although interesting, the 54 studies included in the analysis did not use a common exercise program, so the analysis could not reveal optimal exercise regimens. Furthermore, most studies are of limited duration so the long-term effects of exercise were not evident. However, the American College of Sports Medicine has published a position statement on hypertension and the role of exercise as a prime preventive strategy. Based on the currently available data, the following exercise prescription is proposed for those with hypertension:

Frequency: on most, preferably all, days of the week.

Intensity: moderate intensity (40% to < 60% of VO₂R).

Time: 30 minutes of continuous or accumulated physical activity per day.

Type: primarily endurance physical activity supplemented by resistance exercise. (Pescatello et al., 2004, p. 533)

EFFECTS OF EXERCISE ON METABOLISM

Exercise has been shown to affect both glucose and lipid metabolism. The demands of working muscles are met by increased glucose utilization and lipid mobilization. Furthermore, individuals who are fit and exercise regularly are leaner and generally have better plasma lipid profiles than those who do not.

Exercise Effects on Lipid Metabolism

Two major forms of cholesterol are of concern to clinicians: low-density lipoprotein cholesterol (LDL-C) and high-density lipoprotein cholesterol (HDL-C). Total cholesterol (TC) content of plasma is the sum total of LDL-C and HDL-C. Recent research has demonstrated the elemental role LDL-C has in the development of cardiovascular disease. Biochemists have identified a number of LDL-cholesterol structures that participate in plaque formation, but total LDL-C measures are the clinical markers used to assess overall risk. As a category, these lipoproteins bind to specific receptors on the intima of the arteries and disrupt smooth muscle growth. The net effect is histological transformation of the normal intima to an atheroma. The HDL-C, on the other hand, is protective of the cardiovascular system. These molecules bind to specific receptors in the liver and facilitate removal of cholesterol from peripheral tissues. The proportion of HDL-C to TC levels is inversely proportional to the risk of cardiovascular disease. That is, the greater the percentage of TC that is of HDL-C, the lower the risk of cardiovascular disease. In 2001, the third report of the National Cholesterol Education Program was released (U.S. Department of Health and Human Services, 2001). The expert panel concluded that LDL-C was a critical clinical factor to be considered in making decisions about treatment for hypercholesteremia, marking a shift in the way clinicians should evaluate cholesterol profiles and treatment. Early intervention by modification of dietary intake of cholesterol and saturated fats will help to lower cholesterol levels and lower weight. Investigators compared plasma lipid profiles to the histologic characteristics of atheroma in individuals undergoing coronary artery bypass grafting (Craig et al., 1999). The findings were consistent with the presumption that high LDL-C, low HCL-C, and elevated fasting blood glucose was associated with plaque formation. Persons with high LDL-C or those with multiple cardiovascular risk factors will be treated with drugs to lower cholesterol levels. Exercise is an important component of therapy because, unlike some drugs, exercise induces increases in HDL-C cholesterol.

Evaluation of plasma lipid levels is an important variable in identifying persons at risk to develop cardiovascular disease. Table 12.1 summarizes the findings of the National Cholesterol Education Program's Expert Panel on Detection, Evaluation and Treatment of High Cholesterol in Adults (U.S. Department of Health and Human Services, 2001). In this report, recommended

12.1 | Recommended Cholesterol Norms

	OPTIMAL	NEAR /ABOVE OPTIMAL	BORDERLINE HIGH	HIGH	VERY HIGH
Total cholesterol	< 200 mg/dL[a]	n.a.	200 mg/dL to 239 mg/dL	≥ 240 mg/dL	n.a.
Low-density lipoproteins	≤ 130 mg/dL	100 mg/dL to 129 mg/dL	130 mg/dL to 159	160 mg/dL to 189 mg/dL	≥ 190 mg/d/L
High-density lipoproteins[b]	≥ 60 mg/dL[b]			≤ 40 mg/dL	

Note. These values are taken from the *Third Report of the Expert Panel on Detection, Evaluation, and Treatment of High Blood Cholesterol in Adults (Adult Treatment Panel III),* by U.S. Department of Health and Human Services, National Cholesterol Education Program, 2001, http://www.nhlbi.nih.gov/guidelines/cholesterol/atglance.htm. In this edition (November 19, 2002), greater emphasis has been placed on the impact of LDL cholesterol level on cardiovascular disease risk.
[a] Premenopausal women and men 35 years of age or younger.
[b] Higher concentrations of high-density lipoprotein cholesterol are associated with lower risk of cardiovascular disease.

lipid levels for premenopausal women and men younger than 35 years are lower than for older men and postmenopausal women. The report strongly encourages all clinicians to evaluate exercise patterns and other lifestyle risk factors for cardiovascular disease. The inclusion of regular exercise is key to prevention and treatment of hyperlipidemia, but is not a cure for critically high levels of lipoproteins in blood. Optimal blood levels should be viewed as levels to be maintained by exercise and diet rather than as therapeutic outcomes of a new or more rigorous program. The panel concluded that blood lipid protein levels are one of many risk factors to be weighed when determining an individual's treatment plan.

LDL-C is the critical factor. The panel recommended a substantive change in the way that clinicians evaluate cardiovascular risk and treatment selection. On the Web site of the National Institute of Heart Lung and Blood, clinicians will find the *Adult Treatment Panel III (ATP III) At-A-Glance: Quick Desk Reference* (http://www.nhlbi.nih.gov/guidelines/cholesterol/dskref.htm), which contains the new guidelines for assessment of lipidemia and recommended standards of care and criteria that may be used to make decisions about drug treatment. LDL-C is the critical factor in determining long-term risk of cardiovascular disease. The categories for evaluation of LDL-C have been expanded to five from three. Optimal levels of LDL-C are below 100 mg/dL. Levels higher than that warrant further evaluation. Clinicians should ascertain the presence or degree of coronary heart disease present and evaluate other major risk factors, including smoking, hypertension, low HDL-C, family history of coronary heart disease, and age. Clinicians should then assess the 10-year risk category based on the Framingham table (U.S. Department of Health and Human Services, 2001). Treatment should be started in those individuals with LDL-C concentration of equal to or greater than 100 mg/dL *and* Coronary Heart Disease (CHD) *or* equal to or greater than 20% 10-year risk of CHD based on the Framingham table. Those persons with LDL-C concentrations of 130 mg/dL *and* two or more risk factors *or* equal to or greater than 20% 10-year risk of CHD based on the Framingham table should be treated as well. Treatment options include lifestyle changes to reduce LDL-C and drugs that reduce total cholesterol. Three elements of the Therapeutic Lifestyle Change (TLC) program are diet, weight control, and increased exercise. Drug therapy should be initiated if TLC fails to lower or maintain LDL-C concentrations below 130 mg/dL.

Studies in both women and men demonstrate that a program of moderate exercise maintained over time effectively lowers blood cholesterol levels. Kelley, Kelly, and Tran (2005) reported the results of a meta-analysis of studies conducted between 1955 and 2003 of aerobic exercise effects on lipid profiles in women. The analysis revealed that triglyceride levels, total cholesterol, and LDL-C were lowered by exercise, while HDL-C increased. However, the studies were of relatively short duration and used a variety of exercise protocols. Despite the limitations of the meta-analytic methodology, the results provide direction for clinicians relative to the effectiveness of aerobic exercise to control lipidemia.

Studies of the long-term effects of exercise are rare due to the challenges of retaining participants and the cost of longitudinal studies. However, Kemmler and colleagues (2004) reported on the effects of a 26-month program of exercise on lipid profiles in early postmenopausal women. Fifty women participated in the exercise intervention, and 33 women were in the nonexercising control group. The intervention consisted of two group training sessions and two training sessions completed at home per week for 26 months. At the end of the study, TC levels for the women in the exercise group decreased by 5% from baseline, while the TC levels for the nonexercising women increased by 4.1%. The effects on triglycerides were even more remarkable: the exercise group experienced a 14% decrease, while the nonexercising control group's triglycerides levels increased by 23%. These results not only demonstrate the potency of exercise in preventing increases in cardiovascular risk factors. They also indicate how rapidly these changes occur after menopause.

Ardern et al. (2004) reported on the relationship between exercise-induced changes in lipid profiles in a large group of men and women of diverse ethnicity. The authors found no differences in exercise-related changes due to gender or to race, but that body fat was a powerful mediator. At baseline, higher TC, LDL-C, and triglycerides levels were associated with higher body fat. Furthermore, the positive effects of exercise, lowered total cholesterol, LDL-C, and triglycerides were greater in those individuals who lost weight as well as exercised.

The challenge for clinicians is to prescribe a program of exercise of sufficient intensity and duration to positively affect lipid metabolism, but is also acceptable to the client. Lifestyle modification is difficult for most people to adhere to and to maintain. Thus, several investigators have explored lifestyle–compatible exercise programs. Boreham and colleagues (2004) evaluated the effects of stair climbing on blood lipid levels in a group of sedentary young women. Participants in the exercise group walked up flights of stairs daily. The numbers of flights of stairs climbed per day progressed from one during week 1 to five flights during week 7. Compared to the control group, who continued their usual level of activity, the experimental group exhibited a 5% reduction in LDL-C at the end of the study. There were no statistically significant differences in TC, HDL-C, or triglycerides levels. Failure to show statistical significance is not surprising in young women with fairly healthy lipid profiles at baseline. Furthermore, the sample size was small and the effect may not be robust enough to be detected in this sample. The significant reduction in TC along with improved VO$_2$max suggests that repeated episodes of endurance-type exercise can have a therapeutic effect. Integrating activities such as stair climbing may be more acceptable and therefore a more effective intervention than treadmill work, aerobic dance, or bicycling for sedentary individuals.

The degree to which exercise effectively reduces cholesterol depends on the state of the individual at the outset of the therapy. Individuals with the worst lipid profiles have the greatest need for improvement and respond rather quickly to intervention. However, significant improvement in very high-risk individuals may take several months. Ideally, TC levels should be maintained below 200 mg/dL with a high percentage of HDL-C. Triglycerides and LDL-C levels should be reduced as much as possible. Estrogen levels play an important role in modifying lipid metabolism, particularly related to HDL-C production (see Table 12.1). Sex steroid levels, primarily estrogen, mediate sex differences in lipid metabolism. Premenopausal women have higher concentrations of HDL-C than age-matched men. Women who smoke effectively eliminate any positive effect of estrogen on cholesterol levels and increase their risk of cardiovascular disease to that of men. Postmenopausal women have cholesterol profiles similar to those of men. Since progesterone levels influence lipid metabolism, increased risk of cardiovascular disease has been associated with the use of high-dose progesterone contraceptive pills. Reformulation of oral contraceptives to contain lower doses of progesterone has eliminated risks previously associated with use of the pill. Women who take high doses of progesterone are at risk to develop hypercholesterolemia. Nurses and other health care providers should monitor plasma lipid levels and encourage healthy lifestyles including regular moderate exercise (D'eon & Braun, 2002).

The importance of understanding the interaction among estrogen levels, lipid metabolism, and exercise is underscored by a study of 26 highly trained women athletes (Lamon-Fava et al., 1998). Very well-trained women are at risk for amenorrhea. The precise mechanisms underlying exercise-induced amenorrhea are not well understood, but amenorrheic women have low levels of estrogen. Nine of the women runners had exercise-induced amenorrhea. Normally menstruating women runners demonstrated significantly better lipid profiles than the control nonexercising women and the amenorrheic runners. Normally menstruating athletes had lower TC levels and higher HDL-C to TC ratios and lower LDL-C and triglyceride levels. In contrast, the amenorrheic runners demonstrated lipid profiles comparable to those of the nonexercising control group. They also demonstrated lower estradiol (a metabolite of estrogen) levels than the menstruating runners. Thus, amenorrhea accompanied by decreased endogenous estrogen negated the positive effects of strenuous exercise on lipids.

Effects of Exercise on Glucose Metabolism

Glucose utilization can increase as much as 20-fold over basal rates during exercise and accounts for 25% to 40% of the energy used. Despite this remarkable demand, exercise does not result in marked reduction in blood glucose levels. Increased demands for fuel by skeletal muscles during exercise are met by activation of several mechanisms to provide carbohydrates and fats as metabolic substrates. At the onset of exercise, the primary fuel used by the cell is stored glycogen. Because this reserve is limited, continued exercise requires that the supply of glycogen and glucose be replenished. An additional source of energy is supplied by the mobilization of lipids from adipose tissue for conversion to glucose and subsequent catabolism in the cell.

The liver plays a key role in the maintenance of adequate supplies of glucose during exercise. Initially, increased glucose is provided to the cells by increased production of glucose from hepatic stores of glycogen. These stores are limited, and prolonged exercise results in an accelerated rate of production of glycogen to replenish supplies. Gluconeogenesis utilizes pyruvate, lactate, and some amino acids to produce glycogen, which is then converted to glucose by glycogenolysis. Conversion of lipids and fatty acids to glucose and subsequent metabolism of it by the cell contributes to two major positive effects of exercise on reducing cardiovascular risk factors: weight loss and reduced plasma concentrations of lipoproteins and triglycerides.

Depletion of glycogen stores in both the muscles and the liver stimulates production of enzymes, which increase non–insulin-dependent uptake of glucose by skeletal muscle cells (Chibalin et al., 2000; Koval et al., 1999). Increased activity persists for up to 48 hours after strenuous exercise stops. Evidently, during this time, depleted cellular stores of glycogen are replenished. Highly trained athletes are reported to have lower resting insulin levels and enhanced tolerance to glucose loading, which may reflect increased use of noninsulin glucose utilization mechanisms.

At rest, glucose metabolism depends on adequate supplies of insulin. Exercise has been shown to increase glucose uptake by skeletal muscles (Arciero, Vukovich, Holloszy, Racette, & Kohrt, 1999; Koval et al., 1999) while plasma levels of insulin fall. Reductions in plasma insulin levels are related not only to increased non–insulin-dependent skeletal muscle uptake of glucose (thereby reducing the demand for insulin), but also because of increased insulin receptor activity. The combination of these two mechanisms facilitates delivery of glucose to the muscle cell; however, for the diabetic, special consideration must be given to maintenance of glucose metabolism during exercise.

Several investigators have considered exercise-induced changes in carbohydrate metabolism in the context of the pathophysiology of diabetes mellitus. Type 1 or insulin-dependent diabetes (IDDM) results from severe insulin deficiency associated with failure to produce insulin. Treatment requires supplementing endogenous insulin with various injected forms of the hormone. Adequate control of carbohydrate metabolism is difficult in IDDM. Increased non–insulin-dependent uptake of glucose consequent to vigorous exercise may require modification of the usual insulin dose (Draznin & Patel, 1998). The need for large amounts of glucagon during prolonged exercise presents several challenges in the care of individuals with IDDM as well. IDDM individuals usually have diminished glycogen stores. Dietary modification may also limit the availability of other carbohydrates, fats, and proteins for conversion to glycogen. In general, a reduction in insulin dosage and the added ingestion and continual availability of carbohydrates are wise precautions (Draznin & Patel, 1998). These aspects must be considered when prescribing or supervising a program of exercise for IDDM patients.

Type 2 or non–insulin-dependent diabetes mellitus (NIDDM) is associated with decreased availability of biologically active insulin. Treatment of this condition includes dietary regulation, weight loss, and oral hypoglycemic drugs. Several investigators have considered the effects of exercise on glucose metabolism in these individuals as possible preventive measures or treatments for NIDDM. The effect of exercise most intriguing to these investigators is the apparent effect of exercise in increasing insulin receptor activity. One characteristic of type 2 diabetes may be that the insulin receptor becomes insensitive or resistant to the effects of insulin. Increasing the activity of the receptor thus reduces resistance to insulin and normalizes insulin-mediated glucose metabolism (Chibalin et al., 2000; Koval et al., 1999). Arciero and colleagues (1999) explored this model in a small group of obese, hyperglycemic men and women. They reported a marked increase in glucose disposal after exercise training, despite lower insulin levels, suggesting that short-term exercise effectively enhances insulin action in individuals with abnormal glucose tolerance.

Childhood onset of type 2 diabetes was virtually unknown until the past several years. The epidemic of childhood obesity has resulted in the diagnosis of this disorder in children. A major risk factor for insulin resistance is abdominal obesity and a sedentary lifestyle (Aylin, Williams, & Bottle, 2005; Lee, Okumura, Davis, Herman, & Gurney, 2006). A discussion of childhood insulin resistance and diabetes 2 is beyond the scope of this chapter. However, parents shape a child's eating habits and lifestyle. Thus, clinicians caring for parents of overweight children could council them regarding the risks for future illness.

The Diabetes Prevention study was designed to evaluate the effectiveness of an intensive diet and exercise intervention in delaying or preventing type 2 diabetes. Five hundred and twenty-three overweight participants with impaired glucose tolerance were randomly assigned to a control group or an intervention group. Those in the intervention group received seven sessions about diet and received individualized guidance about increasing physical activity as ways of preventing diabetes. The control group received one session describing lifestyle modification that could prevent diabetes and were urged to have annual follow-up visits with their care provider. Preliminary evidence after 1 year demonstrated that the intervention group members lost weight, increased glucose tolerance, and improved lipid profiles. These data suggest that interventions aimed at lifestyle modifications can influence elements of cardiovascular risk associated with NIDDM (Eriksson et al., 1999).

Increasing endurance exercise could have a profound effect on the prevalence, morbidity, and mortality of cardiovascular disease. The challenge for clinicians is to prescribe a program of exercise that the client will follow. Lifestyle modification is a difficult process for most. Therefore, intervening early in life may be the most effective approach to preventing cardiovascular disease. Some strategies may be more palatable than others. Recent evidence that endurance exercise embedded within the usual daily activities have positive cumulative effects is promising. However, the most effective intervention is exercise paired with dietary control of fat and calories to maintain optimal weight.

EFFECTS OF EXERCISE ON BONES AND JOINTS

Weight-bearing exercise has been shown to play a significant role in the development and maintenance of the skeletal system. During growth, loads exerted by body weight and muscle forces model bone strength and mass. In young adulthood, these forces plateau and bones strengthen. Muscle strength wanes with age, inducing disuse loss of bone strength. Experiments conducted by NASA on the effects of weightlessness on muscle function and bone changes have demonstrated that even short periods of non–weight-bearing inactivity can result in profound demineralization of the bone. Loss of mineral content of bone (osteoporosis) has been associated with aging in both women and men, with a higher incidence among postmenopausal women (Sheth, 1999). Clinical problems associated with osteoporosis include greater incidence of fractures (particularly of the hip) and severe pain from osteoporosis of the spine.

Estrogen plays a significant role in maintenance of bone density. The mechanisms regulating the role of estrogen in the maintenance of bone density are not well understood. Animal studies suggest that estrogen influences the rate of bone turnover. Turner reported that ovariectomized rats experienced increased bone loss. Treadmill exercise reduced the rate of loss and immobility enhanced it. Administration of estrogen slowed the rate of bone turnover in the immobile rats and lowered the exercise load needed to reduce bone turnover in exercised rats (Turner, 1999). In women, aging is a well-characterized risk factor for bone loss. Women also are at risk for bone loss as their menstrual periods become irregular prior to menopause (see chapter 6). Women at risk include those who are athletes who experience training-related amenorrhea or menstrual irregularity (Green, Crouse, & Rohack, 1998). Grinspoon and colleagues (1999) compared bone density parameters in estrogen-deficient women with hypothalamic amenorrhea and women with anorexia nervosa. Both groups demonstrated significant bone loss. Bone density was less in the anorexic group. These data demonstrate the importance of estrogen in maintaining bone density but also illustrate the importance of nutrition.

In contrast, several investigators have investigated the efficacy of exercise in maintaining bone density in postmenopausal women. Studies of both aerobic and strength training exercise have been shown to prevent bone loss (Bemben, 1999). Strength training has the advantage of increasing coordination and balance as well as strength and may reduce risk of falls in elders. Lewis and Modlesky (1998) have argued that supplementing calcium and vitamin D intake in elders is an important adjunct to strength training or other exercise in prevention of osteoporosis. A National Institutes of Health Report on Osteoporosis Expert Panel (2001) concluded that "regular exercise, especially resistance and high-impact activities, contributes to development of high peak bone mass and may reduce risk of falls in older persons" (p. 785). However, there is scarce evidence that exercise alone can restore bone mass in women and men with osteoporosis.

Recent advances in drug therapy for osteoporosis provide clinicians with powerful tools to arrest bone loss. These drugs may be combined with exercise programs to minimize bone loss. Emphasis on strength training may be especially useful because of the benefits of added coordination and agility. Caution must be used when prescribing exercise for individuals with osteoporosis because of the increased risk of bone fracture. Also, consideration of strength and postural stability must be included when recommending increased activity for elderly or frail persons. Clinicians should keep in mind that, for exercise therapy to affect bone density, adequate nutritional intake of calcium and vitamin D must be assured. Individuals at risk for osteoporosis or those taking bone-building drugs should be supplementing their diets with one of several over-the-counter combined preparations available (Gass & Dawson-Hughes, 2006).

EFFECTS OF EXERCISE ON MOOD AND AFFECT

Regular aerobic exercise has positive effects on psychological factors such as well-being and depression. Positive effects have been reported in elders, women during the postpartum period and persons with chronic fatigue syndrome and arthritis (Clapp et al., 1999; Tsutsumi et al., 1998; Williams, Bullen, McArthur, Skrinar, & Turnbull, 1999). However, studies in highly trained individuals result in some fascinating paradoxical findings. Overtraining, as might be required for endurance athletes, has been reported to be associated with mood disturbances. Further, some individuals may become "addicted" to vigorous exercise (Scully, Kremer, Meade, Graham, & Dudgeon, 1998).

Recently, there has been greater interest in the effects of exercise on mood and affect. Improved mood may motivate some to engage in exercise. Sakuragi and Sugiyama (2006) evaluated mood at baseline and following a 4-week program of walking. The intervention was sufficiently robust to induce statistically significant increases in VO$_2$max. Mood significantly improved with a lower score on the anger and hostility scale of the Profile of Mood States. Sarsan, Ardic, Ozgen, Topuz, and Sermez (2006) reported a significant reduction in scores on the Beck's Depression Inventory in a group of obese women after a 12-week training period. The mechanistic bases for the change in mood are not known, but, when supporting individuals through lifestyle modification interventions, quantifying affective changes could be used to motivate continuation in the program.

EXERCISE, THE MENSTRUAL CYCLE, AND PREGNANCY

Modulation of the endocrine mechanisms regulating the menstrual cycle has been associated with athletic training in some women (Green et al., 1998). Although the mechanisms associated with this phenomenon are not clear, the effects of stress and vigorous aerobic exercise on menstrual function suggest some possibilities.

The menstrual cycle is regulated by the hypothalamic-pituitary-ovarian (HPO) axis. The HPO axis is regulated by neuronal input from limbic structures in the brain. The basal medial hypothalamus serves as a transducer that integrates signals from the brain and the endocrine system to regulate regular menstrual cycles. Cyclicity, menstruation, and fertility are maintained by precise secretory patterns of gonadotropin releasing hormone (GnRH). Corticotropin-releasing hormone seems to exert an inhibitory effect on GnRH at the level of the hypothalamus (Van Vugt, Piercy, Farley, Reid, & Rivest, 1997). Although the exact mechanisms are unclear, GnRH-secreting neurons and CRH neurons are anatomically proximal. Infusion of CRH into the third ventricle of ewes during proestrus resulted in reduction of immunoreactive GnRH in the median eminence of the hypothalamus. This finding suggests that CRH exerts regulatory control of GnRH release and synthesis (Polkowska & Przekop, 1997). Thus, the effects of exercise as a stressor on hypothalamic-pituitary-adrenal (HPA) and HPO axis regulation are important to consider.

Exercise-induced amenorrhea and fertility problems have been reported in well-trained women athletes. The mechanisms governing these disturbances are not known. Studies of basal levels of stress and gonadal axis hormones are inconsistent. Harber and colleagues (1997) reported wide variability in plasma β-Endorphin (β-END) levels among sedentary and athletic eumenorrheic women and amenorrheic athletes. Both groups of athletes had slightly higher plasma β-END levels, but no apparent cycle differences. Elevated resting plasma β-END levels have been widely reported and probably reflect an adaptation to training. Other hypothetical explanations for exercise-induced menstrual difficulties focus on nutritional health and adiposity (Kopp-Woodroffe, Manore, Dueck, Skinner, & Matt, 1999; Manore, 1999; Meyer, Muoio, & Hackney, 1999).

Effects on Menstrual and Menopausal Symptoms

Although theoretical evidence exists to suggest that exercise should have a positive effect on premenstrual symptoms, few studies have been done to validate its usefulness. Some research groups reported difficulty in recruiting and maintaining a participant pool for a study designed to evaluate exercise treatments for premenstrual syndrome (Grinspoon et al., 1999; Miller, McGowen, Miller, Coyle, & Hamdy, 1999; Pescatello et al., 1999). Perhaps women who engage in exercise or who are amenable to regular exercise do not experience premenstrual changes. Despite the lack of empirical data demonstrating the efficacy of the treatment, several articles in journals targeted to clinicians include exercise as a recommended intervention. Because exercise in moderation represents minimal risk to otherwise healthy young adults and those of middle age, continued inclusion in the therapeutic plan for premenstrual symptoms is appropriate. However, without well-conducted studies, the basis of the therapeutic effect and potential adverse events remain unknown.

Studies of exercise in menopausal women, on the other hand, are more plentiful. Most focus on the effects of the treatment on cardiovascular risk factors, including adiposity, and osteoporosis. Ivarsson, Spetz, and Hammar (1998) investigated the association between exercise patterns and reports of hot flashes. Only 5% of 1,323 Swedish women reported severe hot flashes compared to 14% of sedentary respondents. Controlled clinical trials of exercise to reduce menopausal symptoms have not been reported, but clinical articles have been published that support alternative therapies including exercise, herbal remedies, and vitamins (McKee & Warber, 2005; McMillan & Mark, 2004). Despite the lack of empirical evidence, some anecdotal reports from women who have tried exercise to alleviate hot flashes have been positive. The evidence that increased physical activity has positive health benefits on cardiovascular health, weight control, and metabolism is substantial, so all women, regardless of age, should be encouraged to exercise.

Exercise in Pregnancy and Lactation

Pregnancy and lactation are events in some women's lives that require special considerations regarding the amount and type of exercise. Consideration of cardiovascular changes associated with pregnancy includes increased cardiovascular load due to increased weight and vascular volume. Some have suggested that to superimpose vigorous aerobic exercise could overtax the cardiopulmonary system and cause problems for the mother as well as the fetus. However, the overwhelming evidence suggests that if the woman engaged in regular aerobic exercise prior to her pregnancy, she may safely continue through her pregnancy. Studies of the relationship between onset of labor, duration of labor, and rate of spontaneous vaginal deliveries suggests a positive relationship. Women who exercise regularly have shorter labors and fewer operative deliveries (Sternfeld, 1997). These results were supported by the work of Oken and colleagues (2006). The only contraindication to aerobic exercise for the woman experiencing a normal pregnancy is associated with pregnancy-related compromise of the cardiovascular system. Late in pregnancy, the position of the baby may interfere with respiratory reserves. Dempsey, Butler, and Williams (2005) reported that regular exercise during pregnancy might reduce the risk of gestational diabetes.

In general, a commonsense approach to exercise during pregnancy should prevail. If a woman has been exercising regularly prior to pregnancy, there is little risk associated with continuing with it. However, changes in balance due to added body weight and changes in posture might influence one's ability to continue to perform certain actions. Activities that require agility may result in greater risk for falling and injury during pregnancy. Aquatic exercise may be a very safe alternative for pregnant women (Hartmann & Bung, 1999). Generally, women who are pregnant should monitor their responses to and comfort during all activities and avoid those that are uncomfortable.

Special thought should be given to the type of exercise program initiated during pregnancy. Women should be advised to be very cautious, because injury is more likely during initiation of a program of regular exercise. Changes in the physiological function associated with pregnancy may influence exercise capacity. Increased circulating blood volume and weight gain may result in increased challenge to the cardiopulmonary system during exercise. Activities that were easily tolerated prior to pregnancy may be too much during pregnancy (Wolfe, Preston, Burggraf, & McGrath, 1999). The best program of exercise for formerly sedentary women during pregnancy is conservative and includes regular monitoring of the mother and the fetus.

There is no evidence to suggest that exercise negatively affects lactation. One study reported that lactating women who exercised regularly produced more milk. In addition to lactation, postpartum exercise may have a positive effect on mood, reducing the risk of postpartum depression and perhaps reducing the fatigue reported to accompany the postpartum period (Daley, Macarthur, & Winter, 2007; Koltyn & Schultes, 1997).

EXERCISE PATTERNS AND PRESCRIPTIONS

Mikkelsson and colleagues (2006) reported on a cohort of 45 individuals who performed a series of fitness tests as adolescents and were evaluated again 25 years later. For the 25 females in the cohort, body mass index, sit-up test, and the flex-arm hang were predictive of physical fitness levels as adults. These data support the assertion that fitness is a lifelong enterprise. The epidemic of obesity and the appearance of type 2 diabetes in school-aged U.S. children foretell a significant increase in cardiovascular disease among the next generation. Much of the problem has been attributed to high-fat diets and lack of physical activity. Parents have a significant role to play in reversing these alarming trends. All clinicians, those caring for adults and for children, have a major responsibility to counsel parents about that role.

Kimm and colleagues (2006) reported on the exercise habits and barriers to exercise described in a survey of adolescent girls who participate in a National Heart, Lung, and Blood Institute Growth and Health Study. The incidence of sedentary respondents increased with age. Sixty percent of the respondents classified as sedentary reported that they did not have time to exercise despite no differences in the numbers of hours worked or household chores performed when compared to the active group. Other barriers cited were lack of interest and feeling too tired. Body mass index and reported preference to do other things were most predictive of barriers to exercise. Work, parental education, TV watching, and childbirth were not associated with barriers to exercise. The probability is that these attitudes will persist into adulthood. The trend toward less physical activity as age progresses has been reported and seems to be profound among women.

REFERENCES

Arciero, P. J., Vukovich, M. D., Holloszy, J. O., Racette, S. B., & Kohrt, W. M. (1999). Comparison of short-term diet and exercise on insulin action in individuals with abnormal glucose tolerance. *Journal of Applied Physiology, 86*(6), 1930–1935.

Ardern, C. I., Katzmarzyk, P. T., Janssen, I., Leon, A. S., Wilmore, J. H., Skinner, J. S., et al. (2004). Race and sex similarities in exercise-induced changes in blood lipids and fatness. *Medicine & Science in Sports & Exercise, 36*(9), 1610–1615.

Aylin, P., Williams, S., & Bottle, A. (2005). Obesity and type 2 diabetes in children, 1996–7 to 2003–4. *British Medical Journal, 331*(7526), 1167.

Barlow, C. E., LaMonte, M. J., Fitzgerald, S. J., Kampert, J. B., Perrin, J. L., & Blair, S. N. (2006). Cardiorespiratory fitness is an independent predictor of hypertension incidence among initially normotensive healthy women. *American Journal of Epidemiology, 163*(2), 142–150.

Belza, B., & Warms, C. (2004). Physical activity and exercise in women's health. *Nursing Clinics of North America, 39*(1), 181–193.

Bemben, D. A. (1999). Exercise interventions for osteoporosis prevention in postmenopausal women. *Journal of the Oklahoma State Medical Association, 92*(2), 66–70.

Boekholdt, S. M., Hack, C. E., Sandhu, M. S., Luben, R., Bingham, S. A., Wareham, N. J., et al. (2006). C-reactive protein levels and coronary artery disease incidence and mortality in apparently healthy men and women: The EPIC-Norfolk prospective population study 1993–2003. *Atherosclerosis, 187*(2), 415–422.

Bond, V., Millis, R. M., Adams, R. G., Oke, L. M., Enweze, L., Blakely, R., et al. (2005). Attenuation of exaggerated exercise blood pressure response in African-American women by regular aerobic physical activity. *Ethnicity & Disease, 15*(4 Suppl. 5), S10, S13.

Boreham, C. A., Ferreira, I., Twisk, J. W., Gallagher, A. M., Savage, M. J., & Murray, L. J. (2004). Cardiorespiratory fitness, physical activity, and arterial stiffness: The Northern Ireland Young Hearts Project. *Hypertension, 44*(5), 721–726.

Brindle, P., Beswick, A., Fahey, T., & Ebrahim, S. (2006). Accuracy and impact of risk assessment in the primary prevention of cardiovascular disease: a systematic review. *Heart, 92*(12), 1752–1759.

Brindle, P. M., McConnachie, A., Upton, M. N., Hart, C. L., Davey Smith, G., & Watt, G. C. (2005). The accuracy of the Framingham risk-score in different socioeconomic groups: A prospective study. *British Journal of General Practice, 55*(520), 838–845.

Bruce, I. N. (2005). "Not only . . . but also": Factors that contribute to accelerated atherosclerosis and premature coronary heart disease in systemic lupus erythematosus. *Rheumatology, 44*(12), 1492–1502.

Camarri, B., Eastwood, P. R., Cecins, N. M., Thompson, P. J., & Jenkins, S. (2006). Six minute walk distance in healthy participants aged 55–75 years. *Respiratory Medicine, 100*(4), 658–665.

Campos, G. E., Luecke, T. J., Wendeln, H. K., Toma, K., Hagerman, F. C., Murray, T. F., et al. (2002). Muscular adaptations in response to three different resistance-training regimens: Specificity of repetition maximum training zones. *European Journal of Applied Physiology, 88*(1–2), 50–60.

Chibalin, A. V., Yu, M., Ryder, J. W., Song, X. M., Galuska, D., Krook, A., et al. (2000). Exercise-induced changes in expression and activity of proteins involved in insulin signal transduction in skeletal muscle: Differential effects on insulin-receptor substrates 1 and 2. *Proceedings of the National Acadademy of Science U S A, 97*(1), 38–43.

Clapp, L. L., Richardson, M. T., Smith, J. F., Wang, M., Clapp, A. J., & Pieroni, R. E. (1999). Acute effects of thirty minutes of light-intensity, intermittent exercise on patients with chronic fatigue syndrome. *Physical Therapy, 79*(8), 749–756.

Courbon, A., Calmels, P., Roche, F., Ramas, J., Rimaud, D., & Fayolle-Minon, I. (2006). Relationship between maximal exercise capacity and walking capacity in adult hemiplegic stroke patients. *American Journal of Physical Medicine & Rehabilitation, 85*(5), 436–442.

Craig, W. Y., Rawstron, M. W., Rundell, C. A., Robinson, E., Poulin, S. E., Neveux, L. M., et al. (1999). Relationship between lipoprotein- and oxidation-related variables and atheroma lipid composition in participants undergoing coronary artery bypass graft surgery. *Arteriosclerosis, Thrombosis & Vascular Biology, 19*(6), 1512–1517.

D'Amore, S., & Mora, S. (2006). Gender-specific prediction of cardiac disease: Importance of risk factors and exercise variables. *Cardiology in Review, 14*(6), 281–285.

D'Eon, T., & Braun, B. (2002). The roles of estrogen and progesterone in regulating carbohydrate and fat utilization at rest and during exercise. *Journal of Women's Health & Gender-Based Medicine, 11*(3), 225–237.

Daley, A. J., Macarthur, C., & Winter, H. (2007). The role of exercise in treating postpartum depression: A review of the literature. *Journal of Midwifery & Women's Health, 52*(1), 56–62.

Dempsey, J. C., Butler, C. L., & Williams, M. A. (2005). No need for a pregnant pause: Physical activity may reduce the occurrence of gestational diabetes mellitus and preeclampsia. *Exercise & Sport Sciences Reviews, 33*(3), 141–149.

DiPietro, L., Dziura, J., Yeckel, C. W., & Neufer, P. D. (2006). Exercise and improved insulin sensitivity in older women: Evidence of the enduring benefits of higher intensity training. *Journal of Applied Physiology, 100*(1), 142–149.

Draznin, M. B., & Patel, D. R. (1998). Diabetes mellitus and sports. *Adolescent Medicine, 9*(3), 457–465, v.

Dwyer, G. B., & Shala, E. (Ed.). (2005). *American College of Sports Medicine's health-related physical fitness assessment manual.* Philadelphia: Lippincott Williams & Wilkins.

Eriksson, J., Lindstrom, J., Valle, T., Aunola, S., Hamalainen, H., Ilanne-Parikka, P., et al. (1999). Prevention of type II diabetes in participants with impaired glucose tolerance: The Diabetes Prevention Study (DPS) in Finland. Study design and 1-year interim report on the feasibility of the lifestyle intervention programme. *Diabetologia, 42*(7), 793–801.

Franco, V., Oparil, S., & Carretero, O. A. (2004). Hypertensive therapy: Part I. *Circulation, 109*(24), 2953–2958.

Gass, M., & Dawson-Hughes, B. (2006). Preventing osteoporosis-related fractures: An overview. *American Journal of Medicine, 119*(4 Suppl. 1), S3–S11.

Green, J. S., Crouse, S. F., & Rohack, J. J. (1998). Peak exercise hemodynamics in exercising postmenopausal women taking versus not taking supplemental estrogen. *Medicine & Science in Sports & Exercise, 30*(1), 158–164.

Grindrod, D., Paton, C. D., Knez, W. L., & O'Brien, B. J. (2006). Six minute walk distance is greater when performed in a group than alone. *British Journal of Sports Medicine, 40*(10), 876–877.

Grinspoon, S., Miller, K., Coyle, C., Krempin, J., Armstrong, C., Pitts, S., et al. (1999). Severity of osteopenia in estrogen-deficient women with anorexia nervosa and hypothalamic amenorrhea. *Journal of Clinical Endocrinology Metababolism, 84*(6), 2049–2055.

Harber, V. J., Sutton, J. R., MacDougall, J. D., Woolever, C. A., & Bhavnani, B. R. (1997). "Plasma concentrations of beta-endorphin in trained eumenorrheic and amenorrheic women." *Fertility & Sterility, 67*(4), 648–653.

Hartmann, S., & Bung, P. (1999). Physical exercise during pregnancy—Physiological considerations and recommendations. *Journal of Perinatal Medicine, 27*(3), 204–215.

Hawkins, M. N., Raven, P. B., Snell, P. G., Stray-Gundersen, J., & Levine, B. D. (2007). Maximal oxygen uptake as a parametric measure of cardiorespiratory capacity. *Medicine & Science in Sports & Exercise, 39*(1), 103–107.

Huxley, V. H. (2007). Sex and the cardiovascular system: The intriguing tale of how women and men regulate cardiovascular function differently. *Advances in Physiology Education, 31*(1), 17–22.

Ivarsson, T., Spetz, A. C., & Hammar, M. (1998). Physical exercise and vasomotor symptoms in postmenopausal women. *Maturitas, 29*(2), 139–146.

Jani, B., & Rajkumar, C. (2006). Ageing and vascular ageing. *Postgraduate Medical Journal, 82*(968), 357–362.

Jonsdottir, S., Andersen, K. K., Sigurosson, A. F., & Sigurosson, S. B. (2006). The effect of physical training in chronic heart failure. *European Journal of Heart Failure, 8*(1), 97–101.

Kaminsky, L. A., & Kimberly, A. (Eds.). (2006). *American College of Sports Medicine* (5th ed.). Philadelphia: Lippincott Williams & Wilkins.

Kelley, G. A., Kelley, K. S., & Tran, Z. V. (2005). Aerobic exercise and lipids and lipoproteins in women: A meta-analysis of randomized controlled trials. [Erratum appears in *Journal of Women's Health, 14*(2), 198.] *Journal of Women's Health, 13*(10), 1148–1164.

Kemmler, W., Lauber, D., Weineck, J., Hensen, J., Kalender, W., & Engelke, K. (2004). Benefits of 2 years of intense exercise on bone density, physical fitness, and blood lipids in early postmenopausal osteopenic women: Results of the Erlangen Fitness Osteoporosis Prevention Study (EFOPS). *Archives of Internal Medicine, 164*(10), 1084–1091.

Kimm, S. Y., Glynn, N. W., McMahon, R. P., Voorhees, C. C., Striegel-Moore, R. H., & Daniels, S. R. (2006). Self-perceived barriers to activity participation among sedentary adolescent girls. *Medicine & Science in Sports & Exercise, 38*(3), 534–540.

Kirk, S., Scott, B. J., & Daniels, S. R. (2005). Pediatric obesity epidemic: Treatment options. *Journal of the American Dietetic Association, 105*(5 Suppl. 1), S44–S51.

Koenig, W., Khuseyinova, N., Baumert, J., Thorand, B., Loewel, H., Chambless, L., et al. (2006). Increased concentrations of C-reactive protein and IL-6 but not IL-18 are independently associated with incident coronary events in middle-aged men and women: Results from the MONICA/KORA Augsburg case-cohort study, 1984–2002. *Arteriosclerosis, Thrombosis & Vascular Biology, 26*(12), 2745–2751.

Koh, K. K., Han, S. H., & Quon, M. J. (2005). Inflammatory markers and the metabolic syndrome: Insights from therapeutic interventions. *Journal of the American College of Cardiology, 46*(11), 1978–1985.

Kokkinos, P., Pittaras, A., Manolis, A., Panagiotakos, D., Narayan, P., Manjoros, D., et al. (2006). Exercise capacity and 24-h blood pressure in prehypertensive men and women. *American Journal of Hypertension, 19*(3), 251–258.

Koltyn, K. F., & Schultes, S. S. (1997). Psychological effects of an aerobic exercise session and a rest session following pregnancy. *Journal of Sports Medicine & Physical Fitness, 37*(4), 287–291.

Kopp-Woodroffe, S. A., Manore, M. M., Dueck, C. A., Skinner, J. S., & Matt, K. S. (1999). Energy and nutrient status of amenorrheic athletes participating in a diet and exercise training intervention program. *International Journal of Sport & Nutrition, 9*(1), 70–88.

Koval, J. A., Maezono, K., Patti, M. E., Pendergrass, M., DeFronzo, R. A., & Mandarino, L. J. (1999). Effects of exercise and insulin on insulin signaling proteins in human skeletal muscle. *Med Sci Sports Exerc, 31*(7), 998–1004.

Lamon-Fava, S., Fisher, E. C., Nelson, M. E.,Evans, W. J., Millar, J. S., Ordovas, J. M., et al. (1998). Effect of exercise and menstrual cycle status on plasma lipids, low density lipoprotein particle size, and apolipoproteins. *Journal of Clinical Endocrinology & Metabolism, 68*(1), 17–21.

Lee, J. M., Okumura, M. J., Davis, M. M., Herman, W. H., & Gurney, J. G. (2006). Prevalence and determinants of insulin resistance among U.S. adolescents: A population-based study. *Diabetes Care, 29*(11), 2427–2432.

Lewis, R. D., & Modlesky, C. M. (1998). Nutrition, physical activity, and bone health in women. *International Journal of Sport & Nutrition, 8*(3), 250–284.

Libby, P. (2006). Inflammation and cardiovascular disease mechanisms. *American Journal of Clinical Nutrition, 83*(2), 456S–460S.

Lloyd-Jones, D. M., Liu, K., Tian, L., & Greenland, P. (2006). Narrative review: Assessment of C-reactive protein in risk prediction for cardiovascular disease. *Annals of Internal Medicine, 145*(1), 35–42.

Manore, M. M. (1999). Nutritional needs of the female athlete. *Clinical Sports Medicine, 18*(3), 549–563.

Matthews, K. A., Sowers, M. F., Derby, C. A., Stein, E., Miracle-McMahill, H., Crawford, S. L., et al. (2005). Ethnic differences in cardiovascular risk factor burden among middle-aged women: Study of Women's Health Across the Nation (SWAN). *American Heart Journal, 149*(6), 1066–1073.

McKee, J., & Warber, S. L. (2005). Integrative therapies for menopause. *Southern Medical Journal, 98*(3), 319–326.

McMillan, T. L., & Mark, S. (2004). Complementary and alternative medicine and physical activity for menopausal symptoms. *Journal of the American Medical Womens Association, 59*(4), 270–277.

Meyer, W. R., Muoio, D., & Hackney, T. C. (1999). Effect of sex steroids on beta-endorphin levels at rest and during submaximal treadmill exercise in anovulatory and ovulatory runners. *Fertility & Sterility, 71*(6), 1085–1091.

Mikkelsson, L., Kaprio, J., Kautiainen, H., Kujala, U., Mikkelsson, M., & Nupponen, H. (2006). School fitness tests as predictors of adult health-related fitness. *American Journal of Human Biology, 18*(3), 342–349.

Miller, M. N., McGowen, K. R., Miller, B. E., Coyle, B. R., & Hamdy, R. (1999). Lessons learned about research on premenstrual syndrome. *Journal of Women's Health & Gender-Based Medicine, 8*(7), 989–993.

Motohiro, M., Yuasa, F., Hattori, T., Sumimoto, T., Takeuchi, M., Kaida, M., et al. (2005). Cardiovascular adaptations to exercise training after uncomplicated acute myocardial infarction. *American Journal of Physical Medicine & Rehabilitation, 84*(9), 684–691.

Murphy, M. H., Murtagh, E. M., Boreham, C. A., Hare, L. G., & Nevill, A. M. (2006). The effect of a worksite based walking programme on cardiovascular risk in previously sedentary civil servants [NCT00284479]. *BMC Public Health, 6*(136).

Napoli, C., Lerman, L. O., de Nigris, F., Gossl, M., Balestrieri, M. L., & Lerman, A. (2006). Rethinking primary prevention of atherosclerosis-related diseases. *Circulation, 114*(23), 2517–2527.

National Cholesterol Education Program. (2007a). *Estimate of 10-year risk for coronary heart disease Framingham point scores.* http://www.nhlbi.nih.gov/guidelines/cholesterol/risk_tbl.htm#women

National Cholesterol Education Program. (2007b). *Risk assessment tool for estimating 10-year risk of developing hard CHD (myocardial infarction and coronary death).* http://hp2010.nhlbihin.net/atpiii/calculator.asp?usertype=prof

National Institutes of Health Consensus Development Panel on Osteoporosis Prevention. (2001). Osteoporosis prevention, diagnosis, and therapy. *Journal of the American Medical Association, 285*(6), 785–795.

Noonan, V., & Dean, E. (2000). Submaximal exercise testing: Clinical application and interpretation. *Physical Therapy, 80*(8), 782–807.

Oken, E., Ning, Y., Rifas-Shiman, S. L., Radesky, J. S., Rich-Edwards, J. W., & Gillman, M. W. (2006). Associations of physical activity and inactivity before and during pregnancy with glucose tolerance. *Obstetrics & Gynecology, 108*(5), 1200–1207.

Paffen, E., & DeMaat, M. P. (2006). C-reactive protein in atherosclerosis: A causal factor? *Cardiovascular Research, 71*(1), 30–39.

Palaniappan, L., Anthony, M. N., Mahesh, C., Elliott, M., Killeen, A., Giacherio, D., et al. (2002). Cardiovascular risk factors in ethnic minority women aged < or = 30 years. *American Journal of Cardiology, 89*(5), 524–529.

Patterson, S. L., Forrester, L. W., Rodgers, M. M., Ryan, A. S., Ivey, F. M., Sorkin, J. D., et al. (2007). Determinants of walking function after stroke: Differences by deficit severity. *Archives of Physical Medicine & Rehabilitation, 88*(1), 115–119.

Pearson, T. (2002). New tools for coronary risk assessment: What are their advantages and limitations? *Circulation, 105*(7), 886–892.

Pescatello, L. S., Franklin, B. A., Fagard, R., Farquhar, W. B., Kelley, G. A., Ray, C. A., et al. (2004). American College of Sports Medicine position stand. Exercise and hypertension. *Medicine & Science in Sports & Exercise, 36*(3), 533–553.

Pescatello, L. S., Miller, B., Danias, P. G., Werner, M., Hess, M., Baker, C., et al. (1999). Dynamic exercise normalizes resting blood pressure in mildly hypertensive premenopausal women. *American Heart Journal, 138*(5 Pt. 1), 916–921.

Physical activity and health: A report of the Surgeon General, executive summary. (1999). Washington, DC: U.S. Department of Health and Human Services.

Polkowska, J., & Przekop, F. (1997). The effect of corticotropin-releasing factor (CRF) on the gonadotropin hormone releasing hormone (GnRH) hypothalamic neuronal system during preovulatory period in the ewe. *Acta Neurobiologiae Experimentalis, 57*(2), 91–99.

Prior, B. M., Lloyd, P. G., Yang, H. T., & Terjung, R. L. (2003). Exercise-induced vascular remodeling. *Exercise & Sport Sciences Reviews, 31*(1), 26–33.

Prior, B. M., Yang, H. T., & Terjung, R. L. (2004). What makes vessels grow with exercise training? *Journal of Applied Physiology, 97*(3), 1119–1128.

Reardon, J. Z., Lareau, S. C., & ZuWallack, R. (2006). Functional status and quality of life in chronic obstructive pulmonary disease. *American Journal of Medicine, 119*(10 Suppl. 1), 32–37.

Reynolds, K., & He, J. (2005). Epidemiology of the metabolic syndrome. *American Journal of the Medical Sciences, 330*(6), 273–279.

Reynolds Risk Score: Preventing heart disease in women. (2007). Retrieved March 2007, from http://www.reynoldsriskscore.org/default.aspx

Ridker, P. M., Buring, J. E., Rifai, N., & Cook, N. R. (2007). Development and validation of improved algorithms for the assessment of global cardiovascular risk in women: The Reynolds Risk Score. *Journal of the American Medical Association, 297*(6), 611–619.

Rosamond, W., Flegal, K., Friday, G., Furie, K., Go, A., Greenlund, K., et al. (2007). Heart disease and stroke statistics—2007 update: A report from the American Heart Association Statistics Committee and Stroke Statistics Subcommittee. *Circulation, 115*(5), 69–171.

Sakuragi, S., & Sugiyama, Y. (2006). Effects of daily walking on subjective symptoms, mood and autonomic nervous function. *Journal of Physiol Anthropology, 25*(4), 281–289.

Sarsan, A., Ardic, F., Ozgen, M., Topuz, O., & Sermez, Y. (2006). The effects of aerobic and resistance exercises in obese women. *Clinical Rehabilitation, 20*(9), 773–782.

Scully, D., Kremer, J., Meade, M. M., Graham, R., & Dudgeon, K. (1998). Physical exercise and psychological well being: A critical review. *British Journal of Sports Medicine, 32*(2), 111–120.

Shaw, L. J., Bairey Merz, C. N., Pepine, C. J., Reis, S. E., Bittner, V., Kelsey, S. F., et al. (2006). Insights from the NHLBI-sponsored Women's Ischemia Syndrome Evaluation (WISE) study: Part I: Gender differences in traditional and novel risk factors, symptom evaluation, and gender-optimized diagnostic strategies. *Journal of the American College of Cardiology, 47*(3 Suppl.), S4–S20.

Sheth, P. (1999). Osteoporosis and exercise: A review. *Mt Sinai Journal of Medicine, 66*(3), 197–200.

Staffileno, B. A., Minnick, A., Coke, L. A., & Hollenberg, S. M. (2007). Blood pressure responses to lifestyle physical activity among young, hypertension-prone African-American women. *Journal of Cardiovascular Nursing, 22*(2), 107–117.

Sternfeld, B. (1997). Physical activity and pregnancy outcome. Review and recommendations. *Sports Medicine, 23*(1), 33–47.

Stewart, K. J., Ouyang, P., Bacher, A. C., Lima, S., & Shapiro, E. P. (2006). Exercise effects on cardiac size and left ventricular diastolic function: Relationships to changes in fitness, fatness, blood pressure and insulin resistance. *Heart, 92*(7), 893–898.

Stisen, A. B., Stougaard, O., Langfort, J., Helge, J. W., Sahlin, K., & Madsen, K. (2006). Maximal fat oxidation rates in endurance trained and untrained women. *European Journal of Applied Physiology, 98*(5), 497–506.

U.S. Department of Health and Human Services. (2001). *Third report of the expert panel on detection, evaluation, and treatment of high blood cholesterol in adults (Adult Treatment Panel III).* Retrieved January 15, 2008, from http://www.nhlbi.nih.gov/guidelines/cholesterol/atglance.htm

TopEndSports.com (2007). VO2 max norms. Retrieved March 2007, from http://www.topendsports.com/testing/vo2norms.htm

Tsutsumi, T., Don, B. M., Zaichkowsky, L. D., Takenaka, K., Oka, K., & Ohno, T. (1998). Comparison of high and moderate intensity of strength training on mood and anxiety in older adults. *Perceptual & Motor Skills, 87*(3 Pt. 1), 1003–1011.

Tune, J. D., Richmond, K. N., Gorman, M. W., & Feigl, E. O. (2002). Control of coronary blood flow during exercise. *Experimental Biology & Medicine, 227*(4), 238–250.

Turner, R. T. (1999). Mechanical signaling in the development of postmenopausal osteoporosis. *Lupus, 8*(5), 388–392.

Van Vugt, D. A., Piercy, J., Farley, A. E., Reid, R. L., & Rivest, S. (1997). Luteinizing hormone secretion and corticotropin-releasing factor gene expression in the paraventricular nucleus of rhesus monkeys following cortisol synthesis inhibition. *Endocrinology, 138*(6), 2249–2258.

Warburton, D. E., Nicol, C. W., & Bredin, S. S. (2006). Health benefits of physical activity: The evidence. *Canadian Medical Association Journal, 174*(6), 801–809.

Whelton, S. P., Chin, A., Xin, X., & He, J. (2002). Effect of aerobic exercise on blood pressure: A meta-analysis of randomized, controlled trials. *Annals of Internal Medicine, 136*(7), 493–503.

Williams, N. I., Bullen, B. A., McArthur, J. W., Skrinar, G. S., & Turnbull, B. A. (1999). Effects of short-term strenuous endurance exercise upon corpus luteum function. *Medicine & Science in Sports & Exercise, 31*(7), 949–958.

Wolfe, L. A., Preston, R. J., Burggraf, G. W., & McGrath, M. J. (1999). Effects of pregnancy and chronic exercise on maternal cardiac structure and function. *Canadian Journal of Physiology & Pharmacology, 77*(11), 909–917.

Wormald, H., Waters, H., Sleap, M., & Ingle, L. (2006). Participants' perceptions of a lifestyle approach to promoting physical activity: Targeting deprived communities in Kingston-upon-Hull. *BMC Public Health, 6*, 202.

Zahner, L., Puder, J. J., Roth, R., Schmid, M., Guldimann, R., Puhse, U., et al. (2006). A school-based physical activity program to improve health and fitness in children aged 6–13 years (Kinder-Sportstudie KISS): Study design of a randomized controlled trial [ISRCTN15360785]. *BMC Public Health, 6*, 147.

Zehnder, M., Ith, M., Kreis, R., Saris, W., Boutellier, U., & Boesch, C. (2005). Gender-specific usage of intramyocellular lipids and glycogen during exercise. *Medicine & Science in Sports & Exercise, 37*(9), 1517–1524.

13

Mental Health

Anne Hopkins Fishel

Mental illnesses occur across all cultures and nations, though cultural differences exist in symptom presentation and prevalence estimates (Ballenger et al., 2001). The good news is that the proportion of people who sought help for a mental health problem in the United States is higher now at 17% than it was a decade ago, at 13% (National Institute of Mental, 2005b). The expansion is explained by more primary care physicians providing psychiatric services, even though the adequacy of treatment is best if provided by a mental health practitioner (National Institute of Mental Health, 2005b). The elderly, racial/ethnic minorities, and those with low income or without insurance have the greatest unmet need for treatment (National Institute of Mental Health, 2005b).

Even when psychological symptoms don't reach diagnostic threshold, they are associated with impaired functioning and play a role in current health status. The number of young people who suffer from psychiatric symptoms and illness is much higher than is currently recognized because they do not report these symptoms to their health care providers (Potts, Gillies, & Wood, 2001). Half of all lifetime cases of mental illness begin by age 14, and there are long delays between first onset of symptoms and when people seek and receive treatment (National Institute of Mental Health, 2005b). College women who reported experiencing stalking by an intimate or dating partner reported significantly more mental health symptoms and lower perceived physical health status than individuals who did not (Amar, 2006). In a study by Ott and Lueger (2002), they noted a dramatic change in overall mental health of recent widows during the beginning phases of bereavement; at 24 months after the death, participants had not attained the same level of mental health as the general population.

Stigma and uninformed consumers prevent many women from seeking treatment. The barriers are even greater for minorities. Former U.S. Surgeon General David Satcher noted that when a history of racism, discrimination, and economic impoverishment is combined with mistrust and fear, members of minority populations may be deterred from using [mental health] services (U.S. Department of Health and Human Services, 2001). The stigma about mental illness also prevents many professionals from making appropriate referrals and treatment decisions. Revealed in a recent survey of psychiatric residents was the belief that, while psychotherapy did not carry stigma, psychotropic medications did have stigma (Fogel, Sneed, & Roose, 2006).

This chapter focuses on the management of mental health problems prevalent among women. Included are mood disorders (major depressive disorder, dysthymia, bipolar disorder, and premenstrual dysphoric disorder) and anxiety disorders (generalized anxiety disorder, panic disorder, social phobia, obsessive-compulsive disorder, and post-traumatic stress disorder). Although eating disorders and borderline personality disorder also are more prevalent among women, they are not discussed in this chapter. Approximately 75% of people diagnosed with borderline personality disorder are women (American Psychiatric Association, 2000; Osborne & McComish, 2006). The incidence of eating disorders (discussed in chapter 11) is growing and is twice as common among women as men. A discussion about future directions for mental health promotion of women concludes the chapter.

PREVALENCE OF MENTAL ILLNESS

An estimated 26.2% of Americans (57.7 million people) aged 18 and older—about one in four adults—suffer from a diagnosable mental disorder in a given year (Kessler, Chiu, Demier, & Walters, 2005). In the United States and Canada for people ages 15 to 44 years, mental disorders are the leading cause of disability (World Health Organization, 2004).

Approximately 20.9 million American adults (9.5%) ages 18 and older have a depressive disorder, and the median age of onset is 30 years (Kessler et al., 2005). Approximately 14.8 million (6.7%) have major depressive disorder, 5.7 million (2.6%) have bipolar disorder, and 3.3 million (1.5%) have dysthymic disorder (Kessler et al., 2005). In 2004, 32,439 people died by suicide in the United States (Centers for Disease Control and Prevention, 2004). Premenstrual dysphoric disorder affects between 5% and 10% of fertile women (Eriksson et al., 2000).

Approximately 40 million American adults ages 18 and older—or about 18.1% of people in a given year—have at least one anxiety disorder (Kessler et al., 2005). Approximately 19.2 million (8.7%) have some form of phobia, and 7.7 million (3.5%) have post-traumatic stress disorder—which can develop at any age and frequently occurs after violent personal assaults such a rape or domestic violence. Approximately 6.8 million (3.1%) have generalized anxiety disorder, 6 million (2.7%) have panic disorder, and 2.2 million (1.0%) have obsessive compulsive disorder in a given year (Kessler et al., 2005).

PREVALENCE OF MENTAL ILLNESS IN WOMEN

Patterns of mental illness vary for women and men. The National Comorbidity Survey Replication (2005) study of more than 9,000 respondents found a lifetime prevalence of several mental disorders (including major depressive disorder, panic disorder, specific phobia, generalized anxiety disorder, and post-traumatic stress disorder) about twice as prevalent for women as men. Although men commit suicide more often than women, women attempt suicide two to three times more often than men (National Institute of Mental Health, 2006). Women who have high impulsivity are at highest risk for suicide (McGirr et al., 2006). Major depression and dysthymia affect twice as many women as men (National Institute of Mental Health, 2005a). Depression is the leading cause of disease-related disability in women (Noble, 2005).

Even though the overall incidence of bipolar disorder is equal between women and men, women with bipolar disorder have more frequent episodes of depression than men, and the depressive episodes are more likely to be lengthy and resistant to treatment (Freeman, Arnold, & McElroy, 2002). In addition, women generally have a later age of onset than men (fifth decade of life is more common with women). Rapid cycling is more common in women than in men and may be more resistant to standard treatments (Freeman et al., 2002; National Institute of Mental Health, 2005a). Bipolar II disorder is more common in women (Miller, 2006), and these women may be at increased risk of developing subsequent episodes in the immediate postpartum period (American Psychiatric Association, 2000).

High depression scores were more than four times more likely to occur during a woman's menopausal transition, compared with when she was premenopausal (Freeman, Sammel, Lin, & Nelson, 2006). A diagnosis of depressive disorder was two and a half times more likely to occur in the menopausal transition compared with when the woman was premenopausal. There are cultural aspects of depression that affect incidence. In a Hispanic population of women, 26.6% at time of delivery and 27.7% at 6 weeks postpartum were classified with depressive symptoms (Malek, Connolly, & Knaus, 2001).

Women are more likely than men to have an anxiety disorder. From the National Comorbidity Survey Replication study, the authors reported that women were statistically more likely than men to evidence panic attacks, panic disorder, and panic disorders with agoraphobia (Kessler et al., 2006). Although women are exposed to proportionately fewer traumatic events in their life time than men, they have a higher lifetime risk of post-traumatic stress disorder (Seedat, Stein, & Carey, 2005).

During pregnancy, some psychiatric disorders, such as panic disorder, may improve or abate; in contrast, obsessive-compulsive disorder appears to be more prevalent during pregnancy, with one study citing that more than 25% of women reported symptom onset during pregnancy (Schatzberg & Nemeroff, 2004). In a review of 21 research articles, the prevalence of depression during pregnancy was cited as being 7.4% during the first trimester, 12.8% during the second trimester, and 12% during the third trimester (Bennett, Einarson, Toddio, Koren, & Einarson, 2004).

In the postpartum period, mental disorders have implications for the mother, the newborn, and the entire family (Logsdon, Wisner, & Pinto-Foltz, 2006). Less than 33% of women with substantial postpartum depression or anxiety symptoms were detected by routine care (Coates, Schaefer, & Alexander, 2004). A study of postpartum Hispanic women in three U.S. cities revealed that 42.6% of participants were depressed (Kuo et al., 2004). Approximately 3% to 5% of women develop panic disorder or obsessive-compulsive disorder (American Psychiatric Association, 2000). The postpartum period is also a common trigger for the onset of depressive symptoms, with postpartum depression occurring in 10% to 15% of new mothers (Kornstein & Wojcik, 2002). The risk of a subsequent postpartum episode may exceed 50%. Remission of maternal depression over 3 months of treatment was significantly associated with independently assessed children's psychiatric diagnosis. There was an 11% decrease in rates of diagnoses in children of mothers with remitting depression and an 8% increase in rates of diagnoses in children of mothers whose depression persisted (Weissman, Pilowsky, & Wickramaratne, 2006).

WHY GENDER DIFFERENCES?

Young, Korszun, and Altemus (2002) report an increased adrenocorticotropic hormone response to stress in women compared with men. This has important implications for our understanding of stress responsiveness in women and women's susceptibility to stress-associated disorders such as depression and anxiety. Women's increased resistance to glucocorticoids, compared with men's, could exaggerate stress responsiveness in a number of physiological systems. Estrogen and progesterone antagonism of glucocorticoid feedback mechanisms, and the increased stress responsiveness of women, may contribute to the increased prevalence of anxiety disorders and autonomic hyperarousal in women compared with men (Young et al., 2002). The potential for dysregulation of a wide variety of brain neurochemical systems may be enhanced because women have much greater and repetitive fluxes in reproductive hormones over the life span (Young et al., 2002). Recent research suggests that the effect of gender in depressive vulnerability may be related to differential sex effects in monoaminergic function (Moreno, McGahuey, Freeman, & Delgado, 2006). In addition, it has been theorized that women who develop depression during the menstrual cycle, after parturition, and during menopause may be especially susceptible to changes in hormonal balance, which in turn are believed to affect the activity of certain neuronal systems—particularly the serotonin-specific ones (Noble, 2005).

Sociocultural and psychological issues are also important in understanding why women have more depression and anxiety disorders than men. Paying attention to the context of women's lives—their roles and relationships—is essential in providing effective mental health care for women. All of the following factors may contribute to women's vulnerability for mental illnesses:

- Gender socialization favoring males over females (Casey, 2002).
- Stressors of marriage, parenting, and divorce (Lasswell, 2002).
- Work place issues such as dual-career role conflicts or role overload and sexual discrimination (Shrier, 2002).
- Trauma experienced in interpersonal relationships with men (Brand, 2002).
- Stressful experiences of women of color (Al-Mateen, Christian, Mishra, Cofield, & Tilton, 2002).
- Aging (Holroyd, 2002).

Risk factors for common mental disorders in women were assessed in India. Results revealed that risk was related to poverty, being married as compared to being single, use of tobacco, experiencing abnormal vaginal discharge, reporting a chronic physical illness, and having high psychological symptom scores (Patel, Kirkwood, Pednekaer, Weiss, & Mabey, 2006).

MOOD DISORDERS

Depression is more common in women than in men, particularly during the childbearing years. Depression in women can surface in association with specific points during the reproductive cycle, such as during the premenstrual period, during pregnancy and the postpartum period, and during the perimenopausal years. Although pregnancy does not increase the risk for depression, women with past histories of depression are at risk for recurrent episodes or relapse if antidepressant medications are discontinued during pregnancy (Burt & Stein, 2002).

Diagnostic Classifications

Specific criteria for each of the depression diagnoses are documented in the *Diagnostic and Statistical Manual of Mental Disorders* (*DSM-IV-TR*) (American Psychiatric Association, 2000). Major depressive disorder is characterized by one or more major depressive episodes (includes postpartum onset). Dysthymic disorder is characterized by at least 2 years of depressed mood, but is less severe than major depressive disorder. Bipolar disorder is characterized by one or more manic episodes usually accompanied by major depressive episodes (American Psychiatric Association, 2000). Premenstrual dysphoric disorder differs from premenstrual syndrome in its characteristic pattern of symptoms, symptom severity, and the resulting impairment (American Psychiatric Association, 2000).

Etiology

Even though scientists recognize the dysregulation of brain neurotransmitters to be involved, exact mechanisms remain unclear. The increased incidence of depression in women cannot be attributed to women's tendency to seek help or to biased diagnostic criteria (Kornstein & Wojcik, 2002). Although genetic vulnerability is critical to the development of depression, the incidence of depressive disorders is low in the absence of environmental stressors. The following biological, developmental, and environmental factors contribute to the development of depression in women.

Hormonal Factors

Estrogen and progesterone have been shown to affect neurotransmitter, neuroendocrine, and circadian systems that have been implicated in mood disorders (Young et al., 2002). They influence the synthesis and release of both serotonin and norepinephrine (Kornstein & Wojcik, 2002). The luteal phase of the menstrual cycle, which is a period of estrogen and progesterone withdrawal, is frequently associated with dysphoric mood changes as well as the onset or worsening of a major depressive episode (Kornstein & Wojcik, 2002).

The postpartum period is also a common trigger for the onset of depressive symptoms—up to 80% of women experience postpartum blues. Postpartum depression occurs in 10% to 15% of new mothers, and the rates are higher in those with a prior history of mood disorder (Kornstein & Wojcik, 2002). The perimenopausal period is a time of increased risk for recurrence in women with a history of major depressive disorder. Other hormonal factors that may contribute to women's vulnerability to mood disorders include gender differences related to the hypothalamic-pituitary-adrenal axis and to thyroid function (Kornstein & Wojcik, 2002).

Genetic Factors

More than two-thirds of people with bipolar disorder have at least one close relative with the disorder or with unipolar major depression, indicating that the disease has a heritable component (National Institute of Mental Health, 2003). Although genetic transmission plays an important role in the etiology of depression, researchers have reported similar heritability in men and women (Kornstein & Wojcik, 2002).

Gender-Specific Socialization and Coping Styles

Parents and teachers tend to have different expectations of girls and boys, which may result in girls becoming more nurturing and more concerned with the evaluations of others, and in boys developing a greater sense of mastery and independence. Such stereotypical gender socialization is hypothesized to lead to differences in self-concept and vulnerability to depression (Kornstein & Wojcik, 2002). Nolen-Hoeksema (1995) demonstrated a self-focused, ruminative style of coping in women in response to feelings of sadness; men tend to use distracting strategies. Positive emission tomography also indicated sex differences in processing of emotional stimuli (Nolen-Hoeksema, 1995). This difference in coping styles may contribute to longer and more severe depressive episodes in women.

Stressful Life Events

Across the life cycle, women are more likely than men to experience the onset of depression following a stressful life event, particularly in response to stressors that involve children, housing, and reproductive problems (Kornstein & Wojcik, 2002). They are also more likely to report a stressful life event in the 6 months preceding a major depressive episode. In addition, the stressors that may precipitate depression in women may involve events not only in their own lives but also in the lives of those around them (Kornstein & Wojcik, 2002).

Major Life Trauma

A history of sexual abuse is more common in women and is a major risk factor for depression; as many as 69% of abused women develop depression (Kornstein & Wojcik, 2002). However, researchers have not been able to demonstrate a difference in depression rates between women who have and have not experienced life trauma.

Social Status and Roles

More women than men live in poverty, and women achieve lower educational attainment than men and face fewer opportunities and salary inequities in the work place (Shrier, 2002). Marriage is less protective for women than men. A good marriage can decrease the risk of depression in both genders; however, married women continue to experience higher rates of depression. In unhappy marriages, women are much more likely than men to become depressed (Kornstein & Wojcik, 2002). Women with extensive social support have a decreased incidence of depression (Kornstein & Wojcik, 2002). However, gender role–related differences in response to events occurring to friends and family may represent a cost of caring for women that translates into elevated levels of depression.

Occupational status and children may influence the risk of depression in women. A satisfying job may help to decrease a woman's risk of depression, but only if she has chosen to work rather than being forced to do so by financial pressures (Kornstein & Wojcik, 2002). The presence of young children is a risk factor for depression in women, especially if child care is a problem for women working outside the home (Kornstein & Wojcik, 2002).

Societal homophobia and discrimination pose additional stresses for gay women. Lesbians are 2.5 times more likely to report an attempted suicide sometime in the past than are heterosexual women (McGrath, Keita, Strickland, & Russo, 1990).

Future research on mood disorders must incorporate study of a variety of factors unique to women's lives such as reproductive, hormonal, genetic or other biological factors, abuse and oppression, interpersonal factors, and certain psychological and personality characteristics (National Institute of Mental Health, 2005a). Until we have more definitive explanations about the etiology of depression in women, treatment will continue to be nonspecific with unpredictable outcomes.

Diagnostic Criteria for Types of Mood Disorders

Major Depressive Disorder (296.xx)

For the diagnostic codes for major depressive disorder (MDD), the first three digits are 296. The fourth digit is either 2 (single episode) or 3 (recurrent major depressive episodes). The fifth digit indicates the current severity: 1 for mild, 2 for moderate, 3 for severe without psychotic features, 4 for severe with psychotic features, 5 for in partial remission, 6 for in full remission. For major depression to be diagnosed, at least five of the following symptoms must have been present during the same 2-week period and represent a change from previous functioning; at least one of the symptoms is either depressed mood or loss of interest or pleasure (American Psychiatric Association, 2000):

- Depressed mood most of the day, nearly every day (feels sad or empty).
- Markedly diminished interest in all activities.
- Significant weight loss (when not dieting) or weight gain, insomnia, or hypersomnia.
- Psychomotor agitation or retardation.
- Fatigue or loss of energy.
- Feelings of worthlessness or inappropriate guilt.
- Diminished ability to think or concentrate.
- Recurrent thoughts of death, recurrent suicidal ideation with or without a suicidal plan, or a suicide attempt (American Psychiatric Association, 2000).

In elderly individuals, it can be difficult to determine whether cognitive symptoms (disorientation, apathy, difficulty concentrating, memory loss) are better accounted for by a dementia or by a major depressive episode. This differential diagnosis may be informed by a thorough general medical evaluation and consideration of the onset of the disturbance, temporal sequencing of depressive and cognitive symptoms, course of illness, and treatment response. In dementia, there is usually a premorbid history of declining cognitive function, whereas the individual with major depressive disorder is much more likely to have a relatively normal premorbid state and abrupt cognitive decline associated with the depression (American Psychiatric Association, 2000).

Dysthymic Disorder (300.4)

The essential feature of dysthymic disorder is a chronically depressed mood that occurs for most of the day more days than not for at least 2 years. At least two or more of the following symptoms are present:

- Poor appetite or overeating.
- Insomnia or hypersomnia.
- Low energy or fatigue.
- Low self-esteem.
- Poor concentration or difficulty making decisions.
- Feelings of hopelessness.

Dysthymic disorder and major depressive disorder are differentiated based on severity, chronicity, and persistence. They share common symptoms, but dysthymic disorder is characterized by chronic, less severe depressive symptoms that have been present for many years (American Psychiatric Association, 2000).

Bipolar I Disorder (296.xx)

The diagnostic codes for bipolar I disorder are selected as follows: The first three digits are 296, and the fourth digit is 0 if there is a single manic episode. For recurrent episodes, the fourth digit indicates the nature of the current episode: 4 if the current episode is a hypomanic or manic, 5 if it is a major depressive episode, 6 if it is a mixed episode, and 7 if the current episode is unspecified. The fifth digit indicates the severity of the current episode: 1 for mild severity, 2 for moderate severity, 3 for severe without psychotic features, 4 for severe with psychotic features, 5 for in partial remission, 6 for in full remission (American Psychiatric Association, 2000).

The distinctive criteria for bipolar disorder is the presence of a manic episode, defined as a distinct period of abnormally and persistently elevated, expansive, or irritable mood, lasting at least 1 week (American Psychiatric Association, 2000). During the period of mood disturbance, three or more of the following symptoms have persisted:

- Inflated self-esteem or grandiosity.
- Decreased need for sleep (e.g., feels rested after only 3 hours of sleep).
- More talkative than usual or pressure to keep talking.
- Flight of ideas or subjective experience that thoughts are racing.
- Distractibility (i.e., attention too easily drawn to unimportant or irrelevant external stimuli).

- Increase in goal-directed activity (either socially, at work or school, or sexually) or psychomotor agitation.
- Excessive involvement in pleasurable activities that have a high potential for pain consequences (e.g., engaging in unrestrained buying sprees, sexual indiscretions, or foolish business investments).

Bipolar II Disorder (296.89)

The major differentiating feature between bipolar I and bipolar II is that the episodes in bipolar II are hypomanic instead of manic. In hypomania, the episode is not severe enough to cause marked impairment in social or occupational functioning or to necessitate hospitalization, and there are no psychotic features.

Postpartum Onset Specifier

The specifier with postpartum onset can be applied to major depressive or bipolar I or bipolar II disorders if the onset is within 4 weeks after childbirth (American Psychiatric Association, 2000). Postpartum depression occurs in a variety of countries, though the manifestations may vary by culture (Posmontier & Horowitz, 2004). Symptoms that are common in postpartum-onset episodes among U.S. women include:

- Fluctuations in mood.
- Mood lability.
- Preoccupation with infant well-being (may range from over concern to frank delusions).

The presence of severe ruminations or delusional thoughts about the infant is associated with a significantly increased risk of harm to the infant (American Psychiatric Association, 2000). Postpartum-onset episodes can present either with or without psychotic features. Infanticide is most often associated with postpartum psychotic episodes that are characterized by command hallucinations to kill the infant or delusions that the infant is possessed, but it can also occur in severe postpartum mood episodes without such specific delusions or hallucinations (American Psychiatric Association, 2000). In the rarest of cases, a disturbed mother may kill her infant, other family members, and/or herself (Lehmann, 2004). Even without the homicide/suicide risk, postpartum depression exerts a moderate to large effect on the interaction of mothers and infants (Logsdon et al., 2006). A study in the United Kingdom reported that infants of depressed mothers had significantly poorer weight gain (O'Brien, Heycock, Hanna, Jones, & Cox, 2004).

Postpartum depression is an intense and pervasive sadness with severe and labile mood swings and is more serious and persistent than postpartum blues. Occurring in approximately 10% to 15% of new mothers, these symptoms rarely disappear with outside help

(Herrick, 2002). The majority of these mothers do not seek help from any source, and only about 20% consult a health professional.

Many women feel especially guilty about having depressive feelings at a time when they believe they should be happy. They may be reluctant to discuss their symptoms or their negative feelings toward the child. A prominent feature of postpartum depression is rejection of the infant, often caused by abnormal jealousy (American Psychiatric Association, 2000). The mother may be obsessed by the notion that the offspring may take her place in her partner's affections. Attitudes toward the infant may include disinterest, annoyance with care demands, and blaming because of her lack of maternal feeling. When observed, she may appear awkward in her responses to the baby. Obsessive thoughts about harming the child are very frightening to her. Often she does not share these thoughts because of embarrassment, but when she does, other family members become very frightened (Fishel, 2007).

The occurrence of postpartum depression among teenage mothers was more than two and a half times that for older mothers (Herrick, 2002). African American mothers were twice as likely as White mothers to experience postpartum depression. Younger mothers (younger than 20 years old) and those with less than a high school degree were significantly less likely to seek help and had higher rates of postpartum depression (Herrick, 2002). Mothers who had no one to talk to about their problems after delivery had a high rate of postpartum depression and a low rate of help-seeking.

Based on her research, Beck (2002) identified 13 risk factors for postpartum depression, with those having the greater effect size listed first: prenatal depression, low self-esteem, stress of child care, prenatal anxiety, life stress, lack of social support, marital relationship problems, history of depression, "difficult" infant temperament, postpartum blues, single status, low socioeconomic status, and unplanned or unwanted pregnancy. Other research reported that fatigue also is an important predictor of postpartum depression (Bozoky & Corwin, 2001).

A postpartum depression screening scale developed by Cheryl Beck is available from Western Psychological Services (e-mail: custsvc@wpspublish.com). Administered in 5 to 10 minutes, the brief self-report instrument provides an overall severity score and scores for seven symptom areas. A cutoff score of 10.5 is recommended when using the Postpartum Depression Predictors Inventory-Revised during pregnancy; cutoff scores have not been determined yet for use during the postpartum period (Beck, Records, & Rice, 2006).

Premenstrual Dysphoric Disorder

Although premenstrual dysphoric disorder (PMDD) is included in the *DSM-IV*, it is only proposed as a new category for possible inclusion in the future. Criteria are still being refined. Approximately 3% to 8% of U.S. reproductive-age women, numbering 2 to 5 million, have symptoms of sufficient severity to be classified as PMDD (Mishell, 2005). In a large national community based sample, PMDD was associated with lower education, history of major depression, and current cigarette smoking (Cohen et al., 2002).

The hallmark feature of PMDD is the predictable, cyclic nature of symptoms or distinct on/offness that begins in the late luteal phase of the menstrual cycle and remits shortly after the onset of menstruation (Steiner et al., 2006). Five of the following symptoms must be present, but they must begin to remit within a few days after the onset of the follicular phase, and are absent in the week post menses. At least one of the symptoms must be one of the first four listed below:

■ Markedly depressed mood, feelings of helplessness, or self-deprecating thoughts.
■ Marked anxiety, tension, feelings of being keyed up or on edge.
■ Marked affective lability (e.g., feeling suddenly sad or tearful or increased sensitivity to rejection).
■ Persistent and marked anger or irritability or increased interpersonal conflicts.
■ Decreased interest in usual activities (e.g., work, school, friends, hobbies).
■ Subjective sense of difficulty in concentration.
■ Lethargy, easy fatigability, or marked lack of energy.
■ Marked change in appetite, overeating, or specific food cravings.
■ Hypersomnia or insomnia.
■ A subjective sense of being overwhelmed or out of control.
■ Other physical symptoms, such as breast tenderness or swelling, headaches, joint or muscle pain, a sensation of bloating, weight gain.

PMDD has an adverse impact on a woman's quality of life (especially her relationships with others) and productivity and leads to increased direct and indirect medical costs (Mishell, 2005). The proposed etiology is multifaceted and includes an underlying genetic predisposition that makes a woman more susceptible to changes in gonadal hormones that interact with neurotransmitters and the neurohormonal systems, resulting in symptoms that occur only in the luteal phase of the menstrual cycle (Halbreich, 2003).

Assessment of Depression

Diagnosing depression requires the nurse to match the patient's symptoms with the diagnostic criteria in the *DSM-IV*. Sometimes it is helpful to administer standardized tools. The advantage of using instruments is that one can evaluate more objectively the outcome of interventions to reduce depression. The most widely used self-report measurement designed explicitly for depression is the Beck Depression Inventory (Beck, 1995). The 21-item scale can be completed and scored quickly and easily, with or without the aid of an interviewer.

The Center for Epidemiological Studies Depression Scale is a self-report scale with 20 items selected from previously validated scales (Radloff, 1977). Its advantages include simple, clear language and the availability of general population norms. The Hamilton Rating Scale for Depression (Hamilton, 1960) has frequently been used as a measure of severity once depression has been identified. A trained rater or professional must complete it, and the interview may require 30 minutes. The Young-Mania Rating Scale is used in many research projects to measure the effects of treatment in patients with bipolar disorder, manic phase.

Another depression screening tool is the visual analogue scale. The patient is asked how depressed he or she feels on a scale from 1 to 10. You can draw a ladder with 10 steps or use stairs or whatever visualization is helpful.

Bipolar disorder can be assessed using the Mood Disorder Questionnaire (Hirschfeld et al., 2000). It is a single-page self-report questionnaire that can be easily scored by a clinician. In a large community sample, Hirschfeld and colleagues (2003) reported that about one-third of persons who screened positive for bipolar disorder had been misdiagnosed as having major depressive disorder, and 49% had never received any diagnosis at all. Misdiagnosis of bipolar disorder is common, because most patients seek treatment during their depressive episode (Miller, 2006). Antidepressant monotherapy in an undiagnosed bipolar patient can have devastating effects. For example, restlessness, insomnia, racing thoughts, and agitation can occur within a few weeks of initiation (Miller, 2006). Monotherapy can precipitate mania—a psychiatric emergency.

Gender Role Assessment

A gender role analysis is an important part of the assessment for depression. One should ask, "Which of these symptoms are primarily exaggerations of this woman's feminine gender role? Has this woman had experiences of interpersonal victimization? Are role strains and poverty contributing to her distress? Do parenting responsibilities overwhelm her?"

Suicide Assessment

All depressed patients should be assessed for risk of suicide. Use direct questions such as, "Sometimes when people feel depressed as you do, they think about hurting themselves or ending their life. Have you had any of these thoughts?" If the reply is yes, then assess the degree of danger for self-harm.

There are four criteria to measure in assessing the seriousness of a suicidal plan: method, availability, specificity, and lethality (Stuart, 2005c). Has the client specified a method? Is the method of choice available to her? How specific is the plan? If the method is concrete and detailed, with access right at hand, the suicide risk increases. How lethal is the method? The most lethal method is shooting, with hanging a close second. The least lethal is slashing one's wrists. Although women formerly relied on pills (lethality dependent on type and amount), they are increasingly more apt to use highly lethal methods.

Some characteristics place people at high risk for suicide. These include multiple high-lethality suicide attempts, family history of suicide attempts, hostility toward self or others, alcohol or substance abuse, psychosis, isolation, and feeling that no one cares (Stuart, 2005c).

If the person is at immediate risk, a family member, friend, responsible adult, or health care provider takes the woman to an appropriate mental health professional or an emergency department. If the person is deemed to be at moderate risk, the nurse can make an appointment with a mental health professional, use a no-suicide contract, give community resource information, identify sources of support, identify reasons not to take self-destructive action, and educate the client about depression and treatment success.

The repetition of suicidal behavior is common and occurs quickly. Risk factors for repetition include most importantly a previous suicidal behavior, but also include psychiatric treatment, being unemployed or registered sick, self-injury, alcohol misuse, and reporting suicidal plans or hallucinations (Kapur et al., 2006). The most important strategies to reduce repetition might include primary prevention of suicidal behavior, targeting psychiatric illness, and tackling social factors such as unemployment.

When more resources are available to the client, the crisis can be managed more easily. Even with these guidelines, the nurse is often in a position of trying to predict what the combination of signs says about the actual suicide risk now and in the future. The nurse has to make decisions about when and to whom to refer for mental health counseling, which family and community resources to utilize, and whether to initiate hospitalization.

Management

Depression is frequently underdiagnosed and undertreated in primary care settings. An important role for the nurse is to recognize the signs of depression and educate women clients that depression is an illness that responds to treatment. Much education is needed about the benefits of psychotherapy and psychotropic medications.

In addition to case finding, educating, and medicating, the nurse may refer women clients to self-help activities or groups and to other mental health professionals. Specialized treatment for resistant depression, a diagnosis of bipolar disorder, and the need for psychotherapy are three reasons to refer to mental health professionals.

Pharmacotherapy and Psychotherapy

Selecting appropriate treatments for individual patients is a complex dilemma. Treatment preferences (antidepressant medication and/or counseling) were assessed among primary care patients with depression (Lin et al., 2005). Participants who preferred medication were older, were in worse physical health, and were more likely to already be taking antidepressants. Overall, 72% of participants in this study were matched with their preferred treatment; matched participants demonstrated more rapid improvement in depression symptoms than unmatched participants (Lin et al., 2005).

In a meta-analysis of studies on efficacy of pharmacotherapy and psychotherapy for depression, remission did not differ between psychotherapy (38%) and pharmacotherapy (35%) (DeMaat, Dekker, Schoevers, & De Jonghe, 2006). Both treatments performed better in mild than in moderate depression. At follow-up, relapse in pharmacotherapy (57%) was higher than in psychotherapy (27%). They concluded that psychotherapy and pharmacotherapy appear equally efficacious in depression. Both treatments have larger effects in mild than in moderate depression (DeMaat et al., 2006).

Research suggests that psychotherapy may play an important role in enhancing the effects of antidepressant drug therapy and improving patients' long-term prognosis (Petersen, 2006). Neuroimaging data suggest that psychotherapy and pharmacotherapy target different primary sites of the cortical-limbic pathway with differential top-down and bottom-up effects, resulting in modulation of critical common targets and facilitation of disease remission (Peterson, 2006). The use of adjunctive psychotherapy in the acute phase of antidepressant drug treatment appears to provide only a modest increase in response rates, but the sequential use of psychotherapy after remission with acute drug therapy may confer a better long-term prognosis for preventing relapse. For some women, psychotherapy alone may be a viable alternative to maintenance medication therapy (Petersen, 2006).

General Guidelines for Medication Treatment

Clients need to know that they must take the medicines as prescribed and that it normally takes 2 to 4 weeks to get a response. Educating clients about side effects and working with them to deal with side effects usually results in higher success in treating the depression. Antidepressants are among the most frequently prescribed medications in the United States (Weilburg, Stafford, O'Leary, Meigs, & Findelstein, 2004). Advanced practice nurses prescribe antidepressants. This privilege carries tremendous responsibility. The nurse needs to establish a caring, hopeful relationship and see the patient weekly for the first month to 6 weeks. Without this support, many patients will discontinue medication before it has had a chance to work.

When prescribing any psychotropic medication, starting low on the dosage and going slowly in increasing the dosage helps to prevent side effects. Never abruptly discontinue antidepressant medications, because withdrawal symptoms can be severe. Be sure to caution patients about not discontinuing medications on their own.

A black box warning about the potential of suicide is now included for most antidepressants. A meta-analysis of randomized controlled trials reported that selective serotonin reuptake inhibitors (SSRIs) increase suicide ideation compared with placebo, but the SSRIs do not increase suicide risk more than older antidepressants. If SSRIs increase suicide risk in some patients, the number of additional deaths is very small, because ecological studies have generally found that suicide mortality has declined as antidepressant use has increased (Hall & Lucke, 2006). In another meta-analysis, it was found that antidepressants may cause a small short-term risk of self-harm or suicidal events in children and adolescents with major depressive disorder (Dubicka, Hadley, & Roberts, 2006).

Antidepressant therapy may influence driving safety. In a recent study, about 16% of depressed patients discharged from hospital to outpatient treatment were found to be unfit to drive, and 60% performed at a questionable level of fitness for driving (Brunnauer, Laux, Geiger, Soyka, & Moller, 2006). The data revealed an advantage for patients treated with SSRIs or mirtazapine when compared with tricyclic antidepressants (TCSs) or venlafaxine.

Unless there is a concern about cost, SSRIs are the first choice of antidepressants (DiPiro et al., 2005). There are few guidelines, however, to determine which specific medications to select for the individual patient. Considerations include prior positive response, responses in family members, short- and long-term side effects, interaction with other medications, patient preferences, patient age, cost of medication, concurrent medical disorders, and concurrent psychiatric disorders. If the patient or a family member has a history of bipolar disorder, bipolar disorder may be presenting as depression. In such cases, an antidepressant should not be started, because a manic episode could be triggered. Most women with bipolar disorder need to be managed by a psychiatric specialist.

After starting a patient on an antidepressant medication, she should be monitored every 1 to 2 weeks for the first few months. Assess response at week 6, and,

if clearly better, continue treatment for 6 more weeks; if there is complete remission after 6 weeks, continue for at least 4 to 9 months. If the patient is somewhat better at week 6, continue treatment or adjust the dosage and monitor every 1 to 2 weeks. Assess response at week 12, and, if no better, refer to a psychiatrist or advanced practice psychiatric nurse practitioner (DiPiro et al., 2005). Initial depression severity and receiving adequate pharmacotherapy predict early recovery in individuals with major depression seeking outpatient treatment (Meyers et al., 2002). These authors also reported that only 45% of the subjects in their study met criteria for adequate pharmacotherapy. In a groundbreaking 20-year naturalistic study, other researchers reported that subjects treated with higher levels of antidepressant treatment were almost twice as likely to recover as those who received no somatic treatment; therefore, depression should be treated more aggressively (Leon, Solomon, & Mueller, 2003).

Hirschfeld (2001) wrote that depression, which only a few decades ago was considered to be a short-term illness requiring short-term treatment, is now recognized as a recurrent, sometimes chronic, long-term illness. He reported that approximately one-third to one-half of patients successfully stabilized in acute-phase treatment will relapse if medication is not sustained throughout the continuation period. Only 10% to 15% will relapse if medication is continued. For maintenance-phase therapy, approximately 60% of patients at risk will experience a recurrent episode of depression within 1 year if untreated, whereas those who continue in treatment will have a recurrence rate between 10% and 30% (Hirschfeld, 2001).

Selective Serotonin Reuptake Inhibitors

Six SSRIs are currently available in the United States, including two in generic versions (fluoxetine and fluvoxamine) (see Table 13.1). They act by inhibiting the reuptake of serotonin, one of the key neurotransmitters implicated in depression (DiPiro et al., 2005). Other neurotransmitters are also affected, such as muscarinic and norepinephrine receptors for paroxetine and dopamine receptors for sertraline. The SSRIs are more expensive than older antidepressants such as tricyclics (TCAs). The efficacy of SSRIs is superior to placebo and equal to TCAs in treating adults with major depression (DiPiro et al., 2005). Fluoxetine and sertraline are efficacious for treating adults with dysthymia. SSRIs are generally better tolerated than TCAs and are a first-line treatment option for major depressive disorder and dysthymia (Wagstaff, Cheer, Matheson, Ormrod, & Goa, 2002).

Early side effects include activation (restlessness, insomnia, anxiety), sedation (somnolence, dizziness), autonomic (sweating, dry mouth), and gastrointestinal symptoms (anorexia, constipation, diarrhea, nausea)

13.1 | Antidepressants: Selective Serotonin Reuptake Inhibitors (SSRIs)

GENERIC NAME	TRADE NAME	USUAL DOSAGE AND DIAGNOSIS
Citalopram	Celexa	20–60 mg per day
Escitalopram	Lexapro	10–20 mg per day
		10 mg per day for elderly
Fluoxetine	Prozac	20–60 mg per day for depression
		20–80 mg per day for obsessive-compulsive disorder
		20 mg per day for panic disorder
	Serafem	20 mg per day
	Prozac weekly	90 mg per week
Fluvoxamine	Luvox	50–150 mg per day for obsessive-compulsive disorder
Paroxetine	Paxil	20–50 mg per day for depression and generalized anxiety disorder
20–60 mg per day for obsessive-compulsive disorder		
	Paxil, CR	25–62.5 mg per day for depression
		12.5–75 mg per day for panic disorder
		10–60 mg per day for panic disorder
Sertraline	Zoloft	20–200 mg per day for depression, obsessive-compulsive disorder, panic disorder, post-traumatic stress disorder, social anxiety disorder
		50–150 mg per day for premenstrual dysphoric disorder

(DiPiro et al., 2005). Troubling persistent side effects may include sexual dysfunction and weight gain. Duloxetine-treated patients had a mean decrease in weight of 0.5 kg compared with an increase of 0.2 kg for patients receiving placebo (Hudson et al., 2005). Fluoxetine is the most activating; fluvoxamine and paroxetine have higher incidences of sedation; and paroxetine has higher rates of anticholinergic effects such as dry mouth, blurred vision, and constipation (DiPiro et al., 2005).

Abruptly discontinuing SSRIs can cause a rebound syndrome for many patients (Baldwin, Montgomery, Nil, & Lader, 2005; Bhanji, Chouinard, Kolivakis, & Margolese, 2006). A review of 46 case reports and 3 studies revealed that the most common minor new withdrawal symptoms included physical (headache, dizziness, visual disturbances, vertigo, gait instability, tremor, nausea, emesis, and diarrhea); affective (anxiety and irritability); and psychomotor (agitation and parasthesias) (Bhanji et al., 2006). Symptoms generally commenced within 48 hours and lasted approximately 1 week. Women are at higher risk than men, and those with underlying anxiety and dysthymic disorders and earlier age of onset of dysthymia are at greater risk.

Discontinuation profiles differ between antidepressants of the same class (Baldwin et al., 2005). Paroxetine is the most problematic SSRI because it has the shortest half-life and the most anticholinergic activity; fluoxetine has the fewest reported cases of withdrawal and the longest half-life (Bhanji et al., 2006). The decreased availability of synaptic serotonin and down-regulated serotonin receptors may explain the symptoms associated with SSRI withdrawal. This information should caution clinicians to gradually taper SSRIs when stopping pharmacotherapy.

Although the SSRIs have been called miracle drugs, nurses should be on the alert for an adverse side effect called *serotonin syndrome*. This syndrome occurs mostly as the result of an interaction between an SSRI and other serotonergic agents, although it can occur when a patient is taking only an SSRI. The syndrome is caused by the inhibition of specific cytochrome P-450 isoenzymes, which results in significant elevations in drug concentrations and reduction in drug clearance (DiPiro et al., 2005).

Patients with serotonin syndrome typically present with altered mental status, agitation, myoclonus, hyperreflexia, diaphoresis, shivering, tremor, diarrhea, incoordination and hyperthermia and hyperthermia (Christensen, 2005). As the syndrome progresses, patients may develop lead-pipe muscle rigidity, acute dystonias, and movement disorders. Older patients are particularly vulnerable to neuromuscular symptoms. Lab work might show progressive and markedly elevated serum creatine phosphokinase, elevated white blood cell count and transaminases, and the serum bicarbonate level may be low. Treatment begins by taking the patient off the offending medication and observing closely. Most cases resolve within 24 hours once the serotonergic agents have been removed. Lorazepam (1 to 2 mg slow IV push every 30 minutes) may alleviate symptoms and possibly shorten the clinical course (Christensen, 2005).

To decrease the risk of serotonin syndrome, a drug washout period of 2 or more weeks is recommended when patients change antidepressant medication—or when any changes involving an SSRI and a serotonergic agent are being considered. Patients need to be informed about the possibility of this syndrome, especially if SSRIs are combined with one or more other SSRIs, monoamine oxidase inhibitors (MAOIs), TCAs, tryptophan, St. John's wort, or other serotonin agonists such as buspirone (DiPiro et al., 2005).

Clinical data warns about the current use of SSRIs with warfarin (Coumadin®). Abnormal bleeding has been reported, and most reports appear to be associated with fluoxetine and sertraline (Lam, 2002).

Novel Antidepressants

The most frequently used novel antidepressants are bupropion, venalafaxine, mirtazapine, and trazadone (see Table 13.2). Bupropion has a mild effect on the reuptake of norepinephrine and serotonin, and its most potent neurochemical action is blockade of dopamine (DiPiro et al., 2005). Also used for smoking cessation (Zyban®), bupropion is contraindicated in patients with seizure disorders, bulimia, and anorexia. The common side effects are agitation, insomnia, gastrointestinal upset, and headache. Bupropion has a low incidence of sexual side effects and weight gain. Because it may interfere with sleep, it is usually taken in the morning.

Venlafaxine (Effexor®) is a serotonin and norepinephrine reuptake inhibitor. The most common side effect is nausea, but tolerance is usually built over a few weeks (DiPiro et al., 2005). Other side effects include somnolence, dry mouth, dizziness, insomnia, constipation, nervousness, sweating, sexual dysfunction, and anorexia. Note that 2% to 5% of patients will experience

13.2 | Antidepressants: Novel Agents

GENERIC NAME	TRADE NAME	USUAL DOSAGE AND DIAGNOSIS
Novel		
Buproprion	Wellbutrin	100 mg three times per day
	Wellbutrin SR	150 mg twice per day
	Zyban	150 mg twice per day for 7 to 12 weeks
	Bupropion	100 mg three times per day
Maprotiline	Ludiomil	75–150 mg per day
	Marpotiline	25–75 mg twice per day to three times per day
Mirtazapine	Remeron	15–45 every bedtime
Nefazodone	Serzone	150–300 mg twice per day
Trazadone	Desyrel/Trazadone	50–100 mg twice per day to three times per day
Serotonin/norepinephrine reuptake inhibitors		
Duloxetine	Cymbalta	20–30 mg twice per day
Venlafaxine	Effexor	37.5–75 mg twice per day to three times per day
	Effexor XR	75 mg per day for depression
		75–225 mg per day for generalized anxiety disorder and social anxiety disorder
Noradrenalin reuptake inhibitors		
Reboxetine	Vestra	Not FDA approved

elevation of blood pressure, so venlafaxine should be used with caution and blood pressure should be closely monitored with patients who have hypertension (DiPiro et al., 2005). Venlafaxine has been found to be especially useful in treatment-resistant depression (Howland, 2006c). In one study, a more rapid response and higher remission rates were noted with venlafaxine compared to the SSRIs (Kornstein & Wojcik, 2002).

Mirtazapine acts by stimulating the release of norepinephrine and serotonin and blocks serotonin receptors. Adverse effects include somnolence, increased appetite, cholesterol increase, weight gain, and dizziness. Mirtazapine improves sleep, reduces anxiety, and has minimal sexual side effects or gastrointestinal upsets. It appears safe for medical patients taking multiple medications because it doesn't interfere with metabolism of other medications (DiPiro et al., 2005).

Trazadone inhibits the reuptake of serotonin and blocks serotonin, histamine, alpha 1, and alpha 2 receptors. The major advantage of trazadone is that it treats insomnia, which may accompany SSRIs and other antidepressants. Because of the histamine blockade, anticholinergic side effects do occur. The potential side effect of priapism with men does not affect women (DiPiro et al., 2005).

A recent drug alert about liver damage with *nefazodone* (Serzone®) has limited its usefulness. *Reboxetine* is the first truly selective noradrenaline reuptake inhibitor. Common side effects include tachycardia and sexual dysfunction and anticholinergic side effects. Reboxetine is

FDA approved in the United States. *duloxetine*, a new dual-action serotonin/norepinephrine reuptake inhibitor antidepressant works to relieve anxiety and physical symptoms such as headache and muscle and joint pain in depressed patients. Nausea, dry mouth, and somnolence were the most common adverse events; no significant incidence of hypertension or weight gain was noted (Brown University, 2002). Female sexual dysfunction with duloxetine was comparable to paroxetine.

Tricyclic Antidepressants

Unless cost is a prohibiting factor, TCAs are not usually used until after SSRIs and the novel antidepressants have failed. Although they are equally efficacious to the SSRIs, they do cause significant side effects and can cause death in overdose because of cardiotoxicity (DiPiro et al., 2005). *Imipramine* is the oldest of the TCAs and is often used as the research comparative in clinical trials of newer antidepressants (see Table 13.3).

All of the TCAs block H1, Ach, alpha1, and serotonin receptors. Tertiary amines also inhibit the reuptake of serotonin, and the secondary amines also inhibit the reuptake of norepinephrine. This extensive manipulation of synaptic activity causes a myriad of side effects such as sedation/drowsiness; hypotension; weight gain; anticholinergic effects (dry mouth, blurred vision, difficulty voiding, constipation, sweating); postural hypotension; dizziness; tachycardia; memory problems; and sexual dysfunction (DiPiro et al., 2005). Suicidal patients

13.3 | Antidepressants: Tricyclics and Monomamine Oxidase Inhibitors

GENERIC NAME	TRADE NAME	USUAL DOSAGE AND DIAGNOSIS
Tricyclics (tertiary amines)		
Amitriptyline	Elavil	not available
	Amitriptyline	50–100 mg per day
Clomipramine	Anafranil/Clomipramine	150–250 mg every bedtime
Imipramine	Tofranil/Imipramine	150-300 mg every bedtime
Doxepin	Sinequan/Doxepin	150–300 mg every bedtime for depression and anxiety
Tricyclics (secondary amines)		
Desipramine	Norpramin/Desipramine	100–200 mg every morning
Nortriptyline	Pamelor/Nortriptyline	50–150 mg every bedtime
Monoamine oxidase inhibitors		
Phenelzine	Nardil	15 mg three times per day
Tranylcypromine	Parnate	30 mg per day

should never be given more than a 1-week prescription because of the potential of overdose.

Patients are usually begun on a low or modest dose of a TCA; gradually the dosage is increased until undesirable side effects appear or until clinical improvement occurs. Orthostatic hypotension usually can be avoided if the dosage is increased slowly. If no improvement is noted in 4 to 6 weeks, the patient's blood level of the drug can be checked (DiPiro et al., 2005). The client may be metabolizing the drug too rapidly or absorbing it poorly. If so, the dosage can be increased, or another antidepressant drug may be tried.

Most tricyclic antidepressants are given at bedtime because they tend to have a sedative effect. Alternately, *desipramine* is generally less sedative and therefore better administered during the day. When higher dosages are being administered, an electrocardiogram is usually obtained to ensure that the drug is not interfering with cardiac conduction.

Common complaints of patients on TCAs and the MAOIs include weight gain; *amitriptyline* and *doxepin* are most likely to cause weight gain, and many women thus refuse to take them. Reducing the amount of sweets ingested and substituting no- or low-calorie drinks is usually necessary to help contain weight gain. Dry mouth can be managed by chewing sugar-free gum and eating sugar-free hard candy.

Another nursing concern for patients on TCAs is constipation. Constipation can be corrected in most cases by use of a bulking agent such as Dulcolax®. Consumption of foods high in fiber (such as Fiber One® cereal), increased water intake (about 10 glasses per day), and increased exercise are useful measures to alleviate constipation.

There are numerous concerns about prescribing TCAs for elderly patients, especially the increased likelihood of falls due to orthostasis (DiPiro et al., 2005). Eye pain should be reported immediately, because it could signal an acute glaucoma attack.

Monoamine Oxidase Inhibitors

The main concern with MAOI drugs, which has limited their clinical use, is the risk of hypertensive crisis caused by dietary and drug interactions (Howland, 2006b). However, an argument can still be made that MAOIs are particularly effective in treating atypical, anxious, bipolar, and treatment refractory types of depression (DiPiro et al., 2005). The action of the MAOIs is unique because they inhibit the enzymatic action of monoamine oxidase, which in turn increases norepinephrine, serotonin, and dopamine in the presynaptic neuron. It also inhibits monoamine oxidase in the liver, which can cause drug interaction problems (DiPiro et al., 2005). The side effects are similar to the TCAs, with the addition of hypertensive crisis (see Table 13.3).

Patients should be taught to watch for signs of hypertensive crisis—throbbing occipital headache, stiff neck, chills, nausea, flushing of head and face, retro-orbital pain, apprehension, pallor, sweating and fever, chest pain, and palpitations (DiPiro et al., 2005). The nurse will also observe extremely high blood pressure and dilated pupils.

This crisis is brought on by the patient eating foods that contain tyramine (a sympathomimetic pressor amine), which normally is broken down by the enzyme monoamine oxidase. Because antidepressant drugs inhibit monoamine oxidase, patients who take MAOIs without limiting their intake of tyramine can rapidly develop hypertensive crisis (DiPiro et al., 2005). Tyramine restriction begins the day the patient takes the first dose and continues for 2 weeks after the last dose. Many foods have to be avoided (see Exhibit 13.1).

Hypertensive crisis also can be caused by drug interactions, including with demerol, sympathomimetics, antihypertensives, central nervous system depressants, antidepressants, general anesthetics, ginseng and over-the-counter cold preparations (DiPiro et al., 2005). Patient need to inform all medication prescribers about being on a MAOI medication. The treatment for hypertensive crisis is 10 to 20 mg of oral nifedipine or 5 mg of phentolamine IV (DiPiro et al., 2005).

Nonprescriptive Products

Hypericum (St. John's wort) is more effective than placebo for the short-term treatment of mild to moderate

---

EXHIBIT 13.1 FOODS CONTAINING TYRAMINE

Alcoholic beverages (beer, ale, and Chianti wine)
Dairy products (aged cheese, yogurt, and sour cream)
Fruits and vegetables (avocados, bananas, canned figs)
Meats (bologna, chicken liver, dried fish, meat tenderizer, pickled herring, salami, sausage)
Other foods (caffeinated beverages, chocolate, licorice, soy sauce, yeast)

Note. From *Pharmacotherapy,* by R. DiPiro, R. Talbert, G. Yee, G. Matzke, B. Wells, and M. Posey, 2005, New York: McGraw-Hill.

depression (Leerubier, Clere, Didi, & Kieser, 2002); however, it is not more effective than an SSRI in the treatment of moderately severe major depression (Davidson et al., 2002). Although rates of side effects are low (see Table 13.4), the following cautions exist for interactions with other drugs. St. John's wort may reduce the efficacy of digoxin, and cardiac patients who are taking digoxin are advised to avoid this herbal product. In addition, decreased pharmacologic effects with the blood thinner or anticoagulant warfarin (Coumadin®) as a result of concurrent St. John's wort therapy have been reported (Xuemin et al., 2004). There was no evidence of ovulation during low-dose oral contraceptive and St. John's wort combination therapy, but intracyclic bleeding episodes increased, which might adversely affect compliance to contraceptives (Pfrunder et al., 2003).

In a meta-analysis of 11 research studies, the authors concluded that there may be a role for the dietary supplement S-adenosyl-L-methionine (SAM-e) in the treatment for depression (Williams, Girard, Sabina, & Katz, 2005). A disadvantage is that it is expensive in dosages needed to treat depression, and it is not covered by insurance.

Gender Differences in Pharmacologic Treatment

A growing literature demonstrates gender differences in pharmacokinetics, including differences in drug absorption and bioavailabiltiy, drug distribution, and drug metabolism and elimination (Kornstein & Wojcik, 2002).

> For example, women have a slower gastric emptying time, lower gastric acid secretion, higher percentage of body fat, decreased hepatic metabolism, and lower renal clearance compared to men. Such differences in pharmacokinetics may lead to higher plasma levels and longer half-lives of drugs, as well as a greater sensitivity to side effects in women. In addition, medication levels in women may be altered by hormonal changes associated with the menstrual cycle, pregnancy, menopause, as well as by the use of exogenous hormones, such as oral contraceptive or hormone replacement therapy. (Kornstein & Wojcik, 2002, p. 155)

Depressed men and women also respond differently to pharmacologic treatment. Men were found to respond significantly greater than women to treatment with imipramine (a TCA), and women had significantly greater response than men to SSRIs (Khan, Brodhead, Schwartz, Kolts, & Brown, 2005; Kornstein, 2003). In a study comparing paroxetine and imipramine for the treatment of major depressive disorder, paroxetine-treated women had a significantly greater decrease in Hamilton Rating Scale for Depression scores compared with imipramine-treated women (Kornstein, 2003). In another study of 635 patients, significantly fewer women than men responded to imipramine, and significantly fewer men than women responded to sertraline. Women with dysthymia had a much more robust response to sertraline than did men (Kornstein, 2003). Younger women responded better for fluoxetine than to maprotiline (Kornstein & Wojcik, 2002).

The research to date suggests that the TCA imipramine is not as effective for the treatment of depression in women as SSRI drugs such as paroxetine and sertraline. In a study of menopausal women, those receiving estrogen and sertraline treatment experienced a greater improvement than women who received sertraline only (Kornstein, 2003).

Pregnancy

No antidepressants are currently approved by the U.S. Food and Drug Administration (FDA) for use during pregnancy. Many scientists are reluctant to do research on the effects of psychotropic medications on fetuses. Because the majority of women are not aware of their

13.4 | Herbal Preparations and Dietary Supplements

NAME	USUAL DOSAGE AND DIAGNOSIS
St. John's wort	300 mg three times per day for depresion
Ginkgo	60–240 mg twice per day for reverse sexual dysfunction
S-adenosylmethionine (SAMe)	800 mg twice per day for depression
Valerian	400–900 mg at bedtime for anxiety
Kava	100 mg three times per day for anxiety

Note. From *Pharmacist's Letter/Prescriber's Letter Natural Medicines Comprehensive Database*, by F. Jellin, P. Gregory, H. Batz, and colleagues, 2002, Stockton, CA: Therapeutic Research Faculty.

pregnancy until at least 6 weeks' gestation, psychotropic medications may be discontinued after the period of greatest potential risk to the fetus has passed (Schatzberg & Nemeroff, 2004). The largest databases are on the TCAs, fluoxetine, sertraline, and paroxetine. In one landmark study, Nulman and colleagues (1997) reported that in utero exposure to fluoxetine or TCAs did not affect either neurodevelopment or behavior in preschool-age children. However, some studies have reported higher rates of prenatal complications (low maternal weight gain, premature birth, and delayed fetal growth rate) associated with third-trimester use of fluoxetine (Hendrick & Altshuler, 2002). In a study comparing 17 SSRI-exposed and 17 nonexposed newborns, the women who used SSRIs during pregnancy had healthy infants; however, they also showed disruptions in a wide range of neurobehavioral outcomes (Zeskind & Stephens, 2004). In reviewing 93 cases of SSRI-induced neonatal withdrawal syndrome, paroxetine (Paxil) caused the most (64 babies), followed by fluoxetine (Prozac®; 14 14), sertraline (Zoloft®; 9), and citalopram (Celexa®; 7) (Sanz et al., 2005).

Although nonpharmacologic treatment is preferable in milder cases, in a severely depressed pregnant woman, the risks of nontreatment versus possible risks to the fetus must be weighed carefully. In one study, 75% of women who discontinued antidepressant medications relapsed during pregnancy; the majority occurred in the first trimester, and relapse was more prevalent in women with histories of more chronic depression (Cohen et al., 2004). Depression may lead to poor prenatal care, substance use, suicide, obstetric complications, and postpartum depression (Kornstein, 2003). Untreated depression may have adverse effects on the developing fetus, including preterm birth, small head circumference, and low Apgar scores (Pigarelli, Kraus, & Potter, 2005).

Another treatment for severe or delusional depression is electroconvulsive therapy, which can be a safe and beneficial treatment for depressed, pregnant women. A telecare intervention with postpartum depressed mothers was reported to significantly lower depression scores (Ugarriza & Schmidt, 2006).

Sexual Dysfunction and Treatment

Even though antidepressants do cause sexual dysfunction, a careful evaluation is necessary because other factors may be involved, such as depression itself, concomitant general medical illness, other medications, or premorbid sexual dysfunction. Symptoms of sexual dysfunction include decreased libido, impotence, painful erections, decreased vaginal lubrication, and impaired orgasmic function.

Men taking SSRIs report higher rates of sexual side effects than women; however, women seem to experience more severe sexual dysfunction (Hensley & Nurnberg, 2002). In patients with previously normal sexual function, 1,022 (610 women) were interviewed using the Psychotropic Related Sexual Dysfunction Questionanaire (Montejo, Llorea, Izquierdo, & Vico-Villademoros, 2001). The overall incidence of sexual dysfunction was 59.1%. Among the SSRIs, patients taking citalopram reported the highest incidence (72.7%) of sexual dysfunction, with other SSRIs following close behind (see Table 13.5). Antidepressants with the lowest incidence of sexual dysfunction are bupropion, nefazodone, mirtazapine, and reboxetine (Hensley & Nurnberg, 2002). Patients using Cymbalta® had significantly better sexual functioning compared with those who were treated with fluoxetine (Paxil®) or Lexapro (Delgado et al., 2005).

Management strategies for sexual dysfunction include wait and hope sexual functioning will return, reduce the current dose, take a drug holiday (skip antidepressant the day of planned sexual activity), use adjunctive pharmacotherapy (bupropion, amantadine, yohimbine, buspirone, sildenafil citrate, cyproheptadine, mirtazapine), or switch antidepressants. Bupropion can be prescribed 75 mg 30 minutes before sex or 100–150 mg each

13.5 | Incidence of Sexual Dysfunction With Antidepressant Medications

NAME OF DRUG	PERCENTAGE OF PATIENTS WHO EXPERIENCE SEXUAL DYSFUNCTION
Citalopram	72.7
Paroxetine	70.7
Venlafaxine	67.3
Sertraline	62.9
Fluvoxamine	62.3
Fluoxetine	57.7

day. Subjects treated with bupropion SR up to 300 mg daily for 7 weeks reported improvement of all sexual side effects for 46% of women and 75% of men (Gitlin, Suri, Altshuler, Zuckerbrow-Miller, & Fairbanks, 2002). Most of the improvement occurred within the first 2 weeks and at low dose.

Treatment Resistance

Successful treatment of depression means complete restoration of psychosocial functioning. Before an antidepressant trial can be declared a failure, several initial steps should be taken: review carefully the diagnosis, evaluate the patient's adherence to the prescribed medication regimen, and maximize current antidepressant dosage (Bailey, 2003). After initial steps, the clinician has three options: switch to a different antidepressant, augment the current antidepressant with an agent from another class (such as thyroid, lithium, antipsychotic), or combine another antidepressant with the current one (Bailey, 2003).

Several augmentation strategies to enhance antidepressant response have shown possible advantages in women. Augmentation with triiodothyronine, specifically L-thyroxine (T4), may be more beneficial in women than in men (Bauer et al., 2002; Kornstein & Wojcik, 2002). Estrogen replacement therapy may enhance response to SSRIs (fluoxetine/sertaline) in postmenopausal women (Kornstein, 2003). In addition, lithium and stimulants may be more effective as augmenting agents in women (Kornstein & Wojcik, 2002).

Efficacy of Psychotherapy in Major Depression

Studies have shown that women with depression do better with psychotherapy and pharmacological treatment than with medication alone, especially patients with more severe depression (Frank, et al., 2000) and women over age 50 (Kornstein & Wojcik, 2002). Psychotherapy targets specific symptoms associated with relapse (such as guilt, hopelessness, negativity, and low self-esteem) that antidepressants may not affect and that frequently are identified in depressed women (Petersen, 2006). Of particular concern is that use of psychotherapy remains uncommon among depressed older adults despite its widely acknowledged efficacy (Wenhui, Sambamoorthi, Olfson, Walkup, & Crystal, 2005).

The psychotherapy treatment for depression that has been most widely studied and most widely regarded by proponents of clinical trial methodologies is cognitive-behavioral therapy (CBT). Other psychotherapy modalities found efficacious are behavioral or cognitive therapy as separate models, and interpersonal therapy (IPT). In a large National Institute of Mental Health (NIMH) multisite collaborative research program for the treatment of

depression, patients were assigned to a psychotherapy, imipramine, or placebo treatment group (Sotsky, 2006). Differential treatment outcomes were identified:

- Low social dysfunction predicted superior response to IPT.
- Low cognitive dysfunction predicted superior response to CBT and to imipramine.
- High work dysfunction predicted superior response to imipramine.
- High depression severity and impairment of function predicted superior response to imipramine and to IPT.

Two additional findings were reported in the NIMH study. The therapeutic alliance had a significant effect on clinical outcome for both psychotherapies and for active and placebo pharmacotherapy (Krupnick et al., 2006). Among those with a history of early childhood trauma (loss of parents at an early age, physical or sexual abuse, or neglect), psychotherapy alone was superior to antidepressant monotherapy (Nemeroff et al., 2005). Moreover, the combination of psychotherapy and pharmacotherapy was only marginally superior to psychotherapy alone among the childhood abuse cohort. The researchers conclude that psychotherapy may be an essential element in the treatment of patients with chronic forms of major depression with a history of childhood trauma (Nemeroff et al., 2005).

Cognitive-Behavioral Therapy

The evolution of CBT took place in three stages. Initially, behavior therapy emerged in independent but parallel developments in the United Kingdom and the United States between 1950 and 1970. The second stage, the growth of cognitive therapy, took place in the United States in the mid-1960s, mostly because of the work of Aaron Beck (1974), when it was recognized that behavior therapy was not as successful with depression as it was with anxiety disorders. The third stage was the merging of the two and took place in the late 1980s. Today, most therapists practice CBT instead of either cognitive therapy (CT) or behavioral therapy (BT), but much of the earlier research was done on the two modalities separately.

The theory explains that depressive symptoms arise from dysfunctional beliefs and thought processes as a result of early learning experiences (Ebmeier, Donaghey, & Steele, 2006). Therapy aims to identify these cognitive distortions and correct them through reality testing. Research has not always supported the efficacy of CBT as superior to other therapies in acute treatment; however, in a review of studies, CBT was found to be a more effective long-term approach than the use of TCAs alone (Ebmeier et al., 2006). In a randomized control trial consisting of a new-age use of telephone-administered

CBT (as compared to supportive emotion-focused psychotherapy) for depression, patients showed significant improvements in depression and positive affect during and following the treatment (Mohr et al., 2005).

In a rigorous and classic experimental study to compare the relative effectiveness of the components of CBT, researchers reported that all treatment conditions were equally effective for treating depression (Jacobson et al., 1996). The comparison involved randomly assigning 150 outpatients with major depression to one of three treatment groups. The groups were (1) behavioral activation alone, (2) behavioral activation and CT, and (3) a full CBT treatment that included both behavioral activation and CT as well as treatment to address core schema of depression.

Cognitive Therapy

Cognitive therapy is often helpful with depressed women. Cognitive therapy is standardized and brief (15 to 20 sessions) and is characterized by highly specific learning experiences; each session consists of a review of reactions to and results of the previous session, planning specific tasks, and assignment of homework (Karasu, 1990). The therapist is continually active and deliberately interacting with the woman. The therapy is based on the maladaptive cognitions theory that people (especially women) behave on the basis of misconceptions and unrealistic thought patterns. The therapist allies herself with the client against the depressive symptoms that afflict the client. Beck and Greenberg (1974) note three approaches, described below.

1. The nurse helps the client learn to recognize idiosyncratic thoughts, and this process may help regulate the depression. The client must learn to distance herself emotionally from her thoughts (that is, to view them objectively) with the critical perspective that will enable her to judge whether the thoughts are realistic or justified. A homemaker who sought help because of global feelings of depression, apathy, and inertia was instructed to pay close attention to her thoughts from the time she woke in the morning and throughout the day. After a day or so, she realized that when she began her household chores she would think, "I'm an incompetent housekeeper; I'll never be able to get this done." This is an example of reacting to a single, isolated failure by overgeneralization. The homemaker in the example was directed to look objectively at what she was a failure at (she did not wash her husband's favorite shirt by the time he wanted it); she came to recognize that one mistake did not constitute total failure. Another woman assumed that her friends no longer cared about her because no one telephoned for a day or two. She was helped to weigh the evidence on which her spontaneous conclusions were based and to consider alternative explanations. Actually, of her two best friends, Mary was sick and Joan was out of town. Another client was overly absorbed in the negative aspect of her life. When she was required to write down and report back positive experiences, she recognized her selective attention to the negative (Beck & Greenberg, 1974).

2. The nurse calls attention to the client's stereotyped themes that influence thinking. The automatic thoughts that constitute the woman's immediate reaction to an event may be cognitive shorthand for elaborate ideas deeply rooted in past experiences that are no longer relevant. A woman who reported that she made a fool of herself in a job interview recognized that this assessment reflected not her actual performance but her tendency to see herself as a subject of humiliation. In reviewing her actual behavior, the nurse was able to shed doubt on the client's perception. In continuing to evaluate new experiences, the woman not only got a more realistic perspective of herself, but also learned new skills to cope with confirmed areas of difficulty (Beck & Greenberg, 1974).

3. The nurse observes that the client holds misconceptions, prejudices, and even superstitions that need to be exposed and evaluated. One university faculty member experienced intense depression when her promotion to full professor was denied. She was helped to see that she held a set of interlocking beliefs, such as, "If I don't become a full professor, my work and life are meaningless." The faculty member was helped to discover other areas of her academic role and was reminded of the family and friends who were rich sources of gratification. Subjecting her basic premises to a process of validation helped her to stop worrying about recognition and to get more enjoyment out of her work. Meanwhile, she looked at the criteria for promotion and readjusted her priorities to do more publishing. Sometimes, idiosyncratic cognitions take a pictorial rather than a verbal form. A woman who felt depressed following a dinner party told the nurse that she had a spontaneous fantasy during the evening in which her husband left the party with another woman. This woman felt inferior and believed her husband would leave her. With help, she was able to recognize that she was, in fact, unusually accomplished and attractive, and her husband was exceptionally devoted; with this recognition, her depression lifted. Clients can also learn to substitute pleasant fantasies for unpleasant ones. One woman who was depressed because her child

required a minor operation was somewhat relieved when she pictured him in a year, playful and happy and without disability (Beck & Greenberg, 1974).

Behavioral Therapy

Behavioral therapy treatments of depression encompass a broad spectrum of strategies and techniques derived from behavioral principles. The idea is that behavior influences feelings, and if the woman changes her behavior, she will feel less depressed. Some of the treatments include training in social skills, assertiveness, relaxation, and increasing the number of pleasant activities in one's life. Graded task assignments also may be used. A depressed homemaker, for instance, may be given a series of tasks starting with simple jobs at which she has a good chance of succeeding and progressing to more complicated tasks. At first, she may be asked only to make beds. In several days, she also can cook breakfast. When she has clearly succeeded at a task, however simple, her lethargy decreases and she is motivated to try more.

The effectiveness of assertiveness training was researched in the 1970s and has been well documented (Wolpe, 1958). Assertiveness training is aimed at reducing maladaptive anxiety that prevents a person from expressing herself directly, honestly, and spontaneously. The training involves the practice of assertive responses.

Behavioral therapy may include the following strategies (Jacobson et al., 1996):

- Monitoring daily activities for impact on mood.
- Assessing pleasure that is achieved by various activities.
- Assigning increasingly more difficult activities that have potential of enhancing pleasure.
- Using cognitive rehearsal of anticipated activities to anticipate obstacles.
- Discussing specific problems such as insomnia and prescribing behavior therapy techniques to deal with them.
- Performing interventions such as assertiveness training to ameliorate deficits in social skills.

Important research by Morin & Azrin (1988) suggests that geriatric insomnia can be treated with psychological interventions and that behavioral procedures are more beneficial than cognitive procedures. The effective behavioral intervention strategy included:

- Going to bed only when sleepy at night.
- Using the bed only for sleep and sex.
- Getting out of bed and going in another room whenever the patient is unable to fall asleep or return to sleep.
- Repeating this last procedure as often as necessary.

- Rising in the morning at the same time regardless of the amount of sleep obtained during the night.
- No napping during the day.

Imagery training, such as imagining a sequence of six neutral objects (candle, hourglass, kite, stairway, palm tree, and light bulb) was also successful but not as successful as the behavioral technique. With their eyes closed, participants concentrated on the image of each object for about 2 minutes. They were instructed to practice the visual-imagery exercises once during the day and whenever they were unable to fall asleep or return to sleep at night.

Interpersonal Therapy

There are few systematic reviews and randomized controlled trials on IPT; however, a sequential treatment strategy in women with recurrent major depression was investigated to look at the efficacy of adding antidepressant medication (imipramine) to IPT in those who did not remit with ITP alone (Ebmeier et al., 2006). They reported that adding antidepressant pharmacotherapy to IPT could be highly effective. For treatment of recurrent depression, the combination of an antidepressant with IPT was the optimum treatment condition (Ebmeier et al., 2006).

In a landmark study for which meta-analysis was feasible (Elkin et al., 1989), the efficacy of IPT exceeded that of cognitive therapy by 13.2%, that of placebo plus clinical management by 22.6%, and that of imipramine by 12.3%, based on the Beck Depression Inventory as the outcome measure. However, only 26% of the IPT patients recovered and stayed well throughout follow-up; this figure was similar to the rates obtained in cognitive therapy (30%), pharmacotherapy (19%), and placebo (19%) (Elkin et al., 1989).

Interpersonal therapy may be especially helpful for women because it focuses on issues currently viewed as central to the psychology of women—that is, that relationships are the core of a woman's self-esteem. For women, more so than for men, social isolation, relationship loss, and dysfunctional family relationships may precipitate, contribute to, or prolong depression.

Interpersonal therapy is a brief treatment designed by Klerman and Wiesmann (1984) in the early 1980s to reduce symptoms and improve social functioning in depressed patients. The focus is on current interpersonal problems that are secondary to unresolved grief, difficult role transitions, interpersonal role disputes, and social skill deficits. Nurses will recognize this approach as the basis for relationship therapy formulated by Peplau (1952) and based on Sullivan's (1953) interpersonal theories. IPT is intense and uses the relationship between the client and therapist as a variable. The focus is on relationships in the here and now and on facilitating the client to develop more effective ways of relating. The goal is not insight but symptomatic relief.

IPT facilitates recovery from the acute depression by (1) relieving the depressive symptoms and (2) helping the patient develop more effective strategies for dealing with current interpersonal problems associated with the onset of symptoms (Klerman & Weismann, 1984). The first goal is achieved by helping patients understand that their experiences are part of a depressive syndrome. Often the patient is instructed to read educational literature written in lay language. The second goal is to help the patient develop more successful patterns for dealing with current social and interpersonal problems that were associated with the onset of the current depression. IPT tries to change the way the patient thinks, feels, and acts in problematic interpersonal relationships. Confrontation is gentle and timely, and the therapist is careful to foster the patient's positive expectations of the therapeutic relationship. The therapist is optimistic and supportive as well as active in helping the patient focus on bringing about improvement in current interpersonal problems.

Self-Help Strategies to Alleviate Depression

Aerobic exercise at a dose consistent with public health recommendations is an effective treatment for major depressive disorder of mild to moderate severity (Dunn, Trivedi, Kampert, Clark, & Chambliss, 2005). Respite for full-time mothers is also helpful. Suggestions include arranging at least half a day or evening each week for herself, maintaining at least one personal interest, planning one evening a month to be out with her significant other, getting information on free or low-cost entertainment (especially the type offering free child care), deepening friendships with other women, and remembering that vacations are for mothers as well.

Self-help groups appear to be especially helpful for persons experiencing grief reactions, such as to divorce, becoming widowed, or being parents of babies who were victims of sudden infant death syndrome. Other self-help groups for widows have stressed coping skills such as auto mechanics, how to travel alone, how to manage as a single parent, how to do taxes, and how to get a job, in addition to providing support for loneliness.

Newer Strategies to Alleviate Depression

In one study, vagus nerve stimulation was reported to show improvement in 30% of depressed patients, with 15% achieving full remission (Howland, 2006d). VNS involves the surgical implantation of a pacemaker-like device in the left upper chest and an electrode lead wire attached to the left vagas nerve in the neck area (Howland, 2006e). In a RCT, acupuncture was not efficacious as a medication monotherapy for MDD (Allen et al., 2006).

Postpartum Depression

A favorable outcome of postpartum depression is associated with a good premorbid adjustment, adequate treatment, and a supportive family network (Kaplan & Sadock, 2005). From a community-based sample, only 12% of women with postpartum depression received psychotherapy, and fewer received psychopharmacologic treatment (Horowitz & Cousins, 2006). Postpartum psychosis is a psychiatric emergency, and the mother will probably need psychiatric hospitalization.

The pharmacological management of this disorder is similar to that for non-postpartum depression, except for considerations of infant safety during breast-feeding. All antidepressants are excreted into breast milk, although levels in infants are usually undetectable (Pigarelli et al., 2005). If the mother is breast-feeding, some sources recommend that no pharmacologic agents should be prescribed, but other sources advise caution while prescribing some agents (Kaplan & Sadock, 2005). The limited data currently available show no adverse effects on infants, and the possible risks of treatment must be weighed against the risks of leaving the illness untreated, not only for the mother and infant but also for the patient's family (Kornstein, 2003). Begin with an antidepressant to which the woman has responded in the past in order to maximize response. If she is has not used medication previously, a drug with a short half-life and some demonstrated safety data during lactation should be used (Pigarelli et al., 2005). Doses should be kept as low as possible, and, if possible, the dosing and feeding schedules should be arranged so as to minimize the infant's exposure to the drug. If pharmacological treatment is necessary in a depressed, breast-feeding mother, the SSRIs seem to be a relatively safe option, although more research is clearly needed (Kornstein, 2003).

Bipolar Disorder

At this time, there is no cure for bipolar disorder; however, treatment can decrease the associated morbidity and mortality (American Psychiatric Association, 2003). About one in three patients will remain free of symptoms by taking mood-stabilizing medication throughout life (Miller, 2006). Misdiagnosis is common because most patients seek treatment during their depressive episode (Miller, 2006). Clinical evaluation of a patient presenting with depression should always include an assessment for bipolar depression. Hirschfeld and colleagues (2000) developed the Mood Disorder Questionnaire that can be used as a screening instrument in the primary care setting. Management includes assessing the patient's safety and level of functioning, establishing and maintaining a therapeutic alliance, monitoring the patient's psychiatric status, providing education, enhancing medication treatment compliance, promoting regular patterns of activity and of sleep, anticipating stressors, identifying new episodes early, and minimizing functional impairments (American Psychiatric Association, 2003).

Mood-stabilizing drugs are the primary treatment for bipolar disorder (Thase, 2005) (see Tables 13.6 and 13.7). Unsatisfactory treatment outcome is more likely to result when antidepressant medications are used (Grunze, 2005). Use of antidepressants can cause mood instability and trigger episodes of hypomania. The highest relative risk of mood switches occurred with venlafaxine and the lowest risk with bupropion (Leverich et al., 2006). Lithium has been the best studied treatment, and it has been found to reduce the risk of suicide attempts and completed suicide (Kessing, Sondergard, Kvist, & Anderson, 2005).

Divalproex (Depakote®) is now used more commonly than lithium as a mood stabilizer in bipolar disorder although its effectiveness as an antidepressant has not been well studied or well established (Howland, 2006a). The use of alternative anticonvulsant agents is growing. Lamotrigine (Lamictal®) has been shown to be effective for acute and maintenance treatment of bipolar depression and does have antidepressant effects (American Psychiatric Association, 2003; Howland, 2006a).

Mood Stabilizers

The *lithium* ion substitutes for the sodium ion, thereby compromising the ability of neurons to release, activate, or respond to neurotransmitters. Its effects on the second messenger system probably account for

13.6 | Mood Stabilizers: Antimanic and Anticonvulsants

GENERIC NAME	TRADE NAME	USUAL DOSAGE AND DIAGNOSIS
Antimanic		
Lithium	Eskalith/Lithium	900–1,200 mg per day for bipolar disorder
		600 mg three times per day for acute mania
	Eskalith CR	450 mg twice per day for bipolar disorder
Anticonvulsants		
Carbamazepine	Tegretol/Carbamazepine	800–1,200 mg per day, divide dose
Lamotrigine	Lamictal	not FDA approved for bipolar disorder
		150–250 mg twice per day
Gabapentin	Neurontin	not FDA approved for bipolar disorder 900–1,800 mg per day, divide dose
Topiramate	Topamax	not FDA approved for bipolar diorder
Valproic acid	Depakene	10–15 mg/kg per day for mania, divide dose

13.7 | Atypical Antipsychotic Medications

GENERIC NAME	TRADE NAME	USUAL DOSAGE AND DIAGNOSIS
Risperidone	Risperdal	1–4 mg once per day for schizophrenia
Olanzapine	Zyprexa	5–20 mg once per day for bipolar disorder
Quetiapine	Seroquel	50–250 mg three times per day for psychosis
Ziprasidone	Geodon	20–80 mg twice per day for schizophrenia
Aripiprazole	Abilify	10–15 mg once per day for schizophrenia

its therapeutic profile. The efficacy of lithium in the treatment of acute mania has been well documented (DiPiro et al., 2005). The major disadvantage is that improvement is slow, and antipsychotic agents such as olanzapine or benzodiazepines such as lorazepam may be necessary to achieve rapid control of psychotic or agitated behavior. One advantage of lithium is that it is inexpensive.

Common side effects include nausea, dry mouth, diarrhea, and thirst. Drowsiness, mild hand tremor, polyuria, weight gain, bloated feeling, sleeplessness, and headaches are other relatively common side effects. Lithium may be associated with development of goiter. Dermatological reactions such as acne may occur. Many patients have gastrointestinal complaints—burning sensations and persistent indigestion (DiPiro et al., 2005). Lithium has a narrow therapeutic window, and therapeutic serum levels should be maintained between 0.6 and 1.2 mEq/L. Lithium levels should be checked every month to 3 months until stable and then every 6 to12 months for long-term maintenance (DiPiro et al., 2005). At serum levels above 1.5 mEqL, adverse reactions usually occur, such as diarrhea, vomiting, drowsiness, muscular weakness, and lack of coordination. At higher levels, ataxia, giddiness, tinnitus, and blurred vision occur. At levels above 3.0 mEq/L, the patient will experience coma and death.

Lithium is an ion interchangeable with sodium. An increase in salt intake increases lithium elimination, and a decrease in salt intake decreases lithium elimination. Thus, it is important to maintain a balanced diet and sodium intake. Any condition that alters fluid and electrolyte balance such as diarrhea or vomiting can alter lithium levels. Because nonsteroidal anti-inflammatory drugs NSAIDs can cause lithium retention, they should be avoided.

Valproic acid (Depakote®) is indicated for the primary treatment of mania and has a rapid onset. It causes relatively few serious side effects (DiPiro et al., 2005). Some gastrointestinal symptoms may occur, but prescription of the enteric-coated form reduces discomfort. Disadvantages include transient hair loss, weight gain (up to 50% of patients taking valproic acid gain weight), tremors, dose-related thrombocytopenia, and hepatotoxicity (rare). Patient education should include instructions to: take valproic acid with food if the gastrointestinal tract upset occurs, swallow tablets whole to prevent irritation of the mouth and throat, take the drug at bedtime, and notify those monitoring for diabetes because valproic acid may give false positive blood and urine ketone values (DiPiro et al., 2005).

Atypical antipsychotics are preferred over typical antipsychotics because of their more benign side effect profile, with most of the evidence supporting the use of olanzapine (Zyprexa®) or risperidone (resperidal) (American Psychiatric Association, 2003; Hussain &

Normal, 2002). Zyprexa® seems to be more effective than Symbyax® (combination of Zyprexa® and fluoxetine). Two large, placebo-controlled studies of quetiapine (Seroquel®) have found it effective for the acute treatment of bipolar disorder (Calabrese, Elhaj, Gajwani, & Gao, 2005). Studies of other atypical antipsychotic agents such as ziprasidone (Geodon®) and aripiprazole (Abilify®) are ongoing, and results have not been reported. Short-term adjunctive treatment with a benzodiazepine also may be helpful.

Other Therapies Useful With Bipolar Disorder

In patients with life-threatening situations, suicidality, or psychosis, electroconvulsive therapy is a reasonable alternative (American Psychiatric Association, 2003). The likelihood of antidepressant treatment precipitating a switch into a hypomanic episode is probably lower in patients with bipolar II depression than in patients with bipolar I depression (American Psychiatric Association, 2003). Types of psychotherapy beneficial to individuals with bipolar disorder include CBT, IPT, and social rhythm therapy (American Psychiatric Association, 2003; Miller, 2006). Family-focused psychoeducational therapy has been shown to decrease depressive symptoms, improve treatment adherence, and reduce the risk of illness relapse and hospitalization (Vieta, 2005).

Gender Considerations With Treatment for Bipolar Disorder

The management of two presentations of bipolar disorder that are more common in women—rapid cycling and mixed states—is challenging. Carbamazapine and valproic acid may be superior to lithium in reducing the frequency of episodes in rapid-cycling bipolar disorder. The use of risperidone (an antipsychotic) is associated with hyperprolactinemia, which may result in galactorrhea, amenorrhea and menstrual cycle irregularities, anovulation and infertility, and sexual dysfunction (Freeman et al., 2002). Atypical antipsychotics such as clozapine, olanzapine, and quetiapine are less frequently associated with hyperprolactinemia and thus are better tolerated by women.

There are important drug interactions to consider. Carbamazepine and topiramate lower the efficacy of oral contraceptives; gababentin, lamotrigine, valproate, and lithium do not affect the efficacy of oral contraceptives. There is some concern about a relationship between valproate and polycystic ovaries, so valproate should not be used in young women with bipolar disorder (Freeman et al., 2002).

The treatment of women with bipolar disorder during the childbearing years includes education of the woman and her partner about family planning, the heritability of bipolar disorder, and the course of illness and treatment options during pregnancy. Women with mild symptoms (one past manic episode or long periods of affective stability) may elect to taper and discontinue medication prior to conception because of the relatively low risk of relapse. Women with moderate illness (two to three episodes of mania or depression) also may choose to taper and discontinue medication prior to conception. Because the risk of relapse is greater in this group, however, they may elect to continue medication until early confirmation of pregnancy, prolonging the period of time on preventative medication (Freeman et al., 2002). Once a woman is pregnant, a medication can be tapered in the 2 weeks prior to the establishment of the placental-fetal circulation, before the fetus is susceptible to teratogens.

Women with mild to moderate illness who elect to discontinue medications should be educated about identifying early signs of relapse and followed closely for recurrence of target symptoms. Women with severe illness (four or more episodes of mania or depression) have a high rate of relapse, and the risks to a mother and fetus from the disorder may exceed the risk of medication treatment. In many cases, these women may not be able to safely discontinue medication treatment during pregnancy (Freeman et al., 2002).

For women who continue psychotropic treatment for bipolar disorder during pregnancy, lithium, valproic acid, and carbamazepine all have potential teratogenic effects on the fetus. Cardiovascular malformations with lithium exposure (particularly Epstein's anomaly) is 10 to 20 times the risk in the general population. With carbamazepine and valproic acid, there is increased risk of spina bifida. The use of higher doses of anticonvulsants and multiple anticonvulsants may increase the risk of neural tube defects. Fetal exposure to the mood stabilizers carbamazepine and valproic aicd, even late in pregnancy, is associated with craniofacial abnormalities and cognitive dysfunction. Lithium use throughout pregnancy has been associated with "floppy baby" syndrome, characterized by cyanosis, hypotonicity, and lethargy; infants also may have cardiac murmurs, arrhythmias, respiratory distress, and poor sucking reflex (Freeman et al., 2002).

Women who have taken mood stabilizers during the first trimester have the option of receiving a level II ultrasound at 18 to 20 weeks' gestation to detect cardiac abnormalities and a screening ultrasound for detection of spina bifida at 16 to 19 weeks' gestation. There have been no reports of major malformations with the use of olanzapine (an atypical antipsychotic) during pregnancy (Freeman et al., 2002).

The American Academy of Pediatrics (1994) considers lithium to be contraindicated during breast-feeding. The data are sparse, and infants treated with valproic acid are at risk for hepatotoxicity; however, both valproic acid

and carbamazepine are considered to be usually compatible with breast-feeding by the American Academy of Pediatrics (1994). Mothers may elect to collect breast milk over a 24-hour period to be analyzed for drug concentration. With this information, a mother may store milk expressed during nonpeak concentration times and discard milk from peak times. The mother may also minimize drug exposure to the nursing infant by taking medication just after she has breast-fed and just before the infant has a lengthy sleep period (American Academy of Pediatrics, 1994).

Premenstrual Dysphoric Disorder

First-line treatment for PMDD is an SSRI medication or venlafaxine (Halbreich, 2005). One theory is that SSRIs work by indirectly increasing synthesis of allopregenolone from preogesterone; the binding of allopregenolone to GABA receptors would account for the rapid relief of PMDD symptoms by SSRIs (Elliott, 2002). The selective preference between SSRIs (such as sertraline, paroxetine, fluoxetine, and citalopram) or venlafaxine is by clinician's experience and personal preference (Halbreich, 2005). Intermittent luteal dosing has been demonstrated to be as effective as continuous dosing (Halbreich, 2005). In a placebo-controlled study with citalopram, intermittent treatment was more effective than continuous treatment, and this was subsequently confirmed using sertraline (Eriksson, Andersch, Ho, Landen, & Sundblad, 2002). In one randomized controlled trial, sertraline was the most effective treatment, with 65% of the subjects responding to treatment (Freeman et al., 1999). In another clinical trial, luteal phase dosing with both 12.5 mg and 25 mg of paroxetine CR was found to be effective and generally well tolerated (Steiner et al., 2005). Non–serontonin-enhancing antidepressants like bupropion or the TCAs are not effective (Elliott, 2002).

Nonpharmacological approaches to caring for patients with PMDD include:

- Patient education.
- Social support.
- Calcium carbonate (1,000–1,200 mg/d), multivitamins with A and E, vitamin B_6 (100–150 mg/d), magnesium (300–400 mg/d), increased intake of complex dietary carbohydrates and fiber, decreased caffeine intake, and decreased simple sugars and salt.
- Lifestyle changes such as increased aerobic exercise, identification and avoidance of stress triggers, attending stress management/relaxation/biofeedback program.
- Cognitive behavioral therapy or relaxation therapy (Elliott, 2002; Frackiewicz & Shiovitz, 2001; Halbreich, 2005).

ANXIETY DISORDERS

Anxiety is a common experience for most women. Although uncomfortable, anxiety symptoms are as necessary to the emotional system as pain is to the physical system. Anxiety alerts us that we must attend to what is happening to us. The continuum of anxiety ranges from this normal response to threats to severe anxiety disorders.

Diagnostic Classifications

Specific criteria for each of the anxiety diagnoses are documented in the *Diagnostic and Statistical Manual of Mental Disorders* (American Psychiatric Association, 2000). Anxiety disorders include: (1) disorders in which anxiety is the dominant problem (generalized anxiety disorder and panic disorder with or without agoraphobia); (2) disorders in which anxiety is experienced if the person attempts to confront the threatened situation (specific or social phobia); (3) disorders whereby anxiety is experienced if the person attempts to resist the thoughts and feelings (obsessive-compulsive disorder); and (4) disorders in which anxiety is reexperienced after an unusual, traumatic event (post-traumatic stress disorder) (American Psychiatric Association, 2000).

Etiology

Although the exact cause for anxiety disorders is unknown, most theorists agree that persons with anxiety disorders have some kind of neurophysiologic abnormality that results from genetic and psychological vulnerability. From a biological perspective, dysfunction in multiple systems—particularly GABA, norepinephrine, and serotonin regulation and transmission—is implicated. Although the GABA system is the major target for research in anxiety disorders, the part of the brain that manufactures norepinephrine, the locus ceruleus, controls the response to anxiety-producing stimuli and may play a critical role in responsiveness to changes in the internal and external environment (Stuart, 2005a). Neurotransmitter pathways connect the locus ceruleus to other structures of the brain (such as the amygdala, the hippocampus, and the cerebral cortex), which are probably implicated in anxiety. Also, the transmission of serotonin in the midbrain may play a role in the etiology of panic attacks, and patients experiencing panic may have hypersensitive serotonin receptors. Genetic vulnerability has been supported by increased incidence of anxiety disorders in first-degree relatives.

Psychological theories about the origin of anxiety abound. Less popular now are the ideas that women's role expectations in society make them more vulnerable to anxiety disorders. The interpersonal view (Sullivan, 1953) suggests that anxiety occurs when a person perceives that she will be viewed unfavorably or will lose the love of the person she values. A person who is easily threatened or has a low level of self-esteem is more susceptible to anxiety. Women who are homemakers with few job skills and are dependent on husbands for their livelihood may be more vulnerable. Behavioral theorists propose that anxiety is learned and that it is the product of frustration caused by anything that interferes with attaining a desired goal (Stuart, 2005a). Anxiety also may arise through conflict that occurs when the person experiences two competing drives and must choose between them. Because anxiety disorders are related to biological, psychological, and sociological factors, the treatment is often multidimensional.

Assessment

Because so many of the symptoms of anxiety mimic symptoms of physical illness, particular vigilance is necessary in the differential diagnostic process. Ruling out other illnesses is the priority. The next step is to match the patient's symptoms with the diagnostic criteria in the *DSM-IV*. Sometimes it is helpful to administer standardized tools. The advantage of using instruments is that one can evaluate more objectively the outcome of interventions to reduce anxiety. Probably the most widely used standardized instrument is the Spielberger State Trait Anxiety Inventory (Spielberger, Gorsuch, & Lushene, 1983). Trait anxiety is the general tendency of an individual to experience anxiety, whereas state anxiety is transient in nature and responds to intervention. The reliability and validity of this tool are well established. Other standardized instruments are the Agoraphobic Cognition's Questionnaire and the Body Sensations Questionnaire (Chambless, Caputo, & Bright, 1984). The Yale-Brown Obsessive-Compulsive Scale is specific for diagnosing and evaluation of treatment with patients experiencing obsessive-compulsive disorder. Another tool is the visual analogue scale. Simply ask the patient how anxious (or nervous) she feels on a scale from 1 to 10. You can draw a ladder with 10 steps or use stairs or whatever visualization is helpful.

Diagnostic Criteria for Types of Anxiety Disorders

Generalized Anxiety Disorder (300.02)

The essential feature of an anxiety disorder is excessive anxiety and worry (apprehensive expectation) about a number of events or activities (such as work or school performance). The person finds it difficult to control the worry. The anxiety and worry are associated with three (or more) of the following six symptoms for at least 6 months (American Psychiatric Association, 2000).

■ Restlessness or feeling keyed up or on edge.
■ Being easily fatigued.
■ Difficulty concentrating or mind going blank.
■ Irritability.
■ Muscle tension.
■ Sleep disturbance (difficulty falling or staying asleep or restless, unsatisfying sleep).

The anxiety, worry, or physical symptoms cause clinically significant distress or impairment in social, occupational, or other important areas of functioning. The disturbance is not due to the direct physiological effects of a substance or a general medical condition (e.g., hyperthyroidism) (American Psychiatric Association, 2000).

Generalized anxiety disorder (GAD) affects women more frequently than men and prevalence rates are high in mid-life (prevalence in women over age 35 is 10%) and older subjects (Wittchen, 2002). The natural course of GAD can be characterized as chronic with few complete remissions, a waxing and waning course of GAD symptoms, and the occurrence of substantial comorbidity, particularly with depression (Wittchen, 2002).

Patients with GAD demonstrate a considerable degree of impairment and disability that is similar to those with major depression. GAD is associated with a significant economic burden owing to decreased work productivity and increased use of health care services, particularly primary health care (Wittchen, 2002). Complicated GAD is much more likely to occur in women than in men, and women are more likely to seek treatment than men (Pigott, 2002). Genetic factors may be more important than environment factors in mediating the expression of GAD.

Panic Disorders With (300.21) or Without Agoraphobia (300.01)

Panic disorder accounts for more emergency department visits than any other psychiatric illness. Conditions to rule out in differential diagnosis include cardiac disorders, drug reaction or intoxication, endocrine disorders, neurologic disorders, and respiratory problems.

Diagnostic criteria for panic disorder include recurrent, unexpected panic attacks followed by a month of at least one of the following symptoms: persistent fear of having additional attacks, worry about the consequences of the attack (e.g., losing control, "going crazy," having a heart attack) and a significant change in behavior related to the attacks (American Psychiatric Association, 2000). The essential feature of a panic attack is a discrete period of intense fear or discomfort in the absence of real danger that is accompanied by at least four of the following symptoms, which develop abruptly and reach a peak within 10 minutes (American Psychiatric Association, 2000):

■ Palpitation, pounding heart, or accelerated heart rate.
■ Sweating.
■ Trembling or shaking.
■ Sensations or shortness of breath or smothering.
■ Feeling of choking.
■ Chest pain or discomfort.
■ Nausea or abdominal distress.
■ Feeling dizzy, unsteady, lightheaded, or faint.
■ Derealization (feelings of unreality) or depersonalization (being detached from oneself).
■ Fear of losing control or going crazy.
■ Fear of dying.
■ Paresthesias (numbness or tingling sensations).
■ Chills or hot flushes.

There are three characteristic types of panic attacks: unexpected (uncued), situationally bound (cued), and situationally predisposed. When agoraphobia is present, the person experiences anxiety about being in places or situations from which escape might be difficult (or embarrassing) or in which help may not be available in the event of having an unexpected or situationally predisposed panic attack or panic-like symptoms. Agoraphobic fears typically involve being outside the home alone; being in a crowd or standing in a line; being on a bridge; and traveling in a bus, train, or automobile (American Psychiatric Association, 2000).

Agoraphobia meets the criteria for panic disorder and, in addition, includes a fear of being in places or situations from which escape might be difficult or embarrassing or in which help might not be available. As a result of this fear, the person restricts travel, needs a companion when away from home, or endures agoraphobic situations despite intense anxiety (American Psychiatric Association, 2000).

Prevalence rates of agoraphobia were two to four times higher in women than in men. Women with panic disorder report more individual panic-related symptoms and a greater level of phobic avoidance than men (Pigott, 2002). These findings may explain the greater levels of dependence and functional impairment detected when panic disorder occurs in women in comparison to men (Pigott, 2002).

Social Phobia (300.23) and Other Phobias (300.29)

The essential feature of social phobia, formerly known as social anxiety disorder, is a marked and persistent fear of social or performance situations in which embarrassment may occur (American Psychiatric Association, 2000). Exposure to the social or performance situation almost invariably provokes an immediate anxiety response.

The person recognizes that the fear is excessive or unreasonable, and the feared situations are avoided or else are endured with intense anxiety. Lifetime prevalence rates range from 12% to 14% (Stein, 2006).

Social phobia is associated with an increased risk for depression and a more malignant course, characterized by increased likelihood of suicide attempts and greater disease chronicity (Stein, 2006). This illness has a chronic course and a greater adverse impact on social functioning than do depressive symptoms or chronic medical illnesses (Keller, 2006). Half of these patients have onset by age 13 and 90% by age 23; however, it is rarely diagnosed or treated by pediatricians (Stein, 2006). Early diagnosis and treatment is extremely important. The Mini-SPIN self-rated screening instrument for social phobia was found to possess 90% accuracy (when all questions were answered yes) in diagnosing the presence of social phobia in a managed care population ($N = 7,165$) (Conner, Kobak, Churchill, Katzelnick, & Davidson, 2001). The three questions are:

- Are you fearful in social settings?
- Are you easily embarrassed or humiliated?
- Do you avoid social/performance situations?

The essential feature of specific phobia is marked and persistent fear of clearly discernible, circumscribed objects or situations (e.g., flying, heights, and animals, receiving an injection, seeing blood) (American Psychiatric Association, 2000). Exposure to the phobic stimulus almost invariably provokes an immediate anxiety response, and the person recognizes that their fear is excessive or unreasonable. Most often the phobic stimulus is avoided, although it is sometimes endured with dread. Animal phobias are two to three times more common in women (Pigott, 2002).

Obsessive-Compulsive Disorder (300.3)

The essential features of obsessive-compulsive disorder (OCD) are recurrent obsessions or compulsions that are severe enough to be time consuming (i.e., they take more than 1 hour a day) or cause marked distress or significant impairment (American Psychiatric Association, 2000). The person recognizes that the obsessions or compulsions are excessive or unreasonable. Obsessions are defined by:

- Recurrent and persistent thoughts, impulses, or images that are experienced as intrusive and inappropriate and that cause marked anxiety or distress.
- The thoughts impulses or images are not simply excessive worries about real-life problems.
- The person attempts to ignore or suppress such thoughts, impulses, or images or to neutralize them with some other thought or action.

- The person recognizes that the obsessional thoughts, impulses, or images are a product of his or her own mind (American Psychiatric Association, 2000).

Compulsions are defined by:

- Repetitive behaviors (e.g., hand washing, ordering, checking) or mental acts (e.g., praying, counting, repeating words silently) that the person feels driven to perform in response to an obsession or according to rules that must be applied rigidly.
- The behaviors or mental acts are aimed at preventing or reducing distress or preventing some dreaded event or situation; however, these behaviors or mental acts are not connected in a realistic way with what they are designed to neutralize or prevent, or they are clearly excessive.

There is a dramatic increase in prevalence rates for OCD in females after the onset of puberty (Pigott, 2002). This occurrence provides support for the importance of female reproductive hormones in the etiology of this illness. Aggressive obsessions and cleaning compulsions occur more frequently in women than men with OCD (Pigott, 2002).

Post-Traumatic Stress Disorder (309.81)

Sexual assault, childhood abuse, and individual assessment of threat during the occurrence of trauma may represent the strongest predictors of post-traumatic stress disorder (PTSD) development in women (Pigott, 2002). The essential features of PTSD are the development of characteristic symptoms following exposure to an extreme traumatic event in which the person experienced, witnessed, or was confronted with an event that involved actual or threatened death of serious injury, or a threat to the physical integrity of self or others; and the person's response involved intense fear, helplessness, or horror (American Psychiatric Association, 2000). The event is persistently reexperienced in at least one of the following ways:

- Recurrent and intrusive distressing recollections of the event, including images, thoughts, or perceptions.
- Recurrent distressing dreams of the event.
- Acting or feeling as if the traumatic event were recurring.
- Intense psychological distress at exposure to internal or external cues that symbolize or resemble an aspect of the traumatic event.
- Physiological reactivity on exposure to internal or external cues that symbolize or resemble an aspect of the traumatic event.

Persistent avoidance of stimuli associated with the trauma and numbing of general responsiveness is indicated by three or more of the following:

■ Efforts to avoid thoughts, feelings, or conversations associated with the trauma.
■ Efforts to avoid activities, places, or people that arouse recollections of the trauma.
■ Inability to recall an important aspect of the trauma.
■ Markedly diminished interest or participation in significant activities.
■ Feeling of detachment or estrangement from others.
■ Restricted range of affect.
■ Sense of a foreshortened future.

Persistent symptoms of increased arousal (not present before the trauma) as indicated by two (or more) of the following:

■ Difficulty falling or staying asleep.
■ Irritability or outbursts of anger.
■ Difficulty concentrating.
■ Hypervigilance.
■ Exaggerated startle response.

The disturbance causes clinically significant distress or impairment in social occupational, or other important areas of functioning, and it is present for at least 1 month (American Psychiatric Association, 2000).

Because significant proportions of women still do not report a rape incident, nurses should be alert to a syndrome called silent rape trauma. As a part of the assessment, ask, "Have you ever been pressured or forced to have sexual activity of any kind?" A diagnosis of silent reaction to rape trauma should be considered when a nurse observes any of the following symptoms during an evaluation interview:

■ Increasing signs of anxiety as the interview progresses, such as long periods of silence, blocking of associations, minor stuttering, and physical distress.
■ Patient reports of sudden marked irritability or actual avoidance of relationships with men or marked change in patient sexual behavior.
■ A history of sudden onset of phobic reactions.
■ Persistent loss of self-confidence and self-esteem and attitude of self-blame.

Management

Because etiology is so multidimensional, treatment of anxiety disorders is usually a combination of medications, interpersonal psychotherapy, cognitive behavioral psychotherapy, education, and sensory interventions. There is growing evidence that CBT produces favorable alterations in brain function (Nutt, 2005).

Acute Anxiety States and Panic Attacks

Benzodiazepines (see Table 13.8) are the drug of choice for acute anxiety states, especially brief, situational-induced anxiety (DiPiro et al., 2005). Benzodiazepines are preferable to barbiturates or meprobamate in terms of safety (in case of overdose), abuse liability, and probably the risk of physical dependence (DiPiro et al., 2005). In general, benzodiazepines are prescribed only for a few weeks and then withdrawn gradually to deter physical dependence. Their use in anxiety disorders is usually limited to an environmentally induced crisis. When medical illness or medical procedures are associated with uncomfortable levels of anxiety, short-term use of benzodiazepines is highly effective and not to be withheld due to fears regarding dependency. They are also highly effective in treating alcohol withdrawal.

The treatment of choice for long-term pharmacotherapy is *antidepressants* (Nutt, 2005). Antidepressants may actually worsen anxiety at the start of therapy; therefore, they must be initiated at lower doses than are generally used in depression, and gradually increased (Nutt, 2005). An alternative strategy is to coadminister a benzodiazepine with the antidepressant and gradually reduce the benzodiazepine over several weeks after the patient experiences symptom relief (DiPiro et al., 2005).

Benzodiazepines enhance GABA binding to postsynaptic receptor sites, rendering them less sensitive to stimulation. Patients generally like the calming effect of these medications and feel the effects within an hour. The most serious effect is tolerance—physiological dependence and psychological habituation that interferes with ability to adapt, adjust, and develop coping skills. Because of the dependence issue, short-term use is recommended. Common side effects include sedation with drowsiness and decreased mental acuity; decreased coordination, occupational efficiency, and productivity with increased risk for accidents; and decreased awareness of body in environment (Kirkwood & Melton, 2005).

Use of benzodiazepine may cause driving to be unsafe. In a double-blind, crossover study, 1 mg of alprazolam or placebo was administered to participants 30 minutes before breakfast and 1 hour before a driving test (Verster, Volkerts, & Verbaten, 2002). Six of the 20 participants were unable to complete their driving test after taking alprazolam because of seriously unsafe driving—all six of them fell asleep, and four of the six were women. The authors explained that women are more sensitive to drug-induced sedation than men because women have a different balance between fat and muscle. When the drug is metabolized, the drug molecules bind to fat. Women also generally weigh less than men, so they are more affected (Verster et al., 2002). Women should be warned about the potentiation of benzodiazepine by alcohol and should be cautioned against operating complex machinery, including automobiles.

13.8 | Antianxiety Medications

GENERIC NAME	TRADE NAME	USUAL DOSAGE AND DIAGNOSIS
Benzodiazepines		
Lorazepam	Ativan/Lorazepam	0.5–2 mg every 6 to hours for anxiety
		2–4 mg qhs for insomnia
Clonazepam	Klonopin/Clonazepam	0.25–0.5 mg twice to three times per day for anxiety
		0.5–1 mg twice per day to three times per day for panic disorder
Chlordiazepoxide	Librium/Chlordiazepoxide	5–10 mg three to four times per day for mild anxiety
		20–25 mg three to four times per day for severe anxiety
Clorazepate	Tranxene SD/Chlorazepate	15–60 mg once per day for anxiety
Diazepam	Valium	2–10 mg three to four times per day for anxiety
Alprazolam	Xanax	0.5–0.5 mg three times per day for anxiety
		0.5–3 mg three times per day for panic disorder
Xanax XR	3–6 mg once per day for panic disorder	
Alprazalam	0.25–0.5 mg three times per day for anxiety	
		0.5–3 mg three times per day for panic disorder
Nonbenzodiazepines		
Buspirone	BuSpar/Buspirone	20–30 mg per day, divide dose
Propranolol	Inderal	unapproved for stage fright
		10 mg before peformance

The potential teratogenicity of benzodiazepine taken during pregnancy remains controversial, but a meta-analysis suggested a two-fold increase in the risk of orofacial clefts (Ward & Zamorski, 2002). Benzodiazepine use during pregnancy is not advised—particularly during the first trimester (Kirkwood & Melton, 2005). Nurses should educate women about the dangers of benzodiazepine during pregnancy, assess for use during pregnancy, help pregnant women find other ways to handle their anxiety and insomnia, or refer them to a psychiatrist who specializes in psychiatric disorders in pregnancy.

Benzodiazepines have a great potential for abuse, and benzodiazepine withdrawal syndrome is potentially serious. Risks and benefits must be carefully assessed and discussed with the patient if benzodiazepines are being considered (Nutt, 2005). Patient education for nonpregnant women should include the following instructions (Kirkwood & Melton, 2005):

- Benzodiazepine should not be used in response to minor stresses of everyday life.
- Over-the-counter drugs may potentiate the actions of benzodiazepine.

- Driving should be avoided until tolerance develops.
- Alcohol and other central nervous system depressants potentiate the effects of benzodiazepine.
- Benzodiazepine should not be discontinued abruptly.

Buspirone is an antianxiety medication that is not a benzodiazepine and therefore has several advantages. There is no impairment of memory or motor coordination, no addiction or withdrawal symptoms, and minimal side effects such as headache, nausea, nervousness, dizziness, lightheadedness, and fatigue (Kirkwood & Melton, 2005). One disadvantage is that it takes 3 to 6 weeks for maximum effects, and patients who are accustomed to the immediate relief from benzodiazepines might not be willing to wait for the effect. Buspirone works best with women who have not taken benzodiazepines. Other disadvantages, in comparison to benzodiazepines, are that buspirone needs to be taken in divided doses and has no euphoria/muscle relaxing properties (Kirkwood & Melton, 2005). Anxiety is controlled as distinguished from the sedative and euphoric actions of the benzodiazepines. The action of buspirone is uncertain, but it probably is a partial agonist at serotonin 5HT receptor postsynaptically and a full agonist at the presynaptic receptors (DiPiro et al., 2005). If a patient is being switched from a benzodiazepine to buspirone, the benzodiazepines must be gradually tapered (over 4 to 6 weeks) while buspirone therapy is being initiated. Recently, *levetiracetam*, an anticonvulsant, was found to be well tolerated with minimal side effects, and patients demonstrated significant improvement in panic attack frequency, anxiety, and global severity of anxiety (Papp, 2006).

For performance anxiety, beta blockers such as *propranolol*, can be used. Propranolol blocks beta-nonadrenergic receptors centrally and in the peripheral cardiac and pulmonary systems, thereby decreasing the physiological symptoms of anxiety, especially tachycardia (DiPiro et al., 2005). Propranolol decreases tremor and heart rate and is useful in women whose anxiety manifests itself in shakiness and palpitations. Propranolol is widely used for performance anxiety by musicians and actors and students who are about to take examinations, even though that use is not approved by the FDA.

Herbal preparations such as kava and valerian can decrease anxiety (see Table 13.4). Kava is a beverage prepared from the rhizome of the kava plant and has been shown in numerous clinical trials to be efficacious (Ernst, 2004). A recent alert warned about possible liver damage with use of kava. Some researchers believe that the liver damage is the result of nontraditional ways of production of commercially available kava supplements (Ernst, 2004). German physicians now recommend kava as an herbal anxiolytic at a dose of 120 to 210 mg kavapyrone per day; length of medication should be limited to 1 to 2 months, and liver enzymes should be checked before and during kava medication (Ernst, 2004). Caution is still advised until knowledge is more complete. In a randomized controlled trial, researchers reported a modest hypnotic effect for a valerian-hops combination and diphenhydramine relative to placebo (Morin, Koetter, Bastien, Ware, & Wooten, 2005). Both treatments appeared safe and did not produce rebound insomnia upon discontinuation. Side effects include mild headache or upset stomach, and valerian should not be used with antianxiety or other sleep aids. The FDA does not control herbal preparations and only reliable products should be used.

Panic Disorder With or Without Agoraphobia

The combined use of pharmacological agents and psychotherapy is used to treat panic disorders. Medications are used to block panic attacks and calm the anticipatory anxiety, and psychotherapy is used to alleviate the underlying cause of anxiety and help the individual deal with the psychosocial effect of the disorder.

Pharmacotherapy. The selective serontonin reuptake inhibitors are the first-line pharmacological treatment for panic disorders because of data supporting their efficacy, the minimal need for dosage titration, the overall favorable side-effect profile, and the length of available clinical experience (Kirkwood & Melton, 2005; see Table 13.1). First-line pharmacologic treatment includes SSRIs such as citalopram (20–60 mg/day), escitalopram (5–20 mg/day), and paroxetine (10 mg/day, increasing to 50 mg/day) (Nutt, 2005). Second-line pharmacologic treatment includes the TCAs such as clomipramine (150 mg/day), imipramine (150 mg/day), and phenelzine (30–60 mg/day) (Nutt, 2005). Drug treatment of panic disorder has been shown to normalize anxious cognitions (Nutt, 2005). In a randomized controlled trial with primary care patients with panic disorder, a combination of cognitive-behavioral therapy and pharmacotherapy resulted in sustained and gradually increasing improvement relative to treatment as usual (Roy-Byrne et al., 2005). In addition, there was a significantly greater improvement in World Health Organization disability scales.

The time for maximum beneficial effect for the SSRIs is about 4 to 6 weeks, so education and support is essential for patients to continue to take the medication while waiting to feel better. Supplementation with the benzodiazepine alprazolam (30–60 mg/day) is usually necessary until the SSRI has had time to take effect, then the benzodiazepine can be gradually tapered. Because of the sensitivity for anxiety-like side effects in patients with panic disorder, medications should be initiated at the lowest dose possible and titrated slowly (Kirkwood & Melton, 2005).

Psychotherapy. Accumulated studies suggest substantial efficacy for cognitive-behavioral therapy in panic disorders. After reviewing 11 research papers on treatments for panic disorder, DeRubeis and Crits-Christoph (1998) concluded that cognitive therapy was superior to supportive psychotherapy, pharmacotherapy, and wait-list. Applying CBT, Wilson (1996) has written an excellent book, appropriate for both patients and therapists, in which he describes specific approaches to deal with panic attacks.

EXHIBIT 13.2 TREATMENT OF ANXIETY DISORDERS

The selective serontonin reuptake inhibitors are the first-line pharmacological treatment for most anxiety disorders because of data supporting their efficacy, the minimal need for dosage titration, the overall favorable side-effect profile, and the length of available clinical experience.

Situation in vivo exposure substantially reduces symptoms in panic disorder with agoraphobia (Stuart, 2005a). In vivo exposure therapy has the patient contact fear-eliciting stimuli in real-life situations. The rate of exposure to fearful stimuli can be gradual, starting on the least fearful end of a fear hierarchy and slowly working up, or it can be extremely rapid, by starting with the most feared situations (Stuart, 2005a). For patients experiencing panic and agoraphobia, exposure therapy reduces avoidance but not panic; cognitive therapy reduces panic but not avoidance. An integrated approach using both CBT and pharmacologic approaches is successful for most patients experiencing panic disorder with agoraphobia.

For many years, agoraphobia has been a closet disorder. Culturally disempowered people, especially agoraphobic women, have come to accept the notion that they exist as solitary freaks unable to cope with the world or even simple tasks in any normal, productive fashion. Group experiences with other women with similar problems demand a personal paradigm shift. It no longer becomes possible to believe that one is entirely alone when confronted by other people experiencing a similar phenomenon.

Insight or understanding is not enough for overcoming agoraphobia. Individuals must behaviorally confront the situations and feelings that terrify them. From a behavioral perspective, exposure to the feared situations causes extinction of the conditioned response. The group often evolves into several subgroups, or buddy systems (Brehony, 1987). For example, one woman who could drive but could not eat out in a restaurant paired up with another woman who found restaurants to be no problem but could not drive. They recognized the need to confront the fears and organized strategies so that they could confront them together.

As a larger goal of empowerment, it is important that the agoraphobic woman learn that there are a number of things she can do to control panic attacks. Three panic management techniques are: (1) diaphragmatic breathing—taking a deep breath, holding it to the count of five, and slowly exhaling; (2) staying in the present with what's happening now—anxiety is almost always a "what if" experience, and this is particularly true of agoraphobic panic ("what if it gets worse and I embarrass myself?"); and (3) stopping negative thoughts (thought-stopping techniques were illustrated by one woman who pretended the thoughts came from someone else whom she named the Ms. Busybody; she would tell Ms. Busybody she wasn't listening anymore).

Social Phobia

Social phobia is influenced by multiple genetic and environmental factors (Mathew & Ho, 2006).

Pharmacotherapy. SSRIs are the favored first-line pharmacologic treatment for social phobia (Davidson, 2006).

Currently the FDA has approved paroxetine (20–50 mg/day), sertraline (50–200 mg/day), and venlafaxine XR (75–225 mg/day) for treatment of social phobia; however, clinical studies indicate that fluvoxamine (50 mg/day) and escitalopram (10 mg/day) can also be effective treatments, although they are not FDA approved for social phobia (Davidson, 2006). A multicenter randomized controlled trial reported that fixed-dose paroxetine (20 mg/day) significantly improved performance on the Liebowitz Social Anxiety Scale compared with placebo (Liebowitz et al., 2002). Full effects may not be seen until 8 weeks after initiation of treatment.

There are many choices for second-line therapies, including the benzodiazepines clonazepam and bromazepam, while the calcium channel blockers gabapentin and pregabalin may possibly provide benefit (Davidson, 2006). Atypical antipsychotics also may be helpful (Davidson, 2006). A study revealed that mirtazapine was an effective agent in the treatment of social phobia in women and in the improvement of their health-related quality of life (Moritz, 2005).

Psychosocial Therapies. Exposure therapy is a set of techniques that helps patients confront their feared objects, situations, memories, and images (Foa, 2006). In vivo exposure deliberately places patients in feared real-life situations that include information that would be incompatible with the patient's maladaptive, unrealistic expectation of outcome. For example, women who panic in grocery stores can discover with repeated exposure that they did not have a heart attack at the store and then realize that what they were afraid of is unrealistic (Foa, 2006).

With other phobias, implosive therapy may be used. Implosive therapy involves the presentation of highly anxiety-provoking imagery (individualized for each phobic patient) in as vivid a manner as possible. The therapist discourages the person from escaping the scene to avoid the stimuli. Reinforced practice allows the client to make gradual repeated approaches toward the phobic situation with permission to turn back whenever the level of anxiety becomes too high (Foa, 2006). Relaxation tapes may be used, and the therapist is very liberal with praise about the client's increasing autonomy. The client also may be asked to record phobic occurrences during the week, what was done to overcome fears, and what triggered them. In addition, patients can be taught to identify their anxiety-evoking stimuli and to develop a hierarchy or stimuli map. Then they choose an initial item from the hierarchy and designate an exposure task to confront this stimulus.

Group CBT is moderately effective with social phobia. However, individual CBT, focusing on using videotaped feedback, eliminating safety behaviors, and incorporating exposure exercises, is superior to group CBT (Foa, 2006).

Generalized Anxiety Disorder

Generalized anxiety disorder is a chronic and recurrent disorder and may be the least likely anxiety disorder to result in long-term remission. The risk of relapse is lower when patients are treated for at least 6 months, and, for many patients, drug therapy should be ongoing and recommended for a life time. First-line pharmacologic treatment includes venlafaxine XR (a serotonin norepinephrine reuptake inhibitor, 75–150 mg/day) and the SSRIs paroxetine (20 mg/day) and escitalopram (10 mg/day) (Nutt, 2005; Thase, 2006). Second-line treatment includes imipramine (150 mg/day) and buspirone (15–30 mg/day) (Nutt, 2005). A research study revealed that pregabalin (400 mg/day), a relatively new anxiolytic, is an effective treatment for GAD (Pohl, Feltner, Fieve, & Pande, 2005). Pregabalin acts as a presynaptic inhibitor of the release of excessive levels of excitatory neurotransmitters by selectively binding to the [alpha]2-[delta] subunit of voltage-gated calcium channels.

A short course of psychological therapy, regardless of whether it was accompanied by active medication, was an effective treatment for patients diagnosed as having severe symptoms of GAD (Bond, Wingrove, Curran, & Lader, 2002). This clinical trial included 60 patients and used buspirone or placebo. Adequate evidence exists for concluding that cognitive-behavioral therapy, exercise, and applied relaxation are efficacious treatments for GAD (Stuart, 2005a).

Obsessive-Compulsive Disorder

As with other anxiety disorders, both pharmacological and CBT are effective in treating obsessive-compulsive disorder. In a large naturalistic study, 62% of participants receiving recommended doses of SSRIs rated themselves as very much or much improved; relatively few participants received the recommended course of CBT, but, of those who did, 67% rated themselves as very much or much improved (Mancebo et al., 2006).

First-line pharmacologic treatments for OCD are the SSRIs (fluoxetine (20–60 mg/day), fluvoxamine (50–300 mg/day), paroxetine (20–40 mg/day), and sertraline (50–200 mg/day)) (Nutt, 2005). Quality of life was significantly improved following both paroxetine and venlafaxine treatments (Tenney, Denys, vanMegen, Glas, & Westenberg, 2003). The second-line treatment is clomipramine (Nutt, 2005). Although efficacious, clomipramine usefulness is limited by significant sedative, anticholinergic, sexual, and orthostatic side effects (DiPiro et al., 2005). If a patient with OCD does not respond to the average dosage of an SSRI within 4 weeks, the dosage should be gradually increased to its maximum level by 8 weeks after therapy initiation. Partial responders should be treated for 10–12 weeks before changing medication or augmenting with another agent. If another SSRI is not effective, then augmentation can include addition of clomipramine, clonazepam, second-generation antipsychotics such as aripiprazole, buspirone, risperidone, or a second SSRI (DiPiro et al., 2005). In a retrospective chart review of treatment-resistant patients with OCD who responded to the addition of an antipsychotic and then later discontinued the antipsychotic drug, 15 of the 18 patients relapsed after antipsychotic discontinuation (Maina, Albert, Ziero, & Bogetto, 2003). These authors advised that antipsychotic augmentation has to be maintained for patients who respond to this strategy. The experts recommend attempting to use CBT alone for patients who are pregnant or who also have medical complications (National Institute of Mental Health, 2003).

With patients who have obsessive-compulsive disorder, CBT involves compensatory skills training consisting of a detailed explanation of the occurrence and maintenance of obsessive thoughts, exposure to obsessive thoughts, response prevention of all neutralizing strategies, cognitive restructuring, and relapse prevention. Behavior therapy, which entails repeated exposure to the stimulus that sets off the ritualistic acts, is also effective. For example, if a patient has a compulsion that causes her to wash her hands 20 or 30 times a day, her hands may be deliberately dirtied, after which she is prevented from washing them. Although such treatment may sound cruel, it has proved to be effective in severe cases in which traditional forms of medication and psychotherapy have failed.

Teaching the client that physiological processes, rather than mismanaged emotions, contribute to the disorder will enable the client to accept OCD as an illness rather than as evidence of personal failure. Support through nursing's caring presence in the client's daily activities, with a focus on the present, will facilitate cooperation in interventions aimed at reducing symptoms through medication or, at the least, increasing the client's ability to control them through behavior therapy. Foa and Wilson (1991) have written an excellent book, appropriate for both patients and therapists, in which they describe specific approaches for dealing with OCD.

Post-Traumatic Stress Disorder

Post-traumatic stress disorder is a highly prevalent, disabling illness. Although women are exposed to proportionately fewer traumatic events in their life time than men, they have a higher lifetime risk of PTSD (Seedat et al., 2005). In addition to higher rates of rape and sexual assault and greater exposure to intimate partner violence, the preponderance of PTSD in women may be attributable to factors other than trauma type, such as sensitization of stress hormone systems in response to early adverse experiences, inherent neuroendocrine factors, subjective interpretation of the event, and peritraumatic association (Seedat et al., 2005). Women with PTSD experience a greater symptom burden, longer course of illness, and have worse quality-of-life outcomes than men. Randomized controlled studies conducted in large samples of women with chronic PTSD indicate that SSRIs have efficacy on clusters of PTSD, and CBT strategies (e.g., prolonged exposure treatment and cognitive processing) are effective in sexually and non–sexually assaulted women (Seedat et al., 2005). Emerging empirical data suggest the potential usefulness of anti-adrenergic agents and preventive CBT treatments in managing acute trauma reactions stemming from the emergence of PTSD.

Pharmacotherapy. SSRIs are considered first-line medication treatment for PTSD, with sertraline (50–200 mg/day), paroxetine (20–50 mg/day), and fluoxetine (20–60 mg/day) being the most studied (Robert, Hamner, Ulmer, Lorberbaum, & Durkalski, 2006). More limited but favorable data suggest that citalopram may also have a role in the treatment. Recent research indicates that escitalopram is both efficacious and well tolerated in PTSD patients (Robert et al., 2006). Treatment should be continued for at least 12 months, if not indefinitely.

Psychosocial Therapies. A systematic review of randomized controlled trials of all psychological treatments (except eye movement desensitization and reprocessing) revealed that individual trauma-focused cognitive-behavioral therapy (TFCBT), stress management, and group TFCBT are effective in the treatment of PTSD (Bisson, 2006). Other generic psychological treatments did not reduce PTSD symptoms as significantly. Some evidence indicated that individual TFCBT was superior to stress management several months following treatment (Bisson, 2006). No published evidence exists that eye movement desensitization and reprocessing is as effective as standard exposure treatments.

CBT research also has focused on the treatment of nightmares. Those in a treatment group were instructed in imagery rehearsal, in which they learned in a waking state to change a nightmare and visualize a new set of images (Krakow et al., 1995). Treated patients showed significant and clinically important decreases in nightmares in terms of both nights per week and actual number of nightmares. They also experienced a significant improvement in their self-rated quality of sleep.

Volunteers have been very effective in rape trauma syndrome, because the victim is considered normal and one who was managing adequately in her life prior to the crisis. Telephone counseling programs are also an effective intervention tool. The telephone is effective because it provides quick access to the victim, places the burden on the counselor to seek out the victim rather than on the victim to seek help, allows the victim considerable power in the situation, encourages the victim to resume a normal lifestyle as quickly as possible, is cost-effective, and provides a way to discuss difficult issues other than face-to-face.

Establishing an alliance with a rape victim is difficult but very important. The goal of the counseling interview is to discuss the victim's emotional reactions and her thoughts and feelings about what happened. This cannot happen without a trusting relationship. During the working phase, the therapist will try to get as complete a picture of the event and its aftermath as possible (Burgess, 1985). The assault must be described in terms of when and where the victim was approached. Who did it? Was he known to the victim? What kind of conversation occurred between the victim and assailant prior to the rape? Did the assailant try to charm her? Did he threaten her or make humiliating comments? What did she say to him?

The sexual details may be the most difficult for the victim to discuss. It is generally the topic the victim wishes to forget. However, the sexual details are apt to be the ones that will keep recurring in the victim's mind. Until the victim is able to talk about the details and is somewhat settled within her when talking about the incident, the details will continue to haunt her and will influence her relationships with other men. It is important to ask about threats and violence. Did the assailant have a weapon? What type of violence was inflicted? It is important to find out how she feels about her struggle or lack thereof. At the time of a rape, many victims decide not to struggle in hopes of saving their lives. The therapist can confirm this universal strategy and help to alleviate guilt. What does the sexual assault mean to her? Was this a first sexual experience? What are her feelings about sex now? Has she been raped before? (Burgess, 1985).

A crucial factor in the treatment of sexual trauma is the nurse's own attitude toward the victim. If the nurse finds herself or himself judging the victim rather than trying to understand the situation the victim has experienced, all therapeutic leverage will be lost. Nurses have to come to grips with their own prejudices regarding sexuality and violence if they are to be effective in treating a victim of sexual assault.

McArthur (1990) wrote about the effectiveness of using reality therapy in a group context with rape victims. Members have an opportunity to learn how others with similar experiences have been able to recover from similar problems. The peer support from members gives an individual a sense of hope. Rape has an effect on the sense of self, affecting a loss of self-esteem, creation of guilt and shame, mistrust in interpersonal relationships, and distorted perceptions of self-worth. Because of the massive injury to the self, rape victims may very quickly become isolated and lonely.

Reality therapy treats the sense of self by offering the victim opportunities to regain self-esteem and resolves guilt and shame by changing the point at which value judgments are made. When the victim develops a passive lifestyle because of chronic feelings of helplessness and powerlessness, the group confronts this in a warm, supportive manner. The group does not allow excuses for acting out or isolative behavior. The responsibility for the victim's behavior is not with a family who does not understand or with her assailant. The opportunity for making a success of her life—for becoming a survivor instead of a victim—is hers. Members of a rape victim support group form a common bond around their experience and realize that they are able to help others because they understand each other's problems. In helping others, they find a sense of purpose and belonging that restores their own self-esteem.

If a pregnancy is a result of rape, the woman may be extremely ambivalent about the baby. If the rape occurred some time ago, the whole experience of pregnancy with prenatal examinations can trigger memories of the original trauma. She may avoid prenatal examinations because of the anxiety triggered by bodily touch and vaginal examinations. Some pregnant women with PTSD may feel more comfortable with a woman nurse or physician. The nurse can verbalize appreciation of the patient's anxiety and reassure her about what is about to happen.

Other Strategies to Decrease Anxiety

Anxiety is contagious and is communicated interpersonally. Nurses must monitor their own anxiety levels and reduce their anxiety before they can help patients. Most of the measures discussed next are effective for professionals as well as patients.

Using Peplau's theory (1963), a nurse would ask the woman to describe one situation in which she felt anxious, including what preceded the feelings. Focus next would center on what the client expected to happen and what happened instead. Anxiety occurs when one's needs or expectations are not met. After helping the client clarify which needs were not met, it is necessary to think of ways the client can express her needs more clearly to others or change the nature of her needs if they are unreasonable. For example, women may expect men to meet all of their needs. Not only is that unrealistic, but often men are not aware of what women need because women have not been able to express themselves; even when they do, men do not always understand them. As women become more clear about what they need from people and as they experience some success in expressing their needs, anxiety can be prevented.

Reviewing with women their coping skills can facilitate problem solving about what else might be healthier and more effective. For example, helping a patient substitute meditation for drinking beer after work would be a healthier coping skill.

Education. Patients with anxiety disorders must be reassured that their symptoms are part of a real illness and that this illness is treatable. Because the most frightening aspect of panic disorder is the somatic symptoms, many women believe that they have a severe physical illness such as cardiac or neurological disorder. The biologic explanation of anxiety must be explained, "You have a dysfunction of the sympathetic nervous system, in which bursts of chemicals called catecholamines are released into the peripheral circulation, causing symptoms such as . . . ." A further analogy about panic attacks is, "They are similar to the fight-or-flight response to dangerous situations, but you are having this danger response at inappropriate times when there is only minimal actual danger" (Fishel, 1998). These explanations enable patients to make realistic interpretations of body symptoms (i.e., "this is anxiety, not a heart attack, that is making my heart pound; it will go away in a few minutes").

Women need specific information about their anxiety disorder. Pamphlets that are available through national organizations and Web sites can be given to clients to supplement patient teaching (see Table 13.9).

Empowerment. One of the most frightening psychological symptoms is a fear of losing control. The nurse must covey the expectation that the patient can learn to control anxiety. Listening to women clients and helping them to sort through their fears and expectations encourages them to take charge of their lives. Teaching them strategies to use to decrease anxiety is very empowering.

Sensory Interventions. Suggesting such activities as a massage, warm bath, hot shower, and a heating pad can facilitate relaxation. *Music therapy* is another effective strategy (Hernandez-Ruiz, 2005; Joske, Rao, & Kristjanson, 2006; Slawson, 2005). Music affects the right side of the brain and causes the pituitary gland to release endorphins that, in turn, relieve pain. The level of catecholamine decreases, which causes a reduction in blood pressure and heart rate (Henry, 1995). Headphones are especially helpful. Some music therapists prefer music with primarily string composition, with low-pitched sound, a simple and direct musical rhythm, and a tempo of approximately 60 to 70 beats (Henry, 1995). Examples are Beethoven's "Moonlight Sonata," Brahms's "Lullaby," Pachelbel's "Canon in D," George Winston's "Autumn" and "December," the soundtrack from *The Sound of Music*, and the Mormon Tabernacle Choir singing "The Old Beloved Songs." A study of agitated elderly reported that, when patients chose their brand of music, the impact on anxiety reduction was greater than with a classical music selection (Gerdner, 2000). *Aromatherapy*, especially lavender, can be very relaxing. Burning a scented candle or applying a dab of essential oil on one's pillow at night can enhance restful sleep.

Behavioral Interventions and Breathing Exercises. To lower anxiety, Knowles (1981) recommends round breathing. With mouth closed, breathe in and out in such a fashion that there is no pause at the beginning or end of each respiration. Another technique is breath holding—patients

13.9 | Patient Resources on Anxiety Disorders

NAME OF ORGANIZATION	ADDRESS
Anxiety Disorders Association of America	6000 Executive Boulevard, Suite 513 Rockville, MD 20852
National Anxiety Foundation	3135 Custer Drive Lexington, KY 40517-4001
National Institute of Mental Health: Publications list	5600 Fishers Lane Rockville, MD 20857
National Mental Health Association	1210 Prince Street Alexander, VA 22314-2971
Web sites	
National Panic & Anxiety Disorder News	www.npadnews.com
The Anxiety Panic Internet Resource	www.algy.com/anxiety

take a very deep breath and hold it for the count of three; then, as they slowly release this breath, they say to themselves, "relax." More in-depth breathing exercises can be demonstrated with patients. If the nurse makes a tape recording of the relaxation exercise, the woman can take it home with her to use whenever she needs it. The sound of the nurse's familiar voice on the tape can be reassuring. Deep abdominal breathing is another technique. Instruct the patient to breathe in through the nose and fill the lungs so that the diaphragm pushes down and the abdomen pushes out. Exhale through the mouth, moving the diaphragm up and the abdomen in. Many people are shallow breathers and use only their upper chest, which means that only their shoulders move up and down. The patient may want to count the breaths going in and out at a rate of three counts in and five counts out and rest. The patient can be encouraged to say to herself, "breathe in calmness, breathe out anxiety."

Progressive Muscle Relaxation. This exercise involves systematically tensing and slowly releasing each muscle group, and usually follows several minutes of breathing exercise. When teaching this activity, the nurse may want to start with the toes and work up, or start the greatest distance away from the uncomfortable area. Instruct the patient at every phase; for example, "tighten your toes, very tight, hold it, now relax your toes and don't forget to breathe, deep breath in and blow it out." Gradually move all over the body until all muscles have been tightened and relaxed. This exercise helps many women fall asleep.

Prayer, Meditation, and Guided Imagery. Other techniques that may be helpful include prayer, meditation, and guided imagery. In guided imagery, patients practice 5 to 10

minutes of deep breathing and then they are asked to close their eyes and imagine a pleasant scene. Ask them to engage all of their senses, to hear the ocean, smell the flowers, taste the honey, feel the warm sun, see the mountain view. Before you create an imagery exercise, find out in what kind of place the patient feels most relaxed. Also, think about whatever event is worrisome and make that go away in the exercise.

Cognitive Strategies. Cognitive-behavioral therapy is well respected as a psychotherapeutic strategy. However, all nurses can use CBT principles in their interactions with patients. CBT is based on the maladaptive cognitions theory; that is, people (especially women) behave on the basis of misconceptions and unrealistic thought patterns (Beck & Greenberg, 1974). The nurse allies herself with the client against the symptoms. Self-statement training consists of three steps: (1) the identification of negative self-statements; (2) recognition of the role that negative self-statements play in influencing self-concept, behavior, and mood; and (3) replacing negative self-statements with positive self-statements that help the patient cope with high levels of anxiety (e.g., "anxiety won't kill me") (Stuart, 2005a).

Reframing. Reframing allows patients to adjust themselves psychologically in such a way that events formerly perceived as threatening are seen in a more positive light. Instead of disparaging oneself for high levels of anxiety, thoughts are reframed; for example, "how lucky I am that I have such a sensitive system for protection." Instead of focusing on the symptoms of a panic attack, encourage the patient to think about a time they were feeling anxious and did not have an attack. Ask how she prevented it, and encourage her to do more of that. Some patients like using videos, books, or how-to manuals to build skills to cope with anxiety and to learn relaxation, breathing exercises, positive self-talk, and nonnegative thinking patterns.

FUTURE DIRECTIONS FOR IMPROVING WOMEN'S MENTAL HEALTH

Gender-Related Research

More research is needed to achieve a comprehensive understanding of the basis for women's increased vulnerability to depression and anxiety (Kornstein & Wojcik, 2002; Pigott, 2002). Lundberg (2005) concludes that gender roles and psychological factors are more important than biological factors for the sex differences in stress responses. However, an integrated theoretical approach is warranted to account for the full complexity of gender differences (Kornstein & Wojcik, 2002).

There is a need for additional studies examining gender differences in clinical features of depression and anxiety and differences in response to various types of pharmacotherapy, psychotherapy, and combination treatments, as well as issues of tolerability and treatment strategies for nonresponders and patients with comorbid disorders (Kornstein & Wojcik, 2002). More research is needed on gender-related issues in the long-term management of mental illness in women; the effect of reproductive cycle events, and prevention and early detection in young women (Kornstein & Wojcik, 2002).

Gender differences in bipolar disorder are clinically important and require more study; especially needed are improved treatments for rapid cycling and mixed states—two presentations that are more common in women (Freeman et al., 2002). More research is needed on the use of psychotropic medications during pregnancy and lactation. What impact do psychotropic medications have on the future health of the fetus and newborn?

Access to Treatment

Removing the stigma about treatment and making mental health services more accessible is necessary. Major depressive disorder is common among impoverished women in the rural South. They seldom get treated because of a paucity of treatment available, their inability to pay for services because of not having insurance, and the distance they must travel to reach care (Hauenstein, 2003). Even if treatment was available, impoverished rural Southern women are unlikely to seek services because of cultural and social prohibitions.

In Taiwan, one solution to improving access to mental health services was to set up a mental health clinic in the gynecologic outpatient department (Hsiao, Lie, Chen, & Hsieh, 2002). Of the patients referred and evaluated in the on-site mental health clinic, the most common diagnosis was major depressive disorder (36.0%), followed by generalized anxiety disorder (29.4%), premenstrual dysphoric disorder (16.2%), and dysthymic disorder (14.7%). Providing advanced practice psychiatric nurses in nurse practitioner offices and gynecology clinics could provide nonstigmatized access to mental health services.

Women's Role Stress

Ever since women surged into the work place in the 1970s, their economic power has grown steadily. Women now make up 47% of the work force; they're awarded 57% of all bachelor's degrees, and about 30% of working women now earn more than their husbands (Deveny, 2003). However, women have legitimate gripes. Most two-income couples without children divide up the household chores pretty evenly (Deveny, 2003). After the kids come, however, men do less around the house; 55% of new fathers spend more time at work after a child is born. Work place stress may be one reason why retirement at age 60 was associated with an improvement in mental health, particularly among high socioeconomic groups of women (Mein, Martikainen, Hemingway, Stansfeld, & Marmot, 2003).

Research participants with more marital concerns reported greater stress throughout the day, showed an attenuated cortisol increase following waking, a flatter cortisol slope over the day, and had elevated blood pressure over the middle of the day (Barnett, Steptoe, & Garteis, 2005). In today's society, which is characterized by high demands, a frantic pace of life, and demands for efficiency and competitiveness, the associated lack of rest, recovery, and restitution that accompanies this lifestyle is a greater health problem than the absolute level of stress.

Motherhood

Is motherhood good for women? Having fewer children in the family predicted less stress for parents; however, household income and an interaction between child behavior problems and work interest were significant predictors of maternal parenting role stress, but not for fathers (Warfield, 2005). Kirkley (2000) asserted that it is time to question this assumption that motherhood is biologic destiny for women. In the early 1970s, some feminist writers theorized that the only hope for women's emancipation was to be freed from the responsibility of bearing and raising children. A decade later, the promothering faction within the feminist community believed that the answer was not to reject the role but rather to reconstruct the resources available and expectations placed on mothers. Child care was acknowledged as a serious need, and grassroots groups of mothers formed cooperative nurseries and marched on Washington for changes in child care laws (Kirkley, 2000).

Child Care

The lack of high-quality, affordable child care prevents many women from entering the labor force and prevents many more from holding well-paying full-time jobs. In France, children can attend free prekindergarten starting at age 2, and their education is free until they graduate from college. For many years, policies in United States have emphasized the need for the government or private sector to support child care for poor women as a necessary prerequisite for women to work. Some private industries have developed on-site child care programs, and kindergarten is now provided as part of public-school education. But we have been slow to respond.

An equal division of child care responsibilities among both parents would help decrease the overload felt by women. The school system could also share the responsibility for child care. Far too many children are staying at home unsupervised because school ends earlier than a typical work day. The school could provide after-school programs with scheduled activities and supervised play until the usual work day ends. For middleschool–aged children, a study hall in the school library after the regular school day likely would be helpful to both parents and children.

Friendship

A landmark study by researchers at the University of California, Los Angeles, suggests that friendships between women are quite unique, shaping who we are and who we are yet to be (Taylor et al., 2000). Friendships have been known to soothe women's tumultuous inner world and fill the emotional gaps in marriages. Hanging out with women friends can counteract the kind of stomach-quivering stress most experience on a daily basis (Taylor et al., 2000).

When oxytocin is released as part of the stress responses in a woman, it buffers the fight-or-flight response and encourages her to tend children and gather with other women instead. When she engages in this tending or befriending, more oxytocin is released, which further counters stress and produces a calming effect (Taylor et al., 2000). This may explain why women consistently outlive men. The Harvard Nurses' Health Study (Taylor et al., 2000) found that the more friends women had, the less likely they were to develop physical impairments as they aged and the more likely they were to be leading a joyful life. Even after the death of their spouse, women who had a close friend and confidante were more likely to survive the experience

without any new physical impairments or permanent loss of vitality.

Yet if friends counter the stress that seems to swallow up so much of women's lives, if they keep women healthy and even add years to their lives, then why is it so hard to find time to be with friends? Usually, when women become overly busy with work and family, the first thing they let go of is friendships with other women. That's a mistake, because women are a source of strength to each other, and they nurture one another. Women need to have unpressured space in which they can do the special kind of talk that women do when they're with other women. It's a very healing experience (Taylor et al., 2000). A woman's sense of self is intimately related to her connections to others.

Social Support

Fifty women receiving welfare for their dependent children in a rural community were interviewed about their work experiences (Taylor, 2001). The findings indicated that the majority of participants were connected to the labor force and expressed positive attitudes about work. Further, barriers to employment identified included a lack of available jobs, child care, transportation, and inconvenient office hours. Perceived social support was negatively related to depression symptoms and positively related to self-efficacy and self-esteem.

Gray and Carson (2002) conducted another study that highlighted the importance of social support in women's lives. After interviewing women with HIV infection, they found that social support and spirituality were significantly correlated with the women's mastery over their stress. Interpersonal conflict was significantly negatively correlated with mastery over stress.

Mental Health Promotion

Within the last decade, a national prevention research, training, and practice agenda on mental health has been established to address the epidemiological increases in mental disorders and associated emotional and financial costs to the American people (Magyary, 2002). A positive mental health orientation—inclusive of health promotion processes—contributes to the national prevention agenda in four ways: (1) prevention of mental disorders in the general public; (2) prevention of secondary comorbid conditions, disabilities, negative consequences, and relapses in psychiatric populations; (3) reduction of risk factors and the enhancement of protective factors in the general public as well as specific psychiatric populations; and (4) the enhancement of a sense of well-being and productivity at the individual, family, and community level (Magyary, 2002).

Mental health promotion focuses on: (1) helping women to avoid stressors or cope with them more adaptively and (2) changing the resources and governmental policies so that they no longer cause stress but rather enhance women's functioning (Stuart, 2005b). Women who are poor, less educated, unemployed, and from minority populations are more likely to experience depression. Prevention programs designed to immunize women against depression need to take into consideration the emergence of risk and protective factors during the early developmental years of life.

For many adults, primary care may be the initial and only source of mental health services. In the next decade, we may see a change toward a service delivery model that integrates mental and general health services with the point of entry being controlled by the general health practitioner (Magyary, 2002). In these integrated practices, in addition to detection of mental disorders, mental health promotion should be emphasized. At this point, however, we know little about how to promote mental health. Research needs to address the short- and long-term effectiveness and efficacy of preventive intervention programs implemented in real-world settings that reflect diverse populations, organizations, and financial structures (Magyary, 2002). Financial and accessible parity between mental health and physical health services must be accomplished. The discrimination and stigmatization associated with mental health must be eliminated (Magyary, 2002).

Summary of Directions for Improving Mental Health

The mental health of women is profoundly affected by the social, economic, physiological, and psychological context of their lives. Policy changes have been recommended by professional and lay groups alike as ways to promote women's mental health. These changes include:

- Eliminating sexism, racism, and ageism.
- Decreasing poverty through work opportunities.
- Educating health care practitioners about efficacious treatment models for women.
- Supporting women in dealing with dual career role conflicts.
- Supporting friendships among women.
- Ensuring adequate child care.
- Teaching advantages of egalitarian roles for couples (home and child-rearing responsibilities) in the public school system.
- Eliminating domestic violence and abuse against females of all ages.
- Assuring financial and accessible parity between mental health and physical health.
- Sponsoring research on effective mental health promotion strategies for women of all ethnicities and social classes.

- Sponsoring research on anxiety and mood disorders that explicitly incorporates the study of gender in relation to genetic contributions, environmental and psychological factors, and biological factors.
- Sponsoring research on the impact of pharmacological treatment on women, including hormonal changes associated with menstrual cycle, pregnancy and lactation, and menopause.

However, policy recommendation is insufficient; policies must be implemented. In 1978, the President's Commission on Mental Health (1978) developed recommendations to change the social status of women and thereby lessen their need for mental health services; most of these recommendations have not been implemented 30 years later.

REFERENCES

Allen, J., Schnyer, R., Chambers, A., Hitt, S., Moreno, F., and Manber, R. (2006). Acupuncture for depression: A randomized controlled trial. *Journal of Clinical Psychiatry, 67*(11), 1665–1673.

Al-Mateen, C. S., Christian, F., Mishra, A., Cofield, M., & Tildon, T. (2002). Women of color. In S. Kornstein & A. Clayton (Eds.), *Women's mental health* (pp. 568–583). New York: Guilford Press.

Amar, A. (2006). College women's experience of stalking: Mental health symptoms and changes in routines. *Archives of Psychiatric Nursing, 20*(3), 108–116.

American Academy of Pediatrics, Committee on Drugs. (1994). The transfer of drugs and other chemicals into human milk. *Pediatrics, 93*, 137–150.

American Psychiatric Association. (2000). *Diagnostic and statistical manual of mental disorders* (4th ed., text revision). Washington, DC: Author.

American Psychiatric Association. (2003). Practice guideline for the treatment of patients with bipolar disorder (revision). Retrieved from www.psych.org

Bailey, K. (2003). Treating treatment-resistant depression. *Journal of Psychosocial Nursing, 41*(6), 14–20.

Baldwin, D., Montgomery, S., Nil, R., & Lader, M. (2005). Discontinuation symptoms in depression and anxiety disorders. *International Journal of Neuropsychopharmacology, 10*(1), 73–84.

Ballenger, J., Davidson, J., Lecrubier, Y., Nutt, D., Kirmayer, L., Lepine, J., et al. (2001). Consensus statement on transcultural issues in depression and anxiety from the International Consensus Group on Depression and Anxiety. *Journal of Clinical Psychiatry, 62* (Suppl. 13), 47–55.

Barnett, R., Steptoe, A., & Garteis, K. (2005). Marital-role quality and stress-related psychobiological indicators. *Annals of Behavioral Medicine, 30*(1), 36–43.

Bauer, M., Berghofer, A., Bschor, T., Baumgartner, A., Kiesslinger, U., & Hellweg, R. (2002). Supra-physiological doses of L-thyroxine in the maintenance treatment of prophylaxis-resistant affective disorders. *Neuropsychopharmacology, 27*, 620–628.

Beck, A. T. (1995). *Beck depression inventory-II.* San Antonio, TX: Psychological Corporation of Harcourt Brace & Company.

Beck, A. T., & Greenberg, R. (1974). Cognitive therapy with depressed women. In V. Franks & V. Burtle (Eds.), *Women in therapy* (pp. 113–131). New York: Brunner/Mazel.

Beck, C. (2002). Revision of the postpartum depression predictors inventory. *Journal of Obstetric, Gynecologic, and Neonatal Nursing, 31* (4), 394–402.

Beck, C., Records, K., & Rice, M. (2006). Further development of the postpartum depression predictors inventory—revised. *Journal of Obstetric, Gynecologic, and Neonatal Nursing, 35*, 735–745.

Bennett, H., Einarson, A., Toddio, A., Koren, G., & Einarson, T. (2004). Prevalence of depression during pregnancy: Systematic review. *Obstetrics and Gynecology, 103*, 698–709.

Bhanji, N., Chouinard, G., Kolivakis, T., & Margolese, H. (2006). Persistent tardive rebound panic disorder rebound anxiety and insomnia following paroxetine withdrawal: A review of rebound-withdrawal phenomena. *Canadian Journal of Clinical Pharmacology, 13*(1), e69–e74.

Bisson, J. (2006). Psychological treatment of post-traumatic stress disorder (PTSD). *Cochrane Review Abstracts*. Retrieved from www.cochrane.org/reviews

Bond, A., Wingrove, J., Curran, V., & Lader, M. (2002). Treatment of generalised anxiety disorder with a short course of psychological therapy, combined with buspirone or placebo. *Journal of Affective Disorders, 72*(3), 267–271.

Bozoky, I., & Corwin, E. (2001). Fatigue as a predictor of postpartum depression. *Journal of Obstetrical and Gynecological Neonatal Nursing, 31*(4), 436–443.

Brand, B. (2002). Trauma and violence. In S. Kornstein & A. Clayton (Eds.), *Women's mental health* (pp. 542–554). New York: Guilford Press.

Brehony, K. (1987). Self-help groups with agoraphobic women. In C. Brody (Ed.), *Women's therapy groups* (pp. 82–94). New York: Springer Publishing.

Brown University. (2002). Experts debate new clinical data on duloxetine. *Psychopharmacology Update, 13*(8), 1, 4–5.

Brunnauer, A., Laux, G., Geiger, E., Soyka, M., & Moller, H. (2006). Antidepressants and driving ability: Results from a clinical study. *Journal of Clinical Psychiatry, 67*(11), 1776–1781.

Burgess, A. (1985). *Psychiatric nursing in the hospital and the community* (4th ed.). Englewood Cliffs, NJ: Prentice Hall.

Burt, V., & Stein, K. (2002). Epidemiology of depression throughout the female life cycle. *Journal of Clinical Psychiatry, 63*(Suppl. 7), 9–15.

Calabrese, J., Elhaj, O., Gajwani, P., & Gao, K. (2005). Clinical highlights in bipolar depression: Focus on atypical antipsychotics. *Journal of Clinical Psychiatry, 66*(Suppl. 5), 26–33.

Casey, M. B. (2002). Developmental perspectives on gender. In S. Kornstein & A. Clayton (Eds.), *Women's mental health* (pp. 499–514). New York: Guilford Press.

Centers for Disease Control and Prevention. (2004). Web-based injury statistics query and reporting system. http://www.cdc.gov/ncipc/wisqars/default.htm

Chambless, D., Caputo, G., & Bright, P. (1984). Assessment of fear in agoraphobics: The body sensations questionnaire and the agoraphobic cognitions questionnaire. *Journal of Consultation and Clinical Psychology, 52*, 1090–1097.

Christensen, R. (2005). Identifying serotonin syndrome in the emergency department. *American Journal of Emergency Medicine, 23*(3), 406–408.

Coates, A., Schaefer, C., & Alexander, J. (2004). Detection of postpartum depression and anxiety in a large health plan. *Journal of Behavioral Health Services & Research, 31*(2), 117–133.

Cohen, L., Nonacs, R., Bailey, J., Viguera, A., Reminick, A., Altshuler, L., Stowe, Z., & Faraone, S. (2004). Relapse of depression during pregnancy following antidepressant discontinuation: A preliminary prospective study. *Archives of Women's Mental Health, 7*(4), 217–221.

Cohen, L., Soares, C., Otto, M., Sweeney, B., Liberman, R., & Harlow, B. (2002). Prevalence and predictors of premenstrual dysphoric disorder (PMDD) in older premenopausal women. The Harvard Study of Moods and Cycles. *Journal of Affective Disorders, 70*(2), 125–132.

Conner, K. M., Kobak, K. A., Churchill, L. E., Katzelnick, D., & Davidson, J. R. (2001). Mini-SPIN: A brief screening assessment for generalized social anxiety disorder. *Depression & Anxiety, 14*(2), 137–140.

Davidson, J. et al (2002). Effect of hypericum perforatum (St John's wort) in major depressive disorder. *Journal of the American Medical Association, 287*, 1807–1814.

Davidson, R. (2006). Pharmacotherapy of social anxiety disorder: What does the evidence tell us? *Journal of Clinical Psychiatry, 67*(Suppl. 12), 20–26.

Delgado, P. L., Brannan, S. K., Mallinckrodt, C. H., Tran, P. V., McNamara, R. K., Wang, F., Watkin, J. G., & Detke, M. J. (2005). Sexual functioning assessed in 4 double-blind placebo-and paroxetine-controlled trials of duloxetine for major depressive disorder. *Journal of Clinical Psychiatry, 66*(6), 686–692.

DeMaat, S., Dekker, J., Schoevers, R., & De Jonghe, F. (2006). Relative efficacy of psychotherapy and pharmacotherapy in the treatment of depression: A meta-analysis. *Psychotherapy Research, 16*(5), 566–578.

DeRubeis, R., & Crits-Christoph, P. (1998). Empirically supported individual and group psychological treatments for adult mental disorders. *Journal of Consulting and Clinical Psychology, 66*(1), 37–52.

Deveny, K. (2003, June 30). We're not in the mood. *Newsweek*, 40–46.

DiPiro, R., Talbert, R., Yee, G., Matzke, G., Wells, B., & Posey, M. (2005). *Pharmacotherapy*. New York: McGraw-Hill.

Dubicka, B., Haley, S., & Roberts, C. (2006). Suicidal behaviour in youths with depression treated with new-generation antidepressants. *British Journal of Psychiatry, 189*, 393–398.

Dunn, A., Trivedi, M., Kampert, J., Clark, C., & Chambliss, H. (2005). Exercise treatment for depression efficacy and dose response. *American Journal of Preventive Medicine, 28*(1), 1–8.

Ebmeier, P., Donaghey, V., & Steele, J. (2006). A sensible 10-year plan for mental health. *Lancet, 367*(9505), 153–167.

Elkin, I., et al. (1989). National Institutes of Mental Health Treatment of Depression Collaborative Research Program: General effectiveness of treatments. *Archives of General Psychiatry, 46*, 971–982.

Elliott, H. (2002). Premenstrual dysphoric disorder. *North Carolina Medical Journal, 63*(2), 72–75.

Eriksson, E., Andersch, B., Ho, H., Landen, M., & Sundblad, C. (2002). Diagnosis and treatment of premenstrual dysphoria. *Journal of Clinical Psychiatry, 63*(Suppl. 7), 16–23.

Eriksson, E., Sundblad, C., Yonkers, K., et al. (2000). Premenstrual dysphoria and related conditions: Symptoms, pathophysiology and treatment. In M. Steiner, K. Yonkers, & E. Eriksson (Eds.), *Mood disorders in women* (pp. 269–294). London: Martin Dunitz.

Ernst, E. (2004). Kava update: A European perspective. *New Zealand Medical Journal, 117*(1205), 1143–1147.

Fishel, A. (1998). Nursing management of anxiety and panic. *Nursing Clinics of North America, 33*(1), 135–151.

Fishel, A. (1999). Psychosocial and behavioral health care. In C. Shea, L Pelletier, E. Poster, G. Stuart, & M. Verhey (Eds.), *Advanced practice nursing in psychiatric and mental health care* (pp. 185–219). St. Louis, MO: Mosby.

Fishel, A. (2007). Mental health disorders and substance abuse. In D. Lowdermilk & S. Perry(Eds.), *Maternity and women's health care* (9th ed., pp. 900–924). St. Louis, MO: Mosby.

Foa, E. (2006). Social anxiety disorder treatments: Psychosocial therapies. *Journal of Clinical Psychiatry, 67*(Suppl. 12), 27–30.

Foa, E., & Wilson, R. (1991). *Stop obsessing*. New York: Bantam.

Fogel, S., Sneed, J., & Roose, S. (2006). Survey of psychiatric treatment among psychiatric residents in Manhattan: Evidence of stigma. *Journal of Clinical Psychiatry, 67*(10), 1591–1598.

Frackiewicz, E., & Shiovitz, T. (2001). Evaluation and management of premenstrual syndrome and premenstrual dysphoric disorder. *Journal of the American Pharmaceutical Association, 41*(3), 437–447.

Frank, E., Grochocinski, V., Spanier, C., et al. (2000). Interpersonal psychotherapy and antidepressant medication: Evaluation of a sequential treatment strategy in women with recurrent major depression. *Journal of Clinical Psychiatry, 61*, 51–57.

Freeman, A., & McElroy, D. . (2002). Bipolar disorder. In S. Kornstein & A. Clayton (Eds.), *Women's mental health* (pp. 166–181). New York: Guilford Press.

Freeman, E., Rickels, K., Sondheimer, S., et al. (1999). Differential response to antidepresants in women with premenstrual syndrome/premenstrual dysphoric disorder: A randomized controlled trial. *Archives of General Psychiatry, 56*, 932–939.

Freeman, E., Sammel, M., Lin, H., & Nelson, D. (2006). Associations of hormones and menopausal status with depressed mood in women with no history of depression. *Archives of General Psychiatry, 63*(4), 375–382.

Gerdner, L. (2000). Effects of individualized versus classical "relaxation" music on the frequency of agitation in elderly persons with Alzheimer's disease and related disorders. *International Psychogeriatrics, 12*, 49–65.

Gitlin, M., Suri, R., Altshuler, L., Zuckerbrow-Miller, J., & Fairbanks, L. (2002). Bupropion-sustained release as a treatment for SSRI-induced sexual side effects. *Journal of Sex & Marital Therapy, 28*(2), 131–138.

Gray, J., & Carson, C. 2002). Mastery over stress among women with HIV/AIDS. *Journal of the Association of Nurses in AIDS Care, 13*(4), 43–57.

Grunze, H. (2005). Reevaluating therapies for bipolar depression, *Journal of Clinical Psychiatry, 66*(Suppl. 5), 17–25.

Halbreich, U. (2003). The etiology, biology, and evolving pathology of premenstrual syndromes. *Psychoneuroendocrinology, 28*(Suppl. 3), 55–99.

Halbreich, U. (2005). Algorithm for treatment of premenstrual syndromes (PMS): Experts' recommendations and limitations. *Gynecological Endocrinology, 20*(1), 49–57.

Hall, W., & Lucke, J. (2006). How have the selective serotonin reuptake inhibitor antidepressants affected suicide mortality? *Australian and New Zealand Journal of Psychiatry, 40*, 941–950.

Hamilton, M. A. (1960). A rating scale for depression. *Journal of Neurology and Neurosurgery Psychiatry, 23*(1), 56–61.

Hauenstein, E. (2003). No comfort in the rural South: Women living depressed. *Archives of Psychiatric Nursing, 17*(1), 3–11.

Hendrick, V., & Altshuler, L. (2002). Management of major depression during pregnancy. *American Journal of Psychiatry, 159*, 1667–1673.

Henry, L. (1995). Music therapy: A nursing intervention for the control of pain and anxiety in the ICU: A review of the research literature. *Dimensions of Critical Care Nursing, 14*, 295–304.

Hensley, P., & Nurnberg, H. (2002). SSRI sexual dysfunction: A female perspective. *Journal of Sex & Marital Therapy, 28*, 143–153.

Hernandez-Ruiz, E. (2005). Effect of music therapy on the anxiety levels and sleep patterns of abused women in shelters. *Journal of Music Therapy, 42*(2), 140–158.

Herrick, H. (2002). Postpartum depression: Who gets help? Statistical Brief No. 24. Raleigh, NC: Department of Health and Human Services.

Hirschfeld, R. (2001). Clinical importance of long-term antidepressant treatment. *British Journal of Psychiatry, 42*(September suppl.), S4–S8.

Hirschfeld, R., et al. (2000). Development and validation of a screening instrument for bipolar spectrum disorder: The Mood Disorders Questionnaire. *American Journal of Psychiatry, 157*, 1873–1875.

Hirschfeld, R., Calabrese, J. R., Weissman, M. M., Reed, M., Davies, M. A., Frye, M. A., Keck, P. E., Lewis, L., McElroy, S. L., McNulty, J. P., & Wagner, K. D. (2003). Screening for bipolar disorder in the community. *Journal of Clinical Psychiatry, 64*(1), 53–59.

Holroyd, S. (2002). Aging and elderly women. In S. Kornstein & A. Clayton (Eds.), *Women's mental health* (pp. 584–593). New York: Guilford Press.

Horowitz, J., & Cousins, A. (2006). Postpartum depression treatment rates for at-risk women. *Nursing Research, 55*(2 Suppl. 1), S23–S27.

Howland, R. (2006a). Challenges in the diagnosis & treatment of bipolar depression. *Journal of Psychosocial Nursing, 44*(5), 9–12.

Howland, R. (2006b). MAOI antidepressant drugs. *Journal of Psychosocial Nursing, 44*(6), 9–12.

Howland, R. (2006c). Pharmacotherapy strategies for treatment-resistant depression. *Journal of Psychosocial Nursing, 44*(11), 11–14.

Howland, R. (2006d). Vagus nerve stimulation. *Journal of Psychosocial Nursing, 44*(9), 11–14.

Howland, R. (2006e). What is vagus nerve stimulation? *Journal of Psychosocial Nursing, 44*(8), 11–14.

Hsiao, M., Liu, C., Chen, K., & Hsieh, T. (2002). Characteristics of women using a mental health clinic in a gynecologic out-patient setting. *Psychiatry & Clinical Neurosciences, 56*(4), 459–463.

Hudson, J., Wohlreich, M., Kajdasz, D., Mallinckrodt, C., Watkin, J., & Martynov, O. (2005). Safety and tolerability of duloxetine in the treatment of major depressive disorder: Analysis of pooled data from eight placebo-controlled trials. *Human Psychopharmacology: Clinical and Experimental, 20*(6), 327–341.

Hussain, M., & Normal, T. (2002, November). *A long-term evaluation of the treatment of bipolar depression and maintenance of therapy with olanzapine*. Poster session presented at the 52nd annual meeting of the Canadian Psychiatric Association, Banff, Alberta.

Jacobson, N., et al. (1996). A component analysis of cognitive behavioral treatment for depression, *Journal of Consulting and Clinical Psychology, 64*(2), 295–304.

Jellin, F., Gregory, P., Batz, H., et al. (2002). *Pharmacist's letter/prescriber's letter natural medicines comprehensive database*. Stockton, CA: Therapeutic Research Faculty.

Joske, D., Rao, A., & Kristjanson, L. (2006). Critical review of complementary therapies in haemato-oncology. *Internal Medicine Journal, 36*(9), 579–586.

Kaplan, H., & Sadock, B. (2005). *Kaplan & Sadock's comprehensive textbook of psychiatry*. Philadelphia: Lippincott Williams & Wilkins.

Kapur, N., Cooper, J., King-Hele, S., Webb, R., Lawlor, M., Rodway, C., & Appleby, L. (2006). The repetition of suicidal behavior: A multicenter cohort study. *Journal of Clinical Psychiatry, 67*(10), 1599–1609.

Karasu, T. (1990). Toward a clinical model of psychotherapy for depression: II. An integrative and selective treatment approach. *American Journal of Psychiatry, 147*(3), 269–278.

Keller, M. (2006). Social anxiety disorder clinical course and outcome: Review of Harvard/Brown Anxiety Research Project (HARP) findings. *Journal of Clinical Psychiatry, 67*(Suppl. 12), 14–19.

Kessing, L., Sondergard, L., Kvist, K., & Anderson, P. (2005). Suicide risk in patients treated with lithium. *Archives of General Psychiatry, 62*, 860–866.

Kessler, R. C., Chiu, W. T., Demier, O., & Walters (2005). Prevalence, severity, and comorbidity of 12-month DSM-IV disorders in the national comorbidity survey replication. *Archives of General Psychiatry, 62*(6), 617–627.

Kessler, R. C., Chiu, W. T., Jin, R., Ruscio, A., Shear, K., & Walters, E. (2006). The epidemiology of panic attacks, panic disorder, and agoraphobia in the national comorbidity survey replication. *Archives of General Psychiatry, 63*(4), 415–424.

Khan, A., Brodhead, A., Schwartz, K., Kolts, R., & Brown, W. (2005). Sex differences in antidepressant response in recent antidepressant clinical trials. *Journal of Clinical Psychopharmacology, 25*(4), 318–324.

Kirkley, D. (2000). Is motherhood good for women? A feminist exploration. *Journal of Obstetrical, Gynecological and Neonatal Nursing, 29*(5), 459–464.

Kirkwood, C., & Melton, S. (2005). Anxiety disorders I: Generalizxed anxiety, panic, and social anxiety disorders. In J. T. DiPiro, C. L.Talbert, G. C. Yee, G. R. Matzke, B. G. Wells, & L. M. Posey (Eds.), *Pharmacotherapy* (pp. 1285–1305). New York: McGraw-Hill.

Klerman, G, et al. (1984). *Interpersonal psychotherapy of depression.* New York: Basic Books.

Knowles, R. (1981). Dealing with feelings: Managing anxiety. *American Journal of Nursing,* January, 110–111.

Kornstein, S. (2003). Gender, depression, and antidepressant treatment. *Primary Psychiatry, 10*(12), 58–61.

Kornstein, S., & Wojcik, B., (2002). Depression. In S. Kornstein & A. Clayton (Eds.), *Women's mental health* (pp. 147–165). New York: Guilford Press.

Krakow, M., et al. (1995). Imagery rehearsal treatment for chronic nightmares. *Behaviour Research and Therapy, 33*, 837–843.

Krupnick, J., Sotsky, S., Elkin, I., Simmens, S., Moyer, J., Watkins, J., & Pilkonis, P. (2006). The role of the therapeutic alliance in psychotherapy and pharmacotherapy outcome: Findings in the National Institute of Mental Health Treatment of Depression Collaborative Research program. *Focus, 4*, 269–270.

Kuo, W., Wilson, T., Holman, S., Fuentes-Afflick, E., Sullivan, M., & Minkoff, H. (2004). Depressive symptoms in the immediate postpartum period among Hispanic women in three U.S. cities. *Journal of Immigrant Health, 6*(4), 145–153.

Lam, F. (2002). SSRIs, warfarin, diazepam result in fatal bleeding. *Psychopharmacology Update, Supplement on Dangerous Drug Interactions, 7.*

Lasswell, M. (2002). Marriage and family. In S. Kornstein & A. Clayton (Eds.), *Women's mental health* (pp. 515–526). New York: Guilford Press.

Leerubier, Y., Clere, G., Didi, R., & Kieser, M. (2002). Efficacy of St. John's wort extract WS 5570 in major depression: A double-blind, placebo-controlled trial. *American Journal of Psychiatry, 159*, 1361–1366.

Lehmann, C. (2004). House committee briefed on postpartum MH issues. *Psychiatric News, 39*(21), 26.

Leon, A., Solomon, D., Mueller, T. I. et al. (2003). A 20-year longitudinal observational study of somatic antidepressant treament effectiveness. *American Journal of Psychiatry, 160*(4), 727–733.

Leverich, G., Altshuler, L., Frye, M., Suppes, T., McElroy, S., Keck, P., et al. (2006). Risk of switch in mood polarity to hypomania or mania in patients with bipolar depression during acute and continuation trials of venlafaxine, sertraline, and bupropion as adjuncts to mood stabilizers. *American Journal of Psychiatry, 163*, 232–239.

Liebowitz, M., Stein, M., Tancer, M., et al. (2002). A randomized, double-blind fixed-dose comparison of paroxetine and placebo in the treatment of generalized social anxiety disorder. *Journal of Clinical Psychiatry, 63*, 66–74.

Lin, P., Campbell, D., Chaney, E., Liu, C., Heagerty, P., Felker, B., & Hedrick, S. (2005). The influence of patient preference on depression treatment in primary care. *Annals of Behavioral Medicine, 30*(2), 164–173.

Logsdon, M., Wisner, K., & Pinto-Foltz, M. (2006). The impact of postpartum depression on mothering. *Journal of Obstetrical, Gynecological and Neonatal Nursing, 35*, 652–658.

Lundberg, U. (2005). Stress hormones in health and illness: The roles of work and gender. *Psychoneuroendocrinology, 30*(10), 1017–1021.

Magyary, D. (2002). Positive mental health: A turn of the century perspective. *Issues in Mental Health Nursing, 23*, 331–349.

Maina, G., Albert U., Ziero, S., & Bogetto, R. (2003). Antipsychotic augmentation for treatment resistant obsessive-compulsive disorder: What if antipsychotic is discontinued? *International Clinical Psychopharmacology, 18*(1), 23–28.

Malek, L., Connolly, T., & Knaus, D. (2001). Cultural aspects of postpartum depressive symptoms: An urban Hispanic population. *Clinical Journal of Women's Health, 1*(5), 273–278.

Mancebo, M., Eisen, J., Pinto, A., Greenberg, B., Dyck, I., & Rasmussen, S. (2006). The Brown longitudinal obsessive compulsive study: Treatments received and patient impressions of improvement. *Journal of Clinical Psychiatry, 67*, 1713–1720.

Mathew, S., & Ho, S. (2006). Etiology and neurobiology of social anxiety disorder. *Journal of Clinical Psychiatry, 67*(Suppl. 12), 9–13.

McArthur, M. (1990). Reality therapy with rape victims. *Archives of Psychiatric Nursing, 4*(6), 360–365.

McGirr, A., Sequin, M., Renaud, J., Benkelfat, C., Alda, M., & Turecki, G. (2006). Gender and risk factors for suicide: Evidence for heterogeneity in predisposing mechanisms in a psychological autopsy study. *Journal of Clinical Psychiatry, 67*(10), 1612–1617.

McGrath, E., Keita, G., Strickland, B., & Russo, N. (1990). *Women and depression: Risk factors and treatment issues* (Final Report of the APA National Task Force on Women and Depression). Washington, DC: American Psychological Association.

Mein, G., Martikainen, P., Hemingway, H., Stansfeld, S., & Marmot, M. (2003). Is retirement good or bad for mental and physical health functioning? Whitehall II longitudinal study of civil servants. *Journal of Epidemiology & Community Health, 57*(1), 46–49.

Meyers, B., Sirey, J., Bruce, M., Hamilton, M., Raue, P., Friedman, S., Rickey, C., Kakuma, T., Carroll, M., Kiosses, D., & Alexopoulos, G. (2002). Predictors of early recovery from major depression among persons admitted in community-based clinics: An observational study. *Archives of General Psychiatry, 59*(8), 729–735.

Miller, K. (2006). Bipolar disorder: Etiology, diagnosis, and management. *Journal of the American Academy of Nurse Practitioners, 18*, 368–373.

Mishell, D. (2005). Premenstrual disorders: Epidemiology and disease burden. *American Journal of Managed Care, 11*, S473–S479.

Mohr, D., Hart, S., Julian, L., Catledge, C., Honos-Webb, L., Vella, L., & Tasch, E. (2005). Telephone-administered psychotherapy for depression. *Archives of General Psychiatry, 62*(9), 1007–1014.

Montejo, A., Llorea, G., Izquierdo, J., & Vico-Villademoros, F. (2001). Incidence of sexual dysfunction associated with antidepressant agents: A prospective multicenter study of 1022 outpatients. *Journal of Clinical Psychiatry, 62*(Suppl. 3), 10–21.

Moreno, F., McGahuey, C., Freeman, M., & Delgado, P. (2006). Sex differences in depressive response during monoamine depletions in remitted depressive subjects. *Journal of Clinical Psychiatry, 67*(10), 1618–1623.

Morin, C. M., & Azrin, N. H. (1988). Behavioral and cognitive treatments of geriatric insomnia. *Journal of Consulting and Clinical Psychology, 56*(5), 748–753.

Morin, C. M., Koetter, U., Bastien, C., Ware, J. C., & Wooten, V. (2005). Valerian-hops combination and diphenhydramine for treating insomnia: A randomized placebo-controlled clinical trial. *Sleep, 28*(11), 1465–1471.

Moritz, M. (2005). Mirtazapine treatment of social phobia in women: A randomized, double-blind placebo-controlled study. *Journal of Clinical Psychopharmacology, 25*(6), 580–583.

National Comorbidity Survey Replication. (2005). Retrieved March 3, 2007, from http://www.hcp.med.harvard.edu/ncs

National Institute of Mental Health. NIMH. (2003a). *Bipolar disorder.* Retrieved from www.nimh.nih.gov

National Institute of Mental Health. (2003b). *The expert consensus guidelines: Treatment of obsessive-compulsive disorder.* http://psychguides.com/ocgl.html

National Institute of Mental Health. (2005a). *Depression: What every woman should know.* http://www.nimh.nih.gov/publicat/depwomenknows.cfm

National Institute of Mental Health. (2005b). *Mental illness exacts heavy toll, beginning in youth.* http://www.nimh.nih.gov/press/mentalhealthstats.cfm

National Institute of Mental Health. (2006). *Mental health statistics.* Retrieved from http://www.nimh.nih.gov/publicat/numbers.cfm

Nemeroff, S. P. et al., (2005). Differential responses to psychotherapy versus pharmacotherapy in patients with chronic forms of major depression and childhood trauma. *Focus, 3*, 131–135.

Noble, R. (2005). Depression: Genetics, pathophysiology, and clinical manifestations. *Metabolism, 54*(5), 49–52.

Nolen-Hoeksema, S. (1995). Gender differences in coping with depression across the lifespan. *Depression, 3*, 81–90.

Nulman, I., et al. (1997). Neurodevelopment of children exposed in utero to antidepressant drugs. *New England Journal of Medicine, 336*(4), 258–262.

Nutt, D. (2005). Overview of diagnosis and drug treatments of anxiety disorders. *CNS Spectrums, 10*(1), 49–56.

O'Brien, L., Heycock, E., Hanna, M., Jones, P., & Cox, J. (2004). Postnatal depression and faltering growth: A community study. *Pediatrics, 113*(5), 1242–1247.

Osborne, L., & McComish, J. (2006). Borderline personality disorder. *Journal of Psychosocial Nursing, 44*(6), 41–44.

Ott, C. H., & Lueger, R. J. (2002). Patterns of change in mental health status during the first two years of spousal bereavement. *Death Studies, 26*(5), 387–411.

Papp, L. (2006). Safety and efficacy of Levetiracetam for patients with panic disorder: Results of an open-label, fixed-flexible dose study. *Journal of Clinical Psychiatry, 67*(10), 1573–1576.

Patel, V., Kirkwood, B., Pednekar, S., Weiss, H., & Mabey, D. (2006). Risk factors for common mental disorders in women. *British Journal of Psychiatry, 189*, 547–555.

Peplau, H. (1952). *Interpersonal relations in nursing.* London: Macmillan.

Peplau, H. (1963). A working definition of anxiety. In S. Burd & M. Marshall (Eds.), *Some clinical approaches to psychiatric nursing* (pp. 333–338). New York: Macmillan.

Petersen, T. (2006). Enhancing the efficacy of antidepressants with psychotherapy. *Journal of Psychopharmacology, 20*(3), 19–28.

Pfrunder, A., Schiesser, M., Gerber, S., Haschke, M., Bitzer, J., & Drewe, J. (2003). Interaction of St John's wort with low-dose oral contraceptive therapy: A randomized controlled trial. *British Journal of Clinical Pharmacology, 56*(6), 683–690.

Pigarelli, D., Kraus, C., & Potter, B. (2005). Pregnancy and lactation: Therapeutic considerations. In J. T. DiPiro, C. L. Talbert, G. C. Yee, G. R. Matzke, B. G. Wells, & L. M. Posey (Eds.), *Pharmacotherapy* (pp. 1425–1442). New York: McGraw-Hill.

Pigott, T. (2002). Anxiety disorders. In S. Kornstein & A. Clayton (Eds.), *Women's mental health* (pp. 195–221). New York: Guilford Press.

Pohl, R., Feltner, D., Fieve, R., & Pande, A. (2005). Efficacy of pregabalin in the treatment of generalized anxiety disorder: Double-blind, placebo-controlled comparison of bid versus tid dosing. *Journal of Clinical Psychopharmacology, 25*(2), 151–158.

Posmontier, B., & Horowitz, J. (2004). Postpartum practices and depression prevalences: Technocentric and ethnokinship cultural perspectives. *Journal of Transcultural Nursing, 15*(1), 34–43.

Potts, Y., Gillies, M. L., & Wood, S. F. (2001). Lack of mental well-being in 15-year-olds: An undisclosed iceberg? *Family Practice, 18*(1), 95–100.

President's Commission on Mental Health. (1978). *Mental health of women: Task panel reports (Vol. 3).* Washington, DC: U.S. Government Printing Office.

Radloff, L. S. (1977). The CES-D scale: A self-report depression scale for research in the general population. *Applied Psychological Measurement, 1*, 385–401.

Robert, S., Hamner, M., Ulmer, H., Lorberbaum, J., & Durkalski, V. (2006). Open-label trial of escitalopram in the treatment of posttraumatic stress disorder. *Journal of Clinical Psychiatry, 67*, 1522–1526.

Rosenfeld, J. (2001). Depression and premenstrual syndrome. In J. Rosenfeld (Ed.), *Handbook of women's health: An evidence-based approach* (pp. 437–485). Cambridge, MA: Cambridge University Press.

Roy-Byrne, P., Craske, M., Stein, M., Sullivan, G., Bystritsky, A., Katon, W., Golinelli, D., & Sherbourne, C. (2005). A randomized effectiveness trial of cognitive-behavioral therapy and medication for primary care panic disorder. *Archives of General Psychiatry, 62*(3), 290–298.

Sanz, E. et al. (2005). SSRI in pregnancy women and neonatal withdrawal syndrome. *Lancet, 365*(9458), 482–487.

Schatzberg, A., & Nemeroff, C. (Eds.). (2004). *The American Psychiatric Publishing textbook of psychopharmacology.* Washington, DC: American Psychiatric Publishing.

Seedat, S., Stein, D., & Carey, P. (2005). Post-traumatic stress disorder in women: Epidemiological and treatment issues. *Posttraumatic Stress Disorder, 19*(5), 411–427.

Shrier, D. (2002). Career and workplace issues. In S. Kornstein & A. Clayton (Eds.), *Women's mental health* (pp. 527–541). New York: Guilford Press.

Slawson, D. (2005). Complementary/alternative medicine for anxiety. *American Family Physician, 71*(3), 557–558.

Sotsky, S. (2006). Patient predictors of response to psychotherapy and pharmacotherapy: Findings in the NIMH Treatment of Depression Collaborative Research Program. *Focus, 4*, 278–279.

Spielberger, C., Gorsuch, R., & Lusdhene, R. (1983). *SSTAI Manual for the State-Trait Anxiety Inventory.* Palo Alto, CA: Consulting Psychologists Press.

Stein, M. (2006). An epidemiologic perspective on social anxiety disorder. *Journal of Clinical Psychiatry, 6* (Suppl. 12), 3–8.

Steiner, M., Hirschberg, A., Bergeron, R., Holland, F., Gee, M., & Erp, E. (2005). Luteal phase dosing with paroxetine controlled release (CR) in the treatment of premenstrual dysphoric disorder. *General Obstetrics and Gynecology, 193*(2), 352–360.

Steiner, M., Pearlstein, T., Cohen, L. S., Endicott, J., Kornstein, S. G., Roberts, C., Roberts, D. L., & Yonkers, K. (2006). Expert guidelines for the treatment of severe PMS, PMDD, and co-morbidities: The role of SSRIs. *Women's Health (Larchmount), 15*(1), 57–69.

Stuart, G. (2005a). Anxiety responses and anxiety disorders. In G. Stuart & M. Laraia (Eds.), *Principles and practice of psychiatric nursing* (pp. 260–284). St. Louis, MO: Mosby.

Stuart, G. (2005b). Mental health promotion and illness prevention. In G. Stuart & M. Laraia (Eds.), *Principles and practice of psychiatric nursing* (pp. 208–220). St. Louis, MO: Mosby.

Stuart, G. (2005c). Self-protective responses and suicidal behavior. In G. Stuart & M. Laraia (Eds.), *Principles and practice of psychiatric nursing* (pp. 381–401). St. Louis, MO: Mosby.

Sullivan, H. (1953). *The interpersonal theory of psychiatry.* New York: Norton.

Taylor, L. (2001). Work attitudes, employment barriers, and mental health symptoms in a sample of rural welfare recipients. *American Journal of Community Psychology, 29*(3), 443–463.

Taylor, S., Klein, L., Lewis, B., Gruenewald, T., Gurung, R., & Updegraff, J. (2000). Female responses to stress: Tend and befriend, not fight or flight. *Psychological Review, 107*(3), 41–42.

Tenney, N. H., Denys, D. A., vanMegen, H. J., Glas, G., & Westenberg, H. (2003). Effect of a pharmacological intervention on quality of life in patients with obsessive-compulsive disorder. *International Clinical Psychopharmacology, 18*(1), 29–33.

Thase, M. (2005). Bipolar depression: Issues in diagnosis and treatment. *Harvard Review of Psychiatry, 13,* 257–271.

Thase, M. (2006). Treatment of anxiety disorders with venlafaxine XR. *Expert review of neurotherapeutics, 6*(3), 269–282.

Ugarriza, D., & Schmidt, L. (2006). Telecare for women with postpartum depression. *Journal of Psychosocial Nursing, 44*(1), 37–44.

U.S. Department of Health and Human Services. (2001). *Mental health: Culture, race, and ethnicity: A supplement to mental health: A report of the Surgeon General.* Rockville, MD: U.S. Department of Health and Human Services, Substance Abuse and Mental Health Services Administration. http://www.surgeongeneral.gov/library/mentalhealth/cre

Verster, J. C., Volkerts, E. R., & Verbaten, M. N. (2002). Effects of alprazolam on driving ability, memory functioning and psychomotor performance: A randomized, placebo-controlled study. *Neuropsychopharmacology, 27*(2), 260–269.

Vieta, E. (2005). The package of care for patients with bipolar depression. *Journal of Clinical Psychiatry, 66*(Suppl. 5), 34–39.

Wagstaff, A., Cheer, S., Matheson, A., Ormrod, D., & Goa, K. (2002). Paroxetine: An update of its use in psychiatric disorders in adults. *Drugs, 62*(4), 655–703.

Ward, R., & Zamorski, M. (2002). Benefits and risks of psychiatric medications during pregnancy. *American Family Physician, 66*(4), 629–642.

Warfield, M. (2005). Family and work predictors of parenting role stress among two-earner families of children with disabilities. *Infant and Child Development, 14*(2), 155–176.

Weilburg, J., Stafford, R., O'Leary, K., Meigs, J., & Findelstein, S. (2004). Costs of antidepressant medications associated with inadequate treatment. *American Journal of Managed Care, 10,* 357–365.

Weissman, R., Pilowsky, D., Wickramaratne, P., et al. for the STAR*D-Child Team. (2006). Remission of maternal depression and child psychopathology: A STAR*D-child report. *Journal of the American Medical Association, 295,* 1389–1398.

Wenhui, W., Sambamoorthi, U., Olfson, M., Walkup, J., & Crystal, S. (2005). Use of psychotherapy for depression in older adults. *American Journal of Psychiatry, 162,* 711–717.

Williams, A., Girard, C., Sabina, J., & Katz, D. L. (2005). S-adenosylmethionine (SAMe) as treatment for depression: A systematic review. *Clinical Investigative Medicine, 28*(3), 132–139.

Wilson, R. (1996). *Don't Panic.* New York: HarperPerennial.

Wittchen, H. U. (2002). Generalized anxiety disorder: Prevalence, burden, and cost to society. *Depression & Anxiety, 16*(4), 162–171.

Wolpe, J. (1958). *Psychotherapy by reciprocal inhibition.* Stanford, CA: Stanford University Press.

World Health Organization. (2004). *The World Health Report 2004: Changing history,* Annex Table 3: Burden of disease in DALYs by cause, sex, and mortality stratum in WHO regions, estimates for 2002. Geneva, Switzerland: Author.

Xuemin, J., Williams, K., Liauw, W., Ammit, A., Roufogalis, B., Duke, C., Day, R., & NcLachian, A. (2004). Effect of St John's wort and ginseng on the pharmacokinetics and pharmacodynamics of warfarin in healthy subjects. *British Journal of Clinical Pharmacology, 57*(5), 592–595.

Young, E., Korszun, A., & Altemus, M. (2002). Sex differences in neuroendocrine and neurotransmitter systems. In S. Kornstein & A. Clayton (Eds.), *Women's mental health* (pp. 3–30). New York: Guilford Press.

Zeskind, P., & Stephens, L. (2004). Maternal selective serotonin reuptake inhibitor use during pregnancy and newborn neurobehavior. *Pediatrics, 113*(2), 368–375.

14

Women's Sexuality

Catherine Ingram Fogel and
Nancy Fugate Woods

Women have the right to intimate and sexual lives and relationships that are voluntary, desired, pleasurable, and noncoercive (World Health Organization, 2007). When women express concerns regarding sexuality and sexual activity, they have the right to expect that nurses and advanced practice nurses will provide accurate sexual information, counseling, or therapy. The goal of this chapter is to provide a knowledge base from which nurses can assess women's concerns about sexual health and provide sexual health care or make appropriate referrals for their care. This chapter includes a focus on sexuality and sexual health, an overview of the physiological and psychological processes inherent in sexual response, and sexual development across the life span. Consideration of challenges to sexual health and sexual dysfunctions precedes a discussion of sexual assessment and a spectrum of sexual health care.

SEXUALITY AND SEXUAL HEALTH

Sexuality is an integrated, unique type of personal expression that includes physiological and psychological processes inherent in sexual development. A multidimensional construct, human sexuality encompasses a view of oneself as a female and presentation of oneself as a woman, sexual desire, sexual response, and sexual orientation (Fogel, 2006). Further, a woman's sexuality is a basic part of her life and an important aspect of her health throughout the life span. Few women find that sex has not been important at some time in their lives. Through her sexuality, a woman expresses her identity and her need for emotional and physical closeness with others. Women express their sexuality differently at different times—alone, with one partner, or with many—and no two women express sexuality in exactly the same way. Expressed positively, sexuality can bring much pleasure, but it also has the potential to cause great pain. One's sexuality need not be limited by age, attractiveness, partner availability or participation, or sexual orientation.

Dimensions of Women's Sexuality

Sexuality is multidimensional and includes sexual desire, sexual identity, and presentation of self. Women's sexuality can be expressed in a variety of behaviors—including fantasy, self-stimulation, noncoital pleasuring, erotic stimuli other than touch, and communication about needs and desires—and includes the ability to define what is wanted and pleasurable in a relationship. Sexual desire or libido is interest in sexual expression, and, for women, intimacy is a strong influence on desire (Basson, 2000). Although some describe sexual desire as an urge for sexual activity, produced by the activation of specific systems in the brain and experienced as a specific sensation that motivates an individual to seek or respond to sexual experience (Kaplan, 1979), research on women emphasizes the importance of intimacy (Basson, 2000). The amount of sexual desire experienced varies from woman to woman and changes across a woman's life span. Sexual desire is learned by experiencing feelings of pleasure, enjoyment, dissatisfaction, or pain during sexual activity. Sexual desire includes interest in sexual activity, which varies in preferred frequency of activity and gender preference for a sexual partner (Fogel, 2006). Sexual desire is, in part, shaped by the culture into which one is socialized (Amaro, Navarro, Conron, & Raj, 2002).

Sexual identity includes one's view of self as female, presentation of self as a girl or woman, and sexual orientation. This identity is formed in early childhood and evolves throughout a woman's life. A woman's view of herself as female includes her gender identity (sense of self as a woman); her sense of having characteristics customarily defined as female, masculine, or both (gender role); and body image (mental picture of one's body and its relationship to the environment). Although gender identity is influenced by biological or anatomical sex, an individual's gender identity is not necessarily consistent with her biological sex (Alexander & LaRosa, 1994).

Presentation of oneself as a woman (gender role behaviors) includes all the behaviors women use to indicate to society that they are women, such as dress, hair style, speech patterns, and others. Gender role behaviors are a reflection of a woman's internalization of societal and cultural stereotypes and expectations of what a woman's behavior should be (Alexander & LaRosa, 1994). Sex role proscriptions and expectations shape sexual expression. Beliefs about women and men, as well as assumptions regarding appropriate behaviors for both, affect sexual behavior communication patterns and expectations of sexual relationships.

Sexual orientation refers to the preference an individual develops for a partner or the preference for the gender of the person to whom one has an emotional and physical attraction and with whom one wishes to share sexual intimacy. Sexual orientation may be determined before birth. Sexual preferences exist on a continuum ranging from complete orientation to the same sex, through bisexuality, to a complete orientation to the other sex. Sexual practices are not always consistent with sexual orientation.

Sexual lifestyles provide the pattern and context for experiencing one's sexuality (Fogel 2006). While many options exist for women today, not all are equally accepted by society. The most frequently acknowledged pattern for women is heterosexual marital monogamy, and marriage with a monogamous partner is assumed to be most desirable by the majority of society. Serial monogamy refers to an established pattern of having one monogamous relationship followed by another. Women who choose nonmonogamous heterosexual marriage may participate in sexual activity with individuals or couples in addition to their husbands. Women may also choose to have sexual relations with one or more partners without marriage. Single women may be unmarried, divorced, or widowed. This lifestyle is often assumed to be transitional in Western society. Bisexuality refers to women who may partner with either a man or a woman. A bisexual woman's sexual and affectional preferences are directed toward individuals of either sex. Women may be married, have partners of both sexes simultaneously or serially, or have lesbian relationships as well as previous sexual relationships with men. Lesbian lifestyles involve partnering with a woman; sexual and affectional preferences are directed toward women. Lesbians may be coupled or single with one or many partners. The most common pattern among lesbians is serial monogamy. Celibacy is a lifestyle in which women make a conscious choice to abstain from sexual activity. Some women view this choice positively as a means of giving oneself time and energy to devote their attention to other activities, but others may experience nonvoluntary celibacy, for example, when a woman desires to be but is not in a relationship.

Sexual Health

Defining sexual health is challenging, and, for many, it is not noted until it is absent. The World Health Organization (1975) definition of sexual health provides a useful focus for nursing practice: the integration of somatic, emotional, intellectual, and social aspects of sexual beings in ways that are positively enriching and that enhance personality, communication, and love. Essential elements of sexual health include the capacity to enjoy and control sexual and reproductive behavior in accordance with a social and personal ethic; freedom from shame, fear, guilt, misconceptions that inhibit sexual response and harm sexual relationships; and freedom from disease, illness, organic disorders, and deficiencies that interfere with sexual functioning. An acceptance of one's gender identity, body image, sexual identity, and sexual orientation are essential elements of sexual health. The abilities to communicate and feel comfortable with one's sexual feelings, needs, and desires are also important elements. In short, sexual health may be considered the physical and emotional state of well-being that enables us to enjoy and act upon our sexual feelings (Comfort, 1975).

Definitions of sexual health and sexual practices require health professionals to confront the values underlying how they interpret variation in behaviors as well as other dimensions of sexual health. Cultural norms shape our definitions of what is acceptable or normal behavior. Awareness of our personal definitions of normal and abnormal sexual practices is essential before providing appropriate sexual health care. It is not always easy to distinguish between aberrant and merely unconventional practices. The following questions can help focus on the health context of a particular sexual behavior or practice (MacLaren, 1995):

- What does the behavior mean to the woman?
- Does the behavior enrich or impoverish the sexual life of the woman and those with whom she shares sexual relations?
- Is the behavior tolerable to society?
- Is the behavior between two consenting adults?
- Does the behavior cause physical or psychological harm to the woman or her partner?
- Does the behavior involve coercion?

WOMEN'S SEXUAL RESPONSE

Sexual response is one element of a woman's sexual health and involves both capacity (what a woman is capable of experiencing) and activity (what she actually experiences). Emotion, cognition, and physiology are interwoven in a woman's sexual response and together can provide enjoyment, satisfaction, and intimacy. One physiologic framework for thinking about women's sexual response is the sexual response cycle, first characterized by Masters and Johnson (1966) and later revised by Kaplan (1979) and by Basson and colleagues (2000).

Although the physical sensations of sexual response are common to all women, the sequence of physical and emotional sensations are uniquely experienced by each woman, and not every woman experiences each response. A woman may experience different affective and physical responses from cycle to cycle. It is not necessary to progress through each of the phases to achieve sexual fulfilment (Roberts, Fromm, & Bartlik, 1998). Indeed, Basson (2000) asserts that women's experience of sexual response may not progress from anticipation to orgasm in the same linear fashion as has been described for men.

Sexual response can be the same whether the stimulus is self-pleasuring, pleasuring from another woman, from a man, or from intercourse. The physiologic aspects of women's sexual response were described in chapter 4. An integrated summary of the psychosocial and physiological aspects of sexual response is summarized below. Consent is an essential factor in the integration of the biological and psychosocial aspects of sexual response (Chalker, 1994).

Desire Phase

Desire for sexual activity (libido) and sexual fantasy or mental imagery characterizes the first phase of sexual response. All of the thoughts, images, wishes, and imaging that are a part of sexual activity characterize this phase, which prepares a woman for sexual stimulation and excitement (American Psychiatric Association, 1994; Kaplan, 1979).

Excitement Phase

The excitement phase consists of physiologic changes of sexual arousal and is characterized by vaginal lubrication, external genitalia swelling, narrowing of the lower third of the vagina, lengthening of the upper two-thirds of the vagina, and breast tumescence. The clitoris becomes engorged and highly sensitive. Some women may experience a sexual "flush." Systemic responses during this phase include accelerated heart rate and respiration and increased blood pressure.

This phase may be interrupted, prolonged, or ended by distracting stimuli (American Psychiatric Association, 1994; Masters & Johnson, 1966; Roberts et al., 1998).

Orgasm

Orgasm is the height of sexual pleasure and is experienced as a feeling of sexual pleasure followed by an involuntary release of sexual tension and rhythmic contractions of perineal muscles, uterus, and the lower third of the vagina. In addition, heart rate, respiration, and blood pressure continue to be elevated. Orgasms commonly last between 3 and 60 seconds and may vary with each sexual experience and from woman to woman. Women are capable of multiple and frequent orgasms during a single sexual encounter (Chalker, 1994; Darling, Davidson, & Jennings, 1991). Women report that orgasms experienced with sexual intercourse were more satisfying and less intense than those experienced with masturbation (Darling et al., 1991; Davidson & Darling, 1989). Women generally emphasize the emotional and physical aspects of a relationship in addition to the orgasmic experience.

Resolution

With resolution, women experience a sense of general relaxation and well-being. The phase is characterized by a bodily return to the preexcitement state. With adequate stimulation, women may again begin sexual response before complete resolution.

New conceptualizations of women's sexual response assert that important aspects of women's experiences have not been adequately reflected in existing models of human sexual response. Components of satisfaction for women—such as intimacy, trust, comfort with vulnerability, communication, respect, affection, and pleasure associated with sensual touching—merit inclusion in the discussion of women's sexual response (Basson, 2000; Leiblum, 1998; Tiefer, 1991). Moreover, Basson asserts that women's sexual response arises from intimacy more commonly than from desire for physical sexual arousal and that women's sexual arousal arises minimally from awareness of genital vasocongestion. She further asserts that women have a lower biological urge than do men to be sexual for release of sexual tension. Women's motivations are not necessarily linked to sexual rewards or biological urges, but may be linked to intimacy. Women's sexual arousal is related to their subjective mental excitement; genital awareness may or may not be an erotic stimulus for women. Finally, women may or may not experience orgasmic release of sexual tension.

Although the human sexual response as described by Masters and Johnson may represent women's experience in new relationships, other models may be more appropriate for women in long-term relationships. Basson proposes that women's movement from a sexually neutral state to seeking sexual stimuli is contingent on sensing an opportunity to be sexual, a partner's need, or potential benefits of sexual activity. Craving for sexual sensations, desire to experience physical and subjective arousal, and possible release of sexual tension may also occur. Sexual desire, in this model, is a response to context. Arousal and desire may occur after the decision to experience sexual stimulation occurs. Needs other than for sexual release may prompt the choice to engage in sexual activity. Emotional closeness may override the experience of orgasm for some women in some circumstances (Cawood & Bancroft, 1996).

SEXUALITY ACROSS THE LIFE SPAN

Adolescence

Adolescence (age 12 to 19 years) is a period of rapid physical and psychosocial changes. Among these changes are an increasing awareness of and change in sexual feelings. Five dimensions of adolescent sexuality include:

■ Physical changes of puberty and their relationship to self-esteem and body image
■ Learning about normal bodily functions and sensual and sexual responses and needs
■ Developing one's sense of self as a woman (gender identity) and comfort with one's sexual orientation
■ Learning about sexual and romantic relationships
■ Developing a personal sexual value system (Masters, Johnson, & Kolodney, 1995; Zwelling, 1997).

For young women, sexuality is often defined through social activities such as dating. As adolescents develop a capacity for sexual intimacy, sexual curiosity and experimentation are common. Although few girls are sexually active before age 15 (8 in 10 are not sexually experienced), an estimated 40% of all adolescents between 15 and 19 years of age have had sexual intercourse (Singh & Darroch, 1999). An estimated 45% of adolescent girls have had two or more sexual partners in the past year (Hall, Holmqvist, & Sherry, 2004). Young women who begin sexual activity early have greater numbers of lifetime sexual partners (Seidman & Reider, 1994). Adolescents may face peer pressure to be sexually active, and an additional motivation for sexual activity for girls may be a desire for sexual intimacy rather than a wish for the physical act of intercourse. Risks associated with early sexual activity include those related to contracting sexually transmitted infections (including human immunodeficiency virus, HIV) and unintended pregnancies.

Adulthood

In early adulthood, ages 20 to 40 years, many women achieve maturity in a gender role and in the relationship tasks started in adolescence, including developing intimacy with another individual and a long-term commitment to an intimate relationship. This is a period of important work and personal decisions and increasing responsibilities that require balancing relationships, work, and children. Women face choices regarding sexual lifestyles and may experience several before settling into one. During these years, women continue to develop their personal sexual value systems and are exposed to and learn to be tolerant of others' sexual values. At some point during the early adult years, women usually face decisions about childbearing. Throughout these years, frequency of sexual activity typically decreases.

Mid-Life

In mid-life (approximately 40 to 60 years of age) women's sexuality is as varied as are women (Sang, Warshow, & Smith, 1991; Taylor & Sumral, 1993). Some report that sex is very good, possibly the best ever, while others report that sex is not the driving force it once was or that it has become less exciting and gratifying. Although decreased libido can occur at any age, many midlife women report a loss of sexual interest during the menopausal transition and early postmenopause (see chapter 6). Physiologic changes associated with menopause can affect sexual desire, expression, and functioning. Fluctuating levels of estrogen and related vasomotor instability can result in sleep disturbances associated with hot flashes and night sweats. Resulting fatigue can adversely affect sexual desire. In the years immediately before and after menopause, women may report a loss of sexual desire associated with a decrease in pleasure with sexual experiences; these changes may be mediated by decreased vaginal lubrication, vaginal dryness, dyspareunia, painful spasms of the vaginal muscles, loss of clitoral sensations, fewer orgasms, and decreased depth of orgasm (Bachmann & Leiblum, 2004; Northrup, 2001). In contrast, other women may report increased sexual desire, increased clitoral sensitivity, increased responsiveness, and/or an increase in their capacity for orgasms (Northrup, 2001). For some women, release from the worry of becoming pregnant increases sexual desire and lessens inhibitions.

Older Adulthood

As women age into their 60s and beyond, they continue to be sexual and enjoy sexual activity. Although sexual frequency may decrease, sexual enjoyment may increase with age and lifelong patterns of sexual behavior may not change dramatically (Alexander & La Rosa, 1994; Steinke, 1988, 1994). Although a woman's desire for excitement, pleasure, and intimacy does not necessarily decrease with age, availability of a partner may become an important issue and preclude women enjoying their sexuality in a relationship. Health of one's sexual partner, as well as one's own general health may challenge sexual health.

Older women are bombarded by the psychosocial stressors that have been associated with decreased sexual desire in younger women (Butcher, 1999; Klock 1999). Increased responsibilities with the burden of roles such as family caregiving and employment may contribute to fatigue and decreased sexual desire. Satisfaction with one's sexuality and sexual function is influenced by personal expectations, and these, in turn, are a product of social and cultural influences that shape our expectations of aging. Although assumptions about older women's interest in and involvement in sexuality are changing, there remain some negative images of older women as sexual beings.

Age-related physiological changes may contribute to sexual symptoms, and these, in turn, may be associated with reduced sexual desire and activity. Reduced tissue elasticity and thinning of the vaginal tissues may cause irritation or discomfort with penetration, contributing to a reduced desire for sexual activity. Vascular changes associated with sexual arousal and the intensity of muscle contractions with orgasms may diminish (Masters & Johnson, 1966). In addition, loss of fatty tissue of the labia and mons may contribute to tenderness, and these tissues may be easily damaged or abraded with sexual stimulation. Orgasms may decrease in intensity, and, in some women, the contractions become painful. Breast size and contour also may change, and, for some women, these changes produce concerns about body image but do not alter her ability to respond sexually.

Body changes may require that women and their partners alter how they engage in sexual activity. With aging, adaptations in sexual practices to promote pleasure may include use of water-soluble lubricant and vaginal moisturizers, providing time for increased sexual stimulation to produce arousal, experimenting with different sexual positions to promote comfort, and planning intercourse for times when energy levels are highest.

While sexual interest and activity may decrease somewhat with aging, most older women do maintain intimate and sexual relationships if a partner is available. Many older women become celibate due to lack of a partner or having a partner with a sexual dysfunction. The need for human touch and closeness continues throughout the remaining life span.

Childbearing

Sexuality is a concern for many women and their partners during pregnancy and postpartum. Levels of sexual desire and frequency of sexual activity can vary with the trimester of pregnancy. During the first trimester, desire and functioning may be inhibited by nausea and vomiting, breast tenderness, fatigue, and anxiety about the pregnancy. In the second trimester, women often express heightened desire as they feel better, although some may be inhibited by increasing weight and bodily changes. Women may experience diminished sexual desire and activity during the third trimester associated with physical discomfort related to increasing size, especially near term.

The physiologic changes associated with pregnancy can contribute to changes in pregnant women's physical sexual response (Masters et al., 1995). Increased vascularity of the genital area from the pregnancy may produce feelings of increased sexual tension. Generalized vasocongestion of the pelvic viscera occurs by the end of the first trimester and persists throughout pregnancy. Vaginal lubrication develops more rapidly and extensively. Orgasm may be triggered more easily during pregnancy due to increased vascular flow to the genital tissues (particularly clitoral erectile tissues) and muscle tension. Indeed, some women may experience their first orgasm during pregnancy. In the third trimester, women may experience continuous (tonic) uterine contractions with orgasm rather than the typical rhythmic contractions (Zwelling, 1997). The resolution phase may be extended due to increased pelvic vasocongestion that may not be completely relieved by orgasm. Worries about the effect of intercourse on the fetus and sexual restrictions associated with high-risk pregnancy (e.g., preterm labor) may alter sexual activity and affect sexual satisfaction during this period. Some women also confront the reduced sexual interest of their partners during pregnancy.

During the postpartum period, women report lessened sexual desire and decreased sexual activity for up to 6 months. Reasons for decreased desire and activity include physical discomfort, lessened physical strength, dissatisfaction with appearance, and fatigue (Ellis & Hewat, 1985; Fischman, Rankin, Socken, & Lenz, 1986). Early postpartum physical symptoms such as lochia, increased vaginal discharge, and episiotomy pain are not conducive to sexual desire or activity. Once the initial postpartum vaginal discharge has subsided, women may notice vaginal dryness associated with decreased estrogen and progesterone levels. Although the vaginal dryness may be experienced by all postpartum women, it is most common in breast-feeding women (Avery, Duckett, & Frantzich, 2000). Women who experience vaginal dryness may require some form of lubrication to prevent dyspareunia. Finally, motherhood allows little privacy and little rest, both of which are necessary for sexual pleasure.

Infertility

Struggles with infertility and repeated attempts to conceive can compromise sexual self-esteem, sexual expression, activity, and desire. Fertility and virility seem to be inextricably linked in U.S. society. A diagnosis of infertility may negatively affect a woman's sense of sexuality, her self-image, and even her relationship. For women who desire pregnancy, pressure to schedule sexual intercourse to optimize conception may interfere with pleasure and communication. Years of attempting to conceive and/or bear a child makes spontaneous sex difficult to maintain. Women may initiate sexual activity around the time of ovulation even if they are experiencing low or decreased desire. Reacting to a feeling of threat or resentful of "sex on demand," men may experience reactive impotence—or an inability to perform sexually—especially around the time of ovulation.

SOCIOCULTURAL INFLUENCES ON SEXUALITY AND SEXUAL HEALTH

Women experience their sexuality in the context of cultural expectations. Family, society, culture, law, and religion all shape attitudes and behaviors regarding sex.

Families provide early socialization and shape sexual attitudes, values, and behaviors that contribute to later sexual health as well as dysfunction. Restrictive family beliefs, such as the belief that expressions of intimacy or sexuality are shameful, may contribute to a woman's inability to express herself sexually. Poor parent-child interactions can contribute indirectly to sexual problems by decreasing self-esteem and reducing one's ability to cope with intimacy (Sheaham, 1989). Messages that sex is something to endure may inhibit sexual expression or enjoyment.

Society defines what sexual behavior is and the norms for that behavior. Current U.S. cultural values present mixed messages to women: women are to be sexually responsive but stay within well-defined boundaries. Today, women are defined as dysfunctional if they are either "too promiscuous" or if they are not sexual enough (e.g., lack desire for an appropriate partner or do not become aroused/reach orgasm with that partner). A specific behavior may be defined as desirable by one cultural group and undesirable by another. Different views often exist regarding premarital, extramarital, and marital sex; appropriate sexual positions; accepted sexual activities; and duration of coitus.

To the extent that sexual activity is a coerced activity, healthy sexual functioning is unlikely to occur. Coercion exists on a continuum from guilt induced by a partner's hurt feelings if refused to the extreme of rape. Male sexual coercion of females in our society is endemic. In almost all societies, incest is prohibited. Incest contributes to sexual dysfunction, particularly when it involves threat or force, occurs at an older age when guilt is more apt to be present, and is associated with strong negative feelings or is repeated over time (Sheaham, 1989).

In part, women form their ideas of what is sexually appropriate and desirable from years of cultural scripting, and these ideas often are the basis of many of the issues women experience in sexual relationships. Sex role stereotypes that prescribe that men initiate sexual activity while women exercise control restrict the range of acceptable behavior for women. Cultural practices that physically alter sexual response such as clitorectomy will affect sexuality.

Religion also influences sexual attitudes, beliefs, and values and can exert a strong influence throughout a person's life. Religious proscriptions can contribute to sexual concerns or problems. For example, a view that sexual intercourse is acceptable only for procreation may raise concerns when pleasurable sensations are felt. Accepting or rejecting premarital sex, contraception to prevent pregnancy, beliefs about monogamy for men and women, and condoning or rejecting homosexuality are examples of religious influences in a woman's life.

Laws to regulate and control unacceptable sexual behavior are common to most societies. Often periods of societal change are necessary to alter cultural beliefs and change laws. One example of such a period was the 1960s and 1970s, when women began to reclaim and redefine their sexuality for themselves. During this period, women-centered definitions of sexuality that included sensuality, closeness, mutuality, and relationships emerged.

SEXUAL HEALTH CARE

Assessment

Clinicians need knowledge about human sexuality and sexual health, sexual problems and their relationship to illness and therapies, and sexual dysfunction as a foundation for providing sexual health care. In addition, comfort with one's sexuality, awareness of one's biases, and a sincere desire to assist clients are foundational to providing appropriate sexual health care. Ability to communicate comfortably and knowledgeably is essential to obtaining a sexual history and discussing therapeutic options with women. MacLaren (1995) recommends that health professionals reflect on a series of questions about their personal values and attitudes about sex and sexuality as a check on imposing their own values on clients.

Sexual health assessment includes a history, physical exam, and lab studies conducted from an integrative physiological, psychological, and sociocultural framework. The sexual history is the most important aspect of the sexual health care process. Some general guidelines will facilitate history taking. Introducing the topic of sexual health is the responsibility of the clinician. Establishing a positive tone before starting the interview will foster comfort in the woman providing the information. Establishing rapport and trust in the short time allotted for most clinical encounters is challenging but significant before eliciting highly personal information. A private, quite location enhances clients' comfort. Assuring women of strict confidentiality and modifying the history taking to respect the woman's comfort is important. Continually monitoring one's own responses for negativity or embarrassment is essential because these feelings are easily conveyed to clients. Using open-ended questions and allowing a woman to tell her story in the way she is most comfortable will enhance her comfort. Closed questions generally follow to facilitate gathering specific information such as medical history, menstrual history, and drug reactions. Women may need an explanation for why certain questions are being asked. Beginning with the least threatening material such as an obstetrical history and moving to sensitive topics such as current sexual practices also respects the need to create a comfortable encounter. A general guide is to begin with questions about the woman's sexual education history (How did you learn about sex?); proceed to personal attitudes and beliefs about sexuality; and, finally, assess actual sexual behaviors. Avoiding excessive medical terminology during an interview and euphemisms such as "slept with" will facilitate clarity in the history. Statistical questions such as "how many times a week do you have sexual intercourse?" are not helpful because normal practices vary widely. Rather than asking about a particular sexual experience, which people tend to deny, it is better to ask how many times the experience has occurred. Techniques such as universalizing or prefacing questions by comments such as, "Many people . . ." or "Other women have told me . . ." can enhance comfort.

A sexual history can be incorporated into a total health history, or it can be more formal and inclusive. A number of formats are available (Fogel, 2006; Heiman, 2002; MacLaren, 1995; Zwelling, 1997). In most cases, sexual problems can be uncovered by asking a few questions such as the following:

- Are you sexually active? Are you sexually involved? Are you having sexual relations?
- Are you having any sexual difficulties or problems at this time? Do you have any pain?
- Has illness, pregnancy, or surgery interfered with your being a partner? Has any illness, surgery, medication, or treatment changed how you feel about yourself as a woman? Has any disease, surgery, medication, or treatment altered your ability to function sexually?
- Is sex pleasurable for you? Are you having difficulty with lubrication during sex? Are you able to have an orgasm/climax? Do you have any pain or discomfort during sexual activity?
- Are you satisfied and happy with your sexual activity?
- Do you have any sexual problems or questions?
- Do you limit physical contact with your partner because you are afraid it will lead to sex?
- Do you become irritated when your partner initiates sex?
- Do you feel that having sex is an imposition?

Other components of the general health history can be significant for a sexual history. A woman's menstrual history, including age at menarche and characteristics of her menstrual cycle (length, duration of flow, presence of premenstrual symptoms, ovulatory discomfort, and dysmenorrhea) should be obtained. Ask about the presence of vaginal discharge, discomfort, itching, her method of sanitary protection, and her level of satisfaction with the chosen method. If a woman is beyond her childbearing years, ask if/when menopause has occurred and whether she experienced any difficulties such as vaginal dryness with sexual functioning. If problems have occurred, ask how she dealt with them.

A woman's obstetrical history, including number of pregnancies, deliveries, and spontaneous and induced abortions, may be important. Any difficulties she had conceiving and any history of infertility should be noted. Ask about her contraceptive history, including methods used, her satisfaction or dissatisfaction with each, her confidence in the method, and her partner's participation when appropriate. Any history of sexually transmitted diseases, including pelvic inflammatory disease must be recorded. Ask women to describe their usual sexual experiences (her individual sexual response cycle). Ask for clarification when necessary—for example, to clarify the degree of lubrication present during sexual arousal if pain occurs during sexual intercourse. Ask the woman to provide a brief description of her present relationship and to rate her relationship with respect to communication, affection, sexual needs met, and sexual communication.

When it is indicated by the woman's health history, her reason for seeking care, her treatment goals, or the need for referral, a physical examination may be performed. The examination may include determination of vital signs and aspects of a general physical examination, particularly an abdominal and pelvic exam. The pelvic exam should include inspection of the external genitalia and internal genitalia using speculum and bimanual techniques.

Lab Studies

While there are no studies specific to sexual assessment, often tests are indicated when is suspected. Cultures for sexually transmitted diseases may be obtained if there is a history of purulent discharge or discharge is noted at the time of the physical examination; if a bladder infection is suspected when a woman complains of dyspareunia, a clean catch urine specimen for culture and sensitivity should be collected.

SEXUAL HEALTH CARE INTERVENTIONS

General dimensions of providing sexual health care for all nurses include:

- Prevention of illnesses that can adversely affect sexuality and sexual functioning and violence and coercive sexuality and reduction of behaviors that place women at risk for sexually transmitted diseases and unintended pregnancy
- Provision of sexual education, including sexual information and resources
- Nonjudgmental, open, and direct communication regarding sexual matters
- Counseling to improve or sustain current sexual relationships or to solve a particular problem

Framework for Intervention

A simple but effective framework for providing sexual health care interventions is the PLISSIT model developed by Annon (1974). This approach, which is used by many nurses for sexual counseling, comprises four levels of intervention: Permission, Limited Information, Specific Suggestions, and Intensive Therapy. As the complexity of intervention levels increases, additional knowledge and skills are needed. All nurses should be able to provide permission and limited information related to many of the sexual concerns of clients. Many nurses and all advanced practice nurses should be able to intervene at the specific suggestion level. Intensive therapy requires special training in sexuality and sex therapy or that the client be referred to experts in the field of sex therapy.

The permission level is simple and involves giving the client permission to function sexually as she usually does with reassurance that such behaviors are normal and encouraging her to talk with her partner and accept herself and her desires. Permission is given if the behavior is realistic, something with which both partners are comfortable, involves no danger or coercion, and causes no harm. Permission involves answering questions about sexual fantasies, feelings, and dreams and may include permission for such things as self-exploration (self-masturbation), initiation of sexual encounters, and the use of fantasy, erotica, and sexual aids such as oils, vibrators, and feathers. Asking about the effect of developmental changes, illness, or lifestyle alterations on sexuality may be ways of giving a woman permission to be a sexual being. Permission giving is particularly helpful for women who are anxious about their sexual adequacy or for clients with sexual dysfunction related to guilt over enjoyment of sexual practices. Examples of interventions at this level are permission to be sexually aroused by normal feelings; to engage in safe activities that arouse sexual feelings such as masturbation and fantasizing; and to have sexual intercourse as often as desired.

Limited information is often the solution when permission is not enough. The purpose of providing limited information on topics of sexual health for a client may be to prepare her to discuss her specific concerns with the nurse. The information given at this level includes specific facts that are directly related to the woman's area of sexual concern. This level of intervention is helpful in changing potentially negative thoughts and attitudes about specific areas of sexuality and in refuting sexual myths. Any information offered should be immediately relevant and limited in scope. To provide this level of sexual health care, nurses need to be familiar with a range of sexual behaviors, norms, and forms of expression. This level is particularly useful when women have a sexuality knowledge deficit or anxiety associated with sexual misinformation.

Specific suggestions are useful when permission and limited information fail to improve the problem. The suggestions do not need to be exotic, complex, or imaginative; usually, they will be suggested by the situation. Specific suggestions entail giving direct behavioral suggestions to relieve a sexual problem that is limited in scope or of brief duration. The nurse and client agree on specific goals, and the nurse offers specific behavioral suggestions that are followed up on after a short time period.

Numerous suggestions can be made to clients but are always tailored to individual needs and the particular situation. For example, the nurse might suggest to a woman who is concerned because her husband's penis bumps her cervix with penetration and this is uncomfortable that she try using a position that gives her more control over penetration such as being on top. Additional examples of specific suggestions are using a water-soluble lubricant to relieve vaginal dryness and prevent dyspareunia in postmenopausal women; sensate focus exercises (mutual erotic stimulation excluding the genitals); medication to treat a vaginal infection; and alternative ways of sexual pleasuring (oral-genital contact, mutual masturbation, cuddling, holding, massage).

Intensive therapy is used when a client's problems are not relieved with interventions from the first three levels or when the problems are personal and emotional difficulties that interfere with sexual expression. This level of intervention is the most complex and should be offered only by professionals with advanced training in sexual counseling and therapy. Referral to a sexual therapist for further assistance is often the appropriate intervention.

SEXUAL HEALTH CHALLENGES

Many health-related factors can affect sexual health. Experiencing illness and/or living with specific pathologies, having surgery, becoming disabled, and using medications (both prescription and nonprescription) can influence sexual health. As seen in Table 14.1,many diseases or health problems have the potential to affect desire and arousal and orgasm. Similarly, a variety of drugs may affect sexual desire, arousal, and orgasm based on their neuroendocrine, neurovascular, or neurological effects. Treatments that affect the vascular system or that produce nerve damage may alter sexual function (Basson et al., 2007).

Chronic illness with associated fatigue, pain, and stress affects sexual desire and arousal more often than it affects orgasm. In the case of cancer, fatigue associated with the disease and its treatment may interfere with sexual desire. Changes in body image also may have a profound effect on sexuality (Rogers & Kristjanson, 2002). Treatment of gynecologic cancer is associated with less frequent intercourse, sexual excitement, and arousal (Andersen, Anderson, & DeProsse, 1989; Schover, Fife, & Gershenson, 1989). Women with endometrial cancer have stressed the negative effect of symptoms such as vaginal bleeding on sexual expression; further, the fatigue and lethargy associated with cancer treatment adversely influence sexual functioning (Lamb & Sheldon, 1994). Results of studies on the effect of a hysterectomy on sexuality vary considerably (Bernhard, 1992; Katz, 2002). Diabetic women report sexual difficulties, including orgasmic dysfunction, inadequate lubrication, performance anxiety that interferes with sexual functioning, and lower levels of sexual desire than nondiabetic women (LeMone, 1993; Watts, 1994; Young, Koch, & Bailey, 1989). Further, alterations in glucose levels and monilial infections interfere with sexual activity.

In societies in which breasts are considered sexual objects, women with breast cancer may express concerns about their sexuality as a result of their treatment, especially with surgery. Women who dislike their breasts, have a negative self-image, have been sexually abused, lack a support system, or are uncomfortable

discussing personal or sexual concerns may experience more distress (Bernhard, 1995).

Women with sexually transmitted diseases may face challenges. They may need to make drastic changes in their sexual behavior, including choice of partner, use of condoms, and specific sexual practices.

Disability may affect sexuality in a number of ways. People with disabilities sometimes are viewed as asexual by health care providers and the public, and they are not encouraged to express sexual feelings or to be sexually active (Cesario, 2002). The attitude that a disability somehow neuters a woman interferes with her right to sexual feelings and sexual expression (Blackwell-Stratton, Breslin, Mayerson, & Bailey, 1988; Nosek et al., 1994; Sawin, 2003). Most women with disabilities are single (Bernhard, 1995). The length of time a woman has been disabled may affect her sexuality such that women whose disability occurred early in life are less likely to engage in various sexual activities than are those whose disability occurred later in their lives (DeHaan & Wallander, 1988). However, research with women with spinal cord injury found that women injured at an earlier age were more likely to have had sexual intercourse and to have resumed intercourse within 12 months of the injury than were older women (White, Rintala, Hart, & Fuhler, 1994). A critical issue for some women with disability is body image. They may view their bodies as a problem and a source of anxiety rather than pleasure. The reactions of others may suggest that a woman's body is unacceptable or unattractive (Nelson, 1995). Specific physical effects of a given disability on sexual activity differ with the disability. For example, women with spinal cord injuries may experience spasticity with orgasm, and women with a complete spinal cord lesion will not experience clitoral or vaginal sensations or a traditional orgasm (Bernhard, 1989; Kettl et al., 1991; Sawin, 2003).

Many medications can alter sexual functioning and cause sexual dysfunctions, including decreased sexual desire, lack of sexual arousal, inadequate lubrication, and delayed or absent orgasm. These effects are summarized in Table 14.1. Depending on the dosage and the individual's mental and physical state, some medications known to inhibit sexual function may also enhance it. Examples of such drugs include the benzodiazepine tranquilizers and chlorpheniramine (Roberts et al., 1998).

Substance use and abuse can have an adverse effect on sexual functioning and sexuality. Sexual dysfunctions can occur with the use of substances such as alcohol, amphetamine, cocaine, opioids sedatives, and tranquilizers. Chemical dependency in women is associated with issues such as incest and childhood sexual abuse experiences, rape, and violent relationships as adults (Teets, 1990). Women who use illicit

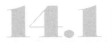

Potential Effects of Illness, Disease, and Drugs on Sexual Desire, Arousal, and Orgasm

ILLNESS OR DISEASE	POSSIBLE EFFECTS ON SEXUAL DESIRE OR AROUSAL	POSSIBLE EFFECTS ON ORGASM
Depression	Low sexual desire in untreated patients; may be linked to sleep disturbance, low self-image, despair, and withdrawal.	
Coronary artery disease, myocardial infarction	Frequency of sexual activity often reduced. May be linked to fear of triggering another cardiac event. Comorbid depression may be a factor.	
Renal failure	Low desire common in those undergoing dialysis; comorbid depression. Desire may not be triggered because of repeatedly painful sexual episodes due to estrogen depletion.	
Lower urinary tract symptoms, including urinary incontinence	Leakage of urine with vaginal penetration reduces sexual motivation.	Orgasm may be delayed or absent.
Diabetes	Low desire reported, and difficulty with vasocongestion and lubrication may be a factor.	
Hyperprolactinemia	Reduced arousal.	Reduced orgasm, dyspareunia.
Postmenopause endocrine changes	Vaginal lubrication may be reduced and vasocongestion reduced; may or may not be perceived in relation to sexual desire.	Orgasm may be painful.
Inflammatory processes		Pelvic inflammatory disease, endometriosis; may perceive pain with orgasm.
Bilateral oophorectomy	Loss of ovarian testosterone and androstenedione precursors to estrogen.	
Adrenal disease	Lack of precursor sex hormones (androstenedione, DHEA).	
Neurological disease	Direct nerve damage in regions involved in processing sexual stimuli.	
Parkinson's disease	Low desire common in women.	
Multiple sclerosis	Low desire in conjunction with other sexual dysfunctions more likely with pontine lesions.	
Head injury	Direct damage to regions involved in processing sexual stimuli.	
Spinal cord injury		Orgasm may be delayed or absent, especially with complete upper motor neuron lesion
Pelvic floor dysfunction		Orgasm delayed or absent.
Pelvic nerve damage		Orgasm may be delayed or absent as a result of radical pelvic surgery.
Drugs		
Antipsychotics	Low desire, possibly linked to reduced dopamine, increased prolaction, alpha blockade, and muscarinic blockade.	Orgasm may be delayed or absent.
Antihypertensives	Selective and nonselective beta blockade.	

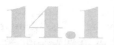

ILLNESS OR DISEASE	POSSIBLE EFFECTS ON SEXUAL DESIRE OR AROUSAL	POSSIBLE EFFECTS ON ORGASM
Antidepressants	Stimulate serotonin receptors, including 5HT3.	Selective serotonin reuptake inhibitors may be associated with delayed or absent orgasm.
Antiandrogens	Suppression of GnRH or LH, antagonism of androgens.	May be associated with delayed or absent orgasm.
Narcotics	Suppression of GnRH.	
Antiepileptics	P450 hepatic enzymes, increase SHBG, decrease testosterone.	

Note. Adapted from Basson, R., & Schultz, W. (2007). Sexual sequelae of general medical disorders. *The Lancet, 369*(9559), Tables 1 and 4; Fogel, C. I. (2006). Sexuality. In K. Schuiling & F. Likis (Eds.), *Women's gynecologic health* (pp. 149–167). Boston: Jones and Bartlett.

drugs have been labeled "crack whores" and described as compulsively exchanging sex for drugs. In reality, contrary to popular folklore that crack is an aphrodisiac, women who use crack cocaine report that the drug has an adverse effect on sexual desire and functioning (Henderson, Boyd, & Whitmarsh, 1995). While crack use reduces sexual desire and physical ability to have sex and have an orgasm, crack use is associated with more frequent sex, trading sex for drugs and money, and having multiple partners.

Sexually transmitted diseases (STDs) including HIV, which are transmitted within the context of a dyadic, interpersonal relationship, have the potential to affect a woman's sexuality and sexual functioning. Women who have been diagnosed with an STD often experience depression, low self-esteem, guilt, lack of trust, and anger.

Adoption of safer sex practices (see the section, Management Strategies for Selected Health Problems Sexually transmitted Diseases, chapter 24) necessitates altered sexual practices. A fundamental characteristic of sexual risk reduction practices is that individuals must give up behavior that is enjoyable, gratifying, highly reinforced, and often long-standing, and replace it with alternatives that are almost always less gratifying, more awkward or inconvenient, and more difficult than current behaviors (Kelly & Kalichman, 1995). Women may decide to be celibate to avoid risk, decrease the number of their partners or avoid certain partners, and change or avoid specific sexual activities that increase risk. The risk of sexual coercion may be greater for women in power-imbalanced relationships with men who resist using condoms. Sex roles and sexual double standards may hinder a woman's ability to ask for safer sex practices and contribute to a man's resistance to implement these practices.

Relationship Issues

Women commonly associate sex with love and commitment, and a woman's subjective perception of sexual pleasure is influenced by her perception of her relationship with her partner. Women have reported that their most pleasurable sexual feelings were in response to intercourse with a partner, though their most profound physical sexual responses occurred in response to masturbation (Darling et al., 1991). Relationship discord may precipitate sexual dysfunction, so much so that many sex therapists believe that sexual dysfunction is a symptom of underlying relationship dysfunction. Open communication of one's sexual preferences, feelings, and desires is essential for sexual satisfaction. One or both partners may experience difficulty after disclosure of sexual activity outside the relationship. Sexual communication difficulties can be exacerbated by distrust, feelings of betrayal, and fear of disease. Sexual dysfunction in one partner may precipitate dysfunction in the other partner; for example, erectile difficulty in men is sometimes accompanied by lack of vaginal lubrication, orgasmic difficulties, and impaired desire disorders in women.

Loss of a Partner

Loss of one's partner can adversely affect opportunities for intimacy as well as sexual expression. Many women define their identity through their relationships; thus, loss of a partner can create a loss of the sense of self. Further, the typical image of a widow is that of a grieving woman whose sexual life has ended. Factors that may be related to a woman's sexuality after the loss of a partner are her extramarital sexual experiences, age, and sexual satisfaction in the marriage (Bernhard, 1995). Remarriage is correlated with age; the older a woman is when she loses a partner, the less likely she is to remarry.

SEXUAL DYSFUNCTIONS

Sexual dysfunction occurs when impaired, incomplete, or absent expressions of typically recurring human sexual desires and responses are associated with distress and discomfort. Sexual dysfunction is defined as the persistent impairment of an individual's usual patterns of sexual interest and response and is inherently subjective (Roberts et al., 1998). Sexual dysfunction may occur:

- in one or more of the phases of the sexual response cycle and is less common in the resolution phase
- during masturbation or during sexual activity with a partner
- throughout a woman's active sexual life (lifelong) or may develop after a period of normal responsiveness (acquired)
- once or repeatedly
- in all situations with all partners (general) or only in certain situations or with certain partners (situational)

Recent research on the prevalence and predictors of sexual dysfunction in the United States indicates that sexual dysfunction is an important public health concern and that emotions contribute to the experience of these problems. In a national probability survey of over 1,700 women aged 18 to 59 years, 43% of women reported a sexual dysfunction. Age and educational attainment were associated with sexual dysfunction, and women of different racial-ethnic groups experienced different problems. Sexual dysfunction was more likely to occur among those with poor physical and emotional health. In addition, sexual dysfunction was associated with negative experiences in sexual relationships and overall well-being (Laumann, Paik, & Rosen, 1999).

Women (and men) reported the following symptoms or problems: lack of desire for sex; arousal difficulties (e.g., lubrication difficulties); inability to achieve climax; anxiety about sexual performance; climaxing too rapidly; physical pain during intercourse; and not finding sex pleasurable. Several questions were asked of women who were sexually active during the prior 12 months. Of 1,486 women reporting data on their interest in sex, about 32% of women reported a lack of interest in sex, regardless of their age, marital status, and educational level. Black women were significantly more likely than White women to report a lack of interest in sex. Of 1,477 women reporting on their ability to achieve orgasm, approximately 26% reported the inability to experience orgasm regardless of their age, marital status, education, or race-ethnicity. Of the

1,479 women reporting on pain during sex, approximately 21% reported pain during sex regardless of their marital status, education, and race-ethnicity. Younger women reported more prevalent pain during sex. Of the 1,479 women reporting on sex as pleasurable, approximately 27% reported sex was not pleasurable regardless of race, marital status, education. Younger women were significantly more likely than older women to report that sex was not pleasurable for them. Of the 1,482 women reporting about anxiety related to sexual performance, approximately 16% reported anxiety regardless of their race-ethnicity; but younger women, women who were not married, and those with less formal education were more likely to be anxious about their performance. Of the 1,475 women reporting on lubrication, approximately 19% reported difficulty with vaginal lubrication regardless of their age, marital status, education. Hispanic women were less likely than White women to report difficulty with lubrication.

Risk factors for sexual dysfunction for women were also explored. Risk factors for low sexual desire included: history of an STD, poor or fair health, emotional problems or stress, decrease in household income, low frequency of sexual activity, infrequent thoughts about sex, and having been forced to have sex by a man. Risk factors for arousal disorder included: history of an STD, urinary tract symptoms, poor to fair health, emotional problems and stress, decreasing household income, liberal attitudes about sex, low sexual frequency, thinking about sex infrequently, having been sexually harassed, having been sexually touched before puberty, and having been forced to have sex by a man. Sexual pain disorders were associated with the following risk factors: urinary tract symptoms, poor to fair health, emotional problems or stress, decrease in household income, and having been sexually harassed. Taken together, these findings indicate the importance of multiple risk factors, including biological changes, socialization, and social circumstances in women's lives, as well as histories of negative experiences of sex. Women with low sexual desire, those with arousal disorders, and sexual pain all experienced lower quality of life, as indicated by low physical satisfaction, low emotional satisfaction, and low general happiness relative to women without these disorders (Laumann et al., 1999).

Recent research on women's sexual dysfunction has been grounded in new frameworks for thinking about women's sexual response. In contrast to men's response—usually described as linear, stage-wise, and genitally focused—women's sexual response is more appropriately described differently. For example, Basson and colleagues (2004a) point out that awareness of sexual desire is not women's most frequent reason for initiating or accepting sexual activity. Sexually healthy women in established relationships may not be aware of spontaneous sexual thoughts. Women may use sexual fantasies as a means to focus on a sexual stimulus, and these may not serve as an indicator of sexual desire. Sexual activities occur in a larger context that is integral to women's sexual functioning. Couples, in contrast to the individual woman, may be the most appropriate focus for assessing sexual dysfunction. Moreover, Basson and colleagues (2004b) point out that the phases of women's sexual response are not discrete and may overlap or occur in a nonlinear order. For example, desire may follow sexual arousal or may occur in its absence. Genital arousal does not correlate well with desire. Women may experience genital arousal and not feel subjective arousal.

Based on a reconceptualization of women's sexual responses, Basson and colleagues (2005) propose the following major categories of sexual dysfunction and associated definitions. Sexual desire and arousal disorders include:

Sexual desire/interest disorder

Combined sexual arousal disorder

Subjective sexual arousal disorder

Genital arousal disorder

Persistent sexual arousal disorder

In addition, orgasmic disorder, vaginismus, and dyspareunia have been redefined based on Basson's model of women's sexual response. Each will be described here.

Sexual Desire/Interest Disorder

This disorder is characterized by absent or diminished feelings of sexual interest or desire, sexual thoughts or fantasies, and responsive desire. There are scarce or absent motivations or incentives for sexual activity. The lack of interest exceeds that typical of life cycle and relationship duration.

Combined Sexual Arousal Disorder

This disorder is characterized by the absence of or reduced subjective sexual arousal—that is, feelings of excitement or pleasure—from any type of stimulation and an absence of or impaired genital arousal (lubrication and vulvar swelling).

Subjective Sexual Arousal Disorder

This disorder is characterized by an absence of or reduced subjective sexual arousal from any type of stimulation. Vaginal lubrication and other signs of arousal (e.g., vulvar swelling) occur.

Genital Arousal Disorder

This disorder is characterized by the absence of or impaired genital sexual arousal (vulval swelling or vaginal lubrication) from any type of stimulation and reduced sexual sensation from caress of the genitalia. Subjective sexual excitement occurs from nongenital sexual stimuli.

Persistent Sexual Arousal Disorder

Characteristics of this disorder are spontaneous, intrusive, and unwanted genital arousal. Women perceive tingling or throbbing when sexual interest or desire is absent. Feelings of arousal persist for hours or days and are relieved by orgasm.

Orgasmic Disorder

Characteristics of this disorder are lack of orgasm from any kind of stimulus or diminished intensity or considerable delay of orgasm in the presence of self-reported high levels of sexual arousal.

Vaginismus

This disorder is characterized by persistent or recurrent difficulty in allowing vaginal entry of a penis, finger, or any other object despite the woman's expressed wish to permit it. Phobic avoidance, anticipation, fear of or experience of pain, and involuntary contraction of the pelvic muscles often occur. Anatomical abnormalities should be ruled out.

Dyspareunia

Characteristics of dyspareunia are persistent or recurrent pain with attempted or completed vaginal entry or penile-vaginal intercourse (Basson, 2005).

These categories significantly change how clinicians think about sexual response. A comparison of the *DSM-IV* diagnostic categories of disorders of sexual dysfunctions with the women-specific categories proposed by Basson and colleagues (2006) is provided in Table 14.2.

The categories of sexual dysfunction for women and definitions proposed by the *DSM-IV* follow.

Hypoactive Sexual Desire Disorder

Women with hypoactive sexual desire disorder have little or no interest in sexual activities, do not become frustrated with lack of sexual activity, and rarely, if ever, initiate sexual stimulation alone or with a partner. Some women may respond to their partner's approaches and experience arousal and orgasm; others may not. Sexual activity occurs infrequently or only in compliance with a partner's wish for sexual activity (Ayers, 1995; Heiman, 2002). Although the cause is unknown, depression, anxiety, and high levels of stress are associated with the disorder. Two common etiologies

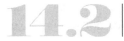

Screening Services: Use of Mammography and Pap Smears by Selected Characteristics, 2003

STAGE OF SEXUAL RESPONSE	BASSON	AMERICAN PSYCHIATRIC ASSOCIATION *(DSM-IV)*
Sexual desire and arousal	Sexual desire/interest disorder Combined sexual arousal disorder Subjective sexual arousal disorder Genital arousal disorder Persistent sexual arousal disorder	Hypoactive sexual desire Sexual aversion disorder Sexual arousal disorder
Orgasm		Inhibited orgasm
Pain disorders	Dyspareunia Vaginismus	Dyspareunia Vaginismus

Note. From Basson 2004; *Diagnostic and Statistical Manual of Mental Disorders* (4th rev. ed.), by the American Psychiatric Association, 1994, Washington, DC: American Psychiatric Press.

are relationship issues that create resentment and hostility and sexual trauma (abuse, assault, incest).

Sexual Aversion Disorder

Sexual aversion disorder is characterized by intense, persistent or recurrent aversion to and avoidance of all or almost all genital contact with a sexual partner. Less common than hypoactive sexual desire disorder, this disorder may be the result of painful intercourse; sexual assault occurring in childhood or earlier in a woman's sexual life; feelings of anxiety, fear, or disgust; or relationship conflicts. Physical factors are usually not involved.

Sexual Arousal Disorder

Sexual arousal disorder is characterized by an inability to attain or maintain an adequate vaginal lubrication and swelling. Additionally, a woman may have little or no sense of sexual excitement, pleasure or arousal. Biological factors may cause insufficient vaginal lubrication, including the hormonal changes associated with pregnancy, postpartum, lactation, and menopause; medications such as antihistamines and anticholinergics; or marijuana use before sexual activity (Ayers, 1995). Chronic vaginal infections such as monilial, bacterial vaginosis, or trichomoniasis also may be associated with inadequate lubrication.

Inhibited Orgasm

Many women report having difficulty achieving orgasm at some time in their lives. The inability to experience an orgasm is defined as a sexual disorder only when a woman reports receiving adequate sexual stimulation without orgasm. Women with this disorder do experience erotic feelings, vaginal lubrication, and genital stimulation. Primary (lifelong, general) orgasmic disorder is rarely caused by a physical condition; rather, factors such as a restrictive home environment, negative cultural scripting, unrealistic performance expectations, inadequate knowledge of female anatomy or sexual response cycles, and current relationship issues are involved. Physical causes of inhibited female orgasm include medications (see Table 14.1); illnesses such as diabetes or hypothyroidism; vaginal damage such as episiotomy scars; any physical cause of dyspareunia; or endometriosis (Morrison, 1995; Seagraves, 1988).

Dyspareunia and Vaginismus

Dyspareunia is recurrent or persistent genital pain associated with attempted or completed sexual intercourse (Schultz et al., 2005). The pain may be deep or superficial. Superficial pain of the introitus may be identified as vula vestibulitis syndrome (VVS) (Schultz et al., 2005). Pain is experienced in the labia, vagina, or pelvis during or after intercourse and may be experienced before, with penetration and/or with thrusting, or after intercourse. Even after the pain is gone, the memory of the pain may continue and interfere with pleasure. The symptoms range from mild discomfort to sharp pain.

Vaginismus involves the involuntary, spasmodic, sometimes painful contractions of the pubococcygeus and other muscles in the lower third of the vagina and introitus (Heiman, 2002; Morrison, 1995). The degree of spasm ranges from partial (penetration is possible but painful) to complete (no penetration is possible). This disorder can occur at any point in sexual response when vaginal entry is attempted. Vaginismus may be associated with other sexual dysfunctions, including lack of desire, arousal, or orgasm. While the incidence of this condition is not known, sex therapists believe it is more common than is documented because women generally do not seek help for it. Women may not seek help until they experience problems in their relationships or wish to become pregnant. Vaginismus may be associated with sexual trauma, phobias about sexual response or intercourse, conservative religious values, or hostile feelings toward one's partner. Although generally medical conditions are not a significant cause of vaginismus, infection or other sources of vaginal mucosa irritation can contribute to the problem. Vaginismus can become repetitive in that a woman may anticipate further pain, and a pain-fear-tension-pain syndrome develops.

Schultz and colleagues (2005) used expert opinion to grade evidence-based medical literature, discussion, public presentation, and debate to develop recommendations concerning knowledge about the assessment and management of women's sexual pain disorders. They found increasing evidence for the role of neuropathic pain mechanisms in these disorders. Their study concluded that: differentiation between vaginismus and dyspareunia using clinical tools is difficult; vaginal spasms have not been identified; physical therapy approaches can differentiate women with vaginismus from controls based on muscle tone and strength differences; evidence is lacking for treatment of women with vaginismus with dilation plus psycho-educational, desensitization therapies; pelvic floor muscle tone/ strength measures for women with vulvar vestibulitis syndrome are intermediate between those of women with vaginismus and controls; and pelvic floor musculature is indirectly innervated by the limbic system and reactive to emotional stimuli and states. On the basis of this review, they suggest pelvic floor therapies for dyspareunia.

Management Strategies for Dyspareunia

Often women do not seek care for care for dyspareunia; thus, the number of women who suffer from this disorder is unknown. Estimates of the prevalence in the general population are about 20%, with a range of 4% to 40%. Some authorities suggest that as many as 60% of women experience dyspareunia at some time in their lives (Glatt, Zinner, & McCormack, 1990). Further, the incidence appears to be increasing; however, it is not clear whether this is a result of the increasing incidence of sexually transmitted diseases, changes in sexual behavior, or women's increased willingness to talk about sexual matters (Sarazin & Seymour, 1991). Most cou-

ples experience one or more mild, transient episodes with only minor interruption in sexual function. Almost 15% of women experience dyspareunia one or more times a year, and about 20% experience lubrication difficulties per year (Smith, 1997). As women age, they also report more dyspareunia associated with changes in the urogenital system after menopause.

Dyspareunia may be classified as primary (pain experienced from first attempt at intercourse) or secondary (pain develops after pain-free intercourse). Causes of dyspareunia are many and diverse (see Table 14.1). Physical causes are the most common and numerous. They include sexually transmitted diseases, bladder disease, diabetes, anatomic defects, and decreased estrogen due to aging. Mechanical causative agents may be excessive douching or the use of irritating soaps or sprays. Dyspareunia also may develop from psychological factors related to family religious taboos or teachings that the vagina should not be touched; traumatic factors such as rape, incest, or previous painful intercourse; or other factors such as a lack of complete arousal and inadequate vaginal lubrication, personal problems, or negative feelings toward one's partner (Heiman, 2002).

A diagnosis of dyspareunia is usually established by self-report; thus, obtaining a careful, accurate history is critical. General points to include in the history are:

- the woman's sexual response and any alterations in phases of sexual response that she has noticed
- attempts to conceive, previous high-risk pregnancy, postpartum difficulties, contraceptive choices, and associated problems
- past and present illness, surgery, medications
- self-concept and body image
- the woman's view of herself as a sexual being and her level of confidence in her ability to function sexually
- past and current psychiatric problems or illnesses, including anxiety and depression, and use of psychotropic medications
- the woman's satisfaction with her current relationship
- any history of sexual abuse
- perceptions of sex-appropriate roles for men and women in relationships
- the woman's perception regarding her ability to fulfill these roles competently
- sexual education, when received, and her reactions to this information (correct and accurate)
- religious affiliation and beliefs and ethnic and cultural belief systems

In addition, a dyspareunia-specific history would include information about the woman's pain (in terms of its quality, quantity, location, duration, and aggravating and relieving factors). A complete medical, surgical, obstetrical, gynecological, and contraceptive history is collected and should include questions about previous vaginal or pelvic surgeries and pelvic trauma such as rape and sexual abuse. Finally, women are asked about medications, douching, and the use of perineal products such as sprays, deodorants, and sanitary pads.

Physical examination is necessary to determine the cause of dyspareunia and may include vital signs, a general physical examination, and an abdominal examination. A pelvic exam always is performed with special attention paid to the external genitalia, observing for irritation, lesions, and discharge. During the bimanual examination, any tenderness in the introitus, vagina, or pelvis and the presence of an unstretched or rigid hymen should be noted (Ayers, 1995). During the speculum examination, cultures, when indicated, are obtained.

The history and physical examination will suggest which diagnostic tests are indicated. There are no tests specific to sexual assessment. Laboratory studies may be indicated when there is evidence of infection.

Treatment for dyspareunia should address the specific cause of dyspareunia; for example, suggesting a water-soluble vaginal lubricant for postmenopausal women, treating the sexually transmitted disease, or providing information about techniques for sexual arousal. Although most of the physical conditions that result in dyspareunia can be managed on an outpatient basis, at times, more extensive treatment is warranted. For example, a woman who has pain with deep pelvic thrusting and other symptoms associated with extensive endometriosis may require a hysterectomy for relief. Emotional care of women and their partners centers on support and specific treatment. Whenever possible, a woman should be reassured about the normalcy of her anatomy, the frequency of this problem in other women, the likelihood of successful therapy, and the probable reason for her problem. Permission may be given to not have intercourse if it is painful and also to try a variety of positions and techniques for stimulation. Limited information and specific suggestions may be given to reduce or eliminate the pain and to address the emotional component of this problem. Referral to mental health professionals may be indicated. Additionally, nurses, particularly advanced practice nurses, may act as consultants to mental health professionals who refer a client with dyspareunia for a physical and gynecological examination (Ayers, 1995).

REFERENCES

Alexander, L. L., & LaRosa, J. H. (1994). *New dimensions in women's health.* Boston: Jones and Bartlett.

Amaro, H., Navarro, A. M., Conron, K. J., & Raj, A. (2002). Cultural influences on women's sexual health. In G. M. Wingood & R. J. DiClemente (Eds.), *Handbook of women's sexual and reproductive health* (pp. 71–92). New York: Kluwer Academic/Plenum.

American Psychiatric Association. (1994). *Diagnostic and statistical manual of mental disorders* (4th rev. ed.). Washington, DC: American Psychiatric Press.

Andersen, B. L., Anderson, B., & DeProsse, C. (1989). Controlled prospective longitudinal study of women with cancer: I. Sexual functioning outcomes. *Journal of Consulting and Clinical Psychology, 57,* 683–691.

Avery, M. D., Duckett, L., & Frantzich, C. R (2000). The experience of sexuality during breastfeeding among primiparous women. *Journal of Midwifery & Women's Health, 45*(3), 227–237.

Ayers, A. (1995). Sexual dysfunction. *Women's primary health care: Protocols for practice.* Washington, DC: American Nurses Publishing.

Bachmann, G. A., & Leiblum, S. R. (2004). The impact of hormones on menopausal sexuality: A literature review. *Menopause: The Journal of the North American Menopause Society, 11*(1), 120–130.

Basson, R. (2000). The female sexual response: A different model. *Journal of Sex & Marital Therapy, 26,* 51–65.

Basson, R., Lieblum, S., Brotto, L., Derogatis, L., Foureray, J., Fugi-Meyer K., et al. (2004a). Revised definitions of women's sexual dysfunction. *Journal of Sexual Medicine, 1*(1), 40–48.

Basson, R., et al. (2004b). Summary of the recommendations on sexual dysfunctions in women. *Journal of Sexual Medicine, 1*(1), 24–34.

Basson, R. (2005). Women's sexual dysfunction: Revised and expanded definitions. *CMA Journal, 172*(10), 1327–1333.

Basson, R. (2006). Sexual desire and arousal disorders in women. *New England Journal of Medicine, 354*(14), 1497–1506.

Basson, R. (2007). Sexuality in chronic illness: No longer ignored. *Lancet, 369,* 350–352.

Basson, R., & Schultz, W. (2007). Sexual sequelae of general medical disorders. *The Lancet, 369*(9559), 409–424.

Bernhard, E. J. (1989). The sexuality of spinal cord injured women: Physiology and pathophysiology. A review. *Paraplegia, 27*(2), 99–112.

Bernhard, L. A. (1992). Consequences of hysterectomy in the lives of women. *Health Care for Women International, 13,* 281–291.

Bernhard, L. (1995). Sexuality in women's lives. In C. I. Fogel & N. F. Woods (Eds.), *Women's health care* (pp. 475–495). Thousand Oaks, CA: Sage.

Blackwell-Stratton, M., Breslin, M. L., Mayerson, A. B., & Bailey, S. (1988). Smashing icons: Disabled women and the disability women's movements. In M. Eine & A. Asch (Eds.), *Women with disabilities: Essays in psychology, culture and politics* (pp. 306–332). Philadelphia: Temple University Press.

Butcher, J. (1999). ABC of sexual health: Female sexual problems: Loss of desire—what about the fun? *British Journal of Medicine, 318,* 41–43.

Cawood, H. H., & Bancroft, J. (1996). Steroid hormones, the menopause, sexuality and well-being of women. *Psychological Medicine, 26,* 925–936.

Cesario, S. K. (2002). Spinal cord injuries: Nurses can help affected women & their families achieve pregnancy, birth. *Association of Women's Health Obstetric and Neonatal Nursing Lifelines, 6,* 224–232.

Chalker, R. (1994). Updating the model of female sexuality. *SIECUS Report, 22*(5), 1–6.

Comfort, A. (1975). The normal in sexual behavior: An ethnological view. *Journal of Sex Education and Therapy, 1,* 1–7.

Darling, C. A., Davidson, J. K., & Jennings, D. A. (1991). The female sexual response revisited: Understanding the multiorgasmic experiences in women. *Archives of Sexual Behavior, 20,* 535.

Davidson, J. K., & Darling, C. A. (1989). Self-perceived differences in the female orgasmic response. *Family Practice Journal, 8*(2), 75–84.

DeHaan, C. B., & Wallander, J. L. (1988). Self-concept, sexual knowledge and attitudes and parental support in the sexual adjustment of women with early- and late-onset physical disability. *Archives of Sexual Behavior, 13,* 233–245.

Ellis, D. J., & Hewat, R. J. (1985). Mother's postpartum perceptions of spousal relationships. *Journal of Obstetric Gynecologic and Neonatal Nursing, 14*(2), 140–146.

Fischman, S. H., Rankin, E. A., Socken, K. L., & Lenz, E. R. (1986). Changes in sexual relationships in postpartum couples. *Journal of Obstetric Gynecologic and Neonatal Nursing, 15*(1), 58–63.

Fogel, C. I. (2006). Sexuality. In K. Schuiling & F. Likis (Eds.), *Women's gynecologic health* (pp. 149–167). Boston: Jones and Bartlett.

Glatt, A. E., Zinner, S. H., & McCormack, W. M. (1990). The prevalence of dyspareunia. *Obstetrics and Gynecology, 75,* 433–436.

Hall, P. A., Holmqvist, M., & Sherry, S. B. (2004). Risky adolescent sexual behavior: A psychological perspective for primary care clinicians. *Topics in Advanced Practice Nursing eJournal, 4*(1), 1–10.

Heiman, J. R. (2002). Sexual dysfunction: Overview of prevalence, etiological factors, and treatments. *Journal of Sex Research, 39*(1), 73–78.

Henderson, D. J., Boyd, C. J., & Whitmarsh, J. (1995). Women and illicit drugs: Sexuality and crack cocaine. *Health Care for Women International, 16,* 113–124.

Kaplan, H. (1979). *Disorders of sexual desire and other new concepts and techniques in sex therapy.* New York: Brunner/Mazel.

Katz, A. (2002). Sexuality after hysterectomy. *Journal of Obstetric Gynecological and Neonatal Nursing, 31*(3), 256–262.

Kelly, J. A., & Kalichman, S. C. (1995). Increased attention to human sexuality can improve HIV-AIDS prevention efforts: Key research issues and directions. *Journal of Consulting and Clinical Psychology, 63*(6), 907–918.

Kettl, P., Zarefoss, S., Jacoby, K., German, C., Hulse, C., Rowley, F., Corey, R., Stedy, M., Bixler, E., & Tyson, K. (1991). Female sexuality after spinal cord injury. *Sexuality and Disability, 9,* 287–295.

Klock, S. (1999). Psychological aspects of women's reproductive health. In K. J. Ryan (Ed.), *Kistner's gynecology and women's health* (7th ed., pp. 534–536). St. Louis, MO: Mosby.

Lamb, M. A., & Sheldon, T. A. (1994). The sexual adaptation of women treated for endometrial cancer. *Cancer Practice, 2*(2), 103–113.

Laumann, E., Paik, M., & Rosen, R. (1999). Sexual dysfunction in the United States: Prevalence and predictors. *Journal of the American Medical Association, 281,* 537–544.

Leiblum, S. R. (1998). Definition and classification of female sexual disorders. *International Journal of Impotence Research, 10,* S102–S106.

LeMone, P. (1993). Human sexuality in adults with insulin-dependent diabetes mellitus. *IMAGE, 25*(2), 101–105.

MacLaren, A. (1995). Comprehensive sexual assessment. *Journal of Nurse-Midwifery, 40*(2), 104–119.

Masters, W., & Johnson, V. (1966). *The human sexual response cycle.* Boston: Little, Brown.

Masters, W. H., Johnson, V. E., & Kolodney, R. C. (1995). *Human sexuality* (5th ed.). New York: Harper-Collins.

Moore, K. A. et al. (1998). *A statistical portrait of adolescent sex, contraception, and childbearing.* Washington, DC: National Campaign to Prevent Teen Pregnancy.

Morrison, J. (1995). *DSM-IV made easy.* New York: Guilford Press.

Nelson, M. R. (1995). Sexuality in childhood disability. *Physical Medicine and Rehabilitation: State of the Art Reviews, 9*(2), 451–462.

Northrup, C. (2001). *The wisdom of menopause.* New York: Bantam Books.

Nosek, M. A., Howland, C. A., Young, M. E., Georgiou, D., Rintala, D. H., Foley, C. C., Bennett, J. L., & Smith, Q. (1994). Wellness models and sexuality among women with physical disabilities. *Journal of Applied Rehabilitation Counseling, 25*(1), 50–58.

Roberts, L. W., Fromm, L. M., & Bartlik, B. D. (1998). Sexuality of women through the life phases. In L. A. Wallis (Ed.), *Textbook of women's health.* Philadelphia: Lippincott-Raven.

Rogers, M., & Kristjanson, L. J. (2002). The impact on sexual functioning of chemotherapy-induced menopause in women with breast cancer. *Cancer Nursing, 25*(1), 57–65.

Sang, B., Warshow, J., & Smith, A. J. (1991). *Lesbians at midlife: The creative transition.* Minneapolis, MN: Spinster's Ink.

Sarazin, S. K., & Seymour, S. F. (1991). Causes and treatment options for women with dyspareunia. *Nurse Practitioner, 16*(10), 30, 35–36, 38, 41.

Sawin, K. J. (2003). Health care concerns for women with physical disability and chronic illness. In E. Q. Youngkin & M. S. Davis (Eds.), *Women's health: A primary care clinical guide* (3rd ed., pp. 861–898). Stamford, CT: Appleton & Lange.

Schover, L. R., Fife, M., & Gershenson, D. M. (1989). Sexual dysfunction and treatment for early stage cervical cancer. *Cancer, 63,* 204–212.

Schultz, W. et al. (2005). Women's sexual pain and its management. *Journal of Sexual Medicine, 2,* 301–316.

Seagraves, R. T. (1988). Psychiatric drugs and inhibited female orgasm. *Journal of Sex and Marital Therapy, 15,* 202–207.

Seidman, S. N., & Reider, R. O. (1994). A review of sexual behavior in the United States. *American Journal of Psychiatry, 151*(3), 330–341.

Sheaham, S. L. (1989). Identifying female sexual dysfunction. *Nurse Practitioner, 14,* 25–26, 28, 30, 32, 34.

Singh, S., & Darroch, J. E. (1999). Trends in sexual activity among adolescent American women: 1982–1995. *Family Planning Perspective, 31*(5), 212–219.

Smith, R. P. (1997). *Gynecology in primary care.* Baltimore: Williams & Wilkins.

Steinke, E. E. (1988). Older adults' knowledge and attitudes about sexuality and aging. *IMAGE, 20*(2), 93–95.

Steinke, E. E. (1994). Knowledge and attitudes of older adults about sexuality in aging: A comparison of two studies. *Journal of Advanced Nursing, 19,* 477–485.

Taylor, D., & Sumral, A. C. (1993). *The time of our lives: Women write on sex after 40.* Freedom, CA: Crossing Press.

Teets, J. M. (1990). What women talk about: Sexuality issues of chemically dependent women. *Journal of Psychosocial Nursing, 28*(12), 4–7.

Tiefer, L. (1991). Historical, scientific, clinical, and feminist criticisms of "the human sexual response cycle." *Annual Review of Sex Research, 2,* 1–23.

Watts, R. J. (1994). Sexual functioning of diabetic and non-diabetic African American women: A pilot study. *Journal of the National Black Nurses Association, 7*(1), 60–69.

White, M. J., Rintala, D. H., Hart, K., & Fuhler, M. J. (1994). A comparison of the sexual concerns of men and women with spinal cord injuries. *Rehabilitation Nursing Research, 3,* Summer, 55–61.

World Health Organization. (1975). Education and treatment in human sexuality: The training of health professionals. Report of WHO meeting. *Technical Report Series, 572.*

World Health Organization. (2007). Gender and reproductive rights. Retrieved January 2007 from http://www.who.int/reproductive-health/gender/glossary.html

Young, E. W., Koch, P. B., & Bailey, D. (1989). Research comparing the dyadic adjustment and sexual functioning concerns of diabetic and non-diabetic women. *Health Care for Women International, 10,* 377–394.

Zwelling, E. (1997). Sexuality during pregnancy. In F. H. Nichols & E. Zwelling (Eds.), *Maternal-newborn nursing theory and practice* (pp. 200–232). Philadelphia: Saunders.

15

Fertility Control

Joellen W. Hawkins, Holly B. Fontenot, and Allyssa Harris

No scientific breakthrough has provided the means to alter women's lives so momentously as the discovery and use of safe, effective contraceptive methods. Margaret Sanger's dream of a safe, available, affordable, and dependable contraceptive method is both realized for some women and still elusive for others, as women around the globe face the opportunities and limitations that fertility imposes.

Fertility regulation information and methods create an available conscious choice, so sexually active women can affect their physical, educational, economic, and social destinies. Regulation of fertility is one of the most value-laden issues with which those interested in and responsible for the health of the human citizens of this planet struggle.

In this chapter, we address the historical, political, social, cultural, and ethical contexts in which women and their partners make decisions about regulating their fertility. We describe the methods presently available to women, although we acknowledge that all methods are not available to all women worldwide. We also describe methods currently in development, in clinical trials, available in countries other than the United States, and/or awaiting approval from the U.S. Food and Drug Administration. Finally, we address the evidence available to guide practice in family planning services.

HISTORICAL AND SOCIAL CONTEXT

No scientific breakthrough has altered as many women's lives so momentously as the development of safe, effective methods for fertility control. Before these methods were available, women suffered chronic illness, fatigue, and even death from unpreventable pregnancy (Cooke & Dworkin, 1979). Multiple pregnancies and unspaced births not only negatively affected women's physical health, but also reduced their economic productivity, leading to increased dependence on others and unfulfilled human potential.

Today, a sexually active, heterosexual, bisexual, or lesbian woman can affect her physical, educational, socioeconomic destiny—and that of her family and significant others and partners—by choosing to use or not to use contraception. By using a highly effective contraceptive method, she reduces the risk of unplanned pregnancy, which enables her to plan her family along with other aspects of her life. When a woman is able to control her fertility, she gains the opportunity to plan and limit family size or to remain childless.

The ability to prevent or defer childbearing allows a woman to pursue educational opportunities and participate in the labor force. A woman's knowledge that she can, if she wishes, control her childbearing, and society's understanding that women can do so, may broaden her outlook when she considers other life opportunities. Because a planned birth can be integrated into a woman's career or job more readily than an unplanned birth, a planned birth has fewer negative effects on her employment or education. Some women use contraceptive methods successfully to take advantage of educational and employment opportunities. Others are not as successful. Instead, they learn by experience that few events change a woman's life as much as the fear of conception or the reality of an unintended pregnancy.

Although information about contraception was available long before Europeans reached North America and other continents, women could not always take advantage of it because of social or political constraints. Such knowledge gave women power and was a threat, changing the roles of women in societies where they had little or no status. However, in societies that were matriarchal or those in which women and men shared power equally, women were able to achieve their full potential, including, but not ruled by, childbearing and childrearing.

Native Americans and Fertility Regulation

There is evidence in the anthropology literature that Native American women in North America did attempt to control their fertility. Oral tradition and history preserved the culture of the Native Americans, Alaskan Natives, and Aleuts. Thus, the information on fertility control practices of these women relies on informants several generations removed from women who first attempted to regulate their childbearing. Native American women used selected herbs and roots, abstained from sex for 9 days following the onset of menses, and prolonged lactation to prevent conception. They occasionally induced abortion (Himes, 1936). In more recent oral histories, Native American women have revealed their knowledge of pregnancy prevention and inducing abortion, usually with plants. For example, Salish women drank a contraceptive made of dogbane roots and water.

Some Native Americans held magical beliefs about conception related to the disposal of the placenta. The Paiute believed that barrenness would result from burying the placenta upside down or allowing it to be eaten by animals. The Lummi believed that further conceptions would be prevented by hurling the placenta into a river or ocean eddy to be twisted by the water (Niethammer, 1977). Once permanent European settlements were established, contamination of information, interjection of so-called Western medicine, and exchanges between women healers from Europe and Native America were inevitable.

The Puritan Ethic

European settlers in the American colonies brought with them the sexual mores and practices of their homelands. For example, the Puritans in Plymouth Colony used coitus interruptus, withdrawal of the penis immediately before ejaculation, to prevent pregnancy. Condoms had been available in Europe for nearly a century before the establishment of Plymouth Colony, but their use for contraception did not occur until the 18th century. Some European settlers brought a Christian morality view of sex as sinful. A perceptive Hopi interpreter of Native American ceremonials for anthropologists confessed that he edited old Hopi stories because "I knew the whites can see more sin than pleasure in sex" (Himes, 1936, p. 213).

Children as an Economic Asset

An economy based on agriculture and a high infant mortality rate curbed interest in birth control for many European settlers. They saw advantages in having large families to help clear the land, plant and tend crops, and process the products into goods for family consumption or to use as currency to purchase imports from Europe. To assure that at least some children would survive to adulthood, women tended to have many children. The price on their health was high. Many women died during childbirth or later from the effects of many pregnancies. When they died, their husbands usually remarried and had more children (Ulrich, 1990).

In some states, slave owners pressured African American women to produce children to work on the plantations or to be sold for profit. The horror of seeing one's child sold motivated many of the women to try to avoid pregnancy. Because magical, medicinal, and mechanical contraceptive methods were practiced in Africa, women slaves may have been aware of these as part of their cultural heritage and used them to prevent pregnancy (Himes, 1936).

Since the time of slavery, African American women have used common folk methods such as vaginal poultices of petroleum jelly and quinine, alum water douches, and plant compounds to control their fertility (Harrison, 1997; Roberts, 2000). The importance of family planning for spacing children and economic and educational improvement was recognized by African American women and community leaders. Despite the undertones of eugenics in Margaret Sanger's birth control movement, African American women found value in supporting it. Civil rights leader W.E.B. DuBois favored family planning programs as a means of improving Black health and "denouncing the argument that blacks should rely on a high birthrate to fight discrimination" (Roberts, 2000, p. 93). The Division of Negro Service, under the Birth Control Federation of America, opened two pilot birth control clinics in Tennessee and South Carolina in 1939 (Roberts, 2000). Many women used these services, but the clinics were not without criticism. Many community leaders of that period felt that Blacks needed to increase their numbers to prevent extinction (Weisbord, 1973), and others feared racial genocide (Thorburn Bird & Bogart, 2005).

Fears of racial genocide, in relationship to family planning, have been noted in the literature. In the popular magazine *Essence*, Grisby Bates (1970) noted, "Since slavery, there have always been those who thought that white America has targeted us for extinction, just as soon as we have outlived our collective usefulness" (p. 79). A long history of individuals believe that family planning programs were targeted to reduce the number of Black Americans. Roberts (2000) quoted the Black nationalist leader Marcus Garvey as being opposed to birth control as a form of "race suicide" (p. 93). In their landmark study, *Family Planning, Race Consciousness and the Fear of Race Genocide*, Darity and Turner (1972) and Turner and Darity (1973) sought to determine to what extent their participants held fears of race genocide and whether the use or nonuse of family planning methods could be attributed to these fears.

Forced sterilization and the eugenics movement gave African Americans reason to mistrust the medical community. Begun in the late 1800s, the eugenics movement was an attempt of its members to improve society. In the United States, proponents embraced the theory that intelligence and other traits were genetically determined and therefore inherited. This idea of rational control of reproduction by individuals considered inferior led to the implementation of policies designed to control the population of races believed to be inferior, including African Americans. Members of White society, using their belief that African Americans were incapable of controlling their sexual urges, castrated men as punishment for certain crimes, including rape, attempted rape, or kidnapping of White women (Roberts, 1997). Castrations were later performed on individuals considered to be "feeble-minded": the poor and ethnic minorities. In 1907, the Indiana State Legislature became the first state body to legalize sterilization of "unwilling and unwitting" people (Rodrigues-Triaz, 1982, p. 147). Thirty states later passed eugenics laws, resulting in forced sterilization of many African American women. According to Rodrigues-Triaz (1982) more than 63,000 people were sterilized between 1907 and 1964 in the United States and its colonies as a result of the eugenics laws. In her book *Killing the Black Body*, Roberts (1997) reported: "It was a common belief among Blacks in the South that Black women were routinely sterilized without their informed consent and for no valid reason" (p. 90). Although most of these laws have been repealed, there are still advocates of sterilization and forced family planning for individuals requiring public assistance. In addition to castration, another method of sterilization is hysterectomy, the surgical removal of the uterus. Hysterectomies were performed on many African American women for reasons other than medical necessity. Rodrigues-Triaz (1982) and Roberts (2000) reported, in the Southern states, this procedure was so commonly practiced that hysterectomies were known as "Mississippi appendectomies."

Victorian America

By the late 19th century, White women had become idealized. Middle-class women, in particular, became "sweet, untouchable guardians of morality, whose distaste for sex led to an explosive increase in prostitution" (Tannahill, 1980, p. 347). Freed from constant work by the industrial revolution, middle- and upper-class women hired servants to do domestic chores and turned their efforts toward moral causes. These women had access to the dozens of treatises on birth control published from 1900 onward. Not so fortunate were their poor sisters who continued to work long hours on farms, in factories, or as domestic servants in homes of the rich.

Illiterate, lower-class women typically obtained contraceptive information by word of mouth. Although most middle-class women could read and use contraceptive information, efforts to disseminate such information were hampered by religious beliefs that abstinence was the only acceptable contraceptive method. Several states had passed legislation that outlawed the dissemination of birth control information and devices (Gieg, 1972). For example, in 1879, Massachusetts law prohibited the sale, loan, or exhibition of any article used to induce abortion or prevent conception, as well as the publication of any information leading to pregnancy termination or prevention (Gieg, 1972). Similar legislation was passed in other states, and it would take until 1967 for the last of these laws to be undone. In 1965, Connecticut struck from its books the anti–birth control law in the landmark case *Griswold v. Connecticut*. Margaret Sanger died one year later—too early to witness the demise of the last of the laws prohibiting distribution of birth control devices and information in Massachusetts.

Margaret Sanger and the Birth Control Movement

In the latter years of the Victorian age, an individual was born who would create for U.S. women a new episode in the contraception drama. Margaret Louise Higgins Sanger, born in Corning, New York, in 1879, dedicated herself to this work after seeing her mother die from tuberculosis and the burden of bearing 11 children, and after observing women in New York's Lower East Side die from childbirth or illegal abortions. She completed nursing school at White Plains Hospital, New York, in 1902.

Inspired by Emma Goldman, the first nurse to lecture on birth control in the United States, in 1912, Sanger began to publish information about women's reproductive concerns. Her first efforts were a series of articles describing puberty and the functions of a woman's body for the *Call*, a socialist newspaper (Gordon, 1990). These articles were the basis for *What Every Girl Should Know*, a pamphlet published in 1915 and later published as a book (Sanger, 1920a). The first issue of *The Woman Rebel* was published in March 1914. In the same year, Sanger prepared the pamphlet *Family Limitation* and organized a committee called the National Birth Control League. She fled to England in October 1914 to avoid prosecution for violating the Comstock Law, federal legislation prohibiting the mailing of obscene material, which included birth control information and devices (Tannahill, 1980). In England, Sanger met C. V. Drysdale, head of the international birth control movement, and Havelock Ellis, author of *Studies in the Psychology of Sex*. An unfortunate consequence of these meetings was Sanger's introduction to the eugenics movement. That association was to affect views of Sanger's work throughout her life. From England, Sanger went to Holland, where she learned how to fit pessaries, now known as contraceptive diaphragms, and studied that country's birth control clinic system.

On October 16, 1916, Sanger and her sister Ethel opened the Brownsville Clinic in Brooklyn, New York, America's first birth control clinic. The clinic provided birth control information and education, although both were illegal at the time. From 1916 to 1934, Sanger established birth control clinics, published birth control articles and pamphlets in defiance of the Comstock Law, worked to change birth control laws, organized the American Birth Control League (1921), attended national and international conferences on birth control, lectured around the world, and was jailed more than once for her activities. In 1922, she engaged Dorothy Bocker to run the Clinical Research Bureau. The next year, she hired James F. Cooper to lecture to physicians across the United States about birth control. She smuggled pessaries into the United States through her husband's factory in Canada until 1925, when she convinced two of her supporters to found the Holland-Rantos Company and begin U.S. production. In 1926, she traveled to London, Paris, and Geneva to prepare for the international meeting in 1927, which led to the formation of the International Union for the Scientific Investigation of Population Problems (Himes, 1936). In 1928, she resigned as president of the American Birth Control League but continued to edit the *Birth Control Review* until 1929, when she withdrew from the League and the paper. In April of that year, police raided the Clinical Research Bureau, because this research was also considered in violation of the Comstock Law, but Sanger did not give up.

The 1930s brought some victories for the birth control movement. In summer of 1930, the Seventh International Birth Control Conference was held under Sanger's leadership. In 1934, Sanger went to Russia to gather data about the birth control movement there. The next year, she attended the All-India Women's Conference, met Mohandas Karamchand (Mahatma) Gandhi, and gave 64 lectures across India. The U.S. Congress finally revised the Comstock Act in 1936, redefining obscenity to exclude birth control information and devices. One year later, the American Medical Association resolved that contraception was a legitimate medical service. By 1938, over 300 clinics were in operation in the United States. In 1939, the American Birth Control League and the Voluntary Parenthood League merged and named Sanger honorary president of what is now Planned Parenthood.

Throughout the 1930s, Sanger continued to promote birth control. In 1952, she persuaded Katherine McCormick, widow of the founder of International Harvester, to fund the research that produced the oral contraceptive. She also traveled to India to help organize the International Planned Parenthood Federation; the next year in Stockholm, Sanger was elected president of this organization. In 1959, the 80-year-old Sanger attended the International Conference on population in New Delhi, where she met Prime Minister Nehru. She died in 1966, in Tucson, Arizona (Douglas, 1970; Gordon, 1990; Gray, 1979; Lader, 1955; Marlow, 1979; Sanger, 1920b, 1931, 1938; Sicherman, Green, Kantor, & Walker, 1980).

The New Feminism

While Sanger was establishing birth control clinics, other U.S. women were working to obtain the vote, which they finally gained with the passage of the 19th Amendment in 1920 (Kerber & De Hart, 1995). The suffrage movement reflected women's growing opportunities for paid employment in nursing, teaching, offices, factories, and other fields.

During this period, some advocates saw birth control as a tool, not only for limiting pregnancies, but also promoting social revolution. They believed the solution for many social ills lay in population control (Gordon, 1990). Thus, most birth control advocates were social radicals; some were also socialists or political radicals.

After World War I, women returned to work in the home, and the birth control movement changed considerably. As health care professionals made birth control an integral part of their practices, they moved it into the mainstream of society. Birth control, which had begun as a radical social movement, shifted decisively into the medical arena, ensuring medical control of contraception. Medical control was synonymous with middle-class and upper-class control, giving contraception a taint of ethnic genocide that survives even today. If contraceptive information and methods had been controlled by radical feminists and socialists, such as Emma Goldman, the story might be told very differently. For example, birth control information and methods might have been in the hands of women users rather than physicians (Gordon, 1990).

Recent efforts of feminists to wrest control of reproduction from the hands of medicine have their roots in the birth control movement of the 1920s and 1930s. In 2007, in the United States, the most effective means of contraception—intrauterine devices (IUDs), oral contraceptives (OCs), hormonal implants, rings, patches, and injectables—remain under health care providers' control. As clinical nurse specialists, nurse practitioners, nurse-midwives, and physician assistants gained prescriptive authority, control of these methods passed to health care professionals other than physicians and into the hands of more women. Interestingly, in many countries, control of these methods rests with the women who use them or with health care professionals who are not physicians. For women in the United States, contraceptive patterns and practices remain tempered by who controls the available methods.

CONTRACEPTIVE PATTERNS AND PRACTICES

Sexual Beliefs and Practices

Since the Kinsey report (Kinsey, Pomeroy, Martin, & Gebhard, 1953) revealed that some women masturbated, had premarital sexual experiences, and were orgasmic, the U.S. public has lived through the baby boom of the 1950s when many middle-class women returned to or stayed home to raise families; the new wave of feminism of the 1960s beginning with Betty Friedan's *Feminine Mystique* (1963); and the sexual revolution of the 1970s.

While the feminist movement of the 1960s was gaining momentum, scientists were developing oral contraceptives, promising freedom from unwanted pregnancy in a pill—a contraceptive method totally disassociated from intercourse. However, physicians controlled this method, as well as abortions legalized in 1973 with *Roe v. Wade*. To counter medical control of women's bodies, the Boston Women's Health Book Collective published the first edition of *Our Bodies, Ourselves* in 1970, and self-help groups sprang up in the 1970s. At the same time, many authors addressed the new sexuality of women, allegedly discovered during the sexual revolution. Thus, while women worked for liberation from feminine stereotypes, they experienced a bombardment of expectations about their sexuality. The role of super woman took on new qualities: not only were U.S. women expected to be faultless wives, mothers, and career women, but they were also supposed to be able to fulfill all their partners' sexual fantasies. However, the sexual revolution did not relieve women of the burden of contraception. Even today, most sexually active fertile women make all decisions about contraception.

Patterns of Contraceptive Use

During the period from 1995 to 2002, the percentage of sexually active women in the United States not using contraception rose from 5.2% to 7.4%, according to the latest data from the National Survey of Family Growth (NSFG) (Mosher, Martinez, Chandra, Abma, & Wilson, 2004).

This increase affects the unintended pregnancy rates and is being studied further. There has been an increase in contraception at first intercourse attributed to the increase in male condom use. In the 1970s, reported contraceptive use was 43%, with 22% of respondents reporting condom use. By 2002, the contraceptive rate at first coitus was 79%, with 67% using condoms (Mosher et al., 2004).

The U.S. Department of Health and Human Services funds periodic cycles of the NSFG. Data collectors use a structured interview format, asking women which contraceptive method or methods they used since their last pregnancy or first intercourse and method(s) they are currently using (Mosher et al., 2004). From these NSFG data, estimates of contraceptive use can be generated. The methods women report using are related to their age, ethnic identity, marital status, and socioeconomic status. Ninety-eight percent of women who are sexually active with a male partner reported having used at least one method of contraception. Oral contraception, sterilization, and condoms, in this order, are the most popular methods in the U.S. The male condom is the leading choice for first intercourse, and the oral contraceptive pill is the preferred method for women under age 30. Female sterilization is the leading choice among women age 35 and older, with Black and Hispanic women more likely than White women to choose this method. However, White women were more likely to rely on male vasectomy. Black and Hispanic women were more likely than White women to have used Depo-Provera®, which is the fifth leading method of contraception. The least used methods included the implant, patch, IUD, diaphragm, natural family planning, sponge, cap, and female condom (Mosher et al., 2004).

The Youth Risk Behavior Surveys, conducted with random samples of youth in the 9th through 12th grades, are another source of data about contraceptive use. Using data from seven surveys conducted between 1991 and 2003, the authors revealed that condom use increased significantly, and use of no method or withdrawal declined. The authors identified a high-risk group of 6.4% of the students who engaged in poorly protected sex (Anderson, Santelli, & Morrow, 2006). Teens also experience unique barriers to access to care in the form of legislation requiring parental involvement and consent (Zavodny, 2004).

Use of the most effective methods of contraception requires access to health care. Because the United States is the only industrialized country without a national health service or national health payment scheme, access to health care depends on ability to pay and proximity to a health care facility. Thus, unintended pregnancies and limited access to health care seem inextricably connected. According to the 2002 NSFG data, 34 million women visited private doctors and 13.5 million visited publicly funded clinics for their family planning needs.

These percentages increased from 33% in 1995 to 42% in 2002 (Mosher et al., 2004).

Access to contraceptive methods influences overall use. According to Ross, Hardee, Mumford, and Eid (2001), couples living in countries that have easy access to all different contraceptive options have the highest level of use. It is important to have access to a variety of contraceptive methods so couples can choose what is best suited for their needs and bodies. To underscore these points, Sangi-Haghpeyker, Ali, Posner, and Poindexter (2006) studied disparities in contraceptive use, knowledge, and attitudes with samples of Hispanic and non-Hispanic White women. These researchers found that Hispanic women had lower levels of social support for and self-efficacy in using contraception. They also reported more religious objections to contraceptive use. Clearly, programs and services need to be tailored to the needs of individuals and groups of patients who share common characteristics. Nearly 50% of family planning services in the United States are covered by Medicaid. In a study of the effects of expanding Medicaid family planning coverage, Lindrooth and McCullough (2007) found that birth rates were lowered, and the expansions were either budget neutral or resulted in cost savings.

Discrimination also plays a role in women's access to contraceptive services. For example, African American women have reported experiencing race-based discrimination in trying to access services. Half of the 326 African American women who completed a telephone survey reported experiences of discrimination, including poorer service and stereotyping by providers (Thorburn & Bogart, 2005). The end result of discrimination, lack of access to services and methods, inappropriate services, and barriers to contraceptive access and use is the occurrence of unintended pregnancies.

Unintended Pregnancies

The U.S. rates of unintended pregnancies and teen pregnancies are among the highest of the Western nations. More than 3 million couples conceive unintentionally each year. Slightly more than half of the women (52%) in 2002 reported no contraception as compared to 47% in 1994 (Finer & Henshaw, 2006). According to the 2002 NSFG, rates of unintended pregnancy were above average for women who were unmarried (particularly cohabiting), had low-income, were a minority, had low education levels, and were ages 18 to 24 years. However, the rates for teens, highly educated, and wealthy women declined (Finer & Henshaw, 2006; Santelli, Lindberg, Finer, & Singh, 2007).

Total teen pregnancy rates in the United States between the years 1995 and 2002 have declined by almost one-quarter (24%). The majority of the decline is a result of teens choosing to use more effective contraceptive methods and multiple methods (86%). For younger teens, ages 15 to 17, a delay in sexual activity played a large role (23%) (Santelli et al., 2007). According to Abma and colleagues (2004), the downward trends in pregnancies and births to teens measured from 1991 are reflective of the trends in contraception. Of the births from 1997 to 2002 to teens ages 17 or younger, 88% were unintended. Barriers to contraceptive use certainly exist even when teens have access to services. Adolescent mothers reported indifference to the possibility of pregnancy, perceived invulnerability to pregnancy, and forgetting to use contraception as barriers to their effective use of contraception (Breheny & Stephens, 2004).

Several researchers have reported on contraceptive use and discontinuation or method changing. Huber and colleagues (2006), using a sample of 369 women visiting a primary care setting, reported that women most often discontinued oral contraceptives due to medical side effects and switched to less effective methods, and over one-quarter of the women on OCs had intercourse on days they missed taking pills. Grady, Billy, and Klepinger (2002) reported rates of method switching of 40% among married women and 61% among unmarried women. These data suggest that method failure may be related to fear of or actually experiencing side effects, switching methods, and incorrect use of methods. Contraceptive decision making is an ongoing process, often requiring input from care providers.

CONTRACEPTIVE DECISION MAKING

From menarche to menopause, women must make decisions about their fertility, including if, how, and when they will regulate it. Women may choose to abstain from heterosexual vaginal intercourse, engage in such intercourse and risk pregnancy, or engage in intercourse and prevent pregnancy by using contraception.

Making a decision about contraception is more than selecting among attractive alternatives. It requires strategies and compromises that satisfy personal, social, cultural, and interpersonal needs influenced by constraints, opportunities, values, and norms. Most often the choice, rather than being a positive choice, is a more negative process, with the woman choosing the method with the fewest negative consequences (Matteson, 1995).

Deciding to Use Contraception

Decision models assume that individuals' choices are determined by beliefs about their consequences and perceptions of their advantages and disadvantages. Although individuals try to make the best possible choices, they can be hampered by the complexity of a situation, conflicting beliefs and motives, misinformation, social constraints, and intrapsychic conflicts

(Adler, 1979). When making a decision, an individual's values and perceptions of probable outcomes and values are valid, even if they are not objective or consistent with cultural values. Some investigators believe that the decision not to use contraception can be sensible even when pregnancy is not intended. In fact, it may be based on a decision model in which a woman decides that benefits associated with not using a contraceptive outweigh the risks associated with pregnancy (Luker, 1978). (Additional information on this topic is found in chapter 19.)

Each decision has antecedents and consequences. Antecedents initiate the decision-making process. These are events or incidents that cause doubt, wavering, debate, or controversy. In turn, these lead to a searching for options, followed by a gathering of information about these options. Before making a decision, the individual examines and evaluates the feasibility of each option and considers the possible risks and consequences of each. Consequences are the events or incidents that result from the decision.

When the individual makes a decision, stabilization occurs because the decision ends the doubt, wavering, debate, or controversy. Then the individual may affirm the decision by implementing it, affirm it but postpone implementation, reverse it, or reconsider it and make new decisions as circumstances and desires change.

For example, a woman is considering switching from an oral contraceptive to a barrier device. She may have used other contraceptive methods in the past and probably will consider those along with the numerous choices for barrier contraception. Then she compares the advantages and disadvantages of the various barrier methods with those of other options. After considering the consequences of using a barrier method—such as its use must be linked to intercourse, the necessity of inserting device in her body, and the need to remove the device in a prescribed time frame—she decides to use this contraceptive method. After choosing the particular barrier method, the woman might consider the consequences of that decision on her relationship with her partner, the need to learn insertion and removal techniques, and other factors unique to her lifestyle and roles.

Before deciding to contracept, a woman must perceive herself as sexually active and at risk for becoming pregnant. A sexual self-concept is strongly correlated with contraceptive use (Winter, 1988). The decision to use contraception is influenced by many factors, such as age, family patterns of health care, advice from health care professionals, the influence of culture (Lethbridge, 1997), socioeconomic status, locus of control, knowledge of pregnancy risks, availability of contraception, approach to risk taking, and relationship with partner (Lethbridge & Hanna, 1997; Mills & Barclay, 2006).

Cultural Influences

Conspiracy theories are not often viewed through the lens of health care. However, these theories can greatly influence a patient's decision making in seeking health care, trusting her provider, and making choices about risky behaviors. In the African American culture, belief in conspiracy theories may play a significant role in health care. Patients often express concern about discrimination, fear of victimization, distrust, and exploitation. Indeed, Lille-Blanton, Brodie, Rowland, Altman, and McIntosh (2000) reported that physician attitudes and interactions with patients are often influenced by the patient's race.

In reference to a particular cultural or social group, Thorburn and Bogart (2005) defined conspiracy theories as beliefs about large-scale discrimination, by the government and health care system, against a group. Conspiracy theories are understood as a class of ethnosociologies: theories ordinary people use to explain social phenomena and social misfortunes by attributing them to the deliberate actions of a particular group of people, often secretly planned (Waters, 1997). Conspiracy theories are common in African American cultural beliefs. Waters (1997) found that African Americans who believe in conspiracy theories are better educated, politically active, and community oriented with closer ties to interethnic conflicts.

In *The Tuskegee Experiment's Long Shadow*, Ruffin (1998) reported that academic scholars think that conspiracy beliefs develop as a reaction to racism as individuals relate their uneasiness to a concrete idea. Some scholars believe that these ideas are useful for political or social change, while others believe that they can be detrimental to the well-being of African American culture. The medical community believes that they threaten the public health of African Americans.

This is one example of beliefs patients bring to the dialogue about contraception. Thus, care providers are challenged to learn about the sociocultural beliefs their patients hold and assist patients to choose methods congruent with their beliefs.

Inadequate or incorrect knowledge about conception leads women to miscalculate or underestimate their risk of pregnancy. Women may obtain this knowledge from friends, classes, books, magazines, family members, or sexual partners. Misinformation from any source places a woman at risk. For example, a woman may risk pregnancy by not using contraception because her partner believes he is infertile.

Communication about sexual and other matters between partners tends to be related to contraceptive use: more communication is associated with more use of contraception, and sometimes use of more effective contraception (Burger & Inderbitzen, 1985). The partner's attitude also may influence contraceptive use in other ways (Lethbridge & Hanna, 1997). For example, one partner might threaten to leave if the woman uses contraception; another might threaten to leave if she becomes pregnant.

Statements from family members and friends may affect a woman's decision. Most adolescents who attend family planning clinics have the support of their friends or mothers in seeking contraception, but few have the support of both (Nathanson & Becker, 1985). Some women feel that family members, friends, or society would disapprove and thus may be less likely to use contraceptives.

Past experiences with contraception can determine what methods a woman will consider. So can the past experiences of family members and friends. Adverse effects from previous methods can affect a woman's choice of contraceptive method, as can the degree to which these effects interfered with her self-image, sexual expression, or lifestyle.

A woman's choice of contraceptive method results from her expectations about the method and her feelings about those expectations (Scott & Glasier, 2006). A woman selects a method because it is available and she believes it will prevent pregnancy. In making her choice, she uses the decision-making process described earlier. She may do this many times during her fertile years. Her partner, too, may be involved in the decision making process. Their satisfaction with a method will determine whether they continue its use, change methods, or discontinue use of contraception altogether (Huber et al., 2006).

A woman's opinions about contraceptive methods may change with her age, relationships, number of children, plans for future children, and experiences with methods (Grady et al., 2002; Huber et al., 2006; Mathias et al., 2006; Mills & Barclay, 2006). For example, a woman who used a barrier method during the years she was actively planning her family may decide on a tubal ligation when her family is complete. A woman who used oral contraceptives during the years she was sure she did not want a pregnancy may switch to condoms and a spermicide while she prepares to attempt conception. At any time, she may stop using a method because it does not meet her expectations, becomes unavailable, or her situation changes.

Some women manage their fertility regulation without the assistance of health care providers. They do not feel a need for educational services or prescription methods. Favorable attitudes toward methods are a prerequisite for contraceptive use and for seeking assistance from a provider when a woman believes she needs such help to choose a method or to access a prescription method. The attitudes of providers affect women's perceptions of methods, especially those requiring a prescription or other assistance in procuring the method (Mills & Barclay, 2006; Thorburn & Bogart, 2005; Wysocki, 2006).

Sometimes women see a health care provider, obtain a contraceptive method, and then never return. If the prescription expires or the method needs replacement, the woman may discontinue it rather than return to the health care provider. Still other women switch from one health care provider to another for various reasons. The quality of the interaction between providers and their patients can positively or negatively affect women's level of contraceptive use over time (Mills & Barclay, 2006; Thorburn & Bogart, 2005).

Deciding Not to Use Contraception

Luker (1978) asserted that women and health care providers make disparate decisions about the need for contraception because of their different perspectives. Health care providers view the risk of pregnancy resulting from unprotected intercourse as a known probability based on theoretical and user statistics on methods and on exposure to pregnancy without contraception. Women view it as an uncertainty or unknown. Using a rational decision-making process, women weigh the advantages and disadvantages of contraception against the advantages and disadvantages of pregnancy. This cost-benefit analysis determines the woman's decision to use contraception or not.

> When a woman cannot completely suppress her wish to become pregnant in spite of important situational constraints, when a woman loses the psychological energy that is continuously required to avoid conception, or when a woman feels the urge to use becoming pregnant as a way of dealing with certain negative feelings about herself, then her contraceptive practice tends to become inconsistent. (Miller, 1986, p. 30)

The woman's perceived risks of conception, her attitudes toward contraception, her interaction with the things and people associated with the method, and her partner's attitude may lead to her decision not to use contraception. Partner disapproval of contraception, in particular, can tip the balance in favor of the decision not to use contraception.

Rates of contraception nonuse and the methods used differ by ethnic identity, income, marital status, and education (Huber et al., 2006; Mathias et al., 2006; Sangi-Haghpeykar et al., 2006). Researchers have suggested, however, that cost is not a cause of contraceptive nonuse; rather, the cause lies with inadequate delivery of contraceptive services and restricted access to the most effective methods (Frost, 2001; Frost, Ranjit, Manzella, Darroch, & Audam, 2001).

Special Considerations for Adolescents

Unintended teen pregnancy continues to be a problem in the United States. During the past decade, teenage birth rates declined and the teenage pregnancy rate dropped, probably due to improved use of contraception

(Santelli et al., 2007). More teens are using contraception at first sex. Teens whose first intercourse occurred after 1990 were more likely to use contraception than those in earlier decades. In 2002, approximately 75% of teen females and 82% of teen males used some sort of contraception during their first intercourse. Older female teens are more likely to use contraception. The most popular method of contraception for teens is the male condom (Abma et al., 2004).

In their attempts to prevent pregnancy, many adolescents continue to depend on over-the-counter methods and natural methods, such as coitus interruptus. They commonly delay seeking contraceptive care from a health care provider who could provide more effective and longer-acting methods because they fear that their confidentiality will not be maintained and their parents will discover their sexual activity (Breheny & Stephens, 2006; Lethbridge & Hanna, 1997).

When an adolescent chooses a health care provider, her criteria are likely to be confidentiality, a staff who care about adolescents, and geographic proximity. However, her chances of finding confidential services may be slim, especially in a community with few alternatives. Health care providers' beliefs may prevent them from condoning the adolescent's sexual behavior. An adolescent expects confidentiality, but that expectation may be modified by her willingness to discuss seeking services with her parents (Lerand, Ireland, & Boutelle, 2007).

When the parent and adolescent come together for care, they may have different agendas. The parent may want the health care provider to stop the adolescent from being sexually active; the adolescent may want to obtain a contraceptive method. The parent may wish to be informed of all findings and treatments, whereas the adolescent may not want her parents to be informed at all (Stevens-Simon, Sheeder, & Harter, 2005).

Finally, adolescents depend heavily on publicly funded family planning services for access to contraception. In regions of the United States where such services do not exist or are geographically remote, teens have little or no access to such care (Frost, 2001; Frost et al., 2001; Herrman, 2006).

The rate of contraceptive nonuse among sexually active adolescents has continued to decline between 1988 and 2003 (Abma et al., 2004; Anderson et al., 2006). Teenagers give several reasons for nonuse: They did not expect to have intercourse; their partners object to contraception; they believe that contraception is wrong or dangerous; they do not know which contraceptive methods exist or where to obtain them; and they feel contraceptives are too difficult or unpleasant to use (Abma et al., 2004; Breheny & Stephens, 2004; Lethbridge & Hanna, 1997). In a study of adolescents who used contraception at first intercourse but who discontinued use as they matured sexually, discovered that

teens did so because of doubts about the need for and desirability of contraceptive use (Kinsella, Crane, Ogden, & Stevens-Simon, 2007). These findings raise important questions for health care providers, including eliciting information from patients about barriers to contractive use and continuation.

Lack of access to family planning services can be an obstacle to the use of contraception for all women. Barriers to access include geographic location, cost, limitations on contraceptive supplies (Nelson, Pietersz, Nelson, & Aguilera, 2007), discrimination, language barriers, and congruence of staff and patient expectations. To create services that are acceptable to women, providers must consider many aspects of the contraceptive decision-making process as well as where women will most readily go for services, who should provide those services, and whether women leave encounters with providers satisfied that their needs have been met.

FAMILY PLANNING SERVICES
Settings

Agencies offering family planning services should provide patients free access to current developments in the field through the use of state-of-the-art media. They should be open at convenient hours for all patients. These agencies should welcome women's and, with the women's permission, their partners' participation in method selection and educational sessions.

The setting should be conducive to teaching and learning. Its waiting and counseling rooms should be large enough to permit various seating arrangements for several persons. To promote teaching and learning, it should have adequate lighting and ventilation. Because individuals have different learning styles and educational backgrounds, providers should use various teaching methods such as one-to-one discussions and group sessions. Patients should be given access to appropriate and up-to-date educational materials, including those available in print, in various media, hands-on displays, interactive computer software, and online access (Tabeek, 1990; Thorburn & Bogart, 2005).

Changing from a technically oriented family planning care delivery system to an educational delivery system with product and nonproduct methods requires fertility awareness education as the basis for all contraception. Increased involvement and control over method selection may increase a woman's use of the method she chooses.

The current system of delivery of family planning services is not meeting the needs of all patients. Drastic change in the system is unlikely, however, unless patients demand more from the system. Patient education may help solve this problem. However, changing the knowledge, attitudes, and behaviors of some family planning providers presents a greater challenge. Addressing the roles of advanced practice nurses in provision of care will also help to individualize care. Fortunately, most providers are enthusiastic about the future of family planning and are eager to participate in new care delivery systems and to integrate of new methods of contraceptive teaching and counseling into their practice (Herrman, 2006; Mills & Barclay, 2006; Tabeek, 1990).

Providers and Their Styles of Interacting

Several types of health care providers offer a range of family planning services such as counseling, prescribing oral contraceptives, the ring or the patch, fitting diaphragms and caps, inserting contraceptive implants or intrauterine devices, administering injectables, and providing family planning education. Specialists and family practice physicians, nurses, nurse practitioners, nurse-midwives, and physician assistants provide these services in private practices; community health centers; hospital-based, public health, and freestanding clinics; and in family planning agencies (Herrman, 2006).

Nurses' roles range from assisting women with decision making to direct hands-on care. Social workers, counselors with various educational backgrounds, health educators, and lay volunteers also participate in family planning programs. All health care providers bring their personal agendas, biases, values, and cultures to the family planning setting, affecting care delivery and interactions with patients. The style of care delivery ranges from giving a method to a woman and assuming she will use it to being a partner in the decision-making process.

Health care providers use a variety of interaction styles when caring for women who are making choices about their health. Providers with a paternalistic style assume they know what is best and make decisions for their patients. They commonly use statements beginning with, "I will . . ." and "You will . . . ." Providers with a maternalistic style attempt to influence the woman's choices and gain her acquiescence by stating consequences of an action rather than the alternatives to it. This approach puts the focus on potential outcomes and the effects of the woman's choice on herself or others. Providers using this approach commonly use statements that begin with, "If you don't . . ., then . . . ." Providers using either style of interaction focus on outcomes and attempt to gain compliance with their own predetermined goals.

Providers using a participatory style demonstrate respect for the woman's autonomy and ability to make decisions. They focus on the process the woman uses to reach a decision, presenting alternatives and encouraging her to participate in the decision. They use statements that begin with "What do you think about . . . ?" or "We can talk about . . . ." The woman's needs and concerns are more likely to emerge in participatory interactions than in maternalistic or paternalistic ones (Schnare & Nelson, 2005; Wysocki, 2006). As Orne and Hawkins (1985) pointed out, "Providers must avoid the temptation to prescribe 'for clients.' Clients must make their own informed choice in collaboration with providers; they should feel supported in their right to choose" (p. 33).

Evidence-Based Family Planning Practice

Evidence from research to guide clinical practice in family planning services is accumulating. For example, Scott and Glasier (2006) delineated evidence-based contraceptive choices using data from electronic databases, a manual literature search, and contact with experts. Helmerhorst and colleagues (2006) reported on a synthesis of best evidence about family planning effectiveness and adverse effects from the Cochrane Fertility Regulation Group. Several authors have published comprehensive reviews of the relationship between combination and progestin-only contraception and bone health (Bahamondes et al., 2006; Curtis & Martins, 2006; Kaunitz, Miller, Rice, Ross, & McClung, 2006; Martins, Curtis, & Glasier, 2006). The World Health Organization (2006) has issued a statement on hormonal contraception and bone health. Burkman, Grimes, Mishell, and Westhoff (2006) published a comprehensive review of the evidence on benefits of contraception to women's health. As more authors scrutinize the research literature and publish the evidence they have gleaned, health care providers will be better informed as they advise women and their partners about the options and engage them in decision making. Because some of the most popular methods have been available for decades, health care providers and researchers have accumulated considerable data to inform practice.

CONTRACEPTIVE METHODS

For most women in the United States, fertility regulation is a major concern. Ideally, young women should be taught about their bodies before menarche, the onset of menses, and learn about the developmental changes of puberty and the signs and symptoms of fertility. After menarche, they may begin the journey along the sometimes-tortuous path of decision making about contraception. During the fertile years, women may decide the number and timing of any pregnancies they choose to have.

Before deciding to use a particular contraceptive method, a woman should weigh the method's effectiveness against its risks (if any), advantages, disadvantages, and adverse effects (Steiner et al., 2006). She should also consider any contraindications that exist for her. The effectiveness among contraceptive methods varies considerably. Each method has a theoretical effectiveness—effectiveness under ideal laboratory conditions, which depends solely on the method and not the human user—and use effectiveness—effectiveness under real-life or human conditions, which allows for the user's carelessness or error as well as method failure. Health care providers often use this information when counseling a woman about contraceptive choices and risks. When a woman seeks assistance with family planning, care may include a detailed personal and family health history and a complete physical examination with a pelvic examination and Papanicolaou (Pap) smear (Association for Women's Health, Obstetric, and Neonatal Nursing & National Association of Nurse Practitioners in Reproductive Health, 2002; Hawkins, Roberto-Nichols, & Stanley-Haney, 2008). Usually this assessment is performed annually, although it may be done more or less frequently for some women. (See chapter 9, "Well-Woman Assessment," for assessment guidelines and recommendations for when to begin having Pap smears and the frequency of testing.) An important component of the initial assessment process is the woman's personal and identifying information.

Natural Family Planning Methods

The cornerstone of fertility regulation, fertility awareness, is the basis for understanding all contraceptive methods, especially the fertility awareness (natural family planning) methods. This information assists the woman in knowing when or if she ovulates. Therefore, the health care provider should explore a woman's awareness of her fertility patterns and provide additional information, if needed, before assisting her with the selection of a contraceptive method (Hawkins, et al., 2008; Tabeek, 1990).

Fertility awareness education refers to imparting information about male and female reproductive anatomy and physiology, primary and secondary signs of fertility, and cyclical changes in these signs. All fertility awareness methods use this information, as well as knowledge of female fertile and infertile phases and their relationship to male fertility and require abstinence from vaginal-penile intercourse during the fertile phase to prevent conception. Because natural family planning (NFP) methods are unmodified by chemical, mechanical, or other artificial means, they represent a natural way to regulate fertility (World Health Organization, 2004). Leonard, Chavira, Coonrod, Hart, and Bay found NFP to be an "appealing family planning alternative" for Hispanic women in their sample (2006, p. 313).

Evidence from ancient times suggests rudimentary knowledge of periods of relative infertility during the menstrual cycle, as well as at other times in a woman's life. East African women believed that avoiding intercourse for a few days after menstruation would prevent pregnancy (Gordon, 1990). Breast-feeding was recognized as a means to prevent pregnancy and was used by Alaska Natives, Native Americans, and ancient Egyptians (Gordon, 1990). This latter method is still practiced and gained in popularity in the 1990s under a new title of lactation amenorrhea method (LAM) (Diaz, 1989; France, 1996; World Health Organization, 2004).

Natural family planning includes the cervical mucus, basal body temperature (BBT), symptothermal, and lactational amenorrhea methods. Except for LAM, these methods use normal signs and symptoms of ovulation and the menstrual cycle to prevent or achieve pregnancy (Finnigan, 2008). The woman is taught the methods and then asked to observe several cycles to best understand and recognize her fertile and infertile phases.

Cervical Mucus Method

The cervical mucus method is based on detecting signs and symptoms of ovulation through consistent observation of the cervical mucus, which is produced by cells in the cervix. Throughout the menstrual cycle, cervical mucus changes. Immediately after the menstrual period, cervical mucus is scant and the woman should notice vaginal dryness for a few days. Then mucus is present for a few days, in which the woman should feel vaginal wetness. After this, the mucus becomes clear (as differentiated from milky white, translucent, or creamy color) and slippery or stretchy, similar to raw egg white. The woman should notice increased wetness or a slippery sensation. The peak day of wetness signals ovulation. During ovulation, cervical mucus nourishes sperm, facilitates their passage into the intrauterine cavity, and probably helps select sperm of the highest quality. However, the peak day is only obvious the day after it occurs, when the mucus becomes less slippery and stretchy. After this day, the mucus starts to lose its slippery, stretchy, wet quality and becomes cloudy and sticky until menses begin. (See chapter 4, "Women's Bodies," for additional information on ovulation and the attendant physical changes.)

To use the cervical mucus method, the woman should check her cervical mucus daily, beginning when menstrual bleeding ends or becomes light enough to allow assessment of the mucus. The woman can check her mucus in several ways, depending on her level of comfort with her body. She can wipe a folded piece of toilet tissue across her vaginal opening, and then feel whether the tissue slides across easily or drags, pulls, or sticks. If mucus is present, she can place it between two fingers and check its wetness and stretchiness (spinnbarkheit). As an alternative, she can check these characteristics by holding the toilet tissue with both hands and pulling it apart (Finnigan, 2008; Tabeek, 2000).

Basal Body Temperature Method

The basal body temperature method is based on the temperature change triggered by the progesterone rise that occurs when the ovum leaves the ovary. To use this method, the woman takes her temperature before she eats, drinks, smokes, and has any physical activity, at the same time every day using a digital basal thermometer, calibrated in 10ths of a degree. Then she documents her daily temperature on a chart, noting any variations. During ovulation, the temperature typically rises up to 1 degree above the preovulatory BBT. To prevent conception, the woman should abstain from intercourse until after 3 days of temperature rise. Infections, illnesses, and other conditions such as fatigue, anxiety, sleeplessness, some medications, use of an electric blanket, or a heated waterbed also can increase the temperature. Therefore, applying the rules for taking and interpreting the BBT are crucial to the effectiveness of this method.

Symptothermal Method

The symptothermal method relies on identifying the primary signs of fertility: changes in cervical mucus; BBT; and the position, consistency, and opening of the cervix. Like cervical mucus and BBT, the cervix changes throughout the menstrual cycle. To receive sperm, as ovulation approaches, the cervix becomes softer and changes position to midline, and the os dilates slightly. After ovulation, it reverts to its preovulatory state. While squatting or standing with one foot on a stool or chair, the woman may place a finger in her vagina and feel for position, softness, or firmness.

The symptothermal method also uses observation for secondary signs of fertility: cyclical breast, skin, hair, mood, and energy changes; vaginal aching; spotting; pelvic pain or aching; and mittelschmerz, the lower abdominal or pelvic pain some women feel during ovulation. By charting the primary and secondary signs, the woman detects her fertile phase with great accuracy and can prevent or achieve conception.

A number of devices to predict ovulation are on the market, including an ovulation calculator. The predictions are based on assessment of lutenizing hormone in urine or saliva. Interactive computer programs also are available to teach fertility awareness methods (Fehring, 2004, 2005; Fehring, Raviele, & Schneider, 2004). Although electronic ovulation detectors and ovulation

detection kits can make natural methods easier to use, they may have some drawbacks. For example, they introduce a profit motive to a natural phenomenon. Their existence suggests that their use will make the method more effective, which is untrue because most women can accurately monitor and make decisions about their fertility without technology (Fehring, 1990, 1991, 1996).

Lactational Amenorrhea Method

After decades of skepticism in the United States, the lactational amenorrhea method is becoming more popular as a fertility awareness method (Arevalo, Jennings, & Sinai, 2003; Fehring, 2004). This method is based on the fact that the length of postpartal amenorrhea is affected directly by the duration of lactation.

Postpartal amenorrhea varies among different populations. In general, it is shorter than the duration of lactation in populations that use prolonged breast-feeding (Diaz, 1989). In the United States, however, breast-feeding patterns—that is, the duration and amount—vary widely and are affected by women's multiple roles, including that of employee. Introduction of solid food or supplementary formula for the infant, which can be influenced by the woman's sociocultural group and culture of origin, also can affect the duration of amenorrhea by affecting how often a mother breast-feeds. Most important to breast-feeding and amenorrhea is the infant's sucking pattern. Rates of pregnancy with LAM appear comparable to those of other methods (Diaz, 1989; Perez, Labbok, & Queenan, 1992). Thus, women who plan to breast-feed can be offered information about LAM to consider along with information about other fertility awareness methods.

Several innovations in natural family planning have resulted from studies of their acceptability by couples in many locations around the globe. Arevalo, Jennings, and Sinai (2002) studied the standard days method of NFP with couples in Bolivia, Peru, and the Philippines. This method requires that users abstain from unprotected intercourse during cycle days 8 through 19. Women follow their cycles using cycle beads and peak day for mucus. They may assess other signs such as position of the cervix, but do not have to do so. Cycle beads were developed by Georgetown University researchers and are an integral part of the standard days method (Fehring, 2002; Georgetown University, 2006; Germano & Jennings, 2006).

Barrier Methods

Although most barrier methods are used with chemical spermicides, the devices also act, in part, as mechanical barriers to sperm trying to reach the uterus. Barrier methods include the diaphragm, Lea's Shield®,

FemCap®, vaginal sponge, and condoms. The prototypes for all of these date from centuries past; their current forms reflect advances in materials and knowledge of fertilization.

Diaphragm

The diaphragm is known to have existed for more than a century. The original rubber diaphragm was invented by Wilde, a German physician, in 1838, but did not gain much of a following until Karl Hasse introduced it into Holland in the late 19th century. Because Hasse used the pseudonym Mensinga to protect his reputation, the diaphragm became known as the Mensinga diaphragm or Dutch cap (Connell, Grimes, & Manisoff, 1989). In the early 1900s, Margaret Sanger introduced the diaphragm to the United States through her birth control clinics. Vulcanization of rubber made the diaphragm more widely available as mass production became practical and affordable. When used with spermicidal jelly that became commercially available in the 1920s, the diaphragm became one of the most popular methods (Glazer, 1965).

Modern diaphragms, which vary most in type of spring and size, are available in four types—flat spring, coil spring, arcing spring, and bow-bend—and in sizes ranging from 50 to 105 millimeters in diameter. Flat spring diaphragms are very difficult to find—a woman may have to try several pharmacies to locate one. The color (white to dark pinkish-beige) and consistency (very thin to thick) of their rubber or silicone varies by type and manufacturer (Diaphragm, 2007).

The diaphragm has two modes of action. It forms a partial mechanical barrier to sperm, and it holds a spermicidal agent against the cervix to stop sperm that circumnavigate around the diaphragm. Therefore, the diaphragm is designed for use with spermicidal jelly, cream, gel, or film. The Milex® diaphragm has a cuff inside the rim, which, according to its manufacturer, enhances the mechanical barrier effect (Hawkins et al., 2008).

As with other contraceptive methods, the diaphragm's use effectiveness is lower than its theoretical effectiveness. This reflects the human involvement required by this method—and the resulting risk of human error. Effectiveness is reduced if the diaphragm is not used each time vaginal intercourse occurs, if it is used without spermicide, if it does not remain in place for several hours after intercourse, if the woman douches, if the diaphragm is dislodged during or after intercourse, or if it has a hole (Hawkins et al., 2008).

Before using the diaphragm, the woman or her partner must prepare it with spermicidal jelly, gel, or cream (1% or 2% spermicide concentration) or vaginal film, insert it correctly to cover the cervix completely, and remove it 4 to 6 hours after the last act of intercourse.

The diaphragm can be left in place for up to 24 hours but should be removed for cleaning and spermicide renewal.

The woman may choose spermicidal cream, gel, jelly, or film according to her preference. Made by several manufacturers, these spermicides come in various flavors and colors, including white cream and clear jelly. The concentration of spermicide also varies by product: for gels, jellies, and creams, concentration ranges from 2% to 4%. Some health care providers recommend application of a tablespoon of spermicide or another vaginal film to the outside of the diaphragm when it has been in place for more than 4 hours before penetration or when intercourse is repeated. The woman can do this with her fingers or an applicator without removing the diaphragm.

Although clinical practice once required the fit of a diaphragm to be checked when the woman loses or gains 10 to 15 pounds, some research and clinical practice experiences suggest that the woman's perception of a change is more likely to predict altered fit. Many providers suggest that the fit be checked annually during the woman's health assessment and Pap test, and once after each pregnancy, but not earlier than 6 weeks after termination of pregnancy or any pelvic surgery.

Lea's Shield

Lea's Shield® is a silicone device similar to a diaphragm that is used to hold spermicide and to provide a partial barrier to sperm when placed over the cervix. It is an elliptical bowl and the posterior end has a reservoir for spermicide. There is a valve in the middle to allow cervical secretions to drain and also to relieve pressure against the cervix. There is a molded loop to aid in removal. Insertion is similar to using a diaphragm. It is rated at 86% effectiveness, but the device has not been in use long, so information is scarce. It may be inserted before intercourse and left in place for up to 48 hours. It is a latex-free device and is reusable for more than a year.

FemCap

The contraceptive FemCap® is a prescription-only contraceptive device that holds spermicide and provides a partial barrier to sperm when placed over the cervix. It is available in three sizes—22 mm, 26 mm, and 30 mm—and needs to be fitted by a health care provider. It has a 96% to 98% effectiveness.

Vaginal Sponge

The vaginal sponge is a modern version of an old contraceptive method. During ancient Egyptian and Roman times, women placed sea sponges soaked with vinegar or lemon juice in the vagina to prevent pregnancy. They also used tampons of cotton or other materials in a similar manner (Glazer, 1965). In 1983, the FDA approved the Today® vaginal sponge (Kafka & Gold, 1983), which is made of polyurethane impregnated with the spermicide nonoxynol-9 and has a loop for easy removal. The sponge was removed from the market in 1995 due to problems in the manufacturing company. In April 2005, the sponge was reapproved by the FDA and is now available over the counter. Advantages of the sponge are convenience, one size fits all, and its ability for continued use over a 24-hour period of time.

Before inserting the Today® vaginal sponge, the woman must wet it to activate the spermicide. Then she places it in the vagina over the cervix. The sponge must be left in place at least 6 hours after intercourse, but can remain in place for up to 24 hours. Because it has enough spermicide to last 24 hours, the woman does not need to apply additional spermicide for repeat intercourse (McClure & Edelman, 1985).

Some women have problems with the sponge. They may have difficulty placing it over the cervix, find it difficult to remove, tear the sponge by pulling too vigorously, or visualize the sponge getting lost in the vagina or uterus. Most of these problems can be resolved by teaching women to squat and bear down when removing the sponge, explaining basic reproductive anatomy, and providing reassurance.

A vaginal sponge called Protectaid® became available over the counter in Canada in 1996 (Murray, 1996). This sponge is made of polyurethane foam and has no loop. Its three spermicides are nonoxynol-9 0.125%, benzalkonium chloride 0.125%, and sodium cholate 0.5%. It does not need to be wet before insertion, is to be left in place at least 6 hours after the last act of intercourse, and can be left in the vagina up to 12 hours.

Many health care providers recommend using a condom with the sponge to increase its contraceptive efficacy. They also suggest that the woman use another method during menses because of the risk of toxic shock syndrome.

Male Condoms

The condom is the only barrier method currently available for men. In 1564, the Italian anatomist Fallopius (discoverer of the Fallopian tubes) first suggested the use of linen covers for the penis as protection against sexually transmitted diseases (STDs). Subsequently, condoms were used not only for protection from infection, but also as badges of rank or honor, for decoration or modesty, or as amulets for fertility (Himes, 1936). By the 18th century, condoms were used to prevent conception. Made of animal membrane, they were waterproof and protected against penetration of sperm and some micro-organisms (Gordon, 1990).

Today's male condoms are generally made of latex, polyurethane, or natural lamb membrane. They are available with or without lubricant or spermicide, ribbing, or a reservoir tip and come in various colors, flavors, and sizes. The new eZ•on® male condom is made of polyurethane—a thin, strong, 100% latex-free material. It is designed to go on in either direction and has no reservoir tip.

The Centers for Disease Control and Prevention (CDC) guidelines (2006) stated that only latex condoms can protect against HIV transmission by vaginal or rectal intercourse. A report on condoms from the National Institutes of Health underscored this recommendation (Cates, 2001). Substitution of nonlatex condoms can be made for persons with latex allergy. Female condoms are also acceptable mechanical barriers against viruses, including HIV. Spermicides are not recommended for STD/HIV prevention in the CDC guidelines, based on recent evidence. Although these barrier methods of protection are not absolute, they are the best available.

Since the advent of oral contraceptives, knowledge about condom use seems less widespread. Yet women purchase more than 40% of condoms, indicating their interest in protecting themselves (Hatcher et al., 2004). Between the years 1982 and 2002, there has been a reported rise in condom use. The percentage of women whose partners have used a male condom rose from 52% in 1982 to 90% in 2002 (Mosher et al., 2004). Therefore, teaching women about condom use may be extremely helpful. (See chapters 24 and 25 on sexually transmitted diseases and HIV/AIDS for related information.)

Vaginal or Female Condoms

The female condom with the brand name Reality® was approved by the FDA in 1993. This barrier device is made of polyurethane and is a soft sheath open at one end and closed on the other. At each end is a flexible ring. One ring is used to insert the device and hold it over the cervix and the other ring remains outside the vagina, covering the labia. The condom is prelubricated, disposable, and intended for one-time use. As a barrier method of contraception, it also offers protection against STDs, including HIV. As with other barrier methods, this protection is relative (CDC, 2006; Soper, et al., 1993; Wisconsin Pharmacal Company, 1994).

Chemical Methods

Several types of chemical methods may be used for contraception. They all may be used alone, but some are designed for use with a barrier method such as the diaphragm, cervical cap, or female or male condom. The latter are not nearly as effective when used without a spermicide.

Spermicidal Jelly, Bioadhesive Gel, Cream, and Foam

All contraceptive jellies, gels, foams, and creams have an inert base or carrier substance and a spermicidal agent, usually nonoxynol-9. The carrier substance may be colored or flavored. One product is a personal lubricant with 2.2% of nonoxynol-9 designed to be used alone or with a condom or diaphragm. Sensitivity to one carrier substance does not preclude use of the method; switching brands may eliminate the problem. The spermicide concentration varies with brand and product from 1% to 5%. Jellies, gels, and creams are inserted in the vagina with a reusable plastic inserter or a disposable plastic or cardboard inserter, prefilled and designed for a single use. They must be put into the vagina no more than 1 hour before intercourse and must be reapplied before each subsequent act of vaginal intercourse. It is important to follow the package directions for each individual product. One exception is the bioadhesive contraceptive gel, designed to maintain its spermicidal efficacy for 24 hours, so it can be applied up to 24 hours in advance.

Spermicidal foams are similar to creams, gels, and jellies, except that they are designed to be used alone, without a barrier method. They all contain nonoxynol-9 in concentrations varying from 8% to 12.5% and are available in prefilled applicators or in canisters with reusable plastic applicators. Although marketed for use alone, foams are most effective when used with a condom. Like creams, jellies, and gels, foam should be applied no more than 1 hour before intercourse and should be reapplied before repeat intercourse.

Other Chemical Methods

Other chemical contraceptive methods include vaginal suppositories, tablets, and film. Of the various contraceptive suppositories sold in the United States, all contain the spermicidal agent nonoxynol-9 in concentrations from 2.3% to 5.6%. Some are waxy and melt in the vagina, releasing the spermicide. Others require a chemical reaction to release it. To ensure that the spermicide is dispersed and effective, users must read and follow the manufacturer's instructions for the particular product, because the waiting time before intercourse can vary.

Vaginal foaming tablets are in use in other parts of the world, and the spermicide in these tablets has been approved for use in the United States. Like some suppositories, the tablets require a chemical reaction in the vagina to activate the spermicide. Some women and their partners complain of a sensation of heat or irritation, which can decrease use of this method.

Vaginal contraceptive film uses a 28% concentration of nonoxynol-9 for its spermicide. The film dissolves within 15 minutes after insertion in the vagina (Hatcher et al., 2004). Dispensed in 5-centimeter squares that are 80 microns thick, the film can be folded, rolled, or placed over a fingertip (finger should be dry) for insertion on or near the cervix (Apothecus, 1989). Some women have used film in diaphragms instead of jelly or cream, although this may affect the diaphragm's effectiveness because the film may not coat the interior thoroughly. The spermicide is effective for 2 hours, after which another film should be inserted.

Hormonal Methods

Hormonal methods include oral contraceptives, the ring, patch, emergency contraceptives, an injectable, a contraceptive implant, and one IUD.

Oral Contraceptives

All oral contraceptives are composed of synthetic hormones. The discovery of progesterone and estrogens in the 1930s and the synthesis of these hormones in the 1950s led to the development of this hormonal method (Kistner, 1968; Rock, 1963).

Two basic types of oral contraceptives have been used in the United States for the past several decades: the combination pill and the progestin-only pill. The combination pill uses one of two types of synthetic estrogen (ethinyl estradiol or mestranol) and one of seven types of synthetic progestin (norethindrone, ethynodiol diacetate, levonorgestrel, norethindrone acetate, norgestimate, norgestrel, or drospirenone). Doses range from 20 mcg to 50 mcg of synthetic estrogen and from 0.05 mg to 2.5 mg of progestin (Dickey, 2006).

Progestin-only oral contraceptives are available in three formulations in the United States. Two have the same synthetic progestin (norethindrone) and the third, norgestrel. These oral contraceptives are taken continuously and come in either 28- or 42-pill packets. Doses of progestin range from 0.075 mg to 0.35 mg. Progestin-only oral contraceptives are a good choice when estrogen is contraindicated (Hawkins et al., 2008).

Progestins and the estrogen in oral contraceptive formulations vary in estrogenic (acting like estrogens, the predominant female hormones) and androgenic effect (acting like androgens, the predominant male hormones). They also vary in their activity on the lining of the uterus—the endometrium—and in their progestational activity—acting like progesterone, a naturally occurring hormone. So if a woman develops side effects from the formulation of one combination oral contraceptive, she may be able to take a different oral contraceptive and decrease or eliminate the side effects.

Combination oral contraceptive formulations vary. Some products contain the same formulation in all 21 pills; others have a biphasic or triphasic formulation.

For example, one biphasic product has 0.5 mg of the progestin in 10 pills and 1.0 mg in 11, creating two phases. In one triphasic product, the first six pills have 0.5 mg of progestin and 30 mcg of estrogen, the next 5 have 0.75 mg and 40 mcg, and the last 10 have 0.125 mg and 30 mcg, respectively. Another formulation has 0.15 mg of progestin in 26 pills, 20 mcg of estrogen in 21 pills, 10 mcg in 5 pills, and 2 inert pills, A regimen of 84 combination pills is packaged in an extended cycle dispenser, meaning the woman has a withdrawal bleed only four times a year (Dickey, 2006; Hawkins et al., 2008). In 2007, an oral contraceptive designed for continuous use was approved by the FDA and released for use (Archer et al., 2006).

These latter regimens represent the several new and unique formulations of oral contraceptives currently on the market. Yasmine® is the first oral contraceptive that contains the progestin drospirenone. Its regimen includes drospirenone 3.0 mg with ethinyl estradiol 30 mcg for 24 days and 4 days of placebo. This new formulation has risks associated with hyperkalemia due to the antimineralcorticoid activity. Therefore, it should not be used in patients with conditions that may predispose them to high serum potassium concentrations, and serum potassium levels should be monitored as recommended. YAZ®, a low-dose version of Yasmin®, was approved by the FDA in March 2006. This 20-mcg ethinyl estradiol pill is effective in treating emotional and physical symptoms of premenstrual dysphoric disorder (Reuters Health Information, 2006).

Mircette® has a unique formulation that includes desogestrel 0.15 mg and 20 mcg of ethinyl estradiol for 21 days followed in the fourth week by 2 days of placebo pills then 5 days of 10 mcg of ethinyl estradiol without progestin. This formulation of shortened placebo interval followed by low-dose estrogen may decrease the likelihood of accidentally prolonging the placebo-free interval and risking breakthrough ovulation (Berga, 2002).

An extended-cycle oral contraceptive, Seasonale®, was approved by the FDA in 2003. Its formulation includes 0.03 mg ethinyl estradiol with 0.15 mg levonorgestrel for 84 days followed by 7 days of placebos. This gives the user only four withdrawal bleeds a year (Anderson, Gibbons, & Portman, 2006; Clark, Barnes-Harper, Ginsberg, Holmes, & Schwarz, 2006; Sulak, Kuehl, Coffee, & Willis, 2006; Willis, Kuehl, Spiekerman, & Sulak, 2006). Seasonique®, approved by the FDA in May 2006, contains levonorgestrel/ethinyl estradiol 0.15 mg/0.03 mg and ethinyl estradiol 0.01 mg. With Seasonique®, instead of the placebo for 7 days, women take the low-dose estrogen.

Loestrin 24 Fe® was approved by the FDA in February 2006. This formulation is the first to have 24 days of active hormones followed by 4 days of ferrous fumarate tablets (Nakajima, Archer, & Ellman, 2007). Lybrel® was approved by the FDA and released in 2007. Each pill is comprised of levonorgestrel 90 mcg and ethinyl estradiol 20 mcg in 28-pill packets (Lybrel, 2007). Archer and colleagues (2006) reported that satisfaction levels remained high for the oral contraceptive users throughout the year, although 21% of subjects continued to have uterine bleeding after 1 year of use, with median of 4 days of bleeding and 3 days of spotting during each month.

Combination oral contraceptives all share the same underlying principle: they suppress ovulation through the combined actions of estrogen and progestin and alter the cervical mucus and endometrium. Progestin-only oral contraceptives suppress ovulation through the action of progestin alone and act on the endometrium and cervical mucus. Protocols for starting an oral contraceptive depend on the manufacturer's recommendation and whether the woman is experiencing regular cycles or recently has given birth or had an abortion. For most formulations, the woman takes one pill at the same time each day for 21 days and then takes no pills for 7 days or takes a placebo or iron pill each day for 7 days. During the last 7 days, the woman experiences withdrawal bleeding, which ranges from spotting to several days of bleeding similar to her regular menses. The endometrial stimulation from the synthetic estrogen and progestin produces sufficient lining to create withdrawal bleeding.

Current oral contraceptive formulations provide much lower hormone doses than the original oral contraceptives. To maintain plasma hormone levels, manufacturers suggest they be taken at the same time each day. Side effects and contraceptive failures are more common when the time varies by more than one hour on either side of the usual dosing time. The most common side effect is breakthrough bleeding that occurs while taking hormone pills. Health care providers should teach the woman the importance of taking the pills on time and what to do if she forgets a pill (Hawkins et al., 2008).

Because each oral contraceptive has a standardized formula, it does not accommodate individual needs. Therefore, a woman may ovulate because the formula does not supply sufficient hormones to suppress ovulation. She is unlikely to become pregnant, however, because the oral contraceptive makes the endometrium relatively unreceptive to implantation and thickens the cervical mucus, inhibiting sperm migration.

The Patch

Similar to combination oral contraceptives, the contraceptive patch, Ortho Evra®, is comprised of a synthetic progestin norelgestromin and a synthetic estrogen, ethinyl estradiol. The patch releases 150 micrograms of the progestin and 20 micrograms of the estrogen daily.

Women apply a patch during menses, usually on a Sunday and 1 week later remove the patch and apply a new one. They repeat this one more time, so the sequence is 3 weeks of wearing a patch and 1 week off. During the off week, the woman will experience a withdrawal bleed, just as on combination oral contraceptives. The actions of the patch, contraindications, dangers, and side effects are those of combination oral contraceptives. Both the patch and the ring may be less effective in women who weigh 198 pounds (90 kg) or more. In November 2005, the FDA approved updated labeling for Ortho Evra®. Stating that the product exposes women to higher levels of estrogen than those in most oral contraceptive formulations, the labeling emphasizes the risk of blood clots from the higher estrogen dose in the patch.

Contraceptive Ring

Like combination oral contraceptives and the patch, NuvaRing® is impregnated with a synthetic progestin, etonogestrel, and a synthetic estrogen, ethinyl estradiol. It releases 0.102 milligrams of progestin and 15 micrograms of estrogen daily for three weeks. Women insert the ring into their vaginas for 3 weeks, remove for 1 week—during which a withdrawal bleed occurs—and then insert a new ring. The data are equivocable on the acceptability of the ring (Fine, Tryggestad, & Sangi-Hagheykar, 2007; Gilliam, Holmquist, & Berlin, 2007; Roumen, 2007). Evidence is accumulating about the safety and convenience of extended use of the ring for 84 days following 7 ring-free days (Barreiros, Guazzelli, Araujo, & Barbosa, 2007). There are also now data on women's acceptance and satisfaction with the quick start of the ring versus oral contraceptives (Schafer, Osborne, Davis, & Westhoff, 2006). Contraindications, dangers, and side effects are the same as for combination oral contraceptives (Ahrendt et al., 2006). Acceptance by women and efficacy of the method have been demonstrated through a 1-year multisite study (Dieben, Roumen, & Apter, 2002).

Because hormonal contraceptives are highly effective in preventing conception, they would be ideal if they posed no dangers. However, they can cause annoying side effects and can be life threatening for some women. Therefore, health care providers and women using hormonal contraceptives should be aware of side effects and absolute and relative contraindications. Discussion of the management of side effects and screening for absolute and relative contraindications is beyond the scope of this book. (For sources of information on this topic, see Dickey, 2006; Hatcher et al., 2004; Hawkins et al., 2008; World Health Organization, 2004).

Hormonal contraceptives pose these cardiovascular risks: thromboembolism, hemorrhagic and embolic cerebrovascular accident, myocardial infarction, hyper-

tension, vascular headaches, and arterial conditions such as subarachnoid hemorrhage and mesenteric artery thrombosis (Dinger, Heinemann, & Kuhl-Habich, 2007; Hatcher et al., 2004; Hawkins et al., 2008; World Health Organization, 2004). The ring, the patch, and combination oral contraceptives increase a woman's risk for venous thromboembolism, so the same precautions apply for each (Jick, Kaye, & Jick, 2007; Rad et al., 2006). Careful screening of candidates for hormonal contraception and monitoring of women using these contraceptive methods can reduce these risks considerably. These risks are several times higher during pregnancy than they are during hormonal contraceptive use, and pregnancy creates other risks for women (Dickey, 2006; Varney, 2004; World Health Organization, 2004). Smoking and age over 30 (and especially over 35) may increase the cardiovascular risks of hormonal contraceptives, although evidence suggests that women 35 and older who do not smoke and have no personal or family history of cardiovascular disease can use hormonal contraceptives safely (Dickey, 2006; Hatcher et al., 2004).

Hormonal contraceptives can also have adverse effects on the liver and gallbladder. Women with a history of liver cancer or active viral hepatitis, severe cirrhosis, known impaired liver function, liver problems, or idiopathic jaundice of pregnancy probably should not use hormonal contraceptives because they induce changes in hepatic excretory function. Hormonal contraceptives also are associated with hepatocellular adenoma, a rare nonmalignant liver tumor (Dickey, 2006). Like pregnancy, hormonal contraceptive use appears to induce gallbladder disease in some women. However, it is unknown whether gallbladder disease would have occurred in these women if they had not been pregnant or used hormonal contraceptives.

Hormonal contraceptives affect carbohydrate metabolism and induce lipid and endocrine changes (Dickey, 2006). Although these alternations are rarely life threatening, they warrant monitoring in any woman using a hormonal contraceptive method. The health care provider and the woman should consider these adverse effects when discussing the appropriateness of such contraceptives. Preexisting condition, such as hypertension or diabetes might contraindicate hormonal contraception or, at least, require close follow-up.

Finally, some questions are being raised about effects of oral contraceptives on bone density. It is reasonable to consider and monitor bone loss with progestin-only oral contraceptives in particular (Vestergaard, Rejnmark, & Mosekilde, 2006).

Benefits of hormonal contraceptives may include relief of dysmenorrhea and menorrhagia and reduced risk of benign breast tumors or lumps, benign and malignant ovarian tumors, endometrial carcinoma, endometriosis, and uterine fibroids. In addition, hormonal contraceptives allow women to control their fertility, have no documented adverse effects on future fertility, improve hirsutism and acne, and may protect against rheumatoid arthritis and osteoporosis (Burkman et al., 2006; Dickey, 2006; Hatcher et al., 2004).

Although hormonal contraceptives reduce the risk of symptomatic pelvic inflammatory disease (PID), this benefit may be offset by an increased incidence among hormonal contraceptive users of unrecognized PID and cervical chlamydial infections (Dickey, 2006; Hatcher et al., 2004; Thurman, Livengood, & Soper, 2007). Hormonal contraceptives also offer no protection against other sexually transmitted diseases. Therefore, clinical management should include screening women at risk for chlamydia and other STDs. Risk factors include age; multiple partners; a partner who is not mutually monogamous; a new partner; a history of STDs, vaginitis, vaginosis, or cervicitis; and clinical symptoms of cervicitis or other STDs (Hawkins et al., 2008).

Weighing risks and benefits against the contraindications and adverse effects is part of the decision-making process for the woman with her health care provider. If she selects a hormonal contraceptive, management includes periodic reassessments. A typical management plan is a follow-up visit after 3 to 6 months to assess for adverse effects and monitor blood pressure, per individual family planning site guidelines, and every 6 months thereafter, with a complete health assessment and Pap smear annually unless recommended less or more frequently (Hawkins et al., 2008). Because hormonal contraceptives are drugs, they can interact with other drugs. Women should be instructed to consult their health care provider about interactions with any prescription or over-the-counter drugs.

Emergency Contraception With Hormones

Administered within 120 hours after unprotected intercourse, combination or progestin-only oral contraceptives are quite effective in preventing pregnancy (Ellertson et al., 2003). In a study of oral contraceptives as emergency contraception (EC), women took two doses, 12 hours apart, of an oral contraceptive that contained 1 mg of progestin and 100 mcg of ethinyl estradiol. Of the 51% who experienced side effects, 30% reported nausea and 20% experienced nausea and vomiting. The failure rate was 2% (Postcoital Pill, 1988). The regimen used in the study, the Yuzpe method, has been used in Canada since 1974.

Hormonal emergency contraception may act by inhibiting or delaying ovulation; interfering with corpus luteum function, thickening the cervical mucus, and possibly altering tubal transport. Okewole and colleagues (2007), from their study of administering a single 1.5-mg dose of levonorgestrel within 72 hours of unprotected coitus, have posited that the mechanism of action is delayed lutenizing hormone (LH) surge and interference with ovulation. Trussell (2006) pointed out that we may never know the true mechanisms, but there is no evidence that EC disrupts an established pregnancy.

Many formulations of combination oral contraceptives now have labeling, approved by the FDA, for use as emergency contraception. These oral contraceptives have from 20 mcg to 50 mcg of estrogen and 0.15 mg to 0.5 mg of progestin. The emergency contraception regimen depends on the amount of estrogen: two oral contraceptive pills with 50 mcg; four pills with 30 or 35 mcg; or five pills with 20 mcg within 72 hours of unprotected intercourse and a second dose 12 hours later.

Progestin-only pills are more commonly used for emergency contraception and appear to be more effective than combination pills. Historically, Ovrette® was used as one of the only available progestin ECs; it contains 0.075 mg of progestin in each pill. The regimen is 20 pills within 120 hours of unprotected intercourse and 20 more 12 hours later (Ogburn, 2006).

The two-pill progestin-only emergency contraception kit, called Plan B®, is now considered the gold standard for emergency contraception (Brunton & Beal, 2006; Gainer, Kenvack, Mboudou, Doh, & Bouyer, 2006). Each pill is equivalent to 20 Ovrette® tablets and contains levonorgestrel (Hatcher et al., 2004; Hawkins et al., 2008). Both pills can be taken at the same time or one and then the other 12 hours later. No differences have been noted in efficacy or side effects (Ngai et al., 2004). Plan B® has been prescribed for women since 1999, and, in August 2006, the FDA approved Plan B® to be sold over the counter to women age 18 years and older (Hoskins, 2006). A prescription will still be necessary for women under 18.

Injectable Contraceptives

The injectable contraceptive Depo-Provera® is a synthetic hormonal substance (depot-medroxyprogesterone acetate) that acts by blocking gonadotropin, thus preventing ovulation from occurring. It also decreases sperm penetration through cervical mucus, decreases tubal motility, and causes endometrial atrophy, preventing implantation. Research on this contraceptive has been conducted in countries around the world for decades.

Depo-Provera® works by suppressing ovulation for 12 weeks through inhibition of gonadotropin production. It offers a reversible method that is long term and disconnected from the act of intercourse. Its administration can be highly confidential, so the woman need not reveal that she is using this method. For women who are estrogen sensitive or have contraindications to methods containing estrogen, Depo-Provera® offers a possible alternative.

As with most chemical methods, there are contraindications to its use. These include known or suspected pregnancy, undiagnosed vaginal bleeding, known breast malignancy, and known sensitivity to Depo-Provera® or any of its ingredients. If a woman has had an allergic reaction to local anesthesia at the dentist, she may also have a reaction to Depo-Provera® because it has the same carrier substance.

Health care providers must use caution and careful monitoring for women with depression, kidney disease, an abnormal mammogram, a planned pregnancy for the near future, hypertension, gallbladder disease, and mild cirrhosis. Women who are mentally handicapped and have menstrual hygiene problems may need special assistance if they experience irregular bleeding patterns on Depo-Provera®. Decisions should be made on a woman-to-woman basis with consultation with the woman's other health care providers as appropriate.

Depo-Provera® is injected intramuscularly in one 150-mg dose every 12 weeks for as long as contraceptive effect is desired (in gluteal or deltoid muscle in the first 5 days of the menstrual cycle [after onset of menses], within 5 days postpartum, or, if breast-feeding, at 4 to 6 weeks postpartum). If time between injections is greater than 13 weeks, a sensitive pregnancy test is done before administration. Women are advised to use a backup contraceptive method for 7 days after the first injection. Depo-Provera® is also available in a subcutaneous formulation with 104 milligrams of depot-medroxyprogesterone acetate. The protocol for use is the same as for the intramuscular version. Depo-Provera® has some side effects, including weight gain or loss, change in appetite, irregular bleeding, depression, tiredness, breast tenderness, skin rash or increased acne, and increased or decreased sex drive (Hatcher et al., 2004; Hawkins et al., 2008; Westhoff, Jain, Milsom, & Ray, 2007).

Because Depo-Provera® does not contain estrogen, health care providers need to counsel women on calcium intake (Albertazzi, Bottazzi, & Steel, 2006; Beksinhska, Kleinschmidt, Smit, & Farley, 2007; Curtis & Martins, 2006; Kaunitz et al., 2006; World Health Organization, 2006). In addition, the FDA in November 2004 issued a black box warning to be added to the labeling describing that the prolonged use may result in significant bone density loss. This loss may be greater the longer a person takes the medication and may not be completely reversible after discontinuing Depo-Provera®.

Contraceptive Implants

First proposed in 1967, contraceptive implants have been tested and received approval by the FDA in 1990, but had been used for more than 40 years in other countries (World Health Organization, 2004). The first FDA-approved product, Norplant®, consisted of flexible,

nonbiodegradable hollow Silastic® tubes filled with the synthetic progestin, levonorgestrel. Norplant® was voluntarily withdrawn from the market in 2002.

Norplant II® (Jadelle®), a two-rod system that was granted FDA approval in 2002. Norplant II® (Jadelle®) differs from Norplant® in the number and character of the implants. It consists of two flexible cylindrical rods made of dimethylsiloxane/methylvinylsiloxane copolymer core that is encapsulated in a silicone tubine. Jadelle's® rods each contain levonorgestrel 75 mg. Each rod is 43 mm long and has a diameter of 2.5 mm (Sivin, Nash, & Waldman, 2002). Jadelle® is currently not being marketed in the United States.

Implanon® was approved by the FDA in July 2006. This matchstick-size one-rod implantable device is effective up to 3 years. It is to be implanted by a health care provider trained in insertion techniques in the inner side of the woman's upper arm. This device has been used worldwide since 1998 and is now available in the United States. Safety and efficacy have been documented in multicenter clinical trials. Investigators have reported side effects of weight gain, bleeding irregularities, emotional lability, depression, headaches, and acne and no effects on body mass index, vital signs, laboratory parameters, or breast-feeding. Major reasons for discontinuation include bleeding disorders (Bitzer, Tschudin, Alder, & the Swiss Implanon Study Group, 2004; Funk et al., 2005; Reinprayoon et al., 2000).

Besides performing a complete health assessment, health care providers should teach women about the method, especially about insertion and removal (Hawkins et al., 2008). Protocols vary depending upon the type of implant.

Intrauterine Methods

Intrauterine contraceptive methods have a long history. Ancient Turks and Arabs put stones in their camels' uteruses to prevent pregnancy. Intrauterine stems, rings, and pessaries were used in Europe during the 19th century and possibly as early as the 11th century (Connell, 1990; Glazer, 1965). However, none of these was a lasting success because of risk of infection.

The IUD first described by Richter in 1909 was a ring-shaped device made of silkworm gut. Since then, various shapes—including rings, loops, spirals, T-shapes and 7-shapes—and materials—including silver, copper, and plastic—have been used (Hatcher et al., 2004). These early IUDs caused problems, such as infection, perforation of the uterus and other pelvic organs, heavy bleeding, cramping, ectopic pregnancy, and infertility. Individual and class action suits against the manufacturer of the Dalkon Shield because it caused infection and other adverse effects resulted in its removal from the market in 1974. The Lippes Loop and Saf-T-Coil were removed in 1984 and 1985, although they still had FDA approval. The Copper T and Copper 7 (Cu-7) were removed from the market in 1986 when their patents expired (Connell, 1990). The Progestasert® was developed next along with a new generation of copper devices replacing the Copper T and the Cu-7. Many of these devices remain in use around the world. IUDs are the most widely used reversible contraceptive method in the world (d'Arcangues, 2007).

IUDs are not abortifacients; they prevent pregnancy through several mechanisms of action. Some may set up a local sterile inflammatory response, changing the cellular composition of the endometrium. These changes may cause phagocytosis of the sperm or the blastocyst, prevent implantation, or disrupt the implantation site. Copper devices may exert a local effect on the endometrium by interfering with various enzyme systems. Devices containing progesterone may stimulate decidual and secretory changes (Connell, 1990).

Progestasert®, the first hormonal device impregnated with synthetic progestin, was available until 2002. Because the progestin lasted only 1 year, this device had to be replaced annually, so demand disappeared. The copper device ParaGard® T380A can remain in place for 10 years (Hawkins et al., 2008). This third-generation, T-shaped device has copper on the stem and both arms, unlike its predecessors the Cu-7 and Copper T, which had copper on the stems only.

Guidelines—for example, those outlined by Hatcher and associates (2004) and the World Health Organization (2004)—have been relaxed considerably for the IUD since the first IUDs came on the market. In a review of contraindications, Nelson (2007) concluded that the only important contraindications are those that exceed the risk of pregnancy and that overly restrictive consideration of those without scientific merit unduly limit women's access to IUDs. Good evidence exists for the use of the levonorgestrel IUD and the copper IUD in nulliparous women (Hubacher, 2007; Prager & Darney, 2007). Women and their health care providers must consider risks and benefits, lifestyle, and the scientific evidence. The woman signs a consent form after this discussion and is given written literature. The cost of an IUD is relatively high, which covers liability insurance. Nevertheless, many women believe the IUD is the best contraceptive choice based on all the factors that they must consider (Hawkins et al., 2008).

In 2001, Mirena®, a hormone-releasing IUD, was released for use. Its current life is 5 years, but it may last as long as 7 years. Mirena® contains levonorgestrel and releases 20 micrograms of the progestin daily. Its action mimics that of other progestin-only hormonal contraceptives, with a similar protocol of precautions and side effects, as well as those associated with an IUD (Hatcher et al., 2004; Hubacher, 2002).

Emergency Contraception With an IUD

Insertion of a copper IUD within 5 to 7 days of unprotected intercourse is an option for women who cannot use combination or progestin-only oral contraceptives for emergency contraception. The health care provider screens the woman for contraindications for IUD use and instructs her on possible adverse effects and danger signs (Hatcher et al., 2004; Hawkins et al., 2008). The advantage of the IUD used as emergency contraception is that the woman then has the potential for 10 years of contraception.

Noncontraceptive Benefits of IUDs

Data are accumulating supporting use of IUDs as a means of delivering hormonal therapy for prevention and treatment of gynecological disorders such as fibroids, endometriosis, hyperplasia of the endometrium, menstrual symptoms, and possibly pelvic infections. Fraser (2007) challenged researchers to explore the possibilities of the IUD for these and other uterine conditions.

Sterilization

The pill and sterilization have been the leading methods of contraception in the United States since 1982. Over 10 million women reported female sterilization as their choice for contraception in 2002 (Mosher et al., 2004). It is considered permanent, although it may be reversed in small percentage of patients. The decision to end one's fertility permanently requires a careful review of all alternatives and full information about risks of surgery.

Female Sterilization

Female sterilization techniques are discussed in chapter 21, "Reproductive Surgery." Sterilization involves a woman's decision to seek a permanent solution to fertility regulation. A woman may seek sterilization because she (a) has used one or more contraceptive methods; (b) is dissatisfied with available methods; (c) has experienced method failure; (d) has medical contraindications for one or more methods; (e) has psychosocial contraindications for one or more methods such as unwillingness to use, fear of use, or method unacceptability to partner; (f) desires to end fertility and have no more children (or no children); (g) is premenopausal and has had no menstrual periods for 1 year or less; or (h) is experiencing problems with one or more methods (Hawkins et al., 2008).

When assisting women with this decision, health care providers should ask about prior use of contraceptive methods; desired family size; cultural beliefs about sterilization; family attitudes toward sterilization; knowledge about sterilization procedures; and history of previous pelvic surgery, such as oophorectomy (removal of one or both ovaries), salpingectomy (removal of one or both fallopian tubes), laparoscopy, or tubal reconstruction.

The provider must have current information on the prerequisites or guidelines used by the medical profession for sterilization. Voluntary sterilization is legal in all 50 states. Guidelines set by the United States Department of Health and Human Services (1978) to ensure informed consent for federally funded sterilizations include the following: a full explanation of the procedures, including risks and benefits, must be provided to the patient; a statement about the permanent nature of the surgery must be presented to the patient; the physician must wait 30 days after the patient has given consent before performing the sterilization; and the consent form must be in the woman's native language or an interpreter must be provided. In addition, there are some restrictions on federal funds for minors (under the age of 21) and mentally incompetent women. Even when federal funds are not used, many hospitals and physicians have similar restrictions.

Although reanastomosis of the tubes (surgical rejoining) is possible, the success rate is not high, so the woman should consider sterilization permanent. The request rate for reanastomosis ranges from 0.1% to 1.0%, but the success rate varies depending on the type of tubal ligation performed and the extent of tubal damage, as does the resulting pregnancy rate and risk of ectopic pregnancy. Many women wishing to have another pregnancy choose assisted reproduction techniques rather than risk tubal reanastamosis. (See chapter 18, "Infertility," for related discussion on this topic.)

Consent procedures vary from state to state and from institution to institution. A husband's consent is not legally required in most states; however, to avoid potential legal actions, many physicians try to obtain the husband's consent. In states where the husband must consent to sterilization of his wife, the reverse is not true. Therefore, the health care provider must be aware of all consent procedures that apply.

Male Sterilization

Male sterilization (vasectomy) involves location and surgical resection of the vas deferens. Although the procedure can be reversed, the success rate varies, so vasectomy should be considered permanent. Several new means of occluding the vas deferens are under investigation and, when approved, may offer a greater chance of successful reversal.

The procedure for male sterilization is much quicker (15 to 30 minutes) than that for female sterilization. It can be done in an ambulatory setting with local anesthesia. Recovery is rapid, and sutures are absorbed in 1 to 2 weeks. A new procedure eliminates the need for an incision, decreasing the time for the procedure and the recovery period. Most protocols require two follow-up visits (usually at 6 and 12 weeks) that include semen analysis to check for aspermia. Until the analysis shows no sperm, the couple should use another contraceptive method for vaginal-penile intercourse.

Death rates from vasectomy remain consistent at 0.1 per 100,000 procedures, compared to 4.0 per 100,000 for tubal ligation, making vasectomy much less risky. Morbidity is also lower, because vasectomy does not require intra-abdominal surgery or general or regional anesthesia.

Future Contraceptive Methods

Barrier, chemical, hormonal, and intrauterine contraceptive methods are under investigation in the United States and around the world. New barrier methods for women and men protect against not only pregnancy but also against STDs.

Male Methods

New male methods of contraception include a water-soluble or spermicidal condom, which is basically a male form of contraceptive film. Gossypol, a cottonseed oil, shows promise in reducing sperm counts by incapacitating sperm-producing cells. Researchers are investigating chemical contraceptive methods, such as enzyme-inhibiting spermicides, as well as substances that coagulate sperm immediately after ejaculation. An oral contraceptive for men has been found to interfere with spermatogenic cell maturation. However, it produces adverse effects such as nephrotoxicity, which had not been reduced with reformulations.

A removable intraluminal device for the vas deferens may be marketed to produce temporary sterility. Under sponsorship from the World Health Organization (2002), investigators are studying effectiveness and reversibility of a no-scalpel vasectomy, a chemical means to block sperm ducts, and plugging ducts with polyurethane.

Testosterone enanthate (TE) injections show potential because they inhibit gonadotropin secretion and decrease sperm counts. The World Health Organization (2002) is studying TE. Depot-medroxyprogesterone acetate, known as the female contraceptive Depo-Provera®, combined with testosterone shows promise for altering fertility. A longer-acting testosterone could lengthen the interval between injections from 1 to 3 months. Combining a new synthetic progestin, cyproterone acetate, with TE appears to produce azospermia. Several other hormonal substances are under investigation as chemical contraceptives for men.

The Population Council (2002) has been investigating a two-implant male contraceptive—one containing gonadotropin-releasing hormone and the other a synthetic androgen. It is also studying an antifertility vaccine for men (Cody, 1998). Several of the new methods under investigation by the Population Council rely on a synthetic steroid resembling testosterone. Methods of delivery for contraception include transdermal gel, patch, and implant.

Female Methods

A number of new hormonal methods of contraception for women are under study. New generations of contraceptive implants for women show promise. Some of the systems have one or two capsules and are biodegradable. Researchers are also testing biodegradable pellets. Several single-implant systems that are not biodegradable are in clinical trials (Cody, 1998). The Population Council (2002) is developing a single-rod implant containing nestorone for women who are lactating.

Additional combination injectables administered monthly are being marketed outside the United States Some injectables under investigation consist of microspheres or microcapsules intended to last 1 to 6 months (Cody, 1998; Hatcher et al., 2004). The World Health Organization (2002) is sponsoring investigation of several hormonal methods. Levonorgestrel butanoate shows promise as a 3-month injectable, offering a lower hormone dose than Depo-Provera®. Another World Health Organization investigation focuses on mifepristone as a once-a-week contraceptive pill.

Transdermal systems under investigation include a gel and patches with new formulations of hormones including nestorone, a steroid that does not affect serum lipoprotein patterns, carbohydrate metabolism, or liver proteins. Nestorone is also being considered with ethnyl estradiol in a combination 1-year contraceptive ring and in a nesterone-only 1-year contraceptive ring for lactating women. A progesterone-only ring for lactating women uses the natural hormone progesterone (Population Council, 2002).

A disposable nonoxynol-9–releasing diaphragm is under study, as is a disposable cervical cap (Cody, 1998). Means to alter cervical mucus so it will inhibit the passage of sperm also hold some promise. A double ring device that fits in the vagina as well as covering the labia and the base of the penis is one idea. One version of this, a female condom, designated WPC-333, is in human subjects testing in the United States at present. The device is also being tested in Europe, where it is known as Femshield.

Several new intrauterine devices, including the CuFix 390, are under study. The CuFix 390 consists of a string of hanging copper rings. This device is already in use in other countries, but its manufacturer may not seek licensure in the United States due to liability (Connell, 1990; Monier & Laird, 1989; Wymelenberg, 1990). The most promising new IUDs are the frameless GyneFix IUD and the FibroPlant levonorgestrel (LNG)-intrauterine system (IUS) (Wildemeersch, 2007). The GyneFix is a nonbiodegradable monofilament string threaded with six 5-mm copper-releasing sleeves. The device is tacked at the uterine fundus with a special inserter. The FibroPlant IUS is another anchored device that releases levonorgestrel. The framed T-shaped Femilis and the Femilis Slim, designed for postmenopausal women, are both levonorgestrel-releasing IUSs (Wildermeersch, 2007). A multiload copper IUD, targeted for nulliparous women, is in development, as is an anti-progestin-releasing IUD (Cody, 1998; Hatcher et al., 2004; Nayak, Slayden, Mah, Chwalisz, & Brenner, 2007).

A unique dual-protection levonorgestrel gel, named Carraguard®, is under investigation as a vaginal contraceptive as well as a microbicide. The active ingredient is carrageenan, known for its antiviral and antibacterial properties. Investigators are examining Carraguard® as a carrier for levonorgestrel in a suspension allowing the LNG to disperse at a slow rate (Sitruk-Ware et al., 2007).

Lastly, new methods of nonsurgical tubal sterilization have been under investigation. In November 2002, the FDA notified Conceptus, Inc. of approval of Essure®. Essure® is a permanent birth control, an alternative to tubal ligation, that occludes fallopian tubes. It does not require incisions or general anesthesia. It is currently marketed in the United States.

Methods for Men and Women

Immunologic methods for both men and women are under study. These vaccines would disrupt one or more of the reproductive processes, such as antibodies against human chorionic gonadotropin and sperm antigens (Cody, 1998; Hatcher et al., 2004).

Although user acceptability of a contraceptive method seems critical to its success, few researchers explore this issue. An interdisciplinary committee on contraceptive development told the FDA: "An expanded understanding of the 'user perspective' is required. Too often methods fail and expose the user to the medical risks associated with pregnancy and childbirth because they are too expensive, too difficult to use, or have unacceptable side effects" (Kaeser, 1990, p. 133). Almost two decades later, this advice is still valid.

REFERENCES

Abma J., Martinez, G., Mosher, W., & Dawson, B. (2004). Teenagers in the United States: Sexual activity, contraceptive use, and childbearing, 2002. National Centers for Health Statistics, *Vital Health Stat, 23*(24). Retrieved January 2, 2007, from www.cdc.gov/nchs/ppt/duc2006/abma_14.ppt

Adler, N. (1979). Decision models and population research. *Journal of Population, 2*(3), 187–202.

Ahrendt, H-J., Nisand, I., Bastianelli, C., Gomez, M. A., Gemzell-Danielsson, K., Urdl, B., et al. (2006). Efficacy, acceptability and tolerability of the combined contraceptive ring, NuvaRing, compared with an oral contraceptive containing 30 ug of ethinyl estradiol and 3 mg of drospirenone. *Contraception, 74,* 451–457.

Albertazzi, P., Bottazzi, M., & Steel, S. A. (2006). Bone mineral density and depot medroxyprogesterone acetate. *Contraception, 73,* 577–583.

Anderson, F. D., Gibbons, W., & Portman, D. (2006). Long-term safety of an extended-cycle oral contraceptive (Seasonale): A 2-year multicenter open-label extension trial. *American Journal of Obstetrics and Gynecology, 195,* 92–96.

Anderson, J. E., Santelli, J. S., & Morrow, B. (2006). Trends in adolescent contraceptive use, unprotected and poorly protected sex, 1991–2003. *Journal of Adolescent Health, 38,* 734–739.

Apothecus. (1989). *Vaginal contraceptive film.* Oyster Bay, NY: Author.

Archer, D., Jensen, J., Johnson, J., Borisute, H., Grubb, G., & Constantine, G. (2006). Evaluation of continuous regimen of levonorgestrel/ethinyl estradiol: Phase 3 study results. *Contraception, 74,* 439–445.

Arevalo, M., Jennings, V., & Sinai, I. (2002). Efficacy of a new method of family planning: The standard days method. *Contraception, 65,* 333–338.

Association of Women's Health, Obstetric, and Neonatal Nurses & National Association of Nurse Practitioners in Women's Health. (2002). *The women's health nurse practitioner: Guidelines for practice and education.* Washington, DC: Author.

Bahamondes, L., Juliato, C. T., Villarreal, M., Sobreira-Lima, B., Simoes, J. A., & dos Fernandes, A. M. (2006). Bone mineral density in users of two kinds of once-a-month combined injectable contraceptives. [JH3]*Contraception, 74,* 259–263.

Barreiros, F. A., Guazzelli, C.A.F., de Araujo, F. F., & Barbosa, R. (2007). Bleeding patterns of women using extended regimens of the contraceptive vaginal ring. *Contraception, 75,* 204–208.

Beksinska, M. E., Kleinschmidt, I., Smit, J. A., & Farley, T.M.M. (2007). Bone mineral density in adolescents using norethisterone enanthate, depot-medroxyprogesterone acetate or combined oral contraceptives for contraception, *Contraception, 75,* 438–443.

Berga, S. (2002). *Contraception: Combined estrogen-progestin contraceptives.* Retrieved January 15, 2007, from http://www.medscape.com/viewarticle/534256

Bitzer, J., Tschudin, S., Alder, J., & the Swiss Implanon Study Group. (2004). Acceptability and side-effects of Implanon in Switzerland: A retrospective study by the Implanon Swiss Study Group. *European Journal of Contraception and Reproductive Health Care, 9,* 278–284.

Boston Women's Health Book Collective. (1970). *Our bodies, ourselves.* Boston: New England Free Press.

Breheny, M., & Stephens, C. (2004). Barriers to effective contraception and strategies for overcoming them among adolescent mothers. *Public Health Nursing, 21,* 220–227.

Brunton, J., & Beal, M. W. (2006). Current issues in emergency contraception: An overview for providers. *Journal of Midwifery & Women's Health, 51,* 457–463.

Burger, J., & Inderbitzen, H. (1985). Predicting contraceptive behavior among college students: The role of communication, knowledge, sexual activity and self-esteem. *Archives of Sexual Behavior, 14*(4), 343–350.

Burkman, R. T., Grimes, D. A., Mishell, D. R., & Westhoff, C. L. (2006). Benefits of contraception to women's health: An evidence-based perspective. *Dialogues in Contraception, 10*(3), 1–8.

Cates, W. (2001). The NIH condom report: The glass is 90% full. *Family Planning Perspectives, 33*(5), 231–233.

Centers for Disease Control and Prevention. (2006). Sexually transmitted diseases treatment guidelines 2006. *Morbidity and Mortality Weekly Report, 55,* No. RR-11.

Clark, L. R., Barnes-Harper, K. T., Ginsburg, K. R., Holmes, W. C., & Schwarz, D. F. (2006). Menstrual irregularity from hormonal contraception: A cause of reproductive health concerns in minority adolescent young women. *Contraception, 74,* 214–219.

Cody, M. M. (1998). New developments in contraception: What's happening. *Clinical Excellence for Nurse Practitioners, 2,* 146–151.

Connell, E. B. (1990). Hormonal contraception. In N. G. Kase, A. B.Weingold, & D. M. Gershenson (Eds.), *Principles and practice of clinical gynecology* (2nd ed., pp. 993–1019). New York: Churchill Livingstone.

Connell, E. B., Grimes, D. A., & Manisoff, M. E. (1989). *The contraceptive diaphragm.* New York: Healthcare Communications.

Cooke, C., & Dworkin, S. (1979). *The MS guide to woman's health.* New York: Anchor Books.

Curtis, K. M., & Martins, S. L. (2006). Progestogen-only contraception and bone mineral density: A systematic review. *Contraception, 73,* 470–487.

d'Arcangues, C. (2007). Worldwide use of intrauterine devices for contraception. *Contraception, 75,* S2–S7.

Darity, W., & Turner, C. (1972). Family planning, race consciousness, and the fear of race genocide. *American Journal of Public Health, 62*(11), 1454–1459.

Diaphragm. (2007). Retrieved July 4, 2007, from http://en.wikipedia.org/wiki/Diaphragm_(contraceptive)

Diaz, S. (1989). Determinants of lactational amenorrhea. *International Journal of Gynecology and Obstetrics* (Suppl. 1), 83–89.

Dickey, R. P. (2006). *Managing contraceptive pill patients* (13th ed.). Durant, OK: EMIS.

Dieben, T.O.M., Roumen, F.J.M.E., & Apter, D. (2002). Efficacy, cycle control, and user acceptability of a novel combined contraceptive vaginal ring. *Obstetrics and Gynecology, 100,* 585–593.

Dinger, J. C., Heinemann, L.A.J., & Kuhl-Habich, D. (2007). The safety of drospirenone-containing oral contraceptives. Final results from the European Active Surveillance study on oral contraceptives based on 142,475 women-years of observation. *Contraception, 75,* 344–354.

Douglas, E. T. (1970). *Margaret Sanger: Pioneer of the future.* New York: Holt, Rinehart & Winston.

Ellertson, C., Evans, M., Ferden, S., Leadbetter, C., Spears, A., Johnstone, K., & Trussell, J. (2003). Extending the time limit for starting the Yuzpe regimen of emergency contraception to 120 hours. *Obstetrics & Gynecology, 101,* 1168–1171.

Fehring, R. J. (1990). Methods used to self-predict ovulation: A comparative study. *Journal of Obstetric, Gynecologic, and Neonatal Nursing, 19,* 233–237.

Fehring, R. J. (1991). New technology in natural family planning. *Journal of Obstetric, Gynecologic, and Neonatal Nursing, 20,* 199–205.

Fehring, R. J. (1996). A comparison of the ovulation method with the CUE ovulation predictor in determining fertile period. *Journal of the American Academy of Nurse Practitioners, 8,* 461–466.

Fehring, R. J. (2002). Standard day method™ found to be effective. *Current Medical Research, 13.* Retrieved January 12, 2007, from http://www.lifeissues.net/writers/nfp/nfp_02standard-day.html

Fehring, R. J. (2004). Simple natural family planning methods for breastfeeding women. *Current Medical Research, 15*(1–2), 1–3.

Fehring, R. J. (2005). New low- and high-tech calendar methods of family planning. *Journal of Midwifery and Women's Health, 50,* 31–38.

Fehring, R. J., Raviele, K., & Schneider, M. (2004). A comparison of the fertile phase as determined by the clearplan easy fertility monitor and self-assessment of cervical mucus. *Contraception, 69,* 9–14.

Fine, P. M., Tryggestad, J., Meyers, N. J., & Sangi-Haghpeykar, H. (2007). Safety and acceptability with the use of a contraceptive vaginal ring after surgical or medical abortion. *Contraception, 75,* 367–371.

Finer, L., & Henshaw, S. (2006). Disparities in rates of unintended pregnancy in the United States, 1994–2001. *Perspectives on Sexual and Reproductive Health, 38*(2), 90–96.

Finnigan, M. (2008). Natural family planning. In J. W. Hawkins, D. Roberto-Nichols, & J. L. Stanley-Haney, *Guidelines for nurse practitioners in gynecologic settings* (pp. 27–29). New York: Springer Publishing.

France, M. (1996). A study of the lactational menorrhea method of family planning in New Zealand women. *New Zealand Medical Journal, 109,* 189–191.

Fraser, I. S. (2007). The promise and reality of the intrauterine route for hormone delivery by prevention and therapy of gynecological disease. *Contraception, 75,* S112–S117.

Friedan, B. (1963). *The feminine mystique.* New York: Dell.

Frost, J. J. (2001). Public or private providers? U.S. women's use of reproductive health services. *Family Planning Perspectives, 33*(1), 4–12.

Frost, J. J., Ranjit, N., Manzella, K., Darroch, J. E., & Audam, S. (2001). Family planning clinic services in the United States: Patterns and trends in the late 1990s. *Family Planning Perspectives, 33*(3), 113–122.

Funk, S., Miller, M. M., Mishell, D. R., Archer, D. F., Poindexter, A., Schmidt, J., et al. (2005). Safety and efficacy of Implanon, a single-rod implantable contraceptive containing etonogestrel. *Contraception, 75,* 319–326.

Gainer, E., Kenfack, B., Mboudou, E., Doh, A. S., & Bouyer, J. (2006). *Contraception, 74,* 118–124.

Georgetown University. (2006). *CycleBeads.* Retrieved January 12, 2007, from www.cyclebeads.com

Germano, E., & Jennings, V. (2006). New approaches to fertility awareness-based methods: Incorporating the standard days and twoday methods into practice. *Journal of Midwifery & Women's Health, 51,* 417–477.

Gieg, D. M. (1972). The birth control movement in Massachusetts: Its early history, 1916–1931. *Essays and Studies by Students of Simmons College, 30*(2), 1–5.

Gilliam, M., Holmquist, S., & Berlin, A. (2007). Factors associated with willingness to use the contraceptive vaginal ring. *Contraception, 76,* 30–34.

Glazer, N. (1965). A history of mechanical contraception. *Medical Times, 93*(8), 865–869.

Gordon, L. (1990). *Woman's body, woman's right.* New York: Penguin.

Grady, W. R., Billy, J.O.G., & Klepinger, D. H. (2002). Contraceptive method switching in the United States. *Perspectives on Sexual and Reproductive Health, 34*(3), 135–145.

Gray, M. (1979). *Margaret Sanger.* New York: R. Marek.

Grisby Bates, K. (1970). Is it genocide? *Essence, 21*(5), 76–81.

Harrison, A. O. (1997). Contraception: Practices and attitudes in the black community. In H. P. McAdoo, (Ed.), *Black families* (3rd ed., pp. 301–319). Thousand Oaks, CA: Sage.

Hatcher, R. A., Trussell, J., Stewart, F., Cates, W., Stewart, G. K., Guest, F., & Kowal, D. (2004). *Contraceptive technology* (19th rev. ed.). New York: Ardent Media.

Hawkins, J. W., Roberto-Nichols, D., & Stanley-Haney, J. L. (2008). *Guidelines for nurse practitioners in gynecologic settings* (9th ed.). New York: Springer.

Helmerhorst, F. M., Belfield, T., Kulier, R., Maitra, N., O'Brien, P., & Grimes, D. (2006). The Cochrane fertility regulation group: Synthesizing the best evidence about family planning. *Contraception, 74,* 280–286.

Herrman, J. W. (2006). Position statement on the role of the pediatric nurse working with sexually active teens, pregnant adolescents, and young parents. *Journal of Pediatric Nursing, 21,* 250–252.

Himes, N. E. (1936). *Medical history of contraception.* New York: Schocken.

Hoskins, I. A. (2006). Over-the-counter emergency contraception: The time has come. *Female Patient, 31,* 47–48.

Hubacher, D. (2002). The checkered history and bright future of intrauterine contraception in the United States. *Perspectives on Sexual and Reproductive Health, 34*(2), 98–103.

Hubacher, D. (2007). Copper intrauterine device use by nulliparous women: Review of side effects. *Contraception, 75,* S8–S11.

Huber, L.R.B., Hogue, C. J., Stein, A. D., Drews, C., Zieman, M., King, J., et al. (2006). Contraceptive use and discontinuation: Findings from the contraceptive history, initiation, and choice study. *American Journal of Obstetrics and Gynecology, 194,* 1290–1295.

Jick, S., Kaye, J. A., & Jick, H. (2007). Further results on the risk of nonfatal thromboembolism in users of the contraceptive transdermal patch compared to users of oral contraceptives containing norgestimate and 35 micrograms of ethinyl estradiol. *Contraception, 76,* 4–7.

Kaeser, L. (1990). Contraceptive development: Why the snail's pace? *Family Planning Perspectives, 22,* 131–133.

Kafka, D., & Gold, R. B. (1983). Food and Drug Administration approves vaginal sponge. *Family Planning Perspectives, 15*(3), 146–148.

Kaunitz, A. M., Miller, P. D., Rice, V. M., Ross, D., & McClung, M. R. (2006). Bone mineral density in women aged 25–35 receiving depot medroxyprogesterone acetate: Recovery following discontinuation. *Contraception 74,* 90–99.

Kerber, L. K., & De Hart, J. S. (Eds.). (1995). *Women's America: Refocusing the past* (4th ed.). New York: Oxford University Press.

Kinsella, E. O., Crane, L. A., Ogden, L. G., & Stevens-Simon, C. (2007). Characteristics of adolescent women who stop using contraception after use at first sexual intercourse. *Journal of Pediatric and Adolescent Gynecology, 20,* 73–81.

Kinsey, A. C., Pomeroy, W. B., Martin, C. E., & Gebhard, P. H. (1953). *Sexual behavior in the human female.* New York: Pocket Books.

Kistner, R. W. (1968). *The pill.* New York: Delacorte.

Lader, L. (1955). *The Margaret Sanger story.* Garden City, NY: Doubleday.

Leonard, C. J., Chavira, W., Coonrod, D. V., Hart, K. W., & Bay, R. C. (2006). Study of attitudes regarding natural family planning in an urban Hispanic population. *Contraception, 74,* 313–317.

Lerand, S. J., Ireland, M., & Boutelle, K. (2007). Communication with our teens: Associations between confidential service and parent-teen communication. *Journal of Pediatric and Adolescent Gynecology, 20,* 173–178.

Lethbridge, D. J., & Hanna, K. M. (1997). *Promoting effective contraceptive use.* New York: Springer Publishing.

Lethbridge, D. J. (1997). The influence of culture and socioeconomic status on contraceptive use. In D. J. Lethbridge

& K. M. Hanna (Eds.), *Promoting effective contraceptive use* (pp. 51–63). New York: Springer Publishing.

Lille-Blanton, M., Brodie, M., Rowland, D., Altman, D., & McIntosh, M. (2000). Race, ethnicity, and the health care system: Public perceptions & experiences. *Medical Care Research & Review, 57,* 218–235.

Lindrooth, R. C., & McCullough, J. S. (2007). *Women's Health Issues, 17,* 66–74.

Luker, K. (1978). *Taking chances: Abortion and the decision not to contracept.* Berkeley: University of California Press.

Lybrel. (2007). Retrieved July 17, 2007, from http://www.drugs.com/lybrel.html

Marlow, J. (1979). *The great women.* New York: Galahad.

Martins, S. L., Curtis, K. M., & Glasier, A. F. (2006). Combined hormonal contraception and bone health: A systematic review. *Contraception, 73,* 445–469.

Mathias, S. D., Colwell, H. H., LoCoco, J. M., Karvois, D. L., Pritchard, M. L., & Friedman, A. J. (2006). ORTHO birth control satisfaction assessment tool: Assessing sensitivity to change and predictors of satisfaction. *Contraception, 74,* 303–308.

Matteson, P. S. (1995). *Advocating for self: Women's decisions concerning contraception.* New York: Harrington Park Press.

McClure, D. A., & Edelman, D. A. (1985). Worldwide method effectiveness of the Today® vaginal contraceptive sponge. *Advances in Contraception, 1,* 305–311.

Miller, W. B. (1986). Why some women fail to use their contraceptive method: A psychological investigation. *Family Planning Perspectives, 18*(1), 27–32.

Mills, A., & Barclay, L. (2006). None of them were satisfactory: Women's experiences with contraception. *Health Care for Women International, 27,* 379–398.

Monier, M., & Laird, M. (1989). Contraceptives: A look at the future. *American Journal of Nursing, 89,* 496–499.

Mosher, W., Martinez, G., Chandra, A., Abma, J., & Wilson, S. (2004). Use of contraception and use of family planning services in the United States: 1982–2002. National Center for Health Statistics. *Vital Health Stat,* Advanced Data No. 350. Retrieved January 2, 2007, www.cdc.gov/nchs/nsfg.htm

Murray, T. (1996). New contraceptive sponge also protects against STDs. *Medical Post, 32*(9), 1.

Nakajima, S. T., Archer, D. F., & Ellman, H. (2007). Efficacy and safety of a new 24-day oral contraceptive regimen of norethindrone acetate 1 mg/ethinyl estradiol 20 ug (Loestrin24® Fe). *Contraception, 75,* 16–22.

Nathanson, C. A., & Becker, M. H. (1985). The influence of client-provider relationships of teenage women's subsequent use of contraception. *American Journal of Public Health, 75*(1), 33–38.

Nayak, N. R., Slayden, O. D., Mah, K., Chwalisz, K., & Brenner, R. M. (2007). Antiprogestin-releasing intrauterine devices: A novel approach to endometrial contraception, 75, S104–S111.

Nelson, A. L. (2007). Contraindications to IUD and IUS use. *Contraception, 75,* S76–S81.

Nelson, A. L., Pietersz, D., Nelson, L. E., & Aguilera, L. (2007). Documented short-term continuation rated for combined hormonal contraceptive in an indigent population with ready access to contraceptive supplies. *American Journal of Obstetrics and Gynecology, 196,* 599.e1–599.e6.

Ngai, S. W., Fan, S., Li, S., Cheng, L., Ding, J. Jing, X., et al. (2004). A randomized trial to compare 24h versus 12h double dose regimen of levonorgestrel for emergency contraception. *Human Reproduction, 20,* 307–311.

Niethammer, C. (1977). *Daughters of the earth.* New York: Collier.

Ogburn, T. (2006). Emergency contraception: Telling the secret. *Female Patient, 31,* 14–19.

Okewole, I. A., Arowojolu, A. O., Odusoga, O. L., Oloyede, O. A., Adeleye, O. A., Salu, J., et al. (2007). Effect of single administration of levonorgestrel on the menstrual cycle. *Contraception, 75,* 372–377.

Orne, R., & Hawkins, J. W. (1985). Reexamining the oral contraceptive issues. *Journal of Obstetric, Gynecologic, and Neonatal Nursing, 14,* 30–36.

Perez, A., Labbok, M. H., & Queenan, J. T. (1992). Clinical study of the lactational amenorrhoea method for family planning. *Lancet, 339,* 968–970.

Population Council. (2002). *Biomedical research and products: Male contraceptive development.* Retrieved November 27, 2002, from www.popcouncil.org/biomed/malecontras.html

Postcoital pill: Rate of success seems high, but side effects common. (1988). *Family Planning Perspectives, 20*(3), 149.

Prager, S., & Darney, P. D. (2007). The levonorgestrel intrauterine system in nulliparous women. *Contraception, 75,* S12–S15.

Rad, M., Kluft, C., Menard, J., Burggraaf, J., de Kam, M. L., Meijer, P., et al. (2006). Comparative effects of a contraceptive vaginal ring delivering a nonandrogenic progestin and continous ethinyl estrdiol and a combined oral contraceptive containing levonorgestre on hemostasis variables. *American Journal of Obstetrics and Gynecology, 195,* 72–77.

Reinprayoon, D., Taneepanichskul, S., Bunyavejchevin, S., Thaithumyanon, P., Punnahitananda, S., Tosukhowong, P., et al. (2000). Effects of the etonogestrel-releasing contraceptive implant (Implanon®) on parameters of breastfeeding compared to those of an intrauterine device. *Contraception, 62,* 239–246.

Reuters Health Information. (2006). *Schering says FDA approves drug to treat PMDD.* Retrieved January 3, 2007, from www.medscape.com/viewarticle/545648.htm

Roberts, D. (1997). *Killing the Black body.* New York: Random House.

Roberts, D. (2000). Black women and the pill. *Family Planning Perspectives, 32*(2), 92–93.

Rock, J. (1963). *The time has come.* New York: Avon.

Rodrigues-Triaz, H. (1989). Sterilization abuse. In R. Hubbard, M. Henitin, & B. Fried (Eds.), *Biological woman—The convenient myth.* Cambridge, MA: Schenkman.

Ross, J., Hardee, K., Mumford, E., & Eid, S. (2001). Contraceptive method choice in developing countries. *International Family Planning Perspectives, 28*(1), 32–40.

Roumen, F.J.M.E. (2007). The contraceptive vaginal ring compared with the combined oral contraceptive pill: A comprehensive review of randomized controlled trials. *Contraception, 75,* 420–429.

Ruffin, P. (1998). The Tuskegee experiment's long shadow. *Black Issues in Higher Education, 15,* 26–28.

Sabatini, R., & Cagiano, R. (2006). Comparison profiles of cycle control, side effects, and sexual satisfaction of three hormonal contraceptives. *Contraception, 74,* 220–223.

Sanger, M. (1920a). *What every girl should know.* New York: Belvedere.

Sanger, M. (1920b). *Woman and the new race.* New York: Truth Publishing.

Sanger, M. (1931). *My fight for birth control.* New York: Maxwell.

Sanger, M. (1938). *Margaret Sanger, an autobiography.* New York: Dover.

Sangi-Haghpeykar, H., Ali, N., Posner, S., & Poindexter, A. N. (2006). Disparities in contraceptive knowledge, attitude and use between Hispanic and non-Hispanic Whites. *Contraception, 74,* 125–132.

Santelli, J., Lindberg, L. D., Finer, L. B., & Singh, S. (2007). Explaining recent declines in Adolescent pregnancy in the United States: The contribution of abstinence and improved contraceptive use. *American Journal of Public Health, 97,* 150–156.

Schafer, J. E., Osborne, L. M., Davis, A. R., & Westhoff, C. (2006). Acceptabilty and satisfaction using quick start with the contraceptive ring versus an oral contraceptive. *Contraception, 73,* 488–492.

Schnare, S. M., & Nelson, A. L. (2005, April). Counseling techniques for contraceptive success. *Female Patient* (Suppl.), 11–14.

Scott, A., & Glasier, A. (2006). Evidence based contraceptive choices. *Best Practice & Research Clinical Obstetrics and Gynaecology, 20,* 665–680.

Sicherman, B., Green, C. H., Kantor, I., & Walker, H. (1980). *Notable American women: The modern period.* Cambridge, MA: Belknap Press of Harvard University Press.

Sitruk-Ware, R., Brache, V., Maguire, R., Croxatto, H., Kumar, N., Kumar, S., et al. (2007). Pharmacokinetic study to compare the absorption and tolerability of two doses of levonorgestrel following single vaginal administration of levonorgestrel in Carraguard® gel: A new formulation for "dual protection" contraception. *Contraception, 75,* 454–460.

Sivin, I., Nash, H., & Waldman, S. (2002). *Jadelle® levonorgestrel rod implants: A summary of scientific data and lessons learned from programmatic experience.* Population Council. Retrieved January 2, 2007, from www.popcouncil.org/pdfs/jadelle_monograph.pdf

Soper, D. E., Shoupe, D., Shangold, G. A., Shangold, M. M., Gutmann, J., & Mercer, L. (1993). Prevention of vaginal trichomoniasis by compliant use of the female condom. *Sexually Transmitted Diseases, 20,* 137–139.

Steiner, M. J., Trussell, J., Mehta, N., Condon, S., Subramaniam, S., & Bourne, D. (2006). Communicating contraceptive effectiveness: A randomized controlled trial to inform a World Health Organization family planning handbook. *American Journal of Obstetrics and Gynecology, 195,* 85–91.

Stevens-Simon, C., Sheeder, J., & Harter, S. (2005). Teen contraceptive decisions: Childbearing intentions are the tip of the iceberg. *Women & Health, 42,* 55–73.

Sulak, P. J., Kuehl, T. J, Coffee, A., & Willis, S. (2006). Prospective analysis of occurrence and management of breakthrough bleeding during an extended oral contraceptive regimen. *American Journal of Obstetrics and Gynecology, 195,* 935–941.

Tabeek, E. (1990). Mainstreaming of natural methods of family planning in selected family planning agencies that receive Title X funding. In J. Wang, P. Simoni, & C. Nath (Eds.), *Proceedings of the West Virginia Nurses Association 1990 Research Symposium* (pp. 423–427). Charleston: West Virginia Association Research Conference Group.

Tabeek, E. (2000). Natural family planning. In J. W. Hawkins, D. Roberto-Nichols, & J. L.Stanley-Haney (Eds.), *Protocols for nurse practitioners in gynecologic settings* (7th ed.). New York: Tiresias Press.

Tannahill, R. (1980). *Sex in history.* New York: Stein and Day.

Thorburn, S., & Bogart, L. M. (2005). African American women and family planning services: Perceptions of discrimination. *Women & Health, 42,* 23–39.

Thorburn Bird, S., & Bogart, L. M. (2005) Conspiracy beliefs about HIV/AIDS and birth control among African Americans: Implications for the prevention of HIV, other STIs, and unintended pregnancy. *Journal of Social Issues, 61*(1), 109–126.

Thurman, A. R., Livengood, C. H., & Soper, D. E. (2007). Chronic endometritis in DMPA users and chlymydia trachomatis endometritis. *Contraception, 76,* 49–52.

Trussell, J. (2006). Mechanism of action of emergency contraceptive pills. *Contraception, 74,* 87–89.

Turner, C., & Darity, W. (1973). Fears of genocide among Black Americans as related to age, sex and region. *American Journal of Public Health, 63*(12), 1029–1034.

Ulrich, L. T. (1990). *A midwife's tale.* New York: Vintage.

U.S. Department of Health and Human Services. (1978). *Sterilization of persons.* Washington, DC: Author.

Varney, H. (2004). *Varney's midwifery.* Sudbury, MA: Jones and Bartlett.

Vestergaard, P., Rejnmark, L., & Mosekilde, L. (2006). Oral contraceptive use and risk of fractures. *Contraception, 73,* 571–576.

Waters, A. (1997) Conspiracy theories as ethnosociologies: Explanation and intention in African American political culture. *Journal of Black Studies, 28*(1), 112–125.

Weisbord, R. (1973). Birth control and the Black American: A matter of genocide? *Demography, 10*(4), 571–590.

Westhoff, C., Jain, J. K., Milsom, I., & Ray, A. (2007). Changes in weight with depot medroxyprogesterone acetate subcutaneous injection 104 mg/0.65 mL. *Contraception, 75,* 261–267.

Wildemeersch, D. (2007). New frameless and framed intrauterine devices and systems—An overview. *Contraception, 75,* S82–S92.

Willis, S. A., Kuehl, T. J., Spiekerman, M., & Sulak, P. J. (2006). Greater inhibition of the pituitary-ovarian axis in oral contraceptive regimens with a shortened hormone-free interval. *Contraception, 74,* 100–103.

Winter, L. (1988). The role of sexual self-concept in the use of contraceptives. *Family Planning Perspectives, 20,* 123–127.

Wisconsin Pharmacal Company. (1994). *Reality female condom status.* Chicago: Author.

World Health Organization. (2002). *Developing new methods of fertility.* Retrieved November 27, 2002, from www.who.int/reproductive-health/publications/biennial_reports/1994-95/7.html

World Health Organization. (2004). *Medical eligibility criteria for contraceptive use.* Geneva, Switzerland: Author.

World Health Organization. (2006). WHO statement on hormonal contraception and bone health. *Contraception, 73,* 443–444.

Wymelenberg, S. (1990). *Science and babies: Private decisions, public dilemmas.* Washington, DC: National Academy Press.

Wysocki, S. (2006). Effective counseling—At the heart of patient care. *Clinical Issues in Women's Health.* Washington, DC: Nurse Practitioners in Women's Health.

Zavodny, M. (2004). Fertility and parental consent for minors to receive contraceptive *American Journal of Public Health, 94,* 1347–1351.

16

Preconceptional Health Promotion: A Focus for Prevention

Merry-K. Moos

Nearly 20 years ago, a movement began in the United States to rethink traditional efforts to address the occurrence of poor pregnancy outcomes (Institute of Medicine, 1985; Merkatz & Thompson, 1990; Moos & Cefalo, 1987). The resulting initiatives, which came to be known as preconceptional health promotion, were stimulated because the incidence of the two leading causes of infant mortality and morbidity in the United States, congenital anomalies and low birth weight, have remained remarkably stable for nearly 80 years. In its argument to change the traditional approach to prevention from a prenatal focus to one that included prepregnancy wellness, the Institute of Medicine (1985) wrote:

> Only casual attention has been given to the proposition that one of the best protections available against low birth weight and other poor pregnancy outcomes is to have a woman actively plan for pregnancy, enter pregnancy in good health with as few risk factors as possible, and be fully informed about her reproductive and general health. (p. 119)

Moving preconceptional health into the mainstream of care was supported when *Healthy People 2000* put forth a target to increase to at least 60% the proportion of primary care clinicians who provide age-appropriate preconception care (U.S. Department of Health and Human Services, Public Health Service, 1990). Supporting rationale for the objective states that "the purpose of preconceptional care and counseling is to ensure that couples are healthy prior to pregnancy and prepared to assume the responsibilities of parenthood, thereby reducing the risk of poor pregnancy outcomes" (p. 199). Preconceptional health promotion is now recognized as an appropriate emphasis for women's health care by leading professional organizations as well as organizations dedicated to the prevention of perinatal morbidity and mortality in the United States. Among those subscribing to preconceptional health promotion are the American College of Obstetricians and Gynecologists (2002), the American Academy of Pediatrics in collaboration with the American College of Obstetricians and Gynecologists (2002), the Association of Women's Health, Obstetrical and Neonatal Nurses (Hobbins, 2001), the March of Dimes (Moos, 2003a), and the Centers for Disease Control and Prevention (2006).

Despite these endorsements, it is difficult to assess the numbers of providers who are including a preconception focus in the care they offer or, more importantly, the percentage of women reached with preconception information through their clinical encounters (Moos, 2002). Indeed, progress in meeting the target for preconception care and counseling is unknown and may be limited. No objective or systematic evidence exists that preconceptional health promotion has become routine in the health care for women of reproductive age. Part of the problem may be that clinicians are unsure of what to do to promote preconception wellness. However, it has been said that, "If you take care of women of reproductive potential, it's not really a question of whether you provide preconception care, rather it's a question of what kind of preconception care you are providing" (Hobbins, 2003, p. 516).

RATIONALE FOR PRECONCEPTIONAL HEALTH PROMOTION

Eighty-four percent of women in the United States initiate prenatal care in the first trimester of pregnancy (March of Dimes, 2007). At the first prenatal visit, a thorough history and a physical exam are completed to assess risk for pregnancy complications, education is offered to promote healthy pregnancy and birth outcomes, and a prescription for prenatal multivitamins is written. However, many poor pregnancy outcomes or their determinants are present before the first prenatal visit—intendedness of the pregnancy, the interpregnancy interval, the occurrence of spontaneous abortion, abnormal placentation, and the majority of congenital malformations.

Birth defects are the leading cause of infant mortality in the United States but the basic perinatal prevention paradigm starts too late to impact their occurrence. Most structural defects occur during the period of organogenesis, which is between 17 and 56 days following fertilization. Since day 17 is only 3 days after the first missed menstrual period, it is highly unlikely that any women, except those being treated for infertility, will be able to secure prenatal care before the most critical window for normal pregnancy development has begun. In many cases, even early prenatal care, defined as starting in the first trimester, commences after organogenesis is complete. Any insult to the developing embryo during this critical period—such as from teratogenic exposures, poor maternal health status, or abnormal nutrient levels—could result in serious birth defects.

Accumulating research underscores the benefits of reaching women with protective interventions before they become pregnant. For instance, it is well accepted that women who have adequate blood folate levels before organogenesis have a 50% to 70% decreased likelihood of having a fetus affected by a neural tube defect than women who do not have optimal levels (Centers for Disease Control, 1992). Because this protection only occurs if adequate folic acid is available to the embryo during organogenesis, the tradition of initiating vitamin supplementation at the first prenatal visit is too late to protect against these frequently devastating and often lethal birth defects. To promote protective levels of folate, the U.S. Public Health Service issued a recommendation in 1992 that "All women of childbearing age in the United States who are capable of becoming pregnant take 0.4 mg of folic acid (400 mcg) per day for the purpose of reducing their risk of having an affected pregnancy" (Centers for Disease Control, 1992). This recommendation is an example of preconceptional health promotion—altering health status before conception in order to affect the outcome of a future pregnancy. Unfortunately, despite widespread public and provider education, only 31% of nonpregnant women of childbearing age were taking folic acid daily in 2005 (Green-Raleigh, Carter, Mulinare, Prue, & Petrini, 2006).

While preconceptional strategies to prevent neural tube defects are perhaps the most recognized example of impacting pregnancy outcomes before conception, there are many others that are evidence-based (Cefalo & Moos, 1995; Moos, 2003a; Centers for Disease Control, 2006). For instance, research has accumulated for over 20 years that supports the dramatic advantages of women with diabetes achieving tight glucose control prior to becoming pregnant. The offspring of women with pregestational diabetes suffer from major congenital anomalies at approximately three times the rate as the offspring of women without the disease. However, when a woman's blood sugar levels are tightly controlled before and during the earliest weeks of pregnancy, her offspring's risk is reduced to that of or below the background rate (Ray, O'Brien, & Chan, 2001).

Other examples of the advantages of preconceptional over prenatal interventions include altering the medication regimens of women with some chronic diseases (e.g., clotting disorders, seizure disorders, thyroid disease); avoidance of drugs known to be teratogens; identification and treatment of sexually transmitted diseases, including HIV/AIDS, chlamydia, and gonorrhea; administering timely immunizations to protect a woman against infectious diseases that are known to be harmful to fetal development (such as rubella) or to both infant and maternal health (such as varicella and hepatitis B); and encouraging women to avoid alcohol (a potent teratogen) as well as tobacco exposures (a major contributor to many pregnancy complications, including low birth weight, prematurity, and abnormal placentation) (Centers for Disease Control, 2006). Another area of women's health that is best addressed prior to pregnancy is obesity. Adverse perinatal outcomes associated with maternal obesity include neural tube defects, preterm delivery, gestational diabetes, operative deliveries, and hypertensive disorders, among others (Centers for Disease Control, 2006).

PROGRESS IN CHANGING THE PREVENTION PARADIGM

The objectives of preconceptional health promotion are to help women and their partners prevent unintended pregnancies, identify risk factors that could negatively affect reproductive outcomes, and begin education and prevention interventions before conception (Moos, 2003a). The overarching goal is to provide women and, if they desire, their partners with the information they need to make informed decisions about their reproductive futures in a timely manner (Moos, 2003a). Jack and Culpepper (1990) recommended that preconceptional care be made available to all women and their partners as an integrated part of primary care; that it become a routine component of initial and annual family planning visits; and that improvements in preconception care skills be supported for all relevant providers, including family practitioners, obstetricians, internists, nurse-midwives, and nurse practitioners. Lack of progress in adopting preconceptional health as a standard of care for all women of childbearing potential can be explained by several attitudes and circumstances (Moos, 2004), including inadequate education of clinicians about preconceptional health; lack of confidence that preconceptional health counseling will make a difference; a belief that women will seek the care appropriate to their needs, perhaps coupled with a lack of awareness that 50% of the pregnancies in the United States are unintended; and concerns about reimbursement coverage for the service. Another contributor might be the lack of a coordinating body to set an agenda for preconceptional health and gather consensus about its dimensions.

In response to the opportunities of preventing poor pregnancy outcomes by promoting women's health status before pregnancy, the Centers for Disease Control and Prevention (2006) convened a Select Panel on Preconception Care in 2005. The panel brought together representatives from 35 national organizations and 22 CDC programs for the purpose of developing a consensus agenda for reframing the perinatal prevention paradigm. Following deliberation, the panel identified preconception care as a critical component of health care for women of reproductive age and defined it as a set of interventions that aim to identify and modify biomedical, behavioral, and social risks to a woman's health or pregnancy outcome through prevention and management. The specific goals set by the panel are to:

- Improve the knowledge, attitudes, and behaviors of men and women related to preconceptional health.
- Assure that all women of childbearing age in the United States receive preconception care services (i.e., evidence-based risk screening, health promotion, and interventions) that will enable them to enter pregnancy in optimal health.
- Reduce risks indicated by a previous adverse pregnancy outcome through interventions during the interconceptional period, which can prevent or minimize health problems for a mother and her future children.
- Reduce disparities in adverse pregnancy outcomes.

To achieve these goals, changes in consumer knowledge, clinical practice, public health programming, health care financing, and data and research activities were identified as critical. The panel's specific recommendations regarding each of these areas are:

- Consumer
  - □ Each woman, man, and couple should be encouraged to have a reproductive life plan.
  - □ Increase public awareness of preconceptional health behaviors and services using age-appropriate

and culturally competent information and tools that have been developed at appropriate literacy levels.
- Clinical
  - □ As part of primary care visits, all women of childbearing potential should receive risk assessment, education, and health promotion counseling appropriate to reducing reproductive risks and improving pregnancy outcomes.
  - □ Timely interventions for high-risk conditions should be available, accessible, and utilized.
  - □ The interconceptional period should be used to provide intensive interventions to women who have had a previous pregnancy that ended in an adverse outcome.
  - □ The prenatal package should be expanded to include one prepregnancy visit for couples/persons planning pregnancy.
- Public Health
  - □ Components of preconception health should be integrated into existing local public health and related programs, including an emphasis on interconceptional services.
- Financing
  - □ Increase public and private health insurance coverage for women to improve access to preventive women's health and preconception and interconception care for all women.
- Research
  - □ Increase the evidence base for preconception health and promote best practices to improve the delivery and impact of services.
  - □ Maximize public health surveillance and related research mechanisms to monitor preconception health.

One common barrier to reaching women and their partners with critical prevention information before pregnancy is the common belief that a new categorical service, the preconception visit, is needed to impart the care. Although a special preconception visit is appropriate for women with complex medical and reproductive risks, there is little to recommend this tactic as a standard approach for all women (Moos, 2006). Such an approach would be expensive, and it would miss all of the women who unintentionally become pregnant each year. Rather, each encounter with a woman of childbearing potential should include assessment of her desires regarding conception in order to promote deliberateness of decisions about becoming pregnant, assessment of personal and reproductive risks, education about identified risks, and counseling for high levels of wellness. It could and should be argued that these same emphases would be appropriate for all men, as well.

Recent writings have stressed that, for the majority of the population, preconceptional health promotion can be achieved at routine well-woman visits (Hobbins, 2001; Moos, 2002, 2003a, 2003b; Reynolds, 1998). According to the American College of Obstetricians and Gynecologists (2003), "periodic assessments" (which might also be called annual exams, well-woman exams, or the yearly exams) provide an excellent opportunity to include screening, evaluation, and counseling based on age and risk factors. At this visit, risks to the woman's health should be identified; these risks can then be evaluated relative to the woman's immediate and long-term health care expectancies as well as those of any offspring that might be conceived in the future (Moos & Cefalo, 2003). Little could be recommended in routine preconceptional counseling that would not benefit the average woman's general health status, irrespective of eventual conceptions.

> For instance, whether the woman plans to become pregnant or not, her smoking habits should be determined at every visit and clear recommendations and strategies for cessation, if needed, offered. To do less is to give poor care relative to the woman's immediate needs; however, in providing this emphasis in each routine visit, not only is the woman's health addressed but also her preconceptional wellness. (Moos, 2002, p. 72)

Similarly, addressing a woman's weight status and dietary intake at her routine wellness visit has the potential to impact not only her immediate and long-term health, but also the health of future pregnancies, should she conceive. Asking women at each visit about their desires for future conceptions not only offers information on which to base contraceptive counseling, but also provides a natural, important, and often overlooked opportunity for education about the benefits of planned pregnancies (Moos, 2002).

A study suggests that providers are not taking advantage of preconceptional health promotion opportunities afforded by routine gynecology visits (Bernstein, Sanghvi, & Merkatz, 2000). In a review of the medical records of 100 women of an inner-city gynecology service, assessments important to medical care, in general, as well as to preconceptional health promotion, in particular, were rarely present. Although 71% of the records noted that family planning methods had been assessed and 72% documented toxic habits had been investigated, other areas traditionally considered components of a routine assessment were not generally present. Less than 30% of the records included documentation of a thorough medical history, over-the-counter drug exposures, domestic violence, nutritional status, and dietary supplementation. Just 30% included evidence that prescription drug use had been explored. The researchers hypothesized that, because preconceptional counseling as a routine component of care for all reproductive age women is a relatively recent emphasis for care, it has

yet to become routine. The results of the study pointed out, however, that issues important to well-woman care, irrespective of the likelihood of future conceptions, were being overlooked (Moos, 2002). Following an educational intervention that included information aimed at heightened awareness of opportunities to integrate preconceptional health information into routine encounters, statistically significant improvements were recorded for all of the health assessments. These improvements reflect better care for women in general, not only women likely to conceive before their next encounter.

CONTENT OF PRECONCEPTIONAL CARE

Table 16.1 identifies areas of importance in a preconceptional assessment—without exception, the same general foci and specific queries are important in the well-woman assessment: medical history, reproductive history, nutritional status, family history, infectious disease risks, and social history. Each annual or well-woman exam for women of reproductive potential should include assessment of the woman's health, desires regarding future conception, and anticipation of risks should pregnancy occur. Risks should be considered for the woman, for the future conceptus, and for the future neonate (Moos, 2003b). For instance, a woman who is on isotretinoin for cystic acne should understand the benefits of this medicine for her condition as well as its serious threat to future pregnancies (because of increased spontaneous abortion rates) and offspring (because isotretinoin is a potent teratogen). Similarly, a woman with chronic hypertension being treated with ACE inhibitors should understand the implications of chronic hypertension on pregnancy, and the fetal/neonatal risks of ACE inhibitors. Women should be encouraged to be deliberate about if and when to become pregnant and be aware that planning for pregnancy in conjunction with their health care providers will reduce reproductive risks for them, their pregnancies, and their offspring.

MOVING THE AGENDA FORWARD

A three-tier approach to achieving the preconception agenda may prove helpful in focusing energies (Moos, 2003a). The tiers are general awareness of the importance of the earliest weeks of pregnancy by both health professionals and the public; a focus on health promotion and disease prevention for all women, with special attention to conditions and behaviors that could pose a risk to a healthy pregnancy for those women who might conceive; and utilization of targeted services for women identified to be at high risk for a complicated antenatal course or poor pregnancy outcome.

16.1 | A Preconception Health Assessment Tool

Medical history	Is the woman under current or former treatment for: ■ Diabetes mellitus? ■ Thyroid disorders? ■ Hyperphenylalaninemia? ■ Asthma? ■ Heart disease? ■ Chronic hypertension? ■ Deep venous thrombosis? ■ Kidney disease? ■ Systemic lupus erythematosus? ■ Epilepsy? ■ Hemoglobinopathies? ■ Cancer? Does the woman handle feline litter boxes or eat raw or very rare meat? Does the woman take any prescribed medications? Does the woman take any over-the-counter medications?
Reproductive history	Has the woman had: ■ Uterine or cervical abnormalities? ■ Two or more pregnancies ending in first-trimester miscarriage without an intervening successful gestation? ■ One or more fetal deaths? ■ One or more preterm deliveries? ■ One or more small-for-gestational age infants? ■ One or more infants requiring care in a neonatal intensive care unit? ■ One or more infants with a birth defect?
Nutrition	Does the woman: ■ Practice vegetarianism? ■ Eat a special diet? ■ Have a history of bulimia or anorexia? ■ Use vitamin supplements in excess of the recommended daily allowance? ■ Have a history of pica? ■ Have a body mass index lower than 19 or higher than 29? ■ Consume adequate folic acid?
Family history	Does the woman, her partner, any of their offspring, or any member of their families have: ■ Hemophilia? ■ Thalassemia? ■ Tay-Sachs trait or disease? ■ Sickle cell disease or trait? ■ Phenylketonuria? ■ Cystic fibrosis? ■ Birth defects? ■ Mental retardation?
Social history	Does the woman: ■ Drink beer, wine, or hard liquor? ■ Smoke cigarettes or use other tobacco products? ■ Use marijuana, cocaine, or other drugs? ■ Use lead or chemicals at home or at work?

(continued)

16.1 | A Preconception Health Assessment Tool (*continued*)

	■ Participate in activities that could result in overheating (e.g., using saunas or hot tubs, demanding exercise in hot, humid conditions)? ■ Have evidence of current or former physical, sexual, or psychological abuse? ■ Have a plan for spacing and timing her pregnancies? ■ Have maternity benefits in her insurance program? ■ Know her employer's policies regarding pregnancy and birth?
Infectious disease risks	Does the woman or her partner have occupational exposures to the blood or bodily secretions of others? Is the woman or her partner at risk for HIV? Is the woman immune to: ■ Hepatitis B? ■ Varicella? ■ Rubella? ■ Tetanus? ■ Pertussis?

Note. Adapted from *Preconceptional Health Care: A Practical Guide* (2nd ed.), by R. C. Cefalo and M. K. Moos, 1995, St. Louis, MO: Mosby.

The first tier, general awareness, can be achieved through basic and continuing education for professionals and through social marketing efforts to introduce and reinforce the importance of healthy life choices throughout the life span to impact healthy futures for the woman, herself, and for any children she might choose to have. Social marketing to promote deliberate decisions about when and if to become pregnant is also part of this first tier. The advantages of well-constructed social marketing efforts could be improvements in the health of men and recognition of the advantages of planning whether and when to have children. The second tier is opportunistic—that is, it takes advantage of every encounter with a woman who might, at some point, become pregnant to assess her health profiles for risks that could pose special challenges to a healthy pregnancy outcome (Moos, 2002). This tier can and should be framed to incorporate the motto used in California for its preconception initiative, Every Woman, Every Time (Cullum, 2003). The third tier requires the availability and coordination of specialty services to address conditions known to present high risks to women in pregnancy or for their offspring. Examples include genetic counseling for the woman/couple with family histories suggestive of genetic abnormalities; endocrine care to help a woman with diabetes achieve good glucose control, and work-ups for women with repeated pregnancy losses.

Nearly 18 years ago, Jack and Culpepper (1990) offered specific recommendations for improving the awareness and availability of preconception care for all women of childbearing potential. Their recommendations, which were informative in the deliberations of the Select Panel on Preconception Care, are as sound today as when they were first offered.

■ Preconception care should be made available to all women and their partners as an integrated part of primary care services.
■ Preconception care should become a routine component of initial and annual family planning visits.
■ Improvement of preconception care skills should be supported for all relevant providers, including family practitioners, internists, obstetricians, nurse practitioners, midwives, and family planning clinic personnel.

It is discouraging that nurses were not specifically identified in the list. Additional steps important to advancing the vision of the Select Panel were offered in 2004 (Moos, 2004):

■ Individual nurses and professional nursing organizations should assume leadership roles in reaching women with the information they need to make informed preconceptional decisions.
■ Basic nursing and medical education should integrate the impact of preconceptional health status on pregnancy outcomes in all relevant curriculum. For instance, study of the mechanisms of disease for diabetes should include the risk of congenital anomalies if a diabetic woman conceives while in poor control;

study of hematologic disorders should include impact on recurrent pregnancy loss and the teratogenic potential of some anticoagulant drugs. Expanding emphasis on the prevention of reproductive casualties beyond the boundaries of courses specific to obstetrics will promote awareness among providers in all specialty areas.

■ The occurrence of unintended pregnancies in the United States and strategies to impact on the rate should be specifically addressed in basic nursing and medical education and in continuing education programs (see chapter 19 for further discussion of unintended pregnancy).

■ Unintended pregnancy should become a recognized and widely reported health indicator comparable to low birth weight and prematurity. To make this a meaningful indicator, the ability to accurately measure its occurrence needs to be refined (Petersen & Moos, 1997).

■ The content of routine preconceptional care needs to be demystified. Routine or annual well-woman visits for all women of reproductive potential should include specific inquiries about intentions regarding future conceptions and when a woman hopes to become pregnant or pregnant again; review of the medical history to identify potential maternal-fetal risks; review of the obstetrical history to identify potential health risks to the woman and to any future pregnancies; and the framing of health care advice that integrates the woman's total health profile into a model that promotes her health, the health of future desired pregnancies, and the health of future offspring, should pregnancy be chosen. Little could be recommended in terms of health behaviors and high levels of personal wellness that would not benefit women's pregnancies should they conceive (Moos, 2003b). This integrated approach to women's wellness care should become the standard of care for all women of reproductive age rather than the exception.

■ Innovations in practice that allow providers to efficiently incorporate preconceptional health information into routine health encounters should be disseminated through innovative continuing education endeavors. Examples of such innovations have begun to surface (Cullum, 2003).

■ Interconceptional care should become a focus of care for all women who have had a pregnancy that ended in a fetal or neonatal loss, a low–birth weight infant, or a congenital anomaly. Often risk factors that may have contributed to a previous poor pregnancy outcome are not considered or addressed until a woman initiates prenatal care in her next gestation (Moos, 2003b). Thus, many women enter prenatal care after those risks have already exercised their influence on the pregnancy's ultimate outcome. In accordance with the recommendations of the Select Panel on

Preconception Care, models for addressing interconceptional risks are surfacing (Biermann, Dunlop, Brady, Dubin, & Brann, 2006; Lu et al., 2006; Loomis & Martin, 2000). Replication of emerging programs and innovations in addressing the interconceptional health care needs of women as well as evaluation of impact are all needed.

Despite the relative paucity of carefully designed studies to prospectively prove the value of general preconceptional health promotion activities, such an emphasis in care should not be discounted. It has the potential to empower women to make informed decisions about future childbearing, and such decisions may result in higher rates of pregnancy intendedness in the United States and in earlier initiation of prenatal care—behaviors that have repeatedly been demonstrated to favorably impact on perinatal outcomes (Moos, 2002). Indeed, much that may be important about including a preconceptional health focus in the routine care of women of childbearing age has probably not yet been measured. Preconceptional health promotion activities well done should increase the level of health for all women of reproductive age, the likelihood that pregnancies are identified as intended, the rate at which our nation's children are born healthy, and the likelihood that women will look back on their behaviors and choices around the time of conception and feel comfortable with the decisions they made (Moos, 2004).

REFERENCES

American Academy of Pediatrics & American College of Obstetricians and Gynecologists. (2002). *Guidelines for perinatal care* (5th ed.). Elk Grove, IL, and Washington, DC: Author.

American College of Obstetricians and Gynecologists. (2002). *Guidelines for women's health care* (2nd ed.). Washington, DC: Author.

American College of Obstetricians and Gynecologists. (2003). ACOG Committee Opinion No. 292: Primary and Preventive Care: Periodic Assessments. *Obstetrics & Gynecology, 102*(5), 117–124.

Bernstein, P. S., Sanghvi, T., & Merkatz, I. (2000). Improving preconception care. *Journal of Reproductive Medicine, 45,* 546.

Bierman, J., Dunlop, A. L., Brady, C., Dubin, C., & Brann Jr., A. (2006). Promising Practices in Preconception Care for Women at Risk for Poor Health and Pregnancy Outcomes. *Maternal and Child Health Journal, 10*(5), S21-S28.

Cefalo, R. C., & Moos, M. K. (1995). *Preconceptional health care: A practical guide* (2nd ed.). St. Louis, MO: Mosby.

Centers for Disease Control. (1992). Recommendation for the use of folic acid to reduce the number of cases of spina bifida and other neural tube defects. *MMWR, 41*(RR-14).

Centers for Disease Control. (2006). Recommendations to improve preconception health and health care—United States. *MMWR, 55*(RR06), 1–23.

Cullum, A. (2003). Changing provider practices to enhance preconceptional wellness. *Journal of Obstetric, Gynecologic, and Neonatal Nursing, 32*(4), 543–549.

Green-Raleigh, K., Carter, H., Mulinare, J., Prue, C., & Petrini, J. (2006). Trends in folic acid awareness and behavior in the

United States: The Gallup Organization for the March of Dimes Foundation Surveys, 1995–2005. *Maternal and Child Health Journal, 10,* S177–S182.

Hobbins, D. (2001). *Preconception care: Maximizing the health of women and their newborns.* AWHONN Practice Monograph. Washington, DC: Association of Women's Health, Obstetric and Neonatal Nurses.

Hobbins, D. (2003). Full circle: The evolution of preconception health promotion in America. *Journal of Obstetric, Gynecologic, and Neonatal Nursing, 32*(4), 516–522.

Institute of Medicine. (1985). *Preventing low birthweight.* Washington, DC: National Academy Press.

Jack, B., & Culpepper, L. (1990). Preconception care. In I. R. Merkatz & J. E. Thompson (Eds.), *New perspectives on prenatal care* (pp. 69–88). New York: Elsevier.

Loomis, L. W., & Martin, M. W. (2000). The Interconception Health Promotion Initiative: A demonstration project to reduce the incidence of repeat LBW deliveries in an urban safety net hospital. *Family & Community Health, 23*(3), 1–16.

Lu, M. C., Kotelchuck, M., Culhane, J. F., Hobel, C. J., Klerman, L. V., & Thorp Jr., J. M. (2006). Preconception Care Between Pregnancies: The Content of Internatal Care. *Maternal and Child Health Journal, 10*(5), S107–S122.

March of Dimes. (2007). *Distribution of prenatal care timing categories: US, 2004.* Retrieved June 27, 2007, from http://www.marchofdimes.com/peristats

Merkatz, I. R., & Thompson J. E. (Eds). (1990). *New perspectives on prenatal care.* New York: Elsevier.

Moos, M. K. (2002). Perceptional health promotion: Opportunities abound. *Maternal and Child Health Journal, 6*(2), 71–3.

Moos, M. K. (2003a). *Preconception health promotion: A focus for women's wellness* (2nd ed.). White Plains, NY: March of Dimes.

Moos, M. K. (2003b). Preconceptional wellness as a routine objective for women's health care: An integrative strategy. *Journal of Obstetric, Gynecologic, and Neonatal Nursing, 32*(4), 550–556.

Moos, M. K. (2004). Preconceptional health promotion: Progress in changing a prevention paradigm. *Journal of Perinatal & Neonatal Nursing, 18*(1), 2–13.

Moos, M. K. (2006). Preconception health: Where to from here? *Women's Health Issues, 16,* 156–158.

Moos, M. K., & Cefalo, R. C. (1987). Preconceptional health promotion: A focus for obstetric care. *American Journal of Perinatology, 4*(1), 63–67.

Moos, M. K., & Cefalo, R. C. (2003). Preconception counseling. In J. Sciarra (Ed.), *Gynecology and obstetrics looseleaf: Vol. 2.* Philadelphia: Lippincott Williams & Wilkins.

Petersen, R., & Moos, M. K. (1997). Defining and measuring unintended pregnancy: A historical background. *Women's Health Issues, 7*(4), 234–240.

Ray, J. G., O'Brien, T. E., & Chan, W. S. (2001). Preconception care and the risk of congenital anomalies in the offspring of women with diabetes mellitus: A meta-analysis. *Quarterly Journal of Medicine, 94*(8), 435–444.

Reynolds, H. D. (1998). Preconception care: An integral part of primary care for woman. *Journal of Nurse Midwifery, 6,* 445–452.

U.S. Department of Health and Human Services, Public Health Service. (1990). *Healthy People 2000.* DHHS Publication No. (PHS); 91–50212. Washington, DC: Author.

PART IV

Threats to Health and Health Problems

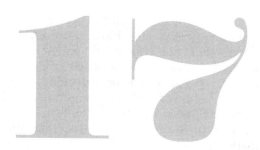

High-Risk Childbearing

Catherine Ingram Fogel and
Julie Smith Taylor

Most expectant mothers will have an uneventful pregnancy with a favorable outcome. Pregnancy itself is not an illness but a normal life event that can sometimes be complicated by illness or medical conditions with approximately 5% to 10% of all pregnancies being categorized as high risk (Dangal, 2008). When a high-risk pregnancy occurs, the challenge to the advanced practice nurse is great. This chapter will present information needed by advanced practice nurses to provide optimal care to clients experiencing any combination of biological, emotional, and social conditions that might pose a threat to the mother or the fetus by (a) defining the concept of high-risk pregnancy; (b) exploring the scope and magnitude of the problem; (c) presenting information about specific risk factors as they are likely to present during the maternity cycle; (d) discussing identification of the high-risk client, including diagnostic procedures for determining the client at risk; and (e) analyzing appropriate nursing interventions.

This chapter is unique in its approach to high-risk pregnancy surveillance in that it not only addresses the biological conditions that can significantly increase the risk of morbidity and mortality for both the mother and the baby, but also identifies the critical points during the childbearing cycle when most problems will arise. Many common complications of pregnancy can predictably present and be identified within a specified time frame during the pregnancy cycle, while others (psychosocial, domestic violence, environmental exposures) may pose a threat at any point during the maternity cycle. Information on how to manage pregnancy complications can be found elsewhere in numerous medical texts and will not be presented in depth in this chapter. According to the *Guidelines for Perinatal Care*

(American Academy of Pediatrics & American College of Obstetricians and Gynecologists [AAP/ACOG], 2007), effective risk identification is a key strategy for managing women and fetuses at risk of morbidity or mortality and improving overall outcome. Therefore, the approach of this chapter is to identify those times during prenatal care and assessment that high-risk complications are most likely to arise and be identified. Ideally, issues related to genetics (advanced maternal age, cystic fibrosis, sickle cell disease), lifestyle behaviors (substance use/abuse, employment), and medical conditions (hypertension, diabetes, thyroid disease) should be identified and addressed prior to conception. During the first trimester, prenatal labs, history, or physical examination may identify a potential or existing problem—such as HIV, anemia, heart murmur, abnormal cervical cytology, or cervical shortening—that can persist throughout the pregnancy and place the mother and/or fetus at risk. Preterm labor, gestational diabetes and Rh isoimmunization are primary concerns of the second trimester. During the third trimester, hypertensive disorders, growth discrepancies, group B strep colonization, and post-term gestation present the greatest risk of morbidity and mortality for the mother and the baby.

DEFINITION AND SCOPE OF THE PROBLEM

Traditionally, a high-risk pregnancy has been defined as one in which the mother or infant (or fetus) has a significantly increased chance of morbidity or mortality when compared with a low-risk pregnancy, in which an optimal outcome is expected for both, either before, during, or after birth. However, a broader definition would allow for consideration of morbidity and mortality resulting from a variety of causative agents—physical, psychological, or sociocultural—that place the mother, fetus, or both at risk during the childbearing cycle. Childbearing carries with it the potential for risk because of the numerous, often catastrophic, factors involved—many of which are impossible to predict or control. The potential for risk exists on a continuum ranging from little or no risk to the woman and her family to the risk of death for the mother and fetus. An understanding of the extent and magnitude of high-risk childbearing may be gained by examining the statistical data available on maternal morbidity and mortality, infant mortality, and perinatal mortality.

Maternal mortality rates declined 99% in the United States over the 20th century, from 850 deaths per 100,000 live births in 1900 to 7.5 deaths per 100,000 live births in 1982 (Chang et al., 2003). However, little progress has been made since that time in reaching the *Healthy People 2010* goal of 3.3 deaths per 100,000 live births (U.S. Department of Health and Human Services, 2000). Historically, most maternal deaths were attributed to hemorrhage, pregnancy-induced hypertension, and infection. Although this triad still accounts for most maternal deaths, medical advances such as antibiotics, safe blood supplies and transfusions, and medical management of hypertension disorders of pregnancy have been credited with the decline in maternal mortality (Centers for Disease Control and Prevention [CDC], 1999a). Moreover, access to adequate prenatal care to manage these and other pregnancy-related complications is a strong predictor of maternal mortality (Maine, 2001). Despite these advances, ethnic discrepancies continue to exist, with women of color having a maternal mortality rate significantly higher than the rate of White women (Koonin, MacKay, Berg, Atrash, & Smith, 1997). The mortality rate is three to six times higher among African American women than among White women (CDC, 1999b). Women are less likely to seek early prenatal care when the pregnancy is unintended (Hulsey, 2001). The breadth of this problem can only be appreciated when one realizes that approximately half of all pregnancies in the United States are unintended (Henshaw, 1998).

It could be argued that childbirth is much safer today if only mortality rates were considered; however, maternal morbidity rates, if they were available, would offer a much more comprehensive view of the entire maternity cycle. Although statistics surface indicating, for example, that 6% to 8% of all pregnancies are complicated by preeclampsia (AAP/ACOG, 2007), the availability of accurate statistics regarding the percentage of women experiencing pregnancy-related complications suffer from a lack of uniformity in reporting even

though we recognize that pregnancy-related complications continue to be a major cause of morbidity and mortality. Furthermore, our definition of high risk is not limited to, or measured in, complications or deaths alone. There are many social, psychological, and economic factors to be considered. These are discussed later in the section on specific risk factors.

In considering the scope of high-risk pregnancy, the infant mortality rate should be reviewed. Despite a significant decline in overall infant mortality during the 20th century, tremendous ethnic and racial disparities persist in infant mortality. This inequitable decrease in infant mortality across all social and ethnic boundaries continues to further make the *Healthy People 2010* national objective of reducing the infant mortality rate to 4.5 or fewer deaths per 1,000 live births even more elusive. Similarly, the fetal mortality rate for non-Hispanic Black women was 2.3 times that of non-Hispanic White women during 2004 (MacDorman, Munson, & Kirmeyer, 2007).

Nearly half of all infant deaths recorded are attributed to three causes: congenital malformations (19.5%), disorders related to preterm birth and low birth weight (16.4%), and sudden infant death syndrome (7%) (CDC, 2005). Despite technological advances over the past few decades and improved quality and access to prenatal care, the incidence of low birth weight, which has a significant impact on the infant mortality rate, has changed very little in the past 30 years. Low–birth weight infants, predominantly the product of high-risk pregnancies, contribute significantly to infant mortality and have greater morbidity in their life times. In 2004, 8.1% of all live births (representing an 18% increase since 1990) were considered to be low birth weight (Martin, Hamilton, Menacker, Sutton, & Mathews, 2004). Today, 7% of all live births in the United States are infants who weigh less than 2,500 grams. In 1997, 65% of infant deaths resulted from the 7.5% of infants born with low birth weight (Kochanek & Martin, 2007). When race is considered, wide discrepancies in infant mortality rates are observed: 5.7% for White infants and 12.7% for African American infants. Deaths for low–birth weight infants in the neonatal period are 30 times more frequent than for infants of normal or average birth weight. It is now widely believed that if birth weight could be improved, infant mortality and morbidity could be substantially reduced.

RISK FACTORS

Obstetricians have long recognized that some women are more likely than others to experience poorer outcomes of pregnancy. While Hippocrates recognized that the outcomes of pregnancy were influenced by intrinsic, extrinsic, and environmental factors, risk factors have traditionally been viewed only within a medical model framework; that is, only medical, obstetrical, or physiological risk factors were considered. However, more recently, health professionals have begun to recognize the need for a more comprehensive model within which to frame high-risk pregnancy. The risk identification model has become a valuable tool for evaluating risk status in pregnancy. In the context of this comprehensive model, pregnant women do not exist in a vacuum free of environmental or social influences; rather, age, parity, environmental influences, and emotional stressors are viewed as equally important factors to consider along with specific disease entities, such as hypertension or diabetes.

With a comprehensive risk identification framework, factors associated with high-risk childbearing can be grouped into broad categories based on specific threats to health and pregnancy outcome. Moreover, timely identification and management of risk factors during the maternity cycle is optimized. Categories of risk include biophysical, psychosocial, sociodemographic, and environmental. Risks that are considered to be biophysical in nature include factors that originate within the mother or the fetus and affect the development or functioning of either. Sociodemographic risks arise from characteristics of the mother and her family that place the childbearing unit at risk. Psychosocial risks involve maternal behaviors and adverse lifestyles that have a negative impact on the health of the mother and the fetus. Internal conflicts, emotional distress, and disturbed interpersonal relationships are likewise considered to be risk factors, as are inadequate social support and unsafe cultural practices. Environmental factors arise from circumstances outside of the woman and her family, including work place hazards and the general environment.

Risk factors are often interrelated and cumulative in their effects. Rarely is serious risk incurred with the presence of a single factor. Usually, high-risk status occurs when several risk factors coexist simultaneously. It is important to remember that risk is incurred within the unit; a threat to the health and well-being of the mother will most often have an adverse effect—direct or indirect—on the fetus. In addition, some threats that arise within the fetus can present a threat to the mother. At times, the mother will be at greater risk, and, in other instances, the fetus will risk the greatest harm. However, when the mother is seriously threatened, the fetus will likewise be in jeopardy. Extending this concept further, pregnancy exists in the context of the family/social unit. Therefore, if the woman and her fetus are threatened, there can be a negative impact on the larger family unit. Conversely, risk to the pregnant woman and her fetus can be intensified by a lack of social support and a worrisome or dangerous family situation.

Biophysical Risk Factors

Genetic

Genetic factors may interfere with normal fetal/neonatal development, result in congenital anomalies, and create difficulties for pregnant women. Defective maternal or paternal genes as well as transmittable inherited disorders can cause genetic disease or anomalies. Deviations in fetal development place the fetus and, at times, the mother at risk. Moreover, known fetal abnormalities and disorders place the mother and family unit at risk of emotional trauma or distress throughout the pregnancy. The most obvious risks are those resulting from chromosomal abnormalities; however, other less aberrant deviations create risk. Multiple gestations carry an increased risk for low–birth weight infants as well as create excessive stress on the woman. Large fetal size can create abnormal labor patterns and birth injuries as a result of dystocia. Certain genetically determined maternal or paternal characteristics can pose a risk in pregnancy. ABO incompatibility (incompatibility of blood types) and Rh incompatibility with its resultant anemia and hyperbilirubinemia in the fetus or newborn are examples of such inherited characteristics. Recessive disorders such as sickle cell anemia, cystic fibrosis, and Tay-Sachs disease are of particular concern if both parents are genetic carriers. Ideally, the potential for familial disorders would be identified preconceptually.

Nutritional Status

Many demographic, sociocultural, and behavioral factors have been associated with weight gain in pregnancy (Varney, Kriebs, & Gegor, 2004). Recommended ranges for weight gain during pregnancy that provide the optimal outcome for the mother and the fetus have been proposed by the Institute of Medicine (2000). Weight gain recommendations during pregnancy are based on prepregnancy weight as follows: for women with a prepregnancy body mass index (BMI) of less than 19.7, the recommended weight gain is 28 to 40 pounds; for women with a BMI of 19.8 to 26, the recommended weight gain is 25 to 35 pounds; for women with a BMI of 26.1 to 29, the recommended weight gain is 15 to 25 pounds); and for women with a BMI of 30 or higher, the recommended weight gain is at least 15 pounds). Fewer than half of pregnant women gain the amount of weight that is necessary to decrease the likelihood of delivering a low–birth weight infant (Varney, Kriebs, & Gegor, 2004). Prenatal care providers have an obligation to educate women about appropriate weight gain during pregnancy and its effect on birth outcomes. Nutritional risk factors present at the beginning of pregnancy include very young age (younger than 15 years); previous poor pregnancy outcomes; three pregnancies in the past two years; tobacco, alcohol, or drug use; inadequate diet due to chronic illness or food fads; and weight less than 85% or greater than 120% of ideal body weight for height. For example, both normal-weight and obese smokers were less likely than their nonsmoking counterparts to gain the recommended amount of weight during pregnancy (Hellerstedt, Himes, Story, Alton, & Edwards, 1997). While inadequate weight gain is associated with low birth weight, excessive weight gain during pregnancy is associated with complications such as macrosomia. Kaiser and Kirby (2001) found, in a study of 1,881 women who delivered between 1994 and 1998, that women with a BMI greater than 29 had a 7.7% cesarean birth rate, while women with a normal BMI (19.8 to 25.9) had a cesarean birth rate of 4.1%. Moreover, short women and obese women were even more likely to deliver by cesarean section. Finally, inadequate or excessive weight gain during pregnancy and a hematocrit of less than 33% are strong predictors of nutritional risk.

Medical and Obstetrical Risk Factors

Medical complications in a previous or the current pregnancy (insulin-dependent diabetes, cardiac disease, hypothyroidism, or obesity), obstetrical complications (hypertensive disorders of pregnancy, preterm delivery, or placenta previa), and recurrent pregnancy losses have long been identified as risk factors and are discussed at length in many standard textbooks. The most common medical and obstetrical complications are given in Table 17.1.

It has long been recognized that obstetrical complications tend to recur in subsequent pregnancies. Furthermore, it has been clearly documented that women with a history of a prior pregnancy loss are at increased risk for future losses. The etiology of this risk factor varies depending on when during the pregnancy it occurs. In early pregnancy, the major risk factors are genetic abnormalities and structural anomalies of the reproductive tract. As pregnancy progresses, obstetrical and chronic medical diseases of the mother become the major risk factor.

Sociodemographic Risk Factors

Although childbearing risk usually is attributed to biophysical factors alone, multiple factors, including sociodemographic characteristics, are associated with increased pregnancy risk in many instances. Sociodemographic characteristics are defined as those factors that dictate lifestyle and influence participation in social behaviors (i.e., substance use and abuse). They are often interdependent and determined by where an individual lives; her access to services and health care; and her family's values, attitudes, and social support system. While many sociodemographic factors that indicate high risk are easily identifiable, it is not possible to determine the specific ways in which these factors will create problems for a given woman. Sociodemographic risk factors most associated with poor pregnancy outcomes are low income, lack of prenatal care, age, parity, residence, and race.

Low Income

For over half a century, it has been noted that the population segment most at risk of complications during childbearing is comprised of the most socioeconomically underprivileged. Poverty underlies many other risk factors intrinsic to the population most at risk

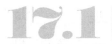 **17.1** | Common Risk Factors Associated with Adverse Pregnancy Outcomes

MEDICAL	OBSTETRICAL	PSYCHOSOCIAL/SOCIODEMOGRAPHIC
Heart disease	Multiple gestation	Low income
Hypertension	Preterm labor	Age extremes
Diabetes	PIH	Parity
Infection	Anemia	Marital status
Collagen vascular disorder	Bleeding disorders	Residence
Anemia	Genetic abnormalities	Ethnicity
Seizure disorder	Recurrent pregnancy loss	Substance use/abuse
		Interpersonal violence
		Insufficient social support
		Maternal role conflict

including race and residence. Inadequate financial resources highly correlate with low birth weight and increased infant mortality. The poor experience increased risk because of poorer general health and nutrition prior to and during pregnancy as well as inadequate or nonexistent prenatal care. Many low-income mothers either seek prenatal care very late in pregnancy, if at all. Moreover, low-income women are more likely to have medical complications that predispose them to increases in perinatal mortality; they experience increased prenatal morbidity with increased risk or mortality; and they more often report a history of prior prenatal loss, which places them at greater risk for fetal loss with a current pregnancy. Likewise, low-income women are considerably more predisposed to illnesses and obstetrical complications during pregnancy. Because these women have either no or minimal prenatal care, their complications tend to be much more progressed than women who are consistently screened for complications throughout their pregnancy. Poverty places an indirect effect on high-risk pregnancy in that other significant risk factors—such as nutritional status, emotional disturbances, and environmental influences—are all affected by socioeconomic status.

Lack of Prenatal Care

Despite the increased availability of prenatal care, the incidence of low birth weight has continued to increase as well during the past two decades. Although the goal of prenatal care has been to readily identify potentially avoidable or treatable conditions associated with poor perinatal outcomes (Gregory & Davidson, 1999), many question the current approach to prenatal care (Moos, 2006). Women who lack access to adequate prenatal care, who underutilize prenatal care, or who initiate prenatal care late in their gestation have an increased risk of morbidity and mortality (CDC, 1999a). Little or no prenatal care places pregnant women and fetuses at greatest risk because the opportunity is lost for early diagnosis and treatment of obstetrical complications. Many complications are easily identifiable early in the pregnancy when corrective measures could be initiated. Women who experience an unintended pregnancy are more likely to initiate prenatal care late in gestation or fail to seek adequate prenatal care (Hulsey, 2001). Research indicates that less than half of women experiencing an unintended pregnancy seek prenatal care during the first trimester (CDC, 1999a). Moreover, research indicates that teenagers and women who initially considered abortion were more likely to initiate prenatal care late or after the first trimester (Hulsey, Laken, Miller, & Ager, 2000). Late initiation of prenatal care minimizes the opportunity to reasonably alter the effects of lifestyle behaviors that pose serious risks to the mother and fetus. Socioeconomic characteristics associated with unintended pregnancy include young age, income, race, and marital status (Henshaw, 1998). Further, women with no prenatal care are more likely to deliver a low–birth weight infant than women with adequate prenatal care. Developing prenatal care services that meet the needs of low-income women as well as recognizing that the reasons for not seeking prenatal care are multifaceted (Sword, 1999) are the first of many steps in the right direction for enhancing the use of health services to improve the health of both mothers and fetuses. Eliminating long waiting times in clinics and providing funding to decrease the cost of care might be reasonable strategies to encourage women to seek care early in their prenatal course (Beckmann, Buford, & Witt, 2000). Nurses need to develop programs of prenatal services that women view as valuable. Mikhail (2000) demonstrated that women who viewed prenatal care as valuable and useful were more likely to attend than those who did not see value in the routine services provided.

Many women do not understand the need for early and continued prenatal care, and there is a trend in many states of more women receiving late or no prenatal care (Park, Vincent, & Hastings-Tolsma, 2007). Their previous orientation to the health care system may have focused on treatment of illness, not prevention and health maintenance. Pregnant women, regardless of their income or background, may not know what type of care is available, how to get an appointment, how early they should present for the first visit, or how to obtain this information. For others, they may feel that they already know how to care for themselves and believe as long as the baby is moving and they feel well, routine prenatal care is unnecessary.

Age

Age has long been considered a crucial variable in determining high-risk pregnancy. Traditionally, women at either end of the childbearing continuum have been considered to be at high risk during pregnancy, because the incidence of poor outcomes increases with both. An examination of statistics reveals that risk and poor outcomes are high in the very young (age 15 and younger), drop to minimal levels during the 20s, and then rise continually until the end of the childbearing years. Research supports the theory that age is related to poor outcomes in some instances but not in others. Some theorize that teenage mothers and their babies may be at more risk of adverse outcomes because they tend to delay seeking prenatal care, are more likely to smoke during pregnancy, and have fewer resources to manage the emotional and financial responsibilities of pregnancy and childbirth (Ventura, Mathews, & Hamilton, 2001); others have found that younger teenage mothers (ages 13 to 17) have a significantly higher risk of adverse pregnancy outcomes, including premature delivery, small-for-gestational-age infants, and low-birth weight infants than women who were 20 to 24 years of age, regardless of other factors. These adverse pregnancy outcomes appear to be independent of confounding sociodemographic variables (Fraser, Brockert, & Ward, 1995). Moreover, Smith and Pell (2001) found that, while first teenage births may not be associated with an increased risk of adverse pregnancy outcomes, second teenage births are at greater risk of preterm delivery and stillbirth. Therefore, the conclusion should not be automatically drawn that women outside the optimal age range are necessarily at an increased risk of adverse outcome. Both physiological and psychological variables need to be considered in assigning risk.

On the other hand, clinicians have traditionally viewed women over the age of 35—especially first-time mothers—as high-risk patients. Risks associated with childbearing at an advanced age do not arise from age alone but rather are affected by numerous lifestyle, historical, social, and demographic factors as well as the number and spacing of previous pregnancies; genetic disposition of the parents; and the medical history, lifestyle, nutrition, and prenatal care of the mother. Socioeconomic factors influencing later childbearing include income, education, housing, and social networks.

Parity

The number of women's previous pregnancies can be a risk factor and is often associated with maternal age. Some authorities consider first pregnancies to be potentially high risk, no matter what the age of the mother. However, more risk is incurred when the first pregnancy is on either end of the childbearing-age spectrum. The incidence of pregnancy-induced hypertension and dystocia is higher in first births; and firstborns have higher rates of morbidity and mortality.

Psychosocial Risk Factors

Certain lifestyle patterns and maternal behaviors can have an adverse impact on pregnancy outcomes. Use of alcohol and tobacco is widely accepted in U.S. society, despite widespread health education efforts to inform the public about the dangers of their use. Many women view the use of tobacco, alcohol, and drugs as habitual or medicinal in nature and do not realize they are consuming biologically active substances that cross the placental barrier. Hellerstedt and colleagues (1998) found that, in comparison to women whose pregnancies were intended, women with unintended pregnancies were less likely to reduce caffeine consumption and usually continued to smoke. Nicotine, caffeine, alcohol, and drugs can influence reproduction either through direct action on the embryo or fetus or indirectly when the maternal equilibrium is disturbed.

Smoking

The Centers for Disease Control (2006) estimate that over 20 million (20.3%) women currently smoke, creating a tremendous health impact for women of reproductive age. In 2003, 10.7% of women smoked during their pregnancy (CDC, 2005); with the highest rate of smoking (23%) reported in the 15 to 19 age group (CDC, 2005). A strong, consistent, causal relationship exists between maternal smoking during pregnancy and reduced birth weight. Women who smoke during pregnancy are at significantly higher risk for premature birth, low–birth weight infants, and higher rates of infant mortality. There appears to be a dose related effect of smoking on the risk of preterm delivery, with the greatest impact resulting from smoking at least 10 cigarettes each day (Kyklund-Blomberg & Cnatingius, 1998). Infants of mothers who smoke weigh less than do infants of nonsmokers at all gestational ages. On average, smokers' babies weigh approximately 350 grams less than nonsmokers' babies (Hamilton, 2001), and twice as many weigh less than 2,500 grams. Moreover, women who are classified as moderate smokers prior to pregnancy deliver infants weighing on average 430 grams less than nonsmokers at equivalent gestational ages (Hamilton, 2001). Eliminating smoking during pregnancy alone could reduce low birth weight by 17 to 26% (CDC, 2000). The influence of smoking during and after pregnancy is noted during the neonatal and infant periods. Neonatal mortality rates for single live births of low–birth weight infants are significantly higher for infants of mothers who smoke. Continued smoking after pregnancy places the neonate at risk of sudden infant death syndrome and inhibits normal lung development that can lead to asthma and recurrent respiratory infections (CDC, 2000). Likewise, studies have documented a direct increase in perinatal morbidity mortality as smoking level increases.

The American College of Obstetricians and Gynecologists (2005) recommends that providers of prenatal services ask all women on their initial presentation about smoking history and habits. This affords providers the opportunity to educate the woman regarding the effects of smoking on the fetus and infant as well as to assess the extent of her smoking behavior and willingness to quit. Similarly, opening the dialogue about the long-term effects of smoking on the fetus allows the woman to participate in the intervention process.

Caffeine

Caffeine, although shown to be teratogenic (cause congenital malformations) in mice, has not been shown to cause birth defects in humans (Narod, de Sanjose, & Victora, 1991). Heavy consumption of caffeine (equivalent to three or more cups of percolated coffee per day) has previously been related to a slight decrease in birth weight (Narod et al., 1991). However, other researchers have concluded that, with normal caffeine use, the overall exposure amount would not exceed a threshold dose capable of causing developmental effects in the fetus (Christian, 2002), nor is caffeine exposure related to reduced birth weight, preterm labor, or intrauterine growth retardation (Clausson et al., 2002).

Alcohol

Sampson and colleagues (1997) suggest that the prevalence of alcohol exposure during pregnancy is astonishingly high: approximately 1 in every 100 live births is affected by fetal alcohol syndrome or alcohol-related neurodevelopmental disorder. Although the precise effects of maternal alcohol use in pregnancy have not been qualified and the mode of action remains unexplained, there is sufficient evidence to suggest that maternal alcohol consumption has various negative reproductive effects. Fetal alcohol syndrome is the leading cause of preventable mental retardation and brain damage in the United States (Sampson et al., 1997). Due to the magnitude and risk of mental deficiency in infants of alcoholic women, any woman who is a chronic alcoholic should be counseled regarding the risk of birth defects if pregnancy occurs, and she should be offered effective birth control measures. Further, if pregnancy does occur in a woman who is an alcoholic, the risks of alcohol exposure should be further stressed and the woman should be offered the option of abortion. New data have shown that women who are social drinkers may have offspring that demonstrate fetal alcohol effects, which can include learning disabilities and hyperactivity. There are no recommendations for a safe amount of alcohol to consume during pregnancy. Interestingly, the women who are most likely to drink during their pregnancy are women who smoke, are single, have some college education or a college degree, and women who live in households with incomes over $50,000 (Ebrahim et al., 1998). Most importantly, fetal mortality was 77% higher when alcohol was consumed during pregnancy (Hoyert, 1996).

Drugs

Most commonly used drugs and medications can be used safely during pregnancy without risk of teratogenic effect. However, some drugs ingested during pregnancy may adversely affect the developing fetus; these drugs may include those prescribed by a health care provider, those bought over the counter, or those commonly abused. Drugs can be teratogenic, cause metabolic disturbances, produce chemical effects, or cause depression and alterations of the central nervous system. When any medication is administered during pregnancy, the benefits must be weighed against the risk. Andrade and colleagues (2004) found that a drug other than a vitamin or mineral supplement had been prescribed during pregnancy to almost 64% of the women who delivered between 1996 and 2000. Prenatal care providers need to be cognizant of the effects of medications on the fetus and prescribe medications that are safe for use during gestation.

Drug abuse during pregnancy is a major problem in the United States. Compounding the effects of the drugs is the fact that women who abuse drugs tend to have inadequate or no prenatal care (Aumed et al., 1990; Kalmuss & Fennelly, 1990). The incidence of maternal complications (especially prematurity and precipitous labor) among women who abuse drugs is markedly higher. In addition, the incidence of sexually transmitted infections is higher in women who abuse drugs (Lipscomb, Gevall, Mercer, & Sibai, 1991). All addictive drugs affect the fetus, with the infant experiencing withdrawal symptoms shortly after birth. The risks involved in multiple drug abuse are more complicated and not clearly understood. Further, the long-term effects of intrauterine drug exposure, neonatal withdrawal syndrome, and subsequent sequelae remain unknown, with the exception of drugs that cause teratogenic effects.

Cocaine is among the most commonly abused drugs in the United States as well as one of the most dangerous of the illicit drugs used during pregnancy. Ingested by sniffing, injection, or smoking (crack cocaine), it causes severe vasoconstriction, followed by rebound vasodilation. Cocaine can cause vaginal bleeding, preterm labor, and abruptio placentae during pregnancy. Dangers to the fetus include asphyxia, meconium-stained amniotic fluid, prematurity, and drug withdrawal after birth, leading to long-term irritability and altered response to caretakers (Chasnoff, 1991; Shiono et al., 1995). Genitourinary tract abnormalities, such as hypospadias and hydronephrosis, have also been reported in infants exposed to cocaine in utero (Chasnoff, 1989). Most studies have failed to find a clear association between cocaine use and many adverse perinatal outcomes. In a meta-analysis, the only two outcomes clearly associated with cocaine exposure were placental abruption and premature rupture of membranes (Addis, Moretti, Ahmed, Einarson, & Koren, 2001). The authors concluded that other adverse outcomes, such as premature delivery and low birth weight, may be related to multiple factors associated with the milieu of drug use. Maternal history has not been shown to be reliable in determining which pregnancies have been exposed to cocaine. Women who use cocaine throughout the pregnancy are less likely to obtain prenatal care, which makes intervention difficult. Lipscomb and colleagues (1991) found that 68% of women with a positive cocaine test at delivery denied any history of use during pregnancy, and many of these women sought no prenatal care. Unfortunately, the effects of in utero exposure to cocaine persists well beyond the neonatal period in very low–birth weight infants. Singer, Hawkins, Huang, Davillier, and Baley (2001) found that very low–birth weight infants with cocaine exposure experienced delays in cognitive, motor, and language development into early childhood.

Women who use intravenous drugs often engage in high-risk behaviors, such as needle sharing and unprotected intercourse with multiple partners. Women heroin and opiate users tend to have irregular menstrual cycles and are thought to ovulate sporadically. However, pregnancy can and does occur. Unfortunately, much of the accepted clinical protocols for managing the pregnancy of women addicted to heroin or other opiates is based on recommendations and not on systematic investigations (Wang, 1999). Thus, no formal guidelines are available to provide advanced practice nurses with the tools necessary to deliver optimal care to these patients. The use of methadone during pregnancy is most effectively managed in a well-coordinated center where women can receive total care; however, there are limited data on the viability of such programs (Wang, 1999). Abrupt withdrawal in the mother can lead to an increased risk of fetal distress and/or fetal demise, while methadone administration may prevent sudden and repeated withdrawal in the fetus (Wang, 1999) as well as decrease the mother's need for drug-seeking behaviors that could put her and the fetus at even greater risk. The methadone program appears to produce superior results in that pregnancy complications are similar to the average obstetrical population with the exception of low birth weight at term. The infant will also experience quite severe and prolonged drug withdrawal following birth when the mother is maintained on methadone (Rayburn & Bogenschutz, 2004).

Psychosocial Status

Childbearing is one of the most critical developmental periods in the life of individuals and families. Even under optimal circumstances, pregnancy, birth, and the postpartum period trigger profound and complex physiological, psychological, and social changes and adjustments. For individuals, it is a period of increased ego vulnerability, whereas for families, it involves extreme change and restructuring. In addition to specific psychological disturbances and destructive lifestyle behaviors such as addiction, the following psychosocial factors may place the mother, infant, or both at risk of pregnancy complications:

■ Maternal, paternal, or familial history of interpersonal violence (child or spouse abuse)

■ Insufficient support systems (inadequate family support systems, families prone to crisis, families unable to fulfill usual functions of the family unit)
■ Family disruption or dissolution (divorce, death, military service, abandonment)
■ Maternal role changes or conflicts (lifestyle alterations, career changes, increased role responsibilities, or conflict about role expectations)
■ Noncompliance with cultural norms (nonmarital pregnancy)
■ Unsafe cultural, ethnic, or religious practices (beliefs regarding blood transfusions or seeking medical care)
■ Situational crisis (unintended or undesired pregnancy)

Environmental Risk Factors

Pregnant women are exposed to a variety of substances that can have an impact on fertility and fetal development, the chance of a live birth, and their children's subsequent mental and physical development. Furthermore, evidence from numerous studies suggests that the following environmental factors are significantly associated with reproductive risk: infections, radiation, chemicals such as pesticides, therapeutic drugs, illicit drugs, industrial pollutants, cigarette smoke, stress, and diet.

Because many women work during pregnancy, potential risk situations in the work environment should be identified and eliminated. Decisions regarding the degree of risk that pregnant women incur in the work place depend on a number of factors: potential risk of exposure to mutagenic and teratogenic agents, increased risk resulting from the interaction of physiological alterations of pregnancy and the demands of a particular occupation, and the mother's general physical condition. A thorough work place history should identify potential risks such as adverse conditions and exposure to hazardous materials. There are few limitations or restrictions on working during pregnancy with the exception of jobs that require prolonged standing or walking. Women who are required to stand or walk for extended periods of time without adequate rest breaks are at risk of preterm labor and intrauterine growth retardation (Gabbe & Turner, 1997). Decisions regarding pregnant women and work should be based on a determination of the degree of risk present to the mother and fetus, the mother's need and desire to continue working, and her access to prenatal care.

IDENTIFICATION OF RISK STATUS AND ONGOING RISK ASSESSMENT

Identification of pregnancies that are at greater than average risk is a basic tenet of prenatal care. It is essential that nurses identify high-risk clients if the hazards of childbearing are to be reduced and nursing strategies aimed at risk reduction developed. The earlier the client is identified, the greater the chances for a favorable outcome. Ideally, potential risk is determined prior to conception. However, in the absence of such an opportunity, risk screening should begin with the initial prenatal visit. Identification of risk status has been approached in various ways, ranging from reiterating the importance of listening carefully to what every woman says about her past and current obstetrical, medical, and social circumstances to formal risk assessment. Risk assessment may be specific to a particular outcome (preterm delivery) or more broadly to general ongoing surveillance. Further, identification of low risk could change over the course of a woman's pregnancy, and a designation of high-risk status does not mean that a battery of tests should be ordered; rather, the usefulness of each modality should be individually evaluated. The importance of performing risk status assessments throughout the maternity cycle cannot be understated. Ongoing and continued risk assessment affords health care providers the opportunity to detect medical and psychosocial complications as well as institute appropriate interventions with the goal of minimizing maternal and fetal morbidity and mortality.

First Trimester

The first trimester of pregnancy is a critical period in the risk assessment process. This is the most opportune time to establish accurate dating of the pregnancy either through history, clinical examination, or diagnostic studies such as ultrasound. Accurate dating of the pregnancy ensures that interventions and testing are initiated at the appropriate time, interventions are not applied unnecessarily, and delivery occurs at the correct gestational age. For example, without correct gestational dating, alphafetoprotein (AFP) screening might be offered too early or too late or a woman may be subjected to treatment for preterm labor when she is actually at term.

Clinical assessment is an essential component of risk status in addition to any formal risk scoring systems that are employed. Clinical assessment of at-risk status is the gathering of data from physical assessment and measurement. Laboratory and diagnostic tests provide additional important information regarding risk status and are useful adjuncts in evaluating pregnant clients. Tests such as clean-catch urine for asymptomatic bacteriuria can be used to screen the total obstetrical population to detect women at risk for increased perinatal loss prior to their developing clinical symptoms associated with pathological processes. Many high-risk factors can be established by asking pregnant women the following questions:

- How old are you?
- How many pregnancies have you had?

- What kinds of complications did you experience during your previous pregnancy?
- How far did you go in school?
- Have you had a previous fetal death?
- What is your marital status?
- Have you had a child that weighed less than 5 pounds at birth?
- What did you weigh when you got pregnant?
- When did you begin prenatal care?

Answers to these questions can serve as a rough screening of pregnant women and alert the health care team to potential risk factors. Many of these questions are asked during a woman's initial prenatal visit; however, the responses may not be adequately placed in the context and perspective of high-risk.

During the first trimester, many women experience bleeding and cramping. This can be frightening for the woman and her partner. In many instances, a definitive etiology of the bleeding may not be found. Women should be offered reassurance and, if available, transvaginal ultrasonography should be performed—especially if the gestation is less than 12 weeks when one would expect to elicit fetal heart tones with a Doppler. Approximately 20% of women are at risk of spontaneous abortion during the first trimester. Women who have experienced a previous miscarriage, undergone cervical treatment (e.g., a LEEP procedure), and women with some medical complications (e.g., systemic lupus erythematosus [SLE]) are at greater risk of spontaneous abortion. Women with Rh-negative blood with first-trimester bleeding should be given RhoGAM®.

A second complication of the first trimester is hyperemesis gravidarum. For many women, this condition can be treated on an outpatient basis; for others, hospitalization will be required to normalize electrolyte and fluid balance. Many women become dangerously dehydrated, which places the mother and fetus at risk. Women who present with intractable nausea and vomiting should be evaluated for ketonuria and dehydration.

Several other medical conditions that exist prior to pregnancy (SLE, thyroid disorder, diabetes mellitus, hypertension) need to be managed aggressively before pregnancy occurs and during the first trimester to ensure that the woman's health remains stable throughout the pregnancy. For example, women with systemic lupus erythematosus should conceive with their disease in optimal control to decrease the potential for fetal wastage (Classen, Paulson, & Zacharias, 1998). Even when the disease process is quiescent, the pregnancy needs to be treated as high risk with frequent (every 1 to 2 weeks) follow-up and close monitoring, because patients with SLE are at increased risk of premature rupture of membrane and premature labor (Johnson, Petri, Witter, & Repke, 1995). Likewise, thyroid disorders are commonly encountered during pregnancy and need close evaluation for optimal outcome. The goal of surveillance and treatment during pregnancy is to keep the woman euthyroid without affecting or compromising the fetus. Women with hypothyroidism will need monthly tests of thyroid-stimulating hormone levels to evaluate their need for increasing doses of levothyroxine as the pregnancy progresses (Mazzaferri, 1997). Once the levels are stabilized, evaluation each trimester should be sufficient. Preeclampsia, thyroid storm, preterm delivery, miscarriage, and stillbirth are all potential complications of inadequately treated hyperthyroidism during pregnancy (Ecker & Musci, 1997). Optimal control of blood sugar in women with diabetes mellitus can be difficult in women during the first trimester because of nausea and inability to eat meals and snacks on a scheduled basis. Moreover, elevated blood sugar values at conception and during the first trimester are associated with an increased risk of congenital malformations (Rosenn, Miodovnik, Combs, Khoury, & Siddiqi, 1994). Although many women manage their diabetes with diet and oral agents, women with preexisting diabetes should be placed on an insulin regime during pregnancy for optimal control. Women with chronic hypertension usually have a decrease in blood pressure during the first and early second trimester due to the physiologic changes associated with pregnancy. If they took medication prior to the pregnancy, their blood pressure should be closely monitored during the first trimester for hypotension. Women who are taking angiotensin-converting enzyme inhibitors should be changed to a more appropriate medication during pregnancy such as methyldopa or labetalol (ACOG, 2001a). Hypertension that persists throughout pregnancy places the woman at risk of intrauterine growth restriction (IUGR), preterm labor, and superimposed preeclampsia. When compared with normotensive women, women with pregnancies complicated by hypertension are at greater risk of having a low–birth weight baby. Further, African American women have a higher prevalence of hypertension than White women; African American women are at greater risk for adverse pregnancy outcomes such as IUGR, low birth weight, prematurity, and perinatal death (Jain, Ferre, & Vidyasagar, 1998). Evaluating for superimposed preeclampsia as well as antenatal fetal assessment to screen for IUGR and fetal compromise will be a focus during the late second and early third trimester.

Screening for infections should be routine during the first trimester and throughout the pregnancy if exposure is noted. Table 17.2 outlines the screening tests that should be considered routine and those that should be initiated following actual or potential exposure. All women should be offered HIV screening during the first trimester or at the initiation of prenatal care (ACOG, 2004). Risk of transmission can be decreased dramati-

cally if HIV status is noted early in the pregnancy. Many regimes are available for treating HIV-positive women during the childbearing cycle. (See chapter 25, "Women and HIV/AIDS" for a discussion of this topic.)

Second Trimester

During the second trimester, most women feel good about themselves and about their unborn babies. The nausea that occurs during the first trimester has usually resolved, and the discomforts traditionally associated with the third trimester have not begun. However, fetal testing during this time can create anxiety for many women. During the early second trimester, most women will be offered screening tests to detect fetal abnormalities. Likewise, many women will undergo invasive diagnostic procedures that may change the outcome of their pregnancies. Finally, health care providers may increase surveillance of the mother and fetus during the latter half of the second trimester to assess for preterm labor, glucose intolerance of pregnancy, or fetal growth abnormalities.

Abnormal AFP screening in the second trimester can produce a stress response in the mother and family unit for concerns over the future well-being of the fetus and pregnancy. Women with abnormal screening will need to receive genetic counseling and be evaluated with targeted ultrasound and/or amniocentesis. This can be a stressful time for the woman while she is waiting to have additional testing performed or waiting for test results. Research indicates that unexplained elevations in AFP are associated with a higher incidence of preterm delivery, premature rupture of membranes, and low–birth weight infants (Simpson et al., 1991). Some authorities have recommended closer surveillance during pregnancy for complications such as IUGR, while others have found that routine screening and obstetrical care are adequate in detecting complications associated with unexplained elevations in AFP (Huerta-Enochian, Katz, & Erfurth, 2001).

Preterm Labor

Initial evaluation and continued monitoring for preterm labor are primary concerns during the second trimester. Effective methods to identify women who are most likely to deliver prematurely combined with validated interventions to prevent birth prior to term might ultimately decrease the preterm delivery rate (Bernhardt & Dorman, 2004). Women who have been identified as high risk for preterm labor may benefit from vaginal examination and vaginal ultrasound to evaluate cervical length. Shortening cervical length may indicate a risk of preterm delivery, especially if cervical length is less than 25 mm at 22 to 24 weeks (Iams, 2003). Although definitions vary, preterm labor is the occurrence of

17.2 | Screening Recommendations for Common Bacterial and Viral Infections During Pregnancy

INFECTIONS AND VIRUSES	ROUTINE SCREENING RECOMMENDED	LAB TESTING AFTER EXPOSURE RECOMMENDED	RECOMMENDED ACTION/TREATMENT
HIV	Yes	Yes	Prophylactic AZT
HbsAg	Yes	Yes	HBIG immunoglobulin Women at risk may receive vaccine during pregnancy
Syphilis	Yes	(Yes) RPR	Treat per CDC guidelines
Chlamydia	No Risk Factor Positive Screening	Cervical culture	Treat per CDC guidelines
Gonorrhea	No Risk Factor Positive Screening	Cervical culture	Treat per CDC guidelines
Herpes Simplex Virus (HSV)	No Symptomatic Screening Only (Ask about history of HSV in patient and partner)	HSV antibody testing	Treat per CDC guidelines
Hepatitis A	No	Little effect on pregnancy	Vaccine recommended before travel to foreign country
Hepatitis C	No	HCV antibodies	MFM referral
Group B Strep (Vertical transmission during labor and delivery)	Yes	N/A	Antibiotic therapy during labor
CMV (transplacental passage of virus)	No	Yes	MFM referral (no vaccine for prevention and no effective treatment for infection available)
Fifth's Disease (Parvo Virus B19)	No	Yes (IgG and IgM antibody titers)	MFM referral (incidence of fetal morbidity/mortality low)
Toxoplasmosis (Protozoan infection—exposure comes from eating inadequately cooked meats and handling feces of infected domestic cats)	No	Yes (IgG and IgM antibody titers initially and repeat in 2–4 weeks)[a]	MFM referral (first trimester exposure results in more severe sequalea, congenital infection more common after maternal infection in the third trimester)
Listeriosis (foodborne transmission)	No	Cervical culture or stool culture	PCN sensitive
Rubella	Yes	Yes (IgG titers, repeat 2 and 4 weeks after exposure)	MFM referral (vaccinate post partum)
Lyme's Disease	No	Yes (IgG and IgM antibody titers)	Treatment recommendation same as nonpregnant individuals
TORCH Titers Toxoplasmosis Other viruses Rubella Cytomegalovirus Herpes Simplex Virus	No	Evaluate each exposure as needed	Refer as needed

[a] Titers may be falsely elevated with rheumatoid factor.
Adapted from American Academy Pediatrics & American College of Obstetricians and Gynecologists (AAP/ACOG). (2007). *Guidelines for perinatal care* (6th ed.). Washington, DC: American College of Obstetrics and Gynecology.

uterine contractions between 20 and 36 weeks of gestation with one or both of the following: cervical change over time or dilation of 2 or more centimeters (ACOG, 2001b; Berkman et al., 2000). The process of identifying women who are at the highest risk for preterm labor must begin with diligent screening at the initial interview. There are known risk factors—such as previous preterm labor and multiple gestation—that predispose women to premature delivery; however, many women experience premature delivery who have been missed with conventional risk assessment measures. Addition risk factors for preterm delivery are non-White race, smoking, low socioeconomic status, and low prepregnancy weight (ACOG, 2001b). Of these risk factors, the most significant is a previous history of preterm labor. A woman who has experienced preterm labor or delivery is at a greater risk of a subsequent preterm labor episode. While preterm labor and delivery are among the most costly high-risk pregnancy complications, leading to the greatest neonatal morbidity and mortality in the United States, few advances have been made in predicting which women will go into preterm labor or how to stop it once it has begun. Moreover, numerous strategies to decrease premature birth have lacked reliable screening methods to identify women at risk (Anderson, 2000; Peaceman et al., 1997). Similarly, many women are subjected to unnecessary treatment because they present with preterm labor symptoms that never progress to premature birth. Iams and colleagues (2002) found that there was no threshold maximum frequency of contractions that would identify women who would inevitably deliver prematurely. They concluded that this lack of consistency is most likely responsible for the failure of ambulatory uterine contraction monitoring to reduce the risk of premature delivery.

Detection of fetal fibrinectin, a trophoblastic protein found in the membranes of the amniotic sac, in the cervical fluids between 22 and 37 weeks of gestation has been shown in numerous studies to assist with identification and management of threatened preterm labor. Fetal fibrinectin testing, approved by the Food and Drug Administration in 1995, has a high negative predictive value (percentage of patients with a negative test who will not have a spontaneous preterm delivery) but a low positive predictive value (percentage of patients with a positive test who will have a spontaneous preterm delivery) (Anderson, 2000). Patients should be questioned regarding intercourse in the previous 24 hours, the presence of ruptured membranes, or vaginal bleeding, all of which can lead to a false positive test (Lukes, Thorp, Euker, & Pahel-Short, 1997). Because of these limitations, the fetal fibrinectin test should be obtained prior to evaluation by pelvic examination or transvaginal ultrasonography. Even in the presence of symptoms, women with a negative test can be reassured that the potential risk for preterm birth is minimal.

Moreover, women are subjected to fewer interventions following a negative fetal fibrinectin test (Peaceman et al., 1997). Unfortunately, none of the traditional testing modalities (routine cervical assessment, home uterine monitoring, or fetal fibrinonectin detection) or risk assessment screening tools can reliably detect or decrease the incidence of preterm labor and delivery (Weismiller, 1999).

Glucose Intolerance of Pregnancy

Gestational diabetes mellitus screening should be offered to all women between the 24th and 26th week of pregnancy regardless of their risk status. It is not known which screening method is the best for detecting gestational diabetes mellitus (Russell, Carpenter, & Coustan, 2007), the single 50-gram load followed by blood glucose evaluation is the most universal method for screening. A blood sugar value of 140 or greater after a 50-gram load of glucose should undergo a 3-hour glucose tolerance test. A diagnosis of glucose intolerance of pregnancy is made if two or more blood sugar values exceed the following: fasting (105), 1-hour (190), 2-hour (165), and 3-hour (145). Women diagnosed with glucose intolerance of pregnancy should immediately be referred for dietary counseling and possibly home glucose monitoring. If diet and exercise do not achieve optimal control of blood sugar, insulin therapy will need to be initiated to prevent the complications associated with macrosomia (large-for-gestational-age fetus). Normalizing maternal blood sugars is the goal of therapy for women with glucose intolerance during pregnancy. However, despite blood sugar normalization, many women with glucose intolerance have large-for-gestational-age babies, which incur risks associated with delivery and postpartum. Further, review of previous studies reveals only about a 50% decrease in macrosomia and a 70% decrease in serious perinatal complications (i.e., shoulder dystocia, nerve injury) with treated gestational diabetes mellitus (Russell et al., 2007). Pregnancies complicated by gestational diabetes are at increased risk of preeclampsia, cesarean delivery, fetal shoulder dystocia, and neonatal hypoglycemia (Dodd, Crowther, Antoniou, Baghurst, & Robinson, 2007). Further, with exposure to excessive blood glucose in utero, the fetus is more likely to develop hypoglycemia during the early neonatal period.

Third Trimester

In a high-risk pregnancy, the third trimester can be quite stressful. Women usually have frequent prenatal visits for increased surveillance of their condition or fetal testing. For women with adequate transportation, financial support, and safe child care for their other children, this can be either inconvenient or reassuring, but, for women without adequate resources, taking time away from their work and family can present many challenges. When possible, care should be coordinated to allow for frequent visits that work around the woman's schedule. Providers should be sensitive to the issues of employment, transportation, and child care. If a woman is at risk of losing her job because of frequent prenatal care visits, she will be less likely to comply with the plan of care. Conversely, involving the woman in the plan of care, including scheduling of tests, will afford her some control in the decision-making process.

Hypertensive Disorders of Pregnancy

While hypertensive disorders affect 6% to 8% of all pregnancies (Peters & Flack, 2004) and have been a leading cause of maternal mortality throughout the ages, much confusion regarding the appropriate terminology continues to exist. The National High Blood Pressure Education Program (2000) has attempted to standardize terminology beginning with replacing the term *pregnancy-induced hypertension* with the term *gestational hypertension*. There are five types of hypertensive disease: gestational hypertension, preeclampsia, eclampsia, preeclampsia superimposed on chronic hypertension, and chronic hypertension. Gestational hypertension is defined as blood pressure of greater than 140/90 that occurs after the 20th week of pregnancy in a woman with previously normal blood pressure. Subsequent development of proteinuria would be classified as preeclampsia. Minimal criteria for diagnosing preeclampsia include blood pressure of 140/90 or higher with proteinuria 300 mg or more per 24 hours or 1+ or greater dipstick. Other findings that may be associated with preeclampsia include physical indicators such as edema, visual changes, or epigastric pain and laboratory indicators such as abnormal liver function studies, decreased platelets, and elevated uric acid levels. Eclampsia is an extension of preeclampsia that includes the new onset of grand mal seizures. Chronic hypertension is defined by an elevation in blood pressure (140/90 or higher) prior to the pregnancy or diagnosed before the 20th week gestation. In women with chronic hypertension, a new onset of proteinuria after 20 weeks changes their diagnosis to superimposed preeclampsia.

Management of hypertensive disorders during pregnancy relies on early detection and consistent follow-up. In some instances, late entry into prenatal care may make the diagnosis more challenging. For example, if a woman does not present for prenatal care prior to the 20th week of the pregnancy, making a diagnosis of chronic hypertension versus preeclampsia becomes more confusing. Most authorities recommend close follow-up of elevations in blood pressure to assess for developing proteinuria and abnormal laboratory values.

Women with chronic hypertension need to be evaluated for worsening hypertension, superimposed preeclampsia, and the development of growth restriction in the fetus. Fetal testing and decisions regarding delivery are made based on how rapidly clinical and laboratory data worsen as well as fetal assessment findings.

There are risk factors associated with developing preeclampsia. A previous history of preeclampsia may predispose a woman to developing preeclampsia during a subsequent pregnancy. However, Li and Wi (2000) found that changing paternity appears to play a significant role in the risk of recurrence of pregnancy-induced hypertension in subsequent pregnancies. In a retrospective study, women who reported a history of preeclampsia during their first pregnancy were 30% less likely to develop preeclampsia during a subsequent pregnancy if they changed partners between pregnancies. Moreover, women without a prior history of preeclampsia were 30% more likely to develop the disease in a subsequent pregnancy if they changed partners between pregnancies.

Post-Term Gestation

Pregnancies that extend beyond the 42nd week (284 days from the last normal menstrual period) are considered post-term and represent about 3% to 12% of all pregnancies (AAP/ACOG, 2007). If accurate gestation dating has been established, post-term gestations present a significant risk to the fetus. Between 41 and 42 weeks of gestation, antepartum fetal surveillance should be initiated to include nonstress testing and ultrasound evaluation of amniotic fluid. With reassuring testing, delivery can be delayed with evaluation repeated at weekly intervals or more frequently depending on the clinical situation. Nonreassuring testing at any point is an indication for delivery by induction.

Maternal Psychological Risk Status

High-risk childbearing women and their families must cope with two distinct crises: the normal developmental crisis of childbearing and the crisis of high-risk status and resulting uncertainty as to the eventual outcome. Pregnancy and illness are uncommon experiences; the usual coping mechanisms normally engaged during a crisis may not work for the woman during this time. Likewise, her coping abilities may become severely overtaxed and overstressed, leaving her with the need to develop new coping skills.

In the past decade, health care professionals have recognized that medically and obstetrically healthy women who have unmet psychosocial needs might become at risk when these needs remain unattended. Women with known medical and obstetrical problems that increase risk in pregnancy or women who give evidence of severe social-emotional dysfunction receive the majority of attention, time, interest, money, and effort of the health care team. The normal patient, who is physically healthy and emotionally and socially stable, may receive substantially less attention. This group can be divided into three types. The first group is composed of women in good physical, social, and emotional equilibrium whose pregnancy progresses normally; they have adequate social support and are not experiencing undue stress. These women are most likely to remain healthy and assume the parental role with minimal support and counseling from the health care team. The second group is comprised of women who are physically healthy but have emotional or social problems that are not identified by the health care practitioner. Many of the women in this group will have needs that are not identified through routine care and counseling. The third group includes women who are not currently stressed but have a background that may place them at risk for potential problems. Ongoing assessment during prenatal care provides the opportunity to identify the latter two groups of women and offer supportive and preventive services to them. Recognition of psychosocial risk allows women the opportunity for positive change and improved outcome.

Accurately assessing a woman's ability to proceed through the developmental tasks of pregnancy is an important focus for prenatal nurses and health care providers. An inability to master the developmental tasks of pregnancy, or pregnancy maladaption, strongly correlates with inadequate identification with the fetus, lack of compliance in therapeutic regimes, difficulties in developing a real perception of the infant, and problems regarding the development of lasting attachment to the child. The mother's mood (her sense of well-being versus depression or anxiety) and maternal reactions to discomfort and body changes should be evaluated. Women must dramatically alter their self-concept and their role definitions as they move through pregnancy. High-risk status may impede successful completion of the maternal developmental tasks of confirming and accepting pregnancy, ensuring safe passage, acceptance of the child by significant others, attachment, and giving of oneself (Rubin, 1984).

All pregnant women must come to believe that their pregnancies are real. Pregnant women who are at high risk or who have had past reproductive failures may have difficulty mastering this task. Although some women with previous high-risk pregnancies or reproductive problems may delay seeking prenatal care, anxiety over the potential outcome for other women may be expressed by intensified physical symptoms or repeated requests for physical examinations or procedures (e.g., ultrasound) in an effort to prove that the pregnancy is real and progressing normally. Ambivalence is common for all women during the time in which pregnancy

becomes a reality to them and their families; resolution usually occurs by the end of the first trimester or when fetal movement is perceived. These feelings are accentuated when negative physical signs indicate a problem or when unanticipated complications disrupt the parents' daily lives. Both parents may experience alternating feelings of love and concern, fear and anger toward the fetus and each other. Although hoping for a positive outcome, the parents may experience negative feelings if the mother's health is in jeopardy. For women who had difficulty conceiving or experienced several pregnancy losses, these feelings may be particularly disturbing and disruptive. Ambivalence frequently makes it difficult for the couple to communicate with each other. Communication becomes strained when each is afraid to express dissatisfaction, anger, fear, or resentment. The partners may not be able to provide each other with the emotional support needed to cope with a high-risk pregnancy. Ambivalence is assessed in terms of how honestly it is expressed and whether it continues past the second trimester.

Another essential psychological task for the pregnant woman is incorporating the fetus into her body image. This may be hard for those with a history of infertility or previous poor outcomes. Fear of loss may prevent attachment to the developing fetus. Helping women to hear fetal heart tones, identifying signs of progressing pregnancy, and pointing out fetal movement can assist women in seeing the pregnancy as real and incorporating the pregnancy into their body image.

Additional indications of pregnancy maladaption include persistent denial of the pregnancy past quickening, inability to develop emotional attachment to the fetus, and inability to see the fetus as a separate individual. Indications of denial of the pregnancy include denial of change in body function or appearance, delaying prenatal care, and failing to keep appointments or noncompliance with suggested health practices, such as weight gain or vitamin supplementation. When faced with a diagnosis of high-risk status, parents may express denial as a defense against attachment to an infant who may not survive. Late in the pregnancy, the woman might dress and act as though she is not pregnant. Lack of attachment can be seen when there is little or no response to quickening or statements such as, "She never stops kicking," "I can't get any sleep," "I wish she'd leave me alone." Absence of nesting behavior in the third trimester, particularly in primigravidas, as evidenced by not choosing names or preparing a room, may indicate a lack of attachment; however, lack of nesting is common when fetal viability is questionable throughout the pregnancy. When evaluating a couple's ability to work through the crisis of a high-risk pregnancy, it is useful to ask about the presence (or absence) of internal strength and social support and whether their anxiety and tension are unbearable or whether they have escape mechanisms available to decrease their anxiety.

Later in the pregnancy, women should begin to view the fetus as a separate entity. Planning for the baby begins with dreams and fantasies and intensifies over time. Women experiencing a high-risk pregnancy may be unable to plan for the baby's arrival and may postpone all preparations for the upcoming delivery and newborn. Women who are concerned about preterm birth are apt to be especially cautious. As labor and delivery become imminent, any doubts the couple may have had about their ability to parent will increase. The woman who delivers early may not have completed her psychological preparation for the transition to parenthood. Likewise, couples who have remained unconvinced that the pregnancy would end in a live, healthy infant may also be unprepared for their role as parents.

Assessment of potential parenting ability is an essential component of maternal psychological risk status assessment. The factors that influence parenting abilities are established long before pregnancy begins. How the woman and her partner were parented, the role models available to them, their beliefs about appropriate methods of childrearing, and their individual personalities all affect their parenting style. Assessment of parental role preparation determines how much the couple desire to be parents, how much preparation they have made, how the couple view themselves in the parenting role, and how much life change they anticipate. The couple relationship should be evaluated to determine the degree of mutuality and interdependency present and what type of social support the expectant mother has experienced in the past. The question, "What kind of mother do you want to be?" should be asked. Answers to the effect of "like my own mother" are a positive sign.

Women at psychosocial high risk may evidence excessive concern over the sex of the unborn infant, suggesting that the mother expects her baby to fulfill her own needs or that she wishes to please her partner by giving him a child of the sex he desires. When an infant or child is expected to meet the needs of a parent and fails, as he or she invariably must, neglect and abuse may result. Family isolation is a frequent cause of psychosocial high risk. Observing who accompanies the woman on her prenatal visits may provide additional clues to poor social support or isolation. The following questions should routinely be included in prenatal assessment to further evaluate social support:

- How long have you lived in this area?
- Where do you live now?
- Where does most of your family live?
- How often do you see your mother or other close relatives?

In a high-risk pregnancy, the usual fears and fantasies of pregnancy are intensified as a woman fears for herself and her infant. Fears of mutilation, death, and deformity—commonly repeated by many pregnant women—may be intense, and concern may be expressed about what the infant will be like and how the infant will be accepted by family and community. Women do not experience childbearing in a vacuum but, rather, within a social support system and community within a cultural framework. The structure of the family system and dynamics of interpersonal relationships are profoundly influenced by high-risk childbearing. A careful evaluation of the family and social system is essential. The support systems, particularly partner and family, are highly significant in assessing stressors, coping abilities, and planning care. Specific areas of assessment that determine the adequacy and influence of partner, family, and social support systems include family composition, support system, and financial situation. Pregnancy is a time of excitement and anticipation; however, high-risk pregnancy can be a stressful time for a woman and her support system as they anticipate a sometimes uncertain outcome.

FETAL EVALUATION IN HIGH-RISK PREGNANCY

When women have been identified as at risk during pregnancy, laboratory data and diagnostic testing can provide information about the intrauterine environment and the well-being of the fetus. Testing performed during early pregnancy may include chorionic villus sampling and amniocentesis for DNA analysis or ultrasound to evaluate fetal anatomy. Antepartal fetal testing is primarily done to evaluate fetal well-being and is customarily performed during the late second and third trimester. Because the goal of antenatal fetal surveillance is to prevent fetal death, testing procedures are indicated in any pregnancy where the risk of fetal demise is increased (ACOG, 1999). Indications for antepartal fetal surveillance are outlined in Table 17.3.

Chorionic Villus Sampling

Chorionic villus sampling (CVS) is a procedure that can be used as an alternative to amniocentesis for prenatal diagnosis of chromosomal abnormalities. The primary advantage is the timing during the pregnancy cycle when the test can be performed. CVS can be performed during the first trimester, which allows for earlier fetal intervention or first-trimester pregnancy termination. With CVS, a small portion of the chorion frondosusm (small projections from the egg sac that later develop into the placenta) is taken and analyzed for chromosome number. New uses for CVS include DNA analyses

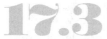 Indications for Fetal Testing

MATERNAL	PREGNANCY RELATED	FETAL
Hypertensive disorders	Multiple gestation	Intrauterine growth restriction
Asthma	Postterm pregnancy	Infection
Seizure disorders	Isoimmunization	Congenital anomalies
Diabetes mellitus	Previous unexplained stillbirth	
Systemic lupus erythematosus	Unexplained elevation of maternal AFP	
Thyroid disorder	Uncontrolled gestational diabetes	
Collagen vascular disease	PIH	
	Polyhydramnios or oligohydramnios	

Adapted from American College of Obstetricians and Gynecologists. (1999). ACOG Practice Bulletin #9: Antepartal fetal surveillance. In 2007 *Compendium* (Vol. 2, pp. 503–513). Washington, DC: American College of Obstetrics and Gynecology.

for diagnosing diseases such as hemophilia, muscular dystrophy, and cystic fibrosis. The rate of spontaneous abortion—a complication of CVS—is similar to that for early amniocentesis. Most recommend that Rh immunoglobulin be administered prophylactically to all Rh-negative women undergoing CVS.

Amniocentesis

Amniocentesis is done between 15 and 20 weeks to detect genetic disorders and diagnose fetal defects, including chromosomal anomalies, skeletal disorders, and central nervous system disorders; amniocentesis is performed at 30 weeks' gestation or later to assess fetal maturity and well-being. The structural chemical compounds and activity of fetal cells in the amniotic fluid can provide valuable information regarding fetal maturity and well-being. Amniotic fluid can be evaluated for color (to detect the presence of meconium) and for the lecithin/sphingomyelin ratio (to determine fetal pulmonary maturity, indicating surface active phospholipids) as well as other chemical compounds and substances.

Amniocentesis is the transabdominal aspiration of amniotic fluid from within the uterine cavity and is performed in an outpatient setting. Although it is a relatively simple and safe procedure, complications include vaginal spotting, amniotic fluid leakage, and infection (Cunningham et al., 2001). Before the procedure, women should receive extensive counseling regarding the potential, albeit limited, risk for complications. As part of the informed consent, women must be very clear that, regardless of the indication, amniocentesis is an optional procedure. The ultimate decision rests with the woman and her family. Likewise, following the procedure, the woman should be observed for a

brief period of time to ensure that the needle site is not bleeding. Most women are reassured that the fetus has not been physically harmed by the needle if they are able to visualize the fetal heart beat and remaining amniotic fluid after the procedure (Cunningham et al., 2001). Finally, health care providers should be cognizant that the woman and her family may be concerned about miscarriage following the procedure and may be anxious awaiting the results (Cederholm, Axelsson, & Sjoden, 1999), especially when the procedure was performed for prenatal karyotyping.

Ultrasonography

Ultrasound or echo sounding has added to the health professional's repertoire of diagnostic techniques that assess the intrauterine environment, fetal growth, and fetal anatomy. The technique consists of sending very short pulses of low-intensity, high-frequency sound waves into the mother's uterus. The returning echo signals are transmitted onto a screen that creates a two-dimensional picture of the intrauterine contents, which can be photographed, videotaped, or stored as a digital image for a permanent record.

Ultrasound provides a useful technique for assessing gestational age for dating pregnancies and determining the estimated date of delivery. This can be particularly beneficial when a woman is uncertain regarding the dates of her last menstrual period, which is traditionally used to calculate the estimated date of delivery. Gestational age is calculated by taking several measurements of the fetus—crown-rump length, biparietal diameter, abdominal circumference, and femur length—and determining ratios. These are then compared to those expected at various gestational ages.

Ultrasound can also document discrepancies in fetal growth patterns. Serial ultrasounds over time (usually at 2- to 3-week intervals) can be used to document fetal growth throughout the pregnancy. When growth aberrations are suspected, serial ultrasounds can be a useful adjunct to management. Ultrasound is also used to evaluate the intrauterine environment and fetal anatomy. During an ultrasound examination, the amount of amniotic fluid, location of the placenta, and fetal behavioral states can be observed.

When a woman is to have an ultrasound early in her pregnancy, she should be encouraged to drink four to six glasses of fluid and not void prior to the procedure to increase bladder fullness. Ultrasound waves will not traverse air; therefore, the fluid-filled bladder displaces the small bowel and provides a medium that can be easily penetrated by sound waves. For most women and their families, having an ultrasound can be an exciting and fun activity during pregnancy. For women with high-risk pregnancies, however, an ultrasound procedure may cause a great deal of anxiety. The health care team needs to be aware of how the woman may be feeling during the procedure.

Fetal Movement

Maternal monitoring of fetal movement is a simple, basic, and inexpensive test that can be used as a screening test to evaluate fetal well-being and can easily be done daily or more often if needed. Fetal movement counting is used routinely as an adjunct to determine when other diagnostic tests might be warranted. During the fetal movement count, the woman identifies the presence and frequency of contractions. Although no standard protocol has been recommended, numerous protocols have been utilized and are deemed acceptable (ACOG, 1999). A vigorous, active fetus is reassuring to both the mother and her health care providers (Christensen & Rayburn, 1999). Women are routinely taught to record the number of fetal movements during a specified period (30 to 60 minutes) two to three times each day. Generally, women are advised to choose a time when relaxation is possible and a time of day when the baby is ordinarily active. She can stimulate movement by lying on her left side, eating a light snack, drinking juice, touching or moving her abdomen, or making a sudden noise by clapping her hands. She can stop counting when she records four to six movements in a 30–60 minute period. If the baby does not move during the allotted hour, she can drink more juice, move around, or massage her abdomen and start recording movements for another hour. In the absence of adequate movement during the 2-hour window, the woman is advised to contact her health care provider for further fetal assessment. All perceived changes in fetal activity warrant further evaluation. At the same time, it is important to remind the woman and her family that wide variations in fetal movement exist between women and between pregnancies.

Nonstress Test

The nonstress test (NST) is designed to evaluate the health of the fetus by assessing the response of the fetal heart rate in relation to fetal movement. As the name implies, the fetus is not subjected to external stressors. The NST may be performed at any point during the second or third trimester, but is most commonly used in the third trimester. Nonstress tests are generally used in situations where the fetus might be expected to be compromised, such as preterm labor, hypertensive disorders of pregnancy, and post-term gestation. The test is performed with an external fetal monitoring device attached to the abdomen very much like that used during labor. The client is placed in the left lateral or semi-Fowler's position to avoid compression of the aorta or vena cava, which can temporarily reduce blood flow and result in an abnormal test. Women are usually advised to eat a snack prior to testing. An NST is considered reactive or reassuring if there are at least two fetal heart rate accelerations of 15 beats per minute over baseline that last for 15 or more seconds within a 20-minute period (ACOG, 1999). If minimal fetal movement is present during the NST, the nurse may have the client touch or rock her abdomen to move the fetus, drink fruit juice (the sugar content of which may stimulate the fetus), or perform 1 to 2 seconds of acoustic stimulation with an artificial larynx on the mother's abdomen. If the fetus continues with inactivity and other reasons for nonreactivity have been ruled out (e.g., smoking prior to testing or normal fetal sleep cycle), further investigation is warranted. Frequency of testing is determined by the clinical indication but is usually performed once to twice each week until delivery.

Biophysical Profile

The biophysical profile (BPP) is a noninvasive test that evaluates fetal behavior and amniotic fluid volume. The biophysical profile combines the nonstress test with four ultrasound observations (Manning, 1999). Scores on a BPP can range from 0 to 10. The components and scoring criteria of this assessment procedure are given in Table 17.4. Each variable receives 2 points for a normal response and 0 points for an abnormal, absent, or insufficient response (ACOG, 1999). Generally, a total score of 8 to 10 is considered normal, and a score of 6 or lower is generally associated with fetal compromise. Substantive decreases in amniotic fluid volume (largest vertical pocket less than 2 cm) is considered ominous regardless the composite BPP score. Since amniotic fluid volume reflects fetal urine output (which

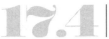

Biophysical Profile Scoring System

COMPONENT	SCORE 0	SCORE 2
Fetal tone	Absence of extension/flexion of an extremity or failure to open and close hand	1 or more fetal extremity extension with return to flexion or opening and closing of fetal hand
Fetal movement	< 3 discrete episodes of body or limb movement	3 or more discrete body or limb movements during 30 minute observation
Fetal breathing movement	< 30 seconds of breathing during 30 minute observation	Sustained episode of breathing movement lasting at least 30 seconds during 30 minute observation
Amniotic fluid volume	Single vertical pocket measuring less than or equal to 2 cm	Single vertical pocket measuring at least 2 cm
Nonstress test	0–1 accelerations in 20–40 minute observation	2 or more accelerations in fetal heart rate of at least 15 beats above baseline, lasting at least 15 seconds during 20–40 minute observation

Adapted from Manning, F. A. (1999). Fetal biophysical profile. *Obstetrics and Gynecologic Clinics of North America, 26*(4), 557–577; Queenan, J. T., Spong, C. Y., & Lockwood, C. J. (2007). *Management of high-risk pregnancy* (5th ed.). Malden, MA: Blackwell Publishing.

indirectly reflects uterine perfusion), some institutions rely on a modified biophysical profile to evaluate fetal health. The modified biophysical profile combines the NST with amniotic fluid assessment. According to the American College of Obstetricians and Gynecologists (1999) guidelines, a reactive NST combined with an amniotic fluid index greater than 5 is considered normal.

Contraction Stress Test

The adequacy of placental respiratory capabilities can be evaluated by the contraction stress test (CST), sometimes referred to as the oxytocin challenge test. The premise of this test is that late decelerations of the fetal heart rate (the decrease in fetal heart rate that begins about 30 seconds after the contraction begins, with the lowest point occurring after the peak of the contraction) indicates fetal compromise, hypoxia, and/or distress. Uterine contractions decrease blood flow and, hence, oxygen transfer to the placenta. If the placenta has adequate oxygen stores, transient decreases in blood flow will not cause changes in the fetal heart rate; however, if the fetus does not have adequate reserve and placental insufficiency is present, the fetal heart rate decreases. Late decelerations observed on the contraction stress test indicate that the fetus possesses inadequate reserves and may not be able to handle further stressors.

The contraction stress test is usually performed during the third trimester to evaluate the fetal heart rate in response to uterine contractions when there is a question of fetal compromise or in the presence of maternal complications or disease. The patient is usually positioned in the semi-Fowler's position with external fetal monitoring equipment applied. Generally, the woman is observed for a period of approximately 10 to 20 minutes to determine whether spontaneous contractions are occurring. If the woman experiences at least three spontaneous contractions of 40-second duration within a 10-minute period, no uterine stimulation is required (ACOG, 1999). However, if the woman is not experiencing spontaneous uterine contractions, either intravenous oxytocin is administered or the woman is asked to stimulate her nipples by gently pulling or twisting on them until uterine contractions occur that meet the criteria (three contractions lasting 40 seconds each during a 10-minute period). The CST is considered positive when late decelerations occur with 50% or more contractions and negative when there are no late or significant variable decelerations. When the test is equivocal or suspicious (intermittent late decelerations or significant variable decelerations) or the test is unsatisfactory (fewer than three contractions during the 10-minute period), the interval for repeat testing depends on the clinical situation and fetal gestational age. Unlike the other modalities for antepartal fetal surveillance (fetal movement counts, BPP, NST), the CST has some risk of labor induction. Therefore, the CST is typically avoided in women with threatened preterm labor, incompetent cervix, or multiple gestations. Other relative contraindications to the contraction stress test include placenta previa, previous uterine rupture, previous classical cesarean delivery, and premature rupture of membranes (ACOG, 1999).

NURSING MANAGEMENT

Even before conception, nurses can be instrumental in preventing high-risk childbearing. The importance of preconceptual care in preventing negative outcomes of a high-risk pregnancy cannot be overemphasized. Although the information presented in this chapter about risk factors, tools for detecting high risk, and understanding the meaning of high risk suggests areas of assessment, it is crucial that nurses listen to their clients regarding their needs, concerns, and stressors. When women assist with directing their care, they are more likely to be responsive to suggestions for improving their overall health and that of their unborn babies.

Optimum care is achieved when the woman and her family are cared for by the same provider at each visit. Developing a helping relationship is essential; trust and continuity of care greatly facilitate nursing care. When the clinic routines and protocols do not allow for one provider to consistently provide care to the patient, accurate and consistent methods of documentation will facilitate continuity of care, better communication, better coordination of procedures, and increased accuracy in evaluating the woman's ability to follow the prescribed recommendations.

In many instances, the nurse will be the teacher, allowing that some nursing care activities be managed by the client herself at home. These activities may include, but are not limited to, fetal movement counting, blood glucose monitoring, and blood pressure monitoring. Nursing roles include teaching and explanation, because it is important that the woman have a thorough understanding of her condition and treatment regime. Without this, she will be unable to participate fully in her care. She must understand the precautions involved in her care, her particular risk factors, and any hospitalization anticipated.

When a woman is diagnosed as having a high-risk pregnancy, many routine choices are taken away from her. Women today are encouraged by popular literature and health care professionals to take charge of their childbirth experience. They are encouraged to interview and choose a provider who shares their philosophy of childbirth and to choose a birthing facility that allows and encourages the things that are most important to them, such as rooming-in, breast-feeding, or early discharge. Women may even consider the option of home birth. Choices about these and many other factors are limited when a woman has a high-risk pregnancy, and the use of a midwife to attend the delivery may be out of the question. Community hospitals and family-centered birthing facilities may not be equipped to provide care to a woman with a known high-risk pregnancy or with a potentially compromised newborn. Prenatal exercise, work, travel, and child care may all

be restricted. Typically, fetal monitoring will be employed continuously, limiting the mother's freedom of movement. Analgesia or anesthesia during labor may be dictated by the woman's medical condition, not the couple's wishes or plans. The option of vaginal delivery may not be available for the high-risk pregnant woman, depending on her condition. For the high-risk pregnant woman, pregnancy may be anything but the normal, natural, healthy time often portrayed by the media, her family, and her friends. Nurses must support high-risk mothers as they cope with loss of choice and control over their childbearing experiences. Nurses can assist their clients in identifying choices they do have and encourage them to take control over these aspects of their care. Women must receive ample explanation regarding the rationales behind the treatments and procedures to which they are subjected. Lengthy discussions and explanations will help the woman understand the rationale behind her course of treatment. By gaining knowledge of the reasons for treatment and knowing what to expect, high-risk pregnant women and their families will gain a sense of control that will enable them to be more informed consumers of the health care services offered during this time.

Women may need to grieve the loss of a fantasized normal pregnancy. A woman may have anticipated pregnancy for years, imagining what it would be like and planning how she and her family would experience the event. Virtually no one plans for a high-risk pregnancy, and a woman will need to release her fantasies before she can fully experience the reality of her pregnancy.

To further compound the problem, hospitalization prior to labor is often necessary. Family separation, unfamiliar hospital routines, and anxiety about the pregnancy contribute to a reluctance to enter or remain in the hospital. At-risk mothers often assume a dependent role. A team approach that involves the woman in her care may reduce the stress of hospitalization and return a measure of control to the client, helping to reduce the stress of separation and disruption of the family unit.

High-risk childbearing brings with it physical, emotional, maturational, situational, and social crises. Demands are enormous for women and their families. Care should be provided in a comprehensive manner to maximize the woman's strengths and minimize her stressors.

CONCLUSION

Managing high-risk pregnancies involves recognizing potential problems for both the mother and the fetus. Prenatal care should focus on education, support, and assessment of the woman and her family. Prenatal care, while focusing on health promotion, is a period of ever vigilant assessment for pregnancy complications. Potential pregnancy complications must first be recognized and identified before they can be managed effectively to ensure the best possible outcome. Prenatal care must be a partnership between the pregnant woman and the health care team. Without commitment and cooperation between the two, optimal outcomes cannot be achieved.

Although many advances have led to lower rates of perinatal mortality, much remains to be accomplished. Many of the proposed interventions focus on altering lifestyle behaviors and access to health care. Further, strategies focused on decreasing unintended pregnancies, decreasing exposure to unhealthy lifestyle behaviors, and increasing the availability and content of culturally sensitive prenatal care for all women will ensure that fewer women and infants will die or experience long-term consequences associated with high-risk pregnancies. For advanced practice nurses providing health care to women, the most important lifestyle behavior modification that they can promote involves preventing obesity. With the increasing rates of obesity in the United States and other developed countries, obesity is rapidly becoming one of the most high-risk complications of pregnancy (Galtier-Dereure, Boegner, & Bringer, 2000). Strategies to increase the overall health of women will produce major changes in the incidence of high-risk pregnancy.

REFERENCES

Addis, A., Moretti, M. E., Ahmed, S. F., Einarson, T. R., & Koren, G. (2001). Fetal effects of cocaine: An updated meta-analysis. *Reproductive Toxicology, 15*(4), 341–369.

American Academy Pediatrics & American College of Obstetricians and Gynecologists (AAP/ACOG). (2007). *Guidelines for perinatal care* (6th ed.). Washington, DC: American College of Obstetrics and Gynecology.

American College of Obstetricians and Gynecologists. (1999). ACOG Practice Bulletin #9: Antepartal fetal surveillance. In *2007 Compendium, Vol. 2* (pp. 503–513). Washington, DC: American College of Obstetrics and Gynecology.

American College of Obstetricians and Gynecologists. (2001a). ACOG Practice Bulletin #29: Chronic hypertension in pregnancy. In *2007 Compendium, Vol. 2* (pp. 609–617). Washington, DC: American College of Obstetrics and Gynecology.

American College of Obstetricians and Gynecologists. (2001b). ACOG Practice Bulletin #31: Assessment of risk factors for preterm birth. In *2007 Compendium, Vol. 2* (pp. 632–639). Washington, DC: American College of Obstetrics and Gynecology.

American College of Obstetricians and Gynecologists. (2004). Committee Opinion #304: Prenatal and perinatal human immunodeficiency virus testing: Expanded recommendations. In *2007 Compendium, Vol. 1* (pp. 353–358). Washington, DC: American College of Obstetrics and Gynecology.

American College of Obstetricians and Gynecologists. (2005). Committee Opinion #316: Smoking cessation during pregnancy. In *2007 Compendium, Vol. 1* (pp. 280–285). Washington, DC: American College of Obstetrics and Gynecology.

Anderson, H. F. (2000). Use of fetal fibrinectin in women at risk for pre-term delivery. *Clinical Obstetrics & Gynecology, 43*(4), 746–758.

Andrade, S. E., Gurwitz, J. H., Davis, R. L, Chan, K., Arnold, F., Fortman, J. A., et al. (2004). Prescription drug use in pregnancy. *American Journal of Obstetrics and Gynecology, 192*(2), 398–407.

Aumed, M. S., Zhou, D., Schoof, T. Spong, C., Sagduyu, K., Agbas, A., & Maulik, D. (1990). Illicit drug use during pregnancy: Effects of opiates and cocaine on human placenta. *NIDA Research Monograph, 105*, 278–279.

Beckmann, C. A., Buford, T. A., & Witt, J. B. (2000). Perceived barriers to prenatal care services. *Maternal Child Nursing, 25*(1), 43–46.

Berkman, N. D., Thorp, J. M. Jr., Hartmann, K. E., et al. (2000). *Management of preterm labor: Evidence Report/Technology Assessment No. 18,* AHRQ Publication No. 01-E021. Rockville, MD: Agency for Healthcare Research and Quality.

Bernhardt, J., & Dorman, K. (2004). Pre-term birth risk: Exploring fetal fibrinectin and cervical length for validating risk. *AWHONN Lifelines, 8*(1), 39–44.

Cederholm, M., Axelsson, O., & Sjoden, P. O. (1999). Women's knowledge, concerns and psychological reactions before undergoing an invasive procedure in prenatal karyotyping. *Ultrasound in Obstetrics & Gynecology, 14*(4), 267–272.

Centers for Disease Control and Prevention. (1999a). Healthier mothers and babies. *Morbidity and Mortality Weekly Report, 48*(38), 849–858.

Centers for Disease Control and Prevention. (1999b). State-specific maternal mortality among Black and White women—United States 1987–1996. *Morbidity and Mortality Weekly Report, 48*, 492–496.

Centers for Disease Control and Prevention. (2005). Youth Risk Behavior Surveillance—United States, 2005. *Morbidity and Mortality Weekly Report, 55*(SS05), 1–106.

Centers for Disease Control and Prevention. (2006). Tobacco use among adults—United States, 2005. *Morbidity and Mortality Weekly Report, 42*(42), 1145.

Chang, J., Elam-Evans, L. D., Berg, C. J., Herndon, J., Flowers, L., Seed, K. A., & Syverson, C. J. (2003). Pregnancy-related mortality surveillance—United States, 1991–1999. *Morbidity and Mortality Weekly Report, 52*(SS02), 1–8.

Chasnoff, I. J. (1989). Cocaine, pregnancy, and the neonate. *Women and Health, 15*(3), 23–35.

Chasnoff, I. J. (1991). Drugs, alcohol, pregnancy, and the neonate: Pay now or pay later. *Journal of the American Medical Association, 266*, 1567.

Christensen, F. C., & Rayburn, W. F. (1999). Fetal movement counts. *Obstetrics and Gynecology Clinics of North America, 26*(4), 607–621.

Christian, M. S. (2002). Caffeine—a human teratogen? *Teratology, 65*(6), 318.

Classen, S. R., Paulson, P. R., & Zacharias, S. R. (1998). Systemic lupus erythematosus: Perinatal and neonatal implication. *Journal of Obstetrical, Gynecological and Neonatal Nursing, 27*(5), 493–500.

Clausson, B., Granath, F., Ekbom, A., Lundren, S., Nordmark, A., Signorello, L., & Cnattingius, S. (2002). Effect of caffeine exposure during pregnancy on birth weight and gestational age. *American Journal of Epidemiology, 155*(5), 429–436.

Cunningham, F. G., Gant, N. F., Leveno, K. J., Gilstrap, L. C., Hauth, J. C., & Wenstrom, K. D. (Eds.). (2001). *Williams Obstetrics* (21st ed.). New York: McGraw-Hill.

Dangal, G. (2008). High-risk pregnancy. *Internet Journal of Gynecology & Obstetrics, 7*(1), 1–8. Retrieved January 8, 2008, from http://www.ispub.com/ostia/index.php?xmlFilePath = journals/ijgo/vol7n1/risk.xml

Dodd, J. M., Crowther, C. A., Antoniou, G., Baghurst, P., & Robinson, J. S. (2007). Screening for gestational diabetes: The effect of varying blood glucose definitions in the prediction of adverse maternal and infant health outcomes. *Australian and New Zealand Journal of Obstetrics and Gynecology, 47*(4), 307–312.

Ebrahim, S. H, Luman, E. T., Floyd, R. L., Murphy, C. C., Bennett, E. M., & Boyle, C. A. (1998). Alcohol consumption by pregnant women in the United States during 1988–1995. *Obstetrics and Gynecology, 92*(2), 187–192.

Ecker, J. L., & Musci, T. J. (1997). Treatment of thyroid disease in pregnancy. *Obstetrics and Gynecology Clinics of North America, 24*(3), 575–589.

Fraser, A. M., Brockert, J. E., & Ward, R. H. (1995). Association of young maternal age with adverse reproductive outcomes. *New England Journal of Medicine, 332*(17), 1113–1117.

Gabbe, S. G., & Turner, L. P. (1997). Reproductive hazards of the American lifestyle: Work during pregnancy. *American Journal of Obstetrics and Gynecology, 176*(4), 826–832.

Galtier-Dereure, F., Boegner, C., & Bringer, J. (2000). Obesity and pregnancy: Complications and cost. *American Journal of Clinical Nutrition, 71*(Suppl.), 1242S–1248S.

Gregory, K. D., & Davidson, E. (1999). Prenatal care: Who needs it and why? *Clinical Obstetrics and Gynecology, 42*(4), 725–736.

Hamilton, B. H. (2001). Estimating treatment effects in randomized clinical trials with noncompliance: The impact of maternal smoking on birthweights. *Health Economics, 10*(5), 399–410.

Hellerstedt, W. L., Himes, J. H., Story, M., Alton, I., & Edwards, L. E. (1997). Effects of cigarette smoking and gestational weight change on birth outcomes in obese and normal-weight women. *American Journal of Public Health, 87,* 591–596.

Hellerstedt, W. L., Pirie, P. L., Lando, H. A., Curry, S. J., McBride, C. M., Grothaus, L. C., & Nelson, J. C. (1998). Differences in preconceptional and prenatal behaviors in women with intended and unintended pregnancies. *American Journal of Public Health, 88*(4), 663–666.

Henshaw, S. K. (1998). Unintended pregnancy in the United States. *Family Planning Perspectives, 30*(1), 24–29, 46.

Hoyert, D. L. (1996). Medical and lifestyle risk factors affecting fetal mortality, 1989–1990. *Vital & Health Statistics. Series 20: Data from the National Vital Statistic System, 31,* 1–32.

Huerta-Enochian, G., Katz, V., & Erfurth, J. S. (2001). The association of abnormal alpha-fetoprotein and adverse pregnancy outcome: Does increased fetal surveillance affect pregnancy outcome? *American Journal of Obstetrics and Gynecology, 184*(7), 1549–1553.

Hulsey, T. M. (2001). Association between early prenatal care and mother's intention of and desire for the pregnancy. *Journal of Obstetrical Gynecological Neonatal Nursing, 30*(3), 275–282.

Hulsey, T. M., Laken, M., Miller, V., & Ager, J. (2000). The influence of attitudes about unintended pregnancy on use of prenatal and postpartum care. *Journal of Perinatology, 20*(8, Pt. 1), 513–519.

Iams, J. (2003). Prediction and early detection of pre-term labor. *Obstetrics and Gynecology, 101*(2), 402–412.

Iams, J. D., Newman, R. B., Thom, E. A., Goldenber, R. L., Mueller-Heubach, E., Moawad, A., Sibai, B. M., Caritis, S. N., Miodovnik, M., Paul, R. H., Dombrowski, M. P., Thurnau, G., & McNellis, D. (2002). Frequency of uterine contractions and the risk of spontaneous preterm delivery. *New England Journal of Medicine, 346*(4), 250–255.

Institute of Medicine. (2000). *Nutrition during pregnancy.* Washington, DC: National Academy Press.

Jain, L., Ferre, C., & Vidyasagar, D. (1998). Racial differences in outcome of pregnancies complicated by hypertension. *Journal of Maternal Fetal Medicine, 7*(1), 23–27.

Johnson, M. J., Petri, M., Witter, F. R., & Repke, J. T. (1995). Evaluation of preterm delivery in a systemic lupus erythematosus pregnancy clinic. *Obstetrics and Gynecology, 86*(3), 396–399.

Kaiser, P. S., & Kirby, R. S. (2001). Obesity as a risk factor for cesarean in a low-risk population. *Obstetrics and Gynecology, 97*(1), 39–43.

Kalmus, D., & Fennelly, K. (1990). Barriers to prenatal care among low-income women in New York City. *Family Planning Perspectives, 22*(5), 215–218, 231.

Kochanek, K. D., & Martin, J. A. (2007). Supplemental analyses of recent trends in infant mortality. National Center for Health Statistics. Retrieved January 2008, from http://www.cdc.gov/nchs/prodcts/pubs/pubd/hestats/infantmort/infantmort.htm

Koonin, L. M., MacKay, A. P., Berg, C. J., Atrash, H. K., & Smith, J. C. (1997). Pregnancy related mortality surveillance—United States, 1987–1990. *Morbidity and Mortality Weekly Report, 46*(4), 17–36.

Li, D. K., & Wi, S. (2000). Changing paternity and the risk of pre-eclampsia/eclampsia in the subsequent pregnancy. *American Journal of Epidemiology, 151*(1), 57–62.

Lipscomb, G., Gevall, D., Mercer, B., & Sibai, B. (1991). A positive urine drug screen in pregnancy: Correlated to adverse pregnancy outcome, but not patient history. *American Journal of Obstetrics and Gynecology, 164*(1), 321.

Lukes, A., Thorp, J., Eucker, B., & Pahel-Short, S. (1997). Predictors of positivity for fetal fibrinectin in patients with symptoms of preterm labor. *American Journal of Obstetrics and Gynecology, 176*(3), 639–641.

MacDorman, M. F., Munson, M. L., & Kirmeyer, S. (2007). Fetal and perinatal mortality, United States, 2004. *National Vital Statistics Report, 56*(3), 1–16.

Maine, D. (2001). How do socioeconomic factors affect disparities in maternal mortality? *Journal of the American Medical Women's Association, 56*(4), 189–190, 192.

Manning, F. A. (1999). Fetal biophysical profile. *Obstetrics and Gynecologic Clinics of North America, 26*(4), 557–577.

Martin, J. A., Hamilton, B. E. Menacker, F., Sutton, P. D., & Mathews, T. J. (2004). Preliminary births for 2004: Infant and maternal health. NCHS Health and Stats. Retrieved January 8, 2008, from www.CDC.gov

Mazzaferri, E. L. (1997). Evaluation and management of common thyroid disorders in women. *American Journal of Obstetrics and Gynecology, 176*(3), 507–514.

Mikhail, B. (2000). Prenatal care utilization among low-income African-American women. *Journal of Community Health Nursing, 17*(4), 235–246.

Moos, M. K. (2006). Prenatal care: Limitations and opportunities. *Journal of Obstetrical, Gynecologic and Neonatal Nursing, 35*(2), 278–285.

Narod, S. A., De Sanjose, S., & Victora, C. (1991). Coffee during pregnancy: A reproductive hazard? *American Journal of Obstetrics and Gynecology, 164*(4), 1109–1114.

National High Blood Pressure Education Program. (2000). Working group report on high blood pressure in pregnancy 2000 update. Retrieved December 2007, from http://hp2010.nhlbihin.net/nhbpep_slds/hbppreg_ss/download/intro.pdf

Park, J., Vincent, D., & Hastings-Tolsma, M. (2007). Disparity in prenatal care among women of colour in the USA. *Midwifery, 23*(1), 28–37.

Peaceman, A. M., Andrews, W. W., Thorp, J. M., Cliver, S. P., Lukes, A., Iams, J. D., Coultrip, L., Eriksen, N., Holbrook, R. H., Elliot, J., Ingardia, C., & Pietrantoni, M. (1997). Fetal fibrinectin as a predictor of preterm birth in patients with symptoms: A multicenter trial. *American Journal of Obstetrics and Gynecology, 177*(1), 13–18.

Peters, R. M., & Flack, J. M. (2004). Hypertensive disorders of pregnancy. *Journal of Obstetrical, Gynecologic and Neonatal Nurses, 33*(2), 209–220.

Queenan, J. T., Spong, C. Y., & Lockwood, C. J. (2007). *Management of high-risk pregnancy* (5th ed.). Malden, MA: Blackwell Publishing.

Rayburn, W. F., & Bogenschutz, M. P. (2004). Pharmacotherapy for pregnant women with addictions. *American Journal of Obstetrics and Gynecology, 191,* 1885–1897.

Rosenn, B., Miodovnik, M., Combs, C. A., Khoury, J., & Siddiqi, T. A. (1994). Glycemic thresholds for spontaneous abortion and congenital malformation in insulin-dependent diabetes mellitus. *Obstetrics and Gynecology, 84*(4), 417.

Rubin, R. (1984). *Maternal identity and the maternal experience.* New York: Springer Publishing.

Russell, M. A., Carpenter, M. W., & Coustan, D. R. (2007). Screening and diagnosis of gestational diabetes mellitus. *Clinical Obstetrics & Gynecology, 50*(4), 949–958.

Sampson, P. D., Streissguth, A. P., Bookstein, F. L., Little, R. E., Clarren, S. K., Dehaene, P., Hanson, J. W., & Graham, J. M. (1997). Incidence of fetal alcohol syndrome and prevalence of alcohol-related neurodevelopmental disorders. *Teratology, 56*(5), 317–326.

Shiono, P. H., Klebanoff, M. A., Nugent, R. P., Cotch, M. F., Wilkins, D. G., Rollins, D. E., Carey, J. C., & Behrman, R. E. (1995). The impact of cocaine and marijuana use on low birth weight and preterm birth: A multicenter trial. *American Journal of Obstetrics and Gynecology, 172*(1), 19.

Simpson, J. L., Elias, S., Morgan, L. D., Anderson, R. N., Shulman, L. P., Sibai, B. M., Mercer, B. H., & Skoll, A. (1991). Does unexplained second trimester (15–20 weeks' gestation) maternal serum alpha-fetoprotein elevation presage adverse perinatal outcome? Pitfalls and preliminary studies with late second and third trimester maternal serum alpha-fetoprotein. *American Journal of Obstetrics and Gynecology, 164*(3), 829–836.

Singer, L. T., Hawkins, S., Huang, J., Davillier, M., & Baley, J. (2001). Developmental outcomes and environmental correlates of very low birthweight, cocaine exposed infants. *Early Human Development, 64*(2), 91–103.

Smith, G. C., & Pell, J. P. (2001). Teenage pregnancy and risk of adverse perinatal outcomes associated with first and second births: Population based retrospective cohort study. *British Medical Journal, 323*(7311), 476.

Sword, W. (1999). A soci-ecological approach to understanding barriers to prenatal care for women of low income. *Journal of Advanced Nursing, 29*(5), 1170–1177.

U.S. Department of Health and Human Services. (2000). *Healthy People 2010* (conference ed., 2 vols.). Washington, DC: Author.

Varney, H., Kriebs, J. M., & Gegor, C. (2004). *Varney's midwifery* (4th ed.). Boston: Jones and Barlett Publishers.

Ventura, S. J., Mathews, M. S., & Hamilton, B. E. (2001). Birth to teenagers in the United States. *National Vital Statistics Reports, 49*(10), 1–24.

Wang, E. C. (1999). Methadone treatment during pregnancy. *Journal of Obstetrical, Gynecologic and Neonatal Nurses, 28*(6), 615–622.

Weismiller, D. G. (1999). Preterm labor. *American Family Physician, 59*(3), 593–602.

18

Infertility

Ellen Olshanky and Catherine Garner

INCIDENCE AND PREVALENCE

Infertility, a condition that is distressing and disruptive to the lives of individuals and families, is very common and affects both men and women. It is estimated that seven million people in the United States experience infertility (Isaacs, 2005)—defined as the inability to conceive a child after a year or more of regular unprotected intercourse (Evers, 2002). Infertility is categorized as primary or secondary, with primary infertility occurring when there has been no history of pregnancy and secondary infertility occurring when there has been a previous pregnancy regardless of the outcome. Recurrent pregnancy loss is defined as two or more miscarriages in the first trimester. Although diagnosis can be made in 90% to 95% of cases and many highly technological therapies are available, only 50% to 60% of these couples can expect to achieve a pregnancy. In addition, infertility treatment is not accessible to all due to lack of insurance coverage for treatment or stigma about the infertility. Fewer than 50% of infertile persons with potential for successful treatment do not seek such treatment (Isaacs, 2005).

Caring for persons who are confronting infertility is challenging to nurses and other health care providers. This challenge includes being able to support various ways of resolving infertility, including caring for those who experience family building through birth or adoption and for those who may eventually choose to be child free. As many as 20% of couples seeking obstetric care may have had infertility problems and have unique needs for nursing care during the maternity cycle. Because infertility is not a life-threatening illness, its profound impact on those persons who are infertile is often dismissed or minimized by health care providers. Research has indicated, however, that infertility is frequently experienced as a major life crisis (Olshansky, 1996a).

TRENDS AND PATTERNS

Looking historically, although the overall incidence of infertility remained relatively unchanged between 1965 and 1983, one age group, married couples in which the women were aged 20 to 24 years, exhibited an increase in infertility from 3.6% to 10% infertile in 1982. This increase may be linked to the rate of sexually transmitted infections (STIs)—specifically gonorrhea in this age group, which tripled between 1960 and 1977 (U.S. Congress, 1988). Women are at higher risk for STIs when they become sexually active at a younger age, have more than one sex partner, and change partners frequently. Untreated STIs can lead to pelvic inflammatory disease (PID), which produces irreparable damage to fallopian tubes, causing infertility and ectopic pregnancies. Currently, there is increasing focus on environmental causes of infertility. Environmental toxins have been implicated in contributing to infertility (Birrittieri, 2005; Ma & Sasson, 2006).

Older women are affected by infertility at significant rates. This is occurring as women delay childbearing to pursue advanced education and careers and is significant because the optimum age for fertility in both men and women is 24. This issue reflects a struggle that women confront in balancing the biological clock with the sociological/career clock. In a society in which more women work outside the home and have careers, they are sometimes blamed for causing the infertility. As noted by Isaacs (2005), current president of Resolve, an infertility support organization, the notion that women cause infertility by waiting to conceive leads to misperceptions that create blame. Women older than age 30 have a higher incidence of ovulation problems, endometriosis, and have a greater length of time to be exposed to STIs and their consequences; however, as noted by Hanson (2003), it may be a misnomer that maternal age older than 35 is a significant factor alone, because it must be placed in the context of the woman's relationship with her partner, various social conditions, and potential physical conditions in the partner. Race is also significant when analyzing the statistical data on infertility. Black couples are one and a half times more likely than White couples to be infertile (Roberts, 1997).

Male fertility declines much more slowly than does female fertility, with no real significant change in sperm count until after the age of 55. Even then, men can father children throughout their life span. Despite these data, male infertility accounts for approximately half of overall infertility problems (Ficorelli & Weeks, 2007).

The number of babies available for adoption in the United States has declined steadily since the early 1970s due to increased availability of effective methods of birth control, legalized abortion, and a sociological trend for single women to keep their babies. International adoption has become more popular as a way of building one's family. Counseling couples about adoption requires that nurses be knowledgeable about many alternative avenues (Hahn, 1991).

There is no evidence that the use of birth control pills or abortion has contributed to the rise in infertility. Although previous research findings have suggested that women who use an intrauterine device (IUD) as a method of contraception are at increased risk for tubal infection, reanalysis of more current data suggests that the risk was overestimated and that IUDs do not increase the risk of PID (Kronmal, Whitney, & Mumford, 1991). The IUDs that are available today are safer than earlier forms, such as the Dalkon Shield, which was taken off the market. Women who are at high risk for PID because of sexual behaviors do have a higher incidence of tubal infertility.

Less is known about infertility worldwide and in differing cultures, particularly regarding incidence and prevalence. In our increasingly global society, more exploration of such information is warranted. Research is beginning to focus on infertility in countries besides the United States.

ASSESSMENT OF AND DIAGNOSTIC APPROACHES TO INFERTILITY

Evaluation of the infertile couple must focus on both partners. Even when the problem seems apparently due to one partner, it is appropriate and essential to evaluate both partners due to the high incidence of multiple problems. The most common problems for women are ovulation disorders, tubal disease, and endometriosis.

Simple problems such as coital frequency can have a significant effect on fertility rates. If a couple has intercourse once a week over 6 months, there is about a 16% chance of pregnancy. If a couple increases this to four times per week around the time of ovulation, this rate increases to 83% over 6 months. Often, simple counseling about the expected time of ovulation and coital frequency can alleviate the problem. Many couples, however, are often anxious and worried about potential infertility and deserve to be listened to and possibly assessed even before 1 year has elapsed. This is particularly true for couples who are at the older end of the childbearing years and who, therefore, have a more finite time available for treatment(s) to be successful.

The nursing diagnosis will depend on the educational level of the couple, the clinical diagnosis, and the treatment decision as well as on the overall goal of the woman and her partner. Many myths still need to be addressed. It is simplistic to assume that the only goal is achievement of pregnancy. For some, the goal is the answer to the question of why the problem is occurring. For others, it will be the achievement of a pregnancy that results from the biological union. For others still, it will be the process of becoming a parent, be it through pregnancy or adoption. The nurse can provide education, facilitate the diagnosis and treatment phases of infertility, assist with the decision-making process, and help with resolution of infertility, either by assisting the grief process or by facilitating parenting.

The infertility evaluation includes six major areas of assessment: (1) ovulation, (2) male factor, (3) sperm-mucus interaction, (4) tubal and uterine anatomy, (5) endometrial sufficiency, and (6) pelvic factors. For pregnancy to occur, the following physiological conditions, which are evaluated in a comprehensive infertility assessment, must function appropriately. Ovulation must, of course, occur for pregnancy to happen. Sufficient motile sperm must be present in the ejaculate, usually at least 20 million motile sperm per cc. At the time of ejaculation, sperm are deposited at the cervix, where the cervical mucus must be well estrogenated to be responsive to the survival of the sperm. An initial vanguard of sperm is in the fallopian tubes within seconds. Numerous sperm remain within cervical mucus crypts, nourished by estrogenic cervical mucus, and are released intermittently until mucus becomes less receptive/hostile to sperm under the influence of progesterone. Fallopian tubes must be patent and normal in anatomy. The endometrium must be sufficiently developed to allow implantation to occur, and the uterus should be free of anatomic defects and growths, such as uterine myomas or fibroids. Finally, the pelvis should be free of conditions that would preclude conception.

The infertility evaluation, by addressing each of these areas, will help to elucidate the causative factor(s) in the infertility, while recognizing that some causes of infertility are not able to be diagnosed because of insufficient technology or lack of scientific knowledge regarding all of the causes of infertility. In some cases, infertility may be caused by a sexual dysfunction.

Testing can and should be organized to evaluate these factors according to the menstrual cycle in the woman who is ovulating. A history of regular menstrual cycles is presumptive of ovulation. Many women keep records of their menstrual cycles by recording their basal body temperature each morning. A biphasic cycle (lower than 98 degrees during the proliferative phase and higher than 98 degrees during the luteal phase) provides indirect evidence of ovulation. A semen analysis can be obtained at any time that can be coordinated with the laboratory. A postcoital test (PCT) is done to evaluate sperm-mucus interaction at mid-cycle around the time of ovulation. A hysterosalpingogram (HSG), or X ray of the tubes, is performed after menstruation but before ovulation. A biopsy of the uterine lining to assess endometrial development is accomplished 1 to 2 days prior to expected menses.

Most of the routine infertility evaluation can be accomplished in one menstrual cycle in the ovulatory woman. It is therefore reasonable to accomplish the evaluation in a systematic manner that facilitates a timeliness in completing the various tests required. Such an approach can help to ease the couple's anxiety over waiting for answers regarding their particular infertility problem. Couples should be given an explanation of the evaluation process and allowed to choose testing intervals. This testing should be done in an efficient and logical sequence to minimize the stress and cost to the couple. The workup of an oligo- or anovulatory woman will require induction of ovulation before the PCT or endometrial biopsy can be performed. However, the semen analysis and HSG should be performed prior to starting ovulation induction medications such as clomiphene citrate.

The next major diagnostic test is a laparoscopy, which is performed to assess the presence of pelvic adhesions or endometriosis. The laparoscopy should not be performed before the other testing is completed unless the woman is in severe pelvic pain or prior to ovulation induction with expensive agents such as certain menotropins.

At the start of the infertility evaluation, nurses can explain the components of the infertility investigation, their purpose, and the reasons for exact timing. The rigid scheduling is often difficult for the couple, particularly if they have to travel some distance and arrange time away from work. Where slight variations in time or date of appointment are reasonable, allowing a couple to choose the day and time of the appointment gives back some measure of control. The assessment process can be reviewed in phases, starting with ovulation disorders that occur in 20% to 30% of infertile women.

CAUSES OF INFERTILITY

This section discusses specific causes of infertility, including the diagnostic tests used to assess the cause and the treatments available.

Ovulation Disorders

Assessment

The only way to document adequate ovulation with certainty is to document pregnancy. Other methods are considered presumptive of ovulation. Regular (every 26–36 days) menstrual cycles with premenstrual symptoms can be considered presumptive of ovulation. Another method to document ovulation is the use of a temperature chart. A woman takes her temperature every morning prior to any activity and records this on the chart. During the first half of the cycle, under the influence of estrogen, the basal body temperature is below 98° F. Within 24 hours after ovulation, under the influence of progesterone, the temperature rises approximately 1 degree. This is called a biphasic temperature chart. Ovulation can be documented only in retrospect. Urinary luteinizing hormone (LH) kits are also used to document the presence of LH in the urine at mid-cycle and are also presumptive of ovulation.

Extensive evaluation is necessary if the woman has had episodes of irregular bleeding, a time lapse of longer than 40 days between periods, amenorrhea, significant weight loss or gain, excessive facial or body hair, or a history of discharge from the breast.

Disorders may originate in the hypothalamus, ovary, or pituitary, or they may be due to congenital anomalies of the reproductive tract. In rare cases, a chromosomal anomaly may first manifest as absence of menses. An evaluation of pituitary function should include follicle-stimulating hormone (FSH), LH, prolactin, and thyroid function tests. Physical examination is necessary to ascertain normal sexual development, which implies a normally functioning ovary and a normal reproductive tract.

An elevated prolactin level is commonly found when evaluating the reproductive-age female for amenorrhea. An elevated prolactin level, with or without galactorrhea, requires further evaluation with computerized axial tomography (CAT scan) or magnetic resonance imaging of the pituitary. The only exception is a woman who has been lactating within the last 6 months. In most cases, the diagnosis will be a benign microadenoma of the pituitary. Less commonly, thyroid dysfunction, macroadenoma, and craniopharyngioma can cause hyperprolactinemia. Treatment for microadenoma is bromocryptine in doses titrated to achieve normal prolactin levels. Prolactin levels should be taken annually, and CAT scans should be taken every 1 to 2 years. Bromocryptine should be started at low doses and gradually increased to therapeutic levels to avoid hypotensive side effects.

Once on bromocryptine, the woman may attempt pregnancy if she begins to ovulate spontaneously, but bromocryptine should be discontinued as soon as pregnancy is confirmed. In cases in which prolactin levels are normal and ovulation does not resume spontaneously, clomiphene citrate is needed to induce ovulation. Baseline visual fields should be documented prior to pregnancy, because monitoring prolactin levels during pregnancy will give no true indication of the growth of the prolactinoma. Excessive enlargement of the prolactinoma during pregnancy may result in visual field changes due to compression of the optic nerve and may be the first indication of complications.

Mullerian anomalies and conditions that obstruct the outflow tract should be ruled out during physical examination. A hysterosalpingogram may be necessary for accurate diagnosis. On rare occasions, genetic disorders may cause amenorrhea.

Elevated FSH and LH levels are indicative of ovarian failure. Ovarian failure before the age of 40 is considered premature, and a thorough reproductive endocrine work-up is indicated, because the incidence of autoimmune disorders is significantly higher in these women. An evaluation is also indicated if menses occurs before age 8 (precocious puberty) or has not occurred by the age of 16.

An elevated LH-to-FSH ratio, with hirsutism and obesity, is indicative of polycystic ovarian syndrome. Further evaluation of testosterone and dehydroepiandrosterone sulfate is indicated to rule out ovarian and adrenal tumors. Women with polycystic ovarian syndrome are often readily susceptible to clomiphine citrate and may require 25-mg doses rather than 50 mg.

Treatment

Proper treatment for an ovulation disorder can be started once a diagnosis is established. If there is an imbalance in the hypothalamic-pituitary-ovarian response or a low FSH and LH, induction of ovulation is usually initiated. Only rarely is ovulation induction successful in a woman with an elevated FSH. Mullerian anomalies and uterine defects may be treated surgically.

Ovulation induction medications are often mistakenly referred to as fertility drugs. These medications simply induce ovulation; they do not enhance fertility. In some cases in which a woman is already ovulating, these drugs can actually decrease fertility due to their antiestrogenic effects. Clomiphene citrate (Clomid,

Serophene) is the drug of choice for initiating ovulation induction. In a normally ovulating woman, a lack of circulating estrogen signals the hypothalamus to release gonadotropin-releasing hormone (GnRH) and initiate the menstrual cycle. It is thought that clomiphene citrate binds to estrogen receptors in the pituitary, blocking them from detecting circulating estrogen. The hypothalamus then releases more GnRH, stimulating pituitary release of FSH and LH, thus initiating a menstrual cycle.

Clomiphene citrate is administered on cycle days 5 through 9 in daily doses of 50 mg. Women can be expected to ovulate approximately 14 days from the start of the clomiphene citrate, or cycle days 17 to 19, with menses occurring days 32 to 34. If the woman fails to ovulate at the 50-mg dose, then the dose can be increased to 100 mg in the next cycle. Most pregnancies that occur as a result of clomiphene citrate occur at doses of 50 mg to 100 mg. Clomiphene citrate can be given in amounts of up to 250 mg per day before considering other therapies. Once ovulation has occurred at a specific dose, there is no advantage in increasing the dose. Once ovulation is established, the PCT and endometrial biopsy should be performed on all women, because the antiestrogenic properties of clomiphene citrate can have an adverse effect on cervical mucus and endometrial development.

Side effects of clomiphene citrate include hot flashes, headaches, ovarian enlargement, and multiple gestation. Other infrequent symptoms include nausea and visual disturbances. These disappear after stopping the medication. Approximately 90% of clomiphene citrate pregnancies result in singleton deliveries. Nearly 10% result in delivery of twins, and less than 1% result in triplets or more. If pregnancy has not resulted in 6 to 12 months of therapy, laparoscopy, to rule out pelvic factors, and the use of other medications should be considered.

Research has raised the possibility of a correlation between use of clomiphene citrate and later development of ovarian cancer. The studies, however, are inconclusive (Goldfien, 1998). Clearly, further research is needed to clarify this potential risk of clomiphene citrate.

Pergonal (human menopausal gonadotropins) is a preparation of FSH and LH in a one-to-one ratio. This therapy is indicated with women who fail to ovulate with clomiphene citrate. Pergonal directly stimulates ovarian follicular development. The dosage is carefully monitored by daily serum estradiol levels and ovarian ultrasound. Once follicular maturation has occurred, ovulation is triggered by administration of human chorionic gonadotropin (HCG). Because Pergonal administration can result in the development of multiple follicles, HCG may be withheld when there are more than three mature follicles to limit the chance of multiple gestation. Although 80% of Pergonal births will be singletons, the multiple gestation rate is 20%, with less than 5% of that being three or more. If the woman becomes pregnant with more than twins, the issue of selective reduction of fetuses must be discussed with the couple. The other serious side effect of Pergonal therapy is ovarian hyperstimulation. This syndrome presents with pelvic distension and weight gain. Early diagnosis and treatment is essential, because death can result if the condition progresses. Metrodin is purified human menopausal gonadotropins, with a resultant mixture of almost pure FSH. Metrodin is also used when amenorrhea is caused by an elevated LH:FSH ratio or by polycystic ovarian syndrome. The use of Metrodin requires the same intensive monitoring as does the use of Pergonal, and it has the same potential side effects.

Nursing care of women undergoing ovulation induction requires adequate patient education regarding the mechanism of action, expected results, and potential side effects. Patient adherence with specified regimens is essential. Ovulation induction with Pergonal or Metrodin can be quite expensive and requires a time commitment due to the necessity of daily monitoring. Couples should be carefully counseled about the prospect of multiple births, and this counseling must be documented in the chart. The drugs used in ovulation induction often have significant side effects. Nurses should educate women and their partners about what to expect and should provide reassurance and support during the cycles. The cost of ovulation induction with Pergonal/Metrodin can run between $1,500 and $3,000 a year.

Cervical Factor

The precise role and relative importance of cervical mucus in human fertilization continues to be controversial. The secretions of the cervical canal serve as a filter for the millions of spermatozoa that are deposited into the vagina. Perhaps as few as 100 sperm pass through the cervical canal into the uterine cavity. Although there is no absolute proof that cervical mucus is necessary for fertilization, poor quantity and quality have been associated with infertility. Although the true incidence of abnormal cervical mucus–sperm interaction is unknown, it is estimated to be a causal factor in between 5% and 15% of infertility cases. Cervical factor infertility is on the rise due to more aggressive treatment of cervical dysplasia associated with the human papillomavirus. Destruction of the cervical mucus glands by cautery or laser vaporization causes permanent destruction of mucus glands.

Assessment

Initial evaluation of the cervical mucus–sperm interaction is the postcoital test. The menstrual cycle is monitored by the woman at home using a urinary LH kit. When the test indicates evidence of the mid-cycle LH surge, couples are asked to have sexual intercourse and come to their health care provider within 24 hours. Cervical mucus is aspirated with a small catheter from the internal os and examined under a microscope for the presence of motile sperm. The results are reported as the number of sperm per high power field. More than five sperm per high power field is considered to be consistent with proven fertility. Sperm that are immotile or observed to shake may indicate the presence of antisperm antibodies.

The most common reason for a poor PCT result is poor timing. There is a window of only 48 to 72 hours when cervical mucus is receptive to sperm. At any other time, cervical mucus serves as a protective barrier. Thus, a careful evaluation of timing in relation to ovulation is important. The urinary LH kits available today to consumers can be used to time this test more accurately and eliminate this factor.

Other reasons for a poor PCT result include coital difficulties, such as premature ejaculation and obesity, which cause the sperm to be deposited in the outer two-thirds of the vagina. Other couples are unable to complete the act of intercourse on demand. If repeated cancellations occur, one should be alert to this possibility. Furthermore, poor cervical mucus can be caused by cervical stenosis, cervical infection, or cervical trauma due to removal of portions of the cervical canal through biopsy, cauterization, or resection. Coital lubricants, such as petroleum jelly, act as spermicides and should be avoided when attempting pregnancy.

Poor PCTs with normal cervical mucus may be due to cervical mucus antisperm antibodies. Antibodies can be found in both women's serum and cervical mucus. Antibodies in women have several proposed mechanisms of action: prevention of mucus penetration, interference with acrosome reaction, activation of macrophages, and impaired sperm-egg interaction.

Treatment

The type of therapy available to couples with repeated poor postcoital testing will depend on the etiology. Highly cellular mucus is indicative of infection, which is treated with doxycycline, 100 mg twice a day for 10 days for both partners, starting on day 1 of menses. The PCT is then repeated in the next cycle. When problems are persistent, sperm are placed directly into the uterus using intrauterine insemination. It is generally recommended that three to four cycles of intrauterine insemination be performed. If the woman has not become pregnant, the couple should consider other therapies, such as in vitro fertilization (IVF) or gamete intrafallopian transfer (GIFT), or consider discontinuing therapy. Repeated inseminations offer no additional advantage for fertility, and repeated failure with inseminations can be very damaging to a couple's self-esteem.

Tubal Factor

Assessment

Damage or blockage of the fallopian tubes is one of the most common causes of female infertility and has been on the increase due to a rise in pelvic infections from chlamydia and gonorrhea. Evaluation of the uterine cavity and fallopian tubes is accomplished with an HSG. X rays are taken from several different angles after the uterus and tube are filled with a contrast media introduced into the uterus through a cannula. If tubal obstruction is present, women may experience moderate to severe discomfort.

Women report varying degrees of pain and cramping with the procedure, and prophylactic analgesia may be indicated. Because serious pelvic infections occur in between 0.3% and 1.3% of patients undergoing HSG, prophylactic antibiotics should be used when there is a history of PID or blocked tubes. Side effects of HSG include uterine cramping, bleeding, nausea, and dizziness. Vagal stimulation may occur with cervical manipulation, resulting in mild bradycardia, hypertension, and diaphoresis. There is a risk of uterine perforation and allergic reaction to the contrast media. Most women report some cervical bleeding after the procedure.

Tubal damage places the woman at much higher risk for ectopic pregnancy should conception occur. Women should be counseled to report for medical observation as soon as they suspect pregnancy. Early monitoring can result in more conservative treatment.

If the HSG shows extensive damage, it is the degree of tubal damage that dictates those therapeutic options available to the woman. Extensive internal damage is rarely able to be treated effectively. If there is limited damage to only a portion of the tube, the damaged portion of the tube may be removed and the healthy part is reanastamosed.

Treatment

Sometimes the HSG, if used with an oil-based dye, is therapeutic in opening up the fallopian tubes slightly. Other times, surgery is necessary. Such microsurgery requires extensive training and experience. The fallopian tubes are delicate organs that, once damaged, never heal. The surgeon's skill is critical in being able to offer a surgical solution to tubal problems. The goals of microsurgery are to correct the anatomic defect and to prevent pelvic adhesions. Any insult to the pelvis may result in further adhesion formation, so tissue handling must be delicate.

IVF was first developed as therapy for women with absent or irreparably damaged tubes and remains one of the primary options to be considered. Women should be counseled about the success rates of tubal surgery and risks of subsequent ectopic pregnancy versus the success rates for IVF.

Disease processes outside the tube that can lead to tubal problems include appendicitis, endometriosis, ruptured ovarian cyst, or peritubular adhesions from abdominal or pelvic surgery. It is suspected that diethylstilbestrol (DES) exposure contributes to ectopic pregnancy because of tubal abnormalities now being documented in DES daughters.

Endometrial Developmental Factors

Adequate development of the endometrium is necessary for normal implantation of an embryo. The endometrial glands and stroma respond to the progesterone secreted by the corpus luteum during the luteal phase. An endometrial factor that can contribute to infertility may be either inadequate progesterone stimulation from the ovarian follicle or an inappropriate response of the endometrium.

Assessment

An endometrial biopsy using a pipelle aspirator or Novak curette is obtained 1 to 2 days prior to expected menses and is used to evaluate the endometrial response. The procedure causes one to two menstrual-like cramps. Discomfort will depend on the individual woman's pain threshold. Women should expect mild cramping and spotting after the procedure. If they experience a fever or severe cramping, however, they should call their health care provider to be sure there is not an infection. Women should be instructed to call with the date of their next menstrual period, because this is essential to the proper interpretation of the biopsy. Occasionally, the endometrial biopsy is done during the cycle of conception, so patients may wish to use barrier contraception during the month of biopsy. If a sensitive urine pregnancy test is available, this should be performed immediately prior to the biopsy.

The biopsy specimen is examined microscopically, and an approximate cycle date is assigned to the endometrial pattern. A biopsy that is out of phase with where it is expected to be must be confirmed by a second biopsy in a subsequent cycle for a diagnosis of luteal-phase inadequacy, because all women occasionally experience an out-of-phase cycle.

Although serum progesterone sampling has been used to document luteal-phase inadequacy, there may be little or no correlation between the serum progesterone and the endometrial response due to the pulsating nature of progesterone secretion. Therefore, it is recommended that endometrial biopsy be obtained to establish a luteal-phase deficiency.

Treatment

Treatment of a luteal-phase defect depends on the etiology. If the defect is present with other conditions, such as elevated serum prolactin or endometriosis, treatment of the underlying disorder may result in correction of the defect.

There is some debate about the treatment of luteal-phase deficiency. Some argue that, because the etiology may involve faulty development of the ovarian follicle, the approach should be to enhance the follicular phase with ovulation induction agents. Others argue that a progesterone deficiency is best treated with luteal-phase progesterone. Both approaches have been successful.

Progesterone supplementation is usually accomplished with progesterone rectal or vaginal suppositories, 12.5 mg to 25 mg every 12 hours. The suppositories are begun 3 days after the mid-cycle rise of basal body temperature and are continued until menstruation, which is rarely delayed beyond 2 days by the progesterone. The dosage is modulated to achieve an adequate endometrial response. The progesterone is absorbed through the vaginal mucosa as the suppository melts, and the use of a sanitary pad may help protect undergarments. Side effects can include local irritation of the vagina and external genitalia. Some patients prefer to self-inject 12.5 mg of progesterone in oil intramuscularly on a daily basis. Oral progesterone has also been used. Should pregnancy occur, the progesterone is continued until an ultrasound scan at 6 to 8 weeks documents a viable pregnancy. At this time, the fetal-placental unit should be able to sustain itself through its own placental progesterone production. The corpus luteum declines at this time.

One-third of recurrent spontaneous abortions are caused by a luteal-phase defect. If this is the indication for the biopsy, the couple should be cautioned to use a barrier method of contraception until the defect has been corrected.

Pelvic Factor

Assessment

Pelvic factors of infertility refer to the health of the intrauterine environment. The pelvic organs are the areas of assessment for problems of infertility that are the result of pelvic factors. Once the initial phases of the infertility evaluation have been accomplished, factors that have been identified should be treated prior to laparoscopy. Ovulation induction should be established and the couple given an opportunity to achieve pregnancy. If pregnancy has not occurred after 6 to 9 months of ovulation, laparoscopy is indicated because direct intra-abdominal visualization may be necessary to establish a diagnosis. Laparoscopy allows direct visualization of the internal organs through a small incision in the umbilicus. A second and occasionally a third incision is necessary to manipulate the pelvic organs for complete evaluation. Six characteristics are noted during diagnostic laparoscopy: the size, shape, surface, color, consistency, and mobility of the uterus, tubes, and ovaries.

Treatment

Much operative work can be accomplished through the laparoscope, including lysis of adhesions, vaporization of endometriosis, and surgical excision of ectopic pregnancy. Postoperatively, many patients report some shoulder discomfort due to the insufflation of carbon dioxide. This usually resolves within 24 hours, and discomfort can be relieved by assuming the knee-chest position. A sore throat from the endotracheal intubation also is common. The degree of abdominal discomfort will depend on the amount of surgical manipulation and the individual's threshold of pain. Nausea and vomiting may occur as a consequence of anesthesia or manipulation of the bowel during surgery.

Hysteroscopy is a similar procedure that examines the inside of the uterine cavity. This may be done at the time of laparoscopy or as a separate procedure. Evaluation and removal of a uterine septum, polyps, or intrauterine adhesions may be accomplished through the hysteroscope. It is particularly valuable for the lysis of adhesions with Ascherman's syndrome, a condition in which there is internal scarring of the uterus.

Endometriosis

Assessment

Endometriosis is commonly observed at laparoscopy. This disease is defined as the presence of endometrial glands and stroma outside the uterine cavity. Endometrial tissue has been found on the ovary, uterine ligaments, pelvic peritoneum, cervix, inguinal area, cul-de-sac, and rectovaginal septum. Endometrial lesions have been found in the vagina, vulva, perineum, bladder, and surgical scars. Some women have lesions of the gastrointestinal tract, usually in the sigmoid. Endometrial implants also have been found in sites far from the pelvic area, such as the thoracic cavity, limbs, gallbladder, and heart. Endometrial lesions contain glands and stroma and respond to cyclic hormones at times similar to the uterine endometrium but often out of phase with it. Blood may flow into endometrial lesions or into their surrounding tissue. Symptoms result from the pathophysiological changes that occur, including bleeding from the lesions, formation of endometriomas (cysts), adhesions, and/or anatomical distortions or obstructions. Pain results from inflammation, irritation, encroachment, and obstruction.

Although its exact incidence is difficult to determine, because it can exist without causing symptoms, a rough estimate is that 10% of all women in the reproductive age group and 25% to 35% of all infertile women have endometriosis (Cramer, 1987). Approximately one-third to one-half of all women having major gynecologic procedures are found to have endometriosis (Clarke-Pearson & Dawood, 1990). At one time it was thought that endometriosis was more prevalent in White middle- and upper-class women; however, racial differences have been found to be nonexistent (Clarke-Pearson & Dawood, 1990). It was also once believed that problems attributed to lower socioeconomic groups, such as tubal blockage caused by gonorrhea, prevented the disease. It is more likely, however, that the symptoms once attributed to PID were actually symptoms of unrecognized endometriosis and that prejudicial attitudes may account for the belief that pelvic pain or other symptoms in Black women were related to PID rather than to endometriosis (Clarke-Pearson & Dawood, 1990). The common belief that endometriosis occurs only in goal-oriented career women who have delayed their childbearing also has been discredited. Traditionally, endometriosis was considered a disease of women in their 30s and 40s; however, endometriosis is more common in adolescents than previously believed. In two series of laparoscopies of teenagers with disabling pain or abnormal vaginal bleeding, a significant percentage were found to have endometriosis. It also had been assumed that nulliparity was a risk factor for endometriosis; however, 30% to 40% of women with the disease are parous (Luciano & Pitkin, 1984). There appears to be a familial tendency to develop endometriosis; research has demonstrated that the incidence of severe endometriosis is higher (61.1%) in the family group than in the nonfamily group (23.8%) (Clarke-Pearson & Dawood, 1990).

Although endometriosis has been recognized as a clinical entity since the mid-1800s and many theories concerning it have been advanced, the etiology and pathology are still poorly understood. One of the most widely accepted, long-debated etiologies is that of retrograde flow of menstrual fluid through the fallopian tubes and subsequent implantation of viable fragments of endometrial tissue within the pelvic cavity. However, this explanation does not account for extrapelvic sites of endometriosis such as the lungs or limbs. Retrograde menstruation alone is unlikely to produce endometriosis; more probably, a genetic factor or susceptibility and a favorable hormonal milieu are needed for implantation and growth of transplanted endometrial tissue (Clarke-Pearson & Dawood, 1990). Other explanations for the development of endometriosis include genetic and immunologic factors, elevated prostaglandin levels, and the luteinized unruptured follicle syndrome, in which a functioning corpus luteum exists but the egg does not leave the follicle.

Careful pain, menstruation, and reproductive histories should provide additional data to support the suspicion. In addition, nurses can obtain a sexual history to document the presence of dyspareunia. Women should be asked if any family members have experienced similar symptoms.

A complete pelvic examination is essential to confirm the diagnosis of endometriosis. In the pelvic exam, the most common indicator of endometriosis is nodularity of the uterosacral ligament. These nodules may be tender. The dyspareunia described by the woman often may be recreated with cervical manipulation that occurs during a pelvic or rectovaginal examination. A rectal examination should be done, because the uterus is often fixed in a retroverted position due to endometriosis, and the endometrial nodules present on the posterior uterine wall, cul-de-sac, and uterosacral ligament may be distinguished well rectally. No specific laboratory tests assess specifically for endometriosis. Definite diagnosis is done by laparoscopy.

Once the diagnosis is made, management is approached from the standpoint of both prevention and treatment. Although absolute prevention of endometriosis is not possible for most women, prophylaxis against some of the more disabling aspects of the disease and decreased fertility may be possible. Clarke-Pearson and Dawood (1990) recommend that women who have a family history of endometriosis and who wish to have children should avoid undue delay in childbearing.

Treatment

Treatment goals for endometriosis include prevention of disease progression, alleviation of pain, and establishment or restoration of fertility. Treatment options include observation alone, medical therapy, surgical therapy, or a combination of medical and surgical options. The woman's age, desire for children, presence or absence of significant adhesions, and severity of symptoms are major considerations in developing a treatment plan.

A young woman with mild endometriosis who wants children and does not have a fixed, retroverted uterus will have as good a chance of becoming pregnant without treatment as with either medical or surgical therapy (Garner & Webster, 1985). Moderate to severe disease with infertility but without significant tubo-ovarian adhesions or endometriosis may be treated medically if the woman is young enough to have time for medical suppression. Women with extensive disease, large endometriomas, or significant distortion of tubo-ovarian anatomy with adhesions will require surgical intervention in most cases.

The aim of medical therapy is to stop the growth of the ectopic tissue and allow regression of the disease. A variety of therapies has been used, including estrogen therapy with DES and progestins. Such therapies are rarely used today, however, because of the significant risk of endometrial hyperplasia and thrombophlebitis associated with estrogen therapy and the numerous side effects associated with progestins. Combination oral contraceptives have been used to produce a state of pseudopregnancy that should induce regression of the disease. When this therapy is stopped, patients experience high rates of recurrence of pain and other symptoms.

Hormonal antagonists such as Danazol and other GnRH antagonists (e.g., buserelinm nafarelin) have been used to suppress ovulation. Danazol acts to produce anovulation and hypogonadotropinism with resultant decreased ovarian secretion of estrogen and progesterone, thus allowing regression of the endometrium. Amenorrhea is seen in most users after 6 to 8 weeks of treatment, and some women experience other symptoms of menopause. The most commonly recommended daily dosage for effective treatment is 800 mg Danazol in four divided doses because of its short plasma half-life (Clarke-Pearson & Dawood, 1990). Symptoms improve in 70% to 93% of women with these regimens, and fertility rates are between 40% and 76% depending on the stage of the disease (Clarke-Pearson & Dawood, 1990), with a recurrence rate of 5% to 15% 1 year after therapy (Garner & Webster, 1985). Side effects usually result from the androgenic and antiestrogenic properties of the Danazol and include weight gain, acne and oily skin, edema, hirsutism, hot flushes, menstrual spotting, and a decrease in breast size. Danazol is contraindicated in women with hepatic dysfunction, severe hypertension, congestive heart failure, or borderline renal function. Usually, Danazol treatment is begun during menses, and women are counseled to wait one normal menstrual cycle after stopping the drug before attempting pregnancy. Danazol is expensive, which may be a problem for many women.

GnRH agonist therapy (Leuprolide, Synarel) is also used to treat endometriosis. GnRH agonists act by inducing down regulation and desensitization of the pituitary. FSH/LH stimulation to the ovary declines markedly and ovarian function diminishes significantly. The hypoestrogenism leads to hot flashes in almost all women. There can be minor bone loss, most of which is reversible within 12 to 18 months after therapy.

Surgery is often necessary for severe, acute, or incapacitating symptoms. Decisions regarding the extent of the surgery depend on age, desire for children, and extent and location of the disease. In women who do not wish to conserve their reproductive capacity, hysterectomy and bilateral salpingo-oophorectomy are the only definitive cures. When the woman is in her childbearing years and wants children, and the disease does not preclude it, reproductive function should be retained through careful removal of all endometrial tissue with retention of ovarian function.

Counseling and education are important components of nursing management of women with endometriosis. A frank discussion of the treatment options and potential risks and benefits is mandatory. Because pelvic pain is a subjective, personal experience that is often frightening, psychological support is important for women with endometriosis. Sexual dysfunction resulting from dyspareunia is common, and referral for psychological counseling may be indicated. Support groups for women with endometriosis are available in some locations, and Resolve, an organization for infertile couples, may also be of help to these women. Continuation or recurrence of pelvic pain may necessitate assisting the woman to manage her chronic pelvic pain and dysmenorrhea. The nursing strategies discussed in the section on dysmenorrhea in chapter 20 are applicable here as well.

Unfortunately, regardless of the form of treatment, endometriosis returns in approximately 40% of cases. Thus, for many, endometriosis represents a chronic disease and will require nursing management of the manifestation of this condition, be it chronic pelvic pain or infertility. Peak fertility after treatment of endometriosis is in the first 12 to 18 months after therapy. This is one of the reasons for correcting other fertility factors prior to laparoscopy.

Male Factor

Assessment

Only recently is male infertility receiving emphasis in research and clinical care of the infertile couple. Yet 40% to 60% of fertility is related to a male factor. Therefore, testing for male factor infertility should be performed before the female partner undergoes any invasive diagnostic or therapeutic procedures. Careful explanation of the components of the evaluation of the man should be provided at the initial exam.

A systematic history of physical development, general health, and sexual habits is necessary to identify potential problems. Because spermatogenesis is an ongoing process, men are much more susceptible to variations in this process. For example, environmental factors, such as drug use and high scrotal temperatures, can adversely affect spermatogenesis. Questions about drug use, illnesses, past episodes of STD, and adequacy of ejaculation are essential to the male fertility assessment.

Alcohol intake and cigarette smoking have been implicated in decreased sperm counts. Medications such as cimetidine (Tagamet) and aldomet can decrease sperm counts. The use of anabolic steroids causes a decline in testosterone and subsequently in sperm production.

Causes of male infertility include pituitary and hypothalamic dysfunction, which can be diagnosed by serum FSH and LH levels. Low FSH and LH may indicate hypothalamic or pituitary dysfunction, whereas elevated gonadotropins (FSH, LH) indicate testicular failure. Hormonal problems at the level of the testes can be detected by serum testosterone levels.

Undescended testes after the age of 2 may result in permanent damage due to high temperature of the testes. Hypospadias, a congenital anomaly in which the urethral outlet is on the shaft of the penis rather than at the end, may result in semen being deposited in the vagina rather than at the cervix. Hyposadias is being reported with increasing frequency in infants born to cocaine-addicted women. Mumps, particularly after adolescence, can result in permanent damage to the testes. Recurrent STD may cause scarring and blockage of the reproductive tract. A low-grade prostate infection also can affect sperm count. Any injury, such as testicular torsion, can result in ischemia to the testes and a decreased sperm count.

Antisperm antibodies may develop and cause fertility problems. Normally the male reproductive tract does not come into direct contact with the circulatory system. When there is a breakdown of the reproductive tract that allows sperm into the general circulation, the immune system forms antibodies to sperm. Conditions that can cause antibody formation include recurrent STD and vasectomy. The titer of antibodies, which can either immobilize or agglutinate sperm, is significant in projecting overall chances of pregnancy. Men should be counseled about obtaining a serum antisperm antibody titer prior to attempting a vasectomy reversal. Men with high antibody titers should be counseled regarding the poor prognosis of pregnancy and the other options available, including adoption and artificial insemination.

Laboratory evaluation of men starts with semen analysis. Traditionally done with a hemocytometer, the introduction of computerized technology is changing the procedure for semen analysis. Normal semen parameters are as follows:

Volume 3 to 5 cc

Count 20 million per cc

Morphology (number of normally shaped sperm) greater than 60%

Motility (number of sperm swimming progressively forward) greater than 60%

No semen analysis will have 100% motility or 100% normal forms. The problem with low motility or abnormally developed sperm is that they are not able to navigate the cervix so that fertilization can occur in the fallopian tubes. Degrees of oligospermia (reduced count) or reduced motility and abnormal morphology will have bearing on the types of therapy available to the couple.

Ideally, the semen sample is collected by masturbation into a sterile container with no fewer than 2 days but no more than 7 days of abstinence. The sample should be examined within 2 hours of collection. Sterile, unlubricated condoms can be used for collection when there are religious or cultural objections to masturbation. Two or more abnormal samples must be obtained before a definitive diagnosis is made. Obtaining serum levels of FSH, LH, and testosterone and a physical examination are then appropriate for further diagnosis.

Additional testing for sperm-mucus interaction, antisperm antibodies, and sperm penetration may be necessary before a prognosis can be given and treatment recommended. The sperm penetration assay is an evaluation of the functional ability of sperm to penetrate hamster eggs. Human eggs are not readily available to test for penetration, but there appears to be a correlation between the ability of sperm to penetrate human eggs and hamster eggs. This test may be used when there is a question about the ability of sperm to fertilize. Although the only true test of sperm is with human eggs, the sperm penetration assay is the best test available at the present time.

A varicocele is a varicose vein in the scrotum and is commonly found on physical exam in men. It is theorized that this causes an elevation in scrotal temperature and thus affects spermatogenesis. The number of fertile men with varicoceles is unknown, but this condition is thought to be associated with male infertility.

Treatment

Treatment will be tailored to the individual problem. Medical therapies for low FSH and LH include clomiphene citrate and tamoxifen citrate, both antiestrogens that stimulate FSH and LH production. Antibiotics are indicated when infection is present. Lifestyle changes may be necessary to correct self-induced fertility factors. Surgical therapy to correct blockages or ligate varicose veins may also be appropriate. Some data indicate that 50% of men will see an improvement in semen parameters after varicocelectomy, but there are no conclusive data that fertility rates are enhanced (Vermeulen & Vandeweghe, 1984). Other therapies, such as artificial insemination and intrauterine insemination of the partner's semen, are directed at manipulation of the semen. Although 20 million motile sperm are required for natural conception, as few as 50,000 to 500,000 sperm are necessary for in vitro fertilization or gamete intrafallopian transfer. The availability of these procedures has led to an increase in couples choosing this because of male factor. These technologies are detailed later in the chapter.

Artificial Insemination

Artificial insemination of a partner's sperm involves collection of the semen sample by masturbation and placing it into the cervix or directly into the uterus. This procedure minimizes semen loss and maximizes motility. Intrauterine insemination allows for direct placement of sperm into the uterus, thus bypassing the cervix when there is a problem with cervical mucus production. The semen sample is processed to remove the seminal plasma and concentrate the motile sperm prior to placement. This procedure is also performed under conditions of low motility and low sperm count, although overall pregnancy rates for male factors are poor.

Both of these procedures require precise timing with menstrual cycles and may be quite taxing to the couple emotionally. Artificial insemination can provoke feelings of inadequacy and abnormality and often interferes with the satisfying sexual relationship of the couple. Nursing sensitivity to these issues is important. Insemination with the partner's sperm can be taught to couples so that this can occur at home. Use of milex clinicap is common.

Therapeutic Donor Insemination

Insemination with donor semen is indicated in cases with severely low sperm count or no sperm (azoospermia), sex-linked genetic diseases, and severe male antisperm antibodies. Couples require extensive counseling regarding this option, because there are a number of psychological issues involved. The couple may need to grieve over the inability to achieve a biological union as well as discuss any religious objections. Most donor insemination programs in the United States are coordinated by nurses, who counsel couples about the procedures, assist them in selecting a donor from a written description of the donor profile, and then perform the inseminations. The nurse must be able to detect problems with the couple's acceptance of the procedure and, ultimately, of the child produced. Nurses must be knowledgeable about the ethical, religious, legal, and medical aspects of the procedure (Hahn, 1991).

More single women who are approaching the end of their reproductive years are considering donor insemination. Frank discussions about the pros and cons of single parenting are an important part of the initial counseling. Single women, more than married couples, will have to address issues related to the societal acceptance of donor insemination and telling a child about donor parentage.

Sperm are usually obtained from a commercial bank that screens donors for STDs, health risk factors, and congenital defects. Sperm must be quarantined for 6 months and the donor retested for HIV prior to release for use, because semen is a route of transmission for HIV. The sample is frozen in liquid nitrogen in the interim. Insemination is accomplished using thawed donor semen by intracervical or intrauterine insemination. An estimated 75,000 babies are born each year through donor insemination.

Unexplained Infertility

There is still much to be learned about human reproduction. In the early 1950s, perhaps 40% to 50% of infertility cases were unexplained. As the knowledge base has expanded, this diagnosis is now applied in less than 5% of cases. With further advances in diagnostic testing, this number will continue to decline.

Unexplained infertility is certainly the most difficult diagnosis for couples to accept. This diagnosis allows for the possibility of subsequent pregnancy but does not pose any specific factor that can be treated. Although many couples with this diagnosis do ultimately become pregnant, there are an equal number who do not. Psychological support is important for these couples.

TREATMENTS FOR INFERTILITY

Assisted Reproductive Technologies

The term assisted reproductive technology (ART) refers to the use of highly technological procedures to treat infertility and is now commonplace in discussions of infertility treatment. Probably the most well known of the ARTs is in vitro fertilization, which evolved as a procedure to assist women with blocked or absent fallopian tubes achieve pregnancy. It has since been used to treat couples with male factor, antisperm antibodies, cervical infertility, and unexplained infertility. Very simply, the ovaries are hyperstimulated using a combination of ovulation-induction agents to obtain a large number of oocytes. Once the ovary has been sufficiently stimulated, oocytes are removed via laparoscopy or vaginal ultrasound-guided aspiration and placed into an incubator with sperm. After 48 hours, if fertilization and division of oocytes has occurred, four to eight cell embryos are transferred into the uterus using a small catheter.

Gamete intrafallopian transfer (GIFT) is a variation of IVF in which oocytes are laparoscopically removed, identified, and then placed back into the ends of the fallopian tubes with the sperm. The woman then recovers, and fertilization occurs naturally. GIFT is an option for women with one normal fallopian tube, unexplained infertility, or recurrent endometriosis. Both IVF and GIFT are performed in women whose male partners have compromised semen analysis, because as few as 50,000 to 100,000 are necessary for IVF and GIFT.

When transfer of embryos or oocytes is accomplished, a major concern is the possibility of multiple births. Many fertility centers limit the number of eggs/embryos transferred to three to significantly decrease the likelihood of multiple gestation. Excess embryos can be frozen (cryopreserved) for indefinite periods of time, then thawed and transferred into the uterus, and progress through normal pregnancy and birth. Couples who do not become pregnant in the initial stimulation cycle can thus return in a subsequent menstrual cycle for a transfer of thawed embryos. When multiple embryos are transferred, the couple must be extensively counseled about the risk of multiple births, and this must be well documented.

The issue of cryopreservation of human embryos presents numerous ethical and religious dilemmas. Couples must be comfortable with their decisions and the lifelong consequences. What happens, for instance, if the couple dies prior to the transfer? Nursing roles focus on education and working through alternatives with couples. The consent form must encompass possibilities such as death, divorce, or simply that the couple does not want the embryo at a later date.

Cost is a significant factor when couples are considering assisted reproductive technologies. The average cycle costs between $5,000 and $7,000, and very few insurance companies cover this procedure. With success rates averaging 15% to 25% for IVF and 20% to 30% with GIFT, this is a significant gamble for many couples. Issues that couples must resolve include the religious acceptance of procedures, feelings about cryopreserving human embryos, and family acceptance of their decision and their child's origins.

Several methods are continuing to be developed to enhance the quality of the male sperm and to optimize the chances for fertilization of the ovum. Intracellular sperm injection is one such method, which involves injecting a sperm into the ovum in vitro and then transferring it into the woman's uterus.

Third-party approaches to infertility involve the use of donor eggs, donor sperm, donor embryos, and surrogates. All of these methods provide options for infertile persons, but also raise a myriad of ethical and legal implications that need to be addressed.

Sandelowski (1999) raised a thought-provoking issue in describing the technology as a kind of cultural expression. She identified a paradox emanating from the technological advances in infertility treatment: while offering more possibilities, these technologies simultaneously reinforce existing sociocultural practices, norms, and values. In other words, while technology offers radical new approaches, this same technology also contributes to a conservative cultural norm wherein parenthood and fertility and pronatalism are emphasized to the exclusion of other approaches.

An important role of the nurse is to assist individuals and couples in making decisions regarding the various options available to them. In this age of technology, several options may be available, creating hope for the couple that they will become parents, but also making it more difficult for them to eventually stop treatment and get on with their lives. They must understand how the various options work, the success rates, and the implications of attempting a particular option. Ultimately, the individual or couple are the only ones who can make a decision; the health care provider can assist them, but it is the person's decision. It is important that the nurse inform the couple of everything that is known and what the unknowns are. Unknowns may include long-term side effects, psychological sequelae, and future legal issues.

HUMAN RESPONSES TO INFERTILITY

The past decade and a half has witnessed an increased amount of research exploring the human responses to infertility, with the goal of understanding better the meaning that infertility has to those persons experiencing it. Woods, Olshansky, and Draye (1991) summarized various theoretical approaches to understanding the human experience of infertility. The notions of chronic sorrow, of grief and eventual resolution, and of infertility taking on a centrality in people's lives have all been described as ways of explaining this experience. Loss of control, being on a roller coaster, and confronting the loss of one's expected life trajectory are all challenges to persons experiencing infertility. Sandelowski and Pollock (1986) addressed the ambiguity associated with dealing with infertility as well as the "otherness" that infertile persons often experience, as they see themselves as different from other, fertile persons. In fact, some infertile persons may perceive themselves as being part of a culture or social world that is infertile and that serves as the context under which they make meaning of their infertility. Olshansky (1996a) found that infertility affects a person's identity/sense of self, a person's meanings of life, and a person's quality of life. In women who become pregnant after infertility, there is a profound effect on their identity, including a greater risk for the development of depression (Olshansky 2003; Olshansky & Sereika, 2005). It is critically important that nurses who care for infertile individuals or couples understand the particular experience of infertility from the perspective of the individuals or couples. The health care provider who is working with an infertile individual or couple would be well served to base interventions on the following three goals, described by Olshansky (1996b): (1) Assist in pushing one's identity as infertile to the periphery; (2) Assist in finding meaning in life and reframing one's meaning away from personal failure; and (3) Assist in improving quality of life through connected relationships with others.

A couple experiencing infertility faces many uncertainties and multiple losses. Malhlstedt (1985) described infertility as a loss of self-esteem, a dream, balance in a relationship, security, and fantasy. Grief follows much the same pattern for infertility as with all losses. Surprise is often experienced first, because few persons ever expect to be infertile. Guilt, anger, and blame may be part of the emotional reaction. Multiple losses can cripple an individual emotionally, and support groups such as Resolve, the national support network for infertile couples, and individual counseling can be beneficial to the individuals involved and to a couple's relationship. Appropriate support is critical.

Managing and coping with the difficulties associated with either unsuccessful individual treatment or the inability to achieve pregnancy requires time and energy. Feelings must be acknowledged to be dealt with openly and honestly. Resolution of infertility takes time. Depression is not uncommon, and significant clinical problems should be referred for appropriate mental health care. Resolution of infertility is not a finite phenomenon. The identity of oneself as an infertile person does not automatically change to that of a fertile person even when pregnancy occurs (Olshansky, 1990, 1996a). After adoption and even after a pregnancy, many couples still describe themselves as infertile. Couples must redefine their relationship and fantasies about the future and must learn to be comfortable living out their lives in a fertile world (Menning, 1988). Some couples cope by becoming proactive. Joining forces through Resolve for community education and legislative efforts are healthy ways to channel feelings and energies. Positive results that affect others experiencing the same difficulty can be tremendously rewarding. Olshansky (1987) described a pattern of integrating infertility into one's career, which can be extended to integrating infertility into one's volunteer efforts, as reflected in those who take such proactive approaches to improving the situation for infertile persons.

Clinical Implications of the Human Responses to Infertility

Based on an understanding of the variety of ways in which infertile individuals and couples respond to and experience infertility, it is possible to systematically develop clinical approaches to help infertile persons cope with and manage their infertility. Olshansky (1996b) described several salient points that should be included in a counseling approach to infertile persons: (1) Assist patients to confront and analyze the choices available to them; (2) assisting patients to focus on and reclaim the successful parts of their lives; (3) assisting patients to move on with their lives; and (4) assisting patients to develop and maintain healthy interpersonal relationships.

An important implication for clinical practice is for nurses to understand the centrality with which individuals and couples approach their infertility. Because infertility often becomes all-encompassing for them, the infertility evaluation and treatment efforts are approached with much drive. Couples may become so centered on solving their infertility problems, that they begin to expect that if they do resolve their infertility, all of their life problems will be solved. It is essential for nurses to assist the couple in putting infertility into perspective by focusing on other important areas of their lives. For couples who do achieve parenthood, it is also essential that the nurse understand that couples may feel some disappointment and then guilt for feeling such disappointment, because they realize that all of their problems in life are not solved. An understanding, empathic approach to these individuals and couples will help them confront and verbalize their feelings without experiencing guilt for having such feelings.

Research Implications of the Human Responses to Infertility

Existing research on infertility has elucidated much important information on the human responses to infertility, as well as responses to the various treatments for infertility. The implications of the findings include the need to develop more systematic interventions for assisting persons as they cope with the distressing aspects of infertility and to pursue further research in a chronological manner, exploring long-term sequelae of infertility, such as women's experiences of pregnancy, parenting, and menopause after infertility. More focus on family members' experiences of infertility would also contribute valuable information. Attention to ethnic and cultural differences in women's and men's experiences of infertility, as well as more focus on gender differences would also yield important information and understanding regarding the complex experiences of infertility.

FUTURE DIRECTIONS

Infertility is a new area for nurse specialists. Reproductive endocrine/infertility nursing was first considered a subspecialty area in the early 1980s. The first certification examination for reproductive endocrinology and infertility was offered by the Nurses' Association of the American College of Obstetricians and Gynecologists (NAACOG) Certification Corporation in 1989. Although there is a paucity of nursing and psychological research in the area, this evolving specialty offers numerous opportunities for research and innovative clinical programs.

The focus of infertility research and practice for the future involves understanding the long-term consequences of infertility. For example, little is known about pregnancy after infertility, although some research has been conducted in this area (Garner, 1985; Olshansky, 1990; Shapiro, 1986). Even less is known about parenting after infertility, despite some research in this area (Bernstein, Mattox, & Kellner, 1988; Dunnington & Glazer, 1991).

Harris, Sandelowski, and Holditch-Davis (1991) studied the emotional impact of spontaneous abortion as well as the transition to parenthood in infertile couples. Couples defined miscarriage as both a loss and a gain. Some of the gains included knowing that a pregnancy was possible for them and having a sense of normalcy.

Much more research is needed on various long-term outcomes after infertility even beyond pregnancy and parenting. For example, how women experience menopause after infertility may yield some interesting and important information for nurses as they assist women through this phase. It would be helpful to understand how families adjust over time to various assisted technology options. With increasing technological means to achieve fertility, there is also more focus on fertility preservation after cancer treatment. This is another area for future research. With increasing technological means, more ethical issues are raised and must be addressed.

REFERENCES

Bernstein, J., Mattox, J. H., & Kellner, R. (1988). Psychological status of previously infertile couples after a successful pregnancy. *Journal of Obstetric, Gynecologic, and Neonatal Nursing, 17*(6), 404–408.

Birrittieri, C. (2005). *What every woman should know about fertility and her biological clock.* Franklin Lakes, NJ: New Page Books.

Clarke-Pearson, D. L., & Dawood, M. Y. (1990). *Green's gynecology: Essentials of clinical practice* (4th ed.). Boston: Little, Brown.

Cramer, D. W. (1987). Epidemiology of endometriosis. In E. A. Wilson (Ed.), *Endometriosis* (pp. 5–22). New York: A. R. Liss.

Dunnington, R. M., & Glazer, R. (1991). Maternal identity in previously infertile and never infertile women. *Journal of Obstetric, Gynecologic, and Neonatal Nursing, 20*(4), 309–318.

Evers, J. L. (2002). Female subfertility. *Lancet, 360,* 151–159.

Ficorelli, C. T., & Weeks, B. (2007). Untangling the complexities of male infertility. *Nursing 2007, 37*(1), 24–25.

Garner, C. H. (1985). Pregnancy after infertility. *Journal of Obstetric, Gynecologic, and Neonatal Nursing, 14*(Suppl.), 58S–62S.

Garner, C. H., & Webster, B. W. (1985). Endometriosis. *Journal of Obstetric, Gynecologic, and Neonatal Nursing, 14*(Suppl.), 10S–20S.

Goldfien, A. (1998). The gonadal hormones and inhibitors. In B. G. Katzung (Ed.), *Basic and clinical pharmacology* (7th ed.). Stamford, CT: Appleton & Lange.

Hahn, S. (1991). Caring for couples considering alternatives in family building. In C. H. Garner (Ed.), *Principles of infertility nursing* (pp. 179–206). Boca Raton, FL: CRC Press.

Hanson, B. (2003). Questioning the construction of maternal age as a fertility problem. *Health Care for Women International, 24*(3), 166–176.

Harris, B. G., Sandelowski, M., & Holditch-Davis, D. (1991). Infertility and new interpretations of pregnancy loss. *The American Journal of Maternal Child Nursing, 16*(4), 217–220.

Isaacs, J. C. (2005). The patient voice in infertility. *AWHONN Lifelines, 9*(5), 363–364.

Kronmal, R. A., Whitney, C. W., & Mumford, S. D. (1991). The intrauterine device and pelvic inflammatory disease: The women's health study reanalyzed. *Journal of Clinical Epidemiology, 44*(2), 109–112.

Luciano, A. A., & Pitkin, R. M. (1984). Endometriosis: Approaches to diagnosis and treatment. *Surgery Annals, 16,* 297–312.

Ma, R., & Sasson, D. A. (2006). PCBs exert an estrogenic effect through repression of the Wnt7a signaling pathway in the female reproductive system. *Environmental Health Perspectives, 114,* 898–904.

Malhlstedt, P. (1985). The psychological component of infertility. *Fertility and Sterility, 43,* 335–346.

Menning, B. E. (1988). *Infertility: A guide for the childless couple* (2nd ed.). New York: Prentice Hall.

Olshansky, E. (1987). Infertility and its influence on women's career identities. *Health Care for Women International, 8*(2,3), 185–196.

Olshansky, E. (1990). Psychosocial implications of pregnancy after infertility. *NAACOG's Clinical Issues in Women's Health and Perinatal Nursing, 1*(3), 342–347.

Olshansky, E. (1996a). Theoretical issues in building a grounded theory: Application of a program of research on infertility. *Qualitative Health Research, 6*(3), 394–405.

Olshansky, E. (1996b). A counseling approach with persons experiencing infertility: Implications for advanced practice nursing. *Advanced Practice Nursing Quarterly, 2*(3), 42–47.

Olshansky, E. (2003). A theoretical explanation for previously infertile mothers' vulnerability to depression. *Journal of Nursing Scholarship, 35*(3), 263–268.

Olshansky, E., & Sereika, S. (2005). Depression and the transition to pregnancy and postpartum in previously infertile women. *Archives of Psychiatric Nursing, 19*(6), 273–280.

Roberts, D. (1997). *Killing the Black body: Race, reproduction, and the meaning of liberty.* New York: Vintage Press.

Sandelowski, M. (1999). Culture, conceptive technology, and nursing. *International Journal of Nursing Studies, 36*(1), 13–20.

Sandelowski, M., & Pollock, C. (1986). Women's experiences of infertility. *Image: The Journal of Nursing Scholarship, 18*(4), 140–144.

Shapiro, C. H. (1986). Is pregnancy after infertility a dubious joy? *Social Casework, 67*(5), 306–313.

U.S. Congress, Office of Technology Assessment. (1988). *Infertility: Medical and social choices.* Washington, DC: U.S. Government Printing Office.

Vermeulen, A., & Vandeweghe, M. (1984). Improved fertility after varicocele correction: Fact or fiction? *Fertility and Sterility, 42,* 249–256.

Woods, N. F., Olshansky, E., & Draye, M. A. (1991). Infertility: Women's experiences. *Health Care for Women International, 12,* 179–190.

19

The Challenge of Unintended Pregnancy

Merry-K. Moos

Confusion surrounds discussions of unintended pregnancy. What is it? Who experiences it? Why? What does it matter? Misunderstandings about unintendedness lead policymakers, opinion leaders, and clinicians to sweeping generalizations and to interventions that, in fact, are unlikely to impact its occurrence. This chapter is offered to suggest that, with an understanding of the factors associated with unintended pregnancies, clinical practice and public policy can evolve that results in more women being able to identify their conceptions as deliberate rather than accidental. This chapter is not intended to educate on the formulations, modes of action, and contraindications of the various methods for contraception because this information is continually changing; to be up to date, women's health providers need access to more current information than a book can guarantee.

UNWANTED, UNINTENDED, AND MISTIMED PREGNANCIES

The terms *unwanted, unintended,* and *mistimed* often are used interchangeably with no clear definition or distinction (Petersen & Moos, 1997). The terms are related but distinct. Two different types of pregnancies combine to form the unintended rate: unwanted and mistimed. Unwanted conceptions are those that occur "when the woman did not want to have any (more) pregnancies at all" (Brown & Eisenberg, 1995, p. 22). Examples of women who would be identified by measurement tools as experiencing an unwanted pregnancy include women who conceived despite tubal ligation or who became pregnant during perimenopause because they believed there was no risk of conception. The other subgroup of unintended pregnancy is classified as mistimed because the woman states she desired to become pregnant at some time but *not at this time.* Typical examples include women who were hoping to space their children a certain distance apart but conceive sooner than hoped due to a failure of their contraceptive method.

Measurement of unintended status is far from a perfect science (Petersen & Moos, 1997). Most national studies ask women to reflect back months to years to remember how they viewed a pregnancy when they found out about it. Such methodology is subject to considerable recall bias. In addition, the distinctions between unwanted and mistimed, as defined above, for an individual woman are fluid and subject to changing life circumstances and perceptions. For instance, a 28-year-old high-powered, single attorney may indicate that she intends never to become pregnant; if asked about her conception, it would be categorized as unwanted. However, upon reflection, the same woman might determine that she wanted to become pregnant sometime, just not at that time, and the very same conception would be categorized as mistimed.

The nation's goal for unintended pregnancies as outlined in *Healthy People 2000* was that the nation reduce the percentage of unintended pregnancies to 30% by the turn of the century (U.S. Department of Health and Human Services, 1991). The goal was not met. Today, nearly 50% of all recognized pregnancies in the United States are identified as unintended (Finer & Henshaw, 2006).

The most recent cycle of the National Survey of Family Growth, which tracks how women who gave birth during the previous five years classify their pregnancies, was completed in 2001 with analysis now being made available (Finer & Henshaw, 2006). According to Finer and Henshaw (2006), 6.4 million pregnancies were recorded in the United States in 2001, which resulted in 4 million births, 1.3 million abortions, and 1.1 fetal losses. Forty-nine percent of the pregnancies were identified by the women as unintended. Of these pregnancies, 44% ended in births, 42% in abortions, and 14% in fetal losses. Of the 3.3 million pregnancies identified as intended, 80% resulted in live birth and the remainder in fetal loss. The likelihood that a woman will experience an unintended pregnancy in her life time is significant. In 1994, 48% of women aged 15 to 44 had experienced at least one unplanned pregnancy sometime in their lives (Henshaw, 1998). Approximately 1 in 20 women of reproductive age had an unintended pregnancy in 2001 (Finer & Henshaw, 2006).

Unintended pregnancies are represented in all populations (with the probable exception of patients being treated for infertility). Contrary to much opinion, unintended pregnancies are not a problem specific to teenagers. Although the great majority (82%) of pregnancies to women younger than 20 years old are unintended (Finer & Henshaw, 2006), adolescent contribution to the total number of unintended pregnancies in the United States is relatively small. In 2001, for instance, 73% of all unintended pregnancies occurred to women older than 19 years of age. Most initiatives to address unintended pregnancy, however, have been targeted toward adolescents.

Who, then, is having these pregnancies? Nearly 60% of conceptions in women ages 20 to 24 are unintended; the only age group that has a proportion of unintended pregnancies less than 30% is women ages 35 to 39 (Finer & Henshaw, 2006). Relative to marital status, 28% of pregnancies occurring in a marital relationship and 74% in a nonmarital relationship are identified as unintended (Finer & Henshaw, 2006).

CONSEQUENCES OF UNINTENDED PREGNANCIES

In 1995, the Institute of Medicine detailed studies examining the effects of unwanted and mistimed pregnancies on children, women, men, and families in a landmark publication, *The Best Intentions: Unintended Pregnancy and Well-Being of Children and Families* (Brown & Eisenberg, 1995). The report concluded that such pregnancies, especially those that are unwanted, carry appreciable risks, many of which burden the nation's health resources. Such pregnancies are positively associated with elective abortions, late entry to prenatal care, low birth weight, child abuse and neglect, and be-

havioral problems in the children. They are also associated with lower educational and economic attainment in young mothers. Separating the impact of intendedness status from other social and environmental influences on these outcomes is, of course, difficult. The greatest impact may be additive rather than causal.

One of the most divisive issues in the political and moral fabric of the United States today is elective termination of pregnancy. The impact of unintended pregnancies is critical to this issue: among women who experienced an unintended pregnancy in 2001, 42% ended in abortion (Finer & Henshaw, 2006). This compares to 54% of such pregnancies ending in abortion in 1994 (Henshaw, 1998). The abortion figure includes both unwanted and mistimed pregnancies.

Public debate becomes confused when all unintended pregnancies are assumed to be unwanted. Too often professionals and the media use the terms unwanted and unintended synonymously. On an individual level, it is destructive for a woman to have her mistimed pregnancy referred to as unwanted. Indeed, it may be a very wanted gestation, but, had things worked out differently, she would have chosen for this wanted pregnancy to occur at a different time. If one asks any gathering of parents whether all of their children are the result of deliberate decisions to become pregnant at a specific time, mistimed conceptions will be represented in plentiful numbers. This is true irrespective of professional training, marital status, age, race, or other demographic features. It is important, as advocates for women's health, that we recognize that unintended does not necessarily mean unwanted; that we teach our colleagues and contacts about the important distinctions in the terms unwanted, mistimed, and unintended; and that we become very deliberate in our own choice of words.

INFLUENCES OF CONTRACEPTIVE EFFECTIVENESS

The idea that the intended status of pregnancy is something that can be affected is relatively recent. Until 1960, when contraceptive pills were approved for general use in the United States, all sexually active women lived continually with the very real possibility of becoming pregnant when they did not want to conceive (Luker, 1999). By 1965, the oral contraceptive pill had transformed the ability to control fertility and was the most commonly used contraceptive among married couples. According to Luker, effective contraception backed up by legally available abortion meant that, for the first time in history, people could decide whether to have a child rather than let nature take its course (Luker, 1999).

Contraceptive options have increased dramatically from the pre-pill barrier methods to modern intrauterine devices, hormonal formulations (including new delivery mechanisms such as injectables, patches, rings, and certain intrauterine devices), and new barrier methods. Two facts have remained constant in the development of modern contraceptives: Their purpose is the intentional prevention of pregnancy, and the general decision and burden of usage almost always rests with the woman (Branden, 1998).

Efforts to decrease the likelihood of unintended pregnancies traditionally have focused on increasing access to contraceptive services and to expanding contraceptive options. However, another major cause of unintended pregnancies is inconsistency and misuse of available contraceptive methods. Computations for 2001 indicate that 48% of the women who had an unintended birth that year used a contraceptive method during the month they became pregnant, as did 54% of those who had abortions (Finer & Henshaw, 2006).

The likelihood of method failure is important and often misunderstood by the public. Table 19.1 compares method effectiveness and use effectiveness of the major contraceptive methods available in the United States. Although method effectiveness and use effectiveness are the traditional terms, new product labeling differentiates failures during "perfect" versus "typical" use. The difference between perfect and typical use can be attributed to several factors that are far more complex than the numbers shown in Table 19.1. Four variables influence these measures for any woman and couple: (1) capacity to conceive; (2) frequency and timing of intercourse; (3) degree of compliance with the method; and (4) the inherent protection of the method (Steiner, Dominik, Trussell, & Hertz-Picciotto, 1996).

Also important are demographic variables: in general, failure rates are highest among cohabiting and other unmarried women, women living at or below 200% of the federal poverty level, and adolescents and women in their 20s. To illustrate, adolescent women who are not married but are cohabiting experience a failure rate of about 31% in the first year of contraceptive use, while the 12-month failure rate among married women aged 30 and older is 7% (Fu, Darroch, Hass, & Ranjit, 1999).

Oakley (1994) has identified eight nondemographic characteristics that place women at risk for contraceptive failures: no future plans; no support for avoiding an unintended pregnancy; previous unintended conceptions; involvement in short-term sexual relationships; lack of previous success with behavior modifications to achieve a specific goal; contraceptive visit not initiated by the patient; cognitive impairment; and ambivalence regarding the desire to postpone pregnancy.

Most, but not all, of the differences between the perfect and typical use rates and between subpopulations can be explained by suboptimal use of the chosen method (Cramer, 1996). Barrier methods, which are event dependent and often require inconvenient behaviors, have the greatest differences in the perfect versus typical failure rates; methods that involve no behavioral choice beyond obtaining the contraceptive (such as intrauterine devices or surgical contraception) have no differences between the two failure rates and, thus, assure the best protection. Between these two extremes of perfect and typical use are oral contraceptives, the most commonly prescribed method of reversible contraception in the United States, and other behavior-dependent hormonal delivery systems such as the patch, ring, and injectables.

EXHIBIT 19.1 MICROBEHAVIORS ASSOCIATED WITH SUCCESSFUL CONTRACEPTIVE PROTECTION FROM ORAL CONTRACEPTIVES

- Obtaining pills
- Taking only one's own pills
- Taking pills in the correct order
- Taking each pill within the appropriate time window
- Abstaining from sex or using a back-up method when necessary
- Obtaining refills on time
- Stopping one cycle and starting the next at the right time
- Interpreting problems correctly—neither under-reacting or over-reacting
- Taking effective actions to resolve problems
- Using contraception continuously, even if there is a method or dosage change

Note. From "Rethinking Patient Counseling Techniques for Changing Contraceptive Use Behavior," by D. Oakley, 1994, *American Journal of Obstetrics and Gynecology, 170,* pp. 1585–1590.

ISSUES IN INITIATION OF AND ADHERENCE TO CONTRACEPTIVE REGIMENS

It might seem obvious to question the motivations of women who do not use their contraceptives as intended and then declare their pregnancies to be unintended. However, adherence to any prescribed routine is complex. A survey of studies to measure compliance with microelectronic systems revealed that, on average, individuals diagnosed with various medical conditions took only 75% of the doses of their medications as prescribed (Cramer, 1995). Nonadherence may be due to poor comprehension of instructions, voluntary refusal because of lack of perceived benefit or fear of complication, or involuntary behaviors such as forgetfulness (Parker, Williams, Baker, & Nurss, 1996). Oral contraceptives and other hormonal delivery systems that depend on regular patient behaviors are no different, except, in some case, they offer less room for error. Current formulations of oral contraceptives minimize the amount of estrogens and progestins, thereby decreasing the likelihood of side effects, but, in so doing, provide a shortened half-life. Therefore, modern oral contraceptives provide little forgiveness for missed pills.

Much of the literature about drug compliance relies on self-report. Oakley and colleagues demonstrated the unreliability of this approach in a study that compared diary reports of oral contraceptive use with the reports of microelectronic pill packs designed to report the time and day that each pill is removed from the pack (Oakley, Potter, deLeon-Wong, & Visness, 1997; Potter, Oakley, deLeon-Wong, & Canamar, 1996). Patients from two family planning clinics and two university health services were studied for 3 consecutive months. Not surprisingly, findings confirmed that self-report is highly unreliable. More surprising was the discovery that compliance in both the low-income and college populations declined over the 3 months. In the first month, perfect compliance was demonstrated by 33% of the sample (meaning no pills were missed); by the third cycle, perfect compliance had dropped to 19%. In addition, the proportion missing three or more pills per cycle increased from 30% to 51% over the same period. Contrary to popular stereotypes, the lack of compliance was not statistically different between the low-income population and the more affluent women attending the universities. Did the declining compliance represent a change in the perceived risk for conception (e.g., less frequent intercourse), a change in desires about becoming pregnant, or a decreased willingness to accept side effects associated with the medication? The answer is unknown.

The 1995 National Survey of Family Growth examined discontinuation rates for various contraceptive methods (Trussell & Vaughn, 1999). Of particular note are the following: 31% of women discontinued their method for method-related reasons within the first 6 months of use; by 24 months, more than 60% of all contraceptive users had quit their method; the implant had better continuation at each assessment point. By 2 years following initiation, nearly 50% of the oral contraceptive users had discontinued them because of method-related reasons. The study revealed that most women who discontinue a method of contraception begin using another method shortly thereafter (68% within 1 month; 76% after 3 months; and 82% within a year) but that the replacement method may have lower method and user effectiveness than the original choice. In addition, the transition between methods may place the patient at risk for conception.

A more recent study (Frost, Singh, & Finer, 2007) used a telephone survey to reach nearly 2,000 women of reproductive age throughout the United States to assess contraceptive patterns in women who had sexual intercourse in the previous 12 months. Only 38% consistently used the same method or methods all year, and 24% switched methods over the same period; 8% of the sample reported themselves to be inconsistent users of contraception, and 15% experienced from 1 to 11 months of nonuse though having sexual intercourse. Women reported method-related difficulties, side effects, infrequent sex, and ambivalence about avoiding pregnancy as reasons for inconsistent contraceptive use.

BARRIERS TO EFFECTIVE CONTRACEPTION

With any prescribed treatment, compliance reflects people's knowledge, attitudes, and behaviors regarding the prescribed therapy (Parker et al., 1996), and these three factors overlap and interact to predict satisfaction and continued use of the treatment. Knowledge, whether it is fact-based or not, can affect attitudes, which result in behaviors other than those prescribed. For instance, knowledge and the related attitudes about the health effects of oral contraceptives may be based on fact or myth, but, whether fact or myth, the resulting attitudes are important predictors of satisfaction and continued use. Expected health effects may be perceived by a woman or her support system as representing serious health risks or as nuisance side effects. Perception is likely to dictate tolerance of the symptoms.

A survey conducted by the Gallup Organization for the American College of Obstetricians and Gynecologists underscored perceptions of risk regarding oral contraceptives. In a telephone interview of 995 women ages 18 and older, more than 50% of women believed oral contraceptives carry substantial and serious health risks; 60% of the sample believed that oral contraceptives were more risky than childbearing; and 29% associated oral contraceptives with an increased risk of cancer. When the findings were compared to a similar Gallup survey conducted in 1985, only slight improvement in knowledge about the risks of oral contraceptives was revealed (Gallup Organization, 1999). More recent data were not located. Coupling an increasing array of contraceptive methods with faster access to factual and nonfactual information through media and electronic sources suggests that knowledge about the risks and benefits of contraception may be no better now than a decade ago.

Some beliefs about health risks may evolve from overgeneralizations about actual risks. For instance, individuals may generalize the risk of oral contraceptives and myocardial infarction in women over 35 who smoke to all women. Similarly, the formerly accepted risk of pelvic infections with the use of certain intrauterine devices may be transferred to current devices. Some beliefs may relate to understandings by previous generations that, despite their lack of credibility, have been passed on to current potential users. A common example is infertility associated with the long-term use of oral contraceptives. What a reported risk actually means is also a source of confusion. For instance, differentiating relative risk from clinical significance is not easily explained or understood. Recent reports of a two-fold increase in thromboembolism associated with the use of the OrthoEvra patch are not understood by most women to represent a very small absolute risk.

Finally, women's understanding of health risks is largely determined by their social networks. In a study of the acceptability and understanding of contraceptive implants among urban adolescent females, it was found that negative media reports about the method were less influential than social circumstances such as peer and partner perspectives and relationships (Kuiper, Martinez, Loeb, & Darney, 1997). Of additional interest in this study was the finding that oral networks propagated misinformation that went unchallenged because of the silence of satisfied users.

Contraceptive side effects have also been identified as a reason women place themselves at risk for unintended pregnancy (Cramer, 1996; Rosenberg & Waugh, 1999); more recent reports, however, indicate that side effects are not a leading reason for poor adherence (Smith & Oakley, 2005; Westoff et al., 2007). Smith and Oakley (2005) used diary cards to assess the self-described reasons for 141 women missing pills over three cycles. The most commonly cited reasons included being away from home and not having the pill pack available, simply forgetting to take one or more consecutive pills, and forgetting or being unable to obtain the necessary refill to continue uninterrupted use.

DECREASING UNINTENDEDNESS BY IMPROVING PATIENT SATISFACTION AND COMPLIANCE

Three approaches or models are commonly used to examine factors associated with nonadherence to contraceptive regimens (Rosenberg et al., 1995). The first is termed *nonspecific* in that a broad range of characteristics, behaviors, and other factors are measured in order to identify those associated with poor compliance. In this approach, attempts are made through statistical techniques to identify patients at risk for poor compliance. Education, age, race, parity, marital status, partner support, cultural values, religiosity, experiences with previous conception, and income are examples of interest. Theoretically, programs could be designed to impact on these influences and, thereby, the incidence of unintended gestations.

The second model is built around *behavioral choices* and what influences cause individuals to make those choices. Oakley (1994) provides a list of 12 potentially relevant behavioral theories ranging from reasoned action to developmental theory. One of the theories that has received particular attention around contraceptive use is the Health Belief Model. The Health Belief Model was originally developed to explain preventive behavior and is based on a conceptual framework whose premise is that the subjective impressions of the patient determine behavior rather than the objective environment surrounding the decisions (Salazar, 1991). Relative to contraception, the Health Belief Model proposes that the likelihood a woman will take action to protect herself against an unintended pregnancy is determined by the perceived benefit of taking an action weighed against the perceived costs or barriers. In this model, important considerations include a woman's estimation of the severity of the consequences of failing to follow a therapeutic plan. If a woman is ambivalent about postponing or avoiding pregnancy or is worried that continuing to follow the therapeutic plan will place her in greater danger because of perceived health risks than would a mistimed pregnancy, she is likely to deviate from the prescribed regimen or discontinue it altogether.

The third model used to explain compliance issues is the *patient-provider model*, which attempts to correlate the quality of the interactions between the woman and her provider with decreased likelihood of unintended conceptions. The attitude of the providers, the directiveness of their counseling, and the involvement of the patient in setting the counseling agenda are examples of variables of interest in this model.

Although the three models have different emphases, they are not necessarily exclusive of one another. If these models explain components of adherence with contraceptive use, then impacting on variables included in the models should affect the occurrence of unintendedness. Although the availability and quality of counseling are commonly cited as influential in individual decisions to use contraception, surprisingly little rigorous evaluation has been undertaken on how to best counsel women (or men) on how to decrease the likelihood of unintended conceptions. In addition, current experiences of women are not well documented. In a recent study by Weisman and colleagues (2002), an attempt was made to examine the contraceptive counseling received by adult women in managed care plans and the relationship between counseling and women's contraceptive attitudes and practices. Their conceptual framework defined contraceptive counseling as a form of interpersonal communication that included information giving as well as opportunities for clients to ask questions and express concerns, values, and preferences. They went on to describe counseling as having three dimensions: (1) *exposure* refers to whether any counseling occurs through any communication channels; (2) *content* refers to the information imparted during counseling; and (3) *personalization* refers to the degree to which women's needs and preferences are addressed. The researchers found that, in their sample of nearly 900 women ages 18 to 44, personalized counseling (as opposed to no counseling or only informational counseling) significantly increased the odds of satisfaction with counseling, current contraceptive use, and intent to use contraception in the following year if at risk for an unintended pregnancy.

The Weisman study (Weisman et al., 2002) is notable because it attempted to study the association between counseling and contraceptive attitudes and practices in adult women. Indeed, few evaluations of any strategies to improve satisfaction and/or compliance with contraceptive use have been reported. Although numerous approaches have been suggested for helping patients improve their compliance once a method has been chosen—including medical diaries, self-care workbooks, contracts signed by both the patient and provider to indicate agreement about a plan, peer-counseling, and computer-based and multimedia educational strategies (Delbanco & Daley, 1996)—none has been adequately evaluated relative to contraceptive behaviors.

A 2003 review of studies published in English between 1985 and early 2000 found almost no experimental or observational literature that could reliably answer whether counseling in the clinical setting could impact unintended pregnancies (Moos, Bartholomew, & Lohr, 2003). The authors concluded that the quality of existing research does not provide strong guidance for recommendations about clinical practice but does suggest directions for future investigations. Similarly, a Cochrane Systematic Review examined randomized

controlled trials and determined that, while good personal communication between clients and providers is generally considered important for successful use of hormonal contraception, little high-quality research exists that demonstrates enhanced counseling improves contraceptive use (Halpern, Grimes, Lopez, & Gallo, 2006). However, these reviewers also found the existing research to have important limitations, including small sample sizes, high losses to follow-up, and lack of comparability across trials. Although the need for research is great, observational and theoretical work complimented by some of the existing small studies may serve to guide program planning and patient interactions.

FRAMEWORKS FOR PROVIDING CONTRACEPTIVE COUNSELING

Choice is not only the first, but the fundamental, element of providing contraceptive services (Moos, 2003). Choice about using contraception and choice about methods are governed by medical and legal ethics and must be governed by informed patient choice. Unfortunately, women often choose methods that are not a good match to their own realities. Recognizing the advantages of a good match between patient desires and personal profile and contraceptive characteristics, the Association of Reproductive Health Professionals has created a computer program to provide education and to suggest contraceptive choices matched to a woman's declared needs and desires. The page can be accessed at www.ARHP.org.

One author has framed contraceptive choice to encompass a broader meaning—the choice to change. She recommends that quality programs seek to impart to the patient two central concepts—*choice* and *change* by emphasizing the following points (Bruce, 1990):

■ There is a choice of methods, and all have distinctive risks and benefits.
■ Choices are provisional (except for sterilization), and the decisions are reversible; acceptance of a method is thus a trial.
■ Patients' needs and preferences often change over time.
■ Discontinuation is not a failure on the part of the user or provider.

It is becoming increasingly accepted that encouraging patients to ask questions, to participate in decision making, and to take part in their own care improves outcomes (Lipkin, 1996). Unfortunately, patient-centered counseling is not the norm. In a study by Lipkin (1996) of 550 return visits at 11 sites involving 126 physicians, only about 8% of the encounters involved what could be construed as a partnership mode of relating. More recent data to suggest that the quality of counseling around contraceptive issues has improved in the last decade are lacking.

If involving the patient in setting the agenda for the contraceptive counseling is an important step in helping women choose contraceptives appropriate to their personal goals and constraints, then processes are needed to guide women in thinking about their goals. One approach for entering into the dialogue has been suggested using the following questions to explore a woman's plans and goals (Moos, 2003):

- How many (more) children, if any, do you hope to have?
- How long would you like to wait until you become pregnant (again)?
- What do you plan to do to delay becoming pregnant until then?
- What can I do to help you achieve your plan?

Counseling techniques for contraceptive users should include assessing both the patient's understanding of the method and her specific concerns: What experiences has she or her friends and family members previously had with the method? What has she heard about problems with the method? What has she heard about advantages? It is most likely beneficial to discuss the potential side effects, dispel method misinformation, and discuss the noncontraceptive benefits of the methods under consideration. It is important that counseling include information about possible side effects, their likely transient nature, and the options available should the patient experience the problem. Many patients believe if they have an adverse experience with one oral contraceptive, for instance, the same experience will accompany all oral contraceptives. In fact, there are more formulations and choices available today then ever before, and the likelihood of finding a medication that minimizes the patient's adverse responses is likely. Finding the most acceptable choice, however, requires patience and a trusting relationship with the provider.

Oakley (1994) argues that most contraceptive counseling deals with method choice and, when the pill is chosen, on one specific behavior: taking a pill every day at the same time. This narrow approach to counseling and education may contribute to unintendedness, because, in fact, many sub- or microbehaviors are necessary for successful contraceptive protection. Microbehaviors related to oral contraceptives are listed in Exhibit 19.1. Similar behaviors attend the successful initiation and continued use of injectables, the patch, and the ring as well as barrier methods. Oakley suggests that using the clinical interaction to help a woman work through strategies to overcome likely barriers to accomplishing the necessary microbehaviors may make

a significant difference in compliance. Oakley (1994) notes that, rather than continuing the current tendency to provide uniform, generalized information to all women regardless of their specific circumstances, the emphasis should be on the client, mobilizing her to plan and implement her own intentions.

Contingency planning—that is, what to do if the best intentions are not realized—is likely to be an important component of the interactions. For instance, it should be anticipated that every woman using oral contraceptives will eventually miss one or more dose. Clear, simple, written guidance on what to do if pills are missed should be a routine complement to every prescription for oral contraceptives. Similarly, at some point, every woman using a patch or ring will fail to achieve perfect use and should know what specific steps to take to reduce the likelihood of conception. Every woman who is likely to have sexual intercourse and who does not desire to become pregnant should be given anticipatory instructions on how to access and use emergency contraception and, if necessary, be given a prescription to be filled if needed.

OTHER INFLUENCES ON CONTRACEPTIVE USE AND ADHERENCE

Do women benefit from obtaining their contraceptive in a clinical setting? Would some or all women do just as well or better with compliance if they could receive their oral contraceptives directly from a pharmacist without a clinical encounter? The current standard of bundling women's preventive health services with access to the most popular reversible method, oral contraceptive, is receiving increasing attention as an important barrier to contraceptive use. To change oral contraceptives to an over-the-counter drug category represents a radical departure from tradition that has strong theoretical advantages and disadvantages. Advantages include eliminating the cost of office visits and professional fees as well as removing the fear or dislike of a pelvic exam as a barrier to initiating the pills. Opponents to this move argue that women's preventive health care would be disadvantaged by not requiring an annual clinic visit for the prescription, because associated clinical assessments such as cervical cancer screening, blood pressure assessment, and cultures for sexually transmitted diseases would not be obtained. Proponents argue that holding women's contraceptive options hostage to well-woman care is somewhat disingenuous—that cancer screenings and other routine preventive health services should be marketed to the public for their own value rather than coupled with access to contraceptive choices. Researchers and physicians, primarily from Europe and the United States, met in Great Britain in 1996 to determine appropriate eligibility criteria for oral contraceptives. According to the resulting consensus document, only two items, assessment of cardiac risk factors and blood pressure are prerequisites for starting combined oral contraceptives (World Health Organization, 1996). Neither of these requires a clinic visit or a pelvic exam. In the third edition of the WHO's Selected Practice Recommendations for Contraceptive Use (2004) the recommendation indicates that even blood pressure assessment can be waived in specific circumstances.

There are many influences on unintended pregnancy beyond those impacted by the actual patient-provider encounter. For instance, access to the chosen method is a barrier for millions of women because contraceptive methods were not covered by most insurers. In 1998, Maryland became the first state to enact a law requiring health insurers to provide coverage for all prescription contraceptives approved for use in the United States. As of June 2007, 26 states require insurers that cover prescription drugs in general to provide coverage of a full range of FDA-approved contraceptive drugs and devises; however, 18 of these states allow employers and insurers to refuse to comply with the mandate (Guttmacher Institute, 2007b). Additional states had passed comparable legislation, but many of these states included a "conscience clause," making it possible for employers purchasing the insurance packages to eliminate contraceptives as a covered service. In some circumstances, methods are covered but not the associated clinical/professional fees. This can be a significant barrier for methods such as intrauterine devices and to affording the frequent clinic visits associated with the use of injectables.

Minors have gained increasing access to contraceptive services over the last 30 years. Twenty-one states allow minors to consent to their own health care related to contraceptive services; 25 states permit access without parental involvement in one or more circumstances; and four states have no explicit policy on minors' authority to consent to contraceptive services (Guttmacher Institute, 2007c). Two exceptions in expanded access to choices for adolescents involve emergency contraception and elective terminations.

Access to emergency contraception has become much easier for women in this country since the FDA, on August 24, 2006, approved Plan B as an over-the-counter medication to prevent conception for women aged 18 and older; younger women, however, require a prescription to obtain this protection. Access for all women, irrespective of age, is still limited in at least eight states that have adopted restrictions on obtaining the medication (Guttmacher Institute, 2007a).

Most states require parental involvement in a minor's access to abortion services. Some states are extremely restrictive, requiring consent or notification of both parents. All of the 35 states that require parental involvement have an alternative process for minors

seeking an abortion who, for a variety of reasons, cannot engage their parent in the process (Guttmacher Institute, 2007e). Beyond the issues involved in an adolescent accessing abortion services for an unwanted pregnancy, policies and access for all women vary tremendously between states. According to the Guttmacher Institute (2007d), "Since the Supreme Court handed down its 1973 decisions in Roe vs. Wade and Doe vs. Bolton, states have constructed a lattice work of abortion law, codifying, regulating and limiting whether, when and under what circumstances a woman may obtain an abortion" (p. 1). To learn more about the various policies and specific state approaches to contraceptive access and abortion services, see www.guttmacher.org.

DEVELOPING A RESEARCH AGENDA

Without doubt, health and social problems resulting from unwanted fertility could be alleviated if the contraceptive technologies that now exist were more broadly available, accessible, and affordable to a wider range of people than those who currently benefit from them (Simmons et al., 1997).

These words were written about approaches to advance fertility control and choices in developing countries, but they also have great applicability to the most developed country in the world. Clearly, with nearly 50% of the pregnancies in the United States identified as unintended, there is much work ahead. What can be done to encourage active decision making about reproductive decisions? Or to decrease the number of pregnancies that are unwanted or mistimed? And to empower women and their partners to obtain and use contraception in a manner that furthers their personal goals? Handing a woman a pack of pills and providing nonpersonalized, rote education about when to start the pills is inadequate; ignoring women's fears about specific methods or discounting their concerns about side effects is to invite unprotected intercourse; counseling women out of the context of their personal realities is to discount their needs and encourage noncompliance; and expecting that women, irrespective of their motivations to avoid pregnancy, will use their contraceptive method without any deviation from perfect use is unrealistic.

According to Weisman and colleagues (2002), while the availability and quality of counseling are believed to influence decisions about the use of contraceptives, no standard definition of contraceptive counseling exists, and little research has addressed the relationship between counseling and contraceptive use, especially among adults. Quality studies on the most efficacious approaches for providing contraceptive counseling and care are scant. Evidence-based research is needed to guide clinical and nonclinical interactions around contraception and fertility choices. Randomized control trials are needed to answer some of the most basic questions about how to help the population avoid unintended conceptions (Moos et al., 2003). Research is needed to:

- Compare and contrast various approaches for matching methods to user profiles.
- Investigate access issues such as the impact of eliminating or postponing the need for pelvic exams prior to dispensing a prescription.

- Determine how various educational strategies about risks, benefits, and side effects of various methods impact on patient choice, satisfaction, and use.
- Evaluate the impact of follow-up strategies, such as hot lines, follow-up visits, computer services, support groups, and mailings on contraception habits, satisfaction, and continuation.
- Determine whether community-based programs such as adolescent pregnancy prevention initiatives

19.1 | Percentage of Women Experiencing an Unintended Pregnancy During the First Year of Typical Use and the First Year of Perfect Use of Contraception

METHOD	% OF WOMEN EXPERIENCING AN UNINTENDED PREGNANCY WITHIN THE FIRST YEAR OF USE	
	TYPICAL USE[a]	PERFECT USE[b]
Chance	85	85
Spermicides	29	18
Periodic abstinence		
Calendar	25	9
Ovulation method		3
Symptothermal		2
Postovulation		1
Cap		
Parous women	32	26
Nulliparous women	16	9
Sponge		
Parous women	32	20
Nulliparous women	16	9
Diaphragm	16	6
Withdrawal	19	4
Condom		
Female (Reality)	21	5
Male	15	2
Pill		
Combined	8	0.3
Intrauterine device		
Copper T 380A	0.8	0.6
LNg 20	0.1	0.1
Depo-Provera	3	0.3
Female sterilization	0.5	0.5
Male sterilization	0.15	0.10

Note. Modified from *Contraceptive Technology* (18th rev. ed.), by R. A. Hatcher, J. Trussell, F. Stewart, W. Cates, G. K. Stewart, F. Guest, and D. Kowal (Eds.), 2004, New York: Ardent Media.
[a] Among *typical* couples who initiate use of a method (not necessarily for the first time), the percentage who experience an accidental pregnancy during the first year if they do not stop use for any other reason.
[b] Among couples who initiate the use of a method (not necessarily for the first time) and who use it *perfectly* (both consistently and correctly), the percentage who experience an accidental pregnancy if they do not stop use for any other reason.

are more effective if they include clear linkages with clinical care services.

- Determine whether the concept of mistimed pregnancies is important to women; there is, indeed, some suggestion that mistimed pregnancies (as opposed to those that are identified as unwanted) are not perceived universally as undesirable (Moos, Peterson, & Meadows, 1997).

Nursing should exercise leadership in moving this important research agenda forward. Studies to understand contributors to contraceptive use and satisfaction are a natural fit for nursing because of its expertise in health promotion, patient education, and counseling for behavioral change (Moos, 2003). Energies on the part of providers, pharmaceutical manufacturers, insurers, legislative bodies, and society can and should coalesce to help women and their partners realize their reproductive goals (Moos, 2003). In so doing, the health of the nation will benefit.

REFERENCES

Branden, P. S. (1998). Contraceptive choice and patient compliance: The health care provider's challenge. *Journal of Nursing-Midwifery, 43,* 471–482.

Brown, S. S., & Eisenberg, L. (Eds.). (1995). *The best intentions: Unintended pregnancy and the well-being of children and families.* Washington, DC: National Academy Press.

Bruce, J. (1990). Fundamental elements of the quality of care: A simple framework. *Studies in Family Planning, 21,* 61–91.

Cramer, J. A. (1995). The relationship between medication compliance and medical outcomes. *American Journal of Health Systems Pharmaceuticals, 52*(Suppl. 3), S27–S29.

Cramer, J. A. (1996). Compliance with contraceptives and other treatments. *Obstetrics and Gynecology, 88,* 4S–12S.

Delbanco, T. L., & Daley, J. (1996). Through the patient's eyes: Strategies toward more successful contraception. *Obstetrics and Gynecology, 88,* 41S–47S.

Finer, L. B., & Henshaw, S. K. (2006). Disparities in rates of unintended pregnancy in the United States, 1994 and 2001. *Perspectives on Sexual and Reproductive Health, 38*(2), 90–96.

Frost, J. J., Singh, S., & Finer, L. B. (2007). U.S. women's one-year contraceptive use patterns, 2004. *Perspectives on Sexual and Reproductive Health, 39*(1), 48–55.

Fu, H., Darroch, J. E., Haas, T., & Ranjit, N. (1999). Contraceptive failure rates: New estimates from the 1995 National Survey of Family Growth. *Family Planning Perspectives, 31*(2), 56–63.

Gallup Organization. (1999). Women's attitudes toward oral contraceptives and other forms of birth control. Survey conducted for the American College of Obstetricians and Gynecologists. Princeton, NJ; as reported in *Dialogues in Contraception, University of Southern California School of Medicine, 6,* 1.

Guttmacher Institute. (2007a). *Emergency contraception.* Retrieved June 11, 2007, from http://www.guttmacher.org

Guttmacher Institute. (2007b). *Insurance coverage of contraceptives.* Retrieved June 11, 2007, from http://www.guttmacher.org

Guttmacher Institute. (2007c). *Minor's access to contraceptive services.* Retrieved June 11, 2007, from http://www.guttmacher.org

Guttmacher Institute. (2007d). An overview of abortion laws. Retrieved June 11, 2007, from http://www.guttmacher.org

Guttmacher Institute. (2007e). *Parental involvement in minor's abortions.* Retrieved June 11, 2007, from http://www.guttmacher.org

Halpern, V., Grimes, D. A., Lopez, L., & Gallo, M. F. (2006). Strategies to improve adherence and acceptability of hormonal methods for contraception. *Cochrane Database of Systematic Reviews, 1,* 1–24.

Hatcher, R. A., Trussell, J., Stewart, F., Cates, W., Stewart, G. K, Guest, F., & Kowal, D. (Eds.). (2004). *Contraceptive technology* (18th rev. ed.). New York: Ardent Media.

Henshaw, S. (1998). Unintended pregnancy in the United States. *Family Planning Perspectives, 30,* 24–29, 46.

Kuiper, H., Martinez, E., Loeb, L., & Darney, P. (1997). Urban adolescent females' view on the implant and contraceptive decision-making: A double paradox. *Family Planning Perspectives, 29,* 167–172.

Lipkin M. Jr. (1996). Physician-patient interaction in reproductive counseling. *Obstetrics and Gynecology, 88,* 31S–40S.

Luker, K. C. (1999). Contraceptive failure and unintended pregnancy: A reminder that human behavior frequently refuses to conform to models created by researchers. *Family Planning Perspectives, 31,* 248–249.

Moos, M. K. (2003). Unintended pregnancies: A call for nursing action. *MCN,* January/February, 23–31.

Moos, M. K., Bartholomew, N., & Lohr, K. (2003). Counseling in the clinical setting to prevent unintended pregnancy: An evidence-based research agenda. *Contraception, 67,* 115–133.

Moos, M. K., Petersen, R., & Meadows, K. (1997). Contributors to unintended pregnancies: Investigation of women's perspectives. *Women's Health Issues, 7,* 385–392.

Oakley, D. (1994). Rethinking patient counseling techniques for changing contraceptive use behavior. *American Journal of Obstetrics and Gynecology, 170,* 1585–1590.

Oakley, D., Potter, L., deLeon-Wong, E., & Visness, C. (1997). Oral contraceptive use and protective behavior after missed pills. *Family Planning Perspectives, 29,* 277–279.

Parker, R. M., Williams, M., Baker, D. W., & Nurss, J. R. (1996). Literacy and contraception: Exploring the link. *Obstetrics and Gynecology, 88,* 72S–77S.

Petersen, R., & Moos, M. K. (1997). Defining and measuring unintended pregnancy: Issues and concerns. *Women's Health Issues 1997, 7,* 234–240.

Potter, L., Oakley, D., de Leon-Wong, E., & Canamar, R. (1996). Measuring compliance among oral contraceptive users. *Family Planning Perspectives, 28,* 154–158.

Rosenberg, M. J., Burnhill, M. S., Waugh, D. A., Grimes, D. A., & Hillard, P. J. A. (1995). Compliance and oral contraceptives: A review. *Contraception, 52,* 137–141.

Rosenberg, M. J., & Waugh, M. S. (1999). Causes and consequences of oral contraceptive noncompliance. *American Journal of Obstetrics and Gynecology, 180,* S176–S179.

Salazar, M. K. (1991). Comparison of four behavioral theories: A literature review. *AAOHN: Official Jornal of the American Association of Occupational Health Nurses, 39,* 128–135.

Simmons, R., Hall, P., Diaz, J., Diaz, M., Fajans, P., & Satia, J. (1997). The strategic approach to contraceptive introduction. *Studies in Family Planning, 28*(2), 79–94.

Smith, J. D., & Oakley, D. (2005). Why do women miss oral contraceptive pills? An analysis of women's self-described reasons for missed pills. *Journal of Midwifery & Women's Health, 50,* 380–385.

Steiner, M., Dominik, R., Trussell, J., & Hertz-Picciotto, I. (1996). Measuring contraceptive effectiveness: A conceptual framework. *Obstetrics and Gynecology, 88,* 24S–30S.

U.S. Department of Health and Human Services, Public Health Service. (1991). *Healthy People 2000: National Health Promotion and Disease Prevention Objectives.* DHHS Pub. No. PHS 91-50212. Washington, DC: Author.

Trussell, J., & Vaughn, B. (1999). Contraceptive failure, method-related discontinuation and resumption of use: Results from the 1995 National Survey of Family Growth. *Family Planning Perspectives, 31,* 64–72, 93.

Weisman, C. S., Maccannon, D. S., Henderson, J. T., Shortridge, E., & Orso, C. L. (2002). Contraceptive counseling in managed care: Preventing unintended pregnancy in adults. *Women's Health Issues, 12*(2), 79–95.

Westhoff, C. L., Heartwell, S., Edwards, S., et al. (2007). Oral contraceptive discontinuation: Do side effects matter? *American Journal of Obstetrics & Gynecology, 196,* 412.e1–412.e7.

World Health Organization. (1996). Improving access to quality care in family planning: Medical eligibility criteria for contraceptive use. Geneva, Switzerland: Author.

World Health Organization. (2004). Selected practice recommendations for contraceptive use. Retrieved March 6, 2008, from http://www.who.int/reproductive-health/publications/spr/spr.pdf

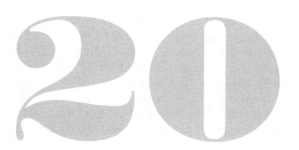

Perimenstrual Symptoms and Syndromes

Diana Taylor, Judith Berg, and
Catherine Ingram Fogel

Symptoms are the most common reason people seek health care and result in the majority of visits to primary health care providers. Symptoms create distress and disrupt social functioning. Management of symptoms and the resulting outcomes often become the responsibility of patients and their families. Many people wonder whether they are doing the right things and whether their symptom management approaches are appropriate. Likewise, health care providers have difficulty developing symptom management strategies that can be applied in both acute and home care settings, because there are few tested models of symptom management.

Symptoms are defined as subjective experiences reflecting changes in a person's biopsychosocial function, sensation, or cognition. In contrast, a sign is defined as any abnormality indicative of disease, detectable by another person or by the individual. Most research on symptoms has been directed toward either a single symptom, such as pain or fatigue, or toward their associated symptoms, such as depression and sleep disturbances (University of California, San Francisco, School of Nursing Symptom Management Faculty Group, 1994).

The symptom experience involves the interaction of a person's perception of the symptom, evaluation of the meaning of a symptom, and response to a symptom (Mechanic, 1995). Perception of symptoms refers to whether an individual notices a change from the way he or she usually feels or behaves. Involving personal appraisal of the interaction between environmental and somatic cues, symptom perception is a conscious, cognitive interpretation of information gathered by the senses in the context of a particular environment or situation. Evaluation of symptoms refers to the judgments people make about their symptoms, such as symptom severity, cause, treatability, and the effects of symptoms. Responses to symptoms include physiological, psychological, and behavioral components (University of California, San Francisco, School of Nursing Symptom Management Faculty Group, 1994). Understanding the interaction of the components of the symptom experience is essential for comprehensive symptom assessment and effective symptom management.

Physicians have traditionally focused on finding and curing the cause of a symptom. While these efforts are essential, persons with noncurable and chronic symptoms need assistance as they try to live with and manage their symptoms. In contrast, nurses have traditionally tried to help individuals and families cope with their symptoms. Although this is a worthwhile endeavor, it is not comprehensive enough to effectively direct individuals toward fully integrated strategies to lessen symptomatology. A broader perspective to symptom management is needed. When both the underlying cause and presenting symptoms are concurrently managed, individuals are more likely to remain in treatment and to benefit from the expertise of health care professionals. People can be guided to use symptoms as cues to indicate appropriate self-management actions.

PERIMENSTRUAL SYMPTOMS

While the menstrual cycle, a normative process, is not a chronic illness, about 10% to 15% of women experience severe recurring symptoms associated with the menstrual cycle that can be considered a chronic illness. Furthermore, most women will experience menstrually related symptoms at some point across their life span that will require professional or self-management. Perimenstrual symptoms, while distressing to some women, are complex gender-specific conditions that require biologic, psychosocial, and cultural assessment and management strategies. The term *perimenstrual symptoms* refers to symptoms in the late luteal phase (prior to menses), menses (bleeding days), and the early follicular phase (a few days following the menstrual bleed). Helping women to identify and manage these menstrually related symptoms can be health protecting and promoting and applied to other women's health problems, such as stress-related conditions (heart disease, arthritis, immune system disorders), psychiatric disorders, or normative menstrual cycle transitions (menarche, postpartum, menopause).

Prevalence of Perimenstrual Symptoms

The most prevalent premenstrual symptoms in a healthy, community-based sample ($N = 193$) of women from a southeastern U.S. city were cramps, mood swings, fatigue, swelling, irritability, tension, skin disorders, headache, depression, backache, painful or tender breasts, weight gain, anxiety, and crying (Woods, Most, & Dery, 1982). In another study of a West Coast population-based, multiethnic sample, the symptoms that 345 women most frequently rated as moderate or extreme during premenses were fatigue (26%), sensation of weight gain (14%), awakening during the night (13%), depression (11%), painful or tender breasts (11%), and bloating (10%). Symptoms were most intense during menses, and the most frequent premenstrual experiences were positive (Woods, Mitchell, Lentz, Taylor, & Lee, 1987). Positive perimenstrual experiences such as increased energy and well-being have received little attention but have been found to be more prevalent (50% to 60%) than negative symptom experiences in a community sample of women. In these studies, when only symptoms that women rated as severe or disabling were considered, the prevalence of symptoms was a much lower 10% to 20%. Approximately 8% to 10% of menstruating women, representing 8 million U.S. women, experience multiple symptoms to a severe degree (Gehlert & Hartlage, 1997; Woods, Most, & Dery, 1982; Woods et al., 1987). Prevalence estimates indicate that 25% to 40% of women in the general population report mild to moderate perimenstrual symptoms (Mitchell, Woods, Lentz, & Taylor, 1991; Severino & Moline, 1995; Woods et al., 1982).

PREMENSTRUAL SYMPTOMS AND SYMPTOM CLUSTERS

Premenstrual symptoms are defined as symptoms of negative affect (sadness, anxiety, irritability, or mood swings), fluid retention, pain and somatic symptoms, and behavioral changes reported to occur during the luteal phase of the menstrual cycle (Richards, Rubinow, Daly, & Schmidt, 2006; Woods, Mitchell, & Taylor, 1999). Perimenstrual symptoms refer to the cyclic symptom experience in relation to menstruation. Few women experience perimenstrual symptoms to such a degree of severity that it would be considered a syndrome.

These cyclic changes may be perceived by a woman as troublesome or problematic, escalate before menstruation, and then subside after menses begin. Premenstrual symptoms, particularly those of low or moderate intensity, usually do not interfere with a woman's ability to function or perform her typical roles (Woods et al., 1999).

Although the most commonly reported perimenstrual symptoms may be complaints of physical discomfort (bloating, skin changes, cramping), the reports of mood change or negative affect symptoms are often the most distressing. Many investigators have confirmed that negative affect symptoms, rapid mood changes, and arousal emerge as the prominent factor accounting for much of the distress experienced by women in the premenstrual and menstrual phases (Abraham, 1980; Futterman, Jones, Miccio-Fonseca, & Quigley, 1992; Halbreich, Endicott, Schacht, & Nee, 1982; Moos, 1969; Taylor, Woods, Lentz, Mitchell, & Lee, 1991; Woods, Dery, & Most, 1982).

With more than 100 reported symptoms attributed to menstrual cyclicity, delineation of symptoms into clusters or subtypes has been an important step in understanding women's perimenstrual symptom experience. Several investigators have focused on identifying symptom clusters—such as negative affect, fluid retention, pain and somatic symptoms, and behavioral changes—using techniques such as factor and cluster analysis (Woods, Mitchell, & Taylor, 1999). Taylor and colleagues (1991) classified symptom clusters of women experiencing severe symptoms using differentiation of perimenstrual symptom subtypes (Abraham, 1980; Halbreich, Endicott, & Lesser, 1985; Moos, 1969; Taylor, 1986; Woods, 1985). The negative affect symptom cluster accounted for 60% of the variance in the factor analytic study. Pain/discomfort and dysphoria were also dominant symptom types for women seeking treatment for severe cyclic symptoms.

LIFE CYCLE VARIATION

Studies of menarche and menstrual changes of young women have been more limited than those of other normative aspects of menstruation in adult women. Nurses have made significant contributions to knowledge about normative experiences of menarcheal girls and young women in the areas of menstrual attitudes, symptoms, and attitudes to adult women's subsequent experiences of symptoms (Menke, 1983; Williams, 1983; Woods, Mitchell, & Taylor, 1999).

In the largest survey of 5,485 menstruating adolescents, Widholm and Kantero (1971) found that 73% of girls had at least one premenstrual symptom, most frequently fatigue and irritability with pelvic cramps reported as the most common symptom associated with menstruation. It is known that young girls learn about symptoms from observing their mothers, sisters, and peers, including their expectations about menstrual experiences and the effects of menstruation on feelings and behavior (Woods, Mitchell, & Lentz, 1999). Some studies have focused on the severity and the consequences of perimenstrual symptoms and changes in younger and older adolescents. In a study of 88 adolescents, 44% reported symptoms severe enough to interfere with school attendance with the most common symptoms reported as fatigue, bloating, breast swelling, food cravings, depression, tearfulness, irritability, moodiness, and loss of self-esteem (Wilson & Keye, 1989). Similar results in a study of 75 adolescents found that older girls, approximately 3 to 4 years postmenarche, experienced more intense symptoms than younger girls (13 to 15 years old); the most commonly reported symptoms were food cravings, breast swelling, abdominal discomfort, mood swings, stressed feeling, and dissatisfactions with appearance (Cleckner-Smith, Doughty, & Grossman, 1998). Although younger age is generally related to increased number and severity of symptoms, some studies found symptom severity peaked in the mid-30s (Logue & Moos, 1986).

Demographic characteristics, such as education, income, employment status, and marital status have demonstrated inconsistent or no relationship to premenstrual symptoms (Johnson, McChesney, & Bean, 1988). However, there is limited evidence that nulliparity, earlier age at menarche, higher body mass index, greater alcohol and caffeine consumption, and higher levels of perceived stress are risk factors for specific, but not all, premenstrual symptoms (Deuster, Adera & South-Paul, 1999; Woods, Most, & Dery, 1982).

SOCIAL CONTEXT AND CULTURAL VARIATION

A woman's social context may contribute to and be affected by her experiences of affective and bodily symptoms, perceptions of and responses to her environments, and perceived personal and behavioral changes associated with her menstrual cycle. Dimensions of a woman's social context include socialization about being a woman or her expectations about how she will experience menstruation. Another important dimension is everyday stresses and strains and women's resources with which to respond to them (Woods, Mitchell, & Taylor, 1999).

Perimenstrual symptoms are not culturally confined although particular symptoms may be reported more frequently in one culture compared to another (Janiger, Riffenburgh, & Kersh, 1972; Severy, Thapa, Askew, & Glor, 1993; World Health Organization, 1981). Although most studies neither support a purely cultural depiction of menstrual experiences nor refute it, clearly, culture has a profound influence on premenstrual and menstrual experiences. However, we need to better understand the variety of societal and cultural influences that can affect women's experiences and how they interpret them.

In the United States, Black and White women have equal frequencies of various premenstrual symptoms, with frequency of symptom reporting peaking in the 25- to 34-year-old group (Steege, Stout, & Rupp, 1985). But in a sample of 1,194 women aged 21 to 45 years in a large health maintenance organization population in northern California, Hispanics reported greater severity of symptoms, and Asians less, relative to Whites (Sternfeld, Swindle, Chawla, Long, & Kennedy, 2002).

PERIMENSTRUAL NORMATIVE EXPERIENCE

Most women who monitor their experiences on a daily basis over more than one menstrual cycle notice changes in their bodies and moods that seem to vary with the course of the menstrual cycle. Studies of nonclinical populations of women have revealed an array of normative menstrual experiences and menstrual symptoms as illness experiences, ranging from perimenstrual changes (before and during menstruation) to premenstrual syndromes (Woods, Mitchell, & Taylor, 1999).

Perimenstrual changes have been attributed to changing ovarian hormone levels and their widespread effects on physiological function. Most women who experience changes such as swelling of their breasts or abdomen, increased sensitivity, menstrual cramps, or bursts of energy do not consider themselves sick or ill. Instead, they view such changes as a natural part of being a woman (Woods et al., 1988). Although most attention has been directed at understanding the changes that women perceive as negative or troubling, it is important to notice that some women describe positive experiences associated with menstrual cyclicity, including an increasing energy level that enables them to accomplish more work or to be more creative (Chrisler, 1995; Woods et al., 1987; Woods, Mitchell, & Lentz, 1999). The most common perimenstrual changes and symptoms described by women across their menstrual life span are related to bleeding, pain, and premenstrual symptoms.

PERIMENSTRUAL SYNDROMES

This discussion includes a newer classification of perimenstrual symptoms called cyclic perimenstrual pain and discomfort (CPPD), cyclic pelvic pain (dysmenorrhea), premenstrual syndrome (PMS), premenstrual magnification (PMM), and premenstrual dysphoric disorder (PMDD). Biological, psychosocial stressors and sociocultural factors must be considered for each diagnosis.

Cyclic Perimenstrual Pain and Discomfort

An interdisciplinary group has proposed a more precise classification of perimenstrual symptoms: cyclic perimenstrual pain and discomfort. This term encompasses a broader perspective that includes pelvic pain, cyclic mood symptoms, and physical discomforts (Association of Women's Health, Obstetric and Neonatal Nurses, 2003). This validates additional distressing symptoms and enables development of treatment guidelines based on research evidence as well as personal evidence from women's own experiences (Taylor, Schuiling, & Sharp, 2006).

Cyclic perimenstrual pain and discomfort includes symptom clusters that occur both before and after menstruation begins (Taylor et al., 2006). The primary feature is that symptom clusters occur cyclically and may include pain, discomfort, and mood symptoms (Collins-Sharp, Taylor, Kelly-Thomas, Killeen, & Dawood, 2002). To recognize CPPD, the clinician must consider each woman as an expert at her own symptom recognition, because self-report of symptom perception and severity are essential to accurate assessment and diagnosis (Taylor et al., 2006).

Dysmenorrhea

Dysmenorrhea is pain experienced during menstruation and is categorized as primary or secondary. Mittelschmerz is a commonly used term to describe mid-cycle pain or pain that occurs with ovulation. Whereas dysmenorrhea is more common than mittelschmerz, women will sometimes describe this symptom in the absence of oral contraceptives or other hormone use that suppresses ovulation.

Dysmenorrhea has been defined as excessive pain experienced during menstruation. Classically there are two types: primary dysmenorrhea, in which there is no evident organic pathophysiology in the uterus, fallopian tubes, or ovaries; and secondary dysmenorrhea, usually associated with organic gynecologic pathology, including endometriosis and pelvic inflammatory disease, accounting for about 20% of all pelvic pain (Kinch & Robinson, 1985). However, dysmenorrhea is more than painful menstrual cramps. It is a syndrome with numerous associated symptoms, including abdominal cramps, headache, leg ache, backache, general body aches, continuous abdominal pain, nausea, vomiting, appetite change, diarrhea, constipation, dizziness, fainting, fatigue/lethargy, sleeping disorders, blemishes, bloating/swelling, breast tenderness, nervousness, depression, irritability, excessive menstrual flow, clot formation, difficulty concentrating, and difficulty with normal activities (Dawood & Ramos, 1990).

Primary dysmenorrhea, painful menstruation beginning shortly after menarche, affects approximately 90% of menstruating women (i.e., 9 million to 55 million women) in the United States (Dawood, 1990). As well as being painful to those women afflicted with the syndrome, dysmenorrhea can result in significant absenteeism (i.e., 1 to 5 days per month) from work or school with an estimated $2 billion loss of productivity in the U.S. work place (Dawood, 1988).

Women typically experience severe abdominal cramps that start either just before or at the onset of bleeding. The severity of the cramps varies directly with the heaviness of the menstrual flow, particularly if clots are passed. The cramps are situated in the suprapubic region, usually in both right and left lower quadrants, and they tend to radiate down the front of the thighs. These cramps may last 6 to 24 hours and may be extremely incapacitating. The pain is often associated with one or more of the symptoms listed above (Kinch & Robinson, 1985). Studies indicate that approximately 50% of postpubescent females suffer from primary dysmenorrhea and 10% of women with primary dysmenorrhea suffer severely enough to render them incapacitated for 1–3 days each month (Dawood, 1990).

Premenstrual Syndrome

Premenstrual syndrome is a diagnostic term used to indicate cyclical recurrence of distressing physical, affective, and behavioral experiences that affect interpersonal relationships and personal health. There is disagreement among clinicians about whether PMS is a distinct disease entity (Taylor et al., 2006) because the term is used in contemporary women's descriptions of their menstrual experiences. This popular use contradicts medical classification of PMS as an illness. Nevertheless, a PMS symptom pattern can be discerned by the absence of symptoms or low severity symptoms after menses followed by an escalation of premenses symptom frequency and severity. PMS is experienced by a minority of menstruating women up to 2 weeks before their menstrual periods, but not at other times (Ford, Lethaby, Mol, & Roberts, 2007). The hallmark of PMS is the repeated occurrence of behavioral, somatic, and mood symptoms with sufficient degree of severity to impair social and work-related functioning perimenstrually (Mitchell, Woods, & Lentz, 1994). Although the symptom pattern is distinct with no or low severity of symptoms after menses, cycle profiles indicate an escalation in both frequency and severity of symptoms in the premenstrual period (Mitchell et al., 1994). Other aspects of the syndrome include emotional and physical feelings of stress, including anticipatory stress prior to symptom occurrence (Taylor et al., 1991; Woods, Lentz, Mitchell, Taylor, & Lee, 1992). Some researchers have identified the occurrence of behavioral patterns such as angry outbursts or low impulse control that may stimulate interpersonal conflict (Woods, Mitchell, & Lentz, 1999). PMS management begins with an assessment of symptom clusters, cluster severity, and impact on functional status (Taylor et al., 2006).

Premenstrual Magnification

Premenstrual magnification is a variant of the premenstrual syndrome pattern in which women experience moderately severe symptoms postmenses and more severe symptoms premenses (Mitchell et al., 1994). Generally the term refers to the exacerbation of somatic or mood symptoms in the late luteal or menstrual phase of the cycle (Harrison, 1985). Commonly identified conditions that may have heightened symptoms in the late luteal phase include depressive disorders, eating disorders, substance abuse, panic or anxiety disorders, migraines, seizure disorders, irritable bowel syndrome, asthma, chronic fatigue syndrome, and allergies (Mitchell et al., 1994; Taylor et al., 2006). Like PMS, PMM includes symptom patterns that may interfere with women's usual functioning. It should be noted that women may experience PMM at the same time as CPPD, and this should be considered a dual diagnosis (Taylor et al., 2006).

Premenstrual Dysphoric Disorder

Premenstrual dysphoric disorder is a severe form of premenstrual syndrome characterized by affective and behavioral symptoms, including depressed and/or irritable mood; anhedonia; changes in sleep, energy, and appetite; and physical symptoms such as bloating and breast pain (American Psychiatric Association, 2000). There is no question that some women experience a more severe form of PMS, but many question the legitimization of PMDD or severe PMS as a psychiatric disorder. Moynihan (2004) found little evidence to support PMDD as a separate classification from severe PMS.

The etiology for cyclic perimenstrual physical and mood discomforts (PMS or PMDD) is unclear. Some research has focused on neuroendocrine etiologies such as hormonal imbalances, sodium retention, nutritional deficiencies, or abnormal hypothalamic-pituitary-adrenal axis function (Backstrom et al., 1983; Keye, 1989; O'Brien, 1987; Reid & Yen, 1981). But additional research suggests a complex etiology that links genetics, environmental stressors, and hormonal processes with individual vulnerabilities (Endicott, 2001; Halbreich, 1997, 1999; Taylor et al., 1991). A few well-designed studies have tested the hypothesis that biologic and psychosocial variables interact to affect vulnerability to mood and behavioral changes across the menstrual cycle (Taylor et al., 2006). Resultant knowledge suggests the effect of stressors and stress response was direct but also operated through general distress mediated by poor health behaviors (Taylor et al., 2006). Taylor and colleagues (2006) purport that, although PMS and PMDD have been regarded as biologically based illnesses, there is evidence that life stress, stress response, history of sexual abuse, and cultural socialization are essential determinants of perimenstrual symptoms and syndromes. This would suggest women with PMS and PMDD are more sensitive to normal hormonal shifts and, as a result, develop symptoms that are not reported by most menstruating women.

PERIMENSTRUAL SYMPTOM ASSESSMENT

The goal for assessment is to understand each individual woman's perimenstrual symptom experience and to help her to define and manage the symptoms and their concomitant problems. Of the women who seek professional help with a self-made diagnosis of PMS, 30% to 40% will have a relatively classic form of PMS, 30% to 40% will have a premenstrual exacerbation of an underlying disorder (PMM), and 20% to 30% will have a chronic problem without a premenstrual exacerbation. It is critical to listen to the woman's story—her description of symptoms, symptom clusters, symptom severity, symptom patterns, as well as the effect of the perimenstrual symptom experience on her life, her personal functioning, and her environment (relationships, family, work). Most women who seek professional help will come with the self-made diagnosis of PMS. However, many women will be uncertain as to the nature of their problems.

General characteristics of women seeking professional help for perimenstrual symptoms:

- Early to mid-30s.
- One or more children.
- Working outside the home.

- Experiencing high levels of stress and distress.
- Experiencing significant marital discord.
- Diminished libido during premenstrual phase.

Although the majority of women experience one or more symptoms around the time of menstruation, they do not experience distress or disability associated with these symptoms.

Obtaining a premenstrual symptom history will provide general information about the woman's symptom experience, but prospective ratings are critical to precise diagnosis and to rule out other chronic illness. Retrospective symptom severity reports are likely to overestimate severity and do not provide data about symptom patterns. Ask whether the woman has monitored her symptom severity using a calendar or a symptom checklist.

Perimenstrual Symptom Calendar

A perimenstrual symptom calendar (Figures 20.1 and 20.2) is useful for women who are able to describe their unique symptoms and symptom clusters across the menstrual cycle, as well as to visualize symptom severity patterns. Women fill in their most distressing symptoms beginning on the first day of their last menstrual period using a 5-point rating scale (0 = no severity, 1 = minimal severity, 2 = mild severity, 3 = moderate severity, and 4 = extreme severity).

Clinical assessment includes:

1. History: symptom, personal, medical, sexual, family.
2. Health risk assessment.
3. Functional assessment.
4. Physical assessment/exam.
5. Lab/diagnostics.

Comprehensive Perimenstrual Symptom and Health History

If a woman does not identify herself as having PMS, then begin by asking the woman about the nature of her symptoms:

1. Which symptoms are the most severe or distressing?
2. Timing of the symptoms throughout the menstrual cycle.
3. Does anything worsen or alleviate the symptoms?
4. Presence of symptoms during or after menstruation.
5. Time and events surrounding onset or exacerbation of symptom.

In addition to the usual health history data, specific historical data that assists with perimenstrual symptom classification includes:

1. Menstrual regularity and whether a woman has been diagnosed with a luteal phase defect (shortened luteal phase or disrupted basal body temperatures).
2. Marked fluctuations in weight in the nonpregnant state.
3. Premenstrual alcohol intolerance.
4. Positive feelings or changes associated with menstruation or the menstrual cycle.
5. Mother's and sister's experiences with perimenstrual symptoms.
6. Intolerance to oral contraceptives, symptoms associated with sterilization procedure
7. Postpartum symptoms and perimenstrual symptoms associated with pregnancy.
8. Menstrual cycle variation related to any chronic condition, such as upper respiratory or allergy symptoms, asthma, arthritis symptoms, migraines, dermatologic conditions, eating disorders, depression, vulvovaginitis, fibroids, endometriosis, or chronic pelvic inflammatory disease.

A complete personal function, lifestyle and health status history (e.g., well-being, sleep, exercise, stress, nutrition) will include the following topics:

1. Current health status: how healthy have you felt in the past 6 months (on a scale from 1 to 10)?
2. General level of well-being by menstrual cycle phase, season, or life events.
3. Sleep patterns: sleep onset, difficulty falling asleep, difficulty staying asleep, early morning awakening, use of sleeping medications or remedies, feeling rested, naps.
4. Physical activity: level of physical activity, type and amount of exercise or physical activity.
5. Stress: general level of stress over the past 3 months (on a scale from 1 to 10), types of stressors (personal health, work, family life, personal life), level of stress created by the stressors, stress management strategies.
6. Nutrition: weight, perception of weight, diet patterns, use of stimulants, vitamins or nutritional supplements, food cravings, eating binges, how often does food control your life?

Using the perimenstrual symptom calendar, ask the woman's partner or spouse to rate her symptoms for one complete cycle. Using this component of the evaluation reveals both the involvement of the partner in

Menstrual Cycle Day	1	2	3	4	5	6	7	8	9	10	11	12	13	14	15	16	17	18	19	20	21	22	23	24	25	26	27	28	29	30	31	32
Month ___ Date ___																																
Menstrual Cycle Phase																																
Bleeding (H, M, L, S, *)																																
Weight																																
SYMPTOMS (0 – 4)																																
1.																																
2.																																
3.																																
4.																																
5.																																
6.																																
7.																																
8.																																
9.																																
10.																																
Well-being (+ / -)																																
Stress (+ / -)																																
Life Events (+ / -)																																
SELF-CARE																																
1.																																
2.																																
3.																																

TRACKING INSTRUCTIONS:

Menstrual Cycle Day: Begin with the first day of menstrual flow and end with the last day of your menstrual cycle.

Month & Date: Write in the month then the corresponding date in the box under each menstrual cycle day.

Menstrual Cycle Phase: At the end of the cycle, divide it into phases by drawing a vertical line down after the day before menstrual bleeding starts; count back 14 days and draw another vertical line—write *premenstrual phase* in the space; next, draw a vertical line down after the last day of your period and write in *menstrual phase*; write in *post-menstrual phase* in the remaining space.

Bleeding: Record your menstrual flow or vaginal bleeding as (H) Heavy, (M) Moderate, (L) Light, (S) Spotting, or blank if no bleeding. Note the last day of your menstrual flow with an asterisk (*).

Weight: Record your weight (weigh yourself about the same time every day).

Symptoms: List your most bothersome or distressing symptoms taken from the Symptom Severity Chart with your worst or most distressing symptom in the #1 space, followed by your second most bothersome symptom, and so on, up to 10 symptoms. Rate these symptoms or behavior changes daily as 0-absent, 1-mild, 2-moderate, 3-severe, or 4-extreme throughout the cycle.

Well-being: Rate your feelings of well-being—including increased energy, creativity or generally feeling good—as (+) High, (/) Moderate, or (-) Low.

Stress: Rate your overall stress level as (+) High, (/) Moderate, or (-) Low.

Life Events: Rate any significant events as (+) Positive, (/) Neutral, or (-) Negative.

Self-Care: List anything you did to relieve your symptoms and place a check in the corresponding menstrual day.

Figure 20.1 PMS tracking chart.

© Diana Taylor, RNP, PhD. From www.takingbackthemonth.com

Menstrual Cycle Day	1	2	3	4	5	6	7	8	9	10	11	12	13	14	15	16	17	18	19	20	21	22	23	24	25	26	27	28	29	30	31	32
Month Sept/Oct Date	9/25	26	27	28	29	30	10/1	2	3	4	5	6	7	8	9	10	11	12	13	14	15	16	17	18	19	20	21	22	23			
Menstrual Cycle Phase	Menstrual Phase						Post-Menstrual Phase									Pre-Menstrual Phase																
Bleeding (H, M, L, S, *)	S	H	H	M	L	*																								S		
Weight	135	134	134	134	133	133									133										133	133	134	134	135	135		
SYMPTOMS (0 – 4)																																
1. Irritability	3	1	0	0	0	0	0	0	0	0	0	0	0	0	0	1	1	1	1	1	2	2	2	3	3	4	4	4	3			
2. Anxiety	4	2	0	0	0	0	0	0	0	0	0	0	0	0	0	2	2	2	2	2	2	2	2	2	2	3	3	3	3			
3. Over-Sensitive	3	2	0	0	0	0	0	0	0	0	0	0	0	0	0	1	2	2	2	2	2	2	2	3	3	3	3	3	3			
4. Cry Easily	3	1	0	0	0	0	0	0	0	0	0	0	0	0	0	0	0	0	0	0	0	1	1	2	2	2	2	3	3			
5. Out of Control	4	2	0	0	0	0	0	0	0	0	0	0	0	0	0	1	1	1	2	2	2	2	2	2	3	3	3	3	3			
6. Act Out	3	1	0	0	0	0	0	0	0	0	0	0	0	0	0	0	0	1	1	1	2	1	1	2	2	2	3	3	3			
7. Bloating	4	3	2	1	0	0	0	0	0	0	0	0	0	0	0	0	0	0	0	0	0	1	2	2	2	3	4	4	4			
8. Swelling	3	3	1	0	0	0	0	0	0	0	0	0	0	0	0	0	0	0	0	0	1	1	2	2	3	3	3	3	3			
9. Difficulty Fall Asleep	3	1	1	0	0	0	0	0	0	0	1	0	0	1	0	0	1	1	0	1	0	1	2	2	2	2	2	3	3			
10. Confusion	2	2	0	0	0	0	0	0	0	0	0	0	0	0	0	0	0	0	0	0	0	0	0	0	0	0	2	2	2			
Well-being (+ / -)	/	/	+	+	+	+	+	+	+	+	+	+	+	+	+	+	+	+	/	/	/	/	/	/	/	/	-	-	-			
Stress (+ / -)	/	/	-	-	-	-	-	-	-	-	-	-	-	-	-	-	-	/	/	/	/	/	+	+	+	+	+	+	+			
Life Events (+ / -)	/	/	+	+	+	/	+	/	/	/	/	/	/	/	/	/	/	/	/	/	/	/	/	/	/	/	/	/	/			
SELF-CARE																																
1. Left Work/Stay Home	√																															
2. Take a walk	√	√																						√		√	√	√				
3. Call my friend			√																							√			√			

TRACKING INSTRUCTIONS:

Menstrual Cycle Day: Begin with the first day of menstrual flow and end with the last day of your menstrual cycle.

Month & Date: Write in the month then the corresponding date in the box under each menstrual cycle day.

Menstrual Cycle Phase: At the end of the cycle, divide it into phases by drawing a vertical line down after the day before menstrual bleeding starts; count back 14 days and draw another vertical line—write *premenstrual phase* in the space; next, draw a vertical line down after the last day of your period and write in *menstrual phase*; write in *post-menstrual phase* in the remaining space.

Bleeding: Record your menstrual flow or vaginal bleeding as (H) Heavy, (M) Moderate, (L) Light, (S) Spotting, or blank if no bleeding. Note the last day of your menstrual flow with an asterisk (*).

Weight: Record your weight (weigh yourself about the same time every day).

Symptoms: List your most bothersome or distressing symptoms taken from the Symptom Severity Chart with your worst or most distressing symptom in the #1 space, followed by your second most bothersome symptom, and so on, up to 10 symptoms. Rate these symptoms or behavior changes daily as 0-absent, 1-mild, 2-moderate, 3-severe, or 4-extreme throughout the cycle.

Well-being: Rate your feelings of well-being—including increased energy, creativity or generally feeling good—as (+) High, (/) Moderate, or (-) Low.

Stress: Rate your overall stress level as (+) High, (/) Moderate, or (-) Low.

Life Events: Rate any significant events as (+) Positive, (/) Neutral, or (-) Negative.

Self-Care: List anything you did to relieve your symptoms and place a check in the corresponding menstrual day.

Figure 20.2 PMS tracking chart (filled in).

© Diana Taylor, RNP, PhD. From www.takingbackthemonth.com

the therapeutic process and the impact of the perimenstrual symptom experience on the relationship. Having the partners or spouses complete their own evaluations provides some privacy if they are reluctant to directly communicate their assessment.

1. Discrepancies between the partner/spouse assessments can be used to query the woman about particular symptoms or behavior (e.g., alcohol and drug use, sexual response or behavior, and marital discord).

2. Many partners experience higher levels of distress and marital discord related to the patient's perimenstrual symptom experience in comparison to the patient, herself.

3. The partner's assessment can be used to develop a complete treatment plan that may need to include marital counseling.

4. It is important to first describe this process to the patient as a usual component of the evaluation process. If the partner/spouse is not present for the evaluation then send the forms home with the patient with specific instructions for how to fill out the menstrual calendar.

Diagnostic Criteria for Premenstrual Syndromes

Three professional groups have suggested diagnostic criteria for clinical assessment of perimenstrual symptoms. Thorough symptom assessment is common to all. The guidelines of the Association of Women's Health, Obstetrical and Neonatal Nurses (AWHONN, 2003) emphasize attention to the interaction of medical, psychological, sociocultural, and lifestyle factors. These guidelines include a need for focused health history data, physical examination, plus distinguishing perimenstrual symptoms and discomfort patterns across at least three menstrual cycle phases. In the AWHONN guidelines, the premenstrual phase is up to 14 days prior to the onset of menses, the menstrual phase is the days during menses, and the postmenstrual phase is after menses and before ovulation (AWHONN; Mitchell, 1991; Mitchell et al., 1991).

Exhibit 20.1 details three to four common classifications of cyclic pain and discomfort patterns as described by Taylor and colleagues (2006). These classifications can only be identified by tracking symptom patterns across one or two menstrual cycles.

The American College of Obstetricians and Gynecologist's (2000) key criteria for diagnosis of PMS are listed in Table 20.1. Research criteria for PMDD from the *Diagnostic and Statistical Manual of Mental Disorders* are given in Table 20.2.

SYMPTOM MANAGEMENT

Both the clinician and patient must work together to set goals and outcome criteria before embarking on treatment (Taylor et al., 2006). In this way, individual and

---

EXHIBIT 20.1 FOUR COMMON CLASSIFICATIONS OF CYCLIC PAIN AND DISCOMFORT PATTERNS

- **Low severity of perimenstrual pain and discomforts**
  - □ Few bothersome symptoms of low to mild severity in the menstrual or premenstrual phases or one or two symptoms that are rated as moderate to severe but last only 1 to 2 days.
- **Classic cyclic pelvic pain or dysmenorrhea**
  - □ Multiple pain symptoms that are rated as moderate or severe for 1 day premenstrually and 3 to 5 menstrual days.
  - □ Symptoms completely subside after menses but might include cyclic headaches and physical discomforts such as bloating.
- **Classic premenstrual syndrome pattern or cyclic perimenstrual mood and physical discomforts**
  - □ Includes symptoms rated as moderate to extreme severity for up to 2 weeks before onset of menses.
  - □ Symptoms subsequently disappear or become much milder with 1 to 4 days of onset of menses.
- **Premenstrual magnification**
  - □ Symptoms that are cyclic in that they are present during the postmenstrual (follicular) and early premenstrual (luteal) phases, but often increase in severity during the premenstrual phase.
  - □ These women need careful evaluation to determine whether they are experiencing a premenstrual exacerbation of another disorder such as depression, anxiety, substance abuse, headaches, allergies, asthma, irritable bowel syndrome, or chronic pelvic pain.

20.1 | Diagnostic Criteria for Premenstrual Syndrome

Premenstrual syndrome can be diagnosed if the patient reports at least one of the following affective and somatic symptoms during the 5 days before menses in each of the three prior menstrual cycles:

- ■ Affective symptoms
  - ☐ Depression
  - ☐ Angry outbursts
  - ☐ Irritability
  - ☐ Anxiety
  - ☐ Confusion
  - ☐ Social withdrawal
- ■ Somatic symptoms
  - ☐ Breast tenderness
  - ☐ Abdominal bloating
  - ☐ Headache
  - ☐ Swelling of extremities
- ■ The symptoms are relieved within 4 days of the onset of menses without recurrence until at least cycle day 13.
- ■ The symptoms are present in the absence of any pharmacologic therapy, hormone ingestion, or drug or alcohol use.
- ■ The symptoms occur reproducibly during two cycles of prospective recording.
- ■ The patient suffers from identifiable dysfunction in social or economic performance.

Note. Reprinted with permission from the *ACOG Practice Bulletin #15, Premenstrual syndrome.* by the American College of Obstetricians and Gynecologists, 2000, Washington, DC: Author.

combination treatments can be evaluated for effectiveness. Setting goals should include health-related outcomes, functional status, and economic concerns. Clinical research suggests that a combination of treatments is more satisfactory than a single treatment (Keye, 1988; Taylor, 1988, 1999; Taylor et al., 1991). In a clinical trial of multimodal symptom management strategies for women experiencing severe PMS, Taylor (1999) found that women prefer to select multiple strategies for symptom management, perimenstrual symptom severity will decline markedly within the first few months, and this effect will be maintained over the long term. In this discussion, symptom management is divided into pharmacotherapies and self-management strategies. Ideally, women combine strategies to create a tailored protocol that best alleviates and/or manages cyclic symptoms associated with the menstrual cycle. It should be noted that management strategies for severe PMS and PMDD rarely differ.

Treatment for Dysmenorrhea

Pharmacologic management of dysmenorrhea centers on the use of nonsteroidal anti-inflammatory drugs (NSAIDs). With the observations of elevated prostaglandin levels in menstrual fluid, endometrial extracts, and plasma prostaglandin levels in dysmenorrheic women and the accumulated evidence that NSAIDs inhibit prostaglandin synthesis, clinical trials based on the rational use of NSAIDs in dysmenorrhea began in the mid-1970s (Chan, 1983). It is clear from the large number of clinical trials that administration of NSAIDs reduces uterine and menstrual prostaglandin levels and is associated with decreased pain and relief of symptoms associated with dysmenorrhea (Tolman, McGuire, Rosenthale, 1985). However, Chan and Dawood (1980) reported that the effectiveness of NSAIDs in relieving dysmenorrhea ranges from 65% to 100%. Jamieson and Steege (1996) reported that 90% of 581 women surveyed in a primary care clinic had a history of dysmenorrhea or pelvic pain, with about half of the women reporting that they received less than optimal relief. While NSAIDs effectively decrease pain and symptom severity associated with dysmenorrhea, 10% obtain no relief from any of the currently available treatment options (Dawood, 1988). In addition, NSAIDs have side effects and may be contraindicated or not tolerated by some women. Consultation and comanagement is recommended because these women are likely to need additional evaluation (laparoscopy, pelvic imaging). Dosing with nonsteroidals is variable by product, but ibuprofen 500 mg to 1,000 mg per day is FDA approved for dysmenorrhea and may relieve mastalgia. It should be taken with food. Use recommendations are for days 17 through 28 of the menstrual cycle.

Acupuncture has been described as a treatment for acute and chronic pain, including dysmenorrhea. Helms (1987) studied 43 women suffering from dysmenorrhea randomized to four treatment groups: real acupuncture, sham acupuncture, standard controls (no intervention), and visitation controls (visits to a treating physician). The women were free to take their previously used pain medications during the 3-month treatment period and a follow-up period. Almost all of the women in the real acupuncture treatment group (91%) showed improvement, compared to 36% of the women in the sham acupuncture group, 18% of the women in the standard control group, and 10% of the women in the visitation control group. The real acupuncture group had a 41% decrease in use of pain medication compared to no change in pain medication use in the three other groups. Improvement beyond the end of the active treatment period persisted only in the real acupuncture group. Although the results of this study were promising, serious adverse reactions have been attributed to

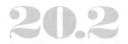 Research Criteria for Premenstrual Dysphoric Disorder

A. In most menstrual cycles during the past year, five (or more) of the following symptoms were present for most of the time during the last week of the luteal phase, began to remit within a few days after the onset of the follicular phase, and were absent in the week postmenses, with at least one of the symptoms being either (1), (2), (3), or (4):

   1. Markedly depressed mood, feelings of hopelessness, or self-deprecating thoughts
   2. Marked anxiety, tension, feelings of being keyed up or on edge
   3. Marked affective lability (e.g., feeling suddenly sad or tearful or increased sensitivity to rejection)
   4. Persistent and marked anger or irritability or increased interpersonal conflicts
   5. Decreased interest in usual activities (e.g., work, school, friends, hobbies)
   6. Subjective sense of difficulty in concentrating
   7. Lethargy, easy fatigability, or marked lack of energy
   8. Marked change in appetite, overeating, or specific food cravings
   9. Hypersomnia or insomnia
  10. A subjective sense of being overwhelmed or out of control
  11. Other physical symptoms, such as breast tenderness or swelling, headaches, joint or muscle pain, a sensation of bloating, weight gain

B. The disturbance markedly interferes with work or school or with usual social activities and relationships with others (e.g., avoidance of social activities, decreased productivity and efficiency at work or school).

C. The disturbance is not merely an exacerbation of the symptoms of another disorder, such as major depressive disorder, panic disorder, dysthymic disorder, or a personality disorder (although it may be superimposed on any of these disorders).

D. Criteria A, B, and C must be confirmed by prospective daily ratings during at least two consecutive symptomatic cycles. (The diagnosis may be made provisionally prior to this confirmation.)

Note. Reprinted with permission from the *Diagnostic and Statistical Manual of Mental Disorders-IV-TR,* by American Psychiatric Association, 2000, Washington, DC: APA Press.

misuse of acupuncture needles including transmission of infection, trauma, and allergic reactions.

Treatment for PMS

Johnson (2004) suggested a hierarchical approach to match women's symptom severity to the type of treatment approach (see Exhibit 20.2 for details).

A wide range of therapeutic agents has been used to manage PMS and PMDD by targeting perceived aspects of the underlying pathophysiology of the conditions (Halbreich et al., 2006). The two main pharmacological strategies are to (1) eliminate hormonal cyclicity via suppression of ovulation and (2) target central nervous system processes thought to contribute to premenstrual mood symptoms. Other hypothesized mechanisms involved in premenstrual symptoms are targeted via dietary and nutritional changes and aldosterone blockade (Halbreich et al., 2006).

Suppression of Ovulation

Bilateral surgical oophorectomy is a drastic solution that appears beneficial in alleviating emotional and physical premenstrual symptoms (Casper & Hearn, 1990). How-

ever, this surgery should be recommended only in cases of severe, disabling symptoms that have not responded to pharmacological treatment.

Medical oophorectomy that is reversible can be accomplished using gonadotrophin-releasing hormone (GnRH) agonists. Yet long-term use is expensive and potential side effects include those associated with hypoestrogenism, demineralization of bone and increased cardiovascular risk (Johnson, 2004; Rapkin, 2003). To counteract side effects, some clinicians add to the therapy by using estrogen/progestin hormone therapy to reduce risks. However, this may only result in recurrence of premenstrual symptoms (Schmidt et al., 1998). Danazol, a synthetic androgen with some antiestrogen effect, and high-dose continuous estrogen or oral contraceptives are other ovulation suppressors used for PMS and PMDD management. These, too, have adverse side effects, such as increased cardiovascular risk and endometrial hyperplasia and cancer for unopposed estrogen use. Some have used transdermal estradiol patches in high enough doses to suppress ovulation with addition of progestin to protect the endometrium in women with intact uteri. Combined oral contraceptives used continuously and transdermal patches are considered appropriate for first-line long-term management strategies

EXHIBIT 20.2 HIERARCHICAL APPROACH TO TREATMENT OF PREMENSTRUAL SYNDROME AND PREMENSTRUAL DYSPHORIC DISORDER

Level 1: Mild to moderate premenstrual syndrome

- Lifestyle: Aerobic exercise, nutritional changes (reduce caffeine, salt, alcohol; increase complex carbohydrates).
- Choose from among the following over-the-counter drugs:
  - ☐ Calcium (1,000 g) or magnesium (400 g) daily supplements
  - ☐ Chaste berry fruit (4–20 mg per day)

Level 2: Premenstrual syndrome, when physical symptoms are the predominant problem. Choose based on specific symptom that's problematic:

- ☐ Spironolactone (Aldactone) (20–50 mg per day)
- ☐ Oral contraceptives (regular or long cycle) or depomedroxyprogesterone acetate for breast pain, cramps, and other abdominal pain
- ☐ Nonsteroidal anti-inflammatory drugs in the luteal phase for most physical symptoms (follow product dosing instructions)

Level 3: Premenstrual syndrome and premenstrual dysphoric disorder, when mood symptoms are the predominant problem

A. Intermittent dosing of selective serotonin reuptake inhibitors (SSRIs), such as symptom-day only (starts on the first day of typical symptoms or luteal phase therapy (starts 2 weeks before expected first day of menses). Fluvoxamine 20 mg per day, paroxetine 10–30 mg per day, maprotiline 25–150 mg per day, fluoxetine 20–60 mg per day, and sertraline 50–150 mg per day have been utilized.

B. Daily SSRI

C. If the initial SSRI is ineffective or not tolerated, try at least two other SSRI agents before abandoning this type of agent.

D. Buspirone 5 mg twice daily in the luteal phase

Level 4: Premenstrual dysphoric disorder not responsive to therapy described in Levels 1 through 3

A. Continuous high-dose progestin (e.g., oral medroxyprogesterone acetate 20–30 mg daily or depomedroxyprogesterone acetate 150 mg every 3 months)

B. Gonadotropin-releasing hormone (GnRH), dosing variable by product

C. Bilateral oophorectomy (only if GnRH is ineffective and there are no other options)

---

for treatment of PMS and PMDD (Halbreich, 2005). A few studies have prospectively examined the use of different combined oral contraceptives to treat PMS and PMDD, and findings have been mixed (Freeman, Kroll, Rapkin, et al., 2001; Graham & Sherwin, 1992; Pearlstein et al., 2005; Yonkers et al., 2005). This suggests the steroidal composition has bearing on overall results (Halbreich, 2005).

GnRH agonists that are used to suppress ovulation include leuprolide, histrelin, goserelin, and buserelin. These agents have been shown beneficial in alleviating both behavioral and physical premenstrual symptoms; no consistent pattern of symptoms responsive to them are noted in the literature (Halbreich et al., 2006). In a study of daily nasal buserelin (400 mg/day for 3 months), there was a significant improvement of swelling, decreased cheerfulness, tension, irritability, fatigue, depression,

and breast tenderness (Hammarback & Backstrom, 1988). Lower doses appear to be less effective. There is evidence that leuprolide (3.75 mg/month for 3 cycles) significantly reduced both physical and behavioral symptoms of PMS—especially irritability, neurological symptoms, breast tenderness, fatigue, and bloating—in over 50% of patients (Brown et al., 1994); however, it is the least effective in women with severe premenstrual depression (Freeman, Sondheimer, & Rickels (1997). Depot goserelin (3.6 mg/month over 3 months) reduced cyclical mood swings but had a stronger effect on physical symptoms, such as breast discomfort and swelling than on mood symptoms (West & Hillier, 1994). However, when an estrogen-progestin regime was added back to counteract symptoms associated with hypoestrogenism, mixed results have been reported (Leather et al., 1999; Mortola, Girton, & Fischer, 1991).

Danazol in high doses (more than 200 mg/day) achieves anovulation but is associated with more adverse effects and long-term risks (Halbreich et al., 2006). Data suggest danazol is more effective than placebo in relieving premenstrual symptoms, particularly mastalgia.

Estrogens as well as antiestrogens appear to be of no benefit and may actually aggravate premenstrual symptoms (Dhar & Murphy, 1990). However, in a study of women with severe premenstrual mastalgia, tamoxifen 10 mg per day from cycle day 5 to 24, six consecutive cycles eliminated mastalgia in 89% of patients (Messinis & Lolis, 1988). Continuous estrogen therapy with 7 to 10 days of luteal phase progestin administered transdermally in a sufficient dose to suppress ovulation significantly decreased dysphoric mood plus physical symptoms of PMS (Magos, Brincat, & Studd, 1986; Messinis & Lolis, 1988).

Combined oral contraceptives induce anovulation by inhibiting GnRH secretion through the combined activity of their estrogenic and progestogenic components on the hypothalamus-pituitary ovarian axis (Halbreich et al., 2006). Although combined oral contraceptives have been shown to reduce physical symptoms associated with PMS and PMDD, they do not reliably ameliorate mood symptoms, and negative mood symptoms may be a side effect of oral contraceptive use (Sanders et al., 2001; Walker & Bancroft, 1990). However, two studies of a monophasic combined oral contraceptive containing ethinylestradiol 20 μg and drospirenone 3 mg taken in cycles of 24 consecutive days followed by 4 hormone-free days demonstrated significantly greater improvements in a wide range of physical and mood-related symptoms compared to placebo (Pearlstein et al., 2005; Yonkers et al., 2005). Preliminary evidence indicates that a new oral contraceptive pill (Yasmin) containing low-dose estrogen and the progestin drospirenone (a spironolactone analog) instead of a 19-nortestosterone derivative can reduce symptoms of water retention and other side effects related to estrogen in women with PMS and PMDD (Rapkin, 2003).

Progesterone treatment for PMS has been widely studied despite the lack of evidence confirming progesterone deficiency as a causal mechanism for PMS. Nevertheless, large doses of progesterone have a sedative effect for both men and women. Anecdotal reports of progesterone treatment suggest dramatic relief of perimenstrual negative affect. In a systematic literature review, Ford, Lethaby, Mol, and Roberts (2007) examined two clinical trials of women aged 18 to 45 years to find participants benefited more from progesterone than placebo to decrease premenstrual symptom severity. However, when data were re-analyzed using the intention-to-treat model, there were no statistically significant differences between oral progesterone, vaginally absorbed progesterone, and placebo (Ford, Lethaby, Mol, & Roberts, 2007). No conclusions can, therefore, be made regarding progesterone effectiveness.

Micronization of progesterone for oral use increases the surface area contact between the steroid molecule and the mucosa. Proponents assert that, because of the human-identical structure of micronised progesterone, the drug is generally well tolerated, does not produce the same unacceptable adverse effect profile as synthetic compounds, and provides similar therapeutic benefits. However, oral failed to show improvement compared with placebo for overall PMS symptoms or for mood and behavioral symptom clusters (Dennerstein et al., 1986; Freeman et al., 1995). While numerous over-the-counter progesterone creams have become available through health retail outlets, the types and concentrations of the available progesterone contained in such products vary greatly. As a result, women may receive a subclinical dose and erroneously conclude that progesterone is ineffective.

Central Nervous System–Targeting Agents

Reduced serotonergic activity has been implicated in PMS and PMDD (Rapkin, 2003). Some researchers have identified a luteal phase reduction in central nervous system serotonergic function that may contribute to PMS and PMDD in vulnerable women (Johnson, 2004; Rapkin, 2003). Therefore, selective serotonin reuptake inhibitors (SSRIs) have become a first-line pharmaceutical choice for PMS and PMDD management. Halbreich and colleagues (2006) reviewed clinical trials of the effect of SSRIs on PMS and PMDD and found that the therapeutic effect occurs more quickly after treatment onset than in patients with acute or chronic depression. This allows for intermittent use from ovulation to onset of menses (Ericksson et al., 1995), yet intermittent treatment appears to be less effective than continuous treatment in reducing somatic complaints (Sundblad, Hedberg, & Eriksson, 1993). SSRIs are most effective for irritability and anxiety symptoms, with lesser efficacy for atypical premenstrual symptoms (Halbreich et al., 2006). Clinical trials of SSRI antidepressants have demonstrated effectiveness for women with severe cyclic depression compared with a placebo, yet many women experience significant side effects (Freeman et al., 2004; Halbreich et al., 2002; Miner et al., 2002; Steiner et al., 1995; Steiner et al., 2005). In a study of fluoxetine or Prozac, 42% of the women did not complete the 6-menstrual cycle protocol due to drug side effects or lack of efficacy. Although most of the side effects were associated with the 60 mg fluoxetine dose, only slightly more than half of all treatment cycles showed moderate improvement in symptoms (Steiner et al., 1995).

Treatment for PMS and PMDD may include noradrenergic agonists and anticholinergics. An inhibitor of both serotonin and noradrenaline reuptake, venlaflaxine has demonstrated greater improvement than placebo on emotion, function, pain, and physical symptoms, but not on appetite in individuals with PMDD (Freeman, Rickels, Yonkers, et al., 2001). Desipramine, a selective noradrenaline reuptake inhibitor, and the anticholinergic methylscopolamine both improved premenstrual symptoms (low mood/loss of pleasure, lability, atypical depression, hysteroid behavior, hostility/anger, social withdrawal, anxiety, impulsivity, general physical discomfort, fatigue, and impaired social function) in women with PMDD. In this same study, desipramine significantly improved fluid retention compared with baseline (Taghavi et al., 1995). In another clinical trial, sertraline was significantly more effective than desipramine or placebo in improving irritability, anxiety or tension, depression, feeling hopeless or guilty, and feeling out of control (Freeman et al., 1999).

Alprazolam is a GABAergic compound administered intermittently to treat PMS and PMDD (Halbreich et al., 2006), usually in the luteal phase of the menstrual cycle. However, individuals with anxiety disorders are subject to addiction with long-term use of alprazolam, and withdrawal of the drug may exacerbate anxiety and physical manifestations such as shakiness, palpitations, and tremors. In one trial, short-term administration during the luteal phase did not cause any addiction, and discontinuation after the onset of menses didn't result in withdrawal symptoms (Harrison, Endicott, & Nee, 1990). The efficacy of alprazolam with PMS and PMDD is mixed. Harrison, Endicott, and Nee found evidence that it significantly reduced depression, anxiety, irritability, low mood, mood lability, hysteroid behavior, social withdrawl, impulsivity, fatigue, and impaired social function. Berger and Presser (1994) found it alleviated tension, irritability, anxiety and feeling out of control relative to placebo but didn't reduce depression. But Schmidt, Grover, and Rubinow (1993) reported no therapeutic benefit of alprazolam over placebo in women with PMS.

Because there is evidence for a relationship between increased prolactin levels and mastalgia, dopamine agonists such as bromocriptine and lisuride have reduced prolactin levels and effectively treated cyclical premenstrual breast pain (Graham et al., 1978; Halbreich et al., 1976). Evidence suggests that luteal phase treatment with bromocriptine results in improvement in edema/bloating, weight gain, depression, insomnia, anxiety, and irritability in some women (Elsner et al., 1980; Graham et al., 1978; Meden-Vrtovec & Vujic, 1992). In other work, lisuride 0.2 mg daily throughout the menstrual cycle significantly reduced mastalgia over 2 months of treatment, and this correlated with prolactin level reduction (Kaleli et al., 2001).

Conflicting evidence exists for the efficacy of spironolactone (an aldosterone antagonist) given during the luteal phase (Halbreich et al., 2006). Two studies have demonstrated that spironolactone 100 mg daily taken for 6 to 8 days before the onset of menses improves mood symptoms (Aslaksen & Falk, 1991; O'Brien et al., 1979). In another study where spironolactone 100 mg daily was given from day 12 of the menstrual cycle through to menses, general bloating was significantly improved compared to placebo, but depression, tension, sadness, libido, lethargy, anxiety, aggression, headache, breast tenderness, swollen abdomen, and swollen feet did not improve (Vellacott et al., 1987). However, in another study of spironolactone 100 mg per day during the 14 premenstrual days, women in the treatment group had significant reductions in irritability, depression, feeling of swelling, breast tenderness, and sweets cravings, but not in tension/anxiety, fatigue, decreased energy, decreased well-being and headache than those receiving placebo (Wang et al., 1995).

Health Promotion Behaviors

Nutrition

Support for a nutritional etiology for PMS is lacking in the scientific literature; however, nutritional therapy for PMS remains common (dietary modification, vitamin and mineral supplementation) (Halbreich et al., 2006). Increasing complex carbohydrates was found to significantly reduce self-reported premenstrual depression, anger, confusion, and food cravings in 24 women with confirmed PMS enrolled in a double-blind, crossover study (Sayegh et al., 1995). PMS severity, especially irritability and insomnia, has been associated with caffeine consumption, with a 30% increased severity with 1 cup of a caffeine-containing beverage per day to as high as a 7-fold increase with 8 to 10 cups per day (Rossignol & Bonnlander, 1990). Decreasing salt intake and increasing fluids premenstrually often is recommended as a way to minimize bloating and physical symptoms but has not been confirmed by research. Pyridoxine (vitamin B_6) has been shown to be effective for symptoms of depression, irritability, and fatigue (Abraham & Hargrove, 1980), yet high doses have been found to cause neurotoxicity (Kleijnen, Ter-Riet, & Knipschild, 1990). Thys-Jacobs (2000) and associates (1989) found that calcium supplementation was more effective than a placebo for perimenstrual symptom management and decreased both mood and somatic symptom severity by 48%.

Physical Activity

The popular literature has promoted the use of exercise for PMS relief, suggesting it is helpful for relieving pain symptoms (backache, pelvic cramps) and negative affect symptoms (crying, anxiety). Evidence from aerobic exercise studies indicates that women who exercise regularly report fewer physical symptoms as well as lower levels of depression, anxiety, hostility, and anger across the menstrual cycle (Aganoff & Boyle, 1994). Prior et al. (1987) showed a positive relationship between conditioning exercise and PMS relief (decreased fluid retention, breast symptoms, and premenstrual depression) in two small studies. Exercise physiologists report that exercisers have increased self-esteem as a result of being more physically competent, regardless of whether they had a difficult or easy workout (Sonstroem & Morgan, 1989). Other researchers have described the therapeutic aspects of aerobic dance participation by women (Estivill, 1995); the immune-enhancing function of moderate, regular exercise (LaPierre et al., 1990); and that exercise regularity or frequency, rather than exercise intensity, is related to PMS relief (Steege & Blumenthal, 1993).

Relaxation Therapy

Considerable evidence has accumulated that relaxation therapy can facilitate recovery from stress arousal (Titlebaum, 1998). Investigators have correlated relaxation and other stress-reduction techniques with the alleviation of hypertension, headaches, chronic pain, anxiety, emotional distress, insomnia, depression, and gastrointestinal disorders (Ewart, Taylor, Kraemer, & Agras, 1984; Raskin, Johnson, & Rondestvedt, 1973; Taylor, Farquhar, Nelson, & Agras, 1977; Titlebaum, 1998). Others have found relaxation therapy to be immunoenhancing (Green & Green, 1987). In a clinical trial of the use of relaxation for treatment of PMS, investigators found a 58% reduction in premenstrual negative affect symptoms after a 3-month use of daily relaxation compared to 17% to 27% improvement in two control groups (Goodale, Domar, & Benson, 1990). Kirby (1994) compared the effects of an experimental cognitive-behavioral coping skills training program with a nonspecific treatment (reading) or a waiting-list treatment in women experiencing severe PMS. The training program reduced the negative effects of premenstrual symptoms by 60%, and these effects were maintained over time. In two studies, Van Zak (1994) demonstrated the effectiveness of biofeedback, cognitive control, and relaxation for PMS symptom relief.

Support Groups

Support groups have been described as helpful in relieving PMS severity (Robertson, 1991; Taylor & Bledsoe, 1985); however, most women find the peer support helpful only after initiation of treatment (Taylor, 1988; Taylor & Bledsoe, 1985). The use of support groups has been described as a mode of intervention for people with chronic conditions such as AIDS, multiple sclerosis, and chemical dependencies, or survivors of stressful or traumatic events or disasters. However, these groups usually have been separate from medical treatments or professional therapies. Muhlenkamp and Sayles (1986) found that women who had access to social support had higher levels of self-esteem, which in turn increased the likelihood of a health-promoting lifestyle. In a few studies, self-help and clinical treatments for chronic disease management have been linked (Beck et al., 1997; Cole, O'Connor, & Bennett, 1979; Conte, Brandzel, & Whitehead, 1974).

Traditional Chinese Medicine

Both herbs and acupuncture are used separately or in combination to treat health conditions that result from disruptions in qi or chi, which is the body's vital energy. Studies by the National Institutes of Health have found acupuncture, the ancient Chinese art of needle placement, helpful in treating menstrual cramps, low back pain, joint pain, headaches, and severe PMS.

Herbal Therapies, Dietary Supplements, and Other Treatments for PMS

Vitex

In the first placebo-controlled tirial to demonstrate the herb's effectiveness in treating PMS, women taking 20 mg of Vitex (agnus castus, chaste tree berry, monks pepper) reported a 52% overall reduction in PMS symptoms compared with 24% for those taking placebo (Berger, Schaffner, Schrader, Meier, & Brattstrom, 2000). Side effects have been rare, with 5% of women experiencing mild symptoms such as acne, skin rash, and bleeding between periods. None of these was responsible for women dropping out of the study. Other clinical trials have shown that chaste tree berry extract keeps the overproduction of progesterone from occurring and effectively reduces breast pain associated with menses (Schellenberg, 2001). Chaste tree berry extracts are best not used in conjunction with birth control pills or other hormone therapies without professional guidance from a health care provider. They should also not be used during pregnancy because they can stimulate premature lactation (Taylor et al., 2006).

Evening Primrose Oil

Several investigators have reported on the potential use of evening primrose oil, including studies of its beneficial use for PMS (American Botanical Council, 2003). However, two clinical trials failed to demonstrate beneficial effects, perhaps due to small sample size. Budeiri and colleagues (1996) found evening primrose oil supplements

EXHIBIT 20.3 SYMPTOM MANAGEMENT PROGRAM FOR PREMENSTRUAL SYNDROME THERAPY

Elements of Effective Symptom Management

Self-monitoring: Self-awareness of symptom severity and symptom patterns is the first step to treatment. Methods for symptom self-monitoring has been described previously.

- For some women, self-monitoring alone may be enough to assist them to make the necessary therapeutic changes.
- Monitoring stress in relationships and work and the individual's reaction to stressors is as important as symptom self-monitoring.

Personal choice: Symptom management includes the use of multiple nonpharmacologic treatments that will involve time and energy on the part of the woman experiencing premenstrual syndrome (PMS). Previous studies indicate that women want to be in control of their treatment by choosing two or more types of nonpharmacologic therapy. Allowing choice among treatments provides the woman with control over treatments that may be time-consuming.

- An individualized treatment plan should be established initially and updated regularly until PMS severity is reduced and stabilized.
- The treatment plan provides a treatment contract between the health care provider and the patient and should include evaluation criteria.

Self-modification: Clinical evidence suggests a relationship among dietary changes, vitamin supplementation, exercise, and relief from PMS. These approaches involve a modification of personal behaviors: dietary change, nutritional supplementation, physical activity and/or exercise.

1. Diet and nutritional therapy: Lack of certain vitamins, minerals, and nutrients has been found to be related to menstrual cycle hormones. Although there is little proof that dietary change alone reduces PMS severity, a healthy diet promotes general good health and minimizes other stressors and diseases. Furthermore, a typical American diet includes a great deal of simple sugars, processed foods, additives, salt, and stimulants, which further deplete the natural stores of vitamins and minerals. General recommendations include:
   a. Consuming a diet high in fruits, vegetables, and complex carbohydrates
   b. Maintaining a low-sodium diet in the premenstrual phase
   c. Reducing intake of all sugars including sucrose, fructose, glucose, honey, and brown sugar
   d. Avoiding alcohol completely or in the premenstruum
   e. Reducing caffeine intake, especially premenstrually
   f. Selecting snacks high in nutrients and low in sugars, salt, and fat
   g. Selecting whole foods (not refined or processed) such as whole-grain breads, brown rice, nuts, seeds
   h. Reducing fats by decreasing meat intake, using unsaturated fats such as cold pressed unhydrogenated vegetable oils, and using low-fat dairy products in moderation
   i. Drinking 1 to 2 quarts of water daily, along with fruit juices and herbal teas
   j. Eating small, frequent meals during the premenstruum (every 2 hours)
   k. Women experiencing severe perimenstrual negative affect (PNA) should reduce all forms of caffeine (chocolate, cola, black tea, coffee), especially during the premenstrual phase
      i. Avoid caffeine withdrawal symptoms by gradually reducing caffeine or by mixing decaffeinated coffee with caffeinated coffee.
      ii. Women experiencing depressive symptoms may find caffeine therapeutic and can tolerate moderate amounts of caffeine, which may improve their mood.
2. Sugar, candy, and chocolate can act in the same way as caffeine, exacerbating symptoms.
3. Nutritional supplements: Vitamins, minerals, amino acids, and PMS-formula supplements have been suggested as nutritional therapy for PMS. Vitamin B_6 and magnesium have been studied more thoroughly than other supplements.

a. Vitamin B_6 (pyridoxine): This vitamin is involved in converting the amino acid tryptophan to serotonin and DOPA to dopamine. Both dopamine and serotonin are related to mood and affect. Two double-blind studies of B_6 found opposite effects when compared with a placebo; however, one study used a 500-mg dose, and the other study used a 100-mg dose (Abraham & Hargrove, 1980; O'Brien, 1987). Some authors have recommended up to 800 mg of B_6, which can be considered a drug rather than a coenzyme. Unfortunately, B_6 is not a harmless placebo, but can cause irreversible nerve damage and sensory neuropathy at 500 mg daily dosage (Schaumberg, et al., 1983). For women who want to try using vitamin B_6, the following recommendations should be followed:
   i. Start with 100–200 mg per day, mid-cycle to menses.
   ii. Do not take more than 500 mg per day and take only cyclically.
   iii. Side effects of B_6 excess are numbness and tingling in the arms and legs, shooting pain, headaches, fatigue, dizziness, and weakness.
   iv. Take with a multiple vitamin or PMS-formula vitamin (see below).
b. Magnesium: Although the theory that women with PMS suffer from a magnesium deficiency has not been substantiated, increasing magnesium has been found to be helpful in reducing premenstrual constipation. Constipation will increase premenstrual pelvic pain and abdominal bloating.
   i. Food sources high in magnesium include whole grains, seeds, and vegetables.
   ii. Magnesium supplements can be taken at 100- to 250-mg doses during the premenstrual week along with increasing amounts of water.
c. Other vitamins: No other individual vitamin has been found to be effective in reducing PMS severity. Vitamin A, while having no effect on PMS, may be useful in acne treatment. Vitamin E (tocopherol) is present in evening primrose oil has had mixed results as an individual treatment for PMS.
d. Amino acids: Amino acids are precursors to brain neurotransmitters like dopamine and serotonin; therefore, amino acid supplements have been suggested to decrease perimenstrual negative affect and depression. Tryptophan, an amino acid precursor to serotonin, has received the most attention. Dosages as high as 8 to 10 g have been studied with mixed results, however most recently irreversible blood dyscrasias have been associated with tryptophan use (Jones, 1987).
   i. Increasing foods high in tryptophan is the recommended method for attempting to increase tryptophan (turkey, complex carbohydrates, low-fat dairy products).
   ii. Increasing these foods is most appropriate for PNA symptom severity because they have a mild tranquilizing effect.
e. Multivitamin and mineral supplements, PMS formulas: A variety of PMS supplements are on the market. Some contain extremely high levels of vitamins or require a woman to take 10 to 15 pills daily to reach the recommended level. However, many women find it easier to take a vitamin and mineral supplement that contains B_6, magnesium, and a combination multivitamin. A few cautionary recommendations can help women choose an appropriate supplement:
   i. Choose a PMS supplement that contains no more than 200 mg to 300 mg of B_6 in four to six pills per day.
   ii. Avoid supplements that have excessive amounts of fat-soluble vitamins (vitamin A, E).
   iii. Take PMS-formula vitamins for half of the month, switching to a regular multivitamin for the remainder of the month.
4. Exercise: Research on exercise and the neuroendocrine system suggests that biopsychosocial benefits of a regular exercise program may directly alleviate some of the symptoms of PMS, as well as indirectly mediate symptoms through healthy coping behavior. Most studies have investigated aerobic exercise as a treatment for PMS (Canty, 1984; Prior et al., 1987), and one study indicated a lowered incidence of PMS among women who ran 1 to 1.5 miles per day (Jones, 1987).
a. Aerobic exercise: While daily exercise is good for all-around health, increasing activity levels 1 to 2 weeks premenstrually is helpful for women experiencing PNA because moving muscles prompts the brain to produce endogenous opiates.
   i. Assessing current forms of aerobic exercise and pleasurable forms of physical activity are critical to success of this symptom management strategy.
   ii. Set realistic goals, both short- and long-term goals.
   iii. Plan for warm-up or cool-down periods (one or both depending on the type of exercise).

(*continued*)

EXHIBIT 20.3 SYMPTOM MANAGEMENT PROGRAM FOR PREMENSTRUAL SYNDROME THERAPY (*CONTINUED*)

  iv. Plan for types of aerobic exercise such as walking, walk-jog, jogging, swimming, bicycling, rope-skipping.
   v. Recommend three to five 20-minute sessions per week.
  vi. Plan time of day, specific place to exercise, and keep exercise log initially.
  b. Exercise modification and nonaerobic exercise: Many women find it difficult to continue aerobic exercise during the premenstruum due to breast tenderness, abdominal bloating, or cyclic headaches. One of the easiest and most effective modifications is yoga, a series of gentle poses that involves stretching, breathing, and visualization.
   i. Videotapes and classes are often available in the community to help women learn yoga.
   ii. Specific yoga poses, such as the sponge, the bow, and the plow are particularly helpful for PNA symptoms as well as the physical symptoms accompanying menstruation.
   iii. Yoga or stretching exercises can also be incorporated into an aerobic exercise plan.

Self-Regulation: Although little is known about stress management and PMS, extensive evidence exists on the effects of stress reduction strategies and psychophysiologic response. Therapeutic effects of cognitive and behavioral stress reduction activities have been demonstrated for headaches, sexual problems, neurodermatitis, hypertension, cardiac disease, depression, anxiety, cancer, and Raynaud's disease (Hamberger & Lohr, 1984). A clinical trial of the use of relaxation for treatment of PMS found a 58% reduction in PNA after a 3 month use of daily relaxation (Goodale, Domar, & Benson, 1990). Both cognitive and behavioral stress reduction strategies have been found to be important for self-regulation in women (Taylor, 1988; Taylor, 1994).

1. Behavioral strategies for stress reduction
   a. Assess specific areas of stress for each individual.
   b. Counter-conditioning to avoid physiologic arousal
      i. Progressive relaxation using tension-relaxation
      ii. Progressive relaxation without use of tension
   c. Combine nonaerobic exercise with counter-conditioning exercise.
   d. Instructions for these exercises can be found in Pender (1987) and Scandrett-Hibden and Vecker (1992).
2. Cognitive strategies for stress reduction: Many women have difficulty relaxing using behavioral stress reduction strategies because of cognitive tension. Women will describe their mind racing or feeling as if they can't stop certain thoughts. To take advantage of the physiologic effects of the behavioral stress reduction strategies, these women will need instruction on cognitive stress reduction.
   a. Identify negative thought patterns and critical self-assessments.
   b. Introduce thought-stopping exercises.
   c. Change critical or negative self-images by introducing positive images.
   d. Enhance self-esteem as a method of cognitive stress reduction.
   e. Identify real versus ideal body image and performance.
      i. Identify positive self-image.
      ii. Visualize high and low self-esteem.
   f. Thought-stopping exercises for down-comparisons and perfectionist thinking.
   g. Prioritizing and goal-setting for change.

Environmental modification: Stress is complex and usually includes external as well as personal aspects. Focusing only on the woman may emphasize her role as a "victim" or as "sick." A combination of personal and environmental change is usually necessary to reduce the effects of stress.

1. Physical or structural environment: Women sometimes have difficulty saying no to requests or needs from their family, friends, and coworkers. Or they may not pay attention to stress-inducing situations. Recommendations for changing stress related to daily activities include:
   a. Minimize the frequency of stress-inducing situations.
   b. Stabilize daily routines.
   c. Assess responsibility for stress (self or others).
   d. Schedule change to minimize stress-inducing situations.
   e. Set specific goals for change.

EXHIBIT 20.3 SYMPTOM MANAGEMENT PROGRAM FOR PREMENSTRUAL SYNDROME THERAPY (*CONTINUED*)

2. Social and relationship environment: Relationships with family members, intimates, or coworkers have been identified as major sources of stress for most women. This area of stress reduction includes enhancement of personal and social competency.

   a. Assess relationships.
   b. Identify areas of stress in particular relationships.
   c. Identify standards for certain relationships (marital, intimate, friendships).
   d. Assess relationship patterns and choices.
   e. Assess communication patterns.
   f. Assess verbal and nonverbal expressions of feeling.
   g. Assess stress in particular feeling expressions.
   h. Identify strategies for healthy expression of feeling.
   i. Practice assertive behaviors.
   j. Balance work, family, and love, and identify areas of importance in these areas.
   k. Demonstrate time-management strategies, and prioritize time in each area.
   l. Modify social, relationship, and work environments.
      i. Identify areas of personal control in work and social situations.
      ii. Prioritize change strategies and set goals.

Peer support and professional guidance: Previous studies of women with severe PMS have found that peer support groups alone are not satisfactory for reducing PMS severity (Taylor, 1988, 1994). Women with a long duration of severe PMS report a lack of trust in other women with similar symptom severity. Professional guidance is necessary in the early phases of treatment. Furthermore, much of the symptom management education can be administered in a group format with individual follow-up. Once women have begun to individualize their symptom management regimen, they can continue in a peer support group to further individualize and reinforce treatment success. Specific components of professional guidance and peer support include:

1. Professional guidance: Before being able to access support from other women experiencing PMS, women need professional expertise and information combined with caring and facilitation of an individualized treatment program. Women seeking professional help have identified these factors.

   a. Education begins with the evaluation and self-monitoring process. By monitoring daily health and perimenstrual symptoms, women become aware of internal and external processes over the course of their menstrual cycle. For some women, treatment consists of only symptom management and self-monitoring. However, for most women, education in the form of verbal, written, or audiovisual information will follow the diagnosis.
   b. Providing women with written and verbal information about the specific diagnosis (PMS, premenstrual magnification) is the next step in the education process. Explain to the woman that this is followed by an individualized treatment plan and preliminary contract starting with the use of the symptom management strategies. Development of the treatment program will take two or more sessions, which can also be accomplished through a group format.
   c. Books and audiotapes can be important supplements to the education process. A good publication on PMS self-help is Bender (1989). Stress management audiotapes are helpful to some women.

2. Peer support: Once a woman has begun the treatment process and experiences symptom relief, then she is able to take advantage of help from other women suffering from PMS. Factors identified as important to peer support include mutual nurturance, emotional attachment, reassurance of self-worth, and practice at social integration and behavior change.

   a. Education in a group format is an efficient method for introducing the symptom management strategies. The self-modification strategies can be introduced at one session with each woman completing her own self-modification plan. Subsequent group sessions can add the self-regulation and environmental modification strategies with practice time. A final session can be used to develop an individualized treatment plan and personal contract.

Note. From "Taking Back the Month: A Personalized Solution to Managing PMS and Enhancing Your Health," by D. Taylor and S. Colino, 2002, New York: Taylor & Francis.

decrease premenstrual mood symptoms, breast pain, and fluid retention. Approximately 2% of those who take evening primrose oil may experience stomach discomfort, nausea, or headaches (Taylor et al., 2006).

SAM-e

S-adenosylmethionine, or SAM-e, is a molecule manufactured in the body from methionine, an amino acid, during metabolism and has been discovered to be related to metabolic disturbances in patients with psychiatric and neurologic disorders (Taylor et al., 2006). SAM-e has been shown to be safe and effective in treating depression and is comparable to tricyclic antidepressants (Bressa, 1994). In a clinical trial, no difference was found between 1600 mg of SAM-e and 400 mg of imipramine, except that SAM-e was more easily tolerated (Delle Chiaie, Pancheri, & Scapicchio, 2002).

SAM-e has been found to be helpful in reducing joint pain associated with osteoarthritis and has been used as an alternative for those who cannot tolerate the side effects from NSAIDs. Its reported side effects have been transient insomnia, nervousness, lack of appetite, constipation, headaches, heart palpitations, nausea, dry mouth, sweating, and dizziness. As well, SAM-e is expensive, requires storage at proper temperatures due to rapid degradation, and has no standardized dose.

Because SAM-e is converted into homocysteine in the body, it is not known whether rising levels of homocysteine secondary to SAM-e metabolism increases the risk of heart disease. Instructions for taking SAM-e include taking with a daily multivitamin and consuming a diet high in fruits and vegetables. These measures can lower the homocysteine levels that SAM-e elevates, because each has three of the B vitamins (folic acid [B_3], B_6, and B_{12}; Taylor et al., 2006).

Light Therapy

Several studies have found a link between PMS and seasonal affective disorder, a cyclical mood disorder characterized by recurrent episodes of major depression in the fall and winter with remission in the spring and summer (Portella, Haaga, & Rohan, 2006). Exposure to full-spectrum light, including ultraviolet light, in highly sensitive women has been found to decrease the moodiness and depressive symptoms of PMS (Lam et al., 1999; Parry, Rosenthal, Tamarkin, & Wehr, 1987). It is hypothesized that bright light corrects disturbances in the sleep-wake cycle linked with PMS or that light promotes the effects of the feel-good brain chemical serotonin (Taylor et al., 2006). Light therapy may be considered a viable option for women who experience depression all month during the fall and winter and experience increased severity of premenstrual mood symptoms during these seasons (Taylor et al., 2006).

Increased exposure to daylight, particularly morning light, may be beneficial (Brown & Robinson, 2002; Taylor & Colino, 2002).

A Research-Based Program for Symptom Management for PMS

Not all women require pharmacologic intervention for PMS. Indeed, only women with the most extreme manifestations are likely to require pharmacologic therapy. A biopsychosocial approach to PMS treatment can often result in a complete or marked reduction to bothersome perimenstrual symptoms. If pharmacologic treatment is necessary, a nonpharmacologic approach can be complementary and decrease the dose and duration of the pharmacologic therapy. Perimenstrual symptom management is one such biopsychosocial, nonpharmacologic approach to PMS therapy. The self-help strategies described here can be found in a science-based self-help book for women that includes step-by-step strategies for self-assessment and self-management of perimenstrual symptoms, PMS, and stress (Taylor & Colino, 2002). Exhibit 20.3 details a symptom management program for PMS therapy that includes self-monitoring, personal choice, self-modification elements, self-regulation, environmental modification, peer support, and professional guidance.

REFERENCES

Abraham, G. (1980). Premenstrual tension. *Current Problems in Obstetrics & Gynecology, 3*(12), 7–23.

Abraham, G., & Hargrove, J. (1980). Effect of vitamin B_6 on premenstrual symptomology in women with premenstrual tension syndrome: A double-blind crossover study. *Infertility, 3*, 155.

Aganoff, J., & Boyle, G. (1994). Aerobic exercise, mood states and menstrual cycle symptoms. *Journal of Psychosomatic Research, 38*, 183–192.

American Botanical Council. (2003). *The ABC guide to herbal medicines.* Austin, TX: Author.

American College of Obstetricians and Gynecologists. (2000). *ACOG Practice Bulletin (No. 15): Premenstrual syndrome.* Washington, DC: Author.

American Psychiatric Association. (1994). *Diagnostic and statistical manual of mental disorders.* Washington, DC: Author.

American Psychiatric Association. (2000). *Diagnostic and statistical manual of mental disorders* (4th ed., text revision). Washington, DC: Author.

Aslaksen, K., & Falk, V. (1991). Spironolactone in the treatment of premenstrual tension: A double-blind study of spironolactone versus bendroflumethiaxide and placebo. *Current Therapy Research, 49*, 120–130.

Association of Women's Health, Obstetrical and Neonatal Nurses. (2003). *Evidence-based clinical practice guideline: Nursing management for cyclic perimenstrual pain and discomfort.* Washington, DC: Author.

Backstrom, T., Sanders, G., Leask, R., Davidson, D., Warner, P., & Bancroft, J. (1983). Mood, sexuality, hormones, and the menstrual cycle: II. Hormone levels and their relationship to premenstrual syndrome. *Psychosomatic Medicine, 45*, 503–507.

Beck, A., Scott, J., Williams, P., Robertson, B., Jackson, D., Gade, G., et al. (1997). A randomized trial of group outpatient visits for chronically ill older HMO members: The cooperative health care clinic. *Journal of the American Geriatric Society, 45*, 543–549.

Bender, S. (1989). *PMS Positive Program.* New York: Perigee Trade.

Berger, C., & Presser, B. (1994). Alprazolam in the treatment of two subsamples of patients with late luteal phase dysphoric disorder: A double-blind, placebo-controlled crossover study. *Obstetrics & Gynecology, 84*(3), 379–385.

Berger, D., Schaffner, W., Schrader, E., Meier, B., & Brattstrom, A. (2000). Efficacy of Vitex agnus castus L. extract Ze 440 in patients with pre-menstrual syndrome (PMS). *Archives of Gynecology & Obstetrics, 264*(3), 150–153.

Bressa, G. (1994). S-adenosyl-l-methionine (SAMe) as antidepressant: Meta-analysis of clinical studies. *Acta Neurologica Scandinavica Supplement, 154*, 7–14.

Brown, C., Ling, F., Andersen, R., et al. (1994). Efficacy of depot leuprolide in premenstrual syndrome: Effect of symptom severity and type in a controlled trial. *Obstetrics & Gynecology, 84*(5), 779–786.

Brown, M., & Robinson, J. (2002). *When the body gets the blues.* New York: Rodale.

Budeiri, D., Li Wan Po, A., & Dornan, J. (1996). Is evening primrose oil of value in the treatment of premenstrual syndrome? *Controlled Clinical Trials, 17*(1), 60–68.

Canty, A. (1984). Can aerobic exercise relieve the symptoms of premenstrual syndrome? *Journal of Occupational Health, 54*, 410–411.

Casper, R., & Hearn, M. (1990). The effect of hysterectomy and bilateral oophorectomy in women with severe premenstrual syndrome. *American Journal of Obstetrics & Gynecology, 162*(1), 105–109.

Chan, W. (1983). Prostaglandins and nonsteroidal anti-inflammatory drugs in dysmenorrheal. *Annual Review of Pharmacology & Toxicology, 23*, 131–149.

Chan, W., & Dawood, M. (1980). Prostaglandin levels in menstrual fluid of nondysmenorrheic and of dysmenorrheic subjects with and without oral contraceptive or ibuprofen therapy. *Advances in Prostaglandin and Thromboxane Research, 8*, 1443–1447.

Chrisler, J. (1995). *Broadening our vision: Class and cultural issues in women's health.* Montreal, Canada: Society for Menstrual Cycle Research.

Cleckner-Smith, C., Doughty, A., & Grossman, J. (1998). Premenstrual symptoms: Prevalence and severity in an adolescent sample. *Journal of Adolescent Health, 22*, 403–408.

Cole, S., O'Conner, S., & Bennett, L. (1979). Self-help groups for clinic patients with chronic illness. *Primary Care, 6*, 325–339.

Collins Sharp, B., Taylor, D., Kelly-Thomas, K., Killeen, M., & Dawood, M. (2002). Cyclic premenstrual pain and discomfort: The scientific basis for practice. *Journal of Obstetric, Gynecological and Neonatal Nursing, 31*, 637–649.

Conte, A., Brandzel, M., & Whitehead, S. (1974). Group work with hypertensives. *American Journal of Nursing, 74*, 910–912.

Dawood, M. (1988). Nonsteroidal anti-inflammatory drugs and changing attitudes toward dysmenorrhea. *American Journal of Medicine, 84*(5A), 23–29.

Dawood, M. (1990). Dysmenorrhea. *Clinical Obstetrics & Gynecology, 75*, 168–178.

Dawood, M., & Ramos, J. (1990). Trancutaneous electrical nerve stimulation (TENS) for the treatment of primary dysmenorrheal: A randomized, crossover comparison with placebo TENS and ibuprofen. *Obstetrics & Gynecology, 75*, 656–660.

Delle Chiaie, R., Pancheri, P., & Scapicchio, P. (2002). Efficacy and tolerability of oral and intramuscular S-adenosyl-L-methionine 1,4-butanedisulfonate (SAMe) in the treatment of major depression: Comparison with imipramine in 2 multicenter studies. *American Journal of Clinical Nutrition, 76*(5), 1172S–1176S.

Dennerstein, L., Morse, C., Gotts, G., et al. (1986). Treatment of premenstrual syndrome: A double-blind trial of dydrogesterone. *Journal of Affective Disorders, 11*(3), 199–205.

Deuster, P., Adera, T., & South-Paul, J. (1999). Biological, social, and behavioral factors associated with premenstrual syndrome. *Archives of Family Medicine, 8*, 122–128.

Dhar, V., & Murphy, B. (1990). Double-blind randomized crossover trial of luteal phase estrogens (Premarin) in the premenstrual syndrome (PMS). *Psychoneuroendocrinology, 15*(5–6), 489–493.

Elsner, C., Buster, J., Schindlr, R., et al. (1980). Bromocriptine in the treatment of premenstrual tension syndrome. *Obstetrics & Gynecology, 56*(6), 723–726.

Endicott, J. (2001). The epidemiology of perimenstrual psychological symptoms. *Acta Psychiatrica Scandinavica, 104*, 110–116.

Eriksson, E., Hedberg, M., Andersch, B., et al. (1995). The serotonin reuptake inhibitor paroxetin is superior to the noradrenaline reuptake inhibitor maprotiline in the treatment of premenstrual syndrome. *Neuropsychopharmacology, 12*(2), 167–176.

Estivill, M. (1995). Therapeutic aspects of aerobic dance participation. *Health Care for Women International, 16*, 341–350.

Ewart, C., Taylor, C., Kraemer, H., & Agras, W. (1984). Reducing blood pressure reactivity during interpersonal conflict. *Behavior Therapy, 15*, 473–484.

Ford, O., Lethaby, A., Mol, B., & Roberts, H. (2007). Progesterone for premenstrual syndrome. *Cochrane Collaboration, 1.*

Freeman, E., Kroll, R., Rapkin, A., et al. (2001). Evaluation of a unique oral contraceptive in the treatment of premenstrual dysphoric disorder. *Journal of Women's Health and Gender-Based Medicine, 10*(6), 561–569.

Freeman, E., Rickels, K., Sondheimer, S., et al. (2004). Continuous or intermittent dosing with sertraline for patients with severe premenstrual syndrome or premenstrual dysphoric disorder. *American Journal of Psychiatry, 161*(2), 343–351.

Freeman, E., Rickels, K., Sondheimer, S., et al. (1995). A double-blind trial of oral progesterone, alprazolam, and placebo in treatment of severe premenstrual syndrome. *Journal of the American Medical Association, 274*(1), 51–57.

Freeman, E., Rickels, K., Sondheimer, S., et al. (1999). Differential response to antidepressants in women with premenstrual syndrome/premenstrual dysphoric disorder: A randomized controlled tiral. *Archive of General Psychiatry, 56*(10), 932–939.

Freeman, E., Rickels, K., Yonkers, K., et al. (2001). Venlafaxine in the treatment of premenstrual dysphoric disorder. *Obstetrics & Gynecology, 98*(5, Pt. 1), 737–744.

Freeman, E., Sondheimer, S., & Rickels, K. (1997). Gonadotropin-releasing hormone agonist in the treatment of premenstrual symptoms with and without ongoing dysphoria: A controlled study. *Psychopharmacology Bulletin, 33*(2), 303–309.

Futterman, L., Jones, J., Miccio-Fonseca, L., & Quigley, M. (1992). Severity of premenstrual symptoms in relation to medical/psychiatric problems and life experiences. *Perception and Motor Skills, 74*, 787–799.

Gehlert, S., & Hartlage, S. (1997). A design for studying the DSM-IV research criteria of premenstrual dysphoric disorder. *Journal of Psychosomatic Obstetrics Gynecology, 18,* 36–44.

Goodale, I., Domar, A., & Benson, H. (1990). Alleviation of premenstrual syndrome symptoms with the relaxation response. *Obstetrics & Gynecology, 75,* 649–655.

Graham, J., Harding, P., Wise, P., et al. (1978). Prolactin suppression in the treatment of premenstrual syndrome. *Medical Journal of Australia, 2*(Suppl. 3), 18–20.

Graham, C., & Sherwin, B. (1992). A prospective treatment study of premenstrual symptoms using a triphasic oral contraceptive. *Journal of Psychosomatic Research, 36*(3), 237–266.

Green, R., & Green, M. (1987). Relaxation increases salivary immunoglobin A1. *Psychological Reports, 61,* 623–629.

Halbreich, U. (1997). Menstrually related disorders—Towards interdisciplinary international diagnostic criteria. *Cephalgia, 17,* 1–4.

Halbreich, U. (1999). Premenstrual syndromes: Closing the 20th century chapters. *Current Opinions in Obstetrics and Gynecology, 9,* 147–153.

Halbreich, U. (2005). Algorithm for treatment of premenstrual syndromes (PMS): Experts' recommendations and limitations. *Gynecologic Endocrinology, 20*(1), 48–56.

Halbreich, U., Ben-David, M., Assael, M., et al. (1976). Serum-prolatic in women with premenstrual syndrome. *Lancet, II*(7987), 1095–1098.

Halbreich, U., Bergeron, R., Yonkers, K., et al. (2002). Efficacy of intermittent, luteal phase sertraline treatment of premenstrual dysphoric disorder. *Obstetrics & Gynecology, 100*(6), 1219–1229.

Halbreich, U., Endicott, J. & Lesser, J. (1985). The clinical diagnosis and classification of premenstral changes. *Canadian Journal of Psychiatry—Revue Canadienne de Psychiatrie, 30*(7), 489–497.

Halbreich, U., Endicott, J., Schacht, S., & Nee, J. (1982). The diversity of premenstrual changes as reflected in the premenstrual assessment form. *Acta Psychiatrica Scandinavica, 62,* 177–180.

Halbreich, U., O'Brien, S., Eriksson, E., Backstrom, T., Yonkers, K., & Freeman, E. (2006). Are there differential symptom profiles that improve in response to different pharmacological treatments of premenstrual syndrome/premenstrual dysphoric disorder? *CNS Drugs, 20*(7), 523–547.

Hamberger, K. & Lohr, J. (1984). *Stress and Stress Management: Research and Applications.* New York: Springer Publishing.

Hammarback, S., & Backstrom, T. (1988). *Acta Obstetrica et gynecologica Scandinavica, 67,* 159–166.

Harrison, M. (1985). *Self-help for premenstrual syndrome* (2nd ed.). New York: Random House.

Harrison, W., Endicott, J., & Nee, J. (1990). Treatment of premenstrual dysphoria with alprazolam: A controlled study. *Archives of General Psychiatry, 47*(3), 270–275.

Helms, J. (1987). Acupuncture for the management of primary dysmenorrhea. *Obstetrics & Gynecology, 69*(1), 51–56.

Jamieson, D., & Steege, J. (1996). The prevalence of dysmenorrhea, dyspareunia, pelvic pain, and irritable bowel syndrome in primary care practices. *Obstetrics & Gynecology, 87,* 55–58.

Janiger, O., Riffenburgh, M., & Kersh, M. (1972). A cross-cultural study of premenstrual symptoms. *Psychosomatics, 13,* 226–235.

Johnson, S. (2004). Premenstrual syndrome, premenstrual dysphoric disorder, and beyond: A clinical primer for practitioners. *Obstetrics & Gynecology, 104*(4), 845–859.

Johnson, S., McChesney, C., & Bean, J. (1988). Epidemiology of premenstrual symptoms in a nonclinical sample. Prevalence, natural history and help-seeking behavior. *Journal of Reproductive Medicine, 33,* 340–346.

Jones, J. (1987). Nutritional therapies for PMS. In *The Melpomene Report* (pp. 10–14).

Kaleli, S., Aydin, Y., Erel, C., et al. (2001). Symptomatic treatment of premenstrual mastalgia in premenopausal women with lisuride maleate: A double-blind placebo-controlled randomized study. *Fertility and Sterility, 75*(4), 718–723.

Keye, W. (1988). Premenstrual syndrome: Seven steps in management. *Postgraduate Medicine, 83*(3), 167–173.

Keye, W. Jr. (1989). The biomedical model of premenstrual syndrome: Past, present and future. In A. Voda & R. Conover (Eds.), *Proceedings of the 8th Conference of the Society for Menstrual Cycle Research* (pp. 589–600). Salt Lake City, UT: Society for Menstrual Cycle Research.

Kinch, R., & Robinson, G. (1985). Premenstrual syndrome—Current knowledge and new directions. *Canadian Journal of Psychiatry, 30*(7), 467–468.

Kirby, R. (1994). Changes in premenstrual symptoms and irrational thinking following cognitive-behavioral coping skills training. *Journal of Consulting and Clinical Psychology, 62,* 1026–1032.

Kleijnen, J., Ter-Riet, G., & Knipschild, P. (1990). Vitamin B_6 in the treatment of the premenstrual syndrome—A review. *British Journal of Obstetrics and Gynaecology, 97,* 847–852.

Lam, R., Carter, D., Misri, S., Kuan, A., Yatham, L., & Zis, A. (1999). A controlled study of light therapy in women with late luteal phase dysphoric disorder. *Psychiatric Research, 86,* 185–192.

LaPerriere, A., Antoni, M., Schneiderman, N., Ironson, G., Klimas, N., Caralis, P., et al. (1990). Exercise intervention attenuates emotional distress and natural killer cell decrements following notification of positive serologic status for HIV-1. *Biofeedback and Self-Regulation, 15,* 125–131.

Leather, A., Studd, J., Watson, N., et al. (1999). The treatment of severe premenstrual syndrome with gosrelin with and without "add-back" estrogen therapy: A placebo-controlled study. *Gynecologic Endocrinology, 13*(1), 48–55.

Logue, C., & Moos, R. (1986). Perimenstrual symptoms: Prevalence and risk factors. *Psychosomatic Medicine, 48,* 388–414.

Magos, A., Brincat, M., & Studd, J. (1986). Treatment of the premenstrual syndrome by subcutaneous estradiol implants and cyclical oral norethisterone: Placebo controlled study. *British Medical Journal, 292,* 1629–1633.

Mechanic, D. (1995). Sociological dimensions of illness behavior. *Social Science & Medicine, 41*(9), 1207–1216.

Meden-Vrtovec, H., & Vujic, D. (1992). Bromocriptine (Bromergon, LEK) in the management of premenstrual syndrome. *Clinical Experience in Obstetrics & Gynecology, 19*(4), 242–248.

Menke, E. (1983). Menstrual beliefs and experiences of mother-daughter dyads. In S. Golub (Ed.), *Menarche* (pp. 133–137). New York: Lexington.

Messinis, I., & Lolis, D. (1988). Treatment of premenstrual mastalgia with tamoxifen. *Acta Obstetrica et Gynecologica Scandinavica, 67*(4), 307–309.

Miner, C., Brown, E., McCray, S., et al. (2002). Weekly luteal-phase dosing with enteric-coated fluoxetine 90 mg in premenstrual dysphoric disorder: A randomized, double-blind, placebo-controlled clinical trial. *Clinical Therapeutics, 24*(3), 417–433.

Mitchell, E. (1991). Identification of recurrent symptom severity patterns across multiple menstrual cycles. *Proceedings of the 9th Conference of the Society for Menstrual Cycle Research* (pp. 73–82). Seattle, WA: Society for Menstrual Cycle Research.

Mitchell, E., Woods, N. F., & Lentz, M. (1994). Differentiation of women with three premenstrual symptom patterns. *Nursing Research, 43*(1), 25–30.

Mitchell, E., Woods, N. F., Lentz, M., & Taylor, D. (1991). Recognizing PMS when you see it: Criteria for PMS sample selection. In D. L. Taylor & N. F. Woods (Eds.), *Menstruation in Health and Illness* (pp. 89–102). New York: Hemisphere.

Moos, R. (1969). Typology of menstrual cycle symptoms. *American Journal of Obstetrics & Gynecology, 103,* 390–402.

Mortola, J., Girton, L., & Fischer, U. (1991). Successful treatment of severe premenstrual syndrome by combined use of gonadotropin-releasing hormone agonist and estrogen/progestin. *Journal of Clincial Endocrinology and Metabolism, 72*(2), 252A–252F.

Moynihan, R. (2004). Controversial disease dropped from Prozac product information. *British Medical Journal, 328,* 365.

Muhlenkamp, A., & Sayles, J. (1986). Self-esteem, social support, and positive health practices. *Nursing Research, 35,* 334–338.

O'Brien, P. (1987). Controversies in premenstrual syndrome: Etiology and treatment. In B. Ginsburg & B. Carter (Eds.), *Premenstrual syndrome: Ethical and legal implications in a biomedical perspective* (pp. 3177–3328). New York: Plenum.

O'Brien, P., Craven, D., Selby, C., et al. (1979). Treatment of premenstrual syndrome by spironolactone. *British Journal of Obstetrics & Gynaecology, 86*(2), 142–147.

Parry, B., Rosenthal, N., Tamarkin, L., & Wehr, T. (1987). Treatment of a patient with seasonal premenstrual syndrome. *American Journal of Psychiatry, 144,* 762–766.

Pearlstein, T., Bachmann, G., Zacor, H., et al. (2005). Treatment of premenstrual dysphoric disorder with a new drospirenone-containing oral contraceptive formulation. *Contraception, 72*(60), 414–421.

Pender, N. (1987). *Health promotion in Nursing Practice. (2nd edition).* Norwalk, CT: Appleton & Lange.

Portella, A., Haaga, D., & Rohan, K. (2006). The association between seasonal and premenstrual symptoms is continuous and is not fully accounted for by depressive symptoms. *Journal of Nervous and Mental Disease, 194,* 833–837.

Prior, J., Vigna, Y., Sciarretta, D., Alojado, N., & Schulzer, M. (1987). Conditioning exercise decreases premenstrual symptoms: A prospective controlled 6-month trial. *Fertility and Sterility, 47,* 402–408.

Prior, J. (1997/1998). Perimenopause: The ovary's frustrating grand finale. *A friend indeed: For women in the prime of life, 14*(7), 1–4.

Rapkin, A. (2003). A review of treatment of premenstrual syndrome and premenstrual dysphoric disorder. *Psychoneuroendocrinology, 28*(Suppl. 3), 39–53.

Raskin, M., Johnson, G., & Rondestvedt, J. (1973). Chronic anxiety treated by feedback-induced muscle relaxation. *Archives of General Psychiatry, 28,* 263–267.

Reid, R., & Yen, S. (1981). Premenstrual syndrome. *American Journal of Obstetrics & Gynecology, 139,* 85.

Richards, M., Rubinow, D., Daly, R., & Schmidt, P. (2006). Premenstrual symptoms and perimenopausal depression. *American Journal of Psychiatry, 163*(1), 133–137.

Robertson, M. (1991). A survey of multidisciplinary and interdisciplinary approaches to premenstrual syndrome. In D. L. Taylor & N. F. Woods (Eds.), *Menstruation, health and illness* (pp. 129–142). Washington, DC: Hemisphere.

Rosignol, A., & Bonnlander, H. (1990). Caffeine-containing beverages, total fluid consumption, and premenstrual syndrome. *American Journal of Public Health, 80,* 1106–1110.

Sanders, S., Graham, C., Bass, J., et al. (2001). A prospective study of the effects of oral contraceptives on sexuality and well-being and their relationship to discontinuation. *Contraception, 64*(1), 51–58.

Sayegh, R., Schiff, I., Wurtman, J., Spiers, P., McDermott, J., & Wurtman, R. (1995). The effect of a carbohydrate-rich beverage on mood, appetite, and cognitive function in women with premenstrual syndrome. *Obstetrics & Gynecology, 86,* 520–528.

Scandrett-Hibdon, S. & Uecker, S. (1992). Rexation training and cognitive reappraisal. In Bulecheck, G. & McCloskey, J. (Eds.). *Nursing Interventions: Essential Nursing Treatments (2nd edition).* Philadelphia: Saunders.

Schaumberg, H., Kaplan, J., Windebank, A., Vick, N., Rasmus, S., Pleasure, D., et al. (1983). Sensory neuropathy from pyridoxine abuse: A new megavitamin syndrome. *New England Journal of Medicine, 309,* 445–447.

Schellenberg, R. (2001). Treatment for the premenstrual syndrome with agnus castus fruit extract: Prospective, randomized, placebo-controlled study. *British Medical Journal, 322*(7279), 134–137.

Schmidt, P., Grover, G., & Rubinow, D. (1993). Alprazolam in the treatment of premenstrual syndrome: A double-blind, placebo-controlled trial. *Archives of General Psychiatry, 50*(6), 467–473.

Schmidt, P., Nieman, L., Danaceau, M., et al. (1998). Differential behavioral effects of gonadal steroids in women with and in those without premenstrual syndrome. *New England Journal of Medicine, 338*(4), 209–216.

Severino, S., & Moline, M. (1995). *Premenstrual syndrome.* New York: Guilford.

Severy, L., Thapa, S., Askew, I., & Glor, J. (1993). Menstrual experiences and beliefs: A multicountry study of relationships with fertility and fertility regulating methods. *Women and Health, 20,* 1–20.

Sonstrom, R., & Morgan, W. (1989). Exercise and self-esteem: Rationale and model. *Medicine and Science in Sports and Exercise, 21,* 329–337.

Steege, J., & Blumenthal, J. (1993). The effects of aerobic exercise on premenstrual symptoms in middle-aged women: A preliminary study. *Journal of Psychosomatic Research, 37,* 127–133.

Steege, J., Stout, A., & Rupp, S. (1985). Relationships among premenstrual symptoms and menstrual cycle characteristics. *Obstetrics & Gynecology, 65,* 398–402.

Steiner, M., Hirschberg, A., Bergeron, R., et al. (2005). Luteal phase dosing with paroxetine controlled release (cR) in the treatment of premenstrual dysphoric disorder. *American Journal of Obstetrics & Gynecology, 193*(2), 352–360.

Steiner, M., Steinberg, S., Stewart, D., Carter, D., Berger, C., & Reid, R. (1995). Fluoxetine in the treatment of premenstrual dysphoria. *New England Journal of Medicine, 332,* 1529–1534.

Sternfeld, B., Swindle, R., Chawla, A., Long, S., & Kennedy, S. (2002). Severity of premenstrual symptoms in a health maintenance organization population. *Obstetrics and Gynecology, 99*(6), 1014–1024.

Sundbland, C., Hedberg, M., & Eriksson, E. (1993). Clomipramine administered during the luteal phase reduces the symptoms of premenstrual syndrome: A placebo-controlled trial. *Neuropsychopharmacology, 9*(2), 133–145.

Taghavi E., Menkes, D., Howard, R., et al. (1995). Premenstrual syndrome: A double-blind controlled tiral of desipramine and methylscopolamine. *International Clinical Psychopharmacology, 10*(2), 119–122.

Taylor, C., Farquhar, J., Nelson, E., & Agras, W. (1977). Relaxation therapy and high blood pressure. *Archives of General Psychiatry, 34,* 339–342.

Taylor, D. (1986). Development of premenstrual symptom typologies. *Communicating Nursing Research, 19,* 168.

Taylor, D. (1988). *Nursing interventions for premenstrual syndrome: A longitudinal therapeutic trial.* PhD dissertation, Seattle, University of Washington.

Taylor, D. (1994). Evaluating therapeutic change in symptom severity at the level of the individual woman experiencing severe PMS. *Image: Journal of Nursing Scholarship, 26,* 27-35.

Taylor, D. (1999). Effectiveness of professional-peer group treatment: Symptom management for women with PMS. *Research in Nursing & Health, 22*(6), 496-511.

Taylor, D., & Bledsoe, L. (1985). PMS, stress and social support: A pilot study and therapeutic hypotheses. In V. Oleson & N. Woods (Eds.), *Culture, society, and menstruation.* Washington, DC: Hemisphere.

Taylor, D., & Colino, S. (2002). *Taking back the month: A personalized solution to managing PMS and enhancing your health.* New York: Taylor & Francis.

Taylor, D., & Woods, N. (Eds.). (1991). *Menstruation, health & illness.* New York: Taylor & Francis.

Taylor, D., Schuiling, K., & Sharp, B. (2006). Menstrual cycle pain and discomforts. In K. Schuiling & F. Likis (Eds.), *Women's gynecologic health* (pp. 469-505). Boston: Jones & Bartlett.

Taylor, D., Woods, N., Lentz, M., Mitchell, E., & Lee, K. (1991). Premenstrual negative affect: Development and testing of an explanatory model. In D. Taylor & N. Woods (Eds.), *Menstruation, health and illness.* New York: Hemisphere.

Thys-Jacobs, S. (2000). Micronutrients and the premenstrual syndrome: The case for calcium. *Journal of the American College of Nutrition, 19,* 220-227.

Thys-Jacobs, S., Ceccarelli, S., Bierman, A., Weisman, H., Cohen, M., & Alvir, J. (1989). Calcium supplementation in premenstrual syndrome: A randomized crossover trial. *Journal of General Internal Medicine, 4,* 183-189.

Titlebaum, H. (1998). Relaxation. *Alternative Health Practitioner, 4,* 123-146.

Tolman, E., McGuire, J., & Rosenthale, M. (1985). Pharmacology of nonsteroidal anti-inflammatory drugs and their use in dysmenorrheal. In M. Y. Dawood, J. L. McGuire, & L. M. Demers (Eds.), *Premenstrual syndrome and dysmenorrhea* (pp. 159-176). Baltimore and Munich: Urban & Schwarzenberg.

University of California San Francisco, School of Nursing Symptom Management Center Group. (1994). A model for symptom management. *Image: Journal of Nursing Scholarship, 26,* 172-176.

Van Zak, D. (1994). Biofeedback treatments for premenstrual and premenstrual affective syndromes. *International Journal of Psychosomatics, 41,* 53-60.

Vellacott, I., Shroff, N., Pearce, M., et al. (1987). A double-blind, placebo-controlled evaluation of spironolactone in the premenstrual syndrome. *Current Medical Research Opinion, 10*(7), 450-456.

Walker, A., & Bancroft, J. (1990). Relationship between premenstrual symptoms and oral contraceptive use: A controlled study. *Psychosomatic Medicine, 52*(1), 86-96.

Wang, M., Hammarback, S., Lindhe, B., et al. (1995). Treatment of premenstrual syndrome by spironolactone: A double-blind, placebo-controlled study. *Acta Obstetrica et Gynecologica Scandanavica, 74*(10), 803-808.

West, C., & Hillier, H. (1994). Ovarian suppression with the gonadotropin-releasing hormone agonist goserelin (Zoladex) in management of the premenstrual tension syndrome. *Human Reproduction, 9*(6), 1058-1063.

Widholm, O., & Kantero, R. (1971). A statistical analysis of the menstrual patterns of 8,000 Finnish girls and their mothers. *Acta Obstetricia et Gynecologica Scandinavica,* Suppl. 14, 1-36.

Williams, E. (1983). Beliefs and attitudes of young girls regarding menstruation. In S. Golub (Ed.), *Menarche* (pp. 133-137). New York: Lexington.

Wilson, C., & Keye, W. (1989). A survey of adolescent dysmenorrhea and premenstrual symptom frequency. *Journal of Adolescent Health, 10,* 317-322.

Woods, N. (1985). Relationship of socialization and stress to perimenstrual symptoms, disability, and menstrual attitudes. *Nursing Research, 34,* 145-149.

Woods, N., Dery, G., & Most, A. (1982). Stressful life events and perimenstrual symptoms. *Journal of Human Stress, 8,* 23-31.

Woods, N. F., Laffrey, S., Duffy, M., Lentz, J., Mitchell, E., Taylor, D., & Cowan, K. (1988). Being healthy: Women's images. *Advances in Nursing Science, 11*(1), 36-46.

Woods, N. F., Lentz, M., Mitchell, E., Taylor, D., & Lee, K. (1992). Perimenstrual symptoms and the health-seeking process. In A. Dan & L. Lewis (Eds.), *Menstrual health in women's lives* (pp. 155-167). Urbana: University of Illinois Press.

Woods, N. F., Mitchell, E., & Lentz, M. (1999). Premenstrual symptoms: Delineating symptom clusters. *Journal of Women's Health and Gender-Based Medicine, 8,* 1053-1062.

Woods, N. F., Mitchell, E., & Taylor, D. (1999). From menarche to menopause: Contributions from nursing research and recommendations for practice. In I. Hinshaw, S. Feetham, & J. Shaver (Eds.), *Clinical Nursing Research: Vol. 1* (pp. 485-507). New York: Saunders.

Woods, N., Mitchell, E., Lentz, M., Taylor, D., & Lee, K. (1987). Premenstrual symptoms: Another look. *Public Health Reports,* July-August (Suppl.), 106-112.

Woods, N. F., Most, A., & Dery, G. (1982). Prevalence of perimenstrual symptoms. *American Journal of Public Health, 72,* 1257-1264.

World Health Organization. (1981). A cross-cultural study of menstruation: Implications for contraceptive development and use. *Studies in Family Planning, 12,* 3-16.

Yonkers, K., Brown, C., Pearlstein, T., et al. (2005). Efficacy of a new low-dose oral contraceptive with drospirenone in premenstrual dysphoric disorder. *Obstetrics & Gynecology, 106*(3), 492-501.

Reproductive Surgery

Deitra Leonard Lowdermilk

During their life times, many women will face a recommendation for gynecologic surgery. Prior to the 1970s, surgical procedures performed on women were often excessive and unnecessary, and alternatives were not always offered. Today, there is still concern that a number of surgical interventions, especially hysterectomies, are not necessary. Hysterectomy continues to be a common surgery with more than 600,000 procedures performed each year in the United States. In fact, it is second only to cesarean delivery in incidence (National Women's Health Information Center, 2006). This fact is concerning because technological advances have introduced new diagnostic and surgical procedures that provide alternatives to major surgery. More than half of all gynecologic surgery can now be performed as outpatient procedures in surgical centers and physician offices with little or no anesthesia necessary (National Women's Health Resource Center, 2005). Nurses need to be knowledgeable about the most current management for reproductive problems requiring surgical intervention as well as when medical or other alternatives may be applicable. In this way, nurses can help women be truly informed consumers as they make decisions about their care. This chapter focuses on the most common reproductive surgical procedures performed; alternative procedures are discussed where applicable. Conditions and problems that necessitate the decision to have surgery are discussed elsewhere in this text.

WOMEN AT RISK

The nurse must recognize women who are at risk for reproductive surgery and the factors that influence this at-risk state so as to inform clients of the potential risk and to counsel them about ways in which the health care system can meet their needs.

The most common signs and symptoms of reproductive problems that may require surgical intervention are vaginal bleeding, pelvic pain, and pelvic or abdominal masses. The significance of these symptoms varies with the woman's age and race (Stenchever, Droegemueller, Herbst, & Mishell, 2001). During the adolescent years (age at onset of menses to age 19), bleeding problems related to menstruation can lead to diagnostic surgery such as dilation and curettage (D&C). The reproductive years (ages 20 to 44) may involve a number of surgical procedures in addition to operative procedures associated with pregnancy (e.g., cesarean birth, ectopic pregnancy). Many sterilizations are performed on women 25 to 35 years of age; surgery for infertility problems is also prevalent in this age group. Furthermore, women in their childbearing years are at risk not only for problems related to menstruation but also for benign tumors and cervical cancer. These latter conditions might lead to hysterectomy. During the perimenopausal and postmenopausal years, women are at risk for uterine fibroids, dysfunctional bleeding related to changing ovarian function, and malignancies, especially endometrial cancer (American Cancer Society, 2006; Stenchever et al., 2001). Finally, there is a high incidence of pelvic surgery in older women (60 to 69 years of age). This fact is correlated with the increased longevity of women and the concomitant increased risk of gynecologic cancer and pelvic relaxation.

Regular health screening to identify health problems is an essential part of the care of women. A record of obstetric and gynecologic problems can facilitate data collection. (See chapter 9, "Well-Woman Assessment," for information regarding obtaining a gynecologic history.)

DIAGNOSIS

Prior to the 1980s, gynecologists relied on bimanual examination, exploratory laparotomy, or laparoscopy to obtain the information needed to make a diagnosis. Today, accurate assessment of pelvic problems can be made without the disadvantages of surgery through the use of diagnostic radiologic procedures. These procedures include intravenous pyelograms, barium studies, ultrasonography, colposcopy, hysteroscopy, computer tomography, magnetic resonance imaging, laboratory tests (e.g., Pap test, pregnancy tests, complete blood count), and X rays. These and other diagnostic procedures that may be used prior to surgery need to be explained to the client to facilitate her decision making and to encourage her to be an active participant in treatment. For all diagnostic procedures, the woman needs to be informed about what to expect during the procedure, why it is being done, what preparations she can expect (i.e., dietary restrictions, enemas), where the procedure will be performed (clinic, physician's office, or hospital), the cost, and whether third-party payers will pay for the procedure (National Women's Health Information Center, 2005).

CONSULTATIONS AND INFORMED DECISION MAKING

Once a diagnosis has been made, it is important that the health care team thoroughly inform the woman about the disease or condition requiring surgery. This dialogue should include family members if possible and should be explained at the woman's level of understanding.

The health care provider should discuss the indications for surgery, the potential risks involved, advantages and disadvantages, and any available alternatives to the surgery. The reasons why the particular treatment has been chosen, the predicted outcome of the surgery, and possible complications must also be discussed during the consultation (National Women's Health Information Center, 2005). Time should also be set aside for the woman to ask any questions she has concerning the surgery. The nurse practitioner can complement the physician's explanations to make sure the woman understands what has been said by reemphasizing important points and making further explanations when necessary. The nurse emphasizes the woman's right to control her body and her right to make informed decisions.

Some women have general concerns about surgical procedures that may influence their decision to have surgery. These include fear of death or disability, fear of postoperative pain, and concerns about anesthesia—loss of control with general anesthesia or feeling pain if awake under regional anesthesia; length of hospitalization and the recovery period; welfare of the family during hospitalization; and financial concerns (especially if surgery means loss of income or paying for surgical costs not covered by third-party payers). The nurse listens to the concerns, answers questions, and refers the client to other resources when necessary to address unanswered concerns (Lindberg & Nolan, 2001).

Women also may have specific concerns about gynecologic surgery that may need to be discussed. Reproductive surgery can affect a woman's self-concept and may be seen as a threat to her femininity, particularly if a woman's self-esteem is related to her ability to bear children (Wade, Pletsch, Morgan, & Menting, 2000). The woman should be informed about whether the surgery will affect her childbearing ability or alter her sexual performance. Often clients have misconceptions about these topics that can be cleared up prior to sur-

---

EXHIBIT 21.1   QUESTIONS TO ASK TO ASSURE INFORMED CONSENT

Why is this procedure proposed for my condition/problem?
What are the risks and benefits of the proposed surgery?
Are there alternatives to this surgery? If so, what are the risks and benefits of these alternatives?
How many times have you performed this surgery?
How long will I be hospitalized? (or Can the procedure be done in an outpatient setting?)
How long will it take to recover?
What types of anesthesia can be used?
How will the surgery affect me—for example, any physical changes, sexual function, childbearing ability?

Sources: Lindberg, C., & Nolan, L. (2001). Women's decision-making regarding hysterectomy. *Journal of Obstetric, Gynecologic and Neonatal Nursing,* 30(6), 607–616; National Women's Health Resource Center. (2005). *Hysterectomy: Questions to ask.* Retrieved January 13, 2007, from http://www.healthywomen.org/healthtopics/questionstoask; Wade, J., Pletsch, P., Morgan, S., & Menting, S. (2000). Hysterectomy: What do women need and want to know? *Journal of Obstetric, Gynecologic and Neonatal Nursing, 29*(1), 33–42.

gery. Health care providers should inform the woman of her right to consult other health care providers prior to consenting to surgery. Many third-party plans require second opinions for major gynecologic surgery or costs may not be covered. Referral to another physician for a second opinion can be requested from the woman's physician, from the health insurer, from family or friends who have had success with a physician, or from a local or national medical registry of specialists (National Women's Health Information Center, 2006).

Prior to surgery, a woman is asked by the physician to sign a written consent that legally authorizes the surgery and acknowledges the information explained to her. Exhibit 21.1 lists questions that the woman can ask during this session.

MANAGEMENT STRATEGIES

After the decision for surgery has been made, the nurse must plan the woman's pre- and postoperative care on the basis of identified needs. In the following discussion of surgical procedures, attention is given not only to the usual techniques but to alternative procedures as well. The goals of nursing care are to meet the physiological and emotional needs of women undergoing the procedures.

DIAGNOSTIC AND THERAPEUTIC PROCEDURES

Several procedures have both diagnostic and therapeutic uses for reproductive problems. Indications, complications, technique descriptions, and nursing care are described in the following section for dilation and curettage, biopsy, cryosurgery, electrocautery, laparoscopy, and hysteroscopy.

Dilation and Curettage

Indications

Dilation of the cervix and curettage (D&C) of the endometrium is one of the most frequently performed uterine operative procedures. Indications for this procedure include diagnosis of uterine malignancy, evaluation and control of dysfunctional uterine bleeding, incomplete abortion, therapeutic abortion, evaluation of causes of infertility, and relief of dysmenorrhea. The diagnostic purpose of endometrial curettage is to differentiate abnormal bleeding related to hormonal function from bleeding related to malignancy. The therapeutic value of curettage is to control abnormal bleeding by removing the endometrium (Stenchever et al., 2001).

Technique

D&C is often done as an outpatient procedure, but it is commonly performed as a day surgery in a hospital or ambulatory surgery center. Preoperatively, the woman may be given nonsteroidal anti-inflammatory agents such as ibuprofen or a local anesthetic; however, brief general anesthesia or regional anesthesia is generally used if a thorough internal examination is needed (Nichols & Clark-Pearson, 2000). For the D&C, the woman is placed in a lithotomy position. A bimanual examination is done to determine the position of the uterus. A speculum is inserted into the vagina to expose the cervix. A sound (elongated instrument) is introduced into the uterus to measure the uterine cavity, and the cervix is gradually dilated with metal dilators. A curette is then introduced into the uterine cavity, and the endometrium is scraped away. Suction curettage may be used instead of a curette. The specimen is sent to a pathology laboratory for analysis and confirmation of the preoperative diagnosis.

Complications

Secondary hemorrhage, lacerations of the cervix, perforation of the uterus, and infection are risks after a D&C (Nichols & Clark-Pearson, 2000).

Nursing Care

Usually, there is no preoperative preparation except that the client consumes nothing by mouth past midnight the day of the surgery if general anesthesia is planned. The woman should void before surgery.

Postoperatively, the nurse should check vital signs every 15 minutes until they are stable. The amount of vaginal bleeding and/or pad count should also be assessed. Mild analgesics may be given for pain, and diet is usually dictated by the client's wishes. Someone should be available to drive the woman home.

Prior to discharge, the nurse informs the woman about the following facts and procedures:

- Slight bleeding is normal. If bleeding is as heavy as your normal period or if bleeding lasts more than 2 weeks, call your health care provider.
- Abdominal cramping is not unusual during the first few days following discharge. For relief, you can take mild analgesics, such as acetaminophen (Tylenol), or nonsteroidal anti-inflammatory agent, such as ibuprofen (Motrin), or place a heating pad or hot water bottle on the abdomen.
- Temperature should be taken once a day for 2 days. If your temperature is more than 100° F (38° C), call your health care provider.
- Sexual intercourse, tub bathing, and the use of tampons should be avoided for 2 weeks to allow healing and to prevent infection (Novak, 2006).

Biopsy of the Cervix or Endometrium

Indications

A *cervical biopsy* is recommended whenever there is a need to investigate suspicious cervical tissue as seen with colposcopy to diagnose or rule out cervical cancer in its earliest stages. Conization is indicated if atypical squamous cells are found in cytology smears and colposcopy examinations. An *endometrial biopsy* is widely used to diagnose infertility problems, to evaluate abnormal bleeding, and to detect uterine malignancies (Lowdermilk, 2007b).

Techniques

Cervical tissues may be obtained by several methods. A *punch biopsy* is a technique in which a needle is inserted into tissue to remove a column of tissue when a lesion is clearly visible. This procedure is almost painless and is usually performed as an office procedure without anesthesia. If bleeding occurs after the biopsy, cauterization of the biopsy site with a silver nitrate stick will usually control bleeding. Cervical tissues can also be obtained by *conization*. This procedure can be performed under local, regional, or general anesthesia in office or hospital settings. A colposcopy is used to visualize the lesion for the procedure. The size of the cone of tissue to be removed by a scalpel is determined by the extent of the lesion.

Endometrial biopsy is usually performed in an office or clinic setting and may require anesthesia. The procedure is used to obtain a cytological specimen of endometrium with a curette or a suction device. If performed for infertility studies, the biopsy is scheduled for the last half of the menstrual cycle (Lowdermilk, 2007a). It is done in the immediate premenstrual phase to evaluate menstrual disturbances and at any time for postmenopausal evaluations (Lowdermilk, 2006).

Complications

Secondary hemorrhage, cervical stenosis, and cervical infection can occur after cervical and endometrial procedures. Uterine perforation is rare.

Nursing Care

Women should be informed about what to expect during the procedure and postoperatively. Women may be anxious before the procedure, especially if it is being done to evaluate a potential malignancy, and they may need time to express their feelings. During the procedure, use of relaxation and breathing techniques may relieve discomfort caused by uterine cramping.

Follow-up care instructions will vary with each procedure. After a conization, the woman may have profuse or prolonged menstrual periods for several cycles. Bleeding that is more than a normal period for the woman as well as signs of infection (fever, severe abdominal pain, foul-smelling vaginal discharge) should be reported. Douching, use of tampons, and sexual intercourse should be avoided until the biopsy site has healed (at least 1 week). After endometrial biopsy, the woman should report any signs of infection or excessive bleeding to the physician and avoid sexual intercourse until bleeding has stopped (Lowdermilk, 2006).

Cryosurgery

Indications

Cryosurgery is used in the treatment of chronic cervicitis, endocervicitis, erosions, and nabothian cysts. It is also used as a preventive measure to treat cervical dysplasia (cervical intraepithelial neoplasia) (Stenchever et al., 2001).

Technique

Treatment is usually performed in the clinic or physician's office and without anesthesia. A nonsteroidal anti-inflammatory agent (ibuprofen) may be given 1 hour before surgery to decrease the pain. During the procedure, a large speculum is inserted into the vagina. Nitrous oxide is circulated through a special cryoprobe that is placed on the area to be treated. Nitrous oxide causes local freezing, allowing necrosis of the affected or diseased tissues to occur. The tissues slough off and the remaining healthy tissue heals cleanly (Stenchever et al., 2001). Cryosurgery is best performed 1 week after the end of a menstrual period. Performing the surgery at this time avoids freezing a uterus with an early pregnancy and permits the most active phase of cervical regeneration to take place prior to the onset of the next menstrual period (Lowdermilk, 2007b).

Complications

Occasional spotting and cervical stenosis (hardening) with resultant infertility may occur. Injuries to normal tissue can occur if touched by the probe.

Nursing Care

The woman will need to know that she must remain in a lithotomy position until the tissues are frozen because movement can cause damage to normal tissues. After the treatment, the woman can expect to have a profuse watery vaginal discharge for 2 to 3 weeks. Perineal pads are usually necessary. The woman is advised to call her physician if she experiences excessive bleeding, purulent or foul-smelling vaginal discharge, a fever, or abdominal pain. Avoidance of sexual intercourse, douching, use of tampons, tub bathing, or swimming for up to 2 weeks also may be recommended to allow for healing. Follow-up visits may be necessary if the cryosurgery was performed for cervical intraepithelial neoplasia (Lowdermilk, 2007b).

Loop Electrosurgical Excision Procedure

Indications

Another treatment that has become standard for treating cevical dysplasia is the loop electrosurgical excision procedure (LEEP). LEEP is also used to remove small fibroids in the uterus (see later discussion of myomectomy).

Technique

The LEEP procedure uses a wire loop electrode to excise and cauterize cervical tissue with minimal tissue damage. It is usually performed under local anesthesia in an outpatient setting, although no anesthesia may be needed for cervical application.

Complications

Possible complications include bleeding heavier than a normal menstrual period, infection, cervical stenosis, infertility, and loss of cervical mucus (Stenchever et al., 2001).

Nursing Care

Preoperative care is similar to that for cryosurgery. Postoperatively, the woman is observed for a brief time before being discharged. Instructions for home care include to expect that cramping may be present; brownish vaginal discharge may be experienced for up to 2 weeks; bleeding may occur up to a week; douching, tampon use, and intercourse should be avoided for up to 4 weeks; and heavy lifting and strenuous exercise should be avoided until vaginal discharge has stopped (Lowdermilk, 2006).

Laparoscopy

Indications

Laparoscopy is a procedure by which the pelvic organs are visualized and examined by insertion of a laparoscope through the abdominal wall. Laparoscopy can be used instead of an exploratory laparotomy to diagnose endometriosis, malignancy, and ectopic pregnancy. It is invaluable for infertility evaluations in which tubal patency and ovulation need to be determined. This approach also can be used for surgery using mechanical, suction, laser, or electrocautery instruments.

Technique

Although laparoscopy can be performed as an inpatient procedure, it is most often performed as an outpatient procedure. Short-acting general anesthesia or local or regional anesthetic agents may be used. Usually, women can go home within 2 hours after surgery.

During the laparoscopic procedure, the woman is placed in a modified Trendelenburg position. A small (2- to 3-cm) incision is made in the skin of the lower rim of the umbilicus. A needle attached to an insufflation apparatus is inserted. Carbon dioxide or nitrous oxide is used to distend the abdomen and separate the organs; the endoscope is then inserted into the incision for visualization. Often, a second instrument is inserted into an incision made in the area above the symphysis pubis to allow the surgeon to visualize the whole pelvic cavity and to perform operative procedures such as removal of tubal adhesions and tubal ligation. After the surgery is completed, as much gas as possible is expelled from the peritoneal cavity. Clips or sutures are used to close the puncture sites.

Complications

Insufflation can cause pulmonary embolism or cardiac or respiratory problems. In addition, hemorrhage and infection are always risks. If electrocautery is used, burns to the abdominal and bowel tissue can occur, leading to necrosis and peritonitis (Stenchever et al., 2001).

Nursing Care

Preoperatively, the woman usually consumes nothing by mouth past midnight on the day of surgery. Postoperatively, her vital signs are usually taken frequently during the first hour or until they are stable. Prior to discharge, instructions should be given regarding convalescence. The woman may have a sore throat from intubation and discomfort at the incision site; mild analgesics may alleviate the pain. The greatest discomfort will likely be from transient shoulder pain caused by residual gas in the peritoneal cavity. This will usually disappear within 48 hours. The woman should observe the incision for signs of infection or bleeding, and the bandage over the incision should be changed as needed. If the woman is concerned about body image, she should be informed that the incision scar will barely be noticeable. Showers are recommended over tub baths until the incision has healed. No heavy lifting or strenuous exercise should be done for at least 1 week after the surgery (Lowdermilk, 2006). Sexual intercourse is usually not restricted.

Hysteroscopy

Indications

Hysteroscopy is a procedure that allows direct visualization of the endometrium using an endoscope and light source inserted vaginally. It can be used to diagnose causes of abnormal bleeding, infertility, endometriosis, recurrent pregnancy loss, and malignancy. Surgical uses include removal of intrauterine devices, small fibroids, and polyps and endometrial ablation (see later discussion) (Sutton, 2006).

Technique

Diagnostic hsyteroscopy is usually an office procedure performed under local anesthesia. Pretreatment with diazepam or nonsteroidal anti-inflammatory agents is common, especially for anxious clients. Surgical procedures are usually performed under local or general anesthesia in an ambulatory surgery unit or as a day surgical procedure in the hospital. Prior to the procedure, the uterus is expanded with a medium such as dextran, dextran and water, or carbon dioxide. Surgery can be performed with instruments similar to those described for laparoscopy; additionally, a form of LEEP can be performed for endometrial ablation (Stenchever et al., 2001).

Complications

Complications include uterine perforation, infection, bleeding, burns, and complications related to the media used to expand the uterus during the procedure (Bradley, 2002; Sutton, 2006).

Nursing Care

Preoperatively, the nurse can assist the woman to use relaxation techniques if the procedure is to be performed under local anesthesia. Postoperatively, the woman is observed for complications related to the medium used to expand the uterus (fluid overload, pulmonary embolism, anaphylactic shock) before being discharged home. Discharge instructions vary, depending on the procedure done. The woman can expect a small amount of vaginal bleeding, mild cramps, and possibly shoulder pain (if carbon dioxide was used). She should be told that her next menstrual period may be irregular. She should call her physician if she has heavy bleeding or signs of infection. She should avoid putting anything into her vagina for 2 weeks (Lowdermilk, 2006).

TUBAL SURGERY

Sterilization and infertility procedures are the primary reasons for tubal surgery, but surgery also may be performed for malignancy, infection, and tubal pregnancy.

Tubal Sterilization

Female sterilization is the most popular method of birth control for couples over the age of 35 in the United States and is reportedly the most widely used contraceptive method in the world (Pollack, Carignan, & Jacobstein, 2004). (See chapter 15, "Fertility Control," for additional information on this topic.)

Methods and Selection of Procedures

Several techniques for tubal sterilization have been developed to interrupt ovum transport through the uterine (fallopian) tube. The choice of technique depends on the woman's life situation and specific needs. For example, sterilization can be performed within 24 to 72 hours after a vaginal birth, at the time of a cesarean birth, after abortion, and as an interval procedure (e.g., 6 weeks after a birth, anytime between pregnancies, or anytime for women who have never been pregnant). More than 50% of all procedures are performed immediately after a pregnancy (Pollack et al., 2004).

Techniques

Sterilization can be performed abdominally or vaginally using traditional surgical techniques or endoscopic approaches (Nardin, Kulier, & Boulvain, 2003). The most popular abdominal approach in the United States is the laparoscopic approach using electrocauterization to seal the tube. Laparoscopic procedures are commonly performed as interval procedures and can be compared to vasectomy in terms of safety and efficacy (Pollack et al, 2004). The failure rates (pregnancy) are low (less than 1%, but, because of tissue destruction, potential for reversibility is also low (Pollack et al., 2004). Mechanical devices that obstruct the uterine tubes, such as plastic clips or rings, also can be used with laparoscopy. These devices have a higher potential for reversibility, and failure rates are reportedly only slightly higher (Pollack et al., 2004). The minilaparotomy (a subumbilical or suprapubic incision) is more commonly performed in the immediate postpartum period. Methods of tubal occlusion with this abdominal approach are ligation and/or removal of a segment of the uterine tubes (Stenchever et al., 2001).

Vaginal surgical approaches are seldom used. However hysteroscopic techniques can be used for sterilization. A hysteroscope is inserted vaginally through a dilated cervix into the uterus under local or regional anesthesia, and an occlusion technique such as electrocauterization is performed (Chapman & Magos, 2005). Nonsurgical methods of tubal sterilization via the hysteroscopic approach continue to be under investigation. These include chemical blocking agents that cause necrosis and fibrosis of the tubes and silicone plugs that block the tubes (Abbott, 2005; Pollack et al., 2004). In 2002, the U.S. Food and Drug Administration approved a device called Essure that can be used for interval sterilization. This soft metal device consisting of two concentric coils is placed in the proximal ends of the uterine tubes. It works by mechanical occlusion as well as stimulation of growth of fibrous tissue that occludes the tubes by 6 months in almost 100% of women who have these devices inserted (Abbott, 2005; Pollack et al., 2004). The device is inserted as an outpatient procedure under local anesthesia. Long-term efficacy and safety of the device are yet to be determined.

Complications

Complications vary depending on the method used. They include bleeding, infection, uterine perforation, bladder and intestinal injuries, and burns (Pollack et al, 2004).

Nursing Care

Recovery from sterilization procedures is usually fast. If local anesthesia is used and if the sterilization is performed in an outpatient setting, the woman usually can go home within 1 to 2 hours, although she should not drive herself home. Postpartum hospitalization usually is prolonged by only a day. Most women can resume normal activities within 24 to 48 hours after surgery. Women should be taught to monitor for signs of infection at the incision site and to report abnormal signs, such as vaginal or incisional bleeding or severe abdominal pain. Signs of ectopic pregnancy (abdominal pain or vaginal bleeding) should also be taught, because this can also be a late complication after tubal sterilization (Pollack et al., 2004). Mild analgesics are usually suggested to relieve postoperative pain.

Discharge instructions should include an explanation of the physical and emotional changes that may occur following sterilization. The woman should be informed that she will continue to menstruate and that the menstrual period may vary in length of cycle, duration of flow, or amount of flow. These changes will probably be mild, if present at all, and will seldom require treatment. Women continue to ovulate, and the ovum will be reabsorbed. There should be no physiological effect on hormones, weight, or sexual response (Lock, 2007). The woman will need to use a barrier method of contraception during sexual intercourse to be protected from sexually transmitted infections.

Women also should be assessed postoperatively for psychological responses. Studies of women's responses after sterilization report that most women have no regrets after surgery. Many report increased sexual satisfaction because they are no longer worried about getting pregnant. Women who are awake and aware during the procedure report a positive psychological response and attribute this feeling to being able to participate fully with the health care team and to being in control of themselves. Those who expressed regrets included women who had the procedure at a young age (younger than 30 years); those who felt pressured to have surgery; who did not feel fully informed, especially about irreversibility; who had just had a baby or an abortion rather than at a time unrelated to a pregnancy; and those whose marital status changed or whose partners reacted negatively to the sterilization (Mattinson & Mansour, 2006; Pollack et al., 2004).

Salpingectomy

Salpingectomy is the removal of one or both uterine tubes through laparoscopic or abdominal surgery. Reasons for this removal may include malignancy, pelvic inflammatory disease, and sepsis. Salpingectomy may be used as treatment for ruptured ectopic pregnancy, but salpingostomy (incision into the tube to remove its contents) is more likely to be performed because this will allow for the preservation of future fertility (Stenchever et al., 2001). Nursing care for clients having a salpingectomy is similar to care for those undergoing tubal sterilization.

Tuboplasty

There continue to be requests for tuboplasty or tubal reconstruction after sterilization. Most of these requests come from women who have been divorced and remarried and who desire to have a baby by their new spouse. Death of a child, a change in lifestyle, and a change in economic status that allows for a larger family are other factors that motivate requests for reversal of sterilization.

The clip and ring techniques have a greater potential for successful reversibility (up to 90%) because these methods cause less interference with tubal blood supply than cauterization or ligation (Pollack et al., 2004). Fibriectomy (removal of the end of the tube nearest the ovary) usually cannot be reversed. In general, the shorter the tube after reanastomosis, the smaller the chance of pregnancy. Reversal surgery may not be covered by insurance or federally funded medical care.

Another major reason for tuboplasty is for correction of infertility problems related to tubal occlusions. Microsurgery is a technique for both reversal of sterilization and tubal occlusions. During this procedure, the surgeon with special skills uses magnification and microsurgical techniques that allow exact alignment and approximation of the remaining portion of tubes to be reconstructed. Microsurgery appears to offer the best opportunity for restoring tubal patency (Gomel & McComb, 2006). Reformation of adhesions after surgery can interfere with the success of surgery; ectopic pregnancy after reversal of female sterilization may occur.

Nursing care after tuboplasty is similar to care after sterilization.

OVARIAN SURGERY

Oophorectomy

Oophorectomy is the removal of one or both ovaries through an abdominal incision. Reasons for surgery may include ectopic pregnancy, ovarian cysts, pelvic inflammatory disease, and malignancy. Although the ovaries may be removed electively when a menopausal woman has a hysterectomy, removal of the ovaries as a routine procedure should be questioned for women of any age. One reason often given for removal of ovaries in menopausal women is to prevent ovarian cancer, which affects about 1% of American women over the age of 50. Removal of ovaries in premenopausal women without hormone replacement can contribute to increased incidence of osteoporosis and coronary heart disease. Removal of healthy ovaries in premenopausal women usually is not recommended because hormone replacement therapy is inferior to natural hormone production (Stenchever et al., 2001).

Surgical menopause occurs when both ovaries are removed in premenopausal women. Symptoms of surgical menopause may include hot flashes, vaginal atrophy, decreased libido, and decreased vaginal lubrication. These symptoms are often treated with estrogen replacement therapy. (See chapter 6, "Mid-Life Women's Health," for discussion of hormonal replacement therapy.) Complications of oophorectomy include infection and hemorrhage. Women should be informed of the risks and benefits of this therapy, as well as available alternatives, so that they can make informed decisions about accepting therapy.

Nursing care for the woman having an oophorectomy is similar to care of the client having tubal sterilization.

UTERINE SURGERY

Myomectomy and hysterectomy are the most common surgical procedures performed on the uterus. Both can be performed using abdominal and vaginal approaches, through surgical incisions or laparoscopic or hysteroscopic techniques.

Myomectomy

Leiomyomas, or uterine fibroids, are the most common benign tumors of women. They are more common in nulliparas and in African American women. For women in their 40s and 50s, vaginal bleeding is usually the first sign of a fibroid. Symptoms vary with the size of the fibroid but usually include pain and discomfort, increased menstrual flow, or irregular bleeding. For women with small fibroids causing discomfort or infertility who want to maintain their childbearing potential, periodic evaluation of the fibroids, medical treatment that can reduce the size of fibroids and stop the bleeding, or myomectomy (removal of myomas with preservation of the uterus) may be the treatment of choice. Often, fibroids will decrease in size after menopause, and surgical treatment may not be necessary if they are asymptomatic and do not increase in size (Cook & Walker, 2004). If surgery is the best treatment option, and the uterine size is no larger than that at 12 to 14 weeks gestation, myomectomy may be recommended as an alternative to hysterectomy. However, early myomectomy may mean subsequent surgery, because there is a 4% to 51% risk of recurrence of fibroids (Banu & Manyonda, 2005; National Women's Health Resource Center, 2006). About 25% of all women having a myomectomy will subsequently have a hysterectomy (Stenchever et al., 2001).

Myomectomy, if performed via an abdominal surgical incision (laparotomy), is a major surgical procedure with all the risks of such surgery. Gonadotrophin-releasing hormone (GnRH) agonists (e.g., Lupron, Syneral, Zoladex) may be used prior to surgery to reduce the size of the myoma, especially if the woman is experiencing bleeding. The woman may experience hot flashes, vaginal dryness, and decreased libido during GnRH therapy, but these effects are reversed when the therapy is discontinued (National Women's Health Resource Center, 2006). If large myomas are reduced in size, myomectomy can be performed as a laparoscopic or hysteroscopic procedure (Falcone & Bedaiwy, 2002).

Preoperative preparations are similar to those of abdominal hysterectomy if the abdominal approach is used, or to vaginal hysterectomy if the vaginal approach is used (see later discussion). Surgery usually is performed in the proliferative phase (days 5 to 14) of the menstrual cycle to avoid the possibility of unsuspected pregnancy and to minimize blood loss. General, spinal, or epidural anesthesia may be used. The procedure includes a skin incision (if abdominal), an incision into the uterus where the fibroids are located, removal of all fibroids, and reconstruction of the uterus without injury to the uterine tubes and ovaries. Incision into the uterine cavity is avoided except if needed for removal of fibroids. If the uterine cavity is entered, cesarean delivery may be recommended in subsequent pregnancies to avoid the risk of uterine rupture.

The pregnancy rate after myomectomy is approximately 50% (Banu & Manyonda, 2005).

Postoperative nursing care after myomectomy is similar to care after hysterectomy (see later discussion). Postoperative recovery after an abdominal procedure takes up to 6 weeks and 2 weeks if laparoscopic surgery is done (National Women's Health Resource Center, 2006). Postoperative hemorrhage is a significant problem (more than hysterectomy) because the incised uterus can bleed into the peritoneal cavity. If a GnRH agonist is given preoperatively, blood loss will be less. The laser also can be used with surgery to improve hemostasis and decrease the occurrence of postoperative adhesions (Stenchever et al., 2001). Infection is also a possible complication.

Women need counseling regarding the risks and benefits of myomectomy. As previously discussed, it is not a procedure that will benefit all women with fibroids, but it may be an alternative for those who want to maintain their fertility or for other women who desire to preserve their uterus.

Alternative Myomectomy Procedures

Alternatives to laparotomy include laparoscopic and hysteroscopic myomectomy (National Women's Health Resource Center, 2006). Both can be performed under local or general anesthesia. *Laparoscopic myomectomy* usually involves three small abdominal incisions—one at the umbilicus and one in the left and one in the right lower quadrant of the abdomen—to accommodate the laparoscope and other instruments. The fibroids can be removed by electrocautery, other coagulation method, or laser vaporization (Peacock & Hurst, 2006). *Hysteroscopic myomectomy* is performed through the cervix. Fibroids are vaporized or destroyed by electrocautery or cut away using an instrument called a resectoscope. Bleeding, infection, and injury to other organs can occur with these two methods; the fibroids will also eventually grow back. Fertility may be preserved with these methods (DiGregorio, Maccario, & Raspollino, 2002).

MINIMALLY INVASIVE TREATMENTS
Uterine Artery Embolization

Another alternative for treatment of myomas is uterine artery embolization (UAE): a procedure in which a catheter is inserted into the femoral artery and threaded up to the uterine artery. Plastic particles are injected into the catheter and become lodged in diminutive blood vessels, cutting off blood supply to the myomas, thus causing shrinkage and resolution of symptoms (National Women's Health Resource Center, 2006). The procedure is done under local anesthesia and conscious sedation.

An incision is made into the groin, and a catheter is threaded into the femoral artery to the uterine artery. An arteriogram identifies the vessels supplying the fibroid. Most fibroids are reduced in size by 50% within 3 months. Long-term effects of the procedure are unknown; temporary amenorrhea or early menopause can occur (Simsek et al., 2006; Tropeano, 2005).

Preoperative teaching includes advising the woman not to drink alcohol or smoke and not to take aspirin or anticoagulant medications 24 hours before the procedure. The woman is told to expect cramping during injection of the pellets. Postoperative explanations about what to expect include that the woman may have pelvic pain, fever, malaise, and nausea and vomiting caused by acute fibroid degeneration. Pain may be controlled with a morphine patient-controlled analgesia pump. Nursing assessments include checking for bleeding in the groin, taking vital signs, assessing pain level, and checking the pedal pulse and neurovascular condition of the affected leg (Hiller, Miller, & Stavas, 2005; Todd, 2002). Discharge teaching includes signs of possible complications and when to notify the physician, self-care instructions, and follow-up advice (Exhibit 21.2). Most women return to normal activities within 7 to 10 days (Nicholson, 2004). An ultrasound or MRI examination is usually done within 6 weeks after the UAE to determine the effectiveness of the procedure.

More research is needed about this procedure to determine safety and effects on future fertility. Pregnancy rates after UAE are reportedly 50% to 60%. There are reports of pregnant women being at risk for malpresentations, preterm labor and birth, cesarean birth, uterine rupture, and postpartum hemorrhage after uterine artery embolization (Goldberg & Pereira, 2006; Gupta, Sinha, Lumsden, & Hickey, 2006; Topfer & Hailey, 2002). For these reasons, UAE is not recommended for women who desire a future pregnancy (National Women's Health Resource Center, 2006).

Myolyis

This procedure is usually performed laparoscopically as an outpatient procedure. A probe is inserted into the fibroid, and laser, radiofrequency energy, or freezing procedures are used to cut off the blood supply to the fibroid. Postprocedure adhesions and scarring can occur in the uterus. This procedure should not be used in women who wish to become pregnant in the future because there is an increased risk of uterine rupture (National Women's Health Resource Center, 2006).

Another form of myolyis is the use of high-intensity ultrasound waves to increase the temperature of the fibroid tissue to destroy and shrink the fibroid. This procedure is called *magnetic resonance imaging–guided focused ultrasound*. It is more precise, and no incision is needed. Complications my include burns

EXHIBIT 21.2 DISCHARGE TEACHING: UTERINE ARTERY EMBOLIZATION

- Call your health care provider if you have any of the following symptoms:
  - ☐ Pain
  - ☐ Bleeding
  - ☐ Fever of 102.2° F
  - ☐ Urinary retention
  - ☐ Nausea and vomiting
  - ☐ Abnormal vaginal discharge
  - ☐ Swelling or hematoma at the puncture site
- Eat a normal diet and include fluids and fiber.
- Avoid straining during bowel movements.
- Take any medications as prescribed.
- Do not use tampons, douche, or have vaginal intercourse for at least 4 weeks.
- Keep your postoperative follow-up appointment.

Sources: Lowdermilk, D. (2007b). Structural disorders and neoplasms of the reproductive system. In D. Lowdermilk & S. Perry (Eds.), *Maternity and Women's Health Care* (9th ed., pp. 276–312). St. Louis, MO: Mosby; National Women's Health Resource Center. (2006). *Uterine fibroids: Your guide to treatment options.* Retrieved January 13, 2007, from http://www.healthywomen.org

of the bowel (National Women's Health Resource Center, 2006).

Endometrial Ablation

Endometrial ablation is a minimally invasive procedure used for treating abnormal uterine bleeding. Hysteroscopic uterine ablation can be performed under local or general anesthesia. It is usually performed as an outpatient procedure. Medical therapy using GnRH agonists to temporarily control bleeding and to suppress endometrial tissue may be given for 8 to 12 weeks before surgery.

A hysteroscope is used to view the endometrium and to insert an instrument with an electrosurgical tip called a roller ball or laser to ablate (burn away) the uterine lining. Although the uterus remains in place, the vaporization process can cause scarring and adhesions in the uterine cavity and may affect future fertility—a result that should be discussed thoroughly before the woman consents to the procedure (Lefebre et al., 2003; National Women's Health Resource Center, 2006). Risks of the procedure include uterine perforation, hemorrhage, cervical injury, and fluid overload (caused by the leaking into blood vessels of fluid used to expand the uterus during surgery) (Banu & Manyonda, 2005). Postoperatively the woman may experience nausea and vomiting, cramping, and have a slight vaginal discharge for a few days. Discharge teaching includes the following information: the next menstrual period may be irregular; the physician should be called if the woman has heavy bleeding or signs of infection; and use of tampons or vaginal intercourse should be avoided for 2 weeks (Lowdermilk, 2007b).

Nonhysteroscopic Endometrial Ablation

A number of procedures are available that are considered less invasive techniques to ablate the endometrium. These use controlled application of heat, cold, microwave, or other forms of energy for ablation.

The *uterine thermal balloon catheter endometrial ablation system* uses a soft flexible balloon that is inserted through the cervix into the uterus. The balloon is inflated with sterile fluid that is heated to ablate the uterine lining. This procedure is usually performed under intravenous sedation and paracervical block on an outpatient basis. Risks include uterine perforation, burns of the internal structures, bleeding, and fluid leaking from the balloon. Fertility is also affected by this procedure (Banu & Manyonda, 2005).

Hydrothermablation is another procedure in which free fluid is instilled into the uterine cavity and then is warmed to a temperature that will ablate the endometrium. Risks include vaginal burns (Banu & Manyonda, 2005).

All nonhysteroscopic endometrial ablation methods of treating menorrhagia have shorter surgical times, shorter hospital stays, quicker recovery, and fewer complications than hysterectomy. However, the safety and efficacy of these procedures continues to be investigated (Banu & Manyonda, 2005; Marjoribanks, Lethaby, & Farquhar, 2006; Sharp, 2006).

HYSTERECTOMY

About 5.8 per 1,000 women have a hysterectomy each year in the United States. Twenty million U.S. women have had a hysterectomy (Keshavarz, Hillis, Keike, &

Marchbanks, 2002). Health care professionals, consumer groups, government agencies, and third-party payers all have concerns about this number. With the exception of procedures related to childbirth, it is the most frequently performed major surgery for all women, and most are done on women who are between 40 and 44 years of age (Kesavarz et al., 2002).

The medical necessity of hysterectomy has been challenged as alternative procedures have been developed. However, there is a lack of agreement about what is necessary. The quality of the woman's life before and after surgery and the risks and benefits of having or not having the procedure need to be considered before judging whether a hysterectomy is necessary. Women need to know that there may be alternatives to hysterectomy for certain problems, and they should consider getting a second opinion before making a decision to have surgery.

Because so many hysterectomies are performed, the nurse needs knowledge about the physiological and psychological changes that occur after the surgery so that comprehensive care can be given.

Indications

Although there is some disagreement among physicians about the absolute indications for hysterectomy, certain conditions are usually treated with this procedure. Fibroids are the most frequent problem treated with hysterectomy (National Women's Health Resource Center, 2005). Usually, cancer of the uterine endometrium or ovary is treated with abdominal hysterectomy. Cancer of the cervix may be treated with abdominal or vaginal hysterectomy depending on the stage; however, radiation therapy may be as effective (American Cancer Society, 2006). If there is persistent bleeding or if no further childbearing is desired, abdominal hysterectomy is usually performed for fibroid tumors that are larger than a 12- to 14-week gestation size (Nichols & Clark-Pearson, 2000).

Other conditions that may be treated by abdominal hysterectomy are chronic pelvic infections, life-threatening hemorrhage, and rupture of the uterus if suturing is not possible. Abdominal procedures are usually performed if the ovaries and uterine tubes are to be removed or if the woman has had previous abdominal surgery.

Indications for vaginal hysterectomy generally include uterine prolapse (which usually occurs in older women) and pelvic relaxation due to impaired bladder or rectal supports (common in multiparous women). It can also be used to treat severe dysfunctional bleeding, although alternatives should be tried first (Nichols & Clark-Pearson, 2000). Hysterectomy is usually not considered justifiable as a method of sterilization in women without pelvic pathology (Stenchever et al., 2001).

The woman must understand all options for treatment. Preoperative counseling should include information about whether the alternative procedures will be as beneficial as hysterectomy; information about hospital admission, the procedure, anesthesia, postoperative care, convalescence, and resumption of activities must also be provided. If the ovaries are to be removed, an explanation of surgical menopause and information about hormone therapy is warranted (National Women's Health Resource Center, 2005). Making sure the woman is fully informed about risks, benefits, and alternatives is a step toward eliminating unnecessary hysterectomies. Another step is to have the woman get a second opinion from a physician about the need for the hysterectomy. In many instances, this step is required by third-party payers. Exhibit 21.3 lists some Web sites that provide information about hysterectomy that may be useful in decision making.

Techniques

When hysterectomy is indicated, it can be performed abdominally or vaginally; abdominal procedures account for more than 60% of all hysterectomies. In both

---

EXHIBIT 21.3 INTERNET RESOURCES FOR INFORMATION ABOUT HYSTERECTOMY

Agency for Healthcare Research and Quality
www.ahrq.gov/consumer
American College of Obstetricians and Gynecologists
www.acog.org
Fibroid Treatment Collective
www.fibroid.org
National Women's Health Information Center
www.womenshealth.gov
National Women's Health Resource Center
www.healthywomen.org

the vaginal hysterectomy and the abdominal hysterectomy the procedure consists of removing the uterus from its supporting ligaments. These ligaments (broad, round, and uterosacral) are attached to the vaginal cuff so that normal depth of the vagina is maintained.

Total hysterectomies (removal of the entire uterus) account for more than 95% of all procedures. *Subtotal hysterectomy,* in which the cervix is not removed, is uncommonly performed, but some practitioners believe it results in better bladder, bowel, and sexual function than a total abdominal hysterectomy (Keshvarz et al., 2002). In a *radical hysterectomy,* the lymph nodes are dissected and may be removed along with the upper third of the vagina and the parametrium. This procedure may be done if uterine malignancy is present (Lowdermilk, 2007b). *Panhysterectomy,* or total abdominal hysterectomy with bilateral salpingo-oophorectomy, refers to the removal of the uterus, uterine tubes, and ovaries and is often seen abbreviated as TAH-BSO in client charts. The ovaries are not usually removed in premenopausal women, because oophorectomy is surgical castration and causes menopause (Stenchever et al., 2001).

Laparoscopic assisted vaginal hysterectomy (LAVH) has been used since the late 1980s to convert an abdominal procedure to one performed vaginally with assistance from viewing instruments in the abdomen. When compared to abdominal hysterectomy, results showed that LAVH took longer, cost about the same, required less postoperative pain medication, and had a quicker recovery than abdominal hysterectomy (American College of Obstetricians and Gynecologists, 2005; Johnson et al., 2006). Complications associated with LAVH include bleeding, adhesions, and injury to the bowel or bladder (National Women's Health Resource Center, 2005).

Laparoscopic supracervical hysterectomy uses the laparoscopic technique to remove the uterus but leave the cervix intact. Although there is some risk that cervical cancer could occur, there may be some benefits to leaving the cervix, including a reduced risk of vaginal prolapse and less effect on the pleasure of sexual intercourse (National Women's Health Resource Center, 2005).

Robotic or computer-assisted surgery also can be used to perform the hysterectomy procedure. Up to four small incisions are made, and instruments and a camera are inserted through the abdomen. The surgeon directs the procedure from a console that provides a magnified view of the surgical area. Safety and efficacy of this procedure in comparison to other surgical procedures continues to be investigated (National Women's Health Resource Center, 2005).

Most hysterectomies are performed as inpatient procedures; however, a growing number of hysterectomies are being performed as outpatient or short-stay procedures. The woman can usually go home within 8 hours of surgery if she is stable, able to walk, take clear liquids, and void spontaneously (Nichols & Clark-Pearson, 2000). If the woman remains hospitalized, she is usually discharged within 72 hours.

Anterior and Posterior Repairs

As noted, uterine prolapse and pelvic relaxation are two major indications for vaginal hysterectomy. Repair of the anterior and posterior vaginal walls is included when there is displacement of one or more of the pelvic organs, including the urethra, bladder, uterus, and rectum. Displacement of these organs usually results from weakening of the pelvic supporting structures by repeated childbearing, obstetric injury, or age (Stenchever et al., 2001). Most pelvic relaxation problems are seen in perimenopausal women because of a decline in estrogen. Complaints include heaviness in the pelvis and a bearing-down sensation (Lowdermilk, 2007b).

A specific complaint related to weakening of bladder support is loss of urine whenever there is increased intra-abdominal pressure, such as that produced by laughing or coughing (stress urinary incontinence). Weakening of the rectal wall causes constipation and difficult defecation. These symptoms are distressing, and women are often embarrassed to describe them to their physician. An alert nurse can assess these problems during history taking and physical examination.

An anterior colporrhaphy or anterior repair can tighten up the pelvic muscles for better bladder support. Alternatives to surgery for mild cases of stress urinary incontinence include performing Kegel exercises to increase pelvic tone, use of vaginal tampons or pessaries to support the bladder neck, and weight reduction in obese women (Dwyer & Kreder, 2005; Kielb, 2005; Klausner, 2005; Sampselle, 2003).

A posterior colporrhaphy or posterior repair can correct rectal displacement, strengthen pelvic supports, and reduce bulging. Alternatives to surgery for these conditions focus on promoting bowel elimination through high-fiber diets, stool softeners, or laxatives. Fecal incontinence is relieved only by surgical repair (Nichols & Clark-Pearson, 2000).

Complications

Nurses should be aware of women who are at risk for postoperative complications. Women older than 65 are at risk for all complications. Obese women are at risk especially for thrombophlebitis. Women who have a history of medical problems such as diabetes or cardiac or pulmonary problems are at a higher risk for complications. These complications include the following

(Lowdermilk, 2007b; Nichols & Clark-Pearson, 2000; National Women's Health Resource Center, 2005):

- Hemorrhage. Hemorrhage may be early (within 24 hours) or late (10 to 30 days postoperatively) and internal or external. Hemorrhage is more frequently seen with vaginal hysterectomy.
- Urinary tract complications. Urinary tract infections, such as cystitis or pyelitis, or urinary retention occur more frequently with vaginal hysterectomies and may not appear for up to 6 months after surgery.
- Infection. Wound infection is more frequent after vaginal hysterectomy. An elevated temperature (100° F or 38° C) is often the first sign, with redness and swelling of the wound area also noted.
- Intestinal obstruction or paralytic ileus. Intestinal complications are more common after abdominal hysterectomy. The chief symptoms are constipation and vomiting, followed by abdominal distention. Bowel sounds are absent with paralytic ileus.
- Thromboembolism. Thromboembolism is a late complication involving the deep veins of the lower extremities and is more common after abdominal hysterectomy. Preventive measures as previously described are the best treatment. Bed rest with the leg(s) elevated is also implemented.
- Pulmonary complications. Pulmonary complications occur more often after abdominal hysterectomy, and atelectasis is the most common problem.
- Evisceration. Wound dehiscence occurs more often after abdominal hysterectomy. Secondary closure of the wound may be required.

Nursing Care

The nurse is often responsible for physiological and psychological preparation of the preoperative hysterectomy client. Women may have concerns about surgery in general as well as hysterectomy in particular. Concerns specifically related to hysterectomy depend on the significance of the uterus for the woman. Hysterectomy can be a threat to self-image in several ways. Body image is affected whenever there is a loss of a body part—even though there is no outward change in appearance with hysterectomy, the loss may be felt strongly by the woman.

Many women have misconceptions about the effects of hysterectomy—for example, that it is associated with masculinization, weight gain, and accelerated aging. Hysterectomy also may pose a threat to women's femininity, especially in cultures in which women's roles are primarily childbearing and motherhood (Kim & Lee, 2001; Kjerulff et al., 2000; Sharts-Hopko, 2001).

Physical assessment in the preoperative period includes finding out a woman's knowledge of pre- and postoperative procedures. A guide for preoperative preparation for hysterectomy will depend on the woman's age and clinic or hospital requirements but may include the following (Lowdermilk, 2007b; Nichols & Clark-Pearson, 2000; Wade et al., 2000):

- Signed consent. The nurse should make sure that this is informed consent.
- Laboratory work: complete blood count, hematocrit, type and cross match of blood, urinalysis, chest X ray, electrocardiogram.
- Vaginal examination or complete physical examination.
- Surgical preparation: abdominal mons or perineal shave if ordered.
- NPO (nothing by mouth) past midnight.
- Empty bladder immediately prior to surgery.
- Preoperative medication and intravenous fluids.
- No makeup or nail polish.
- Removal of glasses, dentures, and so on.
- Identification band in place.
- Prophylactic antibiotics that may be given for clients at high risk for complications.
- Teaching postoperative care such as turning, coughing, and deep breathing.

Preoperative care should also include a psychological assessment. The nurse may particularly be alert for a grief reaction. The woman's initial response may be shock and disbelief or denial, especially if the hysterectomy is to be performed as an emergency procedure. The woman may react angrily to having an intrusive procedure that will result in physical loss of childbearing potential or a conceptual loss, such as loss of femininity. Depression can occur preoperatively if the woman is reminded of her impending loss through an encounter with a pregnant woman or if she is worried about losing her attractiveness (Wilmoth & Spinnelli, 2000).

Psychological assessment also includes an assessment of the significance of the loss to the individual woman. Some women will be relieved by the loss of menses, especially if bleeding is a problem; others will be sad if menses is seen as a sign of youth or as a cleansing process. In addition, impaired sexual function can occur in women who feel that their sexuality is dependent on the presence of the uterus (Roussis, Waltrous, Kerr, Robertazzi, & Cabbad, 2004). The woman's support system also must be assessed, because some women fear rejection by their husbands or significant others.

Postoperative assessment begins immediately after surgery and continues until convalescence is complete. Physiological care after abdominal hysterectomy is similar to other abdominal surgery postoperative care. Usual interventions for both vaginal and abdominal hysterectomy clients include monitoring vital signs every

15 minutes until stable and then every 4 hours for at least 48 hours. Maintaining an unobstructed airway is critical. Turning, coughing, and deep breathing should be performed at frequent intervals (every 2 hours) for the first 24 hours. After abdominal hysterectomy, assisting the woman to splint her abdomen with her hands or a pillow as she coughs may be helpful. Incentive spirometry may also be ordered.

Stimulating circulation with leg exercises (passive or active) is done. Antiembolism stockings occasionally may be ordered for the woman to wear until she is walking satisfactorily. These measures will help prevent thrombophlebitis. All clients should be observed for signs of bleeding that can lead to hemorrhage. This is accomplished by assessing the amount of drainage on the abdominal dressing and/or perineal pads. Vaginal bleeding is usually minimal, but a saturated pad in 1 hour should be reported to the physician. A drop in blood pressure, signs of shock, or a decrease in hematocrit or hemoglobin may also indicate bleeding.

When assessing for pain relief, the type of surgery and individual tolerance for pain need to be considered. Analgesics (narcotics) are usually ordered every 3 to 4 hours for the first 24 hours. Patient-controlled analgesia or epidural narcotics are also used after abdominal hysterectomies (Nichols & Clark-Pearson, 2000). As discomfort lessens, the amount and strength of medication is reduced. Nursing measures for pain relief should be used with, or as alternatives to, medications. These may include the use of breathing and relaxation techniques, position changes, guided imagery, and back rubs. Ambulation or application of heat to the abdomen may relieve discomfort produced by intestinal gas. Warm sitz baths, ice packs, or heat lamps may relieve pain after vaginal hysterectomy.

Fluid intake should be carefully monitored. Intravenous fluids and ice chips or clear liquids are given after surgery. Maintenance needs as well as replacement of lost fluids are important. Women who are discharged within 8 hours of surgery should drink at least 6 glasses of fluids within the first 24 hours (Nichols & Clark-Pearson, 2000). Urinary output should be monitored accurately to assess achievement of fluid balance. Foley catheters are usually discontinued after 24 hours or sooner. After surgery for prolapse with repairs, retention of urine is a problem and, often, a catheter (foley or suprapubic) may be left in place until the woman's bladder sphincter is functioning again. These women are at risk for urinary infections and may be given prophylactic antibacterial or antibiotic medications (Nichols & Clark-Pearson, 2000). Bowel sounds and function are also monitored. Stool softeners or mild laxatives usually are not needed unless posterior repair has been done. Enemas are usually not given unless laxative treatment is ineffective.

Early ambulation is encouraged because it improves circulation, muscle tone, lung expansion, and bowel function. Women who have had abdominal hysterectomies are usually encouraged to get out of bed by at least the first postoperative day. Getting up may be delayed if the woman has had extensive surgery or if her condition warrants bed rest. The woman may need to be assisted to get out of bed without straining. To do this, the woman is told to roll on her side, bring her knees up so that her thighs are at right angles to the abdomen, put her feet over the side of the bed, push up on her elbow, and sit up. Women who have had vaginal hysterectomies as short-stay procedures must be able to ambulate before discharge.

Diet usually progresses from clear liquids to solid foods as tolerated. Sugar in foods, milk products, and carbonated beverages tends to cause gas production and may need to be kept to a minimum if the woman is experiencing problems with intestinal gas.

Assessing abdominal and vaginal incisions is another important nursing function following hysterectomy. When abdominal dressings are removed, the incision is assessed for intactness and signs of infection. Clips or sutures usually are removed by the fourth postoperative day. Superficial drains (Hemovacs) may be present the first 24 to 48 hours, especially with radical hysterectomy. With vaginal hysterectomy, sutures are usually absorbable. The vagina is assessed for signs of infection or hemorrhage. Vaginal packing may be used to control bleeding and hematoma formation in the first 24 to 48 hours.

The nurse should continue psychosexual assessments during the postoperative period to identify problems and intervene appropriately. An association between loss of the uterus and psychological problems has been posed for hundreds of years. Although there is controversy about whether hysterectomy is the cause of these reactions, nurses working with women who undergo hysterectomy need to know what responses research studies have attributed to the surgery and the factors affecting these responses.

Depression is the most frequently reported symptom after hysterectomy (Kjerulff et al., 2000). Studies in the 1990s looked at supposed reactions to hysterectomy, including loss of femininity, lessened sex drive, personality changes, and weight gain. More recent studies have not found these reactions to be a major concern. Instead, results suggest that women are usually satisfied, particularly with relief of bothersome symptoms (e.g., bleeding, pain), after their hysterectomy and that their physical well-being may enhance their psychological well-being (Flory, Bissonnette, Amsel, & Binik, 2006; Galavotti & Richter, 2000; Hartmann et al., 2004; Kjerulff et al., 2000; Wade et al., 2000).

No consensus exists about whether hysterectomy causes sexual dysfunction. Sexual problems after hysterectomy that have been reported include dyspareunia related to vaginal shrinkage and decreased lubrication, low libido, and not experiencing orgasm (Dragisic &

Milad, 2004). Sexual dysfunction seems to be more prevalent in women who have declining ovarian hormone function postoperatively, possibly related to decreased vaginal lubrication. Emotional distress can also cause sexual dysfunction (Kjerulff et al., 2000). Studies suggest that frequency of sexual activity increases and problems with sexual functioning decrease after hysterectomy (Dragisic & Milad, 2004; El-Toukhy, Hefni, Davies, & Mahadevan, 2004; Kuscu et al., 2005). Factors proposed to explain the increase in sexual desire include absence of fear of pregnancy and absence of the pain related to the condition requiring hysterectomy.

Possible psychological reactions after hysterectomy should be discussed preoperatively. The woman should be encouraged to express her feelings about the surgery. Partners may be included in these discussions if both the woman and partner agree. Use of support groups as previously discussed can also provide women with opportunities to share their surgical experiences and express their feelings and concerns (Galvotti & Richter, 2000; Wilmoth & Spinelli, 2000).

Specific information about sexual functioning after hysterectomy and repair surgery may need to be provided to assist women and their partners in resuming sexual activity, but there is no one best approach to this counseling. Male sexual partners may have concerns or misconceptions about sexual functioning with a woman who has had a hysterectomy. Often, it is important to include the husband or sexual partner in discussions about sexual functioning, but in other instances, classes for men only or provision of information in written format suffice (Wilmoth & Spinelli, 2000).

In general, nursing interventions after hysterectomy include providing or reinforcing information about the reproductive system and what it means to have part of it removed surgically. Specific information that may assist the woman in sexual adjustment after hysterectomy includes the following:

- Sexual intercourse is usually restricted after abdominal hysterectomy for 4 to 6 weeks; however, it may be several months before the woman is comfortable due to abdominal soreness and a temporary shrinkage of the vagina, which makes it feel narrow and short. Reassuring the couple that coitus will help stretch the vagina is a necessary support measure.
- Decreased sexual response may be caused by both hormonal (if ovaries are removed) and anatomical changes. As many as one-third of women having hysterectomies report decreased orgasm and excitement related to absence of cervical stimulation and decreased pelvic congestion (Wilmoth & Spinelli, 2000).
- Use of foreplay to arouse the woman before penile penetration may be helpful. Also, use of water-soluble lubricants may be helpful for a dry vagina (Katz, 2002; Wilmoth & Spinelli, 2000).

- If the abdomen is tender, positions other than those with the male on top may be more comfortable.
- Intercourse after vaginal hysterectomy may be painful at first, especially if anterior or posterior repair surgery was performed. Sexual functioning is poorly preserved after repair surgery because of narrowing and shortening of the vagina, resulting in stenosis. Resumption of intercourse within 6 weeks will help keep stenosis to a minimum. Use of dilators and lubricants also may relieve some vaginal tightness (Wilmoth & Spinelli, 2000).

Preparation for home care should begin in the early postoperative period. The woman may be discharged as early as 8 hours after surgery if she has had a vaginal hysterectomy in an ambulatory care facility or in 2 to 3 days if she has had abdominal surgery and has not developed complications.

The nurse should be aware of the information needs of the woman postoperatively. The physician is responsible for providing the woman with information relevant to recovery, both physically and emotionally, and the nurse should be available to answer or clarify questions as needed.

Women should be reminded that, following hysterectomy, weakness and fatigue are normal and that they will no longer menstruate and can no longer become pregnant. They should be reassured that masculinization, weight gain, and so on are merely old wives' tales and not supported by research findings. The possibility that they may have phantom pains (uterine cramping) should be mentioned. Numbness around the incision site will be present after an abdominal hysterectomy, and some women will experience a temporary loss of vaginal sensation after vaginal hysterectomy.

Women are cautioned to increase physical activities and exercise slowly. No active sports (e.g., tennis, jogging, aerobics) should be undertaken for 1 month. Heavy housework (vacuuming, hanging out clothes, picking up objects weighing more than 10 to 25 pounds) should be deferred at least 1 month. Driving may be resumed about 2 weeks after discharge (some sources allow driving earlier, but many suggest delaying the activity for longer than 2 weeks). Women are cautioned to avoid sitting for long periods because this can cause pelvic congestion. Women can resume their usual diet when they feel ready to do so; however, foods high in protein, iron, and vitamin C are encouraged because they promote healing and repair of tissues. Increasing intake of fluids and foods that are high in fiber may be helpful if constipation is a problem. Although showers and washing the hair are not restricted, tub baths may be restricted after abdominal hysterectomy, because the difficulty of getting into the tub can cause strain on the sutures (Lowdermilk, 2007b).

Tampons and douching should be avoided for a month. Sexual intercourse may be resumed in 4 to 6 weeks, depending on the woman's degree of comfort, healing, and desire. Suggestions such as using water soluble lubricants and other recommendations previously described can be given to assist in sexual adjustment after surgery. A postoperative checkup may be suggested as early as 1 week, with a follow-up checkup scheduled 1 month to 6 weeks after discharge (Nichols & Clark-Pearson, 2000).

If ovaries are removed in premenopausal women, the women will experience surgical menopause; hormone therapy may be prescribed in these cases. (See chapter 6 for information on hormonal therapy.)

Signs of physical complications should be reviewed, because these can occur after discharge—especially infection, hemorrhage, and bladder problems.

Review of emotional reactions, especially depression, that can occur need to be included in discharge teaching, because reactions can occur 3 months to 3 years after surgery. Women who are identified at high risk for psychological problems may need long-term follow-up or referral to a community agency or support group.

Vaginal screening with cytology (i.e., Pap test) after a total hysterectomy for a nonmalignant reason is no longer recommended (American Cancer Society, 2006; National Comprehensive Cancer Network, 2004). However, general practices will vary depending on the beliefs of the health care provider. Women undergoing subtotal hysterectomy will continue to need Pap tests as recommended by their health care provider.

EXTENSIVE GYNECOLOGIC SURGERY

Extensive gynecologic surgical procedures, such as vulvectomy and pelvic exenteration, are usually reserved for treatment of reproductive malignancies.

Vulvectomy

Carcinoma in situ or preinvasive cancer of the vulva can be treated with one of the following surgical procedures, although laser surgery, cryosurgery, or electrosurgical excision may be used for premalignant lesions.

A local wide excision may be used to remove abnormal tissue, or a *simple vulvectomy* may be used to remove part or all of the vulva, labia majora and minora, and possibly the clitoris. The clitoris can be preserved if there is no cancer present. More radical procedures are performed for invasive cancer of the vulva. A partial radical vulvectomy is the removal of the entire vulva and deep tissues. A complete radical vulvectomy removes skin, labia, clitoris, subcutaneous tissues, and possibly inguinal and femoral nodes (DiSaia & Creasman, 2002).

An alternative to a node dissection is a sentinel node biopsy. The procedure involves injection of a blue dye or radioactive material into the tumor site. A scan is done to identify the first (sentinel) node, which is then removed for study. If no cancer is present, no other nodes are removed; if cancer is present, the rest of the lymph nodes are removed (American Cancer Society, 2006).

Preoperatively, a woman needs extensive explanation of the procedure she is undergoing, information about whether alternatives are possible, encouragement to talk about her fears and concerns about adjustment to physical changes and sexual functioning, and information about pre- and postoperative procedures. Specific preoperative procedures may include a mons or perineal skin shave, enema, and douche.

Interventions for women who have been treated with laser surgery include application of topical steroids, sitz baths, and application of local anesthetic agents or administration of oral pain medications as needed. Postoperative interventions depend on the type of surgery performed but may include care of suction drains to the wound for 7 to 10 days; use of an indwelling bladder catheter for urinary drainage to prevent urethral stenosis and wound contamination; and frequent, meticulous wound care. Wound care is usually done with a solution of one-half strength hydrogen peroxide followed by a rinse with normal saline. Both solutions may be applied with a large bulb syringe or an automatic irrigating device such as a water pic. The wound is dried with the application of a heat lamp or use of a hair dryer on cool setting. Analgesics are usually ordered for postoperative pain and as premedication for wound care. Wound infection and breakdown occur in almost 50% of clients after radical vulvectomy (Lowdermilk, 2007b).

If radical surgery is performed, women may experience discomfort in everyday situations. Sitting for long periods will be uncomfortable due to the loss of perineal fatty tissue. Chronic edema of lower extremities after lymph node dissection can continue for years and may cause problems with mobility. Many women have problems controlling urine flow after surgery if the urethra has been removed or reconstructed.

If a radical vulvectomy is performed, clitoral removal may mean loss of orgasm; dyspareunia can occur due to loss of part of the vagina and introital stenosis. The woman and her partner can be counseled to include alternative measures of giving and receiving sexual pleasure, such as breast stimulation. Vaginal dilators can be used to stretch the remaining vaginal tissues, and water-soluble lubricants and using a side-lying or woman-on-top position can decrease discomforts of intercourse. Performing Kegel exercises can increase perineal muscle tone (Wilmoth & Spinelli, 2000). The woman may need to be encouraged to express her feelings about loss of normal sexual function.

A vulvectomy may affect the woman's self-image. The sudden disfigurement may cause a negative body image or low self-esteem. She may fear rejection by her sexual partner or other significant persons and may withdraw from intimate relationships (Shell, 2001; Wilmoth & Spinelli, 2000). Women and their significant others may need counseling and encouragement to express their fears and concerns. The nurse can use knowledge of the client's beliefs about feminine roles and sexual practices to identify appropriate interventions.

Pelvic Exenteration

Although done rarely, pelvic exenteration is one of the most radical surgical procedures performed. It is performed for recurrent cancer of the cervix and some vaginal and vulvar lesions when the tumor is confined to the pelvis and there is no lymph node involvement (DiSaia & Creasman, 2002). Exenteration procedures can include the anterior, posterior, or whole pelvis. Anterior exenteration includes the removal of the uterus, ovaries, uterine tubes, vagina, bladder, urethra, and pelvic lymph nodes; an ileal conduit is created for urinary diversion. Posterior exenteration includes the removal of the uterus, ovaries, uterine tubes, descending colon, rectum, and anal canal; a colostomy is created for passage of feces. A total exenteration includes removal of all pelvic organs with creation of both ileal conduit and colostomy. With any of these procedures, a neovagina may be constructed.

Preoperative nursing measures include providing the woman with information about physical preparation, postoperative care, and recovery. Specific attention is given to assessing psychological readiness for surgery, including exploration of fears and concerns about surgery, death, and changes in body image and evaluation of support systems. Sexual assessment is critical because of the potential impact of surgery on sexual functioning related to alterations in excretory function and removal of the vagina. If vaginal reconstruction is possible or desired, discussion is needed about this option. Significant others need to be involved in discussions when possible, because their reactions are critical for postoperative adjustment (Wilmoth & Spinelli, 2000).

Preoperative physical preparation begins with extensive tests to rule out spread of cancer outside the pelvis. Extensive bowel preparation (enemas) is performed, and stoma sites are selected. Information is given to the woman regarding immediate postoperative recovery care, because this recovery may take place in an intensive care setting. She is also told what to expect with regard to pain management and invasive procedures (for example, nasogastric suctioning, intravenous lines, arterial catheters) (Lowdermilk, 2007b).

Postoperative nursing care immediately following surgery focuses on stabilizing the woman and assessing for complications. Because of the extent of surgery, the woman is at risk for cardiovascular complications such as shock and hemorrhage; pulmonary complications, such as atelectasis and pneumonia; fluid and electrolyte imbalance; and urinary complications (Otto, 2001). After the woman is stabilized, she returns to the gynecologic/surgical unit for continued postoperative care. Assessments are made for pain, infection, deep vein thrombosis, pulmonary embolus, paralytic ileus or other gastrointestinal complications, and wound dehiscence (Lowdermilk, 2007b). Care of the ileal conduit and colostomy is initiated, as is wound care. The wound is usually cleaned with a solution of one-half hydrogen peroxide and one-half normal saline applied with a large bulb syringe. After cleaning, the wound is dried with a heat lamp or hair dryer on cool setting. Sitz baths may also be used.

The woman may be discharged home and followed by a home health nurse or discharged to an extended-care facility, depending on her rate of recovery and need for nursing care. The woman will need assistance after discharge, because she will not be able to do any strenuous activities for up to 6 months. She will need to be taught colostomy and/or ureterostomy care or have family members or others who are willing to assist with care. She will also require information regarding (a) diet, including foods that promote healing as well as foods that can be tolerated; (b) perineal care; (c) range of motion exercises and physical activities that are permitted by the physician; (d) signs of complications, such as infection or bowel obstruction; and (e) the importance of follow-up care.

Psychosocial adjustment is an integral part of postoperative recovery and adaptation to an altered body image. Usually, the woman expresses grief about her mutilated body. Initially, she may refuse to look at the wound or stoma sites as a form of denial. She may then become angry, hostile, or depressed and withdrawn. As she accepts the changes in her body, she will become active in self-care.

Pelvic exenteration patients will experience sexual disruption. If vaginal reconstruction is not done after anterior or total exenteration, the woman will not be able to have vaginal intercourse. Even with reconstruction surgery, women report decreased vaginal sensation of penile enclosure, increased chronic discharge, or the neovagina being too large or too short. Often a waiting period of 12 to 18 months before resumption of sexual intercourse is advised to allow for healing. Another concern is that the presence of a colostomy or ureterostomy may cause odor or leakage during sexual activities. The bags can be emptied prior to engaging in sexual activity to decrease the chance of an accident. The woman also may be worried about her altered physical appearance. Information about alternative techniques and options for sexual expression may need to be offered. These include touching and fondling other sensitive areas such as breasts and buttocks and bringing her partner to orgasm with hand or mouth stimulation (Shell, 2001). Open communication between partners is essential in resolving problems related to sexual expression, and couples may need further sexual counseling to help promote this communication.

SUMMARY AND IMPLICATIONS FOR RESEARCH

This chapter provides nurse practitioners with a broad knowledge base to use in the care of gynecologic clients facing decisions about and undergoing reproductive surgery. The focus is specifically on the areas of preventive teaching, counseling about surgical procedures and alternatives, and physiological and psychological care. The focus of future research in the area of caring for women who are facing reproductive surgery should be on ways to promote preventive health practices and identifying effective nursing interventions related to preoperative and postoperative care. Specific research needs include identification of interventions that are effective in preventing problems related to pelvic supports, such as pelvic exercises; interventions that promote pyschological well-being after hysterectomy; and interventions that promote sexual adjustment after hysterectomy and other reproductive surgery. Dissemination of research findings to nurses working in women's health care settings continues to be needed so that care given is evidence based.

REFERENCES

Abbott, J. (2005). Transcervical sterilization. *Best Practices and Research, Clinical Obstetrics and Gynaecology, 19*(5), 743–756.

American Cancer Society. (2006). *Cancer facts and figures 2006.* New York: Author.

American College of Obstetricians and Gynecologists. (2005). Appropriate use of laparoscopically assisted vaginal hysterectomy. ACOG Committee Opinion No. 311. *Obstetrics and Gynecology, 105*(4), 929–930.

Banu, N., & Manyonda, T. (2005). Alternative medical and surgical options to hysterectomy. *Best Practices & Research Clinical Obstetrics and Gynaecology, 19*(3), 431–449.

Bradley, L. (2002). Complications in hysteroscopy: Prevention, treatment and legal risk. *Current Opinion in Obstetrics and Gynecology, 14*(4), 409–415.

Chapman, L., & Magos, A. (2005). Currently available devices for female sterilization. *Expert Review of Medical Devices, 2*(5), 623–634.

Cook, J., & Walker, C. (2004). Treatment strategies for uterine leiomyoma: The role of hormonal modulation. *Seminars in Reproductive Medicine, 22*(2), 105–111.

DiGregorio, A., Maccario, S., & Raspollino, M. (2002). The role of laparoscopic myomectomy in women of reproductive age. *Reproductive Biomedicine Online, 4*(Suppl. 3), 55–58.

DiSaia, P., & Creasman, W. (2002). *Clinical gynecologic oncology* (6th ed.). St. Louis, MO: Mosby.

Dragisic, K., & Milad, M. (2004). Sexual functioning and patient expectations of sexual functioning after hysterectomy. *American Journal of Obstetrics and Gynecology, 190*(5), 1416–1418.

Dwyer, N., & Kreder, K. (2005). Conservative strategies for the treatment of stress urinary incontinence. *Current Urology Report, 6*(5), 371–375.

El-Toukhy, T., Hefni, M., Davies, A., & Mahadevan, S. (2004). The effect of different types of hysterectomy on urinary and sexual functioning: A prospective study. *Journal of Obstetrics and Gynaecology, 24*(4), 420–425.

Falcone, T., & Bedaiwy, M. (2002). Minimally invasive management of uterine fibroids. *Current Opinion in Obstetrics and Gynecology, 14*(4), 401–407.

Flory, N., Bissonnette, F., Amsel, R., & Binik, Y. (2006). The psychosocial outcomes of total and subtotal hysterectomy: A randomized controlled trail. *Journal of Sexual Medicine, 3*(3), 483–491.

Galavotti, C., & Richter, D. (2000). Talking about hysterectomy: The experiences of women from four cultural groups. *Journal of Women's Health & Gender-Based Medicine, 9*(Suppl. 2), S63–S67.

Goldberg, J., & Pereira, L. (2006). Pregnancy outcomes following treatment for fibroids: Uterine artery embolization versus laparoscopic myomectomy. *Current Opinion in Obstetrics and Gynecology, 18*(4), 402–406.

Gomel, V., & McComb, P. (2006). Microsurgery for tubal infertility. *Journal of Reproductive Medicine, 51*(3), 177–184.

Gupta, J., Sinha, A., Lumsden, M., & Hickey, M. (2006). Uterine artery embolization for symptomatic uterine fibroids. *The Cochrane Database for Systematic Reviews, (1),* CD005073.

Hartmann, K., Ma, C., Lamu, G., Langenberg, P., Steege, J., & Kjerulff, K. (2004). Quality of life and sexual functioning after hysterectomy in women with preoperative pain and depression. *Obstetrics and Gynecology, 104*(4), 701–709.

Hiller, J., Miller, M., & Stavas, J. (2005). Uterine artery embolization: A minimally invasive option to end fibroid symptoms. *Advance for Nurse Practitioners, 13*(10), 20–26.

Johnson, N., Barlow, D., Lethaby, A., Tavender, E., Curr, E., & Garry, R. (2006). Surgical approach to hysterectomy for benign gynaecological disease. *Cochrane Database of Systematic Review, (2),* CD003677.

Katz, A. (2002). Sexuality after hysterectomy. *Journal of Obstetric Gynecologic and Neonatal Nursing, 31*(3), 256–262.

Keshavarz, H., Hillis, S., Keike, B., & Marchbanks, P. (2002). Hysterectomy surveillance—United States, 1994–1999. *MMWR Surveillance Summaries, 51*(SS05), 1–8.

Kielb, S. (2005). Stress incontinence: Alternatives to surgery. *International Journal of Fertility and Women's Medicine, 50*(1), 24–29.

Kim, K., & Lee, K. (2001). Symptom experience in women after hysterectomy. *Journal of Obstetric Gynecologic and Neonatal Nursing, 30*(5), 472–480.

Kjerulff, K., Langenberg, P., Rhodes, J., Harvey, L., Guzinski, G., & Stolley, P. (2000). Effectiveness of hysterectomy. *Obstetrics and Gynecology, 95*(3), 319–326.

Klausner, T. (2005). The best kept secret. Pelvic floor muscle therapy for urinary incontinence. *Advance for Nurse Practitioners, 13*(7), 43–46, 48.

Kuscu, N., Oruc, S., Ceylan, E., Eskicioiglu, F., Goker, A., & Caglar, H. (2005). Sexual life following total abdominal hysterectomy. *Archives of Gynecology and Obstetrics, 271*(3), 218–221.

Lefebvre, G., Vilos, G., Allaire, C., Jeffry, J., Arneja, J., Birch, C., et al. (2003). The management of uterine leiomyomas. *Journal of Obstetrics and Gynecology, 25*(5), 396–418.

Lindberg, C., & Nolan, L. (2001). Women's decision-making regarding hysterectomy. *Journal of Obstetric, Gynecologic and Neonatal Nursing, 30*(6), 607–616.

Lock, S. (2007). Contraception and abortion. In D. Lowdermilk & S. Perry (Eds.), *Maternity and women's health care* (9th ed., pp. 207–234). St. Louis, MO: Mosby.

Lowdermilk, D. (2006). Assessment of the reproductive system. In D. Ignatavicius & M. Workman (Eds.), *Medical-surgical nursing: Critical thinking for collaborative care* (5th ed., pp. 1768–1790). St. Louis, MO: Elsevier Saunders.

Lowdermilk, D. (2007a). Infertility. In D. Lowdermilk & S. Perry (Eds.), *Maternity and women's health care* (9th ed., pp. 235–254). St. Louis, MO: Mosby.

Lowdermilk, D. (2007b). Structural disorders and neoplasms of the reproductive system. In D. Lowdermilk & S. Perry (Eds.), *Maternity and Women's Health Care* (9th ed., pp. 276–312). St. Louis, MO: Mosby.

Marjoribanks, J., Lethaby, A., & Farquhar, C. (2006). Surgery versus long term hormone treatment for heavy menstrual bleeding. The *Cochrane Database of Systematic Reviews, (2), CD003855.*

Mattinson, A., & Mansour, D. (2006). Female sterilisation: Is it what women really want or are alternative contraceptive methods acceptable? *Journal of Family Planning and Reproductive Health Care, 32*(3), 181–183.

Nardin, J., Kulier, R., & Boulvain, M. (2003). Techniques for the interruption of tubal patency for female sterilization. The *Cochrane Database of Systematic Reviews, (1), CD003034.*

National Comprehensive Cancer Network Inc. (2004). *NCCN practice guidelines in oncology. Cervical screening. Version 1.2005.* Retrieved January 12, 2007, from http://www.nccn.org

National Women's Health Information Center. (2006). *Hysterectomy.* Retrieved January 13, 2007, from http://www.womenshealth.gov.

National Women's Health Resource Center. (2005). *Hysterectomy: Questions to ask.* Retrieved January 13, 2007, from http://www.healthywomen.org/healthtopics/questionstoask

National Women's Health Resource Center. (2006). *Uterine fibroids: Your guide to treatment options.* Retrieved January 13, 2007, from http://www.healthywomen.org

Nichols, D., & Clark-Pearson, D. (2000). *Gynecologic, obstetric, and related surgery* (2nd ed.). St. Louis, MO: Mosby.

Nicholson, T. (2004). Outcome in patients undergoing unilateral artery emboliation for symptomatic fibroids. *Clinical Radiology, 59*(2), 186–191.

Novak, K. (2006). Interventions for clients with gynecologic problems. In D. Ignatavicius & M. Workman (Eds), *Medical-surgical nursing: Critical thinking for collaborative care* (5th ed., pp. 1823–1855). St. Louis, MO: Elsevier Saunders.

Otto, S. (2001). Gynecologic cancers. In S. Otto, *Oncology nursing* (pp. 248–284). St. Louis, MO: Mosby.

Peacock, K., & Hurst, B. (2006). Laparoscopic myomectomy. *Surgical Technology International, 15,* 141–145.

Pollack, A., Carignan, C., & Jacobstein, R. (2004). Female and male sterilization. In R. Hatcher et al. (Eds.), *Contraceptive technology* (18th rev. ed., pp. 531–573). New York: Ardent Media.

Roussis, N., Waltrous, L., Kerr, A., Robertazzi, R., & Cabbad, M. (2004). Sexual response in the patient after hysterectomy: Total abdominal versus supracervical versus vaginal procedure. *American Journal of Obstetrics and Gynecology, 190*(5), 1427–1428.

Sampselle, C., (2003). Behavior interventions in young and middle-aged women: Simple interventions to combat a complex problem. *American Journal of Nursing, 103*(Suppl. March), 9–19.

Sharp, H. (2006). Assessment of new technology in treatment of idiopathic menorrhagia and uterine leiomyomata. *Obstetrics and Gynecology, 108*(4), 990–1003.

Sharts-Hopko, N. (2001). Hysterectomy for nonmalignant conditions. *American Journal of Nursing, 101*(9), 32–40.

Shell, J. (2001). Impact of cancer on sexuality. In S. Otto (Ed.), *Oncology nursing* (pp. 973–999). St. Louis, MO: Mosby.

Simsek, M., Sadik, S., Taskin, O., Guler, H., Onoglu, A., Akar, M., Kursun, S., & Tinar, S. (2006). Role of laparoscopic uterine artery coagulation in management of symptomatic myomas: A prospective study using ultrasound and magnetic resonance imaging. *Journal of Minimally Invasive Gynecology, 113*(4), 315–319.

Stenchever, M. A., Droegemueller, W., Herbst, A., & Mishell, D. (2001). *Comprehensive gynecology* (4th ed.). St. Louis, MO: Mosby.

Sutton, C. (2006). Hysteroscopic surgery. *Best Practice and Research. Clinical Obstetrics and Gynaecology, 20*(1), 105–137.

Todd, A. (2002). An alternative to hysterectomy. *RN, 65*(3), 30–35.

Topfer, L., & Hailey, D. (2002). Uterine artery embolization for the treatment of fibroids. *Issues in Emergency Health Technology, 36*(August), 1–6.

Tropeano, G. (2005). The role of uterine artery embolization in the management of uterine fibroids. *Current Opinion in Obstetrics and Gynecology, 17*(4), 329–332.

Wade, J., Pletsch, P., Morgan, S., & Menting, S. (2000). Hysterectomy: What do women need and want to know? *Journal of Obstetric, Gynecologic and Neonatal Nursing, 29*(1), 33–42.

Wilmoth, M., & Spinelli, A. (2000). Sexual implications of gynecologic cancer treatments. *Journal of Obstetric, Gynecologic and Neonatal Nursing, 29*(4), 413–421.

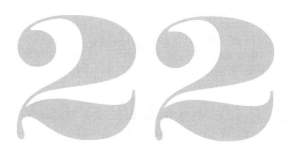

Substance Abuse and Women

Shirley A. Murphy

Healthy, employed women have high prevalence rates of at-risk substance use. Data show that 11% to 19% abuse alcohol, 27% are smokers, and 25% reported using illicit drugs in the previous 6 months (Curry et al., 2000; Manwell, Fleming, Johnson, & Barry, 1998). These use and abuse patterns of substances are detrimental to the individual, family, employer, and society.

An Institute of Medicine (1990) report stated that the early detection and treatment of at-risk drinkers is as important as the identification and treatment of persons who are alcohol dependent. To meet this challenge, *Healthy People 2010* recommended a 75% increase in the number of primary health care providers who screen for substance abuse problems (U.S. Department of Health and Human Services, 2000).

For the purposes of this chapter, primary care is defined as the provision of integrated, accessible health care services by clinicians who are accountable for addressing a large majority of personal health care needs, developing a sustained partnership with clients, and practicing in the context of family and community (Institute of Medicine, 1994). The first section of this chapter addresses the epidemiology, consequences, risk and protective factors, and prevention strategies pertaining to substance use among women. The second section addresses screening, assessment, diagnosis, intervention strategies, specialized treatment, and maintenance of behavioral change. The last section addresses legal and ethical issues and policy implications.

EPIDEMIOLOGY, CONSEQUENCES, RISK AND PROTECTIVE FACTORS, AND PREVENTION OF SUBSTANCE ABUSE

Alcohol, Tobacco, and Other Drug Use Among Women

According to the *National Survey on Drug Use and Health* (Substance Abuse and Mental Health Services Administration [SAMHSA], 2005b), in 2003, 70.1 million (63.4%) of women between 18 and 25 years of age reported using alcohol during the past year, 12.5 million used an illicit drug in the past year, and 5.9% met the criteria for abuse or dependence of alcohol (4.9%) or an illicit drug (1.9%). Alcohol and drug abuse are defined as maladaptive patterns of use leading to clinically significant impairment as manifested by any of the following four criteria in a 12-month period: inability to fulfill life obligations, use in situations that are physically hazardous, legal involvement, and continued use despite consequences (American Psychiatric Association, 1994). Users' drugs of choice vary over time, making it difficult for clinicians to keep current. For example, ecstasy, methamphetamine, steroids, Oxycontin, and Vicodin have replaced the use of other illegal drugs among adolescents and young adults (National Institute on Drug Abuse, 2006).

Women's substance abuse appears to decrease with age. For example, women meeting the abuse/dependence criteria by age groups is as follows: 15.7% among 18- to 25-year-olds; 8.9% among 26- to 34-year-olds;

5.4% among 35- to 49-year-olds; and 1.5% by age 50 (SAMHSA, 2005a).

Demographic data in addition to age are compiled by ethnicity, marital status, and living with children. Rates of abuse/dependence on alcohol and illicit drugs are highest among American Indians (19.9%) followed by Whites (6.3%), Blacks (4.5%), Hispanics (4.4%), and Asians (3.4%). Women aged 18 to 49 years who were married had lower rates of abuse or dependence compared with women who were separated, divorced, or never married. Abuse/dependence criteria were nearly double for women aged 18 to 49 who reported not living with children (12.9%) compared with women living with children (5.5%) (SAMHSA, 2005a).

Tobacco-related morbidity and mortality have increased in women, whereas they have decreased among men. More than 25% of women in the United States smoke cigarettes; 80% begin as adolescents. Tobacco use accounts for more than 400,000 premature adult deaths annually among U.S. women, with lung cancer as the leading cause (American Cancer Society, 1999). Among pregnant women who smoke, low birth weight is often attributed to smoking.

Substance use and abuse among women may go unnoticed for several reasons. First, women are reluctant to report use or misuse, particularly illicit drug use (Manwell et al., 1998), and are more likely to seek health care for a substance-induced health problem rather than seeking treatment for substance abuse per se. For this reason, at-risk women drinkers are detected only about 10% of the time. Second, despite significant increases in substance abuse education over the past two decades, some health care providers state they lack the assessment skills needed; others have negative attitudes toward persons who abuse substances, including the belief that clients will not change substance use behavior; and still other clinicians don't want to get involved in cases where they are required by law to report incidents such as child abuse (SAMHSA, 1997). A national sample of physicians considered a diagnosis of substance abuse only 1% of the time when presented with a vignette describing early symptoms of substance abuse among older women (Center for Substance Abuse, 1998). Despite the reluctance of some clinicians, primary care settings provide opportunities to intervene in the early phases of substance misuse.

Consequences of Substance Abuse on Women

All aspects of women's lives can be affected by substance abuse. This section provides some examples of health, interpersonal, social, and economic costs associated with substance abuse as well as differences in these consequences by age and ethnicity.

Alcohol, Tobacco, and Other Drugs' Impacts on Health Status

Alcohol use is the third leading cause of premature death in the United States. It is well established that when women and men use the same amount of alcohol, women have more severe effects that appear to occur sooner after initiation of use than occurs with men (Randall et al., 1999). A major factor accounting for gender differences is thought to be women's sensitivity to alcohol (Antai-Otong, 2006; Nolen-Hoeksema, 2004). Physiologically, women have higher concentrations of alcohol in the blood compared with men, which is believed to be due to lower body weight, more fatty tissue, and women under the age of 50 having a lesser first-pass effect—that is, lower gastric metabolism and/or alterations in enzymatic processes.

Although all body systems can be affected by alcohol abuse and dependence, the gastrointestinal, cardiovascular, central nervous, immune, musculoskeletal, and endocrine systems appear to be most vulnerable to damage from alcohol and other drugs. Gastrointestinal disturbances include gastritis, pancreatitis, hepatitis, cirrhosis, and colon cancer. Alcohol abuse and dependence depress immune function by altering the distribution and function of lymphoid cells and by disrupting cytokine regulation of lymphoid cell activities that may be a precursor to breast and other forms of cancer (Antai-Otong, 2006; Nolen-Hoeksema, 2004). Menstrual disorders have been reported following both alcohol and illegal drug use (Center for Substance Abuse, 1996).

Illnesses attributable to tobacco use include lung cancer; chronic lung disease; respiratory infections; heart disease; and esophageal, laryngeal, and other oral cancers (American Cancer Society, 1999). Tobacco-related deaths are higher in African American than White women. Women who smoke one pack of cigarettes per day throughout adulthood cut their bone density up to 10% by the time they reach menopause (Center for Substance Abuse, 1998). Smokers also tend to be drinkers—a deadly combination. Individuals who smoke and drink are 38 more times likely to develop mouth and throat cancer compared with those who do not combine the two substances (National Institute on Alcohol Abuse and Alcoholism, 1998).

Marijuana, cocaine, and heroin use are attributed to heart attacks, hypertension, strokes, malnutrition, suppressed immune function, AIDS, sexually transmitted diseases, hepatitis B and hepatitis C infections from intravenous injection sites, amenorrhea, and spontaneous abortion (Boyd, Phillips, & Dorsey, 2003). Much remains to be known about the impact of illicit drugs on women's health.

Prescribed psychoactive substances, particularly benzodiazepines, and when accompanied by alcohol use, puts women at risk for injury (Graham & Wilsnack, 2000). Even when prescribed and used according to directions, psychoactive drugs contribute to falls and are said to be accountable for 14% of all hip fractures in older women (Center for Substance Abuse, 1998).

Interpersonal and Social Consequences

Both alcohol and marijuana heighten the likelihood of unprotected intercourse (Boyd et al. 2003; Nolen-Hoeksema, 2004). Adolescent women who have used alcohol up to five times in the past month or marijuana three times in the past month were twice as likely to be sexually active and 25% less likely to use condoms than non–drug and alcohol users (Center for Substance Abuse, 1996).

The uses of cocaine, heroin, and methamphetamines have led to incarceration among women, particularly those who are poor, non-White, and have young children. Women who commit crimes are more likely to be using drugs at the time of the crime than nonusers (Center for Substance Abuse, 1996). Over 60% of incarcerated women have at least one child and up to 15% are pregnant at the time of incarceration.

The association between mental disorders and substance use is well established; however, some investigators have not documented which disorder is primary and which is secondary. Cyr and McGarry (2002) found that depression was present prior to alcohol abuse 30% of the time in their study sample. These authors also reported that suicide attempts were four times as high in alcoholic women compared with nonalcoholic women. African American women abstain from alcohol more frequently than White women, but, among those who meet dependence criteria and have been victimized as adults, have reported symptoms of post-traumatic stress disorder, panic attacks, and phobias (Boyd et al., 2003).

Consequences Among Pregnant Women and Women With Children of Alcohol, Tobacco, and Other Drugs

Substance abuse among pregnant women results in numerous consequences for both pregnant women and their children. Among pregnant women aged 15 to 44, nearly 10% reported drinking alcohol: 4% reported binge drinking in the past month. Binge drinking is defined as five or more drinks on the same drinking occasion at least 1 day in the past month. Eighteen percent of pregnant women in the survey smoked compared with 30.7% of nonpregnant women. Smoking was heaviest among 15- to 25-year-olds. Secondhand smoke is a significant threat to children (SAMHSA, 2005).

Among the 4 million women who get pregnant each year, rates of fetal alcohol syndrome are estimated at about 12,000 babies per year (National Institute on

Drug Abuse, 1996). Smoking accounts for 20% of all low–birth weight babies born in the United States (National Institute on Drug Abuse, 1996). Illicit drug use in the past month among pregnant 15- to 44-year-olds was 4.3% (SAMHSA, 2005).

Data show that women who use cocaine or heroin during pregnancy give birth to babies who are born prematurely; have lower birth weights; are tremulous, irritable, erratic sleepers; and unable to suck properly (Eyler, et al., 1998). Studies show that, by age two, cocaine-exposed children showed few developmental differences compared with those not so exposed. However, these children become easily overstimulated and function at lower cognitive levels than non-exposed children. These effects have been shown to persist into early childhood. Cocaine-exposed children need to work harder and need help focusing attention, remaining alert, and processing information (Eyler et al., 1998; Mayes, Grillon, Granger, & Schottenfeld, 1998).

Economic Consequences

Financial costs associated with substance abuse include costs associated with accidents and crime; use of emergency, health, and social services; and impaired work productivity. Health care costs to treat medical consequences of alcohol abuse alone costs $26 billion a year (Harwood, 2000). Among employed individuals, it is the problem drinkers rather than heavy drinkers who are responsible for 95% of alcohol-related costs in the work place, including lost productivity, absenteeism, injuries, and aggressive behavior (Frone, 2006; Institute of Medicine, 1990).

Most of the money spent for drug-exposed infants and children comes from their need for hospital care. The average hospital stay is 2 months (Huestis & Choo, 2002; Oei, Feller, & Lui, 2001). It has been estimated that the costs of foster care and special education for neurologic impairments could reach $750,000 per child by the time the child reaches 18 years of age. The costs of caring for children with fetal alcohol syndrome who are developmentally delayed are estimated to be $90 million (U.S. General Accounting Office, 1994).

A study by the Center for Substance Abuse (1998) showed that substance abuse among women over 60 years of age cost over $22 billion in Medicare, Medicaid, and private insurance in 1998. These costs are expected to rise dramatically as baby boomers reach age 60. The Center for Substance Abuse (1998) estimates that, at current rates of substance use, the annual health care cost of substance abuse among mature women will be $100 billion in 20 years.

In summary, the abuse of alcohol, tobacco, and other drugs—including prescription and over-the-counter—has serious consequences for women. Some encouraging findings come from prevention studies conducted over the past decade. However, the challenge of reducing the demand remains. The next section draws on empirical findings regarding risk and protective factors that precede substance use and show how these factors can be used in prevention.

Risk and Protective Factors Associated With Substance Use and Implications for Prevention

Risk factors are attributes of individuals or environments that increase the chances of developing a disorder and contribute to greater severity or longer duration of the disorder (Wheaton, 1985). Protective factors decrease the risk of disorders by reducing exposure to risk factors, disrupting important processes involved in the development of the disorder, and by interacting with the risk factor to reduce its effects (Wheaton, 1985). Three major types of risk and protective factors are biological, psychological, and social/environmental.

Biological risk factors are age, sex, ethnicity, genetic transmission, family history, personality disorders, and psychiatric disorders. Of these, genetic transmission, family history of disorders, and personal history of psychiatric disorders play a prominent role in initiation and continuation of substance use (Hawkins, Catalano, & Miller, 1992; SAMHSA, 2005).

Psychological risk factors are personality and coping styles—that is, sensation seeking, appraisal of substances as having no or minor consequences and even positive benefits, low self-esteem, lack of resistance skills, prior experimentation, and negative life events, such as child abuse, trauma, deaths of significant others (Pentz, 1994). For example, Kilpatrick and colleagues (1998), found that 29% of sexual assaults of women occurred by age 11, and 32% occurred between ages 11 and 17. The risk of lifetime alcohol dependence increased as a function of the number of lifetime assaults experienced. For 50% of the 638 assault victims who participated in the study, first alcohol consumption occurred within a year after the assault.

Older women who do not reduce drinking as they age may have other risk factors, such as friends' approval, engaging in avoidance coping strategies, deaths of significant others, depression, and isolation. These risk factors predict late-life drinking problems (Moos, Schutte, Brennan, & Moos, 2004).

Social Environment Risk Factors

Influences in this category include parental substance abuse, exposure to poor parenting practices, negative peer bonding, poor interpersonal relationships, lack of social support, negative educational experiences, easy access to substances, the changing of social and gender norms, economic and social incentives for drug trafficking, and exposure to drinking environments (Pentz, Bonnie, & Shopland, 1996).

A major risk factor for heterosexual women is their relationships with men who use substances (Henderson & Boyd, 1997), whereas for lesbian women, going to gay bars and clubs is a major influence (Hughes & Wilsnack, 1997). Women who have sex with other women are predicted to have higher injection drug use and higher prevalence of sexually transmitted diseases (Bell, Ompad, & Sherman, 2004) and may be at heightened risk for consequences of drinking (McCabe, Hughes, & Boyd, 2004).

Initiation of substance use may involve all three types of risk factors—biological, psychological, and social/environmental. Early age of onset was one of the most important predictors of movement from smoking and alcohol use to illegal drug use. A frequently mentioned concern in the literature is the narrowing of the gap between boys' and girls' ages of initiation of substance use (Cyr & McGarry, 2002; Greenfield, Manwani, & Nargiso, 2003). Among high school senior girls, crack cocaine users began smoking cigarettes at 10.6 years of age compared with 13.5 years for those who remained exclusively cigarette smokers (Kandel & Yamaguchi, 1993). A second predictor of movement to illegal use is the substance itself. Tobacco and alcohol use among women are important "gateway" substances—that is, those that lead to use of drugs that are costly and obtained illegally (SAMHSA, 2002).

Findings suggest that gender differences for both initiation and heavy substance use are associated with different perceptions of life problems and what the drugs did for the individual. Liu and Kaplan (1996) showed that young women used substances primarily because of personal problems, such as arguments with significant others, anger directed toward someone, and self-medication feelings of worthlessness and inadequacy.

Protective Factors

Mechanisms of protective factors work by decreasing the risk of disorders by reducing exposure to risk factors, disrupting processes involved in the development of the disorder, and interacting with risk factors to reduce their effects (Institute of Medicine, 1990). Differences in gender roles may be protective factors that prevent women from abusing substances at the same rates as men. For example, there are social sanctions against women's substance use; women tend to be more nurturing, less aggressive, and less sensation-seeking than men (Nolen-Hoeksema, 2004).

Events along the life course, such as pregnancy, may be protective factors. For example, a longitudinal study of 100 pregnant women addicted to heroin found that pregnancy led to cessation of drug use. The women had concerns about the development of their unborn babies and concerns regarding losing custody of their children (Nolen-Hoeksema, 2004). One of the protective factors regarding alcohol use is the benefit of moderate drinking among postmenopausal women in lowering the risk of coronary artery disease (Zakhari, 1997).

Linking Known Risk Factors With Prevention Programs

Outcome studies show reductions in substance use—that is, *prevention works* (Eggert et al., 1994, Holder, 1999; Kumpfer, 1998; Pentz, 1994). Changing situational and environmental factors show *how programs work.*

The Institute of Medicine (1994) identified three levels of prevention for alcohol, tobacco, and other drugs: universal, selective, and indicated. Universal prevention programs are "targeted to the general public or a whole population group that has not been identified on the basis of individual risk; i.e., the intervention is desirable for everyone in that group" (p. 24). Public education via the mass media and other sources can focus on the risks and consequences of the use of alcohol, tobacco, and other drugs, including risks to pregnant and childbearing women, such as smoking, which contributes to low–birth weight infants and secondhand smoke damage in children.

Selective prevention programs counteract risk factors and promote individual, social, and environmental protective factors. The hallmark of selective prevention programs is not the type of intervention, but who receives the intervention—that is, high-risk groups (Kumpfer, 1998). For example, a school-based intervention for 12-year-old girls demonstrated a faster increase over time on social assertiveness and a slower increase in initiation of substances (Lillehoj, Trudeau, Spoth, & Wickrama, 2004). Kumpfer (1998) initiated a "strengthening families" program that provides parent training, children's skill training, and family skills training to families who are at risk because of drug-abusing parents.

Prevention programs target those already manifesting known precursors of substance use and who are in need of help. Eggert and colleagues (1994) designed a school-based prevention program that targeted negative peer bonding—that is, encouraging involvement with peers who are successful in school rather than those who are skipping school.

Primary care providers can have roles in all three types of prevention. For example, they can point out television specials that feature risks of teenage drinking and referring clients and/or family members to support groups.

SCREENING, ASSESSMENT, BRIEF INTERVENTION, SPECIALIZED TREATMENT, AND RELAPSE PREVENTION

This section describes assessment and brief intervention techniques and continues with in-depth assessment and specialized treatment. It is organized by the algorithm Client Flow Through Primary Care and Referral (SAMHSA, 1997; see Figure 22.1). The algorithm was designed to exemplify at-risk drinkers, because alcohol abuse is commonly encountered in primary care practice, and treatment can be offered in the form of brief intervention. As Figure 22.1 shows, a positive screen and brief assessment can lead to either brief intervention or in-depth assessment followed by specialized treatment.

The Goal of Substance Abuse Screening

Screening identifies individuals who have begun to develop problems or are at high risk for problems. The goal of screening is to be able to say yes, there is a problem, or no, there is not (Institute of Medicine, 1994). Good screening tools possess understandable directions, are quick to administer, and demonstrate sensitivity (accuracy in problem identification) and specificity (ruling out those not affected) (Institute of Medicine, 1994). Many clinics use a standard health assessment form, but substance use and abuse questions are typically few in number, stated in a way that clients can give yes or no responses (do you drink?), or the questions are so direct that clients are offended by these items and may become defensive or provide untruthful replies.

Screening Techniques

An important contribution to the substance abuse field is the concept of motivational interviewing (Miller & Rollnick, 2002; SAMHSA, 1999). The principles derived from motivational interviewing have been shown to reduce client denial and resistance to change. Nonetheless, clinicians must be aware that they are asking for sensitive information that may be threatening to clients. Cooperation can be obtained by assuring the client of confidentiality, conveying a willingness to listen carefully, and showing respect. Clinicians need to know how to ask about quantity and frequency of substances used and the impact of use on the client's life situation. For example, if the clinician begins with the statement, "Tell me about the last time you drank alcohol," he or she is likely to establish more trust with the client than if she or he asks a series of direct questions, such as "How much beer or wine do you drink in a day? In a typical week?" "How much marijuana do you smoke in

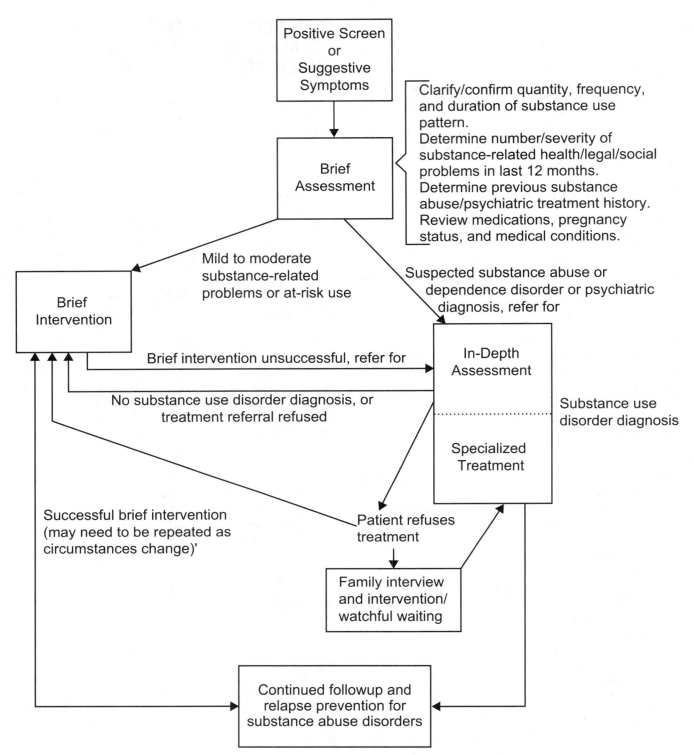

"If situation deteriorates over time, a referral for specialized treatment remain an option.

**Figure 22.1   A decision tree for substance abuse assessment, diagnosis, and
treatment for primary care clinicians.**
Derived from National Institute on Alcohol Abuse and Alcoholism, 1993.

a week?" "Have you ever used crack, heroin, or some form of speed?" If the first open-ended question stated above does not yield the quantity and frequency of substances used and consequences that may have followed, then the clinician can add a statement such as: "Tell me about the last time you were unable to fulfill your responsibilities because of substance use." Some clients will then volunteer information about relationship consequences, arrests for drunk driving, or job loss.

Screening Instruments for Varied Population Groups

A recommended test for adults is AUDIT (Alcohol Use Disorders Identification Test; Babor, de al Fuente, Saunders, & Grant, 1992)—a 10-item scale that can be self-administered or used in an interview. The time required for administration is 2 minutes and time for scoring is 1 minute. A user's manual is available, and AUDIT has been translated into several non-English languages.

A recommended screening instrument for adolescents 12 to 19 years of age is the POSIT (Problem-Oriented Screening Instrument for Teenagers; Gruenewald & Klitzner, 1991). The POSIT has 139 items (10 subscales), the yes/no format takes 20 minutes to administer, and has adequate validity and reliability.

All pregnant women should be asked about substance use, however, standardized tools are lacking. One suggested screening instrument for pregnant women is the TWEAK, a phonetic acronym for five questions: tolerance, worried, eye-opener, amnesia, and cut down (Russell, 1994). These items come from the CAGE questionnaire, which is more appropriate for chronic drinkers. The TWEAK has promising face validity but no tests of reliability.

A suggested screening instrument for older adults is the MAST-G (Michigan Alcoholism Screening Test—Geriatric Version), a 24-item test (Blow et al., 1992). The NIAAA Treatment Handbook Series 4 (National Institute of Alcohol Abuse and Alcoholism, 1998) contains additional suggested brief and in-depth screening instruments.

Brief Assessment

The goals of brief assessment may overlap with screening and are to confirm the intensity and duration of substance use; obtain a past history of substance abuse treatment and psychiatric treatment; and review current medications, pregnancy status, and health conditions (see Figure 22.1). The first goal is typically met by current screening tools, and the other two goals shown on Figure 22.1 are usually part of a primary care health assessment. Some indicators that have led to clients' successful behavior change are: a score of 8 or less on the AUDIT screening instrument and/or individuals with

moderate alcohol use, occasional use of marijuana, or questionable use of mood-altering prescription drugs. If the clinician does not have information about initiation and continuation of substance use, interference with role performance or other adverse consequences, then this information needs to be obtained prior to recommending or beginning brief intervention.

Brief Intervention

The goal of brief intervention is to help clients reduce or eliminate alcohol and drug consumption to prevent addiction to substances and address health problems that may have resulted from substance misuse (see Figure 22.1). Brief interventions can range from a few to 60 minutes, are usually conducted in two sessions, and consist of five steps: (1) Give feedback about screening results and make comparisons with adult drinking norms, risks, and current level of impairment; (2) inform the client about safe alcohol consumption and offer suggestions for change; (3) assess the client's readiness for change; (4) negotiate goals and strategies for change; and (5) arrange for a follow-up session, and, depending on the outcome, refer the client for in-depth assessment or specialized treatment. Some elements shown to enhance the success for each step of brief intervention are provided next.

Give Feedback About Screening Results and Make Comparisons With Adult Drinking Norms, Risks, and Current Level of Impairment

The clinician should interpret the findings of a current health assessment and alcohol, tobacco, and other drug screening for the client. Personalized feedback addresses misperceptions of how the client's substance use compares with that of one's peer group—for example, colleagues. Those receiving this normative feedback may be surprised that their consumption is higher than national norms, because close peers may have similar drinking styles (Anderson & Larimer, 2002). Concerns about potential or actual problems should be presented in a straightforward and nonjudgmental manner, such as, "at your current level of consumption of alcohol, you are at risk for accidents as well as the health problems we've been talking about"; "I'm concerned that your alcohol use is related to the reduction in bone density that we are currently seeing." Even when clinicians present screening results carefully, some clients may react with denial, resistance, anger, or shame. The clinician must be tolerant of the range of client reactions. Risk factors discussed in the previous section can be included in feedback, such as smoking, which should be considered high risk for adolescents and childbearing and child-rearing women.

Inform the Client About Safe Alcohol Consumption and Offer Suggestions for Change

The clinician can use the definition of low-risk drinking provided by the National Institute of Alcohol Abuse and Alcoholism—no more than one drink per day and never more than three drinks on one occasion for women. These guidelines need to be personalized; they need to be related to the woman's age, weight, current prescribed medication use, patterns of use (with or without food), metabolism, and other factors. There are no safe levels of illicit drug use.

Assess the Client's Readiness for Change

Most clients in primary care are in the first three phases of stages of change (Prochaska, DiClemente, & Norcross, 1992). These are precontemplation (client does not see substance use as a problem or does not want to change it), contemplation (client recognizes consequences of use, but is resistant to change), or preparation (willing to discuss options for change).

Negotiate Goals and Strategies for Change

This step assumes that the client is ready for change and that the client and clinician can work together to set goals and strategies. The clinician should first ask the client what seems realistic to her. Clinicians can suggest self-help manuals and should provide daily diary forms to assist clients in meeting goals to cut down on daily consumption or reduce the number of consumption occasions in a week or in a month.

Arrange for a Follow-Up Session, and, Depending on the Outcome, Refer the Client for In-Depth Assessment Or Specialized Treatment

A second session of brief intervention consists of reinforcing what was covered in the first session and monitoring the progress toward change. Depending on whether health status has been affected by substance use, medical conditions and chronic illnesses also need to be monitored.

The Efficacy of Brief Intervention

Findings from numerous empirical studies support the utility of brief, structured interventions in the treatment of alcohol, tobacco, and other drug use across age groups and conducted in primary care settings (Bien, Miller, & Tonnigan, 1993; Fleming et al., 1997, 1999; SAMHSA, 1997). Fleming and colleagues (1997, 1999) showed that two 15-minute physician-delivered counseling sessions significantly reduced excessive drinking, including binge drinking, 6 and 12 months later in a sample of adults from 18 to 60 years of age and in

adults 65 years of age and older. The intervention was more effective for women in the general adult sample and equally effective for both men and women in the study limited to older adults. Similarly, investigators have reported positive results when studying individually each of the five elements of brief intervention as described in the preceding section—for example, personalized feedback given to women (Neighbors, Larimer, & Lewis, 2004) and investigations of readiness to change among women (Brown, Melchoir, Slaughter, & Huba, 2005).

Smoking cessation has been shown to be successful when conducted by primary care providers; however, because many drinkers are also smokers and because nicotine has been shown to be highly addictive, tobacco use may be part of intensive treatment. The most effective interventions are behavioral: identifying high-risk situations; developing self-monitoring; and developing coping skills such as relaxation, exercise, and other diversion therapies (Flemming et al. 1997). Nicotine replacement therapies are also beneficial and include gum, patches, nasal sprays, and inhalers (Andrews & Tingen, 1999; Windsor et al., 1993). In a study of smoking cessation counseling with pregnant women, nurse practitioners and nutritionists in obstetric clinics had higher rates of success than other providers in other settings (Zapka et al., 2000).

In-Depth Assessment

In contrast to screening and brief assessment, in-depth assessment has multiple functions, including problem description; examination of risk factors specific to age, ethnicity, sexual orientation, and pregnancy; differential diagnosis; and motivating clients in the process of treatment decision making and goal setting (see Figure 22.1). The time involved is usually 90 to 120 minutes. In-depth assessment is necessary for clients whose brief assessment suggests compulsion to use substances, impaired control, the presence of personal and social problems, or for those for whom brief intervention was not successful. Referral to qualified substance abuse specialists is recommended unless the primary care health provider has advanced training.

Randall and colleagues (1999) suggested obtaining the following information from women on "landmark events": age of first intoxication, age of first drinking problem, and age of first treatment, if applicable. Saltz and Ames (1996) identified four "novel" indicators that were significant predictors of problems unique to women: having a high capacity for drinking alcohol (i.e., greater tolerance for alcohol without reaching a state of intoxication when compared with other women drinkers), seeking out a "wet" environment (i.e., selecting a restaurant that serves alcoholic beverages), planning opportunities to drink (i.e., if given the choice, going to a party instead of a movie), and the importance of family context (i.e., married to a drinker instead of a nondrinker).

Alcohol, tobacco, and other drug assessment of older women should include social and living situations, alcohol and prescription drug abuse, and the interactions between these classes of drugs and other prescribed medications. (See excellent primer by Weatherman & Crabb, 1999.)

Pregnant women need to be urged to participate in prenatal care and to obtain evaluations for treatment. Pregnant women are also at risk for violence, HIV, and sexually transmitted diseases. Infants born to women who smoke and use drugs also must be assessed carefully for fetal alcohol syndrome, withdrawal symptoms, and ongoing developmental delays (Kaltenbach, Berghella, & Finnegan, 1998; Plessinger & Woods, 1998; Streissguth, 1994).

Ethnicity is an important assessment consideration. For example, data show that Native American women are the heaviest drinkers compared with Whites, Blacks, Hispanics, and Asians (SAMHSA, 2005). Data also show that some African American women are heavy drinkers, are known heavy users of crack cocaine, and some use heroin (SAMHSA, 2005). Therefore, in-depth assessment needs to include screening for unprotected sex, weight loss, malnourishment, pregnancy, partner violence, HIV, sexually transmitted diseases, tuberculosis, hepatitis B, and suppressed immune function.

Assessment of Co-Occurring Disorders

Assessment and differential diagnosis of psychiatric disorders and substance use is an extremely complex process and requires advanced knowledge and skills. Because co-occurring disorders occur across the life span, clinicians must understand the developmental processes of adolescence, young, middle, and older adulthood as well as the substances of choice among each of these age groups by gender, ethnicity, and sexual orientation.

Similarly, clinicians can assess expected outcomes by asking clients about their preferred treatment setting; whether the client's views appear realistic in terms of coping skills, relapse risk, financial status, and life responsibilities; and whether the client's views are congruent with those of significant others. Finally, the clinician is advised to provide this feedback to the client and significant others.

Supplementing Assessment Results

Information supplemental to the client's data can be obtained from several sources discussed next. These sources are typically part of an in-depth assessment.

Significant Others

Clients should be asked to provide the names and contact information of at least one relative or close friend (collaterals). Informants can provide information about current alcohol, tobacco, and other drug use and whether these quantities and frequencies are consistent with the goals and strategies for change agreed upon by the client and clinician.

Physical Examination

Visual examination can reveal hand tremors, needle marks, agitation, and tissue damage associated with prolonged alcohol and other drug use and related trauma. The clinician can then observe clients for scars, bruises, and dislocated bones or joints. Palpitation can identify an enlarged liver.

Laboratory Tests

Potential sources of additional information used for comparison with client self-report are laboratory tests, including blood, urine, and hair. Blood tests include blood alcohol concentration, gamma-glutamyltransferase, and mean corpuscular volume (see Anton, Litten, & Allen, 1995, for a thorough review). Urinalysis provides an index of more recent or concurrent drug use, while hair analysis provides a long-term drug use history. Clients who have used drugs in the past 72 hours prior to assessment will screen positive. Marijuana can be detected in urine for up to 2 weeks prior to the last use (SAMHSA, 1997).

Timing of Assessments

One important aspect of timing involves determining when the last alcohol or other drug use occurred. Allen, Columbus, and Fertig (1995) suggested that measures less likely to be affected by alcohol or drug effects or withdrawal can be collected at the time of initial client contact. These assessment data include client demographic characteristics and legal history. Assessment factors that require a longer period of abstinence (i.e., 10 to 21 days) include mood state, multiple diagnoses, and tests of cognitive impairment. Referral to addiction specialists is necessary when primary care clinicians do not have advanced training and experience with addictions.

In-Depth Assessment Instruments

Currently, one in-depth assessment tool is designed specifically for women: the female version of the Addiction Severity Index (ASI-F; Brown, Frank, & Friedman, 1997). The ASI-F is based on the Addiction Severity

Index (McClellan et al., 1992), which is considered the gold standard of addiction assessment. The ASI-F is very similar to the ASI except that it has a section pertaining to women's issues, albeit mostly reproductive. The ASI-F, like the ASI, is comprehensive. Items include medical, psychiatric, employment, and legal status; family and social relationships; family history of alcohol and other drug use; and current and past history of alcohol and other drug use. The assessment must be conducted in person the first time it is administered. Phone interviews can be conducted thereafter. The person being assessed responds verbally to items. At the end of each section, the clinician administering the ASI-F records what are referred to as clinician confidence ratings. That is, the clinician provides his or her opinion of the client's understanding of the questions in the section being completed and assesses the client's degree of distortion to each response. The ASI has an extensive history of psychometric development.

Diagnosis

The two most commonly used diagnostic systems are the *DSM-IV* (American Psychiatric Association, 1994) and the *ICD-10* (World Health Organization, 1990). Both systems use a syndrome approach, which facilitates dependence being rated along a severity continuum and differentiates dependence from other negative consequences of drug and alcohol use. The syndrome approach considers how central drug use is to the individual, tolerance, withdrawal, the subjective awareness of the compulsive nature of use, and the cycle of relapse/return to use.

Establishing a primary and secondary diagnosis may be helpful for treatment planning as the clinical picture tends to run the course of the primary disorder (Rosenthal & Westreich, 1999).

Specialized Treatment

Specialized treatment can be characterized by duration, setting, and programming. Specialized treatment typically ranges from 30 to 180 days. Most inpatient treatment is 30 days or less, whereas programs for women and children are 180 days and sometimes longer. Settings include outpatient treatment, day treatment, inpatient treatment, long-term residential treatment, therapeutic communities where clients may reside for a year or more, and 12-step programs that are available on a daily basis. Programming has improved dramatically over the past decade. Many programs are manualized, and many treatment programs address multiple components of treatment, such as cognitive therapy, medication, individual counseling, and group therapy that addresses anger management, self-esteem, refusal skills, parenting, and vocational training. Subsequent paragraphs provide a rationale for specialized treatment (as

opposed to brief intervention), provide empirical findings of programs that achieve successful outcomes for clients, and cite some examples of innovation in women's treatment programming.

An initial treatment step for alcohol and other drug dependence is detoxification. Withdrawal from alcohol dependence can be life-threatening and is therefore a serious assessment concern (see Saitz, 1998, for an excellent primer on this topic). In contrast to alcohol, stimulants, opioids, and nicotine are accompanied by a great deal of physical discomfort, but these symptoms are not life-threatening except in cases of drug overdoses and some infections resulting from intravenous injection.

Cognitive-behavioral therapies are synonymous with psychosocial approaches and refer to all nonpharmacological interventions, such as coping and refusal skills training, interpersonal psychotherapy, and relapse prevention training. An advantage of cognitive-behavioral therapies is that they have widespread empirical support. A disadvantage is that not all clients have the motivation or ability to remain in treatment and obtain the known benefits (National Institute on Drug Abuse, 1999).

Medication therapies for both men and women have demonstrated efficacy among persons dependent on alcohol, nicotine, and opiates (Schnoll & Weaver, 1998). There are no known successful medications to treat cocaine addiction. Methadone and levo-alpha-acetylmethadol have become treatments of choice in heroin addiction, with concurrent psychotherapy strongly recommended (National Institute on Drug Abuse, 1999).

Women's Admission to Specialized Addiction Treatment

The following data come from the Drug and Alcohol Services Information System (SAMHSA, 2005) and refer to the year 2002. Women accounted for 30% of substance abuse treatment admissions, compared with 61% reported users of alcohol and illicit drugs for whom treatment would likely benefit. Female admissions were more likely than male admissions to be for treatment for cocaine and opiate abuse; however, alcohol was the primary substance reported by both women and men. Women self-referred themselves for treatment more frequently than men, whereas men were more frequently referred by the criminal justice system. Therefore, primary care practitioners can be instrumental in helping clients select a program that best meets clients' needs. At the time of entry into treatment, only 23% of women were employed full- or part-time. Treatment costs for women came from self-payment, Medicaid or Medicare, and other government payments. Outpatient treatment was the most common setting: 64% for women and 59% for men. Equal percentages (18%) of men and women were admitted to residential treatment.

The Effects of Treatment Completion and Length of Stay (Retention) on Client Outcomes

Treatment completion, regardless of type of treatment, is associated with positive client outcomes and is less costly to society than no treatment (Beutler, Zetzer, & Yost, 1997; Ettner et al., 2006; Knight, Logan, & Simpson, 2001; National Institute on Drug Abuse, 1999). The longer women remain in treatment, the better the outcome, so the goal is to reduce barriers to treatment such as perceived stigma, lack of motivation for treatment, lack of child care, and lack of financial resources (Britt, Knisley, Dawson, & Schnoll, 1995; Knight et al., 2001).

In most cases, the primary client outcome is posttreatment abstinence from alcohol and drugs. This is because clients who enter specialized treatment are more likely to lack control of alcohol use, more likely to be polydrug users, and more likely to have experienced negative outcomes because of substance use than clients for whom brief interventions are successful (Ashley, Mardsen, & Brady, 2003; Greenfield et al., 2004).

Green and colleagues (2004) used the Addiction Severity Index subscale data to predict treatment outcomes by gender. Outcomes for women were more likely to be predicted by social, sociodemographic, and life-history characteristics rather than medical conditions, severity of addiction, and mental health problems. For abstinence outcomes, women who completed treatment were nine times as likely to be abstinent at 7-month follow-up as other women; men who completed were three times more likely to be abstinent than other men.

Women-Only Versus Mixed-Gender Treatment

This has been a controversial issue for two decades without any firm conclusions drawn. Kaskutas and colleagues (2005) conducted a randomized clinical trial comparing treatment programs that were community based, hospital based, mixed gender, and for women exclusively. No significant differences were found between women's and mixed-gender programs, abstinence rates were similar, and the hospital-based programs were twice as expensive as community-based programs. These gender-based studies suggest that it may be program features rather than gender-based treatment per se that facilitates successful treatment outcomes for women.

Sun (2006) reviewed 36 empirical studies to determine treatment factors that led to completion of treatment and abstinence. Six studies showed advantages to women in women-only treatment programs; however, Sun noted methods limitations that prevented her from drawing firm conclusions about gender-based treatment: the lack of randomized controlled designs, lack of consistent definitions for treatment factors and outcomes, small sample sizes, lack of thorough program descriptions, and lack of thorough statistical analyses.

Treatment Programs for Pregnant and Parenting Women

Drug treatment programs for pregnant and parenting women have been a high national priority since the late 1980s. Many women and their children are homeless or live in poverty, psychiatric comorbidity among the mothers is high, and few supports are available. Some children are developmentally delayed and exhibit short- and long-term effects of the teratogenic nature of alcohol and drugs. Identifying and providing prevention services to children through drug treatment facilities that house the mothers has been shown to be highly beneficial for both parents and children (Conners, Bradley, Whiteside-Mansell, & Crone, 2001; Kumpfer, 1998). Parent stress and depression are reduced, parents remain in treatment longer if their children are receiving services, and children have better outcomes than children not receiving services (Kumpfer, 1998). Moreover, the financial costs to society are extremely high among pregnant and parenting women. Retention in treatment appears to be a crucial factor for pregnant and parenting women. Many women entering these programs are ethnically diverse, and many are addicted to cocaine and heroin. In one study, postdischarge abstinence rates for women who remained in a treatment program for 91 to 181 days were 68% to 71%, whereas women who stayed in treatment for 1 to 30 days experienced postdischarge abstinence rates of 21% to 25% (Greenfield et al., 2004).

In a study by Connors and colleagues (2001), many aspects of treatment recommended by the National Institute on Drug Abuse (1999) were included. The authors compared 72 women enrolled in a women's and children's program that involved both preschool and school-age children. Multiple outcomes were examined for both women and children, and follow-up data were collected 3, 6, and 12 months later. Women who completed the program had significantly lower relapse rates and significantly higher parenting skills, family interaction skills, and rates of employment compared with women in the early and late dropout groups. Young children of women who completed the program had lower indications of developmental delay, and older children had significantly higher drug refusal skills when compared to the children of early and late dropouts. Most women were single African American mothers for whom crack cocaine was the drug of choice. Treatment completion, comprehensive programming, follow-up, and testing of multiple outcomes were important features of the study. The results demonstrate that women who are difficult to treat benefit from comprehensive, long-term programming.

Treatment of Co-Occurring Disorders

Prevalence rates for both mental disorders and substance abuse are high: 13.7% nationally. Among those seeking treatment, prevalence rates are even higher:

20% to 50%. Common Axis I and II disorders are borderline personality, depression, and bipolar disorder (Rosenthal & Westreich, 1999). Childhood physical and sexual abuse, interpersonal violence, and other traumatic experiences have all been shown to be antecedents to substance abuse (Stewart, 1996). Both substance abuse and mental disorders must be treated; however, there is controversy about which treatments should come first. According to Stewart (1996), some clinicians view alcohol use as secondary to post-traumatic stress disorder and assume drinking will normalize following treatment for trauma symptoms. Because many women affected by trauma are binge drinkers, other authorities suggest that binge drinking should be treated first. Still others suggest integrated treatment (Rosenthal & Westreich, 1999).

Treatment for Women in the Criminal Justice System

Women of all ages, ethnic backgrounds, and sexual preference with drug use histories are entering the criminal justice system at alarming rates, primarily for criminal activity associated with drug-seeking behavior. Some innovative programs have been proposed, such as relapse prevention, strengthening women's support networks, and follow-up after leaving prison (Grella, Stein, & Greenwell, 2005). Haack and colleagues (2005) are conducting a pilot study using online counseling for court-involved parents who have been charged with child abuse and neglect related to substance abuse. Key family members agree to work with the client in their shared environments and provide feedback on client progress. Online counseling, if shown to be effective, can help fill the gap between those needing (13 million) and those receiving (3 million) treatment.

Adolescent Intensive Treatment

Treatment efficacy data for adolescents is sparse and not gender specific. Predictors of good treatment outcomes for adolescents are motivation; perceived choice in seeking treatment; rapport with treatment staff; provision of educational, vocational, and recreational services; broad-spectrum behavioral substance abuse treatment; and parental involvement (Dennis, 2002). In contrast, early onset of drug use, criminal history, problem severity, and perceived family control are predictors of poor outcomes. Relapse rates are high and vary from 39% for girls and 60% for boys (Dennis, 2002).

Elder-Specific Addictions Treatment

This is an emerging treatment modality that has shown positive results (see Fleming et al., 1999; Graham et al., 1995). Graham and colleagues (1995) found that many elderly respond to the same behavioral strategies that

are successful for young and middle-aged adults—that is, functional analysis of drinking behavior, identification of high-risk situations, drink refusal skills, and self-monitoring skills. However, Graham et al. (1995) also noted that older adults require individual instead of group therapy; management of depression; vastly improved social networks; and attention to physical health status, cognitive skills, motivation, and transportation.

Relapse and Relapse Prevention

Relapse prevention is a self-management program designed to enhance the maintenance phase of the habit change process (Marlatt & Gordon, 1985). Relapse prevention begins during specialized treatment and continues thereafter (see Figure 22.1). Relapse rates typically range from 60% to 80% for most substances, with negative mood states (anger, boredom, frustration, and depression) accounting for 35% of initial abstinence failures. Interpersonal conflict and social pressure each account for about 20% of relapses (Marlatt & Gordon, 1985). Therefore, relapse prevention is an essential component of treatment and begins with helping the client to recognize high-risk situations. Relapse prevention is based on social learning theory that provides information and skill building on the coping response, lifestyle balance, and managing slips and lapses not as major life events, but as part of a journey of learning new behaviors (Marlatt & Gordon, 1985; Marlatt & Donovan, 2005).

Several groups of women at high risk for relapse have been identified. These are women whose partners or spouses continue substance use when the woman is attempting to abstain, women with co-occuring disorders, and lesbian women for whom gay bars and clubs are an important social environment. A history of trauma-related post-traumatic stress disorder increases the risk for relapse because its three-symptom clusters, that is, re-experiencing the event, intrusive thoughts, and hyperarousal, may interfere with recovery.

Relapse risks continue after treatment and when clients have returned to primary care. Primary care clinicians have the opportunity to continue to assess relapse risks and help clients avoid risk-taking behavior. Some collaborative approaches to relapse prevention are self-monitoring, identifying social network support, and encouraging ongoing involvement with women's peer support groups.

LEGAL AND ETHICAL CONSIDERATIONS AND IMPLICATIONS FOR SOCIAL AND HEALTH POLICY

The identification of reportable situations is both a legal and ethical issue. Primary care clinicians are sometimes reluctant to report illegal drug use because the consequence will likely be loss of custody of a child or children. Some clinicians believe that alcohol, tobacco, and other drug problems are incorrigible and that they might not have the skills to facilitate behavior change. Women who are faced with losing custody of children and/or criminal prosecution may accept substance abuse treatment as an alternative.

An ethical issue is whether drug-addicted women use scarce resources and deprive others of needed services. In one national demonstration project, women were recommended for and received more services than men for acute non-HIV-related medical services (31% vs. 21%), nutritional services (45% vs. 33%), immunizations (14% vs. 6%), dental services (12% vs. 7%), and psychiatric services (15% vs. 9%) (Roland, 1999). One argument favoring provision of services to individuals who use drugs is its cost effectiveness. For example, the average cost of 1 year of methadone maintenance treatment is $4,700 per client, whereas 1 year of prison treatment costs $18,000 (National Institute on Drug Abuse, 1999). On the other hand, a cost analysis conducted by the Center for Substance Abuse (1998) showed that Medicare, Medicaid, and private insurance costs for women over the age of 59 who abuse substances was $22.3 billion in 1998.

The implications for social and health policies resulting from the information presented in this chapter are profound. Much remains to be done. Some policy priorities are considered next.

Combat Stigma, Reduce Barriers to Treatment, and Provide More Comprehensive Services

As has been pointed out, social norms make substance abuse far more stigmatizing for women than for men, which affects policies regarding treatment availability. Many programs, particularly those that serve the poor and most disadvantaged, have long waiting lists for admission. Current barriers to treatment include lack of appropriate treatment, cost, lack of child care, and other needed services (Haack, 1997).

Change the Social Construction of How Society Views Women

Both the media and product marketing cater to youth, attractiveness, and the glamorization of alcohol and tobacco. Full-page advertisements particularly for alcoholic beverages found in fashion, gourmet cooking, home decorating, and travel magazines, substantiate this observation.

Educate Health Care Providers

Funds for training providers particularly in primary care need to be available to nursing, medical, social work, and other health professional schools. Licensing and certification bodies need to require substance abuse experience as part of health professional education, including continuing education.

Research

Much has been learned about women's substance use in the past two decades. However, more funding—both public and private—needs to be available for the examination of such topics as smoking and weight loss; polydrug use; the health consequences of alcohol, tobacco, and other drug use; prevention and intervention strategies; and relapse among women with attention to age and ethnicity.

CONCLUSION

Substance abuse is prevalent among women of all ages and is highly detrimental to health and well-being. Some important antecedents such as family history of substance use, early childhood abuse and trauma, and psychiatric conditions put women at high risk for early initiation and continuation of substance use. The necessity and advantages of gender-specific treatment are inconclusive. However, many of the prevention and intervention strategies presented in this chapter have demonstrated efficacy and can be recommended. Nonetheless, much additional research is needed and much remains to be done regarding women's health policy development, implementation, and evaluation.

REFERENCES

Allen, J. P., Columbus, M., & Fertig, J. B. (1995). Assessment in alcoholism treatment: An overview. In J. P. Allen & M. Columbus (Eds.), *Assessing alcohol problems: A guide for clinicians and researchers* (pp. 1–9). Treatment Handbook Series, No. 4. Bethesda, MD: National Institute on Alcohol Abuse and Alcoholism.

American Cancer Society. (1999). *Quitting smoking.* Washington, DC: Author.

American Psychiatric Association. (1994). *Diagnostic and statistical manual of mental disorders* (4th ed.). Washington, DC: Author.

Anderson, B. K., & Larimer, M. E. (2002). Problem drinking and the workplace: An individualized approach to prevention. *Psychology of Addictive Behaviors, 16,* 243–251.

Andrews, J., & Tingen, M. S. (1999). Nicotine addiction: Current treatment options. *Journal of Addictions Nursing, 11*(1), 3–12.

Antai-Otong, D. (2006). Women and alcoholism: Gender-related medical complications: Treatment considerations. *Journal of Addictions Nursing, 17,* 33–45.

Anton, R. F., Litten, R. Z., & Allen, J. P. (1995). Biological assessment of alcohol consumption. In J. P. Allen & M. Columbus (Eds.), *Assessing alcohol problems: A guide for clinicians and researchers* (pp. 31–40). Treatment Handbook Series, No. 4. Bethesda, MD: National Institute on Alcohol Abuse and Alcoholism.

Ashley, O. S, Marsden, M. E., & Brady, T. M. (2003). Effectiveness of substance abuse treatment programming for women. A review. *American Journal of Drug and Alcohol Abuse, 29*(1), 19–53.

Babor, T. F., de la Fuente, J. R., Saunders, J., & Grant, M. (1992). *AUDIT: The Alcohol Use Disorders Identification Test: Guidelines for use in primary health care.* Geneva, Switzerland: World Health Organization.

Bell, A. V., Ompad, D., & Sherman, S. (2004). Sexual and drug-risk behaviors among women who have sex with women. *American Journal of Public Health, 96*(6), 1066–1072.

Beutler, L. E., Zetzer, H., & Yost, E. (1997). Tailoring interventions to clients: Effects on engagement and retention. In L. S. Onken, J. D. Blaine, & J. J. Boren (Eds.), *Beyond the therapeutic alliance: Keeping the drug dependent individual in treatment* (pp. 85–109). NIDA Research Monograph No. 165. Rockville, MD: National Institute on Drug Abuse.

Bien, T. H., Miller, W. R., & Tonigan, J. S. (1993). Brief interventions for alcohol problems: A review. *Addiction, 88,* 315–335.

Blow, F. C., Brower, K. J., Schulengerg, J. E., Demo-Dananberg, L. M., Young, J. P., & Beresford, T. P. (1992). The Michigan Alcoholism Screening Test—Geriatric Version (MAST-G): A new elderly specific screening instrument. *Alcoholism: Clinical and Experimental Research, 16,* 372.

Boyd, M. R., Phillips, K., & Dorsey, C. J. (2003). Alcohol and other drug disorders, comorbidity, and violence: Comparison of rural African American and Caucasian women. *Archives of Psychiatric Nursing, 17*(6), 247–289.

Britt, G. C., Knisley, J. S., Dawson, K. S., & Schnoll, S. H. (1995). Attitudes toward recovery and completion of a substance abuse treatment program. *Journal of Substance Abuse Treatment, 12,* 349–353.

Brown, E., Frank, D., & Friedman, A. (1997). *Supplementary administration manual for the expanded female version of the Addiction Severity Index (ASI) instrument, The ASI-F.* DHSH Publication No. SMA 96-8056. Rockville, MD: Center for Substance Abuse Treatment, Office of Evaluation, Scientific Analysis and Synthesis.

Brown, V. B., Melchior, L. A., Slaughter, R., & Huba, G. J. (2005). Stages of multiple behavior change as a function of readiness for substance abuse treatment among women at risk. *Journal of Addictions Nursing, 16*(1–2), 23–30.

Center for Substance Abuse. (1996). *Substance abuse and the American woman.* New York: Columbia University Press.

Center for Substance Abuse. (1998). *Under the rug: Substance abuse and the mature woman.* New York: Columbia University Press.

Conners, N. A., Bradley, R. H., Whiteside-Mansell, L., & Crone, C. C. (2001). A comprehensive substance abuse treatment program for women and their children: An initial evaluation. *Journal of Substance Abuse Treatment, 21,* 67–75.

Curry, S. J., Ludman, E., Grothaus, L., Donovan, D., Kim, E., & Fishman, P. (2000). At-risk drinking among clients making routine primary care visits. *Preventive Medicine, 31,* 595–602.

Cyr, M. G., & McGarry, K. A. (2002). Alcohol use disorders in women. Screening methods and approaches to treatment. *Postgraduate Medicine, 112,* 31–32, 39–40, 43–47.

Dennis, M. L. (2002, May). Treatment research on adolescent drug and alcohol abuse. *Connections.* Washington, DC: Academy for Health Services Research and Health Policy.

Eggert, L. L., et al. (1994). Preventing adolescent drug abuse and high school dropout through an intensive school-based social network development program. *American Journal of Health Promotion, 8*(3), 202–215.

Ettner, S. L., Huang, D., Evans, E., et al. (2006). Benefit-cost in the California treatment outcome project: Does treatment "pay for itself"? *Health Services Research, 41,* 192–213.

Eyler, F. D., Behnke, M., Conlon, M., Woos, N. S., & Wobie, K. (1998). Birth outcome from a prospective, matched study of prenatal crack cocaine use. Interactive and dose effects on neurobehavioral assessment. *Pediatrics, 101,* 237–241.

Fleming, M. F., Barry, K. L., Manwell, L. B., Johnson, K., et al. (1997). Brief physician advice for problem alcohol drinkers: A randomized controlled trial in community-based primary care practices. *Journal of the American Medical Association, 277,* 1039–1045.

Fleming, M. F., Manwell, L. B., Barry, K. L., Adams, W., & Stauffacher, E. A. (1999). Brief physician advice for alcohol problems in older adults. *Journal of Family Practice, 48*(5), 378–384.

Frone, M. R. (2006). Prevalence and distribution of alcohol use and impairment in the workplace: A U.S. national survey. *Journal of Studies on Alcohol, 67*(1), 147–157.

Graham, K., Saunders, S. J., Flower, M. C., Timney, C. B., White-Campbell, M., & Pietrapaolo, A. Z. (1995). *Addictions treatment for older adults: Evaluation of an innovative client-centered approach.* Binghamton, NY: Haworth Press.

Graham, K., & Wilsnack, S. C. (2000). The relationship between alcohol problems and use of tranquilizing drugs: Longitudinal patterns among American women. *Addictive Behaviors, 25*(1), 13–28.

Green, C. A., Polen, M. R., Lynch, F. L., Dickinson, D. M., & Bennett, M. D. (2004). Gender differences in outcomes in an HMO-based substance abuse treatment program. *Journal of Addictive Disease, 23*(20), 47–70.

Greenfield, L., Burgdorf, K., Chen, X., Pororwski, A., Roberts, T., & Herrel, J. (2004). Effectiveness of long-term residential substance abuse treatment for women: Findings from three national studies. *American Journal of Drug and Alcohol Abuse, 30*(3), 537–550.

Greenfield, S. F., Manwani, S. G., & Nargiso, J. E. (2003). Epidemiology of substance use disorders in women. *Obstetrical Gynecological Clinics of North America, 30*(3), 413–446.

Grella, C. E., Stein, J. A., & Greenwell, L. (2005). Associations among childhood trauma, adolescent problem behaviors, and adverse adult outcomes in substance-abusing women offenders. *Psychology of Addictive Behaviors, 19*(1), 43–53.

Gruenewald, P. J., & Klitzner, M. (1991). Results of a preliminary POSIT analyses. In E. Radhert (Ed.), *Adolescent Assessment/ Referral System Manual* (DHHS Pub. No. [ADM] 91-1735). Rockville, MD: National Institute on Drug Abuse.

Haack, M. R. (1997). Drug-dependent mothers and their children. *Issues in public policy and public health.* New York: Springer Publishing.

Haack, M. R., Burda-Cohee, C., Alemi, F., Harge, A., Dill, R., & Benson, L. (2005). Facilitating self-management of substance use disorders with online counseling: The intervention and study design. *Journal of Addictions Nursing, 16*(1–2), 41–46.

Harwood, H. (2000). *Updated estimates of the economic costs of alcohol abuse in the United States: Estimates, update methods, and data.* Report prepared by The Lewin Group for the National Institute on Alcohol Abuse and Alcoholism, Falls Church, VA.

Hawkins, J. D., Catalano, R. F., & Miller, J. Y. (1992). Risk and protective factors for alcohol and other drug problems in adolescence and early adulthood: Implications for substance abuse prevention. *Psychological Bulletin, 112*(1), 64–105.

Henderson, D., & Boyd, C. (1997). All my buddies was male: Relationship issues of addicted women. *Journal of Obstetric, Gynecologic, and Neonatal Nursing, 26*(4), 469–476.

Holder, H. D. (1999). Prevention aimed at the environment. In B. S. McCrady and E. E. Epstein (Eds.), *Addictions: A comprehensive guidebook* (pp. 573–594). New York: Oxford University Press.

Huestis, M. I., & Choo, R. E. (2002). Drug abuse's smallest victims: In utero drug exposure. *Forensic Science International, 128*(1–2), 20–30.

Hughes, T. L., & Wilsnack, S. C. (1997). Use of alcohol among lesbians: Research and clinical implications. *American Journal of Orthopsychiatry, 67*(1), 20–36.

Institute of Medicine. (1990). *Broadening the base of treatment for alcohol problems.* Washington, DC: National Academy Press.

Institute of Medicine. (1994). *Reducing risks for mental disorders: Frontiers for preventive intervention research.* Washington, DC: National Academy Press.

Kaltenbach, K., Berghella, V., & Finnegan, L. (1998). Opioid dependence during pregnancy. *Obstetrical Gynecological Clinics of North America, 25*(1), 139–151.

Kandel, D. B., & Yamaguchi, K. (1993). From beer to crack. *American Journal of Public Health, 83*, 851–855.

Kaskutas, L. A., Zhang, L., French, M. T., & Witbrodt, J. (2005). Women's programs versus mixed-gender day treatment: Results from a randomized study. *Addiction, 100*(1), 60–69.

Kilpatrick, D. G., Resnick, H. S., Saunders, B. E., & Best, C. L. (1998). Victimization, posttraumatic stress disorder, and substance use and abuse among women. In C. L. Wetherington & A. B. Roman (Eds.), *Drug addiction research and the health of women.* (pp. 285–307). NIH Pub. No. 98-4290. Rockville, MD: National Institute on Drug Abuse.

Knight, D. K., Logan, S. M., & Simpson, D. D. (2001). Predictors of program completion for women in residential substance abuse treatment. *American Journal of Drug and Alcohol Abuse, 27*(1), 1–18.

Kumpfer, K. L. (1998). Selective prevention interventions: The strengthening families program. In R. S. Ashery, E. B. Robertson, & K. L. Kumpfer (Eds.), *Drug abuse prevention through family interventions.* NIDA Research Monograph #177 (pp. 160–297). Rockville, MD: National Institute on Drug Abuse.

Lillehoj, C. J., Trudeau, L., Spoth, R. Wickrama, K. A. (2004). Internalizing, social competence, and substance initiation: Influence of gender moderation and a preventive intervention. *Substance Use and Misuse, 39*(6), 963–991.

Liu, X., & Kaplan, H. (1996). Gender-related differences in circumstances surrounding initiation and escalation of alcohol and other substance use/abuse. *Deviant Behavior: An Interdisciplinary Journal, 17*, 71–106.

Manwell, L. B., Fleming, M. F., Johnson, K., & Barry, K. L. (1998). Tobacco, alcohol, and drug use in a primary care sample: 90-day prevalence and associated factors. *Journal of Addictive Diseases, 17*, 67–81.

Marlatt, G. A., & Donovan, D. (2005). *Relapse prevention: Maintenance strategies in the treatment of addictive behaviors* (2nd ed.). New York: Guilford Press.

Marlatt, G. A., & Gordon, J. R. (1985). *Relapse prevention: Maintenance strategies in the treatment of addictive behaviors.* New York: Guilford Press.

Mayes, L., Grillon, C., Granger, R., & Schottenfeld, R. (1998). Regulation of arousal and attention in preschool children exposed to cocaine prenatally. *Annals of the New York Academy of Sciences, 846*, 126–143.

McCabe, S. E., Hughes, T. L., & Boyd, C. J. (2004). Substance use and misuse: Are bisexual women at greater risk? *Journal of Psychoactive Drugs, 36*(2), 217–225.

McLellan, A. T., Kushner, H., Metzger, D., Peters, R., Smith, I., Grissom, G., Pettinati, H., & Argeriou, M. (1992). The fifth addition of the Addiction Severity Index. *Journal of Substance Abuse Treatment, 9*, 199–213.

Miller, W. R., & Rollnick, S. (2002). *Motivational interviewing: Preparing people for change* (2nd ed.). New York: Guilford Press.

Moos, R. H., Schutte, K., Brennan, P., & Moos, B. S. (2004). Ten year patterns of alcohol consumption and drinking problems among older women. *Addiction, 99*(7), 829–838.

National Institute on Alcohol Abuse and Alcoholism. (1998). *Assessing alcohol problems. A guide for clinicians and researchers.* NIAAA Treatment Handbook Series #4. Rockville, MD: Author.

National Institute on Drug Abuse. (1996). *National pregnancy and health survey: Drug use among women delivering live births, 1992.* Rockville, MD: Author.

National Institute on Drug Abuse. (1999). *Principles of drug addiction treatment. A research-based guide.* NIH Publication No. 99-4180. Rockville, MD: National Institute on Drug Abuse.

National Institute on Drug Abuse. (2006). *Monitoring the future survey.* Bethesda, MD: Author.

Neighbors, C., Larimer, M. E., & Lewis, M. A. (2004). Targeting misperceptions of descriptive drinking norms: Efficacy of a computer-delivered personalized normative feedback intervention. *Journal of Consulting & Clinical Psychology, 72*(3), 434–447.

Nolen-Hoeksema, S. (2004). Gender differences in risk factors and consequences for alcohol use and problems. *Clinical Psychology Review, 24*(8), 981–1010.

Oei, J., Feller, J. M., & Lui, K. (2001). Coordinating outpatient care of the narcotic-dependent infant. *Journal of Paediatric Child Health, 37*(3), 266–270.

Pentz, M. A. (1994). Adaptive evaluation strategies for estimating effects of community-based drug abuse prevention programs. *Journal of Community Psychology, 22*(1), 26–51.

Pentz, M. A., Bonnie, R. J., & Shopland, D. S. (1996). Integrating supply and demand reduction strategies for drug abuse prevention. *American Behavioral Scientist, 39*(7), 897–910.

Plessinger, M. A., & Woods, J. R. (1998). Cocaine in pregnancy. *Obstetrical Gynecological Clinics of North America, 25*(1), 99–118.

Prochaska, J. O., DiClemente, C. C., & Norcross, J. C. (1992). In search of how people change: Applications to addictive behaviors. *American Psychologist, 47*, 1102–1114.

Randall, C. L., Roberts, J. S., Del Boca, F. K., Carroll, K. M., Connors, G. J., & Mattson, M. E. (1999). Telescoping of landmark events associated with drinking: A gender comparison. *Journal of Studies on Alcohol, 60*, 252–260.

Roland, E. J. (1999). Health services needs among male and female methadone treatment clients: Findings from a national demonstration project. *Journal of Addictions Nursing, 11*(2), 61–69.

Rosenthal, R. N., & Westreich, L. (1999). Treatment of persons with dual diagnoses of substance use disorder and other psychological problems. In B. S. McCrady & E. E. Epstein (Eds.), *Addictions: A comprehensive guidebook* (pp. 439–476). New York: Oxford University Press.

Russell, M. (1994). New assessment tools for drinking in pregnancy: T-ACE, TWEAK, and others. *Alcohol, Health, and Research World, 18*(1), 55–61.

Saitz, R. (1998). Introduction to alcohol withdrawal. *Alcohol, Health, & Research World, 22*(1), 5–12.

Saltz, R., & Ames, G. (1996). Combining methods to identify new measures of women's drinking problems. Part II. The survey stage. *Addiction, 91,* 1041–1051.

Schnoll, S. H., & Weaver, M. F. (1998). Pharmacology: Gender-specific considerations in the use of psychoactive medications. In C. L. Wetherington & A. B. Roman (Eds.), *Drug addiction research and the health of women* (pp. 223–227). NIH Pub. No. 98-4290. Rockville, MD: National Institute on Drug Abuse.

Stewart, S. H. (1996). Alcohol abuse in individuals exposed to trauma: A critical review. *Psychological Bulletin, 120,* 83–112.

Streissguth, A. P. (1994). A long-term perspective of FAS. *Alcohol, Health, & Research World, 18*(1), 74–81.

Substance Abuse and Mental Health Services Administration, Office of Applied Studies. (1997). *A guide to substance abuse services for primary care clinicians.* Rockville, MD: Author.

Substance Abuse and Mental Health Services Administration, Office of Applied Studies. (1999). *Enhancing motivation for change in substance abuse treatment.* Rockville, MD: Author.

Substance Abuse and Mental Health Services Administration, Office of Applied Studies. (2002). *National household survey on drug abuse: Population estimates 2000.* Rockville, MD: Author.

Substance Abuse and Mental Health Services Administration, Office of Applied Studies. (2005a). *The DASIS Report for 2000.* Rockville, MD: Author.

Substance Abuse and Mental Health Services Administration, Office of Applied Studies. (2005b). *The National Survey on Drug Abuse and Health for 2003.* Rockville, MD: Author.

Sun, A. P. (2006). Program factors related to women's substance abuse treatment, retention, and other outcomes. *Journal of Substance Abuse Treatment, 30*(1), 1–20.

U.S. Department of Health and Human Services. (2000). *Healthy People 2010: With understanding and improving health and objectives for improving health.* (2nd ed., 2 vols.). Washington, DC: U.S. Government Printing Office.

U.S. General Accounting Office. (1994). *Foster care: Parental drug abuse has alarming impact on young children.* Washington, DC: Author.

Weatherman, R., & Crabb, D. W. (1999). Alcohol and medication interactions. *Alcohol, Research, & Health, 23*(1), 40–54.

Wheaton, B. (1985). Models for the stress-buffering functions of coping resources. *Journal of Health and Social Behavior, 26,* 352–365.

Windsor, R. A., Lowe, J. B., Perkins, L. L., Smith-Yoder, D., Artz, L., Crawford, M., Amburgy, K., & Boyd, N. R. (1993). Health education for pregnant smokers: Its behavioral impact and cost benefit. *American Journal of Public Health, 83*(2), 201–206.

World Health Organization. (1990). *International Classification of Diseases* (10th rev.). Geneva, Switzerland: Author.

Zakhari, S. (1997). Alcohol and the cardiovascular system. Molecular mechanisms for beneficial and harmful action. *Alcohol, Health, & Research World, 21*(1), 21–29.

Zapka, J. G., Pbert, L., Stoddard, A. M., Ockene, S. K., Goins, K., & Bonollo, D. (2000). Smoking cessation counseling with pregnant and postpartum women: A survey of community health center providers. *American Journal of Public Health, 90*(1), 78–84.

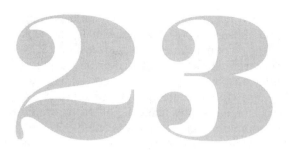

Violence Against Women

Kären Landenburger and
Jacquelyn C. Campbell

Violence against women is pervasive in U.S. society, occurring in all socioeconomic and ethnic groups. The causes, consequences, and remedies of violence must be seen within the context of a society that permits violence and fails to punish adequately those who perpetrate crimes against women—a society that permits treating women as a commodity or an object that must be dominated. Violence against women can be conceptualized as an issue of control of women; each of the forms in which it is seen serves to keep individual women within the control of individual men (Crooks, Goodall, Hughes, Jaffe, & Baker, 2007). Collectively, the sum total of acts of violence against women can be viewed as one of many forms of patriarchal social control. Many levels of complexity exist between the individual act of violence and patriarchal society, and the answer to violence against women is not simply equal status for women (Loseke, 2005; Stark, 2007; Yllö, 2005). However, this overall conceptual framework of violence against women as a form of social control provides the background for understanding the various forms of violence as part of one continuum, ranging from sexual harassment to homicide. All have health care implications and opportunities for nursing interventions.

FORMS OF VIOLENCE AGAINST WOMEN: DEFINITIONS AND INCIDENCE

Homicide

Of all female murder victims, the number of intimate partner homicides declined from 1976 through 1995. In 1995, the incidence increased and then stabilized through 2004. Approximately one-third of adult female homicide victims are killed by an intimate male partner. Although men have a higher incidence of fatal victimizations by both strangers and friends, women have a 25% greater chance than men of being killed by their intimate partner, and a 4% chance of being killed by a family member (Fox & Zawitz, 2006; Zahn, 2003).

Homicide has dropped from 11th to 15th as a leading cause of premature death for women in general (Hoyert, Heron, Murphy, & Kung, 2006). It is the 5th leading cause of death for women between the ages of 25 and 34 and the 8th leading cause of death for women between the ages of 35 and 44 (Centers for Disease Control, 2002). The number of female intimate partner homicides is equivalent for spouses and nonmarried couples. Over 60% of these women are killed by a family member, most often an intimate partner (husband, lover) or ex–intimate partner (Fox & Zawitz, 2006). In most of the murders by male partners, the homicide was preceded by the abuse of women (Sharps, Campbell, Campbell, Gary, & Webster, 2003). Some factors that may have played a role in decreasing the incidence of intimate homicide are a decrease in marriage rates, an increase in women's economic status, warrantless arrest, and increased Aid to Families with Dependent Children (Dougan, Nagin, & Rosenfeld, 2003).

Abuse of Female Partners

Abuse is a multifaceted phenomenon. Abuse of a female partner can be defined as repeated physical, sexual, and/or emotional assault within a context of coercive control by an intimate partner (or ex-partner). A context of coercive control refers to the environment of isolation; denial of economic resources; forced sex; and threats against children, family, and personal property that abusers impose on their female partners. According to the National Violence Against Women Survey, 25% of surveyed women were raped or physically assaulted by their husband, cohabitating partner, date, or boyfriend. In the United States, approximately 55% of women were raped or physically assaulted by an intimate partner sometime in their lives (Tjaden & Thoennes, 2000).

Although women also assault their male partners, such violence is far more frequently done in self-defense, less likely to cause injury, and less often accompanied by coercive control in other sphere of life (Dobash & Dobash, 2004; Loseke & Kurz, 2005). Men claim a lack of control over their behaviors and tend to minimize the violence or shift the responsibility for the violence to women (Dobash & Dobash, 2004). Because abuse of female partners tends to escalate in severity and frequency over time, the minor violence can be expected to increase to serious battering if not recognized as a serious problem and interrupted by health care professionals (Block, 2003; Plichta, 2004). Given the magnitude of the problem, abuse of women constitutes a major national health problem.

Dating Violence

Dating violence is of endemic proportions in our society. Dating violence may start in early adolescence and continues through adult dating relationships. Dating violence, similar to other forms of violence, crosses socioeconomic status and ethnic groups. As in intimate partner violence between adults, young women who experience physical violence also experience significant emotional abuse (Amar & Gennaro, 2005). Risk factors for dating violence in adolescents include violence in family of origin, troubles in school, and alcohol use (Glass et al., 2003). Similar to intimate partner violence in marital relationships, the severity of the physical abuse was positively correlated with an increased level of emotional abuse. Although the incidence of physical dating violence is similar between males and females, females were more likely to suffer more violence in terms of sexual and psychological abuse (Centers for Disease Control, 2006). Alcohol was positively correlated with dating violence in youth (Miller, Naimi, Brewer, & Jones, 2007). In addition, depression was often an outcome of all forms of dating violence for females. Males who were victims of physical abuse were more likely to victimize another individual (Banyard, Cross, & Modecki, 2006).

Girls who grow up in homes where physical violence takes place are at greater risk for depression and low self-esteem and are more likely to be involved in a dating relationship where violence takes place. Feelings of depression and low self-esteem lead to feelings of loss of control, and subsequently the young woman feels unable to take control of the violent relationship (Downs, Capshew, & Rindels, 2006; Schewe, Riger, Howard, Staggs, & Mason, 2006). In addition, childhood experiences of abuse are considered to account, to some degree, on how a woman responds to dating violence. It may be that girls who grow up in a home where physical abuse has occurred despair that change can take place. Blame for the situation in which they are involved may lead to characterological self-blame, where young women think that innate personality flaws are responsible for the abuse (Malik, Sorenson, & Aneshensel, 1997; O'Keefe, 1998).

Societal and individual factors are at the core of violence in dating relationships. Societal roles that frame men as aggressors and women as passive recipients and the belief that women wish to be controlled are factors that support the use of aggressive behavior in dating relationships. Although male-female roles perpetuate intimate partner violence, many factors such as parental conflict, divorce, and lack of support contribute to violence in adolescent dating relationships (Carr & VanDeusen, 2002; Lavoie et al., 2002). Greater focus is being placed on dating violence in youth and prevention of such violence. The prevention of violence against others regardless of gender is a primary principle in these programs.

FEMALE PARTNERS

Approximately 1.3 million or 22 percent of American women are physically assaulted by their male partners each year in the United States (Tjaden & Thoennes, 2000; U.S. Department of Justice, 2006c). The exact prevalence of wife (or intimate partner) abuse varies across ethnic groups. The incidence of intimate partner physical abuse is highest in American Indian and Alaskan Native women. Although the incidence is similar for Hispanic versus non-Hispanic women, Black women are 2 percent more likely to be victims of intimate partner violence than white women (U.S. Department of Justice, 2006c). Research on women and violence has exploded in the last decade. Although there is a greater understanding of intimate partner violence and the context of that violence, the definition of intimate partner violence needs to be more inclusive of the victimization that currently takes place (Stark, 2007; Tjaden, 2004). In a review of the definitions of domestic violence, Tjaden (2004) states that nonviolent acts such as stalking and emotional abuse need to be considered when measuring the incidence of domestic violence. Stark (2007) asserts that we must look more closely at the continuous nature of abuse in a relationship and be more inclusive of psychological abuse such as forced isolation, coercion, and economic abuse. Regardless of how we define abuse, women continue to be victimized by their male partners more often than men, and women report a higher prevalence of lifetime abuse (Stark, 2007). In addition, women continue to be at risk for physical assault and stalking after they leave the abusive relationship (Tjaden & Thoennes, 2000; U.S. Department of Justice, 2006a).

Violence against women has serious long- and short-term physical and mental health outcomes. Over 60% of all women over the age of 18 will have experienced some form of violence, including physical assault, sexual assault, and stalking. Lifetime exposure for violence was slightly higher in African American, Native American, and Hispanic women. Lesbian and bisexual women reported the highest level of lifetime violence (Moracco, Runyan, Bowling, & Earp, 2007). Even though there were differences among groups of women, the overall prevalence of violence against women suggests that economic and educational resources do not necessarily keep women from being abused but rather make it more possible for them to escape or end the violence against them. In other words, poverty is less a risk factor for a woman being with an abusive man than for her becoming trapped in an abusive relationship. Women who have been abused have a higher use of health care and report a higher degree of physical and psychological problems than women who have not been victims of violence (Rivara et al., 2007). Often the symptoms remain untreated because of a lack of proper screening (Richter, Surprenant, Schmelzle, & Mayo, 2003). In addition, McFarlane et al. (2001) suggest that women with disabilities are at greater risk for abuse not only from partners but from caregivers and health care providers. In many cases, there are no signs of physical injury, suggesting that nurses need to conduct routine screening for abuse rather than only asking women who are obviously injured.

Thus, it is clear that at least one-third of women in the United States have experienced physical violence from an intimate partner or prior intimate partner at some time in their lives. Furthermore, nurses should expect that between 1 in 10 and 1 in 20 women that they see in any health care setting has been physically abused by an intimate partner in the past year, and that the percentages will be larger in patient populations of younger and poorer women. Psychological and sexual abuse increases the numbers still further.

Violence also takes place in lesbian relationships. While the abuse that takes place is similar in form to that in heterosexual relationships, it is important to realize that the context of abuse is different. The social context for heterosexual women is that of misogyny, while for lesbians, abuse takes place within a social context of misogyny and homophobia (Girshick, 2002). Unfortunately, much of the research conducted on violence in lesbian relationships has been based on models developed through research in heterosexual intimate partner violence. The use of heterosexual models leads to misunderstandings and myths about lesbian violence that hinders the ability of health care providers to intervene appropriately. Patriarchal power and the intergenerational transmission of violence are considered casual factors for heterosexual violence. Although power may play a part in lesbian violence, it is a myth that the more "masculine" partner is the perpetrator of the violence (Donnelly, Cook, van Ausdale, & Foley, 2005). Sokoloff and Dupont (2005) propose that internalized homophobia may be a factor that contributes to lesbian violence. If internalized oppression leads to low self esteem, feelings of powerlessness, and denial of one's sexual orientation, these feelings, in turn, may lead to aggression against one's female partner.

CHARACTERISTICS OF ABUSE

Abuse of women partners is found in all economic, social, and cultural categories. However, most studies have found higher levels of abuse in relationships where the man's income, occupation, and stability of employment are low (Bograd, 2005; Hines & Malley-Morrison, 2005). Although intimate partner violence is associated with minority ethnicity, most of the increased risk disappears if income is controlled (Moracco et al., 2007). Although abuse may cross ethnic and socioeconomic groups, it is important to acknowledge the differential in resources as one's socioeconomic status decreases. In addition, women who are already marginalized because of race experience multiple forms of oppression that influence their situations and experiences in relation to violence (Bograd, 2005). There is also research support for abuse being related to "status inconsistency" between the partners, such as the husband's having less education or less occupational prestige than his wife (Schewe et al., 2006; Schmidt et al., 2007). In addition, men who feel they should have the final say in decision making (whether they do or not) or otherwise feel their male role is threatened are likely to compensate with aggression toward their female partners (Glass, Laughon, & Campbell, 2004).

Abuse is more likely to occur in couples where there is a great deal of stress from outside occurrences (e.g., job loss, death in family) as well as discord, argument, and verbal aggression between the partners (Hines & Malley-Morrison, 2005). Most studies indicate that men who were exposed to violence in childhood (child abuse or abuse of their mothers) are more likely to assault their wives, but the evidence is mixed as to whether childhood violence increases the risk for women to become abused partners. In fact, few personal or demographic characteristics of women are consistently indicated by research to be predictive of their becoming victims of adult abuse.

An important component of the violent situation is whether alcohol is involved. The Bureau of Justice Statistics reports that 7% of victims reported that their abuser was under the influence of drugs or alcohol (U.S. Department of Justice, 2006b). Evidence suggests that alcohol consumption is related to violent acts between family members. While women use alcohol to cope with depressive symptoms, it appears that chronic alcohol problems in men are predictive of woman battering (Kaysen et al., 2007). Approximately 43% of batterers have problems with alcohol, and, although most experts consider alcohol a factor in abuse, it is not seen as causative (Walton-Moss, Manganello, Frye, & Campbell, 2005). Curing alcohol problems does not necessarily help abuse problems, and both must be treated as separate problems with specific interventions.

Sexual Violence

Sexual violence against women includes rape (date or acquaintance, stranger, and marital), incest, and prostitution.

Rape

Rape is one of the underreported forms of violence against women. One out of six women is a victim of rape. Approximately 17% of women have been a victim of rape at some point in their life, and 54% of victims report rape before the age of 18. In the last decade, the number of rapes reported to law enforcement agencies has decreased, with only a third of victims reporting. Most rapes are perpetrated by an intimate partner, acquaintance, friend, or relative (Tjaden & Thoennes, 2000). Although major strides have taken place in the United States in the treatment of rape victims and in the prosecution of rape, women are still often seen as being responsible for the occurrence of the rape. If a woman's appearance is deemed sensual or she is walking the street at night or otherwise placing herself in a potentially vulnerable situation, she is sometimes seen as complicit in the assault. Generally, society views women as responsible for men's behavior.

Rape outside of marriage can be divided into two categories: date or acquaintance rape and stranger rape. Although both are forms of sexual assault, differences can be seen in how others attribute blame to the victims of rape. Until recently, it was generally believed that if women followed normative social behaviors, they would not be raped. In a sense, women were viewed as the perpetrators of the assault and had to prove that they did not cause the assault. Although women who are raped by a stranger are now more frequently viewed as unwilling victims, women experiencing date rape are often seen either as willing victims or as responsible for the assault.

Date rape among young people has recently gained attention as a threat to women. Women are at high risk for various forms and levels of physical and sexual violence in their dating relationships (Straus, 2004). Amar and Gennaro (2005) claim that 39% of all dating relationships include some form of physical aggression, including date rape. Women who are emotionally abused are more likely to report physical abuse and assault. Women who experienced multiple forms of abuse had a significant increase in health complaints (Amar & Gennaro, 2005). The degree of violence is also considered a factor in whether a young woman acknowledges a rape (Briere & Jordon, 2004). It is also hypothesized that the level of blame a young woman attributes to herself after a rape influences her likelihood of reporting the experience. The greater the amount of self-blame, the less likely she is to report the assault (Briere & Jordon, 2004). Because of the tendency to remain silent about experiences including physical aggression and the difficulty of labeling what constitutes this form of behavior, the exact incidence remains ambiguous.

Schissel (2000) reported that peer pressure influenced the desire of men to be sexually active, contributing to the rape of intimate partners, regardless of whether they had been sexually involved. In addition, submissiveness may be construed by the aggressor as acceptance of force. Women may feel obligated to respond to sexual demand in established relationships, and men may think that they have a right to make these demands. When women are raped in this context, it is generally labeled as sexual coercion. Physical coercion involves rape through physical force. In both forms of coercion, the closeness of the relationship and the intoxication of the victim influence responsibility held for the rape. When a victim has been drinking, she often is seen as responsible for the rape when she is either assaulted by a stranger or by a man she has dated but with whom she does not have a committed relationship. Regardless of the context in which the physical assault took place, the younger a victim, the less likely she is to report the assault. Only a quarter of high school students compared to 92% of college students talked to someone about the abusive episode (Black & Weisz, 2003). Because social norms ascribe to women the role of maintaining relationships, blame is placed on women for the abuse that takes place. Subsequently, the role of the man and his responsibility as the perpetrator of violence becomes a secondary issue. The opposing roles of initiator and gatekeeper set up an adversarial relationship in courtship.

Marital Rape

Approximately 3.2 intimate partner rapes per 100,000 women were committed annually in the United States (Tjaden & Thoennes, 2000). This form of sexual abuse can happen in a marriage that is otherwise nonviolent, but most often occurs with physical battering. In fact, 40% to 45% of battered women are also being raped on an ongoing basis by their partners (Tjaden & Thoennes, 2000). This sexual trauma has specific emotional and physical sequelae separate from and in addition to physical abuse. Women have reported such chronic difficulties as depression, anxiety, substance abuse, and pelvic inflammatory disease (Briere & Jordon, 2004; Champion, Piper, Hoklen, Korte, & Shain, 2004). Physically abused women who are also sexually abused have even lower self-esteem, especially in the area of body image, than do those who are only physically beaten. The male partner who sexually abuses his wife as well as physically abusing her is a particularly violent and dangerous batterer in terms of homicide potential.

The laws of the United States were based on traditional English law that stated that a man had the right to force his wife into sex, that her marriage vow constituted perpetual and irrevocable consent to sex at his desire. As recently as 1980, 45 states recognized this right of men, with marital rape exemptions to sexual misconduct laws. In other words, the sexual assault laws of almost all states applied to all men except husbands. By 1990, 10 states still retained that exception, and even today, 32 states have laws that make husbands less culpable than other men for rape of their wives (Bennice & Resick, 2003). These legal realities are indicative of the vestiges of attitudes that condone violence against women.

Incest

Incest, a matter of common concern in U.S. society, is a sexual act whereby a parent or a significant person whom a child trusts abuses that trust and exerts control over a child. The traditional legal definition of incest is usually limited to sexual intercourse between blood relatives. Finkelhor (1980) has broadened that definition to include explicit sexual contact. Currently, most research conducted on incest is based on Finkelhor's (1986) framework of incest.

The incidence of incest is difficult to determine and is considered underreported (Urbanic, 2004). Some researchers state that 20% to 22% of women have experienced childhood sexual abuse, with approximately 33% to 50% of the abuse being attributed to family members (Finkelhor, 1994; Gorey & Leslie, 1997). Difficulties in obtaining the incidence of incest in U.S. society are a result of societal avoidance of the topic or disbelief that it takes place. Although the reported number of children sexually abused has increased, this number is considered to be a result of an increase in reporting of the abuse rather than an increase in the actual number of cases (Finkelhor, 1994). Children often block from their memories the assaults to cope psychologically with an untenable situation. Usually, children are hesitant to speak of the abuse. They may have been threatened not to speak of the incidents, and often children do not possess the vocabulary to describe what is happening to them. These causes are even more profound in cases of incest in which the perpetrator is someone whom the child trusts and depends on.

Similar to intimate partner violence, incest is seen as an issue of power and control. It often happens in an environment where there are other forms of domestic violence present (Hines & Malley-Morrison, 2005). Many women have kept their experiences of incest a secret until reaching adulthood. Sometimes women have reframed their experiences so that they can deal with the abuse and go on with their lives. Conversely, some women have been unable to heal from the experience, resulting in an avoidance of intimate relationships, leading to social isolation and lack of social support networks (Martsolf & Draucker, 2005). Long-term effects of childhood sexual abuse include depression; social isolation; difficulties in future intimate relationships, especially with men; guilt; and low self-esteem. The child's search for some way to make sense of the incest along with the above symptoms persist into adulthood. The adult's understanding of the experiences and constructing some meaning of the past childhood experiences are essential in recovering from childhood trauma (Hobbins, 2004; Martsolf & Draucker, 2005; Urbanic, 2004).

Other Forms of Violence Against Women

Prostitution and sexual harassment, are widespread forms of violence against women, and they can lead to major health concerns. Prostitution is an institution that economically exploits women. Although economic exploitation is an important factor, sexual domination of women can be viewed as the foundation that supports prostitution in the United States. Many women become involved in prostitution at an early age and are victims of child sexual abuse (Nixon, Tutty, Downe, Gorkoff, & Ursel, 2002). Violence against prostitutes or street walkers is usually hidden from health professionals because of the social stigma attached to the activity (Williamson & Folaron, 2001). Street walkers are at high risk for severe beatings, drug abuse, and sexually transmitted diseases. Because of their need for money, street walkers have a continual conflict between survival and violence (Mallory & Stern, 2000; Williamson & Folaron, 2001). Trafficking of women and children is a major problem worldwide. It is "understood as the recruitment, transportation, transfer, harboring or receipt of persons for the purpose of subjecting them to sexual exploitation, slavery, forced labor or services, peonage or debt bondage (Family Violence Prevention Fund, 2005, p. 5).

Usually, sexual harassment is perpetrated by men against women. Sexual harassment is a form of sex discrimination composed of sexual threats and/or a hostile work environment where an employee is faced with unwanted sexually explicit behavior. Sexual harassment includes gender-specific verbal and nonverbal harassment; inappropriate and offensive sexual advances; and sexual bribery, coercion, and assault (Welsh, 1999). In most cases of sexual harassment, a power differential exists between the victim and the perpetrator. The power one individual has over another can lead to a fear in reporting the events, with the harassment continuing and psychological healing prohibited.

HEALTH CARE CONSEQUENCES AND COSTS

Women who have been abused are more likely to report poor health. Risky behaviors such as smoking and binge drinking are higher in women who are victims of abuse than women who have not experienced abuse (Bonomi et al., 2006). Substance abuse and well-documented physical health problems related to intimate partner violence in addition to injury include chronic pain (head, back, pelvic), neurological problems, and pelvic inflammatory disease (Champion et al., 2004; Meagher, 2004; Rysberg, 2004). Problems specific to reproductive health include urinary tract infections; increased risk of sexually transmitted diseases, including HIV/AIDS; pelvic pain; pelvic inflammatory disease; abortion; and unintended pregnancy (Champion et al., 2004; Plichta, 2004). These diagnoses are undoubtedly related to the forced sex aspects of violent relationships. Sexual violence also increases the risk of HIV. Burke and colleagues (2005) found that women who were victims of abuse and who were HIV positive also had a higher rate of substance abuse. In addition, women who were abused also reported a perception of being at risk for HIV and other sexually transmitted diseases due to male infidelity and sexual control over the women (Raj, Silverman, & Amaro, 2004). Health care consequences specific to abuse during pregnancy include low birth weight and miscarriage (Brokaw et al., 2002; Campbell et al., 2002; Coker, Smith, Bethea, King, & McKeown, 2000; Wingood, DiClemente, & Raj, 2000). Mental health sequelae include depression, post-traumatic stress disorder (PTSD), and substance abuse (smoking, alcohol, and drugs) (Basile, Arias, Desai, & Thompson, 2004; Bonomi et al., 2006; El-Bassel, Gilbert, Wu, Go, & Hill, 2005). Since actual injury is probably the least frequently seen health problem related to intimate partner violence, it is necessary for health care professionals to screen for abuse in all health care settings and to screen all women (McFarlane et al., 2001; Richter et al., 2003; Trautman, McCarthy, Miller, Campbell, & Kelen, 2007).

Because of the stigma involved, women and health care providers are often reluctant to initiate discussion about abuse. However, most battered women say they would have talked about the issue with a health care professional if they were asked (Wyszynski, 2000). Because abuse is usually insidious, starting with minor psychological abuse and building to more severe physical incidents, it sometimes remains unrecognized by victims and health care providers alike until a severe episode forces attention on the situation. Stigma and inadequate assessment lead to women continually seeking health care for a variety of complaints, with the underlying problem being virtually unmentioned.

Violence against women is a significant health care problem. Women seek entrance to the health care setting through multiple venues. Unless providers screen for domestic violence, they may be unaware that they are treating a victim of violence (D'Avolio et al., 2001). When the underlying reason for the health care visit is unrecognized, women receive little or no emotional support or interventions specific to their needs (Campbell, Torres, McKenna, Sheridan, & Landenburger, 2004). It can be surmised that the cost to the health care system is phenomenal, with little or no positive outcome. A cycle persists in which women seek care and receive either no intervention or interventions that are grossly ineffective (D'Avolio et al., 2001). This cycle perpetuates feelings of anger and inadequacy with health care providers, resulting in blame placed on women for their lack of compliance with remedies offered.

THE INTERSECTION OF RACE, SOCIAL CLASS, AND SEXUAL ORIENTATION

Policy, educational services, and resources are essential for all women who are victims of intimate partner violence. Equally important is that all providers are acutely aware of how experiences differ among women according to gender, race, class, and sexual orientation and how that understanding may enhance or inhibit intervention with different cultural groups of women (Bograd, 2005; Landenburger, Campbell, & Rodriguez, 2004; Whitaker et al., 2007). Although many similarities exist among the experiences of different women regardless of background, there are differences because of ethnicity, economic background, religion, and sexual orientation. Language, social class, racial oppression, and homophobia can directly influence the experiences of women, the responses of providers, and the availability of information specific to different groups of women. These differences, in turn, influence the resources women use, the treatment they receive, and ultimately the outcome of a domestic situation (Bograd, 2005). Many women experience multiple forms of discrimination, which severely decreases their access to assistance.

Although the patterns of abuse may be somewhat similar across ethnic groups, women's responses to abuse and the barriers they face in seeking assistance may differ. Cultural issues and language differences may be important factors that influence the decisions a woman may make (Bograd, 2005; Merchant, 2000). Abuse takes place in a society where racism is common. Women of color who seek help may be stigmatized for the abuse and for their racial or ethnic background (Bograd, 2005). Because of these differences, women may feel more comfortable receiving assistance from someone of their own ethnic group.

For many women trying to leave an abusive relationship, an already complex process is compounded by ethnic norms that tie them to their culture. Hassouneh-Phillips (2001) describes the needs of Muslim women living in the United States. For Muslim women to leave their abusive partner, women must initiate a divorce proceeding called *khula.* Obtaining a decree in this manner can be difficult, because there are no Islamic courts in the United States. Asian American women may feel that they have no option to leave an abusive situation, because, in leaving the abuser, they may be stigmatized by their family and the community in which they reside (Tran & des Jardin, 2000). Both Black women and Asian American women may be fearful of the police and, due to fear of recriminations or pressures from the community, may not call on the police for assistance (Weil & Lee, 2004; Weisz, 2005). The criminal justice system sometimes responds inadequately to ethnic minority women because of a lack of understanding of ethnic differences among women and difficulties with communication due to language differences. Immigrant woman may be fearful of deportation if they report abuse. This fear of deportation, loss of their children, or censorship from family and community can prevent women from seeking support (Raj & Silverman, 2002).

Lesbian women who are battered are often invisible to providers. Many providers assume heterosexuality and, through this assumption, silence the victim. In addition, in many discussions of domestic violence, the perpetrators are identified as male. Due to the lack of research on women of color and intimate partner violence and a similar lack examining intimate partner violence and lesbian women, there is a dearth of literature on women of color who are also lesbian (Kanuha, 2005).

CORRELATES OF VIOLENCE AGAINST WOMEN

Cross-cultural and historical research efforts are beginning to identify societal correlates of violence against women that either enhance or deter such practices. These factors are important in both understanding the societal context for such violence and identifying useful prevention and public policy measures.

In a quantitative cross-cultural analysis of family violence using aggregate anthropological data, Cunradi, Caetano, and Schafer (2002) found that the most important predictors of wife beating in ethnic groups were economic inequality between genders, violent conflict resolution, male domestic authority, and divorce restrictions for women. Using more in-depth descriptions from 14 diverse societies with a variety of levels of violence against women, Counts, Brown, and Campbell (1999) found that community-level sanctions against battering and sanctuary for beaten wives was important in preventing occasional wife beating from escalating to ongoing abuse. Definitions of manhood that include an emphasis on toughness and control of women and strong importance of the wife/mother role were predictive of wife abuse. When cultures define the wife/mother role as the primary role for women, women who are hit by their husbands may find it difficult to escape; the same mechanism occurs where divorce is restricted.

Strong cultural gender preference for men is associated with forms of violence against women other than wife beating, as is general low status of women, especially in terms of political power and economic autonomy. Generally, where there are other forms of violence against women, wife beating is also prevalent. As cultural norms regarding women change with political upheaval, the degree and frequency of violence against women can be expected to change also. For instance, the 1990s brought a severe curtailment of women's autonomy in Algeria and Afghanistan, whereas the status of women has been increasing steadily in Zimbabwe since the revolution of the 1980s. Although it is difficult to ascertain exact rates, women in these countries feel that the incidence of violent practices against them increases as autonomy decreases and vice versa. However, it may be that in cultures where women have remained strictly controlled by law and tradition, to keep female autonomy circumscribed, violence against women only needs to be permitted rather than frequently committed (Counts et al., 1999).

THEORETICAL FRAMEWORKS FOR UNDERSTANDING VIOLENCE AGAINST WOMEN

As well as general theories explaining violence against women, specific theories have been posited that attempt to explain the causes and nature of wife abuse. Understanding the environmental, interpersonal, and interactional dynamics that occur during a woman's experiences of abuse assists in determining why women remain in or leave an abusive relationship. The experience of being abused in the context of a significant relationship can be understood by clarifying the views women have of themselves as individual persons and the meaning they attach to their interactions with others and the environment. Because abuse is a multicontextual problem, no one theory can totally explain the dynamics of abusive relationships. The different theories viewed as a whole are helpful in identifying the societal, familial, and individual components that contribute to the existence and continuation of violence against women in U.S. culture.

Theories About Wife Abuse

Theories about violence among intimates can be divided into three groups: intraindividual theories, sociopsychological theories, and sociocultural theories.

Intraindividual Theories

Intraindividual theories focus on individual characteristics. Personality traits inherent in individuals—such as low self-esteem, poor impulse control, and psychopathology—can lead to violent behavior. The difficulty with this approach is that social context is ignored, and perpetrators are relieved from responsibility for their malbehavior. In addition, the majority of abusers cannot be diagnosed with major psychopathology.

In the intraindividual view, alcohol and drug abuse are viewed as mechanisms that break down natural inhibitions against deviant behavior. Although abuse is indeed more prevalent in relationships where one or both individuals misuse alcohol and drugs, it is also present without the use of these chemicals.

Sociopsychological Theories

In sociopsychological theories—such as exchange theory, social learning theory, and attribution theory—the source of violence and the explanations for the behavior of those victimized are located in interpersonal interactions.

Exchange Theory

Exchange theory examines abuse in a costs-rewards framework. Abuse is the result of interactions in which benefits and rewards are exchanged. If rewards are not acquired, the exchange is ended. Rewards for the abuser include increased power and instant gratification of demands. This approach is based on the premise that the exchange is mutual, and there is consent between the players in the interaction. In exchange theory, the well-documented efforts of women to end the abuse are discounted. Blame for the abuse and responsibility for the abuse are placed on the woman as well as on her perpetrator. This supports the myth that women ask for abuse and could end the unwanted behavior if they wished to do so.

Social Learning Theory

Social learning theory claims that abusive behavior is learned from exposure to violence. In this framework, abuse is learned to be a normative means of control that is passed down within the family. Research supports the theory that violence can be learned. The strongest risk factor across studies is a history of either being abused as children or witnessing violence against their mother (Carr & VanDeusen, 2002; Loh & Gidycz, 2006). Although this theory links violence in the family of origin with men who batter, it does not explain why some men who were either indirect or direct victims become abusive but most do not. Research evidence less clearly supports women "learning" to be victims of abuse from childhood experience than men learning to be perpetrators (Purvin, 2003).

Attribution Theory

A woman who is abused is sometimes stigmatized not for the abuse itself but for the role others attribute to her for causing or, more often, not ending the abuse. The responsibility for the abusive situation may be attributed to the woman, offering evidence to her that aspects of her personality or behavior are to blame (Fishwisk, Campbell, & Taylor, 2004). A woman is influenced by attributions of cause and blame for the abuse she sustains. When a woman is labeled by others as being abused, expectations and judgments about her behavior are formulated by others. The internalization of the labels designated by others influences a woman's view of herself and becomes a potentially important part of her subsequent behavior. She also searches for explanations about why this is happening to her. These explanations take the form of a woman questioning her ability to perform the roles of wife and mother regardless of her achievements. She may blame herself for the problems of other family members even though she may not be responsible for these problems. As she continues in the abusive relationship, the sum of the past events and the meaning she makes of the events influence her current view of herself and her life (Campbell et al., 2004).

Research on women who have experienced rape by a stranger suggests that if she blames her own behavior (as contrasted to a personality characteristic) for the attack and subsequently changes that behavior, she may feel less vulnerable to another attack and thereby recover from the rape trauma more quickly (Ullman, Townsend, Filipas, & Starznski, 2007). In addition, women who blamed themselves and their partners (interaction blame) were less depressed and had higher self-esteem than those who blamed their husband or partner alone. However, those who blamed themselves solely were the most depressed. Although these findings suggest that internalizing some responsibility can be useful in assisting women to believe they can control outcomes, if these attributions place most of the blame and responsibility of negative outcomes on women, they can be harmful (Littleton & Breitkopf, 2006). More research is needed to understand these issues.

Sociocultural Theories

Current evidence suggests that it is pressures or social conditions in the external environment that lead to abuse and a combination of external pressures and individual (Hines & Malley-Morrison, 2005). The most salient factor that leads to abuse is the overall acceptance and practice in U.S. society of violence as a means of maintaining, demonstrating, or regaining control. The news media and television are filled with incidents of seemingly acceptable violence. Men are socialized in a manner that holds in esteem acts of aggression and control. Most children grow up surrounded with fairy tales, nursery rhymes, and television shows that depict violence as appropriate behavior. If a child learns that abuse is an acceptable form of behavior through stories and is confronted with actual abuse of self or acts of parental violence, there is a greater likelihood of abuse being a normal mode of behavior for that child in the future (Landenburger et al., 2004). As long as positive social sanctions exist to use physical force to control others, there is a high probability that many individuals will extend this use beyond that which is considered acceptable.

Systems theory has been used to explain family violence, including wife abuse, by Straus and his associates (Fishwick, Campbell, & Taylor, 2004). Although this theoretical framework includes the issues of both societal gender inequality and the domestic control of wives as predictors of wife abuse, its emphasis on stressors and considering all forms of family violence together makes it less explanatory for violence against women.

Certain family conflicts seem to trigger violent outbursts. The demands a woman may make on her husband to attain a better job, to be a better father, or to stop drinking may be seen as criticisms of his role as head of the household and may lower an already shaky self-esteem. In the United States and around the world, a woman's role in the family, more often than not, is subordinate to the man's. Acts of violence are often precipitated by what is seen as a violation of this role. In many incidents, a woman's suggesting that she find a job to help support the family has been met with abuse by her partner. Women working and especially succeeding outside the home are still responded to with jealousy or feelings of inadequacy by many men (Kaukinen, 2004). Conflict over how children should be raised and the timing of pregnancy also have been named as precipitating factors for abuse.

Pearlin (1975) first described the relationship between status equality and stress in marriage. He stated that when there are norms of inequality existing in society and when these norms are considered important within the marriage relationship, there is likely to be conflict between the couple.

Status inconsistency as a precursor of wife abuse is one of the research findings that supports a feminist framework explanation for violence against women. The findings from historical and cultural analyses also generally support the premises that violence against women in all its forms is fundamentally related to the patriarchal structures and attitudes that permeate almost all cultures historically and presently (Kaukinen, 2004; Stark, 2007).

Recent feminist analyses of the behavior of victimized women also contribute to our understanding. Rather than a general emphasis on the pathology of women who have experienced violence, such analyses stress their strengths (Smith, 2005; Weis, Fine, Proweller, Bertram, & Marusza, 2005). Without minimizing the potential and actual health care problems of these women, such an approach can be incorporated into nursing research and practice to their advantage.

Nursing Theories

Several of the broad nursing conceptual frameworks have been applied to the issues of violence against women. Some of the earliest work was conducted by Limandri (1986) when she applied Roy's (1976) framework to help in understanding the nursing role in increasing women's effective adaptation to abuse. Stuart and Campbell (1989) used Rogers's (1970, 1986) framework for research to further identify homicide risk factors in abusive relationships. Parse's (1985) theory was used by Butler and Snodgrass (1991) to direct nursing care of an abusive couple so that they learned to coexist.

Midrange nursing theories have also been introduced. The early nursing research of Ann Burgess (Burgess & Holmstrom, 1974, 1979), which established the notion of a rape trauma syndrome, has been elaborated on by researchers in many different disciplines. Burgess also developed a midrange theory of trauma encapsulation that explains the variety of behavior seen in victims of childhood sexual abuse (Hartman & Burgess, 1988). Children are unable to process the trauma and therefore "encapsulate" it, some almost totally. They may experience indirect effects, such as physical symptoms, but may not fully recall the trauma until adulthood. However, this defense prevents the memory from being processed, depletes psychic energy, and interferes with normal development. Ongoing intervention is needed for these children.

Landenburger (1989, 1998) developed a midrange theory of a process of entrapment and recovering from an abusive relationship. Her research indicated that a woman passes through a cumulative process that includes four phases: binding, enduring, disengaging, and recovering. The binding phase incorporates a description of the initial development of the relationship and the beginnings of abuse in the relationship. The positive aspects of the relationship are the primary focus for the woman, and they overpower the negative aspects of the relationship. When abuse takes place, a woman sometimes assumes the blame and tries to change her behavior to make the relationship run smoothly. During the second phase, enduring, a woman sees herself as putting up with the abuse while she strives to enhance the positive aspects of the relationship. Whereas in the first phase, a woman tended to blame her behavior for the abuse, she now blames her character for the negative aspects of the relationship. Therefore, her solutions focus on how to please her partner, while she tries endlessly to change who she is and, in the process, loses a sense of her self. During the disengaging phase, an identity with other women in her situation begins to form. During this phase, a woman tends to place a conscious label on what is happening to her. She tries to find people who will support her instead of accepting those who question her or blame her for the abuse. She becomes fearful of the abuse and begins to believe that she risks dying if she stays in the relationship or dying if she leaves. This paradox of fear mobilizes her to leave the relationship. The recovering phase contains the period of initial readjustment after a woman has left her abusive partner until she regains a balance in her life. Lutz et al. (2006) identified the process called double binding, where women becoming mothers were simultaneously involved in abusive relationships. In Landenburger's theory, binding is a time when women are trying to end the abuse but not the relationship. They ignore warning signs of the abuse and blame themselves for the abuse that takes place. Lutz found that women who were pregnant and abused also experienced a process of binding with their unborn child. This process could be an impetus to either leave or stay in the relationship. The choice to stay in or leave the relationship was based on women's views of what it meant to be a good mother. Some women left to keep their unborn child safe, and others stayed to offer their unborn child a stable home and a father.

Further development and application of theory specific to nursing roles include assessment and identification of the need specific to this population of women. Nurses must become actively involved in identifying women who are at risk for abuse. Nurses should make it a routine practice to assess all women for signs and symptoms of abuse. Women should be offered information from which they can learn more about abusive relationships and resources available to them. Efforts must center not only on helping a woman, but on conveying to her the effects of an abusive environment on her children.

NURSING RESEARCH

Most nursing research on violence against women has been in the area of intimate partner violence, with some research in sexual abuse. Nursing research has added a unique perspective to knowledge development about violence against women because of its holistic perspective. The literature in most other disciplines tends to concentrate on documenting emotional effects and sociological and psychological contextual factors. Medical research has increased in the area of violence against women and has tended to concentrate on determining the prevalence of abuse and sexual abuse in various medical settings and consequent medical diagnoses. The nursing research to date has been more concerned with responses to and characteristics of the various forms of victimization rather than on causation and medical issues. Most nursing researchers have collaborated with advocacy organizations against wife abuse and sexual assault that has strengthened the use of research results for policy change on behalf of battered women. Two of the early studies that are considered classic examples of groundbreaking quality research in the area of violence against women were conducted by nurses on rape and wife abuse, respectively (Burgess & Holmstrom, 1974; Parker & Schumacher, 1977). Nursing research has provided much of the impetus for the official health care system concern with abuse during pregnancy (Bullock, Bloom, Davis, Kilburn, & Curry, 2006; Curry, Durham, Bullock, Bloom & Davis, 2006; Helton, McFarlane, & Anderson, 1987; McFarlane, Parker, & Soeken, 1996). Campbell, García-Moreno, and Sharps (2004) have provided a challenge to broaden the focus to abuse during pregnancy in developing countries.

A review of nursing research on intimate partner violence has documented an impressive quality and quantity of studies using a variety of methods that has further developed the body of knowledge begun by nursing researchers in the 1980s. Hobbins (2004) has discussed the importance of identifying childhood sexual abuse and its impact on pregnant women. Memories of childhood sexual abuse can impact labor and symptoms of depression in the postnatal period. Nursing has been a leader in research on abuse during pregnancy. Bohn, Tebben, and Campbell (2004) found a significant relationship among education, income, and ethnicity during pregnancy and concluded that abuse is most prevalent among the most disadvantaged women. Martin and colleagues (2004) conducted a study comparing women who had screened positive for abuse with women who had not screened positive for abuse. In relationships where women had not screened positive for abuse, both women and men showed a significantly higher level of psychological aggression during pregnancy compared to before pregnancy. Women who screened positive for abuse were found to have experienced higher levels of sexual coercion and psychological aggression by their male partners. This study supports the ongoing necessity of screening during all stages of pregnancy. Lutz's work (2005) reiterates these findings. She stresses the importance of respectful and empathetic attitudes of health providers when conducting screening.

A review of abuse during pregnancy compared the prevalence of abuse in developing countries with prevalence of abuse in the United States and Canada. The effects of abuse during pregnancy, the importance of screening, and the effectiveness of intervention both during and after pregnancy have been identified in industrialized countries. Replication of this body of research in developing countries is needed so that culturally appropriate interventions are developed and implemented (Campbell, García-Moreno, & Sharps, 2004). The last 10 years have brought a development of research on unintended pregnancy. In a review of this research, Pallitto, Campbell, and O'Campo (2005) stress the importance for women to have the information, means, and power to control fertility. Without this ability to control fertility, cycles of violence and unintended pregnancy are repeated.

Nursing research has continued to demonstrate the detrimental physical and mental health effects of violence against women. Important work by Griffing and colleagues (2006), Bohn (2002), and Henderson (2004) has demonstrated the cumulative effects of lifetime physical and sexual assault on women, a beginning synthesis of the two areas of knowledge with important implications for practice. Further explication of the mental health effects of depression and PTSD have shown both the significant prevalence and persistence among battered women, and that physical and emotional abuse are both important predictors (Torres & Han, 2000; Woods, 2005; Woods & Isenberg, 2001; Woods & Wineman, 2004; Woods et al., 2005). Continuing nursing research has investigated the risk factors for femicide by intimate partners, including abuse during pregnancy, forced sex, and stalking (Burgess, Burgess, Koehler, Dominick, & Wecht, 2005; Campbell, 2004; Campbell et al., 2003; Lewandowski, McFarlane, Campbell, Gary, & Barenski, 2004; McFarlane et al., 2005). Glass and colleagues (2003) conducted a study on femicide perpetration by female partners. Similar to male-perpetrated femicide, physical violence is a risk factor for female-perpetrated femicide.

An emerging area of research is intimate partner violence and women with disabilities. Curry, Hassouneh-Phillips, and Johnston-Silverberg (2001) addressed this gap in the literature through the presentation of an ecological model for identifying factors that place women with disabilities at increased risk for abuse. The marginalization of people with disabilities and the stigma associated with disabilities lead to a compounded vulnerability based on gender and disability. Similar to other women who are abused, women who are disabled tend to be abused by their partner and may also be abused at the hands of various providers who offer them services. Dependence on others for assistance leaves women with disabilities either stranded for assistance or a victim of abuse. Individual and systemic barriers inhibit women from receiving the care they need. Internalized oppression may stop women from seeking the help they need (Hassouneh-Phillips & NcNeff, 2005). Lack of education of police or shelter is a barrier to receiving appropriate and timely assistance. In addition, the lack of licensure for personal caregivers results in an inability to determine whether someone may be abusive (Hassouneh-Phillips & Curry, 2002; Powers, Curry, Oschwald, & Maley, 2002; Saxton et al., 2001).

Building on Torres's (1987) important explication of cultural differences in women's perceptions of abuse, nursing researchers have continued to explore both across and within ethnic group variations. Nursing research on abuse during pregnancy has been noted for its ethnic diversity and exploration of ethnic variations (Campbell et al., 2003; Torres et al., 2000). Authors such as McFarlane and colleagues (2005), Schollenberger and colleagues (2003), and Taylor (2002a) have examined the abuse of African American women, while Weil and Lee (2004) have outlined cultural factors essential to understanding domestic violence in Asian American Pacific Islander families. Lee, Thompson, and Mechanic (2002) have raised the issue of the importance of developing violence prevention strategies particular to all women of color.

As well as the harmful outcomes, nursing research has identified significant strengths of battered women, such as taking care of themselves and their children in most aspects of their lives, indications of normal processes of grieving and recovering, and cultural and social support influences on responses to battering (Hassouneh-Phillips, 2003; Taylor, 2002b).

Despite the many positive aspects of nursing research, there are many gaps and improvements to be made. There are many opportunities to use larger, more culturally diverse samples of women and to document the prevalence of violence against women in each kind of health care setting. More important, there is a need for nursing research to further test theories explaining the responses of women to abuse and nursing interventions designed to be helpful to them.

Campbell and Soeken (1999) and Campbell and Weber (2000) reported the test of a midrange theory of women's responses to battering derived from Orem's (1991) self-care deficit theory using structural equation modeling. The model was originally specified from data from a volunteer community sample of 117 women (55% Anglo or Euro American, 39% African American, 4%

Mexican American and Puerto Rican, and 2% Arab American) either physically or emotionally abused (Campbell & Weber, 2000). The first test supported the hypothesis (derived from Orem's propositions) that self-care agency (ability to care for one's own health) is positively related to physical and mental health, but there were problems in both measurement and model fit. Using improved measurement, a test of the model with a new sample (N = 141; 80% African American) of physically abused urban women demonstrated preliminary support of the model and explained 51% of the variance of health (Campbell & Soeken, 1999). Both direct and indirect (mediated by self-care agency) relationships of severity of battering with the health outcomes were also supported.

Although learned helplessness was a sociopsychological theory frequently used to explain women's responses to battering in the 1980s (e.g., Campbell, 1989), its premises were not supported by findings that the majority of battered women ended either the abuse or the relationship (Rhatigan & Street, 2005; Shurman & Rodriguez, 2006) and more active help seeking over time (Kaukinen, 2004; Lipsky, Caetano, Field, & Larkin, 2006). Instead, more sophisticated theories of trauma response are being used to explain both the perpetration of and the responses to intimate partner violence (e.g., Classen et al., 2002; Woods, 2005; Woods & Isenberg, 2001). Batterers have been found to have significant attachment difficulties and higher rates of PTSD and borderline personality characteristics than in other men probably secondary to direct and indirect experiences of violence in childhood, and high rates of domestic violence have been found among men with PTSD secondary to war (Buttell, Muldoon, & Carney, 2005; White & Gondolf, 2000). High rates of both PTSD symptoms and diagnoses have been documented among both battered women and sexual abuse survivors (rape and incest) (Taft, Murphy, King, Dedeyn, & Musser, 2005; Woods, 2005; Woods & Wineman, 2004). The three clusters of symptoms characteristic of PTSD (trauma re-experience, avoidance and numbing, and hyperarousal) help to explain behavior and problems of survivors of violence that health care providers find problematic. Thus, sleep disturbances and anxiety symptoms can result from re-experiencing; seeming denial and flat affect from avoidance; and jumpiness, short temper, and stress-related physical symptoms from hyperarousal. The increased use of substances by victimized women may be efforts to self-medicate the PTSD symptoms, especially given recent findings of neurophysiologic changes secondary to PTSD.

Nursing Care

Assessment

Assessment for all forms of violence against women should take place—ideally, by nurses—for all women entering the health care system. The assessment should be ongoing and stress confidentiality. A thorough assessment gathers information on physical, emotional, and sexual trauma from violence; risk for future abuse; cultural background and beliefs; perception of the woman's relationships with others; and the woman's stated needs. The assessment should be conducted in private. Other adults who are present could be an abuser and should be directed toward the waiting area and told that it is policy that, initially, women are seen alone. Women should be asked directly if they have been or are currently in an abusive relationship either as a child or as an adult. They also should be asked if they have ever been forced into sex that they did not wish to participate in. Shame and fear often make disclosure difficult. Verbal acknowledgement of the seriousness of the situation and emotional and physical support assist women in talking about past or current circumstances (see Figure 23.1).

Women can be categorized into three groups in terms of abuse: no risk, low risk, or moderate to high risk. Women with no signs of current or past abuse are considered no risk. At the initial assessment, a woman may be hesitant to speak of concerns she may have. Future visits should include questioning a woman about whether there have been any changes in her life or whether she has additional information or questions about topics discussed at previous visits. Education that helps a woman gain perspective on her situation and her needs should be discussed. Resource materials, including group and individual formats, can be suggested. It is important that the nurse is identified as a supportive and knowledgeable person. The risk level should be recorded, and preventive measures and teaching should be documented.

Assessment of moderate to high risk includes evaluation of a woman's fear for both psychological and physical abuse. Lethality potential should be assessed (Campbell, 2004; Campbell et al., 2004). Risk factors for lethality include behavior such as stalking or frequent harassment, threat or an escalation of threats, use of weapons or threat with weapons, excessive control and jealousy, and public use of violence. Statements from an abuser such as, "If I can't have you, no one can" should be taken seriously. In all cases, a history of abuse and alcohol and drug use should be collected on both partners and carefully documented. The determined risk level should be documented, and any past or present physical evidence of abuse from prior or current assault should be either photographed or shown on a body map as well as described narratively. It is important that the assailant be identified in the record, which can be accomplished by the use of quotes from the woman or subjective information. These records can be very important for women in future assault and child custody cases, even if she is not ready to make a police report at the present time.

(Circle YES or NO for each question)

1. **WITHIN THE LAST YEAR**, have you been hit, slapped, kicked, or otherwise physically hurt by someone?   YES   NO

   If YES. by whom? _____

   Total number of times _____

2. **SINCE YOU'VE BEEN PREGNANT**, have you been hit, slapped, kicked, or otherwise physically hurl by someone?

   If YES. by whom? _____

   Total number of times _____

MARK THE AREA OF INJURY ON THE BODY MAP SCORE EACH INCIDENT ACCORDING TO THE FOLLOWING SCALE:

SCORE

1. Threats of abuse including use of a weapon   _____

2. Slapping, pushing: no injuries and or lasting pain   _____

3. Punching, kicking, bruises, cuts and or continuing pain   _____

4. Beating up. severe contusions, burns, broken bones   _____

5. Head injury, internal injury, permanent injury   _____

6. Use of weapon: wound from weapon   _____

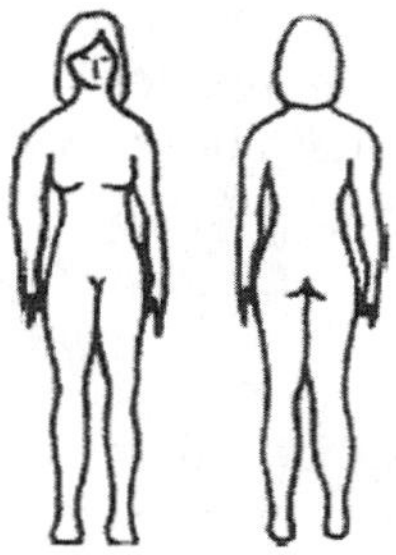

If any of the descriptions for the higher number apply, use the higher number.

YES   NO

3. **WITHIN THE LAST YEAR**, has anyone forced you to have sexual activities?

   If YES. by whom? _____

   Total number of times _____

Developed by the Nursing Research Consortium on Violence and Abuse.
Readers are encouraged to reproduce and use this assessment tool.

Figure 23.1   Abuse assessment screen. From McFarlane, J. (1993).
Abuse during pregnancy: The horror and the hope. *AWHONN'S Clinical Issues in Perinatal and Women's Health Nursing, 4*(3), 350–361

Nursing Interventions

Immediate care for a woman in a potentially harmful or present abusive situation involves the development of a safety plan. Questions that are important to ask include the following: How can we help you be safe? Do you have a place to go? Privacy when asking women about abuse is essential. A woman can be assisted to look at the options available to her. Shelter information, access to counseling, support groups, and legal resources should be discussed. Shoultz, Phillion, Noone, and Tanner (2002) found that women may feel more comfortable about gaining information about domestic violence from groups and activities that are already a part of a woman's life. Some places where a woman may feel freer to follow up on disclosure about domestic violence issues are through local church groups, classes for English as a second language, and craft groups. Dienemann, Campbell, Landenburger, and Curry (2002) suggest the use of a domestic violence survivor form to assist a woman in reviewing her situation and to determine what her needs are at a particular point in time. If a woman wants to return to her partner, she can be helped in the development of plans that can be carried out if the abuse continues or becomes more serious.

Whenever there is evidence of sexual assault within the past 24 to 48 hours—whether by father or father figure, husband, boyfriend, acquaintance, or stranger—a rape kit examination should be performed. In many settings, nurses are conducting these exams with accuracy equal to that of physicians and with better results in terms of rapport with female victims, willingness to spend sufficient time to do a thorough and empathetic exam, and willingness to testify in court when necessary (Hatmaker, Pinholster, & Saye, 2002; Sommers, Schafer, Zink, Hutson, & Hillard, 2001). Advocacy for female victims of violence includes ascertaining who is conducting rape kit exams in hospitals in the nurse's community and working to change policy if necessary so that nurses are conducting the exams.

Women who are survivors of past psychological, physical, and sexual abuse can benefit from survivor groups or individual counseling. Lists of resources such as rape crisis clinics and support groups for survivors of incest or physical and emotional abuse should be made available.

Prevention

Prevention, public policy, and social attitudes are intertwined. U.S. society has taken a major step toward the secondary prevention of abuse and sexual assault through the establishment of programs that encourage women and children to speak about their experiences. We need to support these programs further by trusting the women who confide in us. In the development of laws that punish child and woman abuse, we have given support to the victims of abuse, but often they are again victimized by disbelief of their experiences, the devaluing of the effects of these assaults on their persons, and the focus on assisting the perpetrators of the crimes.

Primary prevention would encompass a total attitudinal change in the values of U.S. society. Both girls and boys would be taught human values of interdependence, respect for human life, and a commitment to empathy and strength in the development of the human species regardless of sex, race, or socioeconomic status. Continued progress would be made toward eliminating the feminization of poverty and ensuring gender parity in the sharing of economic resources. In addition, local communities would make it clear that violence against women is not to be tolerated by eliminating pornography, mandating the arrest of wife abusers, and creating a general climate of nonviolence.

Women who are victimized by violence need assistance in making decisions and taking control of their lives. Nurses are involved with women at key times when they can be screened for the presence or absence of all forms of abuse. Mechanisms for screening women who are either abused or at risk for abuse from male partners

and other intimates are available (D'Avolio et al., 2001; Wyszynski, 2000). To intervene effectively, nurses must understand abuse as a cumulative process that must be examined as a continuum (Landenburger, 1998). During this process, the abuse, the relationship, and a woman's view of self-change, requires time-specific interventions. Research indicates that blame and responsibility for the victimization that is inflicted on the woman by the man is attributed by society to women (Draucker, 2001; Landenburger, 1998). Subsequently, either women are assisted in a manner that discounts their feelings and further devalues them or the abuse is ignored. Through understanding the societal contexts that perpetuate violence and shape a woman's responses to experiencing violence, nursing is in a key position to intervene with individual women. Nurses also can work toward changing public policy in general and specific health care policies so that violence toward women decreases in U.S. society.

REFERENCES

Amar, F. A., & Gennaro, S. (2005). Dating violence in college women: Associated physical injury, healthcare usage, and mental health symptoms. *Nursing Research, 54*(4), 235–242.

Banyard, V. L., Cross, C., & Modecki, K. L. (2006). Interpersonal violence in adolescence: Ecological correlates of self-reported perpetration. *Journal of Interpersonal Violence, 21*(10), 1314–1332.

Basile, K. C., Arias, I., Desai, S., & Thompson, M. P. (2004). The differential association of intimate partner physical, sexual, psychological, and stalking violence and posttraumatic stress symptoms in a nationally representative sample of women. *Journal of Traumatic Stress, 17*(5), 413–421.

Bennice, J. A., & Resick, P. A. (2003). Marital rape: History, research, & practice. *Trauma, Violence & Abuse, 4*(3), 228–246.

Black, B. M., & Weisz, A. N. (2003). Help seeking behaviors of African American middle schoolers. *Violence Against Women, 9*(2), 187–206.

Block, C. R. (2003). How can practitioners help abused women lower her risk of death? *National Institute of Justice Journal, 250*. Retrieved December 28, 2005, from http://www.ojp.usdoj.gov/nij

Bograd, M. (2005). Strengthening domestic violence theories: Intersections of race, class, sexual orientation, and gender. In N. J. Sokoloff (Ed.), *Domestic violence at the margins: Readings on race, class, gender, and culture* (pp. 25–38). New Brunswick, NJ: Rutgers University Press.

Bohn, D. K. (2002). Lifetime and current abuse, pregnancy risks, and outcomes among Native American women. *Journal of Health Care for the Poor and Underserved, 13*(2), 184–198.

Bohn, D. K., Tebben, J. G., & Campbell, J. C. (2004). Influences of income, education, age, and ethnicity on physical abuse before and during pregnancy. *Journal of Obstetric, Gynecologic, & Neonatal Nursing, 33*(5), 561–571.

Bonomi, A. E., Thompson, R. S., Anderson, M., Reid, R. J., Carrell, D., Dimer, J. A., et al. (2006). Intimate partner violence and women's physical, mental, and social functioning. *American Journal of Preventive Medicine, 30*(6), 458–466.

Briere, J., & Jordon, C. E. (2004). Violence against women: Outcome complexity and implications for assessment and treatment. *Journal of Interpersonal Violence, 19*, 1252–1276.

Brokaw, J., Fullerton-Gleason, L., Olson, L., Crandall, C., McLaughlin, S., & Sklar, D. (2002). Health status and intimate partner violence: A cross-sectional study. *Annals of Emergency Medicine, 39*(1), 31–38.

Bullock, L., Bloom, T., Davis, J., Kilburn, E., & Curry, M. A. (2006). Abuse disclosure in privately and Medicaid-funded pregnant women. *Journal of Midwifery & Women's Health, 51*, 361–369.

Burgess, A. W., Burgess, A. G., Koehler, S. A., Dominick, J., & Wecht, C. H. (2005). Age-based factors in femicide. *Journal of Forensic Nursing, 1*(4), 151–157.

Burgess, A. W., & Holmstrom, L. L. (1974). The rape trauma syndrome. *American Journal of Psychiatry, 131,* 981–986.

Burgess, A. W., & Holmstrom, L. L. (1979). *Rape, crisis and recovery.* Bowie, MD: R. J. Brady.

Burke, J. G., Thieman, L. K., Gielen, A. C., O'Campo, P., & McDonnell, K. A. (2005). Intimate partner violence, substance use, and HIV among low-income women. *Violence Against Women, 11*(9), 1140–1161.

Butler, M. J., & Snodgrass, F. G. (1991). Beyond abuse: Parse's theory in practice. *Nursing Science Quarterly, 4*(1), 76–82.

Buttell, F., Muldoon, J., & Carney, M. (2005). An application of attachment theory to court-mandated batterers. *Journal of Family Violence, 20*(4), 211–217.

Campbell, J. C. (1989). A test of two explanatory models of women's responses to battering. *Nursing Research, 38,* 18–24.

Campbell, J. C. (2004). Helping women understand their risk in situations of intimate partner violence. *Journal of Interpersonal Violence, 19*(12), 1464–1477.

Campbell, J., García-Moreno, C., & Sharps, P. (2004). Abuse during pregnancy in industrialized and developing countries. *Violence Against Women, 10*(7), 770–789.

Campbell, J., Jones, A. S., Dienemann, J., Kub, J., Schollenberger, J., O'Campo, P., et al. (2002). Intimate partner violence and physical health consequences. *Archives of Internal Medicine, 162*(10), 1157–1163.

Campbell, J. C., & Soeken, K. (1999). Women's responses to battering: A test of the model. *Research in Nursing & Health, 22,* 49–58.

Campbell, J. C., Torres, S., McKenna, L. S., Sheridan, D. J., & Landenburger, K. (2004). Nursing care of survivors of intimate partner violence. In J. Humphreys & J. C. Campbell (Eds.), *Family violence and nursing practice* (pp. 307–360). Philadelphia: Lippincott Williams & Wilkins.

Campbell, J. C., & Weber, N. (2000). An empirical test of a self-care model of women's responses to battering. *Nursing Science Quarterly, 13*(1), 45–53.

Campbell, J. C., Webster, D., Kozio-McLain, J., Block, C., Campbell, D., Curry, M. A., et al. (2003). Risk factors for femicide in abusive relationships: Results from a multisite case control study. *American Journal of Public health, 93*(7), 1089–1097.

Carr, J. L., & VanDeusen, K. M. (2002). The relationship between family of origin violence and dating violence in college men. *Journal of Interpersonal Violence, 17*(6), 630–646.

Centers for Disease Control. (2002). *Leading causes of death archives: All females by age group.* Retrieved April 10, 2007 from http://www.cdc.gov/women/lcodarch.htm

Centers for Disease Control. (2006). Physical dating violence among high school students—United States 2003. *Morbidity and Mortality Report Weekly, 55*(19). Retrieved February 23, 2007, from http://www.cdc.gov/mmwr/index2006.htm

Champion, J. D., Piper, J., Hoklen, A., Korte, J., & Shain, R. N. (2004). Abused women and risk for pelvic inflammatory disease. *Western Journal of Nursing Research, 26*(2), 176–191.

Classen, C., Nevo, R., Koopman, C., Nevill-Manning, K., Gore-Felton, C., Rose, D. S., et al. (2002). Recent stressful life events, sexual revictimization, and their relationship with traumatic stress symptoms among women sexually abused in childhood. *Journal of Interpersonal Violence, 17*(12), 1274–1290.

Coker, A. L., Smith, P. H., Bethea, L., King, M. R., & McKeown, R. E. (2000). Physical health consequences of physical and psychological intimate partner violence. *Archives of Family Medicine, 9*(5), 451–457.

Counts, D., Brown, J., & Campbell, J. (Eds.). (1999). *To have and to hit: Anthropological perspectives on wife beating.* Chicago: University of Illinois Press.

Crooks, C. V., Goodall, G. R., Hughes, R., Jaffe, P. G., & Baker L. L. (2007). Engaging men and boys in preventing violence against women: Applying a cognitive-behavioral model. *Violence Against Women, 13*(3), 217–239.

Cunradi, C. B., Caetano, R., & Schafer, J. (2002). Socioeconomic predictors of intimate partner violence among White, Black, and Hispanic couples in the United States. *Journal of Family Violence, 17*(4), 377–389.

Curry, M. A., Durham, L., Bullock, L., Bloom, T., & Davis, J. (2006). Nurse case management for pregnant women experiencing or at risk for abuse. *Journal of Obstetric, Gynecologic, & Neonatal Nursing, 35,* 181–192.

Curry, M. A., Hassouneh-Philips, D., & Johnston-Silverberg, A. (2001). Abuse of women with disabilities: An ecological model and review. *Violence Against Women, 7*(1), 60–79.

D'Avolio, D., Hawkins, J. W., Haggerty, L. A., Kelly, U., Barrett, R., Toscano, S. E. D., et al. (2001). Screening for abuse: Barriers and opportunities. *Health Care for Women International, 22,* 349–362.

Dienemann, J., Campbell, J., Landenburger, K., & Curry, M. A. (2002). The domestic violence survivor assessment: A tool for counseling women in intimate partner violence relationships. *Patient Education and Counseling, 46,* 221–228.

Dobash, R. P., & Dobash, R. E. (2004). Women's violence to men in intimate relationships: Working on a puzzle. *British Journal of Criminology, 44*(3), 324–349.

Donnelly, D. A., Cook, K. J., van Ausdale, D., & Foley, L. (2005). White privilege, color blindness, and services to battered women. *Violence Against Women, 11*(1), 6–37.

Dougan, L., Nagin, D. S., & Rosenfeld, R. (2003) Do domestic violence services save lives? *National Institute of Justice Journal, 250.* Retrieved December 28, 2005, from http://www.ojp.usdoj.gov/nij

Downs, W. R., Capshew, T., & Rindels, B. (2006). Relationships between adult women's mental health problems and their childhood experiences of parental violence and psychological aggression. *Journal of Family Violence, 21*(7), 439–447.

Draucker, C. B. (2001). Learning the harsh realities of life: Sexual violence, disillusionment, and meaning. *Health Care for Women International, 22*(1/2), 67–84.

El-Bassel, N., Gilbert, L., Wu, E., Go, H., & Hill, J. (2005). HIV and intimate partner violence among methadone-maintained women in New York City. *Social Science and Medicine, 61,* 171–183.

Family Violence Prevention Fund. (2005). *Turning pain into power: Trafficking survivors' perspectives on early intervention strategies.* San Francisco: Author.

Finkelhor, D. (1980). Risk factors in the sexual victimization of children. *Child Abuse and Neglect, 4,* 265–273.

Finkelhor, D. (1986). *A sourcebook on child sexual abuse.* Beverly Hills, CA: Sage.

Finkelhor, D. (1994). Current information on the scope and nature of child sexual abuse. *The Future of Children: Sexual Abuse of Children, 4*(2), 31–53.

Fishwick, N. J., Campbell, J. C., & Taylor, J. (2004). Theories of intimate partner violence. In J. Humphreys & J. C. Campbell (Eds.), *Family violence and nursing practice* (pp. 29–57). Philadelphia: Lippincott Williams & Wilkins.

Fox, J. A., & Zawitz, M. W. (2006). Homicide trends in the United States. U.S. Department of Justice, Office of Justice Programs, Bureau of Justice Statistics. Retrieved February 26, 2007, from http://www.ojp.gov/bjs/homicide/homtrnd.htm

Girshick, I. B. (2002). No sugar, no spice: Reflections on research on woman-to-woman sexual violence. *Violence Against Women, 8*(12), 1500–1520.

Glass, N., et al. (2003). Adolescent dating violence: Prevalence, risk factors, health outcomes, and implications for clinical practice. *Journal of Obstetric, Gynecologic, & Neonatal Nursing, 32*(2), 227–238.

Glass, N., Laughon, K., & Campbell, J. C. (2004). Theories of aggression and family violence. In J. Humphreys & J. C. Campbell (Eds.), *Family violence and nursing practice* (pp. 3–28). Philadelphia: Lippincott Williams & Wilkins.

Gorey, K. M., & Leslie, D. R. (1997). The prevalence of child sexual abuse: Integrative review adjustment for potential response and measurement biases. *Child Abuse & Neglect, 21*(4), 391–398.

Griffing, S., Lewis, C. S., Chu, M., Sage, R., Jospitre, T., Madry, L., et al. (2006). The process of coping with domestic violence in adult survivors of childhood sexual abuse. *Journal of Child Sexual Abuse, 15*(2), 23–41.

Hartman, C. R., & Burgess, A. W. (1988). Information processing of trauma. *Journal of Interpersonal Violence, 3*, 443–457.

Hassouneh-Phillips, D. (2001). American Muslim women's experiences of leaving abusive relationships. *Health Care for Women International, 22*, 415–432.

Hassouneh-Philips, D. (2003). Strength and vulnerability: Spirituality in abused American Muslim women's lives. *Issues in Mental Health Nursing, 24*, 681–694.

Hassouneh-Philips, D., & Curry, M. A. (2002). Abuse of women with disabilities: State of the science. *Rehabilitation Counseling Bulletin, 45*(2), 96–104.

Hassouneh-Philips, D., & McNeff, E. (2005). "I thought I was less worthy": Low sexual and body esteem and increased vulnerability to intimate partner abuse in women with physical disabilities. *Sexuality and Disability, 23*(4), 227–240.

Hatmaker, D. D., Pinholster, L., & Saye, J. J. (2002). A community-based approach to sexual assault. *Public Health Nursing, 19*(2), 124–127.

Helton, A., McFarlane, J., & Anderson, E. (1987). Prevention of battering during pregnancy: Focus on behavioral change. *Public Health Nursing, 4*, 166–174.

Henderson, A. (2004). Restorative health: Lessening the impact of previous abuse and violence in the lives of vulnerable girls. *Health Care for Women International, 25*(9), 794–812.

Hines, D. A., & Malley-Morrison, K. (2005). *Family violence in the United States: Defining, understanding and combating abuse.* Thousand Oaks, CA: Sage.

Hobbins, D. (2004). Survivors of childhood sexual abuse: Implications for perinatal nursing practice. *Journal of Obstetric, Gynecologic, & Neonatal Nursing, 33*(4), 485–487.

Hoyert, D. L., Heron, M., Murphy, S. L, & Kung, H. C. (2006). Deaths: Final data for 2003. *Health E-Stats.* Retrieved April 10, 2007, from http://www.cdc.gov/nchs/products/pubs/pubd/hestats/finaldeaths03/finaldeaths03.htm

Kanuha, V. K. (2005). Compounding the triple jeopardy: Battering in lesbian of color relationships. In N. J. Sokoloff (Ed.), *Domestic violence at the margins: Readings on race, class, gender, and culture* (pp. 71–82). New Brunswick, NJ: Rutgers University Press.

Kaukinen, C. (2004). Status compatibility, physical violence, and emotional abuse in intimate relationships. *Journal of Marriage and Family, 66*(2), 452–471.

Kaysen, D., Dillworth, T. M., Simpson, T., Waldrop, A., Larimer, M. E., & Resick, P. A. (2007). Domestic violence and alcohol use: Trauma-related symptoms and motives for drinking. *Addictive Behaviors, 32*(6), 1272–1283.

Landenburger, K. (1989). The process of entrapment in and recovery from an abusive relationship. *Issues in Mental Health Nursing, 10*(3), 165–183.

Landenburger, K. (1998). The dynamics of leaving and recovering from an abusive relationship. *Journal of Obstetric, Gynecologic, & Neonatal Nursing, 27*(6), 700–706.

Landenburger, K., Campbell, D. W., & Rodriguez, R. (2004). Nursing care of families using violence. In J. Humphreys & J. C. Campbell (Eds.), *Family violence and nursing practice* (pp. 220–251). Philadelphia: Lippincott Williams & Wilkins.

Lavoie, F., Herbert, M., Tremblay, R., Vitaro, F., Vezina, L., & McDuff, P. (2002). History of family dysfunction and perpetration of dating violence by adolescent boys: A longitudinal study. *Journal of Adolescent Health, 30*(5), 375–383.

Lee, R. K., Thompson, V. L. S., & Mechanic, M. B. (2002). Intimate partner violence and women of color: A call for innovations. *American Journal of Public Health, 92*(4), 530–534.

Lewandowski, L. A., McFarlane, J., Campbell, J. C., Gary, F., & Barenski, C. (2004). "He killed my mommy!" Murder or attempted murder of a child's mother. *Journal of Family Violence, 19*(4), 211–220.

Limandri, B. J. (1986). Research and practice with abused women: Use of the Roy adaptation model as an explanatory framework. *Advances in Nursing Science, 8*(4), 52–61.

Lipsky, S., Caetano, R., Field, C. A., & Larkin, G. L. (2006). The role of intimate partner violence, race, and ethnicity in help-seeking behaviors. *Ethnicity and Health, 11*(1), 81–100.

Littleton, H., & Breitkopf, C. R. (2006). Coping with the experience of rape. *Psychology of Women Quarterly, 30*, 106–116.

Loh, C., & Gidycz, C. A. (2006). A prospective analysis of the relationship between childhood sexual victimization and perpetration of dating violence and sexual assault in adulthood. *Journal of Interpersonal Violence, 21*(6), 732–749.

Loseke, D. R. (2005). Through a sociological lens: The complexities of family violence. In D. R. Loseke, R. J. Gelles, & M. M. Cavanaugh (Eds.), *Current controversies on family violence* (2nd ed., pp. 35–47). Thousand Oaks, CA: Sage.

Loseke, D. R., & Kurz, D. (2005). Through a sociological lens: The complexities of family violence. In D. R. Loseke, R. J. Gelles, & M. M. Cavanaugh (Eds.), *Current controversies on family violence* (2nd ed., pp. 79–95). Thousand Oaks, CA: Sage.

Lutz, K. F. (2005). Abused pregnant women's interactions with health care providers during the childbearing years. *Journal of Obstetric, Gynecologic, & Neonatal Nursing, 34*(2), 151–162.

Lutz, K. F., Curry, M. A., Robrecht, L. C., Libbus, M. K., & Bullock, L. (2006). Double binding, abusive intimate partner relationships, and pregnancy. *Canadian Journal of Nursing Research, 38*(4), 118–134.

Malik, S., Sorenson, S. B., & Aneshensel, C. S. (1997). Community and dating violence among adolescents: Perpetration and victimization. *Journal of Adolescent Health, 21*(50), 291–302.

Mallory, C., & Stern, P. N. (2000). Awakening as a change process among women at risk for HIV who engage in survival sex. *Qualitative Health Research, 10*(5), 581–594.

Martin, S. L., Harris-Britt, A., Li, Y., Moracco, K. E., Kupper, L. L., & Campbell, J. C. (2004). Changes in intimate partner violence during pregnancy. *Journal of Family Violence, 19*(4), 201–210.

Martsolf, D. S., & Draucker, C. B. (2005). Psychotherapy approaches for adult survivors of childhood sexual abuse: An integrative review of outcomes research. *Issues in Mental Health Nursing, 29*, 801–825.

McFarlane, J. M., Groff, J. Y., O'Brien, J. A., & Watson, K. (2005). Prevalence of partner violence against 7,443 African American, White, and Hispanic Women receiving care at urban public primary care clinics. *Public Health Nursing, 22*(2), 98–107.

McFarlane, J., Hughes, R. B., Nosek, M. A., Groff, J. Y., Swedlend, N., & Mullen, P. D. (2001). Abuse assessment screen-disability (AAS-D): Measuring frequency, type, and perpetrator of abuse toward women with physical disabilities. *Journal of Women's Health & Gender-Based Medicine, 10*(9), 861–866.

McFarlane, J., Malecha, A., Gist, J., Watson, K., Batter, E., Hall, I., et al. (2005). Intimate partner sexual assault against women and associated victim substance use, suicidality, and risk factors for femicide. *Issues in Mental Health Nursing, 26*, 953–967.

McFarlane, J., Parker, B., & Soeken, K. (1996). Physical abuse, smoking, and substance use during pregnancy: Prevalence, interrelationships, and effects on birth weight. *Journal of Obstetric, Gynecologic, & Neonatal Nursing, 25*, 313–320.

Meagher, M. W. (2004). Links between traumatic family violence and chronic pain: Biopsychosocial pathways and treatment implications. In K. A. Kendall-Tackett (Ed.), *Health consequences of abuse in the family: A clinical guide for evidence-based practice* (pp. 155–177). Washington, DC: American Psychological Association.

Merchant, M. (2000). A comparative study of agencies assisting domestic violence victims: Does the South Asian community have special needs? *Journal of Social Distress and the Homeless, 9*(3), 249–259.

Miller, J. W., Naimi, T. S., Brewer, R. D., & Jones, S. E. (2007). Binge drinking and associated health risk behaviors among high school students. *Pediatrics, 119*(1), 76–85.

Moracco, K. E., Runyan, C. W., Bowling, J. M., & Earp, J. A. L. (2007). Women's experiences with violence: A national study. *Women's Health Issues, 17*(1), 3–12.

Nixon, K., Tutty, L., Downe, P., Gorkoff, K., & Ursel, J. (2002). The everyday occurrence: Violence in the lives of girls exploited through prostitution. *Violence Against Women, 8*(9), 1026–1043.

O'Keefe, M. (1998). Factors mediating the link between witnessing interparental violence and dating violence. *Journal of Family Violence, 13*(1), 39–57.

Orem, D. E. (1991). *Nursing: Concepts of practice*. St. Louis, MO: Mosby.

Pallitto, C. C., Campbell, J. C., & O'Campo, P. (2005). Is intimate partner violence associated with unintended pregnancy?: A review of the literature. *Trauma, Violence, & Abuse, 6*(3), 217–235.

Parker, B., & Schumacher, D. (1977). The battered wife syndrome and violence in the nuclear family of origin: A controlled pilot study. *American Journal of Public Health, 67*, 760–761.

Parse, R. (1985). *Man, living and health: A theory of nursing*. New York: Wiley.

Pearlin, L. I. (1975). Status inequality and stress in marriage. *American Sociological Review, 40*, 344–357.

Plichta, S. B. (2004). Intimate partner violence and physical health consequences: Policy and practice implications. *Journal of Interpersonal Violence, 19*(11), 1296–1323.

Powers, L. E., Curry, M. A, Oschwald, M., & Maley, S. (2002). Barriers and strategies in addressing abuse: A survey of disabled women's experiences. *Journal of Rehabilitation, 68*(1), 4–13.

Purvin, D. M. (2003). Weaving a tangled safety net: The intergenerational legacy of domestic violence and poverty. *Violence Against Women, 9*(10), 1263–1277.

Raj, A., & Silverman, J. (2002). Violence against immigrant women: The roles of culture, context, and legal immigrant status on intimate partner violence. *Violence Against Women, 8*(3), 367–398.

Raj, A., Silverman, J., & Amaro, H. (2004). Abused women report greater male partner risk and gender-based risk for HIV: Findings from a community-based study with Hispanic women. *AIDS Care, 16*(4), 519–529.

Rhatigan, D. L., & Street, A. E. (2005). The impact of intimate partner violence on decision to leave dating relationships: A test of the Investment model. *Journal of Interpersonal Violence, 20*(12), 1580–1597.

Richter, K. P., Surprenant, Z. J., Schmelzle, K. H., & Mayo, M. S. (2003). Detecting and documenting intimate partner violence. *Violence Against Women, 9*(4), 458–465.

Rivara, F. P., Anderson, M. L., Fishman, P., Bonomi, A. E., Reid, R. J., Carrell, D., et al. (2007). Healthcare utilization and costs for women with a history of intimate partner violence. *American Journal of Preventive Medicine, 32*(2), 89–96.

Rogers, M. E. (1970). *An introduction to a theoretical base for nursing*. Philadelphia: F. A. Davis.

Rogers, M. E. (1986). Science of unitary human beings. In B. M. Malinski (Ed.), *Explorations in Martha Rogers' science of unitary human beings* (pp. 3–8). Norwalk, CT: Appleton-Century-Crofts.

Roy, C. (1976). *An introduction to nursing: An adaptation model*. Englewood Cliffs, NJ: Prentice Hall.

Rysberg, J. (2004). Health care needs of abuse survivors at midlife and beyond. In K. A. Kendall-Tackett (Ed.), *Health consequences of abuse in the family: A clinical guide for evidence-based practice* (pp. 129–149). Washington, DC: American Psychological Association.

Saxton, M., Curry, M. A., Powers, L. E., Maley, S., Eckels, K., & Gross, J. (2001). "Bring my scooter so I can leave you": A study of disabled women handling abuse by personal assistance providers. *Violence Against Women, 7*(4), 393–417.

Schewe, P., Riger, S., Howard, A., Staggs, S. L., & Mason, G. E. (2006). Factors associated with domestic violence and sexual assault victimization. *Journal of Family Violence, 21*(7), 469–475.

Schissel, B. (2000). Boys against girls: The structural and interpersonal dimensions of violent patriarchal culture in the lives of young men. *Violence Against Women, 6*(9), 960–986.

Schmidt, M. C., Kolodinsky, J. M., Carsten, G., Schmidt, F. E., Larson, M., & MacLachlan, C. (2007). Short term change in attitude and motivating factors to change abusive behavior of male batterers after participating in a group intervention program based on the pro-feminist and cognitive-behavioral approach. *Journal of Family Violence, 22*(2), 91–100.

Schollenberger, J., Campbell, J., Sharps, P. W., O'Campo, P., Gielen, A. C., Dienemann, J., et al. (2003). African American HMO enrollees: Their experiences with partner abuse and its effect on their health and use of medical services. *Violence Against Women, 9*(5), 599–618.

Sharps, P., Campbell, J. C., Campbell, D., Gary, F., & Webster, D. (2003). Risky mix: Drinking, drug use, and homicide. *National Institute of Justice Journal, 250*. Retrieved December 28, 2005, from http://www.ojp.usdoj.gov/nij

Shoultz, J., Phillion, N., Noone, J., & Tanner, B. (2002). Listening to women: Culturally tailoring the violence prevention guidelines from the Put Prevention Into Practice program. *Journal of the American Academy of Nurse Practitioners, 14*(7), 307–315.

Shurman, L. A., & Rodriguez, C. M. (2006). Cognitive-affective predictors of women's readiness to end domestic violence relationships. *Journal of Interpersonal Violence, 21*(11), 1417–1439.

Smith, B. V. (2005). Battering, forgiveness, and redemption: Alternative models for addressing domestic violence in communities of color. In N. J. Sokoloff (Ed.), *Domestic violence at the margins: Readings on race, class, gender, and culture* (pp. 321–339). New Brunswick, NJ: Rutgers University Press.

Sokoloff, N. J., & Dupont, I. (2005). Domestic violence at the intersections of race, class, and gender. *Violence Against Women, 11*(1), 38–64.

Sommers, M. S., Schafer, J., Zink, T., Hutson, L., & Hillard, P. (2001). Injury patterns in women resulting from sexual assault. *Trauma Violence and Abuse: A Review Journal, 2*(3), 240–258.

Stark, E. (2007). *Coercive control: How men entrap women in personal life.* New York: Oxford University Press.

Straus, M. (2004). Prevalence of violence against dating partners by male and female university students worldwide. *Violence Against Women, 10*(7), 790–811.

Stuart, E., & Campbell, J. C. (1989). Assessment of patterns of dangerousness with battered women. *Issues in Mental Health Nursing, 10,* 245–260.

Taft, C. T., Murphy, C. M., King, L. A., Dedeyn, J. M., & Musser, P. H. (2005). Posttraumatic stress disorder symptomatology among partners of men in treatment for relationship abuse. *Journal of Abnormal Psychology, 114*(2), 259–268.

Taylor, J. Y. (2002a). Talking back: Research as an act of resistance and healing for African American women survivors of intimate male partner violence. *Women & Therapy, 25*(3/4), 145–160.

Taylor, J. Y. (2002b). "The straw that broke the camel's back": African American women's strategies for disengaging from abusive relationships. *Women & Therapy, 25*(3/4), 79–94.

Tjaden, P. (2004). What is violence against women? Defining and measuring the problem. *Journal of Interpersonal Violence, 19*(11), 1244–1251.

Tjaden, P., & Thoennes, N. (2000) Full report of the prevalence, incidence, and consequences of violence against women: Findings from the National Violence Against Women survey. National Institutes of Justice and the Centers for Disease Control (NCJ 183781). Retrieved February 4, 2006, from http://www.ojp.usdoj.gov/nij/pubs-sum/183781.htm

Torres, S. (1987). Hispanic-American battered women: Why consider cultural differences? *Response, 12,* 113–131.

Torres, S., Campbell, J. C., Ryan, J., King, C., Campbell, D., Stallings, R., & Fuchs, S. (2000). Abuse during pregnancy: An ethnic group comparison. *Violence and Victims, 15*(3), 303–321.

Torres, S., & Han, H. (2000). Psychological distress in non-Hispanic White and Hispanic abused women. *Archives in Psychiatric Nursing, 14*(1), 19–29.

Tran, C. G., & des Jardins, K. (2000). Domestic violence in Vietnamese refugee and Korean immigrant communities. In J. L. Chin (Ed.), *Relationships among Asian American women* (pp. 71–96). New York: Hamilton Printing.

Trautman, D. E., McCarthy, M. L., Miller, N., Campbell, J. C., & Kelen, G. D. (2007). Intimate partner violence and emergency department screening: Computerized screening versus usual care. *Annals of Emergency Medicine, 49*(4), 526–534.

Ullamn, S. E., Townsend, S. M., Filipas, H. H., & Starzynski, L. L. (2007). Structural models of the relations of assault severity, social support, avoidance coping, self-blame, and PTSD among sexual assault survivors. *Psychology of Women Quarterly, 31,* 23–37.

Urbanic, J. C. (2004). Sexual abuse in families. In J. Humphreys & J. C. Campbell (Eds.), *Family violence and nursing practice* (pp. 186–219). Philadelphia: Lippincott Williams & Wilkins.

U.S. Department of Justice, Bureau of Justice Statistics. (2006a). *Homicide trends in the U.S.: Intimate homicide.* Retrieved February 7, 2007, from http://www.ojp.usdoj.gov/bjs/homicide/intimates.htm

U.S. Department of Justice, Bureau of Justice Statistics. (2006b). *Intimate partner violence in the U.S.: Circumstances.* Retrieved February 7, 2007, from http://www.ojp.usdoj.gov/bjs/intimate/circumstances.htm

U.S. Department of Justice, Bureau of Justice Statistics. (2006c). *Intimate partner violence in the U.S.: Victim characteristics.* Retrieved February 7, 2007, from http://www.ojp.usdoj.gov/bjs/intimate/victims.htm

Walton-Moss, B. J., Manganello, J., Frye, V., & Campbell, J. C. (2005). Risk factors for intimate partner violence and associated injury among urban women. *Journal of Community Health, 30*(5), 377–389.

Weil, J. M., & Lee, H. H. (2004). Cultural considerations in understanding family violence among Asian American Pacific Islander families. *Journal of Community Health Nursing, 21*(4), 217–227.

Weis, L., Fine, M., Proweller, A., Bertram, C., & Marusza, J. (2005). "I've slept in clothes long enough": Excavating the sounds of domestic violence among women in the White working class. In N. J. Sokoloff (Ed.), *Domestic violence at the margins: Readings on race, class, gender, and culture* (pp. 227–252). New Brunswick, NJ: Rutgers University Press.

Weisz, A. N. (2005). Reaching African American battered women: Increasing the effectiveness of advocacy. *Journal of Family Violence, 20*(2), 91–99.

Welsh, S. (1999). Gender and sexual harassment. *Annual Review of Sociology,* 25, 169–190.

Whitaker, D. J., Baker, C. K., Pratt, C., Reed, E., Suri, S., Pavlos, C., et al. (2007). A network model for providing culturally competent services for intimate partner violence and sexual violence. *Violence Against Women, 13*(2), 190–209.

White, R. J., & Gondolf, E. W. (2000). Implications of personality profiles for batterer treatment. *Journal of Interpersonal Violence, 15*(5), 467–488.

Williamson, C., & Folaron, G. (2001). Violence, risk, and survival: Strategies of street prostitution. *Western Journal of Nursing Research, 23*(5), 463–475.

Wingood, G. M., DiClemente, R. J., & Raj, A. (2000). Identifying the prevalence and correlates of STDs among women residing in rural domestic violence shelters. *Women and Health, 30*(4), 15–26.

Woods, S. J. (2005). Intimate partner violence and post-traumatic stress disorder symptoms in women: What we know and need to know. *Journal of Interpersonal Violence, 20*(4), 394–402.

Woods, S. J., & Isenberg, M. A. (2001). Adaptation as a mediator of intimate abuse and traumatic stress in battered women. *Nursing Science Quarterly, 14*(3), 215–221.

Woods, S. J., & Wineman, N. M. (2004). Trauma, posttraumatic stress disorder symptom clusters, and physical health symptoms in postabused women. *Archives in Psychiatric Nursing, 18*(1), 26–34.

Woods, S. J., Wineman, N. M., Page, G. G., Hall, R. J., Alexander, T. S., & Campbell, J. C. (2005). Predicting immune status in women from PTSD and childhood and adult violence. *Advances in Nursing Science, 28*(4), 306–319.

Wyszynski, M. E. (2000). Screening women for family violence in the maternal child healthcare setting. *Clinical Excellence for Nurse Practitioners, 4*(2), 76–82.

Yllö, K. (2005). Gender, diversity, and violence. In D. R. Loseke, R. J. Gelles, & M. M. Cavanaugh (Eds.), *Current controversies on family violence* (2nd ed., pp. 19–34). Thousand Oaks, CA: Sage.

Zahn, M. A. (2003). Intimate partner homicide: An overview. *National Institute of Justice Journal, 250.* Retrieved December 28, 2005, from http://www.ojp.usdoj.gov/nij

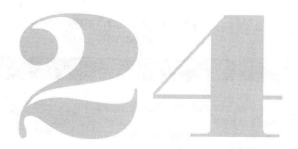

Sexually Transmitted Infections

Catherine Ingram Fogel

Sexual relations are a natural and healthy part of a woman's life and should be free of infection (Hatcher et al., 2004). However, preventing, diagnosing, and treating sexually transmitted infections (STIs) is becoming ever more challenging as an increasing number of persons are infected with more severe infections (Hatcher et al., 2004; Institute of Medicine, 1997). STIs are a "hidden epidemic of tremendous health and economic consequences in the United States" and represent a "growing threat to the nation's health" (Institute of Medicine, 1997, p. 28). Despite the U.S. Surgeon General targeting STIs as a priority for prevention and control efforts (Public Health Service, 1979), these infections are among the most common health problems in the United States today. Rates of curable STIs in the United States are the highest in developed countries and are higher than the rates in some developing countries (Centers for Disease Control and Prevention [CDC], 2005). Individuals with an STI are often undiagnosed regardless of whether they are asymptomatic and are a huge risk for the spread of infection. STIs affect approximately 19 million Americans every year (CDC, 2006a), almost half of which occur in persons ages 15 to 24 (Weinstock et al., 2004). At the current rate, at least one in four—and possibly as many as one in two—Americans will contract an STI during their life time (Gonen, 1999).

Sexually transmitted infections are a direct cause of tremendous human suffering, place heavy demands on health care services, and cost over $15 billion dollars in direct medical costs yearly (CDC, 2006a; Chesson, Blandford, Gift, Tao, & Irwin, 2004). The human costs are equally overwhelming. A diagnosis of cervical cancer or living with chronic pelvic pain can be devastating, and experiencing a preterm delivery or stillbirth can cause prolonged grief and suffering. Couples faced with a diagnosis of infertility due to STIs may require invasive diagnostic procedures and assisted reproductive technology such as in vitro fertilization.

Sexually transmitted infections are a group of contagious diseases commonly transmitted from person to person by close intimate contact (Nelson, 2006). The organisms causing STIs include a wide variety of microorganisms: bacteria, viruses, spirochetes, protozoans, and obligate intracellular organisms that infect the mucosal surfaces of the genitourinary tract as well as ectoparasities (organisms that live on the outside of the body such as lice) and the dozens of clinical syndromes that they cause (Schmid, 2001). These terms have replaced the older designation, venereal disease, which primarily described gonorrhea and syphilis. Common STIs are listed in Table 24.1. The common STIs in women are chlamydia, human papillomavirus, gonorrhea, herpes simplex virus type-2, syphilis, hepatitis B virus, and HIV infection.

In the past, public health efforts were aimed at the control of gonorrhea and syphilis; however, more recently, when it appeared that these diseases were controlled, concern focused on other diseases including chlamydia, herpes simplex virus (HSV), human papillomavirus (HPV), and the human immunodeficiency virus (HIV). Unfortunately, this shifting focus does not mean that gonorrhea and syphilis are no longer a concern, and, in recent years, increases in the number of syphilis and gonorrhea cases and drug-resistant strains of gonorrhea have become increasingly more common (CDC, 2006a). In the Unites States, STIs are among the most common infections, with 5 of the 10 most reported infections being STIs (American Social Health Association, 1998).

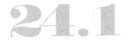

| Sexually Transmitted Infections in Women |

Diseases characterized by genital ulcers
- Chancroid
- Genital herpes simples virus infection
- Granuloma inguinale
- Lymphogranuloma
- Syphilis

Diseases characterized by urethritis and cervicitis
- Chlamydia
- Gonococcal infections
- Mucupurulent cervicitis

Diseases characterized by vaginal discharge
- Bacterial vaginosis
- Trichomoniasis
- Vulvovaginal candidiasis

Human papillomavirus infection

Vaccine-preventable sexually transmitted infections
- Hepatitis A
- Hepatitis B
- Hepatitis C

Ectoparasitic infections
- Pediculosis pubis
- Scabies

Human immunodeficiency virus

Note. From "Sexually Transmitted Diseases Treatment Guidelines 2006," by Centers for Disease Control and Prevention, 2006, *MMWR, 55*(RR-11), 1–94.

IMPACT OF SEXUALLY TRANSMITTED INFECTIONS ON WOMEN

Although, historically, STIs were considered to be symptomatic illnesses usually afflicting men, women and their children have the most severe symptoms and sequelae of these diseases. STIs have a greater and more long-lasting impact on the health of women than on the health of men. STIs in women and children are associated with multiple severe complications and death (see Table 24.2).

Reproductive Health Concerns

Pelvic inflammatory disease (PID), a preventable complication of some STIs such as chlamydia and gonorrhea, is a serious threat to women's reproductive capabilities. More than a million women every year experience an episode of PID and as many as 1 in 7 U.S. women report that they have received treatment for PID (Hatcher et al.,

2004). Further, at least 25% of women who have had PID experience long-term sequelae, including pelvic abscesses, chronic pelvic pain, dyspareunia, ectopic pregnancy due to partial tubal scarring and blockage, tubal infertility, increased need for reproductive tract surgery, and recurring PID (CDC, 2006b; Gonen, 1999). After an episode of PID, a woman is 6 to 10 times more likely to have an ectopic pregnancy compared to women who have not had PID. Ectopic pregnancy occurs in about 2% of all pregnancies; this rate is up 600 percent since 1970. Approximately 10 to 15 percent of all pregnancy-related deaths are attributed to ectopic pregnancy (Planned Parenthood, 2003). Half of all women's infertility is attributable to STIs (Nelson, 2006). At least 15% of infertile U.S. women are infertile because of tubal damage caused by PID, and no more than half have been previously diagnosed with PID. Ectopic pregnancy also substantially increases the risk of tubal-factor infertility. In contrast, STIs rarely cause infertility in men.

Adverse Pregnancy Outcomes

STIs may cause acute complications for pregnant women and their offspring. Pregnant women may transmit the infection to their fetus, newborn, or infant through vertical transmission (through the placenta prior to delivery, during vaginal birth, or after birth through breast-feeding) or horizontal transmission (close physical or household contact). Some of the complications associated with an STI experienced by pregnant women can include spontaneous abortion, stillbirth, premature rupture of membranes, and preterm delivery. Vaginal and cervical STI infections during pregnancy can lead to inflammation of the placental or fetal membranes, resulting in maternal fever during or after delivery, wound and pelvic infections after cesarean section, and postpartum endometritis. Sexually transmitted pathogens that have serious consequences for women tend to have even more serious, potentially life-threatening health conditions in the fetus or newborn. Damage to the brain, spinal cord, eyes, and auditory nerves are of particular concern with STIs in the fetus and infant. For example, severe, permanent central nervous system manifestations or fetal or neonatal death can occur with congenital syphilis. Currently, all transmission of HIV to infants in the United States is attributable to mother-to-infant transmission. Ophthalmia neonatorium can occur when infants of women with vaginal gonorrheal or chlamydial infections are infected during delivery and, if untreated, can result in corneal ulcers and blindness (CDC, 2002a).

Cancer-Related Consequences

Women are far more likely to develop cervical cancer from an HPV infection than are men to develop penile

24.2 | Major Complications of Sexually Transmitted Infections for Women and Children

HEALTH CONSEQUENCES	WOMEN	CHILDREN
Cancers	Cervical cancer Vulva cancer Vaginal cancer Anal cancer Liver cancer T-cell leukemia Body cavity lymphoma	Liver cancer as adult
Reproductive health problems	Pelvic inflammatory disease Infertility Spontaneous abortion	
Pregnancy-related problems	Ectopic pregnancy Preterm delivery Premature rupture of membranes Puerperal sepsis Postpartum infection	Stillborn Neonatal death Prematurity Low birth weight Conjunctivitis Pneumonia Neonatal sepsis Hepatitis, cirrhosis Hepatitis B virus infection Neurologic damage Laryngeal papillomatosis Congenital abnormalities

Neurologic problems	Human T-lymphotropic Virus-associated
	    myelopathy (paralysis)
	Neurosyphilis
		Cytomegalovirus-, herpes simplex virus-, and
		    syphilis-associated neurologic problems

Other health consequences	Chronic liver disease Cirrhosis Disseminated gonococcal infection Septic arthritis Tertiary syphilis (cardiovascular and gumma)	Chronic liver disease Cirrhosis

Note. Adapted from *The Hidden Epidemic: Confronting Sexually Transmitted Diseases,* by Institute of Medicine, 1997, Washington, DC: National Academy Press; "Sexually Transmitted Diseases Treatment Guidelines 2006," by Centers for Disease Control and Prevention, 2006, *MMWR, 55*(RR-11), 1–94.

carcinoma. Several key subtypes of sexually acquired human papillomavirus are associated with the development of cervical and other anogenital cancers (Koutsky et al., 2002). Cervical cancer is the second most common cancer among women worldwide, and about 95% of cervical cancers are associated with 10 to 15 HPV subtypes (Davies, 2000). Further, women with HPV infection of the cervix are 10 times more likely to develop invasive cervical cancer compared to women without HPV (Gall, 2001; Institute of Medicine, 1997). HIV infection may increase the risk that HPV infection will progress to cervical vaginal, vulvular, and anal cancers. Further, hepatitis B virus (HBV) causes hepatocellular carcinoma (Pastorek & Yordan-Jovet, 2001), and human herpes virus type-8 causes Kaposi sarcoma (Cates, Alexander, & Cates, 1998).

Increased HIV Risk

A synergistic relationship appears to exist between HIV and STIs (Cates, 2001). The inflammation or disruption of genital mucosa that can occur with ulcerative and inflammatory STIs is a risk factor for contracting HIV during a sexual encounter (Greenblatt & Hessol, 2001). The increased risk for HIV acquisition in women with genital ulcer diseases and gonococcal and chlamydial cervicitis is estimated to be two- to four-fold (Wang & Celum, 2001). Women with *candida* and trichomonal vaginitis are estimated to have a two- to three-fold increased risk of transmission (Wang & Celum, 2001).

Preventing, identifying, and managing STIs are essential components of women's health care. Advanced practice nurses play an essential role in promoting women's reproductive and sexual health by counseling women about STI risk, encouraging sexual and other risk-reduction measures, incorporating education regarding STI disease prevention in their nursing practice, and being current on management strategies. By doing so, advanced practice nurses can assist women in avoiding STIs and in living better with the sequelae and chronic infections of STIs.

TRANSMISSION OF SEXUALLY TRANSMITTED INFECTIONS

The chance of contracting, transmitting, or suffering complications from HIV and STIs depends on multiple biological, behavioral, social, and relationship risk factors. The Institute of Medicine (1997, p. 1) noted that STIs are "hidden from the public view because many Americans are reluctant to address sexual health issues in an open way and because of the biological and social factors associated with these infections." Microbiological, hormonal, and immunological factors influence individual susceptibility and transmission potential for STIs. These factors are partially influenced by a woman's sexual practices, substance use, and other health behaviors. Health behaviors, in turn, are influenced by socioeconomic factors and other social factors. In general, the prevalence of STIs tends to be higher in those who are unmarried, young (aged 15 to 35 years), and live in urban areas.

Biological Factors

Women are biologically more likely to become infected than are men; for example, the risk of a woman contracting gonorrhea from a single act of intercourse is 60% to 90%, while the risk for a man is 20% to 30%. Further, men are two to three times more likely to transmit HIV to women than the reverse. The vagina has a larger amount of genital mucous membranes exposed and has an environment more conducive for infections than does the penis (Cates et al., 1998). Further, risk for trauma is greater during vaginal intercourse for women than for men (Kurth, 1998). The cervix, particularly the squamocolumnar junction/transformation zone and endocervical columnar epithelial cells, are most susceptible to HIV; however, the virus can invade the vaginal epithelium as well (Futterman, 2001).

More than 50% of bacterial and 90% of viral STIs are asymptomatic and thus likely to be undetected in women. Additionally, when or if symptoms develop, they may be confused with those of other diseases not transmitted sexually. The frequency of asymptomatic and unrecognized infections results in delayed diagnosis and treatment, chronic untreated infections, and complications. Further, it is more difficult to diagnose

STIs in a woman because the anatomy of her genital tract makes clinical examination more difficult. For example, to diagnose gonorrhea in men, all that is needed is a urethral swab and Gram stain; in women, a speculum exam and specific cervical culture are necessary. Lesions that occur inside the vagina and in the cervix are not readily seen, and the normal vaginal environment (warm, moist, enriched medium), is ideal for infection.

Age and gender influence an individual's risk for an STI; specifically, young women (age 20 to 24) and female adolescents (10 to 19 years) are more susceptible than are their male counterparts. STIs tend to occur at a younger age in females than in males (Nelson, 2006). Eighty percent of adolescent girls are sexually active by age 18, with the end result of a large number of young women at risk for STIs (Guttmacher Institute, 2002). Compared to women prior to menopause, female adolescents and young women are more susceptible to cervical infections, such as chlamydial infections and gonorrhea, and HIV because of the ectropion of the immature cervix and resulting larger exposed surface of cells unprotected by cervical mucus. The cells eventually recede into the inner cervix as women age. Postmenopausal women also are at increased risk due to thin vaginal and cervical mucosa. Further, women who are pregnant have higher rates of cervical ectropion (Cunningham et al., 2002).

Other biological factors that may increase a woman's risk for acquiring, transmitting, or developing complications of certain STIs include vaginal douching, risky sexual practices, and use of hormonal contraceptives. Risk for contracting the infections that can lead to PID may be increased with vaginal douching, and risk for PID may increase with greater frequency of douching (CDC, 2006b). Certain sexual practices such as anal intercourse, sex during menses, and "dry sex" (insertive vaginal sex without sufficient lubrication) may predispose a woman to acquiring an STI. This may be because the bleeding and tissue trauma that can result from these practices facilitate invasion by pathogens.

The role of oral contraceptives in the acquisition and transmission of STIs is not fully understood. Several studies have found oral contraceptives to be associated with a decreased risk (10% to 70%) of developing PID (Hatcher, 2004). Cervical ectopy is positively associated with the use of oral contraceptives and with chlamydial infections. A meta-analysis of studies on the effects of oral contraceptives on HIV susceptibility reported that the use of oral contraceptives may be associated with a small increased risk of HIV infection (Wang & Celum, 2001).

Normal vaginal flora may confer nonspecific immunity, and recent data suggest that women with bacterial vaginosis are at increased risk for HIV seroconversion (Wang & Celum, 2001). Both younger and postmenopausal women are at greater risk for acquiring HIV because of a thinner vaginal epithelium and resulting increased friability, thus providing direct access to the bloodstream (Kurth, 1998).

Social Factors

Preventing the spread of STIs and HIV is difficult without addressing individual and community issues that have a tremendous influence on prevention, transmission, and treatment of these diseases. Societal factors such as poverty, lack of education, social inequity, and inadequate access to health care indirectly increase the prevalence of STIs and HIV in risk populations.

Persons with the highest rates of many STIs are often those with the poorest access to health care, and health insurance coverage influences if and where a woman obtains STI services and preventive services. Further, even if a poor woman perceives herself to be at risk for an STI, she may not practice protective behaviors if survival is an overarching concern or if there are other risks that appear to be more threatening or imminent (Mays & Cochran, 1988). The need to secure shelter, food, clothing, safety for self and children, and money may override concerns about preventive health and thus prevent women from changing risky behaviors (Nyamanthi & Lewis, 1991; Stevens et al., 1995).

Social Interactions and Relationships

STIs are the only illnesses whose spread is directly caused by the human urge to share sexual intimacy and reproduce. Because intimate human contact is the common vehicle of transmission, sexual behavior in the context of relationships is a critical risk factor for preventing and acquiring STIs. The gender-power imbalance and cultural proscriptions sometimes associated with sexual relationships make it difficult for women to protect themselves from infection (Miller, Exner, Williams, & Ehrhardt, 2000; Mize, Robinson, Bockting, & Scheltma, 2002). Women may have less say over when and under what circumstances intercourse occurs. Young women are particularly at risk because they may have sex with older men and—because of the power difference in the relationship, feelings of low self-efficacy, and lack of self-confidence—may be unable to negotiate safer sex practices (Jemmott & Brown, 2003; Upchurch & Kusunoki, 2004). Lifestyles of premarital, intermarital, and extramarital sexual activity are common for many women; because of the secrecy and cultural proscriptions surrounding such activities, women often engage in them without preparation, leading to risk for themselves and their partners.

A woman may be dependent on an abusive male partner or a partner who places her at risk by his own risky behaviors (Fisher et al., 2004; Kurth, 1998). The risk of acquiring STIs or HIV infection is high among women who are physically and sexually abused. Past and current experiences with violence, particularly sexual abuse, erode women's sense of self-efficacy to exercise control over sexual behaviors, engender feelings of anxiety and depression, and increase the likelihood of risky sexual behaviors (Maman, 2000). Additionally, fear of physical harm and loss of economic support hamper women's efforts to enact protective practices. Further, past and current abuse is strongly associated with substance abuse, which also increases the risk of contracting an STI.

A woman's risk of acquiring an STI is determined not only by her actions but by her partner's as well. Although prevention counseling customarily includes recommending that women identify the partner who is at high risk because of drugs and medical factors and also determine his sexual practices, this advice may be unrealistic or culturally inappropriate in many relationships. Women who engage in sexual activities with other women only may or may not be at risk for infection. Many women who identify themselves as lesbian have had intercourse with a man at one time by choice, by force, or by necessity. Their female partners may have had intercourse with a man. In addition, lesbians may use drugs and share needles.

Societal Norms

Cultural and religious attitudes regarding appropriate sexual behaviors affect risk at the individual and community levels. Relationships and sexual behavior are regulated by cultural norms that influence sexual expression in interpersonal relationships. Often women are still socialized to please their partners and to place men's needs and desires first and may find it difficult to insist on safer sex behaviors. Traditional cultural values associated with passivity and subordination may diminish the ability of many women to adequately protect themselves.

Power imbalances in relationships are the product of and contributors to the maintenance of traditional gender roles that identify men as the initiators and decision makers of sexual activities and women as passive gatekeepers (Miller et al., 2000). As long as traditional gender norms define the roles for sexual relationships as men having the dominant role in sexual decision making, negotiating condom use by women will remain difficult. Additionally, cultural norms define talking about condoms as implying a lack of trust that runs counter to the traditional gender norm expectations for women. Women may not request condom use because of a need to establish and maintain intimacy with partners. Research has demonstrated that women at risk for HIV place significant importance on and investment in their heterosexual relationships, and these dynamics impact on the women's risk taking and risk management (MacRae & Aalto, 2000). Urging women to insist on condom use may be unrealistic, because traditional gender roles do not encourage women to talk about sex, initiate sexual practices, or control intimate encounters.

Recognition of Risk

Lack of a perception of risk is often given as a reason for not using sexual protective practices. Younger women may incur more STIs because they have less knowledge of reproductive health, less effective skills in communicating and negotiating with their partners about safer sex practices, and more barriers to access to health care services. Taking risks is a universal human element. In the throes of passion, people can make unwise sexual decisions. Further, safer sex is not always perceived to be the most enjoyable sex.

Substance Use

Substance use (alcohol and drugs) is associated with increased risk of HIV and STIs (Wechsberg, Lam, Zule, & Bobshev, 2004), and STI rates are higher in areas where rates of substance abuse are high. For example, in many areas, crack use has paralleled trends in syphilis, gonorrhea, chancroid, and HIV infection. There are several possible reasons for this association, including social factors such as poverty and lack of educational and economic opportunities and individual factors such as risk taking and low self-efficacy. In addition to the risk from sharing needles, use of drugs and alcohol may contribute to risk of HIV infection by undermining cognitive and social skills, thus making it more difficult to engage in HIV-protective actions (Harris, 1995; Substance Abuse and Mental Health Services Administration, 2005). Further, depression and other psychological problems and/or a history of sexual abuse are associated with substance abuse and thus contribute to risky behaviors (Johnson, Cunningham-Williams, & Cottler, 2003). Being high and thus not able or willing to clean drug paraphernalia can be a pervasive barrier to protective practice. Further, drug use may take place in settings where persons participate in sexual activities while using drugs. Cocaine abusers have demonstrated higher levels of sexual risk behaviors than other addict populations (McCoy, McCoy, & Lai, 1998). Finally, women who use drugs may be at higher risk because of the practice of exchanging sex for drugs or money and high numbers of sexual partners and encounters (Dolcini, Coates, Catania, Kegeles, & Hauck, 1995; Wechsberg et al., 2003).

Past and current physical, emotional, and sexual abuses characterize the lives of many, if not most, drug-using women (Kearney, 2001; McFarlane, Parker, & Cross, 2001). For women who have experienced violence, use of alcohol and drugs can become a coping mechanism by which they self-medicate to relieve feelings of anxiety, depression, guilt, fear, and anger stemming from the violence (Grella, Anglin, & Annon, 1996). Women's drug use is strongly linked to relationship inequities and some men's ability to mandate women's sexual behavior. Sexual degradation of women is described as an intimate part of crack cocaine use (Henderson, 1997).

Cultural and religious attitudes and beliefs also affect health care services. The loss of support for safer sex education programs in favor of an abstinence-only program does not protect adolescents (Camampang, Barth, Korpi, & Kirby, 1997). Teens who pledge to remain a virgin until marriage have the same, if not higher, rates of STIs than those who do not commit to abstinence (Brucker & Bearman, 2005). In response to these findings, a more pragmatic abstinence-plus or "ABC" message based on harm-reduction principles has been instituted. The message is Abstinence, Be faithful for married couples or those in committed relationships, and use a Condom for individuals who put themselves at risk for HIV infection. Reflecting a shift from prevention toward treatment, no more than 20% of funding can be spent for HIV prevention programs (Nelson, 2006); further, prevention funds may be appropriated to organizations that are not required to participate in prevention or treatment programs due to religious or moral objections.

PREVENTION

Preventing infection (primary prevention) is the most effective way of reducing the adverse consequences of STIs for women, their partners, and society. With the advent of serious and potentially lethal STIs that are not readily cured or are incurable, primary prevention becomes critical. Prompt diagnosis and treatment of current infections (secondary prevention) also can prevent personal complications and transmission to others. Prevention and control of STIs depend on five major activities: (1) education of persons who are at risk on ways to reduce risky behaviors; (2) preexposure vaccination; (3) identification of asymptomatically infected and symptomatic untreated persons; (4) effectively diagnosing and treating infection and counseling infected persons; and (5) assessment, treatment, and counseling of sex partners of those infected with an STI (CDC, 2006b). Primary prevention of STIs begins with changing those behaviors that place persons at risk for infection. Moreover, treatment of infected individuals is a form of primary prevention of spread within the community in that it reduces the likelihood of transmission of STIs to sexual partners (CDC, 2006b). Further, key to real progress in STI prevention is coordination of prevention programs for unintended pregnancy and HIV with those for other STIs, because all are the consequences of unprotected sexual activity (Cates & Cates, 1998). Risk factors for STIs and HIV are summarized in Exhibit 24.1.

Education

Educational efforts, both population-based and individual, that are gender- and culturally specific and are at an appropriate literacy level are important to STI control. Educational messages about specific infections, personal protective practices, and communication skills should be delivered in age-appropriate, culturally sensitive, appealing formats. Specific patient education messages are found in Table 24.3.

Unfortunately, mass educational efforts in the United States are limited largely to schools and the media. Further, the cultural imposed secrecy surrounding sexual issues prevalent in U.S. society results in a tremendous lack of information about STI prevention. To change risky behaviors, Americans need to become more comfortable discussing sexuality and sexual health issues between health care providers and patients, between sexual partners, and between parents and children (Institute of Medicine, 1997). Comprehensive sexual health education provides information about STIs and HIV transmission, prevention, and treatment and abstinence and protective practice as well as training to build negotiation and communication skills. Although knowledge is essential in preventing STIs and HIV, it is not sufficient to change behavior (Mize et al., 2002).

Individual Counseling

Since the advent of HIV and other incurable viral STIs, counseling individual women has become even more important. As incurable infections have emerged, the role of treatment with cure has lessened, and the need for risk-reduction counseling has increased. Woman-centered counseling to prevent acquisition or transmission of STIs should be a standard component of STI care regardless of where it is provided in the health care system. Counseling skills that are characterized by respect, compassion, and a nonjudgemental attitude toward all patients are essential to obtaining a complete sexual risk history and counseling women effectively about prevention. Specific techniques that have been found to be effective in providing prevention counseling include using open-ended questions (e.g., "What's your experience with using condoms been like?"), using understandable language ("Have you ever had a sore or scab on your

EXHIBIT 24.1 RISK FACTORS FOR SEXUALLY TRANSMITTED INFECTIONS AND HIV

Women who are at increased risk for contracting sexually transmitted infections (STIs) and HIV include:

- Those who have unprotected vaginal, anal, or oral intercourse.
- Those who have multiple sex partners.
- Those who use alcohol or illicit drugs during sexual activity.
- Those with high-risk sex practices, including fisting, oral-anal contact, anal intercourse.
- Those who share sex toys and douching equipment.
- Those who share needles or other drug use paraphernalia.
- Those who have partners who are bisexual men who also have sex with other men.
- Women with a previous history of a documented STI or HIV infection.
- Women with partners who have a previous history of STIs or HIV.
- Women involved in the exchange of sex for drugs or money.
- Women who live in areas with a high STI/HIV incidence or prevalence.
- Women at their initiation of sexual activity.

Note. From "Sexually Transmitted Infections," by C. I. Fogel, 2006, in K. D. Schuiling and F. K. Likis (Eds.), *Women's Gynecological Health* (pp. 421-469), Boston: Jones and Bartlett; *The Hidden Epidemic Confronting Sexually Transmitted Diseases,* by Institute of Medicine, 1997, Washington, DC: National Academy Press; "Sexually Transmitted Diseases Treatment Guidelines 2006," by Centers for Disease Control and Prevention, 2006, *MMWR, 55*(RR-11), pp. 1-94; "Epidemiology of Sexually Transmitted Infections," by G. P. Schmid, 2001, in S. Faro and D. E. Soper (Eds.), *Infectious Diseases in Women* (pp. 395-402), Philadelphia: Saunders; "Sexually Transmitted Diseases," by W. Star, 2004, in W. L. Star, L. L. Lommel, and M. T. Shannon (Eds.), *Women's primary health care* (2nd ed., pp. 13-1–13-59), San Francisco: UCSF Nursing Press.

24.3 | Messages for Patients

Strategies for reducing personal risk
■ Avoiding all sexual contact (abstinence) with others is the only sure way to avoid contracting a sexually transmitted infection (STI).
■ Have sex with only one person who doesn't have sex with anyone else and who is free of STIs.
■ Always use a condom and use it correctly.
■ If you inject needles, always use clean needles and other drug paraphernalia.
■ Prevent and treat all STIs to decrease your susceptibility to HIV infection and to decrease your infectiousness if you are HIV positive.
■ Delay starting to have sex as long as possible because the younger you are when you starting having sex, the greater your risk for catching an STI.
■ Decrease the number of partners you have because the risk of contracting an STI increases with the number of partners you have at one time and over your life time.

If you are sexually active,
■ Always use protection unless you are having sex with only one person who is also monogamous and who has no infection.
■ Have regular checkups for STIs even if you have no symptoms.
■ Always have a checkup when having sex with a new person.
■ Know the symptoms for STIs and see a health care provider if any suspicious symptoms develop, no matter how minor they are.
■ Do not have sex during your menstrual period because you are more susceptible to contracting an STI at that time.
■ Avoid anal intercourse, and use a condom if you have anal intercourse.
■ Do not douche unless prescribed by your health care provider because it removes some of the normal protective bacteria and increases the risk of getting some STIs.

If you are diagnosed with having an STI,
■ Be treated to decrease your risk of transmitting an STI to your partner.
■ Notify all recent sex partners, and urge them to get a checkup and be treated if necessary.
■ Follow all of your health care provider's recommendations.
■ Take all medications as prescribed and take all medications.
■ Have a follow-up test if indicated.
■ Do not have sex during your treatment.

Note. From "Sexually Transmitted Infections," by C. I. Fogel, 2006, in K. D. Schuiling and F. L. Likis (Eds.), *Women's Gynecologic Health* (pp. 421–468), Boston: Jones and Bartlett..

private parts or lips?"), normalizing language ("Some of my patients tell me that it is hard to use a condom every time they have sex. How has it been for you?"), and reassuring the women that treatment will be provided regardless of consideration such as ability to pay, language spoken, or lifestyle (CDC, 2006b).

Assurances of confidentiality are equally important in providing effective risk reduction counseling. Prevention messages should include descriptions of specific actions to be taken to avoid acquiring or transmitting STIs (e.g., refrain from sexual activity if you have STI-related symptoms, be vaccinated against hepatitis B infection) and be tailored to the individual woman with attention given to her specific risk factors.

Safer Sex Practices

Risk-free individual activities aimed at deterring infection include complete abstinence from sexual activities

that transmit semen, blood, or other body fluids or that allow for skin-to-skin contact (Hatcher et al., 2004). Counseling that encourages abstinence from sexual intercourse is critical for women who are being treated for an STI, for women whose partner is being treated for an STI, and for persons wanting to avoid all possible consequences of sex (e.g., STIs, HIV, and unintended pregnancies). Alternatively, involvement in a mutually monogamous relationship with an uninfected partner also eliminates risk of contracting an STI. For women beginning a mutually monogamous relationship, screening for common STIs before beginning sex might decrease the risk for future transmission of asymptomatic STIs (CDC, 2006b). When neither of these options is realistic for a woman, however, the nurse must focus on other, more feasible measures (see Table 24.4).

An essential component of primary prevention is counseling women regarding safer sex practices, including knowledge of her partner, reduction of number

24.4 | Sexual Risk Practices and Preventive Practices

SAFEST	LOW RISK	POSSIBLE RISK	HIGH RISK

Behavior
Abstinence
Self-masturbation
Mutual monogamy
    (both partners monogamous
    and no high-risk activities)
Hugging, touching, massage[a]
Dry kissing
Mutual masturbation
Drug abstinence
 	
Prevention
Avoid all drug and sexual
    high risk behaviors.
	Behavior
	Wet kissing
	Vaginal intercourse with condom
	Fellatio interruptus
	Urine contact with intact skin
	
	Prevention
	Avoid exposure to any potentially
	    infected body fluids.
	Consistently use latex or
	    polyurethane condoms.
		Behavior
		Cunnilingus
		Fellatio
		Mutual masturbation with skin
		    breaks
		Anal intercourse with condom
		
		Prevention
		Avoid anal intercourse.
		Use dental dam, unlubricated
		    male condom cut in half,
		    female condom, or plastic
		    wrap with cunnilingus.
		Use latex gloves with
		    masturbation.
			Behavior
			Unprotected anal intercourse
			Unprotected vaginal intercourse
			Unprotected oral-anal contact
			Vaginal intercourse after anal
			    intercourse without a new
			    condom
			Fisting
			Multiple sex partners
			Sharing sex toys, needles or other
			    drug paraphernalia, or douching
			    equipment
			
			Prevention
			Avoid exposure to potentially
			    infected body fluids.
			Consistent condom use with
			    vaginal and anal intercourse.
			Avoid anal penetration.
			If having anal penetration, use
			    condom with intercourse, latex
			    glove with hand penetration.
			Avoid oral-anal contact.
			Do not share sex toys, drug
			    paraphernalia, or douche
			    equipment.
			Clean needles and drug
			    paraphernalia with bleach and
			    water before and after use.

Note. From "Sexually Transmitted Diseases," by C. I. Fogel, 1995, in N. F. Woods and C. I. Fogel (Eds.), *Women's Health Care* (pp. 571–609), Thousand Oaks, CA: Sage; "Sexually Transmitted Infections," by C. I. Fogel, 2006, in K. D. Schuiling and F. L. Likis (Eds.), *Women's Gynecologic Health,* (pp. 421–468), Boston: Jones and Bartlett; "Sexually Transmitted Diseases Treatment Guidelines 2006," by Centers for Disease Control and Prevention, 2006, *MMWR, 55*(RR-11), 1–94.
[a] Assumes no breaks in the skin.

of partners, low-risk sex, and avoiding the exchange of body fluids. No aspect of prevention is more important than knowing one's partner. Reducing the number of partners and avoiding partners who have had many previous sexual partners decreases a woman's chance of contracting an STI. Deciding not to have sexual contact with a casual acquaintance may be helpful too. Discussing each new partner's previous sexual history and exposure to STIs will augment other efforts to reduce risk. Women must be cautioned that, in any sexual encounter other than a mutually monogamous relationship, safer sex measures are always advisable, even when partners insist otherwise. Critically important is whether male partners resist wearing condoms. This is crucial when women are not sure about their partner's sexual history. Women should be cautioned against making decisions about a partner's sexual and other behaviors based on appearances and unfounded assumptions such as:

- Single people have many partners and risky practices.
- Older people have few partners and infrequent sexual encounters.
- Sexually experienced people know how to practice safer sex.
- Married people are heterosexual, low risk, and monogamous.
- People who look healthy are disease free.
- People with good jobs don't use drugs (Guest, 2006).

Women should be taught low-risk sexual practices and which sexual practices to avoid (Table 24.4). Sexual fantasizing is safe, as are caressing, hugging, body rubbing (frottage), and massage. Mutual masturbation is low risk as long as there is no contact with a partner's semen or vaginal secretions. All sexual activities when both partners are monogamous, trustworthy, and known by testing to be free of disease are safe.

When used correctly and consistently, male latex condoms are effective in preventing sexual transmission of HIV infection and can reduce the risk for other STIs (gonorrhea, chlamydia, and trichomonas). However, because they do not cover all exposed surfaces, they are more likely to be most effective in preventing infections that are transmitted by fluids from mucosal surfaces (gonorrhea, chlamydia, trichomonas, and HIV) than those transmitted by skin-to-skin contact (e.g., herpes simplex virus, human papillomavirus, syphilis, chancroid). Rates of latex condom breakage during sexual intercourse and withdrawal are low (about 2 condoms per 100 condoms used) in the United States (CDC, 2006b). Although nonlatex condoms (e.g., those made of polyuerethane) have higher rates of breakage and slippage than do latex condoms, they can be substituted for persons with latex allergies (CDC, 2006b). The failures of condoms to protect women against STI transmission or unintended pregnancy are usually the result of inconsistent or incorrect use rather than from condom breakage.

Thus, counseling women about correct condom use is critical. Nurses can help to motivate clients to use condoms by first discussing the subject with them. This gives women an opportunity to discuss any concerns, misconceptions, or hesitations they may have about using condoms. The nurse may initiate a discussion of how to purchase and use condoms. Information to be discussed includes importance of using latex or plastic condoms rather than natural skin condoms. The nurse should remind women to use condoms with every sexual encounter, only use them once, use condoms with a current expiration date, and handle them carefully to avoid damaging them with fingernails, teeth, or other sharp objects. Condoms should be stored away from high heat. Contrary to popular myth, a recent study found no increase in breakage after carrying condoms in a wallet for a lengthy period of time (Hatcher et al., 2004). Although not ideal, women may choose to safely carry condoms in wallets, shoes, or inside a bra. Women can be taught the differences between condoms, price ranges, sizes, and where they can be purchased. This information can be found on the Web site of the American Social Health Association (www.ashastd.org) or in any drug store.

Laboratory studies have demonstrated that the female condom (Reality)—a lubricated polyurethane sheath with a ring on each end that is inserted into the vagina—is an effective mechanical barrier to virus, including HIV, and to semen (Drew, Blair, Miner, & Conant, 1990; French et al., 2003). Further, clinical studies have documented its effectiveness in providing protection from recurrent trichomonas (CDC, 2006b). If used consistently and correctly, the female condom should reduce the risk of contracting or transmitting an STI. Information on using male and female condoms is found in Exhibits 24.2, 24.3, 24.4, and 24.5.

Selection of a contraceptive method has a direct impact on STI risk. Many women view condoms first, and perhaps only, as a method of contraception. Women who have another method of birth control such as sterilization or hormonal contraceptives are less likely to use condoms when compared to other women. The effectiveness of contraceptive methods against STIs

---

EXHIBIT 24.2 SUGGESTIONS ON HOW TO USE A MALE CONDOM

Use new condoms every time you perform any vaginal, anal, and oral sex (try flavored).

- Open the package carefully to avoid damage.
- Do not unroll before placing it on the penis.
- Gently press out air at the tip before putting it on.
- Put on when the penis is erect.
- Unroll to cover the entire erect penis.
- If it tears or comes off in the vagina, stop immediately and withdraw. Put on a new one before you continue.
- After ejaculation and before the penis gets soft, withdraw the penis and the condom together.
- Hold on to the rim as you withdraw so nothing spills.
- Gently pull off the penis.
- Discard in waste containers.
- Don't flush down the toilet.
- Never reuse condoms.

EXHIBIT 24.3 QUESTIONS AND ANSWERS ABOUT USING MALE CONDOMS

- **How many condoms will I need?**
  You need to use a new condom every time you have sexual intercourse (however you have it). If you think you might have sex more than once, you should carry several with you. Never reuse the same condom—it won't work. Carry more condoms than you think you might need.

- **Where should I keep my condoms?**
  You need to keep condoms cool and dry (and in the dark), so keep them in the pocket of a jacket or in a bag. Don't keep them in the pocket of your jeans or the glove compartment of your car, because they will get too hot.

- **What do I need to do before I have sex?**
  Make sure the package the condom is sold in looks okay and check the expiration date. Carefully open the condom package at one corner. Don't attack it with your teeth or fingernails (this is the most common reason for a condom to be torn). You might tear a hole in the condom too. The condom will be rolled up ready for use. Make sure you use it the right way around (so the condom rolls down smoothly).

- **What do I need to do before I have intercourse?**
  You need to put the condom on when the penis is erect but before you have made any contact between the penis and any part of your partner's body.

- **How do I put a male condom on?**
  If you have not been circumcised, you will need to roll back your foreskin a bit before putting the condom on. Put the still rolled-up condom over the tip of the hard (erect) penis. If the condom doesn't have a reservoir (the blob at the end, which most condoms do have), you need to pinch half an inch at the end of it to make room for the semen (sperm) to collect. Pinch the air out of the condom tip between your finger and thumb of one hand, and unroll the condom over the penis with the other hand. Roll the condom all the way down to the base of the penis, and smooth out any air bubbles (air bubbles can cause a condom to break).

- **How do I put extra lubrication on a condom?**
  If you want or need to use some extra lubrication, put it on the outside of the condom before you use it. Only use a water-based lubricant, because an oil-based lubricant will dissolve the latex of the condom, making it useless.

- **What if I can't get the condom on?**
  Most of the time (and when you have practiced a bit) condoms will roll down your penis very easily and smoothly. If it is getting stuck or is difficult to roll down, it probably means you are putting it on inside out. You will need to get this condom off by holding its rim. Throw this condom away and start again with a new one.

- **When do I take the condom off?**
  When you are wearing a condom, you need to come out of your partner when your penis is still hard. To make sure that you don't spill any semen (sperm), which will be at the end of the condom, you need to hold the condom against the base of the penis while you pull out. Have a look at the condom to look for tears or spills, and then pull the condom off.

- **What do I do with the used condom?**
  It is best to tie a knot in the used condom and then throw it in a bin (preferably wrapped in some tissue). Do not litter, and don't flush them down the toilet because they are not biodegradable and can be dangerous for marine life.

- **What if I haven't used it perfectly or have found a tear?**
  No one is perfect and accidents happen. If you think the condom you have used might not have been used perfectly or you find a tear in it, don't panic. Tell your partner right away. She might be annoyed at the time, but she will be more annoyed if she gets an infection or misses her next period and finds out she is pregnant. If your partner can get to a family planning clinic, her general practitioner, or a genitourinary medicine clinic soon

(continued)

(preferably within 24 hours), she can get emergency contraception. The earlier she starts to take the emergency contraceptive pills, the more likely they are to prevent a pregnancy. It is still worth going to seek advice up to 5 days after having sex because sometimes a coil intrauterine device can be fitted as a type of emergency contraception. If the condom hasn't worked properly, the sex you have had is unprotected, and you and your partner are both at risk of getting an infection. Get yourselves to a clinic and get checked out.

Note. From Sexual Health Advice Center, How to use a male condom http://www.addenbrookes.org.uk/serv/clin/shac/advice/contraception/types/mcondom.htm

EXHIBIT 24.4 HOW TO USE A CONDOM

- DO use only latex or polyurethane (plastic) condoms.
- DO keep condoms in a cool, dry place.
- DO put the condom on an erect (hard) penis before there is any contact with a partner's genitals.
- DO use plenty of water-based lubricant (like KY® or Astroglide®) with latex condoms. This reduces friction and helps prevent the condom from tearing.
- DO squeeze the air out of the tip of the condom when rolling it over the erect penis. This allows room for the semen (cum).
- DO hold the condom in place at the base of the penis before withdrawing (pulling out) after sex.
- DO throw the condom away after it's been used.
- DON'T use out-of-date condoms. Check the expiration date carefully. Old condoms can be dry, brittle, or weakened and can break easily.
- DON'T unroll the condom before putting it on the erect penis.
- DON'T leave condoms in hot places—like your wallet or in your car.
- DON'T use oil-based products—such as baby oil, cooking oil, hand lotion, or petroleum jelly (Vaseline®)—as lubricants with latex condoms. The oil quickly weakens latex and can cause condoms to break.
- DON'T use your fingernails or teeth when opening a condom wrapper. It's very easy to tear the condom inside. If you do tear a condom while opening the wrapper, throw that condom away and get a new one.
- DON'T reuse a condom. Always use a new condom for each kind of sex you have.

More information

If you have additional questions about the right way to use a condom, call the National STD and AIDS hot lines at 1 (800) 342-2437 or 1 (800) 227-8922. The hot lines are open 24 hours a day, 7 days a week. For information in Spanish, call 1 (800) 344-7432, 8:00 A.M. to 2:00 A.M. Eastern time, 7 days a week. For the deaf and hard-of-hearing, call 1 (800) 243-7889, 10:00 A.M. to 10:00 P.M. Eastern time, Monday through Friday. The hot lines provide referrals and more answers to your questions.

Note. From http://www.ashastd.org/condom/condom_introduction.cfm

EXHIBIT 24.5 FEMALE CONDOMS

What are female condoms?

Female condoms are made of very thin polyurethane. They are already lubricated to help you use them, but they don't have any spermicide (which is useful for people who are allergic to spermicide). Because they are made of a type of plastic, they can be used by people who are allergic to latex. They can also be used with oil-based lubricants and products (but be sure to not use oil-based lubricants with male condoms by mistake).

Where do they go?

Female condoms are placed in a woman's vagina to line it and prevent sperm entering her cervix. It also helps protect her from infections that can be caught by having unprotected sex. (This will also protect her from most infections.) If used perfectly, they can be as effective as other contraceptives. If you use them with the birth control (or contraceptive) pill, they will be even more effective.

EXHIBIT 24.5 FEMALE CONDOMS (CONTINUED)

What are the advantages of female condoms?
- The woman is in control of her contraception.
- Female condoms can protect against infections.
- There are no side effects.
- You don't have to remember to take a pill.
- You can put a female condom in any time before sex.

What makes them less effective?
- If the penis touches the vagina or area around it before a female condom is inserted.
- If the condom splits.
- If the female condom gets pushed too far into the vagina.
- If the penis enters the vagina outside the condom.
- The open end must stay outside the vagina during sex.

How to use female condoms?
A new packet will have full instructions, including diagrams.

1. Check it is new and check the use-by date.
2. You can put one in when you are lying down, squatting, or have one leg on a chair (like using a tampon, find the position that suits you best).
3. Take it out of the packet with care (fingernails and rings can tear polyurethane).
4. Hold the closed end of the condom and squeeze the inner ring (at the closed end) between your thumb and middle finger. If you keep your index finger on the inner ring too, it will help to keep it steady.
5. With your other hand, spread the outer and inner lips (labia), which are the folds of skin around your vagina. Push the squeezed ring into the vagina and as far up as you can (about a long-finger length). Now put your index finger or both your index and middle finger inside the open end of the condom, until you can feel the inner ring at the top. Push the inner ring at the top as far as you can into your vagina. (You will be able to feel the hard front of your pelvis—pubic bone—just in front of your fingers if you curve them forward a bit.)
6. The outer ring should be close against the outside of your vagina (vulva).
7. The female condom is loose fitting, so it is a good idea for the woman to help guide the penis into the ring. It will move about a bit during sex, but you will be protected from pregnancy and most infections as long as the penis stays inside the condom.

How to remove female condoms?
Take hold of the outer ring (the open end), and give it a twist to trap any semen inside it. Pull it out gently.

What to do with used female condoms?
Never reuse a female condom. Wrap it up in a tissue and throw it in a trash bin. Don't put it in the toilet.

How to Use a Female Condom
http://www.addenbrookes.org.uk/serv/clin/shac/advice/contraception/types/fcondom.htm

including HIV is summarized in Table 24.5. Women should be counseled that the contraceptive methods that are most protective against STIs usually are not the most effective pregnancy prevention methods. For example, condoms are the most protective method against STIs and HIV but are not the most effective in preventing pregnancy. Use of dual protection to prevent pregnancy and STIs is critical for women. Because it is unclear how many women understand the need for dual protection, clinicians can play an important role in counseling women in this regard and in the importance of other risk-reduction practices.

Until recently, women were counseled to use spermicides—specifically nonoxynol-9 (N-9)—with condoms for the prevention of HIV and other STIs. Research has found no significant reduction in the risk of HIV and STIs with the addition of N-9 spermicide to condom use. Further, there is some evidence of harm through

24.5 | Effectiveness of Contraceptives Against Sexually Transmitted Diseases

CONTRACEPTIVE METHOD	SEXUALLY TRANSMITTED DISEASE	
	BACTERIAL	**VIRAL (INCLUDING HIV)**
Condoms	Reduces risk; most protective in preventing infections transmitted by fluids	Protective
Sterilization	No protection	No protection
Vaginal spermicides with nonoxynol-9	Not effective in preventing cervical gonorrhea, chlamydia	No protection, possibly increased risk[a]
Diaphragm, cervical cap	Modest protection against cervical infection (gonorrhea, chlamydia)	Questionable
Oral contraceptives	No known protection	Not protective; some studies suggest increased risk for HIV; others do not
Implantable/injectable contraceptives	Not protective	Not protective; some studies suggest increased risk for HIV[b]
Intrauterine device	Associated with pelvic inflammatory disease in first month after insertion[c]	No protection
Natural family planning	No protection	No protection

Note. From *The Hidden Epidemic: Confronting Sexually Transmitted Diseases,* by Institute of Medicine, 1997, Washington, DC: National Academy Press; *Contraceptive Technology* (18th rev. ed.), by R. Hatcher et al., 2004, New York: Ardent Media; "Sexually Transmitted Diseases Treatment Guidelines 2006," by Centers for Disease Control and Prevention, 2006, *MMWR, 55*(RR-11), 1–94.
[a] Frequent use is associated with genital lesions, which may be associated with an increased risk of HIV transmission (Hatcher et al., 2004).
[b] Progestin-only contraceptives cause vaginal thinning, which may increase risk for HIV and may increase viral shedding if the woman has HIV (Hatcher et al., 2004).
[c] Likely due to microbiological contamination at insertion (Hatcher et al., 2004).

increased numbers of genital lesions with N-9 spermicide use and slightly higer rates of urogenital gonorrhea in nonoxynol-9 users (Hatcher, 2004; Roddy, Zekeng, Ryan, Tamoufe, & Tweedy, 2002). Therefore, N-9 cannot be recommended for prevention of HIV and STIs.

The exact risk of HIV transmission through ingestion of male or female sexual secretions is not known definitively; however, a few HIV cases have been linked to transmission through oral sex (Stratton & Alexander, 1997). Hepatitis B and hepatitis C can rarely be spread through saliva, and herpes simplex types 1 and 2, syphilis, gonorrhea, and chlamydia can be spread through oral sex. Therefore, women should use barriers such as dental dams, male unlubricated condoms cut in half, or nonmicrowaveable saran wrap when engaging in cunnilingus or unlubricated condoms for fellatio.

With most of the condoms now available to women in the United States, active male cooperation is essential. A key issue in condom use as a preventative strategy is that, in sexual encounters, men must comply with a woman's suggestion or request that they use a condom. Moreover, condom usage must be renegotiated with every sexual contact, and women must address the issue of control of sexual decision making every time they request a male partner to use a condom. Women may fear that their partner will be offended if a condom is introduced. Some women may fear rejection and abandonment, conflict, potential violence, or loss of economic support if they suggest the use of condoms to prevent STI transmission. For many individuals, condoms are symbols of extra-relationship activity. Introduction of a condom into a long-term relationship where they have not been used previously threatens the trust assumed in most long-term relationships.

Many women do not anticipate or prepare for sexual activity in advance; embarrassment or discomfort in purchasing condoms may prevent some women from using them. Cultural barriers also may impede the use of condoms. Latino gender roles make it difficult for Latina women to suggest using condoms to a partner (Mays & Cochran, 1988). Suggesting condom use implies that a woman is sexually active, that she is available for sex, and that she is seeking sex; these are messages that many women are uncomfortable conveying given the prevailing mores in the United States. In a society that commonly views a woman who carries a condom as overprepared, possibly oversexed, and willing to have sex with any man, expecting her to insist on the use of condoms in a sexual encounter is unrealistic. Finally, women should be counseled to watch out for situations that make it hard to talk about and practice safer sex. These include romantic times when condoms are not available and when alcohol or drugs make it impossible to make wise decisions about safer sex.

Certain sexual practices should be avoided to reduce one's risk of infection. Abstinence from any sexual activities that could result in exchange of infective body fluids will help decrease risk. Anal-genital intercourse, anal-oral contact, and anal-digital activity are high-risk sexual behaviors and should be avoided (Hatcher et al., 2004). Sexual transmission occurs through direct skin or mucous membrane contact with infectious lesions or body fluids. Because mucosal linings are delicate and subject to considerable mechanical trauma during intercourse, small abrasions often may occur, facilitating entry of infectious agents into the bloodstream. The rectal epithelium is especially easy to traumatize with penetration. Sexual practices that increase the likelihood of tissue damage or bleeding such as fisting (inserting a fist into the rectum) should be avoided. Deep kissing when lips, gums, or other tissues are raw or broken also should be avoided (Hatcher et al., 2004). Because enteric infections are transmitted by oral-fecal contact, avoiding oral-anal, rimming (licking the anal area), and digital-anal activities should reduce the likelihood of infection. Vaginal intercourse should never follow anal contact unless a condom has been used and then removed and replaced with a new condom.

Nurses can suggest strategies to enhance a woman's condom negotiation and communication skills. Suggesting that she talk with her partner about condom use at a time removed from sexual activity may make it easier to bring up the subject. Role playing possible partner reactions with a woman and her alternative responses can be helpful. Asking a woman who appears particularly uncomfortable to rehearse how she might approach the topic is useful, particularly when a woman fears her partner may be resistant. The nurse might suggest her client begin by saying, "I need to talk with you about something that is important to both of us. It's hard for me and I feel embarrassed but I think we need to talk about safe sex." If women are able to sort out their feelings and fears before talking with their partners, they may feel more comfortable and in control of the situation. Women can be reassured that it is natural to be uncomfortable and that the hardest part is getting started. Nurses should help their clients clarify what they will and will not do sexually because it is easier to discuss it if they are clear. Women can be reminded that their partner may need time to think about what they have said and that they must paying attention to their partner's response. If the partner seems to be having difficulty with the discussion, a woman may slow down and wait a while. She can be reminded that

if her partner resists safer sex, she may wish to reconsider the relationship. In addition, if a woman indicates fear for her safety if she suggests using a condom, clinicians must provide her with resources for prevention of violence and emphasize that her safety is paramount.

Women may delay seeking care for STIs because they fear social stigma, have limited access to health care services, are asymptomatic, or unaware that they have an infection.

Women who have been diagnosed with an STI also need prevention counseling. Because of their behavior, both the woman and her partner need treatment for their infection and counseling to avoid reinfection. Key aspects to emphasize for women already infected include: (1) responding to disease suspicion by obtaining appropriate assessment promptly; (2) taking oral medications as directed; (3) returning for follow-up tests when applicable; (4) encouraging sex partners to obtain examination and treatment when indicated; (5) avoiding sexual exposure while infectious; (6) preventing future exposure by practicing protective practices; and (7) confidentiality.

SCREENING AND DETECTION

Prompt diagnosis and treatment are predicated on the assumption that any person who believes he or she may have contracted an STI, has symptoms of an STI, has had sexual relations with someone who has symptoms of an STI, or has a partner who has been diagnosed with an STI will seek care. To obtain prompt diagnosis and treatment, clients must know how to recognize the major signs and symptoms of all STIs and obtain health care if they experience symptoms or have sexual contact with someone who had an STI. Nurses have the responsibility of educating their clients regarding the signs and symptoms of STIs. This may be done when a woman comes in for a well-woman examination, seeks contraception, obtains preconceptual care, or comes to her health care provider for prenatal care. Nurses also must ensure that clients know where and how to obtain care if they suspect they might have contracted an STI. Many local health departments have clinics specifically designed to treat STIs, and free treatment sometimes can be obtained at local emergency rooms.

A critical first step detecting STIs is for nurses to routinely and regularly obtain STI histories from their patients. To identify those at risk, specific questions should be asked during the collection of a health history.

Key aspects of obtaining a useful STI history include assurances of confidentiality and a nonjudgmental attitude. It is important that the history be conducted in a private room with the woman fully clothed. Be sure to begin with a rationale for why the questions are being asked, which assures the patient that you are not singling her out for some reason and also reinforces the importance of sexual health as a part of total health. When possible, use nonmedical terminology and be specific—for example, "How many partners have you had in the past month, past year?" Although it is advisable to collect a complete STI history, there may be times when this is not possible. If only a few minutes are available, ask something such as, "What are you doing to protect yourself from AIDS?" or "Thinking about AIDS and other sexual infections, what do you think is the riskiest thing you do?" From the answers to these questions, the clinician can get a sense of STI awareness and safer sex behaviors and can respond with at least one individualized, focused suggestion to add to knowledge and/or skill (Guest, 2006). If it is possible to take a few more minutes, nurses can ask questions that elucidate a fuller history of infection, risk taking, and relationships in more detail. To obtain a comprehensive STI history, the questions in Table 24.6 and Table 24.7 can be used to shape a risk assessment and STI history that is tailored to the cultural and social context of a patient's life and the prevalence of various STIs in a specific area.

Risk assessment depends on a woman's willingness to self-identify risk factors that may be seen as socially unacceptable or stigmatizing. It is possible that women may not reveal such risk factors directly to health care providers but will do so if they are asked to fill out a questionnaire using questions similar to those given in the sexual risk history. Current recommendations (CDC, 2006a) are that all women from age of first sexual act until age 25 should be screened at least yearly for STIs; after age 25, the timing of screening depends on risk factors present and whether the woman is pregnant. All pregnant women must be screened for gonorrhea, syphilis, chlamydia, and HBV. In addition, all pregnant women should be tested for HIV infection as early as possible in pregnancy (CDC, 2006b). Further, any woman who has been diagnosed with an STI should be screened for other STIs, because many of these infections (e.g., chlamydia, gonorrhea, syphilis, hepatitis B) can be asymptomatic in women.

Infected individuals should be asked to identify and notify all partners who might have been exposed. In addition, all persons infected with an STI must be thoroughly and appropriately treated. General procedures for reporting and treating STIs are discussed in the next section, and information specific to screening for individual STIs is presented in subsequent sections devoted to individual STIs.

CARING FOR A WOMAN WITH A SEXUALLY TRANSMITTED INFECTION

Women may delay seeking care for STIs because they fear social stigma, have limited access to health care services, or may be asymptomatic or unaware that they have an infection (Fogel, 1995). In this age of widespread and often sensational media publicity about STIs, being told she has any STI may be terrifying for a woman. She may not understand the difference between one infecting organism and another. Instead, she may hear a diagnosis of illness, possibly incurable. Symptoms such as increased vaginal discharge, malodor, and itching associated with some STIs may be perceived as dirty, and the woman may be embarrassed and concerned that she will offend those caring for her. When a woman is diagnosed with an STI, her reactions may range from acceptance to hurt, disbelief, anger, or concern. These reactions may vary with the expectations in the woman's subculture and personal experience.

Assessment

The diagnosis of an STI is based on an integration of relevant historical, physical, and laboratory data (see Table 24.8). A history that is accurate, comprehensive, and specific is essential for accurate diagnosis. Because many women are embarrassed or anxious, generally the history should be taken first, with the woman dressed. Information should be collected in a nonjudgmental manner, avoiding assumptions of sexual preference. All partners should be referred to as partners and not by gender. It is helpful to begin with open-ended questions that might elicit information that otherwise would be missed; these can be followed with symptom-specific questions and relevant history. Specific areas to address include the reason why the woman has sought care and any symptoms she has noticed; a sexual history, including a description of the date and type of sexual activity; number of contacts; whether she has had contact with someone who recently had an STI; and potential sites of infection (mouth, cervix, urethra, rectum). Pertinent medical history includes anything that will influence the management plan: history of drug allergies, previously diagnosed chronic illnesses, and general health status. A menstrual history, including the date of the client's last menstrual period, must always be obtained so that pregnancy may be ruled out, because certain medications used to treat STIs are contraindicated in pregnancy. When indicated, an HIV-oriented systems review should be conducted (see chapter 25, about women and HIV/AIDS). Any positive answers regarding symptoms should be followed up to elicit information about onset, duration, and specific characteristics such as color, amount, and consistency of discharge.

Before the actual physical examination is performed, the nurse should discuss the exam with her client so that she is prepared for it. The physical examination begins with careful visualization of the external genitalia including the perineum. Erythema, edema, distortions, lesions or trauma from scratching, sexual activity, sports

24.6 | Sexually Transmitted Infection History

Risk Screening
- Are you sexually active? That is, have you engaged in sexual activities (had sex or intercourse) with anyone in the past 6 months? In the past year?
  - If no, Have you engaged in sexual activities in past?
  - If yes,
    - Have your partners been men, women, or both?
    - With how many different people? ___1 ___2–3 ___4–10 ____more than 10
    - How many different people are you having sex with right now?
    - Does your partner have any other partners that you know of?
    - Have you ever had sex with someone who had been in jail or prison?
    - Have you ever had sex with someone whom you were afraid put you at risk for HIV or other sexually transmitted diseases?
      - Someone who had a positive AIDS test?
      - Someone you think might have AIDS?
      - Someone who uses illicit drugs? IV drugs?
      - Someone who might have had sex with a sex worker?
      - Someone who might have had sex with both men and women?
    - Have you ever been told that you had a sexually transmitted infection?
      - ___ Never
      - ___ Chlamydia
      - ___ Gonorrhea
      - ___ Trichomonas
      - ___ Syphilis
      - ___ Other (list):_____
- Have you ever been told that you had a pelvic infection or pelvic inflammatory disease?
- Many women have sex when they have drunk too much alcohol or have been using drugs. Has this happened to you?
- What kinds of drugs do you use?
  - ___Opiods: Types_____ Route of administration_____ Frequency
  - ___Stimulants: Types_____ Route of administration _____ Frequency
  - ___Crack cocaine: Frequency_____ Have you had sex in a crack house?
  - ___Alcohol: Types: _____ Frequency_____
- Have you ever blacked out from alcohol or drugs, especially during sex?
- Have you ever traded sex for drugs, money, food, housing, or anything else?
- Do you ever have sex when you are high?
- Can you tell me the kinds of sex that you have? This will help us figure out what your risks are.

Mouth on penis or vulva	protected ___	unprotected ___
Penis in vagina	protected ___	unprotected ___
Penis in the butt	protected ___	unprotected ___
Mouth on butt	protected ___	unprotected ___

For every sexually active woman, ask
  - Are you worried about catching a sexually transmitted disease or HIV (the AIDS virus)?
  - Do you do anything to prevent catching a disease?
  - Have you had sex without a condom?
  - When did you start using condoms?
  - Have you performed oral sex on a man or woman without a barrier (dental dam, plastic wrap, condom)?

Note. Management Guidelines for Women's Health Nurse Practitioners, by K. Brown, 2000, Philadelphia: F. A. Davis; *Advanced Health Assessment of Women,* by H. A. Carcio, 1999, Philadelphia: Lippincott; *Sexual Health Promotion,* by C. I. Fogel and D. Lauver, 1990, Philadelphia: Saunders; *Women's Health Care,* by C. I. Fogel and N. F. Woods, 1995, Thousand Oaks, CA: Sage; "Promoting Sexual Health in the Age of HIV/AIDS," by A. Kurth, 1998, *Journal of Nurse-Midwifery, 43*(3), pp. 162–181; "Primary Care for Women: Comprehensive Sexual Health Assessment, by A. MacLauren, 1995, *Journal of Nurse-Midwifery, 40,* pp. 104–119; "Women's Health Primary Care: Protocols for Practice," by W. L. Star, L. L. Lommel, & M. T. Shannon, 1995, Washington, DC: American Nurses Publishing.

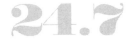

| Menstrual/Gynecologic History Questions to Assess Risk of Sexually Transmitted Infections

Do you experience now or have you ever experienced:
■ Frequent vaginal infections?
■ Unusual vaginal discharge or odor?
■ Vaginal itching, burning, sores, or warts?
■ Sexually transmitted infections? (Ask about individual diseases.)
■ Abdominal pain?
■ Pelvic inflammatory disease or infection of the uterus, tubes, or ovaries?
■ Rape or violent intercourse?
■ Physical, emotional, or sexual abuse?
■ Abnormal Pap smear?
■ Pain or bleeding with intercourse?
■ Severe menstrual cramps occurring at the end of your period?
■ Ectopic pregnancy?
■ HIV testing?
■ STI testing?
■ Immunizations for the prevention of sexually transmitted infections?

activity, or injury are noted. Palpation can locate areas of tenderness. During the speculum exam, the vagina and cervix are inspected for edema, thinning, lesions, abnormal coloration, trauma, discharge, and bleeding. Thorough palpation of inguinal area and pelvic organs; milking of the urethra for discharge; and assessment of vaginal secretion odors are essential. Lesions should be evaluated and cultures obtained when appropriate. Because the speculum is usually not lubricated prior to insertion into the vagina as cultures of vaginal secretions may have to be obtained, insertion may be somewhat uncomfortable. Clients should be informed of this and reassured that every effort will be made to make the speculum exam as comfortable as possible. Appropriate laboratory studies will be suggested, in part, by the history and physical examination results. Because women are often infected with more than one STI simultaneously and many are asymptomatic, additional laboratory studies may be done, including a Pap smear, wet mounts, gonococcal culture, Venereal Disease Research Laboratory (VDRL) or rapid plasma reagent (RPR) for syphilis, and a hepatitis B panel (HbcAB, HBsAg, HBsAb). Cultures for HSV are obtained when indicated by history or physical examination. The woman should be offered HIV testing (see chapter 25, on women and HIV/AIDS). When indicated, a complete blood count, sedimentation rate, urinalysis, or urine culture and sensitivity should be obtained. Further, if history or

physical examination indicates, a pregnancy test should be performed.

Management

The woman with an STI will need support in seeking care at the earliest stage of symptoms. Counseling women about STIs is essential for (a) preventing new infections or reinfection, (b) increasing compliance with treatment and follow-up, (c) providing support during treatment, and (d) assisting patients in discussions with their partner(s). Clients must be made aware of the serious potential consequences of STIs and the behaviors that increase the likelihood of infection.

Exhibit 24.6 outlines necessary client education for all STIs. The nurse must make sure that her client understands what disease she has, how it is transmitted, and why it must be treated. Clients should be given a brief description of the disease in language that they can understand. This description should include modes of transmission, incubation period, symptoms, infectious period, and potential complications. Effective treatment of STIs necessitates careful, thorough explanation of treatment regimen and follow-up procedures. Thorough, careful instructions about medications must be provided, both verbally and in writing. Side effects, benefits, and risks of the medication should be discussed. Unpleasant side effects or early relief of symptoms may discourage women from completing their medication course. Clients should be strongly urged to continue their medication until it is used up regardless of whether their symptoms diminish or disappear in a few days. Comfort measures that decrease symptoms such as pain, itching, or nausea should be suggested. Providing written information is a useful strategy, because this is a time of high anxiety for many clients and they may not be able to hear or remember what they were told. A number of booklets on STIs are already available, or the nurse may wish to develop literature that is specific to her practice setting and clients.

In general, women will be advised to refrain from intercourse until all treatment is finished and a reculture, if appropriate, is done. After the infection is cured, women should be urged to continue using condoms to prevent recurring infections, especially if they have had one episode of pelvic inflammatory disease (PID) or continue to have intercourse with new partners. Women may wish to avoid having sex with partners who have many other sexual partners. All women who have contracted an STI should be taught safer sex practices if this has not been done already. Follow-up appointments should be made as needed.

Addressing the psychosocial component of STIs is essential. It is never easy to tell a woman that she has an STI. Learning that one has an STI may be extremely upsetting, particularly if the STI is serious, has

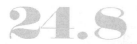 **24.8** | Assessment of the Woman with a Vaginal Discharge, Vaginitis, or Sexually Transmitted Infection

HISTORY	PHYSICAL EXAMINATION	LABORATORY TESTS
Current symptoms Vaginal discharge: onset, color, odor, consistency, amount, constant vs. intermittent, related to sexual contact, relationship to menses Lesions or rashes anywhere on body Genital itching, burning, swelling, rash, sores, or tears Pain: location, intensity, any radiation, associated aggravating or alleviating factors, description Abdominal or pelvic pain Dysuria: internal vs. external Dyspareunia and/or postcoital bleeding Symptoms of generalized infection (myalgia, arthralgia, malaise, fever) Menstrual history Last menstrual period Sexual history Sexual preference Type and time of sexual activity Frequency Areas of contact Partners: number, known partner history, history of new partner in past month Past history of similar problems: dates, times, follow-up, treatment response History of: Previous infection or STD Chronic cervicitis Cervical surgery Abnormal Pap smear DES exposure Unintended pregnancy Death in utero or stillbirth Preterm delivery or low–birth weight delivery Allergies Adult health problems Diet, alcohol, cigarettes, drugs, use of sex toys, stimulants Contraceptive methods used Medications: recent antibiotics, use of vaginal medications (over-the-counter and prescription) Frequency of douching, use of feminine sprays and deodorants, new toiletry products, perfumed toilet tissue Change in laundry soaps, fabric softener, body soap	Vital signs: blood pressure, pulse, respiration, temperature General examination of skin: Alopecia Rash on soles of feet, palms Condyloma lata Inguinal lymph nodes Abdominal examination rebound, bowel sounds, suprapubic tenderness, masses, organomegaly, enlarged bladder, costovertebral angle tenderness External genitalia examination (tenderness, enlargement, discharge, excoriations, erythema, lesions): Bartholin's glands, Skene's glands, sores, rash, genital warts, urethra Vaginal examination (speculum): Vaginal lesions, tears, discharge (color, odor, amount, odor) Cervix: friability, ectropion, cervical erosion, discharge from os, cervical tenderness, color Bimanual examination: Pain on cervical motion (positive Chandelier sign), fullness or pain in adnexa, tenderness of uterus, size of uterus	As indicated by history or finding: Wet prep with potassium hydroxide (KOH), normal saline KOH "whiff" test Gram stain Urinalysis or urine culture Gonorrhea culture Chlamydia culture Herpes culture Cervical culture pH with nitrazine testing HIV testing Serology test for syphillis Hepatitis B and hepatitis C testing Papanicolaou test Complete blood count

Note. From "Sexually Transmitted Diseases," by C. I. Fogel, 1995, in N. F. Woods and C. I. Fogel (Eds.), *Women's Health Care* (pp. 571–609), Thousand Oaks, CA: Sage Protocols for Nurse Practitoiners in Gynecologic Settings (7th ed.), by J. E. Hawkins, D. M. Roberto-Nichols, and J. L. Stanley-Haney, 2008, New York: Tiresias Press; "Sexually Transmitted Diseases Treatment Guidelines 2006," by Centers for Disease Control and Prevention, 2006, *MMWR, 55*(RR-11), pp. 1–94; *Ambulatory Obstetrics* (3rd ed.), by W. L. Star, M. T. Shannon, L. L. Lommel, and Y. M. Gutierrez (Eds.), 1999, San Francisco: UCSF Nursing Press.

EXHIBIT 24.6 PATIENT STI PREVENTION INFORMATION

What can you do to prevent STIs?

The only certain way to prevent STIs is to avoid sexual contact with others. If you choose to be sexually active, there are things you can do to decrease your risk of developing a sexually transmitted infection:

- Have sex with only one person who doesn't have sex with anyone else and who has no infections.
- Always use a condom and use it correctly.
- Use clean needles if you inject any drugs.
- Prevent and control other STIs to decease your susceptibility to HIV infection and to reduce your infectiousness if you are HIV-infected.
- Wait to have to sex for as long as possible. The younger you are when you start having sex for the first time, the more likely are to catch an STI. The risk of acquiring an STD also increases with the number of partners you have over a life time.

Anyone who is sexually active should:

- Always use protection unless you are having sex with only one person who doesn't have sex with anyone else and who has no infections.
- Have regular checkups for STIs even if you have no symptoms and especially when having sex with a new partner.
- Learn the common symptoms of STIs. Seek health care immediately if any suspicious symptoms develop, even if they are mild.
- Avoid having sex during menstruation. HIV-infected women are probably more infectious, and HIV-uninfected women are probably more susceptible to becoming infected during that time.
- Avoid anal intercourse, but, if practiced, use a condom.
- Avoid douching because it removes some of the normal protective bacteria in the vagina and increases the risk of getting some STIs.

Anyone diagnosed as having a STI should:

- Be treated to reduce the risk of transmitting an STI to another person.
- Notify all recent sex partners and urge them to get a checkup as soon as possible to decrease the risk of catching the infection again from them.
- Follow the health care provider's recommendations and complete the full course of medication prescribed. Have a follow-up test if this is necessary.
- Avoid sexual activity while being treated.

complications, or is incurable. Knowledge of an STI may unsettle a sexual relationship. Remember that a woman may be afraid or embarrassed to tell her partner, ask her partner to seek treatment, admit her sexual practices, or she may be concerned about confidentiality. The nurse may need to help the client deal with the effect of a diagnosis of an STI on a committed relationship for the woman who is now faced with the necessity of dealing with uncertain monogamy. In other instances, the women may be afraid that telling her partner may place her in danger of escalating abuse. This potential consequence must be discussed with each client.

For most STIs, sexual partners should be examined; thus, the infected woman is asked to identify and notify all partners who might have been exposed (partner notification). She may find this difficult to do. Empathizing with the client's feelings and suggesting specific ways of talking with partners will help decrease anxiety and assist in efforts to control infection. For example, the nurse might suggest that the woman say, "I care about you and I'm concerned about you. That's why I'm calling to tell you that I have a sexually transmitted infection. My clinician is ____ and she will be happy to talk with you if you would like" (Fogel, 1995). Offering literature and role-playing situations with the client may also be of assistance. It can be helpful to remind the client that, although this is an embarrassing situation, most persons would rather know than not know that they have been exposed. Health professionals who take time to counsel their clients on how to talk with their partner(s) can improve compliance and case finding. In situations when patient referral may not be effective or possible, health departments should be prepared to assist the woman either through contact referral or provider referral. Contract referral is the process by which a woman agrees to notify her partners by a certain time. If her partners do not obtain medical evaluation and treatment within the given time period, then provider referral is implemented. Provider referral is the process by which partners named by identified patients are notified and counseled by health department providers (CDC, 2006b).

Accurate identification and timely reporting of STIs are integral components of sucessful disease control efforts. All states require that gonorrhea, syphilis, and AIDS be reported to public health officials. Chlamydial infection is reportable in most states. The requirements for reporting other STIs differ from state to state. The nurse is legally responsible for reporting all cases of those diseases identified as reportable and should make sure she knows what the requirements are in the state in which she practices. The client must be informed when a case will be reported and told why. Failure to inform the client that the case will be reported is a serious breech of professional ethics. Confidentiality is a crucial issue for many clients. When an STI is reportable, women need to be told that they may be contacted by a health department representative. They should be assured that the information reported to and collected by health authorities is maintained in strictest confidence; in most jurisdictions, reports are protected by statute from subpoena. Every effort, within the limits of one's public health responsibilities, should be made to reassure clients.

The following sections outline the treatments for specific STIs following guidelines of the Centers for Disease Control and Prevention. When available, they also delineate self-help measures and preventive strategies. Instructions specific to individual diseases are given in the appropriate sections.

CERVICITIS

Chlamydia Infection

Chlamydia trachomatis is the most common and fastest spreading sexually transmitted infection in U.S. women, with almost one million cases reported to the Centers for Disease Control and Prevention in 2005 (CDC, 2006a). Because up to 80% of these infections are silent (Faro, 2001) and very destructive, their sequelae and complications can be very serious. In women, chlamydial infections are difficult to diagnose, and the symptoms, when present, are nonspecific.

Acute salpingitis or PID is the most serious complication of chlamydial infections and is a major etiologic factor in subsequent development of tubal factor

infertility, ectopic pregnancy, and chronic pelvic pain (Scharbo-DeHaan & Anderson, 2003). Further, chlamydial infection of the cervix causes inflammation resulting in microscopic cervical ulcerations and thus may increase risk of acquiring HIV infection. Chlamydia infection in pregnancy has been associated with premature rupture of the membranes, preterm birth, stilbirth, and low–birth weight infants. Maternal chlamydial infectious morbidity includes increased risk of postabortion endometritis and salpingitis and postpartum endometritis. Chlamydial infections of neonates results from perinatal exposure to the mother's infected cervix. Initial infections involve the mucous membranes of the eye, oropharnyx, urogenital tract, and rectum. Conjungtivitis usually develops 5 to 12 days after delivery in 20% to 50% of exposed infants. Chlamydia is also a common cause of subacute, afebrile pneumonia in infants aged 1 to 3 months of age (CDC, 2006b).

Chalymidia is more common among adolescents than older women. Sexually active women younger than 20 years are two to three times more likely to become infected with chlamydia than women between 20 and 29 years; women older than age 30 have the lowest rate of infection (CDC, 2006b). Risky behaviors—including multiple partners and nonuse of barrier methods of birth control—increase a woman's risk of chlamydial infection. Lower socioeconomic status may be a risk factor, especially with respect to treatment-seeking behaviors.

Assessment and Diagnosis

In addition to obtaining information regarding the presence of risk factors, the nurse should inquire about the presence of any symptoms. Although usually asymptomatic, some women may experience spotting or post-coital bleeding, mucoid or purulent cervical discharge, urinary frequency or dysuria. Bleeding results from inflammation and erosion of the cervical columnar epithelium. Women who are taking oral contraceptives may also experience breakthrough bleeding. Occasionally, women report lower abdominal pain and dyspareunia.

The 2006 Centers for Disease Control and Prevention STI guidelines have expanded recommendations for chlamydia screening among asymptomatic women. All sexually active women age 25 and younger should be screened for chlamydia at least annually, even if no symptoms are reported (CDC, 2006b) Further, women older than age 25 with risk factors (history of previous STI, inconsistent or incorrect condom use, new or multiple partners) should also be screened. A sexual risk history should always be done and may indicate more frequent screening for some women. The prevalence of chlamydia in pregnancy has been reported to range between 2% and 21% (Faro, 2001). Screening for chlamydia should be done in the third trimester (36 weeks) for women at increased risk. First-trimester screening might prevent the adverse effects of chlamydia during pregnancy; however, evidence for adverse effects in pregnancy is minimal, and, when screening is done only early during the first trimester, a longer period exists for acquiring infection before delivery (CDC, 1998).

Once considered the gold standard for identification of chlamydia, culturing is time-consuming, expensive, and infrequently used today (Faro, 2001). Recommended screening procedures for chlamydial infection (in order of preference) are:

- Nucleic acid amplification test (NAAT) of an endocervical sample (if a pelvic exam is acceptable) or a urine sample (if not acceptable). Endocervical NAAT is preferred because it provides the highest sensitivity of any screening test.
- Unamplified nucleic acid hybridization test, enzyme immunoassay, or direct fluorescent antibody test of an endocervical sample.
- Culture of an endocervical sample (CDC, 2006b).

Genital/pelvic examinations should be done on all women who have a positive urine test to identify complications such as PID. Endocervical (columnar) cells are required; cell scrapings provide better specimens, so the cervix should be swabbed with cotton or rayon swabs prior to collecting the specimen to remove mucus and discharge from the cervical os. Special culture media and proper handling of specimens are important, so the nurse should always know what is required in her individual practice site. Further, chla-mydial culture testing is not always available primarily due to expense. Nucleic acid amplification tests such as ligase chain reaction and polymerase chain reaction are the new gold standard, with sensitivity and specificity near 100%.

There is a high prevalence of reinfection in women who have had chlamydial infections in the preceeding several months, usually from reinfection by a partner who was untreated (CDC, 2002b). Because reinfection rates are high and the risk of complications increases with reinfection, nurses should advise all women, especially adolescents, with a chlamydial infection to be rescreened 3 to 4 months after treatment.

Management

Recommendations for treatment of urethral, cervical, and rectal chlamydial infections are found in Table 24.9. Azithromycin is now the recommended treatment because only one dose is needed; however, expense is a concern with this medication. Repeat culture is not necessary for women who complete treatment with doxycycline or azithromycin unless symptoms persist or reinfection is a possibility. A test of cure may be considered if the woman is treated with erthyromycin.

Doxycycline and ofloxacin are contraindicated for pregnant women; however, clinical experience and preliminary data suggest that azithromycin 1 gm is safe and effective (CDC, 2006b). It has fewer gastrointestinal side effects than does erthromycin and has equivalent cure rate. Women who have a chlamydia infection and are also infected with HIV should be treated with the

---

24.9 | Treatment Regimens for Chlamydial Infections

NONPREGNANT WOMEN	PREGNANT WOMEN	LACTATING WOMEN
Recommended regimens Azithromycin 1 g orally once *or* doxycycline 100 mg orally twice per day for 7 days *Alternative regimens* Erythromycin base 500 mg orally four times per day for 7 days *or* erythromycin ethylsuccinate 800 mg orally four times per day for 7 days *or* ofloxacin 300 mg orally twice per day for 7 days *or* levofloxacin 500 mg orally for 7 days	*Recommended regimens* Azithromycin 1 g orally once *or* amoxicillin 500 mg orally three times per day for 7 days *Alternative regimens* Erythromycin base 500 mg orally four times per day for 14 days *or* erythromycin ethylsuccinate 800 mg orally four times per day for 7 days *or* erythromycin ethylsuccinate 400 mg orally four times per day for 14 days	*Recommended regimens* Erythromycin base 500 mg orally four times per day for 7 days *Alternative regimens* Erythromycin base 250 mg orally four times per day for 14 days *or* erythromycin ethylsuccinate 800 mg orally four times per day for 7 days *or* erythromycin ethylsuccinate 400 mg orally four times per day for 14 days *or* azithromycin 1 g orally once

Note. From "Sexually Transmitted Diseases Treatment Guidelines 2006," by Centers for Disease Control and Prevention, 2006, *MMWR, 55*(RR-11), pp. 39–40; "The CDC 2002 Guidelines for the Treatment of Sexually Transmitted Diseases: Implications for Women's Health Care," by M. Scharbo-DeHaan and D. G. Anderson, 2003, *Journal of Midwifery & Women's Health, 48*(2), 96–104.

same regimen as those who are HIV negative. Because chlamydia is often asymptomatic, the patient should be cautioned to take all medication prescribed. All exposed sexual partners should be treated to avoid reinfection.

Gonorrhea

Gonorrhea is probably the oldest communicable disease in the United States. Reported gonorrheal rates in the United States are the highest of any industrialized country (CDC, 2005), with an estimated 600,000 new cases contracted each year (CDC, 2006b). The incidence of drug-resistant cases of gonorrhea—in particular, penicillinase-producing *Neisseria gonorrhoeae*—has been increasing and is becoming widespread in the United States (CDC, 2007b). Gonorrhea is caused by the aerobic, gram-negative diplococci *Neisseria gonorrhoeae*. Gonorrhea is almost exclusively transmitted by sexual activity, primarily genital-to-genital contact; however, it is also spread by oral-to-genital and anal-to-genital contact. Sites of infection in women are cervix, urethra, oropharynx, Skene's glands, and Bartholin's glands. Gonorrhea can be transmitted to the newborn in the form of ophthalmia neonatorum during delivery by direct contact with gonococcal organisms in the cervix. Although the organism has been recovered from inanimate objects artificially inoculated with the bacteria, there is no evidence that natural transmission occurs this way (Schaffer, 2003).

Age is probably the most important risk factor associated with gonorrhea. The majority of those contracting gonorrhea are under age 20. In a single act of unprotected sex with an infected partner, a teenage woman has a 50% change of contracting gonorrhea. Other risk factors include early onset of sexual activity and multiple sexual partners. Traditionally, the reported incidence of gonococcal disease has been higher in non-Whites. Many of the apparent differences in infection rates can be explained by the disproportionate representation of Blacks among the nation's poor and among inner-city dwellers. Rates of gonorrhea are higher in urban than rural areas, with even higher rates in inner cities.

Common sites of gonococcal infection in women are the endocervix (primary site), urethra, Skene's and Bartholin's glands, and rectum. The main complication of gonorrheal infections is pelvic inflammatory disease and subsequent infertility; women also may have pelvic abscess or Bartholin's abscess. Gonococcal infections in pregnancy potentially affect both mother and infant. Women with cervical gonorrhea may develop salpingitis in the first trimester. Perinatal complications of gonococcal infection include spontaneous septic abortion, premature rupture of membranes, preterm delivery, chorioamnionitis, neonatal sepsis, intrauterine growth retardation, and maternal postpartum sepsis.

Endometritis after elective abortion or chorionic villus sampling procedures may also occur (Star & Deal, 2004a). Amniotic infection syndrome manifested by placental, fetal, and umbilical cord inflammation following premature rupture of the membranes may result from gonorrheal infections during pregnancy. Opthalmia neonatorum, the most common manifestation of neonatal gonococcal infections, is very contagious and, if untreated, may lead to blindness of the newborn.

Disseminated gonococcal infections (DGI) are a rare (0.5% to 3%) complication of untreated gonorrhea. DGI occurs in two stages: the first stage is characterized by bacteremia with chills, fever, and skin lesions and is followed by stage two, during which the patient experiences acute septic arthritis with characteristic effusions, most commonly of the wrists, knees, and ankles (Star & Deal, 2004a). The most common clinical presentation of gonorrhea in pregnancy is DGI, and risk increases in the second and third trimester.

Assessment and Diagnosis

Up to 80% of women are asymptomatic; when symptoms are present, they are often less specific than the symptoms in men. Women may have a purulent, irritating endocervical discharge, but discharge is usually minimal or absent. Menstrual irregularities may be the presenting symptom, or women may complain of pain—chronic or acute severe pelvic or lower abdominal pain or longer, more painful menses. Unilateral labial pain and swelling may indicate Bartholi's glands infection, and periurethral pain and swelling may indicate inflamed Skene's glands. Infrequently, dysuria, vague abdominal pain, or low backache prompts a woman to seek care. Later symptoms may include fever (possibly high), nausea and vomiting, joint pain and swelling, or upper abdominal pain (liver involvement). Gonococcal rectal infection may occur in women following anal intercourse. Individuals with rectal gonorrhea may be completely asymptomatic or, conversely, experience severe symptoms with profuse purulent anal discharge, rectal pain, and blood in the stool. Rectal itching, fullness, pressure, and pain are also common symptoms, as is diarrhea. Gonococcal pharyngitis may appear to be viral pharyngitis; some individuals will have a red, swollen uvula and pustule vesicles on the soft palate and tonsils similar to strep infections. A diffuse vaginitis with vulvitis is the most common form of gonococcal infection in prepubertal girls. There may be few signs of infection; or vaginal discharge, dysuria, and swollen, reddened labia may be present.

Given that gonococcal infections are often asymptomatic, they cannot be diagnosed reliably by clinical signs and symptoms alone. Individuals may present with classic symptoms, with vague symptoms that may be attributed to a number of conditions, or with no symptoms at all. When symptoms are present, they typically are less specific than those seen in men. Cultures are considered the gold standard for diagnosis of gonorrhea because of their ease of testing and the need to test for antibiotic resistance. Cultures should be obtained from the endocervix, rectum, and, when indicated, the pharynx. Thayer-Martin cultures are recommended to diagnose gonorrhea in women. NAAT or nucleic acid hybrization of an endocervical swab specimen may be used if viable organisms cannot be maintained for culture (CDC, 2006b). Any woman suspected of having gonorrhea should have a chlamydial culture and serologic test for syphilis if one has not been done in the past 2 months. A test for gonorrhea should be done at the first prenatal visit (Star & Deal, 2004a). A repeat culture should be obtained in the third trimester for women at risk or women living in an area in which the prevalence is high (American Academy of Pediatrics & American College of Obstetricians and Gynecologists, 1997; CDC, 2002b).

Infants with gonococcal opthalmia should be hosptialized and assessed for signs of disseminated infection (sepsis, arthritis, meningitis). A single dose of ceftriaxone 25–50 mg/kg IV or IM is adequate for gonococcal conjunctivitis. Mothers of infants who have gonococcal infection and the mother's sex partners should be assessed and treated.

Management

Management of gonorrhea is straightforward, and the cure is usually rapid with appropriate antibiotic therapy (see Table 24.10). Single-dose efficacy is a major consideration in selecting an antibiotic regimen for women with gonorrhea. Another important consideration is the high percentage (45%) of women with coexisting chlamydial infections. Penicillin is no longer used to treat gonorrhea because of the high rate of penicillin-resistant strains of the organism. The Centers for Disease Control and Prevention suggest concomitant treatment for chlamydia because coinfection is common. All women with gonorrhea and syphilis should be treated for syphilis according to CDC guidelines (see later discussion of syphilis). All patients with gonorrhea should be offered confidential counseling and testing for HIV infection.

Gonorrhea is a highly communicable disease. Recent (past 30 days) sexual partners should be examined, cultured, and treated with appropriate regimens. Most treatment failures result from reinfection. Women need to be informed of this, as well as of the consequences of reinfection in terms of chronicity, complications, and potential infertility. Women are counseled to use condoms.

Gonorrhea is a reportable communicable disease. Health care providers are legally responsible for reporting all cases to the health authorities, usually the local health department in the client's county of residence. Women should be informed that the case will be reported, told why, and informed of the possibility of being contacted by a health department representative.

Treatment failure in uncomplicated gonorrhea in women who are treated with any of the recommended regimens is rare (less than 5%); therefore, follow-up culture (test of cure) is not essential. A more cost-effective approach is reexamination with culture 1 to 2 months after treatment. This approach will detect both treatment failures and reinfections. Patients also

24.10 | Recommended Treatment Regimens for Gonococcal Infections

NONPREGNANT WOMEN	PREGNANT WOMEN	LACTATING WOMEN
Cefixime 400 mg orally once *or* ceftriaxone 125 mg IM once *or plus (if chlamydia is not ruled out)* azithromycin 1 g orally once *or* doxycycline 100 mg orally twice per day for 7 days Quinolones are not recommended for women younger than 18 years of age	Ceftriaxone 125 mg IM once If cephalosporin allergic, spectinomycin 2 g IM once (not available in the United States) *plus* amoxicillin 500 mg orally TID for 14 days *or* azithromycin 1 g orally once Do not use quinolones or tetracyclines	Ceftriaxone 125 mg IM once *plus* amoxicillin 500 mg orally three times per day for 14 days *or* azithromycin 1 g orally once If cephalosporin allergic, spectinomycin 2 g IM once (not available in the United States) *plus* erythromycin base 500 mg orally four times per day for 7 days

Note. From "Sexually Transmitted Diseases Treatment Guidelines 2006," by Centers for Disease Control and Prevention, 2006, *MMWR, 55*(RR-11), pp. 43–47; "Update to Sexually Transmitted Disease Treatment Guidelines, 2006: Fluoroquinolones No Longer Recommended for Treatment of Gonococcal Infections," by Centers for Disease Control and Prevention, 2007, *MMWR, 56*(14), pp. 332–336; "Treatment of Sexually Transmitted Bacterial Diseases in Pregnant Women, by G.G.C. Donders, 2000, *Drugs, 59*(3), pp. 477–485.

should be counseled to return if symptoms persist after treatment.

PELVIC INFLAMMATORY DISEASE

Pelvic inflammatory disease is a spectrum of inflammatory disorders of the upper female genital tract, including any combination of endometritis, salpingitis, tubo-ovarian abcess, and pelvic peritonitis. Multiple organisms have been found to cause PID, and most cases are associated with more than one organism. In the past, the most common causative agent was thought to be *N. gonorrhoeae*; however, *C. trachomatis* is now estimated to cause one-half of all cases of PID. In addition to gonorrhea and chlamydia, a wide variety of anaerobic and aerobic bacteria such as *streptococcus*, *E. coli*, and *Gardnerella vaginalis* are recognized to cause PID. Because PID may be caused by a wide variety of infectious agents and encompasses a wide variety of pathologic processes, the infection can be acute, subacute, or chronic and has a wide range of symptoms.

Most PID results from an ascending spread of microorganisms from the vagina and endocervix to the upper genital tract. This spread most frequently happens at the end of or just after menses following reception of an infectious agent. During the menstrual period, several factors facilitate the development of an infection: the cervical os is slightly open; the cervical mucus barrier is absent; and menstrual blood is an excellent medium for growth. PID also may develop following an abortion, pelvic surgery, or delivery.

Each year more than 1 million women in the United States will have an episode of symptomatic PID (Hatcher, 2004) and nearly 180,00 hospitalizations. Teenagers have the highest risk for PID associated with their decreased immunity to infectious organisms and increased risk of gonorrhea and chlamydia. Young age at first intercourse, frequency of sexual intercourse, multiple sex partners, and a history of STIs also increase a woman's risk for PID. In addition, cigarette smoking and douching may increase a woman's risk for acute pelvic inflammatory disease. Until recently, it was believed that the use of intrauterine devices (IUDs) increased a woman's risk for acquiring PID. The Centers for Disease Control state that women who use intrauterine devices are probably at increased risk for PID that may not be STI-related, and that most of this risk occurs in the first months after IUD insertion.

Major medical complications are associated with PID. Short-term consequences include acute pelvic pain, tubo-ovarian abscess, tubal scarring, and adhesions. Long-term complications include an increased risk (12% to 16%) of infertility, ectopic pregnancy, chronic pelvic pain, dyspareunia, and recurrent episodes of PID (Ness & Brooks-Nelson, 2000). Because PID caused by chlamydia is more commonly asymptomatic, it more often results in tubal obstruction from delayed diagnosis or inadequate treatment.

Assessment and Diagnosis

Diagnosis of PID is difficult, because the symptoms of PID vary and almost all of the most common signs and symptoms could accompany other urinary, gastrointestinal or reproductive tract problems. Symptoms may mimic other disease processes such as ectopic pregnancy, endometriosis, ovarian cyst with torsion, pelvic adhesions, inflammatory bowel disease, or acute appendicitis. Exhibit 24.7 contains detailed information on diagnosing PID.

History taking must be comprehensive. A menstrual history is useful in establishing the relationship of onset of pain to menses and in identifying any variations from normal in the cycle. Other relevant history includes recent pelvic surgery, delivery, dilation of the cervix, abortion, recent (within 1 month) IUD insertion, purulent vaginal discharge, irregular bleeding, and a longer, heavier menstrual period. A thorough sexual risk history should be obtained—including current or most recent sexual activity, number of partners, and method of contraception—and will assist in identifying possible increased risk for STI exposure. Intestinal and bladder symptoms are important to review. Women may report various symptoms ranging from minimal pelvic discomfort to dull cramping and intermittent pain or severe, persistent, and incapacitating pain. Pelvic pain usually develops within 7 to 10 days of menses, remains constant, is bilateral, and is most severe in the lower quadrants. Pelvic discomfort is exacerbated by Valsalva maneuver, intercourse, or movement. Women with acute PID also may complain of intermenstrual bleeding. Symptoms of an STI in a woman's partner(s) also should be noted.

Vital signs are obtained, and a complete physical examination performed. A fever of 102°F or above is characteristic. Physical examination reveals adnexal tenderness, with or without rebound, and exquisite tenderness with cervical movement (Chandelier's sign). Pelvic tenderness is usually bilateral. There may or may not be a palpable adnexal swelling or thickening. Fever and peritonitis are more characteristic of gonococcal PID than of PID caused by other organisms which are more likely to be "silent."

Subacute PID is far less dramatic, with a great variety in the severity and extent of symptoms. At times, symptoms are so mild and vague that the woman ignores them. Symptoms that suggest subacute PID are chronic lower abdominal pain, dyspareunia, menstrual

EXHIBIT 24.7 DIAGNOSING PELVIC INFLAMMATORY DISEASE

Empiric treatment of pelvic inflammatory disease (PID) should be initiated for sexually active young women and others at risk for STDs if these **minimum criteria** are present and no other cause(s) for the illness can be found:

- Uterine/adnexal tenderness
  or
- Cervical motion tenderness

Additional criteria to support a diagnosis of PID include:
- Oral temperature > 101° F (> 38.3° C);
- Abnormal cervical or vaginal mucopurulent discharge
- Presence of white blood cells on saline microscopy of vaginal secretions
- Elevated erthrocyte sedimentation rate
- Elevated C-reactive protein
- Laboratory documentation of cervical infection with *N. gonorrheae* or *C. trachomatis*

The **most specific criteria** for diagnosing PID are:
- Endometrial biopsy with histopathologic evidence of endometriosis
- Transvaginal sonography or magnetic resonance imaging techniques showing thickened, fluid-filled tubes with or without free pelvic fluid or tubo-ovarian complex
- Laparoscopic abnormalities consistent with PID

Note. From "Sexually Transmitted Diseases Treatment Guidelines, 2006," by Centers for Disease Control and Prevention, 2006, *MMWR, 55*(RR-11), p. 58.

irregularities, urinary discomfort, low-grade fever, low backache, and constipation. Abdominal examination usually reveals no rebound tenderness; there is slight adnexal tenderness with cervical movement; and cervical or urethral discharge, often purulent in nature, may be present.

Essential laboratory studies are a complete blood count with differential, erythrosedimentation rate (highest in chlamydial infections) and cervical cultures for gonorrhea and chlamydia. Laboratory data are useful only when considered in conjunction with history and physical examination findings.

Clinical diagnosis of PID is imprecise; nevertheless, most diagnoses of PID are clinical because laparoscopy and biopsy are too expensive and invasive to be practical screening tools. Because delay in diagnosis and treatment of PID is associated with severe sequelae, the 2002 CDC guidelines established new minimum criteria for beginning treatment. The Centers for Disease Control (2006b) recommend a "low threshold for diagnosing PID" because of the risk of damage to reproductive health. The 2006 guidelines recommend empiric treatment of PID if one or both of two minimum criteria are present and if no other cause(s) of the illness can be identified: (1) uterine or adnexal tenderness or (2) cervical motion tenderness (CDC, 2006b). Further, a diag-

nosis of PID must be considered in a woman with any pelvic tenderness any any sign of lower genital tract inflammation.

Management

Perhaps the most important nursing intervention for PID is prevention. Primary prevention would be education in avoiding acquisition of sexually transmitted infections, whereas secondary prevention involves preventing a lower genital tract infection from ascending to the upper genital tract. Instructing women in self-protective behaviors such as practicing safer sex and using barrier methods is critical. Also important is the detection of asymptomatic gonorrheal and chlamydial infections through routine screening of women with risky behaviors and/or specific risk factors such as age. Partner notification when an STI is diagnosed is essential to prevent reinfection.

In the past, most women with PID were hospitalized so that bed rest and parental therapy could be started. However, today approximately three-quarters of women with PID are not hospitalized (Ness & Brooks-Nelson, 2000) because there are no available data that compare the efficacy of inpatient versus outpatient treatment. The decision of whether to hospitalize should be based on each woman's individual circumstances. To guide clinicians' decision regarding hospitalization, the following criteria have been offered by the CDC (2006b):

- Surgical emergencies (e.g., appendicitis).
- Pregnancy.
- No clinical response to oral antimicrobial therapy.
- Inability to follow or tolerate an outpatient oral regimen.
- Severe illness, nausea and vomiting, or high fever.
- Tubo-ovarian abscess.

There are no current data to suggest that adolescents would benefit from hospitalization for treatment; however, there is some evidence that women older than age 35 are likely to have a more complicated course and thus may benefit from hospitalization (CDC, 2006b). The guidelines recommend that pregnant women with PID be hospitalized and treated with parental antibiotics because of the high risk for preterm delivery, fetal wastage, and maternal morbidity (Scharbo-DeHaan & Anderson, 2003).

Although treatment regimens vary with the infecting organism, a broad-spectrum antibiotic generally is used. Several antimicrobial regimens have proved to be effective and no single therapeutic regimen of choice exists (see Table 24.11). Women with acute PID should be on bed rest in a semi-Fowler's position. Comfort measures include analgesics for pain and all other nursing measures applicable to a patient confined to bed. Minimal pelvic examinations should be done during the acute phase of the disease. During the recovery phase, the woman should restrict her activity and make every effort to get adequate rest and a nutritionally sound diet. Follow-up laboratory studies after treatment should include endocervical cultures for a test of cure.

Health education is central to effective management of PID. Nurses should explain to women the nature of the disease and should encourage them to comply with all therapy and prevention recommendations, emphasizing the necessity of taking all medication, even if symptoms disappear. Any potential problems such as lack of money for prescriptions or lack of transportation to return to the clinic for follow-up appointments that would prevent a woman from completing a course of treatment should be identified, and the importance of follow-up visits should be stressed. Women should be counseled to refrain from sexual intercourse until their treatment is completed. Contraceptive counseling should be provided. The nurse can suggest that the client select barrier methods such as condoms, contraceptive sponge, or diaphragm. A woman with a history of PID should not us an IUD.

Women who suffer from PID may be acutely ill or may experience long-term discomfort. Either takes an emotional toll. Pain in itself is debilitating and is compounded by the infectious process. The potential or actual loss of reproductive capabilities can be devastating and can affect the patient's self-concept adversely. Part of the nurse's role is to help her client adjust her self-concept to fit reality and to accept alterations in a way that promotes health. Because PID is so closely tied to sexuality, body image, and self-concept, women who are diagnosed with it will need supportive care. The woman's feelings need to be discussed and her partner(s) included when appropriate.

ULCERATIVE GENITAL INFECTION
Syphilis

Syphilis, one of the earliest described STIs, is a systemic disease caused by *Treponema pallidum,* a motile spirochete. The disease is characterized by periods of active symptoms and periods of symptomless latency. It

24.11	Treatment of Pelvic Inflammatory Disease

	TREATMENT OF CHOICE	ALTERNATIVES
Parenteral regimen	Cefotetan 2 gm IV every 12 hours *or* cefoxitin 2 gm IV every 6 hours *plus* doxycline 100 mg IV or orally every 12 hours	Clindamycin 900 mg IV every 8 hours *plus* gentamycin loading dose IV or IM (2 mg/kg of body weight), followed by maintenance dose (1.5 mg/kg) every 8 hours; single daily does may be substituted
Oral regimen	Ofloxacin 400 mg orally twice per day for 14 days *plus* metronidazole 500 mg orally twice per day for 14 days	Cefoxitin 2 gm IM *or* cefoxitin 2 g IM plus probenecid 1 gm orally in a single dose concurrently *or* other parental third-generation cephlosporin *plus* doxycline 100 mg orally twice per day for 14 days

can affect any tissue or organ in the body. Transmission is thought to be by entry in the subcutaneous tissue through microscopic abrasions that can occur during sexual intercourse. The disease can also be transmitted through kissing, biting, or oral-genital sex. A single sexual exposure to a person with active mucocutaneous syphilis has up to a 50% risk of acquiring the disease (Jacobs, 2001). Transplacental transmission may occur at any time during pregnancy; the degree of risk is related to the quantity of spirochetes in the maternal bloodstream. Women with early syphilis are most likely to transmit the disease to their infants (Marrazzo & Celum, 2000).

There are an estimated 40,000 cases of primary and secondary syphilis in the United States each year. During 1986 to 1990, an epidemic of syphilis occurred throughout the United States (CDC, 1998). In 1991, syphilis rates began to decline and continued to drop through 2000. However, since 2001, primary and secondary syphilis rates have increased, particularly in women and men having sex with men. Syphilis rates are higher for heterosexual African American and Hispanic women than they are for White women. Much of the rise in cases seen is directly attributable to illicit drug use, particularly crack cocaine; the exchange of sex for drugs or money; reduction in resources for syphilis control programs; and rising poverty rates. Approximately as many women as men have primary or secondary syphilis. Rises in cases of congenital syphilis have paralleled these rates for women. In contrast to other bacterial STIs, which affect mostly teens and adults younger than age 34, syphilis persists into the early 30s in both men and women. Further, as many as 15% of adolescents and adults with syphilis are HIV-positive.

Syphilis is a complex disease that can lead to serious systemic disease and even death when untreated. Infection manifests itself in distinct stages with different symptoms and clinical manifestations (see Table 24.12). *Primary* syphilis is characterized by a primary lesion, a chancre that often begins as a painless papule at the site of inoculation and then erodes to form a nontender, shallow, indurated, clean ulcer several millimeters to centimeters in size. The chancre is loaded with spirochetes and is most commonly found on the genitalia, although other sites include the cervix, perianal area, and mouth. *Secondary* syphilis is characterized by a widespread, symmetrical maculopapular rash on the palms and soles and generalized lymphadenopathy. The infected individual may experience fever, headache, and malaise. Condyloma lata (wart-like infectious lesions) may develop on the vulva, perineum, or anus. If the patient is untreated, she enters a latent phase that is asymptomatic for most individuals. If left untreated, about one-third of patients will develop tertiary syphilis. Cardiovascular (chest pain, cough), dermatologic

(multiple nodules or ulcers), skeletal (arthritis, myalgia, myositis), or neurological (headache, irritability, impaired balance, memory loss, tremor) symptoms can develop in this stage. Neurological complications are not limited to tertiary syphilis; rather a variety of syndromes (e.g., meningitis, meningovascular syphilis, general paresis, and tabes dorsalis) may span all stages of the disease. Evidence has suggested that the disease is shifting from these more traditional symptomatic forms of neurosphyilis to asymptomatic central nerous system involvement with subtler, less well-defined syndromes (Star & Deal, 2004b).

Screening and Diagnosis

Darkfield examination and direct fluorescent antibody tests of lesion exudates or tissue provide definitive diagnosis of early syphilis. Diagnosis is dependent on serology during latency and late infection. Any test for antibodies may not be reactive in the presence of active infection, because it takes time for the body's immune system to develop antibodies to any antigens. A presumptive diagnosis is possible with the use of two serologic tests: nontreponemal and treponemal. Nontreponemal antibody tests such as the VDRL or RPR are used as screening tests; they are relatively inexpensive, sensitive, moderately nonspecific and fast. False-positive results are not unusual with these tests, particularly when conditions such as acute infection, autoimmune disorders, malignancy, pregnancy, and drug addition exist and after immunization or vaccination. A high titer ($>1:16$) usually indicates active disease. A four-fold drop in the titer indicates a response to treatment. Treatment of primary syphilis usually causes a progressive decline to a negative VDRL within 2 years. In secondary, latent, or tertiary syphilis, low titers persist in about 50% of cases after 2 years. Rising titer (four times) indicates relapse, reinfection, or treatment failure (Wallach, 1996). The treponemal tests, fluorescent treponemal antibody absorbed, and microhemagglutination assays for antibody to *T. pallidum* are used to confirm positive results. Test results in patients with early primary or incubating syphilis may be negative. Seroconversion usually takes place 6 to 8 weeks after exposure, so testing should be repeated in 1 to 2 months when a suspicious genital lesion exists. Treponemal antibody tests frequently stay positive for life regardless of treatment or disease activity; therefore, treatment is monitored by the titers of the VDRL or RPR. Sequential serologic tests should be obtained by using the same testing method (VDRL or RPR), preferably by the same laboratory.

Tests for concomitant STIs should be done, HIV testing offered, and, if indicated, wet preps carried out. All pregnant women should be screened for syphilis at the first prenatal visit and again in the late third trimester for high-risk patients. Some states also mandate

24.12 | Stages of Syphilis

	PRIMARY	SECONDARY	EARLY LATENT	LATE LATENT	TERTIARY
Time after exposure	9 to 90 days	6 weeks to 6 months	3 to 12 months	More than 1 year	Years
Duration	Weeks	Weeks	Less than 2 years	More than years	Variable
Infectious	Yes	Yes	No	No	Yes
Clinical symptoms	Chancre Painless lympha- denopathy	Skin lesions; papular rash of soles and palms; patchy alopecia; condylomata Symptoms of systemic illness (fever, malaise, anorexia, weight loss, headache, myalgias)			Symptomatic central nervous system disease Cardiovascular syphilis Skin lesions (gumma) Progressive bone destruction
Laboratory changes	Dark-field serology[a] often negative or rising titers VDRL and FTA-ABS	Dark-field positive; peak antibody titers Seroconversion of FTA-ABS or MHA-TP positive CSF abnormal in up to 50% Proteinuria	CSF VDRL - Falling VDRL titers	CSF VDRL - Falling VDRL titers	CSF: VDRL positive or Increased cells and protein, serum treponemal positive; nontreponemal positive or negative VDRL remains positive indefinitely with declining titer

Note. From Augenbraum, 2007; *Nursing Assessment of the Pregnant Woman: Antepartal Screening and Laboratory Evaluation,* by M. L. Barron, 1998, New York: March of Dimes Birth Defects Foundation; "Sexually Transmitted Diseases Treatment Guidelines 2006," by Centers for Disease Control and Prevention, 2006, *MMWR, 55*(RR-11), pp. 1–94; "Syphilis," by C. H. Livengood, 2001, in S. Faro and D. E. Soper (Eds.), *Infectious Diseases in Women* (pp. 403–429), Philadelphia: Saunders; "Syphilis," by W. Star, 1999, in W. L. Star, M. T. Shannon, L. L. Lommel, and Y. M. Gutierrez (Eds.), *Ambulatory Obstetrics* (3rd ed., pp. 1031–1056), San Francisco: UCSF Nursing Press; *Varney's Midwifery* (4th ed.), by H. Varney, J. M. Kriebs, and C. L. Gegor, 2004, Sudbury, MA: Jones & Bartlett.
[a] Dark field is only useful when examining moist lesions of primary syphilis.

screening of all patients in the third trimester and/or at delivery. No infant should be discharged from the hospital without the syphilis serologic status of its mother having been determined at least once during pregnancy. Any woman who delivers a stillborn infant should be tested for syphilis (CDC, 2002b).

Management

Parenteral penicillin G is the preferred drug for treating patients with all stages of syphilis (see Table 24.13). It is the only proven therapy that has been widely used for patients with neurosyphilis, congenital syphilis, or syphilis during pregnancy. Intramuscular benzathine penicillen G (2.4 million units IM once) is used to treat primary, secondary, and early latent syphilis. Women who have had syphilis for more than a year (late latent or tertiary stage) require weekly treatment of 2.4 million units of benzathine penicillen G for 3 weeks.

While doxycycline, tetracycline, and erythromycin are alternative treatments for penicillin-allergic patients, both tetracycline and doxycycline are contraindicated in pregnancy and erythromycin is unlikely to cure a fetal infection. Therefore, pregnant women should, if necessary, receive skin testing and be treated with penicillin, or be desensitized (CDC, 2006b). Specific protocols for desensitization are recommended by the CDC (2006b, pp. 33–35). Some pregnant women treated for syphilis may experience a Jarisch-Herxheimer reaction. This is an acute febrile reaction to the toxins given off by treponemes when killed rapidly by treatment; the reaction occurs 4 to 24 hours after treatment with penicillin and is characterized by fever up to 105° F, headache, myalgias, and arthralgias which last 4 to 12 hours (CDC, 2006b; Schaffer, 2003). Women treated in the second half of pregnancy who experience a Jarisch-Herxheimer reaction are at risk for preterm labor and delivery. They should be advised to contact their health care provider

24.13 | Treatment of Syphilis

NONPREGNANT WOMEN OLDER THAN 18 YEARS OF AGE	PREGNANT WOMEN	LACTATING WOMEN
Primary, secondary, early latent disease: Benzathine penicillin G 2.4 million units IM once	Primary, secondary, early latent disease: Benzathine penicillin G 2.4 million units IM once	Primary, secondary, early latent disease: Benzathine penicillin G 2.4 million units IM once
Late latent or unknown duration disease: Benzathine penicillin G 7.2 million units total, administered as three doses 2.4 million units IM each at 1-week intervals	Late latent or unknown duration disease: Benzathine penicillin G 7.2 million units total, administered as three doses 2.4 million units each at 1-week intervals	
Penicillin allergy: Doxycycline 100 mg orally four times per day for 28 days or tetracycline 500 mg orally four times per day for 28 days[a]	No proven alternatives to penicillin in pregnancy. Pregnant women who have a history of allergy to penicillin should be desensitized and treated with penicillin.	

Note. From "Sexually Transmitted Diseases Treatment Guidelines 2002," by Centers for Disease Control and Prevention, 2002, *MMWR, 51*(RR-6), pp. 32–36; "Infectious Diseases: Spirochetal," by R. A. Jacobs, 2001, in "Vaginitis and Sexually Transmitted Diseases," by S. D. Schaffer, 2003, in E. Q. Youngkin and M. S. Davis (Eds.), *Women's Health: A Primary Clinical Guide* (3rd ed., pp. 261–290), Upper Saddle River, NJ: Pearson Prentice Hall; "Syphilis," by W. Star, 1999, in W. L. Star, M. T. Shannon, L. L. Lommel, and Y. M. Gutierrez (Eds.), *Ambulatory Obstetrics* (3rd ed., pp. 1031–1056), San Francisco: UCSF Nursing Press.
[a] Use only with close clinical follow-up.

if they notice any change in fetal movement or experience cramping, contractions, or persistent low back pain or pressure.

Monthly follow-up is mandatory so that retreatment may be given if needed. The nurse should emphasize the necessity of long-term serologic testing even in the absence of symptoms. The patient should be advised to practice sexual abstinence until treatment is completed, all evidence of primary and secondary syphilis is gone, and serologic evidence of a cure is demonstrated. Women should be told to notify all partners who may have been exposed. They should be informed that the disease is reportable. Preventative measures should be discussed.

Genital Herpes Simplex Virus Infection

Unknown until the middle of the 20th century, genital herpes is now one of the most common STIs in the United States, especially for women, who contract it far more often than men. Genital herpes is a recurrent, incurable viral disease characterized by painful vesicular eruption of the skin and mucosa of the genitals. Two serotypes of HSV have been identified: herpes simplex virus I (HSV-1) and herpes simplex virus II (HSV-2). HSV-2 is usually transmitted sexually and HSV-1, nonsexually. Although HSV-1 is more commonly associated with gingivostomatitis and oral labial ulcers (fever blisters) and HSV-2 with genital lesions, both types are not exclusively associated with the respective sites.

Although HSV infection is not a reportable disease, it is estimated that approximately half a million cases are diagnosed annually and that at least 55 million Americans are infected with genital herpes. Prevalence is higher in women with multiple sex partners. Most new cases occur in individuals between 15 and 34 years of age.

An initial herpetic infection (primary genital herpes) characteristically has both systemic and local symptoms and lasts about 3 weeks. Women generally have a more severe clinical course than do men. Flu-like symptoms with fever, malaise, and myalgia appear first about a week after exposure, peak within 4 days, and subside over the next week. Multiple genital lesions develop at the site of infection, usually the vulva; other common sites are the perianal area, vagina, and cervix. The lesions begin as small painful blisters or vesicles that become "unroofed," leaving ulcerated lesions. Individuals with primary herpes often develop bilateral tender inguinal lymphadenopathy, vulvar edema, vaginal discharge, and severe dysuria. Ulcerative lesions last 4 to 15 days before crusting over. New lesions may develop up to the 10th day of the course of the infection. Herpes simplex viral cervicitis also is common with initial HSV-2 infections: The cervix may appear normal or be friable, reddened, ulcerated, or necrotic. A heavy, watery to purulent vaginal discharge is common. Extragential lesions may be present because of autoinnoculation. Urinary retention and dysuria may occur secondary to autonomic involvement of the sacral nerve root.

Women experiencing recurrent episodes of HSV infections commonly will have only local symptoms, which are usually less severe than those associated with the initial infection. Systemic symptoms are usually absent, although the characteristic prodromal genital tingling is common. Recurrent lesions are unilateral, less severe, and usually last 7 to 10 days without prolonged viral shedding. Lesions begin as vesicles and progress rapidly to ulcers. Very few women with recurrent disease have cervicitis.

The most severe complication of maternal HSV infection is neonatal herpes, a potentially fatal or severely disabling disease. Infection of the newborn is acquired by exposure to the virus in the maternal genital tract at the time of delivery. Neonates who develop HSV infection usually have severe disseminated or central nervous system infection resulting in mental retardation or death. Most mothers of infants who acquire neonatal herpes do not have a history of clinically evident genital herpes (CDC, 2006b). The risk for transmission to the neonate is high (30% to 50%) among women who have an initial herpetic infection near time of delivery and low (less than 1%) in women who have a history of recurrent herpes at or near term or who acquire genital herpes during the first half of pregnancy.

Screening and Diagnosis

The risk profile for herpes is less clear-cut than in other STIs, and screening for asymptomatic women is not recommended.

Although a clinical diagnosis of genital herpes is both insensitive and nonspecific, a careful history provides much information when making a diagnosis of herpes. A history of exposure to an infected person is important, although infection from an asymptomatic individual is possible. A history of having viral symptoms such as malaise, headache, fever, or myalgia is suggestive. Local symptoms such as vulvar pain, dysuria, itching or burning at the site of infection, and painful genital lesions that heal spontaneously also are very suggestive of HSV infections. The nurse should ask about prior history of a primary infection, prodromal symptoms, vaginal discharge, dysuria, and dyspareunia.

During the physical examination, the nurse should assess for inguinal and generalized lymphadenopathy and elevated temperature. The entire vulvular, perineal, vaginal, and cervical areas should be carefully inspected for vesicles or ulcerated or crusted areas. A speculum examination may be very difficult for the patient because of the extreme tenderness associated with herpes infections.

Although a diagnosis of herpes infection may be suspected from the history and physical, it is confirmed by laboratory studies. Isolation of HSV in cell culture is the preferred virologic test in women who have genital ulcers or other muco-cutaneous lesions. Viral culture has a sensitivity of 70% to 80% (CDC, 2006b; Schaffer, 2003). Culture yield is best if the specimen is taken during the vesicular stage of the disease; however, the sensitivity of a culture declines rapidly as lesions begin to heal. In a primary infection, viral shedding is prolonged and the HSV is more easily isolated.

Because false-negative HSV cultures are common, especially with healing lesions or recurrent infection, type-specific serologic tests are useful in confirming a clinical diagnosis. The POCkit™-HSV-2 assay is a point-of-care test that provides results for HSV-2 antibodies from capillary blood or serum during a clinic visit (CDC, 2006b). Sensitivity varies from 80% to 90%, and false-negative results can occur, especially in early stages of infection. Specificity of the assay is greater than 96%; false-positive results occur in patients with a low likelihood of HSV infection.

Management

Genital herpes is a chronic and recurring disease for which there is no known cure. Antiviral drugs do not eradicate the latent virus and do not affect subsequent risk, frequency, or severity of recurrence after administration. Systemic antiviral drugs partially control the symptoms and signs of HSV infections when used for the primary or recurrent episodes or when used as daily suppressive therapy. However, these drugs do not eradicate the infection nor alter subsequent risk, frequency, or reoccurrence after the drug is stopped. Three antiviral medications provide clinical benefit for genital herpes: acyclovir, valacyclovir, and famciclovir (CDC, 2006b). Treatment recommendations are given in Table 24.14.

Safety and efficacy have been shown clearly in persons taking acyclovir daily for up to 3 years. The safety of acyclovir, valacyclovir, and famciclovir therapy during pregnancy has not been definitively established. However, available data do not indicate an increased risk for major birth defects compared with the general population in women treated with acyclovir in the first trimester. (Stone et al., 2004). The first clinical episode of genital herpes during pregnancy may be treated with oral acyclovir. In the presence of life-threatening maternal HSV infection, acyclovir IV is indicated (CDC, 2006b).

Women in their childbearing years should be counseled regarding the risk of herpes infection during pregnancy. They should be instructed to use condoms

24.14 | Treatment of Genital Herpes

NONPREGNANT WOMEN OLDER THAN 18 YEARS OF AGE	PREGNANT WOMEN	LACTATING WOMEN
Primary infection: Acyclovir 400 mg orally three times per day for 7 to 10 days Treatment may be extended if healing is incomplete after 10 days of therapy. Higher dosages of acyclovir (400 mg orally five times per day) may be used in treatment of first-episode oral herpes simplex virus infection. or acyclovir 200 mg orally five times per day for 7 to 10 days or famciclovir 250 mg orally three times per day for 7 to 10 days or valacyclovir 1 g orally twice per day for 7 to 10 days Recurrent infection: Acyclovir 400 mg orally three times per day for 5 days or acyclovir 200 mg orally five times per day for 5 days or acyclovir 800 mg orally three times per day for 5 days Famciclovir 125 mg orally twice per day for 5 days or valacyclovir 500 mg orally twice per day for 5 days Suppression therapy: Acyclovir 400 mg orally twice per day or famciclovir 250 mg orally twice per day or valacyclovir 250 mg orally twice per day or valacyclovir 500 mg orally once per day or valacyclovir 1,000 mg orally once per day	Acyclovir may be administered orally in first episode or severe recurrent herpes Acyclovir should be administered IV for severe HSV infection Safety of systemic acyclovir, valacyclovir, or famciclovir therapy has not been definitively established in pregnancy	Safety of systemic acyclovir, valacyclovir, or famciclovir therapy has not established

Note. Few comparative studies of valacyclovir or famciclovir with acyclovir; however, results suggest the drugs are comparable in clinical outcomes. From "Sexually Transmitted Diseases Treatment Guidelines 2006," by Centers for Disease Control and Prevention, 2006, *MMWR, 55*(RR-11), pp. 17–20.

if there is any risk of contracting any STI from a sexual partner. If they are using acyclovir therapy, they should be counseled to use contraception due to the potential teratogencity of acyclovir. Women currently breastfeeding should not use acyclovir.

Because neonatal HSV infection is such a devastating disease, prevention is critical. Current recommendations include carefully examining and questioning all women about symptoms at onset of labor (CDC, 2006b). Diagnosis of genital herpes in any pregnant women with active, visible lesions should be confirmed with culture. The results of viral cultures during pregnancy with or without visible herpetic lesions do not predict viral shedding at delivery, and therefore weekly surveillance

cultures for HSV are not indicated for pregnant women who have a history of recurrent genital herpes (CDC, 2006b). All pregnant women should be asked whether they have a history of genital herpes. When a woman is admitted to the labor and delivery unit, she should be carefully questioned about the symptoms of genital herpes, including prodomal symptoms, and all women should be examined carefully for herpetic lesion. For women with no symptoms or signs of genital herpes or its prodrome at onset of labor, vaginal delivery is acceptable. Cesarean delivery within four hours after labor begins or membranes rupture is recommended if visible lesions are present in order to prevent neonatal herpes. However, cesarean delivery does not completely eliminate the risk for HVS transmission to the infant. Any infant who is delivered through an infected vagina should be carefully observed and cultured and followed carefully by a specialist. Some experts recommend presumptive treatment with systemic acyclovir for infants who were exposed to HSV at delivery.

Cleaning lesions twice a day with saline will help prevent secondary infection. Bacterial infection must be treated with appropriate antibiotics. Measures that may increase comfort for women when lesions are active include warm sitz baths with baking soda; keeping lesions warm and dry by using a hair dryer on a cool setting or patting dry with soft towel; wearing cotton underwear and loose clothing; using drying aids such as hydrogen peroxide, Burrow's solution, and oatmeal baths; compresses of cold milk or Domeboro solution; applying cool, wet black tea bags to lesions; and applying compresses with an infusion of cloves or peppermint oil and clove oil to lesions (Star, 2004).

Oral analgesics such as aspirin or ibuprofen may be used to relieve pain and systemic symptoms associated with initial infections. Because the mucous membranes affected by herpes are very sensitive, any topical agents should be used with caution. Ointments containing cortisone should be avoided. Women should be informed that occlusive ointments may prolong the course of infections.

A diet rich in vitamins C, B-complex and B_6, zinc, and calcium is thought to help prevent recurrences. Daily use of kelp powder (2 capsules) and sunflower seed oil (1 tablespoon) also have been recommended to decrease recurrences. The amino acid L-lysine has been used in doses of 750 to 1,000 mg daily while lesions are active and 500 mg during asymptomatic periods. It is thought that L-lysine has an inhibitory effect on the multiplication of the herpes simplex virus (Fogel, 1995).

Counseling and education are critical components of the nursing care of women with herpes infections. Information regarding the etiology, signs and symptoms, sexual and perineal transmission, methods to prevent transmission, and treatment should be provided. The nurse should explain that each woman is unique in her response to herpes and emphasize the variability of symptoms. Women should be helped to understand when viral shedding and thus transmission to a partner is most likely, and that they should refrain from sexual contact from the onset of prodrome until complete healing of lesions. All persons with genital herpes should consistently use condoms with intercourse or oral-genital activity, and women should be encouraged to avoid intercourse when active lesions are present. Women can be encouraged to maintain close contact with their partners while avoiding contact with lesions. Women should be taught how to look for herpetic lesions using a mirror and good light source and a wet cloth or finger

covered with a finger cot to rub lightly over the labia. The nurse should ensure that patients understand that, when lesions are active, sharing intimate articles (e.g., washcloths, wet towels) that come into contact with the lesions should be avoided. Plain soap and water is all that is needed to clean hands that have come in contact with herpetic lesions; isolation is neither necessary nor appropriate.

The nurse should explain the role of precipitating factors in the reactivation of the latent virus and recurrent episodes. Stress, menstruation, trauma, febrile illnesses, chronic illness, and ultraviolet light have all been found to trigger genital herpes. Women may wish to keep a diary to identify which stressors seem to be associated with recurrent herpes attacks for them so that they can then avoid them when possible. Referral for stress reduction therapy, yoga, or meditation classes may be done when indicated. The role of exercise in reducing stress can be discussed. Avoiding excessive heat, sun, and hot baths and using a lubricant during sexual intercourse to reduce friction also may be helpful.

The emotional impact of contracting herpes is considerable. Media publicity regarding this disease has made receiving a diagnosis of genital herpes a devastating experience. No cure is available, and most women will experience recurrences. At diagnosis, many emotions may surface—helplessness, anger, denial, guilt, anxiety, shame, or inadequacy. Women need to be given the opportunity to discuss their feelings and help in learning to live with the disease. A woman can be encouraged to think of herself as a person who is not diseased but rather healthy and inconvenienced from time to time. Herpes can affect a woman's sexuality, her sexual practices, and her current and future relationships. She may need help in raising the issue with her partner or with future partners.

A common misconception that may cause anxiety for women is that HSV causes cancer. This myth should be dispelled because the role of HSV-2 in cervical cancer is at most that of a cofactor rather than a primary etiologic agent (CDC, 2006b).

Chancroid

Chancroid or soft chancre is a bacterial infection of the genitourinary tract caused by the gram-negative bacteria *Haemophilus ducreyi*. The acute localized infection of chancroid is found more often in Asia, Africa, and South America; however, discrete outbreaks do occur in the United States. The disease also is endemic in some areas; for example, the disease appears to be more prevalent among sex workers in areas such as Los Angeles, Boston, Dallas, New York City, and parts of Georgia and Florida. About 10% of persons in the United States who have chancroid are co-infected with HSV or *T. pallidum*. Because chancroid is a genital ulcer, it is a cofactor for

HIV infection. The major way chancroid is acquired is through sexual contact; trauma or an abrasion is necessary for the organism to penetrate the skin.

Chancroid is characterized by a rapidly growing ulcerated lesion formed on the external genitalia. The incubation period is usually 3 to –10 days but may be as long as 3 weeks.

Typically, the client presents with a history of a painful macule on the external genitalia, which rapidly changes to a pustule and then to an ulcerated lesion. Autoinnoculation of fingers or other sites occasionally occurs. The patient may develop enlarged unilateral or bilateral enlarged inguinal nodes know as buboe. After 1 to 2 weeks, the skin overlying the lymph node becomes erythematous, the center necroses, and the node becomes ulcerated.

Assessment and Diagnosis

The combination of a painful genital lesion and tender suppurative inguinal adenopathy suggest the diagnosis of chancroid. A probable diagnosis can be made if all of the following criteria are met: presence of one or more painful genital ulcers; no evidence of syphilis or herpes genitalia infection is present; and the clinical presentation, appearance of genital ulcers, and regional lymphadenopathy are typical for chancroid (CDC, 2006b). Definitive diagnosis of chancroid is difficult because the organism can only be identified by culture on a special media that is not used routinely. A cotton or calcium alginate swab is used to obtain the specimen from the ulcer base after gentle removal of necrotic exudate with saline. Culture sensitivity is less than 80% or lower (CDC, 2006b). Gonorrheal and chlamydia cultures should be obtained, and syphilis and HIV testing should be done at the time of diagnosis and repeated in 3 months.

Management

The recommended treatment for chancroid includes: azithromycin 1 g orally single dose or ceftriaxone 250 mg IM single dose or ciprofloxacin 500 mg orally twice a day for 3 days or erythromycin base 500 mg orally four times a day for 7 days (CDC, 2006b). HIV-infected persons may require retreatment after single-dose therapy. No adverse effects of chancroid on pregnancy outcome or on the fetus have been reported. Ciprofloxacin is contraindicated for pregnant and lactating women. Medications for use in pregnancy include ceftriaxone 250 mg IM single dose or erythromycin base 500 mg orally four times a day for 7 days.

Women should be instructed to have no sexual contact until all medication is taken, and the importance of completing the entire course of medication must be stressed. Comfort measures the nurse can suggest are tepid sitz baths followed by drying carefully with cool

air hair dryer; avoiding tight, restricting clothes; and exposing the perineum to air flow as much as possible (e.g., wear a skirt without underpants when at home).

Patients should be reexamined 3 to 7 days after beginning therapy. If treatment is successful, there should be symptomatic improvement within 3 days of starting therapy. If no clinical improvement is seen, the clinician should consider whether the diagnosis is correct; the patient is coinfected with another STI; the patient is infected with HIV; the treatment was not used as recommended; or the strain causing the infection is resistant to the prescribed antimicrobial (CDC, 2006b). It should be noted that it may take more than 2 weeks for complete healing of the ulcers to occur. All sexual partners who have had sexual contact within 10 days preceding the onset symptoms with a person diagnosed with chancroid should be evaluated regardless of whether symptoms are present.

DISEASES CHARACTERIZED BY VAGINAL DISCHARGE

Vaginal discharge and itching of the vulva and vagina are among the most common reasons a woman seeks help from a health care provider. Indeed, more women complain of vaginal discharge than any other gynecologic symptom. Vaginal discharge resulting from infection must be distinguished from normal secretions. Normal vaginal secretion or leukorrhea are clear to cloudy in appearance and may turn yellow after drying; the discharge is slightly slimy, nonirritating, and has a mild inoffensive odor. Normal vaginal secretions are acidic, with a pH range of 3.8 to 4.2. The amount of leukorrhea present differs with phases of the menstrual cycle, with greater amounts occurring at ovulation and just before menses. Leukorrhea also increases during pregnancy. Normal vaginal secretions contain lactobacilli and epithelial cells. Women who have adequate endogenous or exogenous estrogen will have vaginal secretions.

Vaginitis, an inflammation of the vagina characterized by an increased vaginal discharge containing numerous white blood cells, occurs when the vaginal environment is disturbed, either by a microorganism (see Table 24.15) or by a disturbance that allows the pathogens that are found normally in the vagina to proliferate..

Factors that can disturb the vaginal environment include douches, vaginal medications, antibiotics, hormones, contraceptive preparations (oral and topical), stress, sexual intercourse, and changes in sexual partners (Schaffer, 2003). Vulvovaginitis or inflammation of the vulva and vagina may be caused by vaginal infection; copious amounts of leukorrhea, which can cause maceration of tissues; and chemical irritants, allergens, and foreign bodies, which may produce inflammatory reactions. Bacterial vaginosis, vulvovaginal candidiasis,

24.15 | Conditions Characterized by Vaginal Discharge

	NORMAL DISCHARGE	TRICHOMONIASIS	BACTERIAL VAGINOSIS	VULVOVAGINAL CANDIDIASIS
STI	No	Yes	No	No
Vaginal pH	3.8–4.2	> 4.5	5.0–6.0	< 4.5 (usually normal)
Wet prep	Normal flora	With normal saline: delay results in drying and loss of characteristic shape of protozoan	With saline solution: positive for clue cells, decreased lactobacilli	With potassium hydroxide (KOH): psuedohyphae with yeast buds
Discharge	White/clear Thin/mucoid	Malodorous, copious, frothy or nonfrothy, thin or thick, white/yellow-green/gray	Thin, homogeneous, grayish-white, adherent	Thick white, curd-like; cottage cheese-like, adherent
Amine odor (KOH "whiff" test)	Normal body odor	Unpleasant smell may be present	Present (fishy)	None/yeasty, musty odor
Vulvular puritis	No	Soreness rather than itching, swelling, redness; burning and soreness of thighs and perineum	Mild if present at all	Yes, swelling, excoriation, redness
Genital ulceration	No	No	No	Skin may crack in severe cases
Pelvic pain	No	Yes, in severe cases; severe pelvic pain with tender inguinal lymph nodes	No	No
Dysuria	No	Yes	Occasionally	Severe cases
Dyspareunia	No	Yes	Occasionally	occasionally
Main patient complaint	No	Excessive discharge, vulvar purities, dysuria, vaginal irritation, dypareunia, postcoital bleeding	May be asymptomatic discharge, bad odor, possibly worse after intercourse; may report suprapubic pain	Itching/burning discharge
Risk of pelvic inflammatory disease	No	May develop	Yes	No

Note. From "Sexually Transmitted Diseases Treatment Guidelines 2006," by Centers for Disease Control and Prevention, 2006, *MMWR, 55*(RR-11), pp. 50–55; "Sexually Transmitted Diseases Treatment Guidelines, 2006: An Update," by A. L. Nelson, 2007, *The Forum, 5*(1), 2–3; "The CDC 2002 Guidelines for the Treatment of Sexually Transmitted Diseases: Implications for Women's Health Care," by M. Scharbo-DeHaan and D. G. Anderson, 2003, *Journal of Midwifery & Women's Health, 48*(2), 96–104; *Varney's Midwifery* (4th ed.), by H. Varney, J. M. Kriebs, and C. L. Gegor, 2004, Sudbury, MA: Jones & Bartlett.
[a] Although not usually transmitted sexually, are included in this module because they are often diagnosed in women being evaluated for an STI

and tricamonasis are the most common causes of abnormal vaginal discharge.

Trichomoniasis

Trichomonasis vaginalis vaginitis is sexually transmitted and is believed to facilitate HIV transmission. Trichomoniasis is caused by *Trichomonas vaginalis,* an anaerobic one-celled protozoan with characteristic flagellae. The organism lives in the vagina, urethra, and Bartholin's and Skene's glands in women, and in the urethra and prostate gland in men. It is transmitted during vaginal-penis intercourse, and transmission rates are about 75% (Schaffer, 2003). Although trichomoniasis may be asymptomatic, commonly women experience characteristically yellowish to greenish, frothy, mucopurulent, copious, malodorous discharge. Inflammation of the vulva, vagina, or both may be present, and the woman may complain of irritation and pruritis. Dysuria and dyspareunia are often present. Typically, the discharge worsens during and after menstruation. Often the cervix and vaginal walls will demonstrate the characteristic "strawberry spots" or tiny petechiae, and the cervix may bleed on contact. In severe infections, the vaginal walls, cervix, and occasionally the vulva may be acutely inflamed. Vaginal trichomoniasis has been associated with adverse pregnancy outcomes, especially premature rupture of the membranes, pretem delivery, and low birth weight.

Trichomoniasis is the most common curable STI in the United States and worldwide and is the cause of up to 20% of all vaginitis with discharge occurring in approximately 3 million women annually (Gorroll, 2001; Hatcher, 2004).

Assessment and Diagnosis

In addition to obtaining a history of current symptoms, a careful sexual history including last intercourse and last sexual contact should be obtained, because trichomoniasis is a sexually transmitted infection (see Table 24.8). Any history of similar symptoms in the past and treatment used should be noted. The nurse should determine whether her client's partner(s) were treated and whether she has had subsequent relations with new partners. Additional important information includes last menstrual period, method of birth control, if any, and other medications. The external genitalia should be observed for excoriation, erythema, edema, ulceration, and lesions. A speculum examination always is done, even though it may be very uncomfortable for the woman; relaxation techniques and breathing exercises may help the woman with the procedure. Any of the classic signs may be present on physical examination. The pH is elevated. Diagnosis is usually made by wet prep visualization of the typical one-celled flagellate trichomonads; however, this method has a sensitivity of only approximately 60% to 70% (CDC, 2006b). Microscopic examination of the wet mount may reveal an increased number of white blood cells. Culture is the most sensitive, specific method of diagnosis but is expensive and not widely available. Pap smear results frequently include reports of trichomonads; sensitivity of the method is low (65%). Because trichomonasis is an STI, once the diagnosis is confirmed, gonorrhea and chlamydia cultures, and serology testing for syphilis if history indicates, should be carried out.

Management

The recommended treatment for trichomoniasis (see Table 24.16) is metronidazole 2 g orally in a single dose (CDC, 2006b). Metronidazole (Flagyl) is an antiprotozoal and antibacterial agent. Complementary and alternative therapies for vaginitis are found in Table 24.17.

Until recently, metronidazole was contraindicated in the first trimester of pregnancy; however, multiple studies and meta-analyses have not demonstrated a consistent association between metronidazole use during pregnancy and teratogenic or mutagenic effects in offspring (CDC, 2006b). Symptomatic pregnant women should be treated with 2 grams orally in a single dose. Treatment of pregnant women with asymptomatic trichomoniasis is not indicated, because data have not demonstrated that this strategy is effective in preventing preterm delivery (Klebanoff et al., 2001). The drug is contraindicated when a woman is breast-feeding, because high concentrations have been found in infants. If it is necessary to prescribe metronidazole for a lactating woman, she should suspend breast-feeding temporarily for 12 to 24 hours after taking the medication (CDC, 2006b). Metronidazole is contraindicated in clients with blood dyscrasia or central nervous system disease, because in rare cases it may affect the hematopoietic or central nervous system.

Side effects of metronidazole are numerous, including sharp, unpleasant metallic taste in the mouth, furry tongue, central nervous system reactions, and urinary tract disturbances. When oral metronidazole is taken, the client is advised not to drink alcoholic beverages, or she will experience severe abdominal distress, nausea, vomiting, and headache. Metronidazole can cause gastrointestinal symptoms regardless of whether alcohol is consumed and can also darken urine. The nurse should stress the importance of completing all medication even if symptoms disappear.

Although the male partner is usually asymptomatic, it is recommended that he receive treatment also, because he may harbor the trichomonads in the urethra or prostate. It is important that nurses discuss the importance of partner treatment with clients. If partners are not treated, the likelihood is that the infection will occur.

Women with trichomoniasis need to understand the sexual transmission of this disease. It is important that the client know the organism may be present without symptoms being present, perhaps for several months, and that it is not possible to determine when she became infected. Women should be informed of the necessity for treating all sexual partners and helped with ways to raise the issue with her partner(s).

Bacterial Vaginosis

Bacterial vaginosis (BV)—formerly called nonspecific vaginitis, hemophilus vaginitis, or Gardnerella—is the most common type of vaginal discharge or malodor in childbearing women; however, up to 50% of women with BV are asymptomatic (CDC, 2006b). BV is a clinical

24.16 | Treatment of Vaginal Infections

INFECTION	NONPREGNANT WOMEN	PREGNANT WOMEN	LACTATING WOMEN
Trichomoniasis	Metronidazole 2 g orally in single dose *or* metronidazole 500 mg twice per day for 7 days	Metronidazole 2 g orally in single dose	Metronidazole 2 g orally in single dose Breast milk should be expressed and discarded during treatment. Resume breast-feeding 12 to 24 hours after completing treatment
Bacterial vaginosis	Metronidazole 500 mg orally twice per day & days *or* metronidazole gel 0.75%, one full applicator (5 g) intravaginally once per day for 5 days *or* clindamycin cream 2%, one full applicator (5 g) intravaginally at bed time for 7 days Clindamycin 300 mg orally twice per day for 7 days *or* clindamycin ovules 100 g intravaginally once at bed time for 3 days	Metronidazole 250 mg orally three times per day for 7 days *or* clindamycin 300 mg orally twice per day for 7 days before the 16th week of pregnancy	Metronidazole 2 g orally in a single dose Breast milk should be expressed and discarded during treatment. Resume breast-feeding 12 to 24 hours after completing treatment
Uncomplicated vulvovaginal candidiasis (VVC)	Butoconazole 2% cream 5 g intravaginally x 3 days[a] *or* butoconazole 2% cream 5 g (sustained release) single intravaginal application *or* clotrimazole 1% cream 5 g intravaginally for 7 to 14 days[a] *or* clotrimazole 100 mg vaginal tablet for 7 days *or* clotrimazole 100 mg vaginal tablet, two tablets for 3 days *or* clotrimazole 500 mg vaginal tablet, one tablet in single application *or* miconazole 2% cream 5 g intravaginally for 7 days[a] *or* miconazole 100 mg vaginal suppository, one for 7 days[a] *or* miconazole 200 mg vaginal suppository, one for 3 days[a] *or* nystatin 100,000-unit vaginal tablet, one for 14 days *or* tioconazole 6.5% ointment 5 g intravaginally in a single application *or* terconazole 0.4% cream 5 g intravaginally for 7 days *or* terconazole 0.8% cream 5 g intravaginally for 3 days *or* terconazole 80 mg vaginal suppository, one for 3 days *Oral Agent* Fluconazole 150 mg oral tablet, 1 tablet single dose	Butoconazole 2% cream 5 g intravaginally for 3 days[a] *or* butoconazole 2% cream 5 g (sustained release) single intravaginal application *or* clotrimazole 1% cream 5 g intravaginally for 7 to 14 days[a] *or* clotrimazole 100 mg vaginal tablet for 7 days *or* miconazole 2% cream 5 g intravaginally for 7 days[a] *or* miconazole 100 mg vaginal suppository, one for 7 days[a]	Butoconazole 2% cream 5 g intravaginally for 3 days[a] *or* butoconazole 2% cream 5 g (sustained release) single intravaginal application *or* clotrimazole 1% cream 5 g intravaginally for 7 to14 days[a] *or* clotrimazole 100 mg vaginal tablet for 7 days *or* miconazole 2% cream 5 g intravaginally for 7 days[a] *or* miconazole 100 mg vaginal suppository, one for 7 days[a]

(continued)

24.16 | Treatment of Vaginal Infections (*continued*)

INFECTION	NONPREGNANT WOMEN	PREGNANT WOMEN	LACTATING WOMEN
Complicated vulvo-vaginal candidiasis	*Recurrent VVC Initial therapy* 7 to 14 days of topical therapy *or* 100, 150, or 200 mg dose of fluconazole every third day for a total of three doses (days 1, 4, and 7) *Maintenance therapy* Clotrimazole 500 mg vaginal suppository weekly Ketoconazole 100 mg each day Fluconazole 100–150 mg dose weekly Itraconazole 400 mg once monthly or 100 mg daily *Severe VVC* 7 to 14 days of topical azole *or* fluconazole 150 mg in two sequential doses, second dose 72 hours after initial dose *Nonalbicans VVC* Optimal treatment is unknown. Nonfluconazole azole drug for 7 to 14 days is first-line therapy. For recurrent episodes, 600 mg boric acid in gelatin capsule vaginally once per day for 14 days	*Recurrent VVC Initial therapy* 7 to 14 days of topical therapy *or* 100, 150, or 200 mg dose of fluconazole every third day for a total of three doses (days 1, 4, and 7) *Maintenance therapy* 100, 150, or 200 mg dose of oral fluconazole weekly for 6 months	*Recurrent VVC Initial therapy* 7 to 14 days of topical therapy *or* 100, 150, or 200 mg dose of fluconazole every third day for a total of three doses (days 1, 4, and 7) *Maintenance therapy* 100, 150, or 200 mg dose of oral fluconazole weekly for 6 months

[a] Over-the-counter preparations.

syndrome in which normal H_2O_2-producing *Lactobacilli* are replaced with high concentrations of anaerobic bacteria (*Prevotella* sp. and *Mobiluncus* sp.) *G. vaginalis* and *Mycoplasm hominis*. With the proliferation of anerobes, the level of vaginal amines is raised, and the normal acidic pH of the vagina is altered. Epithelial cells slough, and numerous bacteria attach to their surfaces (clue cells). When the amines are volatilized, the characteristic fishy odor of BV occurs. The cause of the microbial alteration is not completely understood. Bacterial vaginosis is a sexually associated condition but is usually not considered a specific STI (Hatcher, 2004). Further, BV is associated with multiple sex partners, douching, and a lack of vaginal lactobacilli and is rarely found in women who have never been sexually active.

Bacterial vaginosis infection is associated with miscarriage, chorioamnionitis, premature rupture of fetal membranes, preterm labor and delivery, postpartum or postabortion endometritis, and postpartum complications in the infant (CDC, 2006b; Koumans, Markowitz, & Hogan, 2002). In addition, new evidence suggests that BV increases a woman's risk of acquiring STIs and HIV infection and of transmitting HIV infection (Koumans et al., 2002; Taha, Hoover, & Dallabetta, 1998). Further, failure to treat BV infection prior to insertion of an IUD is associated with increased incidence of PID in the first month after insertion.

Women with BV may be asymptomatic or complain of a malodorous discharge. The fishy odor may be noticed by the woman or her partner after heterosexual intercourse as semen releases the vaginal amines. When present, the BV discharge is usually increased, thin and white or gray, or milky in appearance. Some women also may experience mild irritation, vulvar pruritus, postcoital spotting, irregular bleeding episodes, or vaginal burning after intercourse while others complain of urinary discomfort. Many women have no symptoms at all.

Assessment and Diagnosis

A careful history may help distinguish BV from other vaginal infections if the woman is symptomatic. Reports of fishy odor and increased thin vaginal discharge are most significant, and report of increased odor after

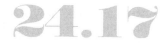 | Alternative Therapies for Vaginitis

INTERVENTION	DOSAGE	ADMINISTRATION	USE
Vinegar (white)	1 T per pint water	Douche or local application	Vulvovaginal candidiasis (VVC)
Acidophilus culture	1 to 2 T per quart water	Douche every five to seven days *or* twice per day for 2 days Douche once or twice per week	VVC Trichomoniasis Bacterial vaginosis (BV)
Vitamin C	500 mg two to four times per day	Orally	VVC
Acidophilous tablet	40 million to 1 billion units (1 tablet) daily	Orally	VVC
Plain yogurt	1 T	Apply to labia or vagina hourly as needed	VVC
Chaparral	Steep 1 handful in 1 quart water for 30 minutes	Douche two to three times per week	Trichomoniasis
Chickweed	Steep 3 T in 1 quart water for 10 minutes, strain	Douche daily	Trichomoniasis
Goldenseal	1 tsp in 3 cups water, strain and cool	Douche	BV
Garlic clove	1 peeled clove wrapped in cloth dipped in olive oil	Overnight in vagina, change daily	BV
Boric acid powder	600 mg in gelatin capsule	Daily in vagina for 14 days	BV
Sassafras bark	Steep in warm water	Compress or insert into vagina	BV, VVC
Cold milk, cottage cheese, plain yogurt		Apply to affected area	Puritis
Gentian violet	Few drops in water, 0.25% to 2%	Douche or local application	VVC

intercourse is also suggestive of BV. Previous occurrence of similar symptoms, diagnosis, and treatment should be asked about because women may experience repeated episodes associated with repeat insults such as antibiotic use, douching, or life stresses.

A speculum examination is done to inspect the vaginal walls and cervix. A microscopic examination of vaginal secretions is always done. Both normal saline and 10% potassium hydroxide smears should be completed. The presence of clue cells (vaginal epithelial cells coated with bacteria) by wet smear is highly diagnostic, because the phenomenon is specific to BV. Vaginal secretions should be tested for pH and amine odor. Nitrazine paper is sensitive enough to detect a pH of 4.5 or greater. The smear should be taken from the lateral walls of the vagina, not the cervix, for accurate pH. The fishy odor of BV will be released when KOH is added to vaginal secretions on the lip of the withdrawn speculum.

Management

Treatment of bacterial vaginosis with oral metronidazole (Flagyl) is most effecive. Treatment guidelines are found in Table 24.16. The CDC 2006 guidelines recommend that regimens in pregnancy be limited to systemic therapy of longer duration rather than a single dose or topical therapy. Intravaginal clindamycin cream is preferred in case of allergy or intolerance to metronidazole. Patients with a known allergy to oral metronidazole should not be given vaginal metronidazole gel (CDC, 2006b). Clindamycin vaginal cream should only be used prior to the 17th week of pregnancy, because research has shown an increased number of low–birth weight infants and neonatal infections in newborns (CDC, 2006b). Treatment of male sexual partners has not been beneficial in preventing recurrent BV infections (CDC, 2006b). A test for BV may be done early in the second trimester for symptomatic pregnant women who are at risk for preterm labor and whenever high-risk women report increased vaginal discharge or symptoms of preterm labor. Treatment of BV in asymptomatic pregnant women who are at high risk may prevent adverse pregnancy outcomes. Therefore, follow-up evaluation 1 month after completing treatment should be considered to evaluate whether therapy was effective (CDC, 2006b).

Vulvovaginal Candidiasis

Vulvovaginal candidiasis (VVC) or yeast infection accounts for 20% to 25% of all vaginal infections and is the second most common type of vaginal infection in the United States. An estimated 75% of women will have at least one episode of VVC in their life times and 40% to 45% will have two or more episodes (CDC, 2006b; Klebanoff et al., 2001). It is difficult to determine the actual incidence of VVC because it is not a reportable condition and the recent availability of over-the-counter treatments prevents many cases from being seen by health care providers (Scharbo-DeHaan & Anderson, 2003). Most (80% to 90%) women who have VVC will have uncomplicated VVC (see Table 24.18). Although vaginal candidiasis infections are common in healthy women, those seen in women with HIV infection are generally more severe and persistent. Genital candidiasis lesions may be painful, coalescing ulcerations necessitating continuous, prophylactic therapy.

The most common organism is *Candida albicans;* it is estimated that 80% to 95% of the yeast infections in women are caused by this organism. However, in the past 10 years, the incidence of non-albicans infections has risen steadily. Women with chronic or recurrent infections, defined as four or more clinically proven infections in 1 year (CDC, 2006b), often are infected with a higher percentage of non-albicans species than are women who are experiencing their first infection or who have few reoccurences.

Numerous factors have been identified as predisposing a woman to yeast infections, including repeated courses of systemic or topical antibiotic therapy, particularly broad-spectrum antibiotics such as ampicillin, tetracycline, cephalosporins, and metronidazole; diabetes, especially when uncontrolled; pregnancy; obesity; diets high in refined sugars or artificial sweetners; use of corticosteroids and exogenous hormones; and immunosupressed states (Varney, Kriebs, & Gegor, 2004). Clinical observations and research have suggested that tight-fitting clothing and underwear or pantyhose made of nonabsorbent materials create an environment in which vaginal fungus can grow.

The most common symptom of yeast infections is vulvular and possibly vaginal pruritis. (see Table 24.15). The itching may be mild or intense, interfere with rest and activities, and occur during or after intercourse. Some women report a feeling of dryness. Others experience painful urination as the urine flows over the vulva; this usually occurs in women who have excoriation resulting from scratching. Most often the discharge is thick, white, lumpy, and cottage cheese–like. The discharge usually is found in patches on the vaginal walls, cervix, and labia. Commonly the vulva is red and swollen, as are the labial folds, vagina, and cervix. Although there is not a characteristic odor with yeast infections, sometimes a yeast or musty smell occurs.

Assessment

In addition to a careful history of the woman's symptoms, their onset, and course, the history is a valuable screening tool for identifying predisposing risk factors. Physical examination should include a thorough inspection of the vulva and vagina. A speculum examination is always done. Commonly saline and KOH wet smear and vaginal pH, are obtained. Vaginal pH is normal with a yeast infection; if the pH is greater than 4.5, trichomoniasis or bacterial vaginosis should be suspected. The characteristic psuedohyphae may be seen on a wet smear done with normal saline; however, they may be confused with other cells and artifacts.

24.18 | Classification of Uncomplicated and Complicated Vulvovaginal Candidiasis (VVC)

UNCOMPLICATED VVC	COMPLICATED VVC	RECURRENT VVC
Sporadic or infrequent VVC or mild-to-moderate VVC or likely to be *C. albicans* or nonimmunocompromised women	Recurrent VVC or severe VVC or nonalbicans candidiasis or women with uncontrolled diabetes, debilitation, or immunosupression or who are pregnant	Four or more episodes of symptomatic VVC in 1 year Predisposing factors are diabetes, immunosuppression, conticosteroid use, use of commercial perineal hygiene or vaginal douche products, greater number of lifetime sexual partners

Note. From "Sexually Transmitted Diseases Treatment Guidelines 2002," by Centers for Disease Control and Prevention, 2002, *MMWR, 51*(RR-6), pp. 32–36; "The CDC 2002 Guidelines for the Treatment of Sexually Transmitted Diseases: Implications for Women's Health Care," by M. Scharbo-DeHaan and D. G. Anderson, 2003, *Journal of Midwifery & Women's Health, 48*(2), 96–104; A *Midwife's Handbook,* by C. Sinclair, 2004, St. Louis, MO: Saunders

Management

A number of antifungal preparations are available for the treatment of *C. albicans* (see Table 24.16). Women must be counseled that the creams and suppositories recommended for treatment of VVC are oil based and may weaken latex condoms and diaphragms. Many of the effective topical azole drugs (e.g., Monistat and Gyne-Lotrimin) are available over the counter (OTC). Self-treatment with OTC preparations should be used only by women who have been previously diagnosed with VVC and are experiencing the same symptoms. Any woman whose symptoms persist or who has a recurrence of symptoms within 2 months should seek medical care (CDC, 2002b). Unnecessary or inappropriate use of OTC preparations is common and can lead to delay in treating other causes of vulvovaginitis. If vaginal discharge is extremely thick and copious, vaginal debridement with a cotton swab followed by application of vaginal medication may be useful.

Women who have extensive irritation, swelling, and discomfort of the labia and vulva may find sitz baths helpful in decreasing inflammation and increasing comfort. Adding Aveeno colloidal oatmeal powder to the bath may also increase the woman's comfort. Not wearing underpants to bed may help decrease symptoms and prevent recurrences. Completing the full course of treatment prescribed is essential to removing the pathogen, and women are instructed to continue medication even during menstruation. They should be counseled not to use tampons during menstruation, because the medication will be absorbed by the tampon. Intercourse should be avoided during treatment; if this is not feasible, the woman's partner should use a condom to prevent introduction of more organisms.

HUMAN PAPILLOMAVIRUS

Human papillomavirus infection, previously named genital or venereal warts, is a sexually transmitted infection that was first described in 25 A.D. and is now the most common symptomatic viral STI in the United States (Hatcher, 2004; Schaffer, 2003; Wiley et al., 2002). Human papillomavirus infections are caused by the human papillomavirus, part of the papovirus family. This double-stranded DNA virus has over 70 known serotypes, of which more than 30 types can infect the genital tract, including the external genitalia, vagina, urethra, and anus (Gall, 2001). Most HPV infections are asymptomatic, subclinical, or unrecognized. The incubation period is at least 1 to 6 months and may be much longer (up to 30 years; Hawkins, Roberto-Nichols, & Stanley-Haney, 2008). Because health care providers are not required to report HPV infections, the true incidence of these infections is not known.

However, approximately 20 million Americans 15 to 49 years of age (approximately 15% of the population are infected with HPV, and it is estimated that as many as 6.2 million new HPV infections occur yearly (CDC, 2007a). It is likely that at least 80% of sexually active young women are infected with HPV. Between 5% and 30% of individuals infected with HPV are infected with multiple types of HPV (Revzina & DeClemente, 2005). Although the period of communicability is unknown, approximately 50% of those with a partner with genital warts will also develop them. In addition to the general risk factors for STIs noted earlier, cigarette smoking has been found to be a risk factor for HPV.

HPV lesions in women are most frequently seen in the posterior part of the introitus; however, lesions also are found on the buttocks, vulva, vagina, anus, and cervix. Typically, the lesions present as small (2–3 mm wide, 10–15 mm high), soft, papillary swellings occurring singularly or in clusters on the genital and anal-rectal region. Infections of long duration may appear as a cauliflower-like mass. In moist areas such as the vaginal introitus, the lesions may appear to have multiple, fine, finger-like projections. Vaginal lesions are often multiple. Flat-topped papules, 1 to 4 mm in diameter, are seen most often on the cervix. These lesions are visualized only under magnification. Women with visible genital warts can be infected with multiple HPV strains, with cervical or vaginal lesions present in up to 70% of women with vulvular lesions (CDC, 2006b). Warts are usually flesh-colored or slightly darker on White women, black on Black women, and brownish on Asian women. Although the lesions are usually painless, they may be uncomfortable, particularly when very large, inflamed, or ulcerated. Chronic vaginal discharge, pruritis, or dyspareunia also can occur.

High-risk, onocogenic, or cancer-associated types of HPV are 16, 18, 31, 33, 35, 39, 45, 51, 52, 56, 58, 59, 69, and 82. HPV 16 is the most common high-risk type, found in almost half of all cervical cancers, and is one of the most common types found in women without cancer. HPV, another common high-risk virus found in squamous lesions and glandular lesions of the cervix, accounts for 10% to 12% of all cervical cancer (Bosch & de Sanjos, 2003). Visible genital lesions are usually caused by HPV types 6, 11, 42, 43, and 44 and are low risk for invasive cancer. Other types (e.g., 31, 33, 35, 51, and 52) have been strongly associated with cervical dyspasia. Cervical infection with oncogenic types of HPV is associated with up to 95% of all cervical squamous cell carcinomas and nearly all preinvasive cervical neoplasms (Schaffer, 2003).

HPV infections seem to be more frequent in pregnant than nonpregnant women, with an increase in incidence from the first trimester to the third. The relative state of immunosupression and hormonal influences during pregnancy contribute to this (Lommel, 1999).

Further, a significant proportion of preexisting HPV lesions enlarge greatly during pregnancy, a proliferation presumably resulting from the relative state of immunosuppression present during pregnancy. Lesions may become so large during pregnancy that they affect urination, defecation, mobility, and fetal descent; cesarean delivery may be indicated for women with genital warts if the pelvic outlet is obstructed or if vaginal delivery would result in excessive bleeding (CDC, 2006b). Initial observation of large growths can be misleading, suggesting that the entire vagina is involved; however, all of the growth may derive from one stalk, and, in such cases, it may be possible to push the large mass to the side, allowing the baby to pass through. HPV infection may be acquired by the neonate during delivery; the frequency of such transmission is unknown. Juvenile laryngeal papillomata (JLP) can occur in children exposed to HPV during delivery. Juvenile laryngeal papillomata can cause mortality or significant morbidity requiring multiple surgical or laser treatments in affected children. The exact incidence of JLP is not known but is thought to be rare. The preventative value of cesarean section is unknown; therefore, cesarean delivery should not be done only to prevent transmission of HPV infection to newborns.

Screening and Diagnosis

A woman with HPV lesions may complain of symptoms such as a profuse, irritating vaginal discharge, itching, dyspareunia, or postcoital bleeding. She also may report bumps on her vulva or labia. History of a known exposure is important; however, because of the potentially long latency period and the possibility of subclinical infections in men, the lack of a history of known exposure cannot be used to exclude a diagnosis of HPV infection.

Physical inspection of the vulva, perineum, anus, vagina, and cervix is essential whenever HPV lesions are suspected or seen in one area. Because speculum examination of the vagina may block some lesions, it is important to rotate the speculum blades until all areas are visualized. When lesions are visible, the characteristic appearance previously described is considered diagnostic. However, in many instances, cervical lesions are not visible, and some vaginal or vulvular lesions may be unobservable to the naked eye. Because of the potential spread of vulvular or vaginal lesions to the anus, gloves should be changed between vaginal and rectal examinations.

Diagnosis is made by careful, thorough clinical examination of visable genital warts or by biopsy of cervical lesions and (rarely) for lesions at other sites if the diagnosis is not clear. It is imperative that women with vulvar HPV or partners with HPV have a cervical examination with Pap smear. Pap smears of the cervical transformation zone are a screening technique, not a di-

agnosis because the sample can miss the lesion. Thus, a negative Pap smear does not indicate absence of disease. It is important that any grossly visible suspicious cervical lesion be biopsied regardless of Pap smear findings. Further, the severity of any cervical lesion identified on a Pap smear is best determined by colposcopy and biopsy. Vinegar solution has been used in the past to highlight early or flat cervical lesions; however, it is important to note that a positive reaction may also be obtained with any inflammatory reaction, after sexual intercourse, and with vaginal trauma. Providers should also test for gonorrhea, chlamydia, and syphilis.

HPV lesions must be differentiated from condyloma lata, molluscum contagiosum, and carcinoma. Molluscum contagiosum lesions are half-domed, smooth, flesh-colored to pearly white papules with depressed centers. Condyloma lata are a form of secondary syphilis and generally are flatter and wider than genital warts. A serologic test for syphilis would confirm the diagnosis of secondary syphilis.

In 2000, the Food and Drug Administration (FDA) approved the use of the HC2 high-risk HPV DNA test to detect the presence of HPV in women with abnormal Pap test results. This test identifies 13 of the high-risk types of HPV associated with cervical cancer. In 2003, the FDA approved expanded use of the HC2 high-risk HPV DNA test for HPV screening, in conjunction with the Pap test, in women over the age of 30 with normal Pap test results.

Management

The primary goal of treatment of visible genital warts is removal of warts and relief of signs and symptoms, not the eradication of HPV (CDC, 2006b). Treatment can induce wart-free periods. If left untreated, visible genital warts may resolve, remain unchanged, or increase in size and number (CDC, 2007a). Currently available treatments for genital warts may reduce but probably do not eradicate HPV infectivity (CDC, 2007). Treatment of genital warts can be very difficult. The client must make multiple office visits; frequently, many different treatment modalities will be used. Eradication of the virus is not considered conclusive even after there is no visible evidence of wart tissue because of the high incidence of reoccurrence.

Treatment of genital warts should be guided by preference of the woman, available resources, and experience of the health care provider. None of the treatments are superior to other treatments, and no one treatment is ideal for all warts. Available treatments are outlined in Table 24.19. Because viable HPV particles have been found in the smoke plume associated with CO_2 laser therapy, it is extremely important to use vacuum suction. Imiquimod, podophyllin, and podofilox should not be used during pregnancy.

24.19 | Treatment of Genital Warts/Condyloma

PATIENT-APPLIED REGIMENS[a]	PROVIDER-ADMINISTERED REGIMENS	ALTERNATIVE REGIMENS
Podofilox 0.5% solution or gel[b] twice per day for 3 days, followed by 4 days of no therapy *or* imiquimod 5% cream[b], once daily at bed time, three times per week for up to 16 weeks	Applied to each wart and air-dried: Cryotherapy with liquid nitrogen or cyro-probe—repeat every 1 to 2 weeks *or* podophyllin[b] resin 10% to 25% in compound tincture of benzoin *or* trichloroacetic acid or bichloroacetic acid 80% to 90% *or* surgical removal by scissor excision, curettage or electrosurgery	Intralesional interferon *or* laser surgery

Note. From "Sexually Transmitted Diseases Treatment Guidelines 2002," by Centers for Disease Control and Prevention, 2002, *MMWR, 51*(RR-6), pp. 32–36; "The CDC 2002 Guidelines for the Treatment of Sexually Transmitted Diseases: Implications for Women's Health Care," by M. Scharbo-DeHaan and D. G. Anderson, 2003, *Journal of Midwifery & Women's Health, 48*(2), 96–104; *Varney's Midwifery* (4th ed.), by H. Varney, J. M. Kriebs, and C. L. Gegor, 2004, Sudbury, MA: Jones & Bartlett.
[a] If possible, the health care provider should apply the initial treatment to demonstrate the proper application technique and identify which warts should be treated.
[b] Do not use during pregnancy.

Women who have cervical warts must be evaluated for dysplasia before treatment is started and should be referred to an expert in the field of gynecological dysplasia. Any concurrent vaginal infections or STIs should be treated. Women who are experiencing discomfort associated with genital warts may find that bathing with an oatmeal solution and drying the area with a cool hair dyer will provide some relief. Keeping the area clean and dry will also decrease growth of the warts. Cotton underwear and loose-fitting clothes that decrease friction and irritation also may minimize discomfort. Women should be advised to maintain a healthy lifestyle to aid the immune system; women can be counseled regarding diet, rest, stress reduction, and exercise. All women who smoke should be counseled in smoking cessation techniques.

Patient counseling is essential; key messages are found in Exhibit 24.8. Women must understand the virus, how it is transmitted, that no immunity is conferred with infection, and that reacquistion of the infection is likely with repeated contact. Women need to know that their partners should be checked even if they are asymptomatic. Because HPV is highly contagious, the majority of women's partners will be infected and should be treated. All sexually active women with multiple partners or a history of HPV should be encouraged to use latex condoms for intercourse to decrease acquisition or transmission of condylomata. Condoms should be used until both partners are lesion free and up to 9 months after appearance of lesions because subclinical condylomata may be infectious.

Detailed instructions for all medications and treatments must be given to the patient. Women should be informed prior to treatment of the possibility of post-treatment pain associated with specific therapies. The importance of proper thorough treatment of concurrent vaginitis or STI should be emphasized. The link between cervical cancer and the need for close follow-up should be discussed. Semiannual or annual health examinations are recommended to assess disease reoccurrence and screening for cervical cancer. Biannual Pap smears should be done for the first 2 years after treatment and annually thereafter on women who have been treated for HPV infections (CDC, 2006b). When the cervix is treated, a Pap test should be done every 6 months until two negative Pap test results are obtained; thereafter, an annual Pap smear can be performed (CDC, 2006b). Women should understand the advisability of treatment before becoming pregnant.

Women with HPV infection may radically alter their sexual practices both from fear of transmission to and from a partner and from genital discomfort associated with treatment, which may have a negative impact on sexual relationships. Unless the partner accepts and understands the necessary precautions, it may be difficult for the woman to follow the treatment regimen. The nurse can offer to discuss feelings that the woman may have, and, when indicated, joint counseling can be suggested.

HPV Vaccine

In 2006, the FDA approved Gardasil, the first vaccine to protect against the four HPV types (6, 11, 16, and 18) that account for up to 70% of cervical cancers and 90%

EXHIBIT 24.8 COUNSELING MESSAGES FOR WOMEN WITH HUMAN PAPILLOMAVIRUS

Based on a new understanding of the life history of the human papillomavirus (HPV), the Centers for Disease Control and Prevention recommend that key counseling points be conveyed to all persons with HPV:

- HPV is a viral infection that is common in sexually active persons and is almost always transmitted through sexual activity.
- Because the incubation period is variable, sexual partners are usually infected when a woman is diagnosed, even though both partners may be asymptomatic.
- Genital warts are usually benign. The types of HPV that cause genital warts are usually not the ones associated with cervical cancer. Recurrence of genital warts within the first several months after treatment is common and usually indicates recurrence rather than reinfection.
- Likelihood of transmission and duration of infectivity after treatment is unknown. Although information on prevention is lacking, the use of latex condoms is associated with a lower rate of cervical cancer.
- Because genital HPV is very common and the duration of infectivity is not known, the value of telling future partners about a past diagnosis of HPV is unclear. At the same time, candid discussions about other STIs is encouraged.

Note. From "Sexually Transmitted Diseases Treatment Guidelines, 2006," by Centers for Disease Control and Prevention, 2006, *MMWR, 55*(RR-11), p. 58; "The CDC 2002 Guidelines for the Treatment of Sexually Transmitted Diseases: Implications for Women's Health Care, by M. Scharbo-DeHaan and D. G. Anderson, 2003, *Journal of Midwifery & Women's Health, 48*(2), pp. 96–104; *Varney's Midwifery* (4th ed.), by H. Varney, J. M. Kriebs, and C. L. Gegor, 2004, Sudbury, MA: Jones & Bartlett.

of genital warts (CDC, 2007a). The vaccine should be administered to 11- to 12-year-old girls and is approved for use in females 9 to 26 years of age. Ideally, the vaccine is administered before onset of sexual activity. It is given through a series of three shots over a 6-month period. The most common side effect is soreness at the injection site. The vaccine is not recommended for pregnant woman (CDC, 2006a). If a woman finds out she is pregnant after she has started the vaccine series, she should complete her pregnancy before finishing the series.

HEPATITIS

Hepatitis is an acute, systemic viral infection that occurs as hepatitis A (HAV); hepatitis V (HBV); non-A; non-B, which includes hepatitis C (HCV), hepatitis G (HGV or GBV-C), hepatitis E (HEV), and hepatitis D (HDV) (see Table 24.20).

Hepatitis A

Hepatitis A, caused by infection with hepatitis A virus (HAV) is the most common form of hepatitis, is highly contagious, self-limiting, and does not result in chronic illness or chronic liver disease. HAV infection is primarily acquired through a fecal-oral route by ingestion of contaminated food—particularly milk, shellfish, or polluted water—or person-to-person contact. Women

living in the western United States, Native Americans, Alaskan Natives, and children and employees in day care centers are at high risk for contracting hepatitis A. Hepatitis A, like other enteric infections, can be transmitted during sexual activity. Many sexual practices facilitate fecal-oral transmission, and unapparent fecal contamination is common with sexual intercourse (CDC, 2006b). Some studies have associated more sexual partners, frequent oral-anal contact, and insertive anal intercourse with HAV infection (CDC, 2006b).

Unlike other persons with STIs, HAV-infected persons are infectious for only a brief period of time. Hepatitis A viral infection is a mild, self-limited disease characterized by flu-like symptoms with malaise, fatigue, anorexia, nausea, pruritis, fever, and upper right quadrant pain; usually, there are no chronic sequelae to infection.

Diagnosis is not done on clinical findings alone and requires serologic testing. The presence of the IgM antibody is diagnostic of acute HAV infection. The IgM antibody is detectable 5 to 10 days after exposure and can remain positive for up to 6 months. Because HAV infection is self-limited and does not result in chronic infection or chronic liver disease, treatment is usually supportive. Women who become dehydrated from nausea and vomiting or who have fulminating hepatitis A may need to be hospitalized. Medications that might cause liver damage or that are metabolized in the liver should be used with caution. No specific diet or activity restrictions are necessary. Immune globulin (IG) or immune-

24.20 | Viral Hepatitis

TYPE	TRANSMISSION	VACCINE	COMPLICATIONS
Hepatitis A virus (HAV)[a]	Person to person (fecal-oral) Contaminated water or food Sexual practices associated with oral-anal contact	Available	Fulminant hepatits
Hepatitis B virus (HBV)[a]	Blood or body fluids Sexually During delivery	Available	Fulminant hepatitis Cirrhosis Cancer Chronic liver disease Hepatitis B carriers
Hepatitis C virus (HCV)	Via blood Transfusion-associated Sexual exposure	Not available	Chronic liver disease Cirrhosis Cancer
Hepatitis D virus (HDV)	Via blood Only in presence of active hepatitis B	Not available	Chronic liver disease Fulminant hepatitis
Hepatitis E virus (HEV)	Fecal-oral	Not available	High mortality in pregnant women

Note. From "Sexually Transmitted Diseases Treatment Guidelines 2006," by Centers for Disease Control and Prevention, 2006, *MMWR, 55*(RR-11); *Varney's Midwifery* (4th ed.), by H. Varney, J. M. Kriebs, and C. L. Gegor, 2004, Sudbury, MA: Jones & Bartlett.
[a] Women who have a laboratory-confirmed HAV or HBV diagnosis and women who have had a previous vaccination for either HAV or HBV are not candidates for concurrent vaccination. If a susceptible woman has never been vaccinated for either HAV or HBV, a combination vaccine (TWINRIX) may be given in a three-dose schedule.

specific globulin is indicated for any pregnant woman exposed to HAV to provide passive immunity through injected antibodies. Perinatal transmission of HAV has not been demonstrated. Two products are available for prevention of hepatitis A: hepatitis A vaccine and immune globulin for IM administration. Inactivated hepatitis A vaccines are available in the United States for any one over age 2. It is administered in a two-dose series and induces protective immunity in virtually all adults following the second dose. A combined hepatitis A and B vaccine is available for adults. Administered on a 0-, 1-, 6-month schedule, its effectiveness is equal to the monovalent vaccine (CDC, 2006b). All household contacts should receive IG. When administered before or within 2 weeks after exposure to HAV, IG is 85% effective in preventing hepatitis A. Persons in the following groups who are likely to be treated in STI clinics should be offered the hepatitis A vaccine: all women who have sex with men having sex with men; illegal drug users (both injecting and noninjecting drugs); and persons with chronic liver disease (CDC, 2006b).

Hepatitis B

Hepatitis B virus (HBV) is a blood-borne pathogen transmitted by exposure to infectious blood or body fluids (e.g., semen, saliva). HBV is approximately 100 times more infectious than HIV and 10 times more infectious than hepatitis C (CDC, 2003). In the United States, about 5% of the general population give evidence of a previous infection, with an estimated 120,000 new cases transmitted sexually each year (Hatcher, 2004) and an estimated 1.25 million persons chronically infected with HBV (CDC, 2006b). Chronically infected persons can transmit the infection and are at 15% to 25% increased risk for premature death from cirrhosis or hepatocellular carcinoma (CDC, 2006b). Women who are infected with HBV can transmit the virus to their neonates during delivery; the risk of chronic infection in the infant is as high as 100% (Drew, 2001). Hepatitis B infection is caused by a large DNA virus and is associated with three antigens and their antibodies (see Table 24.20). Screening for active or chronic disease or disease immunity is based on testing for these antigens and their antibodies.

Overall prevalence of HBV infection differs among racial/ethnic populations and is highest among persons who have emigrated from areas with a high endemicity of HBV infections—that is, Asia, Pacific Islands, Africa, and the Middle East (CDC, 2006b). Factors considered to place a woman at risk for HBV are those associated with STI risk in general (history of multiple sexual partners, multiple STIs, intravenous drug use), behaviors that are associated with blood contact (e.g., work or treatment in a dialysis unit, history of multiple blood transfusions, public safety workers exposed to blood in the work place, health care workers), and persons born in a country with a high incidence of HBV infection. While HBV can be transmitted via blood transfusion, the incidence of such infections has decreased significantly since testing of blood for the presence of HBsAg became possible. Women who abuse drugs and share needles are at risk, as are women with a history of jail or prison experience and/or a history of needle-stick injury, tattoos, or body piercing. Also at risk for HBV are day care workers who are exposed to body fluids and health care workers who are exposed to blood and needle sticks.

HBV infection is transmitted parentally and through intimate contact. Hepatitis B chronic infection affects 5% of the world population, with higher percentages found in tropical areas and Southeast Asia. Hepatitis B surface antigen has been found in blood, saliva, sweat, tears, vaginal secretions, and semen. Perinatal transmission does occur; however, the fetus is not at risk until it comes in contact with contaminated blood at delivery. HBV has also been transmitted by artificial insemination.

HBV infection is a disease of the liver and is asymptomatic in up to one-third of infected persons. In children and adults, the course of the infection can be fulminating and the outcome fatal. Symptoms of HBV infection are similar to those of hepatitis A: arthralgias, arthritis, lassitude, anorexia, nausea, vomiting, headache, fever, and mild abdominal pain. Later, the patient may have clay-colored stools, dark urine, increased abdominal pain, and jaundice. Between 6% and 10% of adults with HBV have persistence of HBsAg and become chronically infected. Up to 25% of chronically infected individuals will die from primary hepatocellular carcinoma or cirrhosis of the liver.

Assessment and Diagnosis

All women at high risk for contracting hepatitis B should be vaccinated. Screening only high-risk individuals may not identify up to 50% of HBsAg-positive women; therefore, current CDC (2006b) guidelines recommend screening for the presence of HBsAg in all women at their first prenatal visit and repeating screening in the third trimester of pregnancy for women with high-risk behaviors.

Components of the history to be obtained when hepatitis B is suspected include inquiry about the symptoms of the disease and risk factors outlined earlier. Women also should be asked about taste and smell peculiarities and intolerance of fatty foods and cigarettes. The nurse should ask about darkened urine and light-colored stools as well. Physical examination includes inspection of the skin for rashes, inspection of

the skin and conjunctiva for jaundice, and palpation of the liver for enlargement and tenderness. Weight loss, fever, and general debilitation should be noted. If the HBsAg is positive, further laboratory studies may be ordered: anti-HBe, anti-Hbc, Sgot, alkaline phosphatase, and liver panel. If the HBsAg is negative in early pregnancy and the woman could be in the "window phase" or if high-risk behaviors continue during pregnancy, a repeat HBsAg should be ordered in the third trimester. HIV testing should be offered if indicated or requested.

Interpretation of testing for hepatitis B is complex (see Table 24.21). Patients with acute hepatitis B generally have detectable serum HBsAg levels in the late incubation phase of the disease, 2 to 5 weeks before symptoms appear. Anti-HBs with a negative HBsAg test signals immunity. Anti-HBs with a positive antigen denotes a chronic state; during this time, the disease can be transmitted. During the recovery phase, the patient may continue to be infectious even though HBsAg can not be detected. This is called the window phase and is identified by anti-HBc in the absence of anti-Hbs. Women should be prepared for repeat testing because HBV screening tests may be used to monitor the progression of the disease.

Management

There is no specific treatment for hepatitis B. Recovery is usually spontaneous in 3 to 16 weeks. Usually pregnancies complicated by acute viral hepatitis are managed on an outpatient basis. Rest and a high-protein, low-fat diet are important. Women should be advised to increase their fluid intake and avoid medications that are metabolized in the liver, drugs, and alcohol. Women with a definite exposure to hepatitis B should be given hepatitis B immunoglobulin IM in a single dose as soon as possible within 7 days after exposure (CDC, 2006b). HB vaccine is indicated for newborns of women who

24.21	Parameters of Hepatitis B Testing
HbsAg	Hepatitis B surface antigen
HbsAb	Hepatitis B surface antibody
IgM HbcAb	Hepatitis B core antibody (IgM class-recent infection)
IgG HbcAb	Hepatitis B core antibody (IgG class-past infection)
HbeAg	Hepatitis B e antigen
HbeAB	Hepatitis B e antibody

have tested positive for HBsAg or who are high risk with unknown status to stimulate the newborn's active immunity. The vaccine should be give as soon as possible after birth up to 7 days and again at 30 and 60 days. The CDC (2006b) recommends routine vaccination of all newborns and vaccination of older children at high risk for HBV infection.

All nonimmune women at high or moderate risk of hepatitis B should be informed of the existence of the hepatitis B vaccine. Vaccination is recommended for all individuals who have had multiple sex partners within the past 6 months (CDC, 2006b). In addition, IV drug users, residents of correctional or long-term care facilities, persons seeking care for an STI, prostitutes, women whose partners are IV drug users or are bisexual, and women whose occupation exposes them to high risk should be vaccinated. Vaccination is not associated with serious side effects and does not carry a risk for contracting HIV. The vaccine is given in a series of three (some authorities recommend four) doses over a 6-month period with the first two doses given within 1 month of each other. In adults, the vaccine should be given in the deltoid muscle, never in the gluteal or quadriceps muscle. The vaccination is not contraindicated during pregnancy.

Patient education includes explaining the meaning of hepatitis B infection, including transmission, state of infectivity, and sequelae. The nurse should also explain the need for immunoprophylaxis for household members and sexual contacts of women with acute or chronic infection. To decrease transmission of the virus, women with hepatitis B or who test positive for HBV should be advised to maintain a high level of personal hygiene: wash hands after using the toilet; carefully dispose of tampons, pads, and adhesive bandages in plastic bags; do not share razor blades, toothbrushes, needles, or manicure implements; have male partner use a condom if unvaccinated and without hepatitis B; avoid sharing saliva through kissing or sharing of silverware or dishes; wipe up blood spills immediately with soap and water. Women with hepatitis B should inform all health care providers of their chronic infective status; all HBsAg-positive pregnant women should be reported to the local and state health departments to ensure that they are entered into a case management system and appropriate prophylaxis is provided for their infants. In addition, household and sexual contacts of HbsAg-positive women should be vaccinated (CDC, 2006b). Newly delivered women should be reassured that breast-feeding is not contraindicated if their infants received prophylaxis at birth and are currently on the immunization schedule.

Hepatitis C

Hepatitis C virus (HCV) infection is the most common chronic blood-borne infection in the United States; an estimated 2.7 million persons are chronically infected (CDC, 2006b). Because up to 70% of patients with HCV infection progress to chronic hepatitis, hepatitis C represents nearly 50% of chronic viral hepatitis. Most infected patients may not be aware of their disease because they are not clinically ill (CDC, 2006b). Hepatitis C is readily transmitted through exposure to blood and much less efficiently via semen, saliva, or urine. Risk factors include a history of intravenous drug use and a history of blood transmissions. Although HCV is not efficiently transmitted sexually, several studies have demonstrated that sexual activity is associated with HCV transmission, particularly with increasing numbers of sexual partners, failure to use a condom, history of STIs such as hepatitis B and HIV, heterosexual sex with a male injection drug user, and sexual activities involving trauma (Page-Shaffer et al., 2002; Terrault, 2002). No association has been documented between HCV and exposure resulting from medical, dental, or surgical procedures; tattooing; acupuncture; ear piercing; foreign travel; or military service (CDC, 2006b).

Most patients with hepatitis C are asymptomatic or have general flu-like symptoms similar to hepatitis A. Nonspecific specific symptoms such as fatigue, nausea, anorexia, and abdominal pain are seen in 20% to 39% of persons (Geller & Herman, 2006). Diagnosis of HCV infection can be made by detecting either anti-HCV or HCV RNA. Anti-HCV is recommended for routine testing of asymptomatic persons. Hepatitis C viral infection is confirmed by laboratory testing; the presence of anti-C antibody is performed with an enzyme immunoassay.

Alpha-interferon-2b, 3–15 million units IM three times a week for 6 to 18 months, is the main therapy for HCV infection. More recently combined interferon/ribavirin therapy has been used with better success than either alpha-interferon or standard interferon plus ribavirin (Cerrato, 2002). Response rates varied from 42% to 82% depending on the genotype of HCV the patient had. However, adverse effects of interferon/ribavirin cause about 10% to 14% of patients to stop treatment. Currently, there is no vaccine for use with hepatitis C. Transmission of HCV through breast-feeding has not been reported.

SEXUALLY TRANSMITTED INFECTIONS DURING PREGNANCY

Perinatal outcomes can be affected by various STIs in that pregnant women may transmit the infection to their fetus, newborn, or infant through vertical transmission (via the placenta, during vaginal birth, or after birth through breast-feeding) or horizontal transmission (close physical or household contact). Some STIs (like syphilis) cross the placenta and infect the fetus in utero. Other STIs (like gonorrhea, chlamydia, hepatitis B, and genital herpes) can be transmitted as the baby passes through the birth canal. The harmful effects of STIs may include stillbirth, low birth weight (less than 5 pounds), conjunctivitis, pneumonia, neonatal sepsis, neurologic damage (such as brain damage or lack of coordination in body movements), blindness, deafness, acute hepatitis, meningitis, chronic liver disease, and cirrhosis. Some of these problems can be prevented if the woman is screened and treated for STIs during pregnancy. Other problems can be treated if the infection is found in the newborn. A pregnant woman with an STI may have early onset of labor, premature rupture of the membranes, and uterine infection after delivery. STI treatment regimens may differ for pregnant women. Clinicians should consult the most current CDC treatment guidelines and selected chapter references for further information about STIs in pregnancy (Star, Lommel, & Shannon, 2004).

CONCLUSION

STIs are among the most common health problems of women in the United States and around the world. Women experience a disproportionate amount of the burden associated with these illnesses, including complications of infertility, perinatal infections, poor pregnancy outcomes, chronic pelvic pain, genital tract neoplasms, and potentially death. Additionally, these infections interfere with one's lifestyle and cause considerable distress, both emotional and physical. Clinicians can help to ameliorate the misery, morbidity, and mortality associated with STIs and other common infections through accurate, safe, sensitive, and supportive care. Nurses should be aware that STI knowledge is constantly increasing and changing with new and improved prevention, diagnostic, and treatment modalities being developed and reported. All clinicians have a responsibility to stay current with these developments through reviewing current journals, attending conferences, and being knowledgeable about recommendations and bulletins from the CDC. Furthermore, it is important that practitioners be aware of policies, recommendations, and guidelines of the state in which they practice, which also may change frequently.

INTERNET RESOURCES

American Social Health Association—www.ashastd.org: A nongovernmental organization that provides accurate, medically reliable information about STIs. Site information follows approved treatment guidelines as recommended by the Centers for Disease Control and Prevention. Includes a sexual health glossary and STI statistics.

The Centers for Disease Control and Prevention—www.cdc.gov: Provides many STI and HIV/AIDS resources, including current STD treatment guidelines and prevention information and educational guides.

CDC Mortality and Morbidity Weekly Report (*MMWR*)—www.cdc.gov/mmwr: Contains in-depth articles, policy statements, recommendations, and guidelines for the prevention, control, and treatment of chronic and infectious disease.

CDC National STD/AIDS Hotline—www.ashastd.org/hotlines/index.html: Provides anonymous, confidential information on STIs, prevention information, and referrals to clinics and other services.

EngenderHealth—www.engenderhealth.org: This Web site has online minicourses about STIs and HIV/AIDS.

Planned Parenthood—www.plannedparenthood.org: Provides reproductive health care and sexual health information to the public. Services include family planning counseling and birth control, gynecological care, and HIV/STI testing and counseling.

REFERENCES

American Academy of Pediatrics & American College of Obstetricians and Gynecologists. (1997). *Guidelines for perinatal care* (4th ed.). Washington, DC: Author.

American Social Health Association. (1998). *Sexually transmitted diseases in America: How many cases and at what cost?* Menlo Park, CA: Kaiser Family Foundation. Retrieved November 2006, from http://wwww.ashastd.org/pdfs/std_rep.pdf

Augenbraun, M. (2007). Syphilis. In J. D. Klausner III & Hook E. W. *Current diagnosis and treatment of sexually transmitted diseases* (pp. 119–129). New York: McGraw-Hill Medical.

Barron, M. L. (1998). *Nursing assessment of the pregnant woman: Antepartal screening and laboratory evaluation.* New York: March of Dimes Birth Defects Foundation.

Bosch, F. X., & de Sanjos, S. (2003). Human papillomavirus and cervical cancer—Burden and assessment of causality. *J Nat'l Cancer Inst Monograph, 3,* 3–13.

Brown, K. (2000). *Management guidelines for women's health nurse practitioners.* Philadelphia: F. A. Davis.

Brucker, H., & Bearman, P. (2005). After the promise: The STD consequences of adolescent virginity pledges. *Journal of Adolscent Health, 36,* 271–278.

Cagampang, H. H., Barth, R. P., Korpi, M., & Kirby, D. (1997). *Family Planning Perspectives, 29,* 271–278.

Carcio, H. (1999). *Advanced health assessment of women.* Philadelphia: Lippincott.

Cates, W. (2001, October). Treating STDs to help control HIV infection. *Contemporary OB/GYN,* 107–115.

Cates, J., Alexander, L., & Cates, W. J. (1998). Prevention of sexually transmitted diseases in an era of managed care: The relevance for women. *Women's Health Issues, 8*(3), 169–186.

Centers for Disease Control and Prevention. (1998). Primary and secondary syphilis—United States, 1997. *MMWR, 47*(24), 493–497.

Centers for Disease Control and Prevention. (2002a). *HIV/AIDS among women.* Retrieved November 2002, from http://www.cdc.gov/hiv/pubs/facts/women.htm

Centers for Disease Control and Prevention. (2002b). Screening tests to detect chlamydia trachomatis and Neisseria gonorrhoeae infections—2002. *MMWR Recommendation Report, 51*(RR-15), 1–38.

Centers for Disease Control and Prevention. (2003). Prevention and control of infection with hepatitis viruses in correctional settings. *Morbidity and Mortality Weekly Review Recommendation Report, 52*(RR1), 1–3.

Centers for Disease Control and Prevention. (2005). *HIV/AIDS surveillance report: Cases of HIV infection and AIDS in the United States, 2004. Vol. 16.* Atlanta, GA: U.S. Department of Health and Human Services. Retrieved November 30, 2007, from www.cdc.gov

Centers for Disease Control and Prevention. (2006a). *Trends in reportable sexually transmitted diseases in the United States, 2005.* Atlanta, GA: U.S. Department of Health and Human Services.

Centers for Disease Control and Prevention. (2006b). Sexually transmitted diseases treatment guidelines 2006. *MMWR, 55*(RR-11), 1–94.

Centers for Disease Control and Prevention. (2007a). *Human papillomavirus: HPV information for clinicians.* www.cdc.gov/std/hpv/hpv-clinician-brochure-htm

Centers for Disease Control and Prevention. (2007b). Update to CDC's sexually transmitted diseases treatment guidelines, 2006: Fluroroquinolones no longer recommended for treatment of gonococcal infections. *MMWR, 56*(14), 332–336.

Cerrato, P. (2002, October). New guidelines for managing hepatitis C. *Contemporary OB/GYN,* 100–103.

Chesson, H. W., Blandford, J. M., Gift, T. L., Tao, G., & Irwin, K. (2004). The estimated direct medical cost of sexually transmitted diseases among American youth, 2000. *Perspectives on Sexual and Reproductive Health, 36*(1), 11–19.

Cummings, S., & Ullman, D. (1997). *Everybody's guide to homeopathic medicines.* New York: Putman.

Cunningham, F. G., MacDonald, P. C., Gant, N. F., Leveno, K. J., Gilstrap, L. C., Hankins, G. D., & Clark, S. L. (2002). *Williams obstetrics 21st.* Stamford, CT: Appleton & Lange.

Davies, J. E. (2000). Hide and seek: Making sure HPV infection doesn't escape detection. *Advance for Nurse Practitioners, 39–40,* 42, 43–44, 49–50, 52.

Dolcini, M., Coates, T. J., Catania, J. A., Kegeles, S. M., & Hauck, W. W. (1995). Multiple sexual partners and their psychosocial correlates: The population-based AIDS in multiethnic neighborhoods (AMEN) study. *Health Psychology, 14*(2), 22–31.

Donders, G. G. C. (2000). Treatment of sexually transmitted bacterial diseases in pregnant women. *Drugs, 59*(3), 477–485.

Drew, W. L. (2001). Hepatitis. In W. R. Wilson & M. A. Sande (Eds.), *Current diagnosis and treatment in infectious diseases* (pp. 431–441). New York: Lange Medical Books/McGraw-Hill.

Drew, W. L., Blair, M., Miner, R. C., & Conant, M. (1990). Evaluation of the virus permeability of a new condom for women. *Sexually Transmitted Diseases, 17,* 110–112.

Faro, S. (2001). Chlamydia trachomatis. In S. Faro & D. E. Soper (Eds.), *Infectious diseases in women* (pp. 451–467). Philadelphia: Saunders.

Faro, S., & Soper, D. E. (2001). *Infectious diseases in women.* Philadelphia: Saunders.

Fisher, J. D., Cornman, D. H., Osborn, C. Y., Amico, R., Fisher, W. A., & Friedland, G. A. (2004). Clinician-initiated HIV risk reduction intervention for HIV-positive persons. *Journal of the Association of Nurses in AIDS Care, 37*(Suppl. 2), S78–S87.

Fogel, C. I. (1995). Sexually transmitted diseases. In N. F. Woods & C. I. Fogel (Eds.), *Women's health care* (pp. 571–609). Thousand Oaks, CA: Sage.

Fogel, C. I. (2006). Sexually transmitted infections. In K. D. Schuiling & F. K. Likis (Eds.), *Women's gynecological health* (pp. 421–469). Boston: Jones and Bartlett.

Fogel, C. I., & Lauver, D. (1990). *Sexual health promotion.* Philadelphia: Saunders.

Fogel, C. I., & Woods, N. F. (Eds.). (1995). *Women's health care.* Thousand Oaks, CA: Sage.

French, P. P., Latka, M., Gollub, E. L., Rogers, C., Hoover, D. R., & Stein, Z. A. (2003). Use-effectiveness of the female vs the male condom in preventing sexually transmitted diseases in women. *Sexually Transmitted Diseases, 30,* 433–439.

Futterman, D. (2001). Adolescents. In J. R. Anderson (Ed.), *A guide to the clinical care of women with HIV 2001 Ed.* (pp. 335–348). Rockville, MD: Womencare.

Gall, S. A. (2001). Human papillomavirus. In S. Faro & D. E. Soper (Eds.), *Infectious diseases in women* (pp. 468–484). Philadelphia: Saunders.

Geller, M. L., & Herman, J. R. (2006). Viral hepatitis. In A. L. Nelson & J. Woodward (Eds.), *Sexually transmitted disease* (pp. 71–98). Totowa, NJ: Humana Press.

Gonen, V. (1999). Confronting STDs: A challenge for managed care. *Women's Health Issues, 9*(2, Suppl. 1), 36S–46S.

Gorroll, A. H. (2001). Approach to the patient with a vaginal discharge. In A. H. Gorroll & A. G. Mulley (Eds.), *Primary care medicine: Office evaluation and management of the adult patient* (pp. 702–707). Baltimore: Williams & Wilkins.

Greenblatt, R. M., & Hessol, N. A. (2001). Epidemiology and natural history of HIV infection in women. In J. R. Anderson (Ed.), *A guide to the clinical care of women with HIV 2001 Ed.* (pp. 1–32). Rockville, MD: Womencare.

Grella, C. E., Anglin, M. D., & Annon, J. J. (1996). HIV risk behaviors among women in methadone maintenance treatment. *Substance Abuse and Misuse, 31,* 277–301.

Guest, F. (2006). Patient-clinician communication and STI care. In A. L. Nelson & J. Woodward (Eds.), *Sexually transmitted diseases* (pp. 279–294). Totowa, NJ: Humana Press.

Guttmacher Institute. (2002). *Facts in brief.* Retrieved August 2004, from http://www.guttmacher.org/

Harris, R. M., & Kavanagh, K. H. (1995). Perception of AIDS risk and high-risk behaviors among women in methadone maintenance treatment. *Substance Abuse and Misuse, 31,* 277–301.

Hatcher, R. et al. (2004). *Contraceptive technology* (18th rev. ed.). New York: Ardent Media.

Hawkins, J. W., Roberto-Nichols, D. M., & Stanley-Haney, J. L. (2008). *Protocols for nurse practitioners in gynecologic settings* (9th ed.). New York: Springer Publishing.

Henderson, D. (1997). *Transition to community for incarcerated addicted women.* 49th Annual Meeting of the American Society of Criminology, November, San Diego, CA.

Institute of Medicine. (1997). *The hidden epidemic: Confronting sexually transmitted diseases.* Washington, DC: National Academy Press.

Jacobs, R. A. (2001). Infectious diseases: Spirochetal. In L. M. Tierney, S. J. McPhee, & M. A. Papadakis (Eds.), *Current medical diagnosis and treatment, 2001* (pp. 205–227). New York: Lange Medical Books/McGraw-Hill.

Jemmott, L. S., & Brown, E. J. (2003). Reducing HIV sexual risk among African American women who use drugs: Hearing their voices. *Journal of the Association of Nurses in AIDS Care, 14*(1), 19–26.

Johnson, S. D., Cunningham-Williams, R. M., & Cottler, L. B. (2003). A tripartite of HIV-risk for African-American women: The intersection of drug use, violence, and depression. *Drug and Alcohol Dependence, 70*(2), 169–175.

Kearney, M. H. (2001). *Perinatal impact of alcohol, tobacco and other drugs* (2nd ed.). White Plains, NY: Educational Services, March of Dimes.

Klebanoff, M. A., Carey, J. C., Hauth, J. C., Hillier, S. F., Nugent, R. D., & Thom, E. A. (2001). Failure of metronidazole to prevent preterm delivery among pregnant women with asymptomatic *trichomonas vaginalis* infection. *New England Journal of Medicine, 345*(7), 487–493.

Koumans, E. H., Markowitz, L. E., & Hogan, V. (2002). Indications for therapy and treatment recommendations for bacterial vaginosis in nonpregnant and pregnant women: A synthesis of data. *Clinical Infectious Diseases, 35,* S152–S172.

Koutsky, L. A., Ault, K. A., Wheeler, C. M., Brown, D. R., Ball, E., Alvarez, F. et al. (2002). A controlled trial of a human papillomavirus type 16 vaccine. *New England Journal of Medicine, 347*(21), 1645–1651.

Kurth, A. (1998). Promoting sexual health in the age of HIV/AIDS. *Journal of Nurse-Midwifery, 43*(3), 162–181.

Livengood, C. H. (2001). Syphilis. In S. Faro & D. E. Soper (Eds.), *Infectious diseases in women* (pp. 403–429). Philadelphia: Saunders.

Lommel, L. L. (1999). Condylomata acuminate. In W. L. Star, M. T. Shannon, L. L. Lommel, & Y. M. Gutierrez (Eds.), *Ambulatory obstetrics* (3rd ed., pp. 959–965). San Francisco: UCSF Nursing Press.

MacLauren, A. (1995). Primary care for women: Comprehensive sexual health assessment. *Journal of Nurse-Midwifery, 40,* 104–119.

MacRae, R., & Aalto, E. (2000). Gendered power dynamics and HIV risk in drug-using sexual relationships. *AIDS Care, 12*(4), 505–514.

Maman, S. C. (2000). The intersections of HIV and violence: Directions for future research and interventions. *Social Science and Medicine, 50,* 459–478.

Marrazzo, J. M., & Celum, C. L. (2000). Syphilis in women. In M. B. Goldman & M. C. Hatch (Eds.), *Women and health* (pp. 302–310). San Diego, CA: Academic Press.

Mays, V. M., & Cochran, S. D. (1988, November). Issues in the perception of AIDS risk and risk reduction activities by Black and Hispanic/Latina women. *American Psychologist,* 949–957.

McCoy, H. V., McCoy, C. B., & Lai, S. (1998). Effectiveness of HIV interventions among women drug users. *Women and Health, 27*(1/2), 49–66.

McFarlane, J., Parker, B., & Cross, B. (2001). *Abuse during pregnancy: A protocol for prevention and intervention* (2nd ed.). White Plains, NY: Educational Services, March of Dimes.

Miller, S., Exner, T. M., Williams, S. P., & Ehrhardt, A. A. (2000). A gender-specific intervention for at-risk women in the USA. *AIDS Care, 13*(3), 603–612.

Mize, S. J. S., Robinson, B. E., Bockting, W. O., & Scheltma, K. E. (2002). Meta-analysis of the effectiveness of HIV prevention interventions for women. *AIDS Care, 14*(2), 163–180.

Nelson, A. L. (2006). Introduction to sexually transmitted infections. In A. L. Nelson & J. Woodward (Eds.), *Sexually transmitted diseases: A practical guide for primary care* (pp. 1–21). Totowa, NJ: Humana Press.

Nelson, A. L. (2007). Sexually transmitted diseases treatment guidelines, 2006: An update. *The Forum, 5*(1), 2–3.

Ness, R., & Brooks-Nelson, D. (2000). Pelvic inflammatory disease. In M. B. Goldman & M. C. Hatch (Eds.), *Women and health* (pp. 369–380). San Diego, CA: Academic Press.

Nyamanthi, A. M., & Lewis, C. E. (1991). Coping of African American women at risk for AIDS. *Women's Health Issues, 1*(2), 53–62.

Page-Shafer, K. A., Cahoon-Young, B., Klausner, J. D., Morrow, S., Molitor, F., Ruiz, J., et al. (2002). Hepatitis C virus infection in young low-income women: The role of sexually transmitted infections as a potential cofactor for HCV women infection. *American Journal of Public Health, 92*(4), 670–676.

Pastorek, J. G., & Yordan-Jovet, R. (2001). Hepatitis A to E. In S. Faro & D. E. Soper (Eds.), *Infectious diseases in women* (pp. 116–127). Philadelphia: Saunders.

Planned Parenthood Federation of America. (2003). Women's health: Ectopic pregnancy. Retrieved February 10, 2003, from http://www.plannedparenthood.org/womenshealth/ectopic.html

Public Health Service. (1979). *Healthy People: The Surgeon General's report on health promotion and disease prevention.* Washington, DC: U.S. Government Printing Office.

Revzina, N. V., & DiClemente, R. J. (2005). Prevalence and incidence of human papillomavirus infection in women in the USA: A systematic review. *International Journal of STD and AIDS, 16*(8), 528–537.

Roddy, R. E., Zekeng, L., Ryan, K. A., Tamoufe, U., & Tweedy, K. G. (2002). The effect of nonoxynol-9 gel on urogenital gonorrhea and chlamydia infection: A randomized controlled trial. *Journal of the American Medical Association, 287,* 1117–1122.

Schaffer, S. D. (2003). Vaginitis and sexually transmitted diseases. In E. Q. Youngkin & M. S. Davis (Eds.), *Women's health: A primary clinical guide* (3rd ed., pp. 261–290). Upper Saddle River, NJ: Pearson Prentice Hall.

Scharbo-DeHaan, M., & Anderson, D. G. (2003). The CDC 2002 guidelines for the treatment of sexually transmitted diseases: Implications for women's health care. *Journal of Midwifery & Women's Health, 48*(2), 96–104.

Schmid, G. P. (2001). Epidemiology of sexually transmitted infections. In S. Faro & D. E. Soper (Eds.), *Infectious diseases in women* (pp. 395–402). Philadelphia: Saunders.

Sexual Health Advice Center. How to use a male condom. Retrieved June 11, 2004, from http://www.addenbrookes.org.uk/serv/clin/shac/advice/contraception/types/mcondom.htm

Sexual Health Advice Center. How to use a female condom. Retrieved June 11, 2004, from http://www.addenbrookes.org.uk/serv/clin/shac/advice/contraception/types/fcondom.htm

Sinclair, C. (2004). *A midwife's handbook.* St. Louis, MO: Saunders.

Star, W. (1999). Syphilis. In W. L. Star, M. T. Shannon, L. L. Lommel, & Y. M. Gutierrez (Eds.), *Ambulatory obstetrics* (3rd ed., pp. 1031–1056). San Francisco: UCSF Nursing Press.

Star, W. (2004). Sexually transmitted diseases. In W. L. Star, L. L. Lommel, & M. T. Shannon (Eds.), *Women's primary health care* (2nd ed., pp. 13-1-3-59). San Francisco: UCSF Nursing Press.

Star, W., & Deal, M. (2004a). Gonorrhea. In W. L. Star, L. L. Lommel, & M. T. Shannon, (Eds.), *Women's primary health care* (2nd ed., pp. 13-17–13-24). San Francisco: UCSF Nursing Press.

Star, W., & Deal, M. (2004b). Syphilis. In W. L. Star, L. L. Lommel, & M. T. Shannon, (Eds.), *Women's primary health care* (2nd ed., pp. 13-50–13-59). San Francisco: UCSF Nursing Press.

Star, W. L., Lommel, L. L., & Shannon, M. T. (1995). *Women's health primary care: Protocols for practice.* Washington, DC: American Nurses Publishing.

Star, W. L., Shannon, M. T., Lommel, L. L., & Gutierrez, Y. M. (Eds.). (1999). *Ambulatory obstetrics* (3rd ed.). San Francisco: UCSF Nursing Press.

Star, W. L., Lommel, L. L., & Shannon, M. T. (2004). *Women's health primary care: Protocols for practice* (2nd ed.). San Francisco: UCSF Nursing Press.

Stevens, J., Zierlier, S., Cram, V., Dean, D., Mayer, K., & DeGroot, A. (1995). Risks for HIV infection in incarcerated women. *Journal of Women's Health, 4*(5), 569–577.

Stone, K. M., Reiff-Eldridge, R. A., White, A. D., et al. (2004). Pregnancy outcomes following systemic prenatal acyclovir: Conclusions from the International Acyclovir Pregnancy Registry, 1984–1999. *Birth Defects Research 7*(Part A), 201–207.

Stratton, P., & Alexander, N. (1997). Heterosexual spread of HIV infection. In D. Cotton & D. Watts (Eds.), *The medical management of AIDS in women* (pp. 115–124). New York: Wiley-Liss.

Substance Abuse and Mental Health Services Administration. (2005). *Substance abuse and HIV/AIDS, January 2005 fact sheet.* Retrieved September 2007 from http://hab.hrsa.gov/history/fact2005/substance_abuse_and_hivaids.htm

Suess, J. A., & Holzman, C. (2000). Vulvular and vaginal disease. In M. A. Smith & L. A. Shimp (Eds.), *20 common problems in women's health care* (pp. 323–352). New York: McGraw-Hill.

Taha, T. E., Hoover, D. R., & Dallabetta, G. A. (1998). Bacterial vaginosis and disturbances of vaginal flora: Association with increased acquisition of HIV. *AIDS, 12,* 1699–1706.

Terrault, N. A. (2002). Sexual activity as a risk factor for hepatitis C. *Hepatology, 36*(Suppl. 1), S99–S105.

Upchurch, D. M., & Kusunoki, Y. (2004). Associations between forced sex, sexual and protective practices, and sexually transmitted diseases among a national sample of adolescent girls. *Women's Health Issues, 14,* 75–94.

Varney, H., Kriebs, J. M., & Gegor, C. L. (2004). *Varney's Midwifery* (4th ed.). Sudbury, MA: Jones & Bartlett.

Wallach, J. (1996). *Interpretation of diagnostic tests.* Boston: Little, Brown.

Wang, C., & Celum, C. (2001). Prevention of HIV. In J. R. Anderson (Ed.), *A guide to the clinical care of women with HIV 2001 Ed.* (pp. 41–76). Rockville, MD: Womencare.

Wechsberg, W. M., Lam, W. K., Zule, W., & Bobashev, G. V. (2004). Reemphasizing the context of women's risk for HIV/AIDS in the United States. *Women's Health Issues, 15*(4), 154–156.

Wechsberg, W. M., Lam, W. K. K., Zule, W. A., Hall, G., Middlesteadt, R., & Edwards, J. (2003). Violence, homelessness, and HIV risk among crack-using African-American women. *Substance Use and Abuse, 38*(3–4), 669–700.

Weinstock, H., et al. (2004). Sexually transmitted diseases among American youth: Incidence and prevalence estimates, 2000. *Perspectives on Sexual and Reproductive Health, 36*(1), 6–10.

Wiley, D. J., Douglas, J., Beutener, K., Cox, T., Fife, K., Moscicki, A. B., et al. (2002). External genital warts: Diagnosis, treatment, and prevention. *Clinical Infectious Diseases, 35,* S210–S224.

Women and HIV/AIDS

Catherine Ingram Fogel
and Beth Perry Black

In the summer of 1981, the Centers for Disease Control (CDC, 1981) reported the occurrence of clusters of several rare illnesses—*Pneumocystis carinii* pneumonia (PCP), *mycobacterium avium intracellulare*, cryptosporidiosis—and tumors (Kaposi's sarcoma, non-Hodgkin's lymphoma) in homosexual and bisexual men in California and New York. This was the beginning of the acquired immune deficiency syndrome (AIDS) pandemic and represented a medical mystery that was solved with the identification of a single infectious agent destroying the immune system of infected persons: the human immunodeficiency virus (HIV). Initially, HIV infection appeared to be associated with homosexual activities, but symptoms of the syndrome were identified in a woman within 2 months of the earliest reports of the disease in men. It soon became clear that heterosexual activity and direct blood contact could also transmit the virus. The first female AIDS case was reported to the CDC in July 1982, and, within the first year of the epidemic, women partners of infected hemophiliacs, female IV drug abusers, and women partners in heterosexual relationships were diagnosed with AIDS. Early misunderstanding of the nature of transmission of HIV led researchers and the medical community to grossly underestimate the numbers of women who were or would become infected with HIV. By 1997, 100,000 AIDS cases in women in the United States had been documented (Stine, 2008). Since the early years of the epidemic, HIV infection and AIDS have spread rapidly throughout the world, affecting millions of persons and resulting in millions of deaths.

Deeply ingrained social and cultural forces that tend to devalue women, and particularly poor women of color, perpetuated the tendency for HIV and AIDS to be underdiagnosed in women, resulting in the delay of treatment. Human immunodeficiency viral infection was long considered to be a men's disease and, more specifically, a disease of homosexual men. The rapid spread of HIV among women, however, is indisputable, with current estimates indicating that almost 18 million women worldwide are living with HIV/AIDS (Bradley-Springer, 2008). In 2006, the CDC estimated that one-fourth of women infected with HIV were unaware of their infection (CDC, 2006a).

At the beginning of the pandemic, researchers and scientists sought to identify the mechanism of infection and to seek a cure. In the ensuing two decades, scientists have identified the means of infection, although a cure remains elusive. However, in contrast to the early days of the epidemic, when HIV infection typically meant premature death from AIDS-related complications, a diagnosis of HIV infection now means a less-certain trajectory toward AIDS and death. With improved antiviral therapy, HIV infection in most persons has evolved into a treatable chronic infection (Jacobson & Hicks, 2000).

In the course of their practice, most advanced practice nurses will likely have occasion to provide care for women infected with HIV. While AIDS is a long-term sequela of unchecked viral replication and immune system damage with its attendant infections, the more salient effect of the HIV epidemic on advanced nursing practice is the management of patients chronically infected with this virus, not those who have developed AIDS. For many women, HIV is treated as a chronic condition, and it may never progress to AIDS (Varney, Kriebs, & Gegor, 2004). Therefore, this chapter will address the issues more closely associated with management of HIV infection rather than AIDS.

Untreated HIV disease progresses relentlessly. In untreated patients, the time between HIV infection and the development of AIDS ranges from a few months to 17 years, with the median interval without treatment being 10 years (CDC, 2006a). The rate of disease progression in an individual is determined by interactions between the host (the infected person), the virus, and the environment (Cohen, 1999). The clinical goal is to minimize viral replication by determining the particular combination of antiretroviral therapies, health-related behaviors, and psychosocial support needed to sustain a woman's health and limit the number of acute illness episodes related to HIV.

EPIDEMIOLOGY OF HIV

The numbers of persons infected with HIV has increased rapidly since the virus was first identified over 20 years ago. In 2006, the CDC estimated that more than one million individuals were living with HIV in the United States (CDC, 2006a). Early in the epidemic, HIV infection and AIDS were diagnosed in relatively few women, although current knowledge suggests that many women were infected but were not diagnosed (CDC, 2007a). The growing number of women living with HIV/AIDS is a dominant feature of the AIDS epidemic today, with women accounting for more than one-quarter of all new HIV/AIDS diagnoses (CDC, 2007a). In 1985, women represented 8% of AIDS diagnoses; by 2005, they accounted for 27% (CDC, 2007a). HIV infection is the fifth leading cause of death among all women aged 35 to 44 years and the sixth leading cause of death among all women aged 25 to 34 years (CDC, 2007).

Women of color, particularly African American women, are disproportionately affected by HIV/AIDS. Although African American and Hispanic women represent less than one-quarter of all women in the United States, almost 80% of women with AIDS in the United States are African American or Hispanic (CDC, 2007b). HIV infection is the leading cause of death for African American women aged 25 to 34 years; it is the sixth leading cause for women overall in this age group. Further, HIV infection is the third leading cause of death for African American women aged 35 to 44 years and the fourth leading cause of death for Hispanic women aged 35 to 44 (CDC, 2007).

Initially, most HIV/AIDS cases in women were located in large cities in the Northeast. However, by 2001, the South accounted for the largest percentage of cases reported in women (46%), followed by the Northeast (36%), West (8%), Midwest (6%), and Puerto Rico and U.S. territories (4%) (Stine, 2008).

Women are more likely to be diagnosed at younger ages than men, with the majority (77%) of women with AIDS diagnosed between the ages of 25 and 44, indicating that many were infected at a young age. In 2004, adolescent girls represented 43% of AIDS cases reported among those aged 13 to 19, and young women aged 20 to 24 represented 33% of cases in their age group (Kaiser Family Foundation, 2006).

The CDC recommends that each state and U.S. territory conduct HIV case surveillance in addition to ongoing AIDS case surveillance (CDC, 1999a). Early in the epidemic, AIDS surveillance data were adequate to allow public health officials to understand and evaluate the impact of the illness and to make programmatic decisions regarding prevention efforts. However, the widespread use of effective antiretroviral therapy has diminished the numbers of AIDS cases, even while the numbers of persons infected with HIV have increased. Therefore, it has become necessary for the CDC to recommend expanded HIV case surveillance to monitor the epidemic and shape policy, prevention, and care services in response to surveillance data.

This is particularly important for women with HIV, because women tend to be under-represented in AIDS surveillance data, as do ethnic minorities. HIV case surveillance is likely to reflect the epidemic in women earlier than AIDS data, which may be reported late in the disease after treatment failure or the onset of serious immunocompromise and health sequelae. The CDC has recommended HIV case surveillance rather than AIDS prevalence reports alone as it can provide a more realistic, useful estimate of the resources needed for patient care and services (CDC, 1999a).

NATURAL HISTORY AND HIV DISEASE PROGRESSION

The human immune system functions to protect the body from invasion by a variety of types of microbes and tumor cells. The immune system is comprised of two arms: humoral immunity, which is involved with antibody production, and cellular immunity, which is effected largely through cytotoxic T-cells. Central components of the cellular arm of the immune system are macrophages and CD4 + T-cells.

HIV is a retrovirus that specifically targets CD4 + T-cells, binding to the cell surface protein known as the CD4 + receptor. The virus affects the cells two ways: first, the absolute numbers of these cells are depleted; second, the function of the remaining cells is impaired, resulting in a gradual loss of immune function. Progressive depletion of CD4 cells in peripheral blood is the hallmark of advancing HIV disease (Hessol, Ganhdi, & Greenblatt, 2005). Unimpeded, HIV can destroy up to one billion CD4 cells per day. In addition to its aggressive destruction, HIV is genetically highly variable, mutating with apparent ease.

Untreated HIV infection is a chronic illness that progresses relentlessly through several characteristic clinical stages. AIDS, the endpoint of HIV infection, results from severe immunologic damage, loss of effective immune response to specific opportunistic pathogens, and tumors. AIDS is diagnosed when one of these specific infections or cancers occurs or when CD4 cell levels are less than 200/mm³.

HIV STAGING AND PROGRESSION

HIV infection causes a wide range of symptoms and clinical conditions reflecting the level of immunologic injury and other predisposing factors. Certain conditions tend to occur at the same time and at specific CD4 cell counts. Staging systems for HIV disease facilitate clinical evaluation and therapeutic intervention, help to determine individual level of infirmary, and information with which to make diagnoses (Hessol et al., 2005). The most widely used system for classifying HIV infection and AIDS in adults and adolescents in industrialized countries was developed by the Centers for Disease Control and Prevention. When a patient has been diagnosed with HIV, clinicians need two important pieces

of data in planning appropriate therapies and in estimating the patient's prognosis: (1) how far the disease has progressed already and (2) how fast the disease is progressing. The CD4+ count provides a clue as to how far the disease has progressed, while the viral load provides a clue as to the rate of progression. Clinically, these data are more relevant to direct appropriate care than are strict categories of illness in which individuals may or may not receive the best care tailored to their own particular state of illness or relative health. However, stages of HIV disease described in general terms are clinically relevant (see Table 25.1).

Initially, women appeared to have a more rapid progression of illness than men and to present with different opportunistic infections. However, current data suggest that the incidence and distribution of HIV-related illnesses are similar in men and women with the exception of Kaposi's sarcoma, which is seen more often in men, and the gynecologic manifestations of HIV. In general, predictors of the rate of HIV disease progression and survival among women are the same as those in men. CD4 cell count depletion and higher HIV RNA level are strong predictors of a woman's

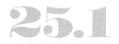 | Stages of HIV

Primary infection	Virus establishes itself in the body; acute HIV syndrome (viral flu-like syndrome) occurs within 2 to 4 weeks of exposure to HIV. Characterized by malaise, lymphadenopathy, fever, chills, fatigue, night sweats, rashes, and other symptoms common in benign viral syndromes. May last for several weeks. May become transiently immunocompromised. Takes 6 to 12 weeks for immune system to produce antibodies. Newly infected individual's blood may not test positive; however, individual may be highly contagious.
Seroconversion	Body begins to produce antibodies to the virus. Occurs 3 to 6 months after infection.
Early to middle-stage infection	Viral load stabilizes. Period of clinical latency with few or no symptoms; however, viral replication in lymphoid tissues continues. The individual is relatively symptom free but may have transient episodes of HIV-related infections. Women may be prone to aggressive cervical dysplasia.
Chronic HIV infection	Relatively mild symptoms not specific to HIV infection, including lymphadenopathy persisting for more than 3 months, fatigue, weight loss, frequent fevers and sweats, persistent and frequent yeast infections (oral and vaginal), persistent skin rashes or flaky skin, pelvic inflammatory disease unresponsive to treatment, short-term memory loss, frequent and severe herpes infection with oral, genital, or anal sores and/or shingles.
Advanced disease	CD4+ count < 200. Patient shows evidence of AIDS-defining illness, such as *pneumocystis carinii* pneumonia. Can respond to aggressive antiretroviral therapy.
Late-stage infection	CD4+ count < 50. Patient is severely ill with extensive organ involvement, aggressive neoplasia (Kaposi's sarcoma), wasting syndromes, severe disseminated infections such as M. tuberculosis, and extra pulmonary histoplasmosis. Death occurs with vascular collapse and organ failure.
Long-term nonprogress	HIV disease does not progress, although the person is infected. May have a genetic predisposition to holding the virus at bay, or may be infected with a less virulent strain.

Note. From Beal, J., & Orrick, J. J. (2006b). *HIV/AIDS primary care guide.* Norwalk, CT: Crown House.

progression and survival. However, recent reports have described sex-based differences in HIV RNA level and in the rate of CD4 depletion, with women having HIV RNA levels 30% to 50% lower than men with comparable CD4 cell counts (Hessol et al., 2005).

TRANSMISSION

Virtually all cases of HIV are transmitted by three primary routes: sexual, parental (blood-borne), and perinatal. Rates of transmission from the infected host to the uninfected recipient vary by mode of transmission and specific circumstances of transmission (Hessol et al., 2005). Because HIV is a relatively large virus, has a short half-life in vitro, and only lives within primates, it is not transmitted through casual contact (i.e., hugging or shaking hands) or surface contact (i.e., toilet seat) or from insect bites. Myths and misconceptions about HIV transmission are found in Table 25.2.

Modes of Transmission

Sexual Activity

The most common mode of transmission involves depositing HIV on mucosal surfaces, especially genital mucosa (Nadler, 2006). Sexual transmission of HIV occurs through male-to-female, female-to male, male-to-male, and female-to-female sexual contact. Receptive anal and vaginal intercourse appears to have the greatest risk of infection; however, insertive anal or vaginal intercourse also is associated with HIV infection. The majority (72%) of HIV infections in women occur through unprotected heterosexual intercourse (National Institute of Allergy and Infectious Diseases, 2006). A much smaller percentage of HIV-infected women report having had sex with women; however, most of these had other risk factors, including injection drug use and sex with men who were infected or who had risk factors for infection (CDC, 2006b). In addition, a few cases of female-to-female HIV transmission have been reported, primarily through acts that may result in vaginal trauma such as sharing sex toys without condoms or digital play with fingers with cuts or sharp nails (Decarlo & Gomez, 1997; Kwakwa & Ghobrial, 2003; Marrazzo, 2007). Assuming that a woman is of very low risk for HIV because she has an expressed sexual preference for women overlooks the fact that many lesbians have a history of sexual intercourse with men or may have other risk factors for HIV infection (Fogel & Black, 2008).

Parental

HIV can reach a person's infectable cells via infected blood or blood products, most commonly through injection drug use and other activities during which HIV is transmitted by skin-piercing instruments such as needles used for injecting drugs, razor blades, or tattoo

| | Myths About HIV Transmission |

MYTH	FACT
HIV is transmitted through casual contact.	HIV is not transmitted through everyday, casual contact, including shaking hands, sharing eating utensils, even when living in close contact.
HIV is transmitted through insect bites.	There is no evidence of HIV transmission through bloodsucking or biting insects, including mosquitoes, flies, ticks, and fleas.
Donating or receiving blood is risky in the United States.	There are numerous safeguards to the U.S. blood supply, including only allowing persons with clean bill of health to donate, drawing blood with sterilized needles, and performing nine screening tests on all donated blood that ensure a safe blood supply.
Pets and other animals can carry HIV and transmit the virus to people.	Humans are the only animal that can harbor HIV. Some animals do carry similar viruses that can cause immune disease in their species; however, these can't be transmitted to humans.
HIV can be transmitted through tears, sweat, and saliva.	Saliva, sweat, tears, and urine either carry no HIV or contain quantities too small to result in infection.

Note. From *The Complete HIV/AIDS Teaching Kit,* by J. J. Card, A. Amarillas, A. Conner, D. D. Akers, J. Solomon, and R. J. DiClemente, 2007, New York: Springer Publishing.

needles. In 2005, approximately 26% of cases of HIV/AIDS in women occurred through injection drug use (CDC, 2007b).

HIV also can be transmitted from person to person through transfusion of blood or blood products; however, strict standards regarding testing of blood and blood products prior to administration have reduced the risk of exposure to HIV through this route. Once the presence of HIV was recognized in the blood supply in the early 1980s, very strict standards for donors regarding behavioral risk factors were set, and testing of donor blood was initiated. Since the institution of these standards, the risk of exposure to HIV through blood and blood product administration is negligible.

Vertical

Perinatal transmission of HIV can occur in utero, during labor and delivery, or postpartum through breast-feeding. Transmission rates vary by maternal stage of disease, use of antiretroviral therapy, duration of ruptured membranes, and breast-feeding (Hessol et al., 2005).

Occupational

Occupational transmission of HIV to nurses and other health care providers is extremely rare. Direct inoculation of HIV via needle-stick injury imposes a risk of infection of 0.3% (3 in 1,000) to the health care worker (CDC, 1998). Casual contact with patients, even those known to be HIV positive, has not been determined to increase one's risk of acquiring HIV. Nurses can care for patients who are HIV positive with the knowledge that their risk of contracting HIV is limited to those contacts identified as being sources of transmission. Nurses need not be afraid to touch HIV-positive patients in the course of providing routine care. The use of standard precautions in caring for all patients minimizes the risk of exposure and infection by HIV and other serious illnesses (see Table 25.3).

Factors Facilitating Transmission

Transmission of HIV infection can be influenced by several factors, including characteristics of the infected

25.3 | Standard Precautions

Standard precautions synthesize the major features of blood and body fluid precautions (designed to reduce the risk of transmission of blood-borne pathogens) and body substance isolation (BSI) (designed to reduce the risk of transmission of pathogens from moist body substances) and applies them to all patients receiving care in hospitals, regardless of their diagnosis or presumed infection status. Standard precautions apply to (1) blood; (2) all body fluids, secretions, and excretions except sweat, regardless of whether they contain visible blood; (3) nonintact skin; and (4) mucous membranes. Standard precautions are designed to reduce the risk of transmission of microorganisms from both recognized and unrecognized sources of infection in hospitals. Use standard precautions, or the equivalent, for the care of all patients.

Handwashing	1. Wash hands after touching blood, body fluids, secretions, excretions, and contaminated items, even if gloves are worn. Wash hands immediately after gloves are removed, between patient contacts, and when otherwise indicated to avoid transfer of microorganisms to other patients or environments. It may be necessary to wash hands between tasks and procedures on the same patient to prevent cross-contamination of different body sites. 2. Use a plain (nonantimicrobial) soap for routine handwashing. 3. Use an antimicrobial agent or a waterless antiseptic agent for specific circumstances (e.g., control of outbreaks or hyperendemic infections), as defined by the infection control program.
Gloves	Wear gloves (clean, nonsterile gloves are adequate) when touching blood, body fluids, secretions, excretions, and contaminated items. Put on clean gloves just before touching mucous membranes and nonintact skin. Change gloves between tasks and procedures on the same patient after contact with material that may contain a high concentration of microorganisms. Remove gloves promptly after use, before touching noncontaminated items and environmental surfaces, and before going to another patient, and wash hands immediately to avoid transfer of microorganisms to other patients or environments.
Mask, eye protection, face shield	Wear a mask and eye protection or a face shield to protect mucous membranes of the eyes, nose, and mouth during procedures and patient-care activities that are likely to generate splashes or sprays of blood, body fluids, secretions, and excretions.

(continued)

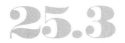 | Standard Precautions (*continued*)

Gown	Wear a gown (a clean, nonsterile gown is adequate) to protect skin and to prevent soiling of clothing during procedures and patient-care activities that are likely to generate splashes or sprays of blood, body fluids, secretions, or excretions. Select a gown that is appropriate for the activity and amount of fluid likely to be encountered. Remove a soiled gown as promptly as possible, and wash hands to avoid transfer of microorganisms to other patients or environments.
Patient-care equipment	Handle used patient-care equipment soiled with blood, body fluids, secretions, and excretions in a manner that prevents skin and mucous membrane exposures, contamination of clothing, and transfer of microorganisms to other patients and environments. Ensure that reusable equipment is not used for the care of another patient until it has been cleaned and reprocessed appropriately. Ensure that single-use items are discarded properly.
Environmental control	Ensure that the hospital has adequate procedures for the routine care, cleaning, and disinfection of environmental surfaces, beds, bedrails, bedside equipment, and other frequently touched surfaces, and ensure that these procedures are being followed.
Linen	Handle, transport, and process used linen soiled with blood, body fluids, secretions, and excretions in a manner that prevents skin and mucous membrane exposures and contamination of clothing and that avoids transfer of microorganisms to other patients and environments.
Occupational health and blood-borne pathogens	1. Take care to prevent injuries when using needles, scalpels, and other sharp instruments or devices; when handling sharp instruments after procedures; when cleaning used instruments; and when disposing of used needles. Never recap used needles or otherwise manipulate them using both hands or use any other technique that involves directing the point of a needle toward any part of the body; rather, use either a one-handed "scoop" technique or a mechanical device designed for holding the needle sheath. Do not remove used needles from disposable syringes by hand, and do not bend, break, or otherwise manipulate used needles by hand. Place used disposable syringes and needles, scalpel blades, and other sharp items in appropriate puncture-resistant containers, which are located as close as practical to the area in which the items were used, and place reusable syringes and needles in a puncture-resistant container for transport to the reprocessing area. 2. Use mouthpieces, resuscitation bags, or other ventilation devices as an alternative to mouth-to-mouth resuscitation methods in areas where the need for resuscitation is predictable.
Patient placement	Place a patient who contaminates the environment or who does not (or cannot be expected to) assist in maintaining appropriate hygiene or environmental control in a private room. If a private room is not available, consult with infection control professionals regarding patient placement or other alternatives.

Note. From Centers for Disease Control and Prevention. (2005). *Universal precautions for the prevention of transmission of HIV and other blood borne infections.* Retrieved November 2007, from www.cdc.gov/ncidod/dhap/bp-universal_precautions.html

host and the recipient, as well as the amount and infectivity of the virus itself.

Infectivity of the Host

There is an association between the amount of virus transmitted and the risk of HIV infection. Transmission is more likely to occur when viral replication is high during the initial stage of infection and in the advanced stages of HIV disease. Individuals with high blood viral loads are more likely to transmit HIV to their sexual partners, persons with whom they share drug paraphernalia, and their offspring. Further, viral load has been found to be the chief predictor of heterosexual transmission risk of HIV-1 (Quinn et al., 2000). Factors that decrease viral load, such as antiretroviral therapy, may decease but not eliminate the risk of HIV transmission. Factors that increase the risk of exposure to blood, such as genital ulcer disease, sexual trauma, and menstruation of an HIV-infected woman during sexual contact, may increase transmission risk (Card et al., 2007; Hessol et al., 2005).

Factors that decrease viral load, including antiretroviral therapy, may decrease but not eliminate the risk of transmission. Persons receiving antiretroviral therapy have shown reduced HIV transmission rates to sexual partners, with studies demonstrating reduced HIV concentration in semen and vaginal secretion (Hessol et al., 2005).

Vasectomy in men does not significantly affect HIV concentration in seminal secretion (Rieg, 2006). Although circumcised men have a lower risk of acquiring HIV than do those who are uncircumcised (Rieg, 2006), circumcision does not appear to decrease risk of transmission to a woman and may increase the risk if sexual activity is resumed before the circumcision wound is completely healed.

Susceptibility of Woman

Women are biologically more vulnerable to HIV infection than men for several reasons. Sexual transmission of HIV is two to four times more efficient from male to female than from female to male (Bradley-Springer, 2008) because HIV in semen is in higher concentrations than in cervical and vaginal infections and because the vaginal area has a much larger mucosal area of exposure to HIV than does the penis. Certain characteristics of an uninfected woman may increase her likelihood of infection. Age and female anatomy are directly related to HIV transmission risk. Younger women have increased exposure of vaginalcervical columnar epithelium, known to be a risk factor in the transmission of other sexually transmitted diseases. Pregnant women also have an increased exposure of columnar epithelium. This tissue is associated with endocervical inflammatory cells and can bleed more easily during intercourse. Normal vaginal flora may confer nonspecific immunity, and recent data suggest that women with bacterial vaginosis are at increased risk for HIV seroconversion (Wang & Celum, 2001). Both younger and postmenopausal women may be at greater risk for acquiring HIV because of a thinner vaginal epithelium, resulting in increased friability and risk of trauma during intercourse, thus providing direct access to the bloodstream (Kurth, 1998; Stratton & Alexander, 1997).

The integrity of the tissues of the female lower genital tract also influences HIV transmission risk. Trauma during intercourse, STI-related inflammation or cervicitis, cervical dysplasia, and an STI ulcer or chancre increase susceptibility to HIV infection. Any activity or condition that disrupts the tissues of the vagina may predispose a woman to infection with HIV. This includes the use of highly absorbent tampons, which are associated with vaginal desquamation with long-term use. Further, higher rates of HIV transmission should be expected in sexual assault cases when trauma to the genital area occurs. Cases of domestic violence and sexual abuse also have been identified as important correlates of HIV in women (Lichtenstein, 2004).

Sexual activity during menstruation may increase a woman's risk of acquiring HIV (Hessol et al., 2005).

Similarly, the disruption of tissues through receptive penile-anal intercourse provides a highly efficient means of HIV transmission (Stratton & Alexander, 1997).

Some contraceptive methods (i.e., barrier methods) may decrease HIV transmission; however, others may afford no protection or increase the risk of transmission. The effect of hormonal contraception on viral shedding is unclear, and these agents may interact with antibiotics and antiretrovirals (Cotter, Potter, & Tessler, 2006). While some research findings suggest that oral contraceptive use increases the risk of cervical ectopy and thus the risk of infection, others do not find this to be the case after adjusting for behavioral risk factors (Cotter, Potter, & Tessler, 2006; Hessol et al., 2005). Use of the vaginal and rectal microbicide, nonxynol-9 provides no protection against HIV acquisition and may even increase susceptibility to infection due to mucosal barrier disruption, particularly with frequent use (Hatcher et al., 2004).

Frequent douching, which can destroy the protective lactobacilli of the vagina, may increase a woman's susceptibility to bacterial vaginosis, STIs (gonorrhea, chlamydia, trichomonias), and HIV-1 (Clark, Theall, Amdee, & Kissinger, 2007). Douching also may dry out the vagina, traumatize vaginal mucosa, and make it more susceptible to tears. In addition, douching after sexual intercourse can push infectious agents further into the genital system, increasing the likelihood of infection.

RISK FACTORS FOR HIV

Unlike many viruses that are easily transmitted through the air, water, food, and/or casual contact, HIV transmission usually requires risky behaviors. Common risky behaviors in women include vaginal, anal, and oral sex without a condom or vaginal barrier, concurrent partners, numerous lifetime partners, substance use or abuse, and a history of intimate partner violence. However, these behaviors do not occur in a vacuum, and biological, behavioral, psychological, demographic, and sociocultural factors all affect the likelihood and consequences of these behaviors (Card et al., 2007).

Cultural and religious attitudes and beliefs also affect health care services. The loss of support for safer sex education programs in favor of an abstinence-only model does not protect adolescents (Cagampang, Barth, Korpi, & Kirby, 1997). Teens who pledge to remain a virgin until marriage have the same, if not higher, rates of STIs than those who do not commit to abstinence (Brucker & Bearman, 2005). In response to these findings, a more pragmatic abstinence-plus or "ABC" message based on harm-reduction principles has been instituted. The message is **A**bstinence, **B**e faithful for married couples or those in committed relationships, and use a Condom for individuals who are or put themselves at risk for HIV infection. Reflecting a shift from prevention toward treatment, no more than 20% of funding can be spent for HIV prevention programs (Nelson, 2006); further, prevention funds may be appropriated to organizations that are not required to participate in prevention or treatment programs due to religious or moral objections—such as condoms.

Biological Factors

Heterosexual transmission of HIV is 12 times more likely from men to women (Paladian, Shiboski, & Jewell, 1990). A number of biological factors make HIV transmission easier or more difficult. These include the presence of sexually transmitted infections, tissue/membrane vulnerability, viral load, and anatomical characteristics (see section on Transmission above).

Demographic Characteristics

Demographic factors such as gender, ethnicity, and age shape HIV risk behaviors and influence social networks, making it more or less likely that an individual who engages in risky behaviors will associate with persons who are HIV positive.

A person's biological sex (i.e., female, male) as well as the social roles associated with biological sex (gender) influence other risk factors for HIV/AIDS. For example, women are more likely to acquire HIV through heterosexual sexual activity than men because of their anatomy. Similar rates of exposure through heterosexual contact are seen in White (65%), Black (74%), and Hispanic (69%) women (CDC, 2007b). The number of persons with heterosexually acquired HIV has significantly increased throughout the epidemic; during 1999 to 2004, 64% of heterosexually acquired HIV infections were in women (Espinoza et al., 2007). HIV can be transmitted through receptive oral sex with ejaculation. Any condition that interrupts the integrity of oral tissues, including periodontal disease, increases the risk of HIV transmission in this manner.

In the United States, the majority of new AIDS cases, persons living with AIDS, and the majority of AIDS deaths are found among racial and ethnic minorities. About 80% of AIDS cases in women are found in Latinas and African Americans (CDC, 2004b), and heterosexual transmission is the leading route for both groups. Further, HIV-infected African Americans and Latinas are more likely than infected Whites to be uninsured, have less access to antiretroviral drugs, and lack access to health care (Card et al., 2007). Closely connected to ethnicity and race is socioeconomic status—one of the most powerful predictors of health and illness. Persons with a lower socioeconomic status are more likely to contract and transmit HIV (Card et al., 2007).

Ethnicity may also be associated with certain contextual factors. Specific factors for African American women include the gender-ratio imbalance and historical and personal victimization.

Social Factors

Societal factors such as poverty, lack of education, social inequity, and inadequate access to health care indirectly increase the prevalence of HIV in at-risk populations. Persons with the highest rates of HIV are often those with the poorest access to health care, and health insurance coverage influences if and where a woman has access to care and whether she can afford antiretroviral medications. Further, even if a poor woman perceives herself to be at risk for contracting HIV, she may not be able to practice protective behaviors if survival is an overarching concern or if there are other risks that appear to be more threatening or imminent (Mays & Cochran, 1988). Survival concerns such as secure shelter, food, safety for self and children, and money may override any concerns about protecting a woman's own health (Card et al., 2007).

Psychological Factors

Recognition of Risk

Beliefs and misconceptions about personal risk can increase an individual's risk for HIV infection. A woman who believes she has no risk factors for contacting a sexually transmitted infection—including HIV—is unlikely to practice any risk-reducing behaviors. In addition, persons who believe they are not at risk for HIV infection are more apt to have risky behaviors. Younger women may be at higher risk because they have less knowledge of reproductive health, less skill in communicating and negotiating with their partners about risk reduction practices, and more barriers to access to health care services. Taking risks is a universal human element. In the throes of passion, people can make unwise sexual decisions. Further, safer sex is not always perceived to be the most enjoyable sex.

Personality Characteristics

Personality characteristics such as low self-esteem, feelings of low self-efficacy, impulsivity, narcissism, tendency to take risks, and tendency to seek out new sensations are related to sexual risk behaviors (Kalichman, 1998). Further, women with a sense of low self-efficacy and lack of self-confidence may be unable to negotiate safer sex practices (Jemmott & Brown, 2003; Jemmott, Jemmott, & O'Leary, 2007; Upchurch & Kusunoki, 2004). Coping strategies such as high-risk sexual behaviors or drug and alcohol use to relieve or escape stress can increase personal risk for HIV infection.

Social Interactions and Relationships

HIV is among the only illnesses whose spread is directly caused by the human urge to share sexual intimacy and reproduce. Because intimate human contact is a common vehicle of HIV transmission, sexual behavior in the context of relationships is a critical risk factor for preventing and acquiring HIV. Cultural and religious attitudes regarding appropriate sexual behaviors affect risk at the individual and community levels. Relationships and sexual behavior are regulated by cultural norms that influence sexual expression in interpersonal relationships. Often women are still socialized to please their partners and to place men's needs and desires first; thus, they may find it difficult to insist on safer sex behaviors. Traditional cultural values associated with passivity and subordination may diminish the ability of many women to adequately protect themselves.

Power imbalances in relationships are the product of and contributors to the maintenance of traditional gender roles that identify men as the initiators of and decision makers about sexual activities and women as passive gatekeepers (Miller, Exner, Williams, & Ehrhardt, 2000). As long as traditional gender norms define the roles for sexual relationships as men having the dominant role in sexual decision making, negotiating condom use by women will remain difficult. Additionally, cultural norms define talking about condoms as implying a lack of trust that runs counter to the traditional gender norm expectations for women (Maman, 2000). Women sometimes do not request condom use due to a need to establish and maintain intimacy with partners. Research has demonstrated that women at risk for HIV place significant importance on and investment in their heterosexual relationships and that these dynamics impact on the women's risk taking and risk management. Urging women to insist on condom use may be unrealistic, because traditional gender roles do not encourage women to talk about sex, initiate sexual practices, or control intimate encounters.

A woman who is dependent upon an abusive male partner or a partner who places her at risk by his own risky behaviors is at higher risk for contracting HIV than are women who are not dependent (Fisher et al., 2004; Kurth, 1998). The risk of acquiring HIV infection is high among women who are physically and sexually abused. Past and current experiences with violence—particularly sexual abuse—erode women's sense of self-efficacy to exercise control over sexual behaviors, engender feelings of anxiety and depression, and increase the likelihood of risky sexual behaviors (Maman, 2000). Additionally, fear of physical harm and loss of economic support hamper women's efforts to enact protective practices. Further, past and current abuse is strongly associated with substance abuse, which also increases the risk of contracting an STI.

The risk of acquiring an STI is determined not only by the woman's actions but by her partner's as well. Although prevention counseling customarily includes recommending that women identify the partner who is at high risk because of drugs and medical factors and also determine his sexual practices, this advice may be unrealistic and/or culturally inappropriate in many relationships. Women who engage in sexual activities with other women only may or may not be at risk for infection. Many women who identify themselves as lesbian have had intercourse with a man at one time by choice, by force, or by necessity or may have used drugs and shared drug paraphernalia such as needles.

Behavioral Risks

Any behavior that increases a woman's contact with bodily fluids of another person increases the likelihood of HIV transmission.

Unsafe Sexual Activity

During sexual activity, infected blood, semen, vaginal fluids, and anal fluids can enter the uninfected woman's body through cuts, tears, and lesions on the penis or labia and in or on the vagina or anus. Cuts and tears are more likely to occur during forced or rough sex, anal sex, dry sex, or when women are very young and their cervixes are not fully developed and thus more likely to rip or tear during sex (Card et al., 2007).

Substance Use

Drug and alcohol use is associated with increased risk of HIV (Wechsberg, Lam, Zule, & Bobshev, 2004). Sharing unclean drug paraphernalia—particularly needles and syringes—increases the risk of HIV transmission, particularly in areas where there is a high incidence of HIV infection among drug users. For example, in many areas, crack use parallels trends of HIV infection. Among several possible reasons for this association are social factors such as poverty and lack of educational and economic opportunities and individual factors such as risk taking and low self-efficacy. In addition to the risk from needle sharing, use of drugs and alcohol may contribute to the risk of HIV infection by undermining cognitive and social skills, thus making it more difficult to engage in HIV-protective actions (Harris & Kavanaugh, 1995). Further, depression and other psychological problems and/or a history of sexual abuse are associated with substance abuse and thus contribute to risky behaviors. Being high and thus not able to clean drug paraphernalia can be a pervasive barrier to protective practice. Further, drug use may take place in settings where persons participate in sexual activities while using drugs. Cocaine abusers have demonstrated higher levels of sexual risk behaviors than other addict populations (McCoy, McCoy, & Lai, 1998). Finally, women who use drugs may be at higher risk because of the practice of exchanging sex for drugs or money and high numbers of sexual partners and encounters (Wechsberg et al., 2003).

Past and current physical, emotional, and sexual abuse characterizes the lives of many, if not most, drug-using women (Kearney, 2001). For women who have experienced violence, the use of alcohol and drugs can become a coping mechanism by which they self-medicate to relieve feelings of anxiety, depression, guilt, fear, and anger stemming from the violence (Grella, Anglin, & Annon, 1996). Women's drug use is strongly linked to relationship inequities and some men's ability to mandate women's sexual behavior. Sexual degradation of women is described as an intimate part of crack cocaine use (Henderson, 1997).

PREVENTION

Primary prevention or preventing the transmission of HIV is the most effective way of reducing the adverse consequences of HIV/AIDS for women, their partners, and society. In addition, the diagnosis, counseling, and treatment of HIV/AIDS infection (secondary prevention) can prevent disease progression and complications for the individual and transmission to others. (Readers are referred to chapter 24, Sexually Transmitted Infections, for a discussion of primary prevention of STIs, including HIV.)

HIV Tests

Beginning in 1985, HIV has been perhaps most associated with antibody testing, either for determination of serostatus or screening blood and tissue donations (Bennett, 2006). In addition, HIV testing includes a number of HIV management assays used to determine disease progression and direct a patient's antiretroviral therapy. Several different types of tests can be used to detect HIV. To date, the enzyme immunoassay or the enzyme-linked immunosorbent assay (ELISA) is the primary antibody screening test (Bennett, 2006). ELISA determines the presence of HIV antibodies in blood or oral fluids (Card et al., 2007). Currently, the available assays can assess HIV-1 and HIV-2 separately or in combination and have a high degree of specificity and sensitivity.

The standard of practice for HIV diagnostic testing requires two tests on the same sample to be reactive for a person to be considered HIV-positive. When an individual shows HIV antibodies on two or more ELISA tests, an independent, highly specific supplemental test—commonly the Western Blot or immunofluorescent-

antibody assay—is used (Bennett, 2006). The Western Blot test is less sensitive than the ELISA test, but rarely is there a false positive result, and therefore it is used for confirming the ELISA test. Rapid HIV tests, saliva- and urine-based antibody tests, and home HIV antibody testing kits that have been approved by the Food and Drug Administration are commercially available (Constantine, 2003). A rapid HIV test can be administered outside of a traditional laboratory, and the results can be available in as soon as 20 minutes (CDC, 2006c). HIV RNA tests are used in research and health care settings to diagnose HIV infections very early after exposure, before antibodies have formed (Constantine, 2003).

HIV Testing

HIV testing is a serious matter with a number of social, ethical, and psychological implications, in addition to the obvious health care issues. Certain persons have histories or clinical indications that warrant HIV testing (see Table 25.4). Counseling for risk factors will help health care providers determine the relative risk of a patient for HIV. Testing for HIV is recommended and should be offered to all women seeking evaluation for and treatment of STIs (CDC, 2006e).

The first guidelines for HIV testing were issued by the U.S. Public Health Service in 1987. In 1993, the CDC expanded the guidelines to include hospitalized patients and individuals receiving health care as outpatients in acute care settings. An important component of these guidelines was HIV counseling and testing as a priority prevention strategy for at-risk persons regardless of

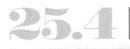 | Indications for HIV Testing

- Physical symptoms consistent with HIV-related illness
- History of multiple sexual partners
- History of crack cocaine, cocaine, or methamphetamine use
- History of injection drug use
- History of sex with an HIV-positive person or one suspected to be HIV-positive
- History of sex with an IV drug user
- History of a direct inoculation with HIV from an occupational exposure (e.g., operating room, emergency room)
- Social history that includes injection drug use or illicit drugs such as crack cocaine
- Pregnancy
- Tattoos or body piercing

Note. From *Sexually Transmitted Infections, Including HIV: Impact on Women's Reproductive Health*, by C. I. Fogel and B. Black, 2008, White Plains, NY: March of Dimes.

the health care setting. Further, the CDC recommended anonymous testing, which allowed persons to find out their status while minimizing their concern that their identities could be revealed. Further, the CDC strongly recommended voluntary HIV testing, preceded by informed consent in accordance with local laws (CDC, 1999a).

As advances in testing technology occurred and knowledge of HIV and its transmission factors increased, the CDC guidelines were revised. The most recent recommendations for HIV testing in primary care settings were released in 2006 (CDC, 2006c). Specific revisions include the following (Burrage et al., 2008; CDC, 2006c):

- HIV screening is recommended for all patients aged 13 to 65 years in all health care settings after the patient is notified that testing will be done unless the patient declines (opt-out screening).
- Persons at risk for HIV infection should be screened for HIV at least annually.
- Separate written consent for HIV testing should not be required; general consent for medical care is considered sufficient to include consent for HIV testing.
- Prevention counseling should not be required with HIV diagnostic testing or as part of HIV screening programs in health care settings.

Additional recommendations for pregnant women include:

- HIV screening should be included in the routine prenatal screening test panel for all pregnant women.
- Repeat screening in the third trimester is recommended in areas with elevated rates of HIV infection in pregnant women.

These revisions are intended to allow a broader testing base, because there is no longer a focus on testing individuals with behavioral risk factors or clinical presentations (Lifson & Rybicki, 2007). Further, these changes are expected to increase early detection of HIV infection and decrease HIV stigma by no longer focusing only on behavioral risk groups (Valdiserri, 2007).

Although a negative antibody test usually indicates that a person is not infected, these tests cannot exclude a recent infection. A patient with a negative test who is at very high risk for contracting the virus should be retested 3 to 6 months after the initial baseline test. A person with a specific exposure to HIV—for example, in an occupational setting or via unprotected sexual contact with a person known to have HIV—should be tested serially: first, at the time of the exposure to determine the baseline serologic status, and then at 3- and 6-month intervals until seroconversion is determined or the person remains seronegative for 1 year.

HIV Counseling

The current CDC recommendation to eliminate pretest prevention counseling might suggest that pretest counseling was ineffective; in fact, research found that interactive client-centered counseling did reduce risk behaviors and the incidence of new STIs (CDC, 2006c) The impact of counseling and testing is likely to be greatest for HIV-positive individuals, because the information gained could be used to avoid transmitting HIV to others (Wohlfeiler & Ellen, 2007). Further, the CDC acknowledges that prevention counseling is desirable for all persons at risk for HIV but also recognizes that counseling may not be feasible in all settings (CDC, 2006c).

Although prevention counseling is no longer required as a part of the HIV screening programs in health care settings, it is strongly encouraged for all persons at high risk for HIV. It is also recommended that easily understood informational materials should be available in the languages of the persons utilizing the health care services.

State laws vary regarding disclosure of a positive diagnosis for HIV to persons other than the patient, such as spouses or sexual contacts. Health care providers must be aware of the regulations governing their practice and should inform the patient of these regulations prior to testing, so that the patient can be fully informed as to the social and legal implications of a positive test. For many women, partner notification may make her vulnerable to abuse and violence in the event she is HIV positive.

Table 25.5 lists the issues that should be addressed in counseling a patient seeking HIV testing. All women seeking HIV-testing should also be tested for hepatitis B.

The posttest visit can be stressful for the patient, regardless of the results; therefore, test results should be disclosed as soon as possible in the visit, because

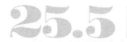 | HIV Test Counseling

- Explain the meaning and implications of negative and positive test results and the meaning of indeterminate results.
- Discuss HIV risk reduction, including behaviors specific to the woman being tested.
- Inform the woman of state-mandated reporting requirements.
- If relevant, explain anonymous versus confidential testing.
- Determine the woman's support system and coping and stress management strategies that may be enlisted based on test results.
- Arrange for a return visit to discuss test results.

Note. From *Sexually Transmitted Infections, Including HIV: Impact on Women's Reproductive Health,* by C. I. Fogel and B. Black, 2008, White Plains, NY: March of Dimes.

the patient may be very anxious regarding the outcome. If the results are positive for HIV, the woman must be given time to accept the message and to react emotionally as needed. She must assimilate a lot of information at the time of this visit. Allowing her to express her feelings prior to discussing issues related to partner notification, treatments, and other issues may help her to take in some of the important information that must be conveyed at this time.

Seropositive patients must understand that, although they may exhibit no signs or symptoms of HIV disease, they are still infectious and will be for life. Basic information regarding minimizing transmission risk must be relayed to the patient at this time. A specific goal is to minimize the risk of transmission of the virus to others; therefore, the patient needs to understand immediately the implications of her HIV seropositivity in terms of transmission risk. Furthermore, the advanced practice nurse must assess the patient's need for further supportive services for psychological and emotional needs of the newly diagnosed HIV-positive patient.

A plan for treatment must be established. Often this requires a referral to an infectious disease health care setting that can provide expert care for the infection. Unless the patient is clearly immunocompromised and needs immediate treatment for an opportunistic infection, there is likely to be an interval between diagnosis and treatment decisions. This time can be used by the woman to begin to emotionally and psychologically integrate her diagnoses. She will need to make decisions about who must be told about her infection and begin to integrate behaviors that are required to minimize her risk of transmitting the virus to others.

The impact of HIV on future childbearing is an important consideration in counseling women with HIV. Many women are diagnosed with HIV during pregnancy. They must be given adequate information regarding vertical transmission and treatment during pregnancy in order to make informed decisions regarding their pregnancy. Most HIV-positive women are diagnosed during their childbearing years. Making the decision to become pregnant or to forego future childbearing should be made only when the woman is fully informed regarding HIV and pregnancy. Perinatal transmission of HIV can be reduced to low levels with the use of ZDV in pregnancy, so women can choose to become pregnant with a relatively small risk of vertical transmission of the virus to the fetus. However, the possibility of a shortened life expectancy due to her HIV may shape a woman's decision to forego any further childbearing. This may be an emotional and personal decision that will require ongoing support.

Unfortunately, many women are diagnosed later after infection than are men and may have more advanced HIV disease at the time of diagnosis. Further, because HIV-positive women are more likely to be African American or Hispanic, they may have diminished economic resources and social support available to them. A comprehensive plan of care that takes into consideration the multiplicity of stressors that HIV-positive women experience has a greater chance at making a healthy impact on their lives.

A patient who is seronegative for HIV should receive counseling and education regarding behavior change to reduce the risk of contracting HIV. The news that one is negative for HIV will be met with relief and an immediate reduction of anxiety. However, it is essential that all women who are tested for HIV based on risky behaviors be counseled regarding the need to be retested at 3 and 6 months given the delay in seroconversion after infection. Women who engage in very high-risk behaviors should be counseled to be tested serially. This is to prevent the ongoing assumption that the woman is seronegative for HIV, when in fact she may have been tested between the time of infection and the development of antibodies.

MANAGEMENT OF HIV/AIDS IN WOMEN

Women infected with HIV manifest a more heterogeneous viral population than do men, which may result in a more diverse immune response (Long, Martin, & Kreiss, 2006). Because women tend to progress to AIDS with viral loads that are significantly lower than men, decisions about beginning antiretroviral therapy should be primarily based on CD4 counts rather than viral load (Cotter et al., 2006).

Women with undiagnosed HIV often seek care for a gynecologic infection or condition. One of the most common symptoms of HIV infection in women is recurrent vaginal candidias. HIV-infected women are also more likely than uninfected women to have abnormal cervical cytology (40%), human papillomavirus infection (58%), more severe pelvic inflammatory disease, and bacterial vaginosis (Brown, 2004; Cotter et al., 2006). In addition, HIV-infected women have higher incidences of toxoplasmosis, herpes, genital ulcerations, and esophageal candidias (Stine, 2007).

The care of HIV-positive persons should be supervised by an expert in infectious disease (Feinberg & Maenza, 2005). Further, current recommendations emphasize using laboratory monitoring of plasma levels of HIV1-RNA (viral load) to direct practitioners in instituting, assessing, and changing antiretroviral therapy .

All women newly diagnosed with HIV should undergo an extensive medical history review, physical examination, and laboratory evaluation. The medical history (see Table 25.6 and Table 25.7) should include inquiries related to sexual behaviors, sexually transmitted diseases (especially syphilis), and chronic illnesses unrelated to but affected by HIV and its treatments, such as heart disease and diabetes mellitus. The history also should include inquiries about illnesses and conditions associated with immunosuppression such as tuberculosis, herpes zoster, and genitorectal herpes; acute and chronic skin disorders such as fungal infections and molluscum contagiosum; severe and repeated episodes of vaginal candidiasis; diarrhea associated with various fungi or bacteria; and frequent bouts of pneumonia and sinusitis (Feinberg & Maenza, 2005). The presence or frequency of these infections not typically found in persons with normal immunological status may help pinpoint the time of infection. In addition, women with HIV should be asked about their gynecological and obstetrical history, including birth control method and plans for future childbearing.

The physical exam for patients with HIV should be very thorough (see Table 25.8). Vital signs should be carefully monitored, especially temperature and weight.

The wide-scale and subtle effects of HIV on various body systems requires careful examination, especially of the mouth, eyes, skin, lungs, heart, lymph nodes, abdomen, genitalia, rectum, and nervous system. HIV may cause subtle or obvious changes in each of these systems. Clinical abnormalities in these systems will give the practitioner evidence of the level of immune system compromise in the patient with HIV. In addition, certain laboratory tests (see Table 25.9) should be included in the initial examination of the HIV-positive woman. Also, all patients should be tested for tuberculosis initially and annually thereafter (Feinberg & Maenza, 2005).

General clinical findings in HIV-positive women are similar to those found in men, with the exception of a high frequency of reproductive tract disorders, including cervical dysplasia and refractory vaginal candidiasis (Feinberg & Maenza, 2005). Women with HIV

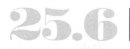 Medical History for HIV-Positive Women

TOPIC	SPECIFIC POINTS TO ADDRESS
HIV diagnosis	When were you first tested? Why were you tested?
HIV treatment history	Pretherapy CD4 count, viral load. Specific antiretroviral treatment history
STI and other infection history	Syphilis; gonorrhea; herpes simplex; pelvic inflammatory disease; anogenital warts; tuberculosis; hepatitis A, B, or C; prior vaccinations; history of chicken pox or shingles
Obstetrical and gynecologic history	Pregnancies and their resolution, menstrual disorders, anovulation, perimenopause, uterine fibroids or polyps, abnormal vaginal discharge, cancer, genital tract infections
Other medical diagnoses	Hypertension, type 2 diabetes mellitus, cardiovascular disease, premalignant or malignant conditions, thyroid disease
Sexual practices	Condoms use; other birth control methods; number of current partners; sexual activity with men, women, or both; history of trading sex for drugs or money; history of anal sex
HIV-associated signs and symptoms	See Table 25.7; bacterial pneumonia, thrush, severe headache, midline substernal discomfort with swallowing, visual changes including flutters or visual filed deficits
Mental health history	Past and current problems, evidence of depression (change in appetite, trouble sleeping, loss of interest in usual activities, anhedonia)
Family history	Age and health of children, including HIV tests if done; HIV in other family members; hypertension; type 2 diabetes; cardiovascular disease; malignancy
Medications	Prescription and over-the-counter; history of and attitude toward regular medication use; use of complementary and alternative therapies; drug allergies
Social history	Place of birth, where raised, who lived with, child care responsibilities, history of interpersonal violence, education and occupational history, travel history, substance use or abuse, illicit drug use
Sources of support	Who has women told of her diagnosis, and what were their reactions? Does she have friends and family members she can talk to? Does she have a job? Does she have health insurance?

Note. From "Primary Medical Care," by J. Feinberg and J. Maenza, 2005, in J. R. Anderson (Ed.), *A Clinical Guide to the Clinical Care of Women with HIV* (pp. 91–166), Rockville, MD: Department of Health and Human Services, HIV/AIDS Bureau; *Sexually Transmitted Infections, Including HIV: Impact on Women's Reproductive Health,* by C. I. Fogel and B. Black, 2008, White Plains, NY: March of Dimes.

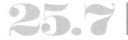 | Signs and Symptoms of HIV

General observation	■ Fatigue
	■ Weight loss
	■ Anorexia
	■ Fever
	■ Sweats
Skin	■ Rashes
	■ Pigmented lesions
	■ Generalized drying
	■ Pruritus
Lymphatics	■ Localized or generalized lymph node involvement
	■ Lymphadenopathy
Head, eyes, ears, nose, and throat	■ Headaches
	■ Nasal discharge
	■ Sinus congestion
	■ Changes in visual acuity
	■ Sore throat
	■ Whitish or painful lesions of the oral mucosa
Cardiopulmonary	■ Cough
	■ Shortness of breath
Gastrointestinal	■ Abdominal pain
	■ Change in bowel habits
	■ Persistent diarrhea
Musculoskeletal	■ Myalgias
	■ Arthralgias
Neurological/psychological	■ Depression
	■ Personality change
	■ Cognitive difficulties
	■ Bowel or bladder dysfunction
	■ Peripheral weakness
	■ Parenthesis
Pain	■ Pain that is not musculoskeletal

Note. From "Primary Medical Care," by J. Feinberg and J. Maenza, 2005, in J. R. Anderson (Ed.), *A Clinical Guide to the Clinical Care of Women with HIV* (pp. 91–166), Rockville, MD: Department of Health and Human Services, HIV/AIDS Bureau; *Sexually Transmitted Infections, Including HIV: Impact on Women's Reproductive Health,* by C. I. Fogel and B. Black, 2008, White Plains, NY: March of Dimes.

should have an initial Pap smear to test for the presence of cervical dysplasia and at least yearly thereafter. Some women will require Pap smears more frequently based on initial findings and gynecological history. For women with cervical dysplasia, referral may be made for follow-up with a gynecologist for colposcopy and treatment.

The management of lower genital tract neoplasia represents a specific treatment issue in the care of women with HIV. Women with HIV are at risk for developing lower genital tract neoplasia, particularly as HIV disease progresses and the woman becomes increasingly immunocompromised. Cervical intraepithelial neoplasia and invasive cervical cancer can be persistent and progressive and difficult to manage effectively in women with HIV. Women with these conditions should be referred to a gynecologist for management.

Appropriate vaccinations will be offered based on patient history and lab findings. Common vaccinations include yearly influenza immunizations, pneumonia immunizations, and the hepatitis A and hepatitis B series, as indicated.

25.8 | Physical Examination for Patients With HIV

General	■ Evidence of wasting
	■ Fat distribution syndromes: buffalo hump, enlarged breasts, truncal obesity, subcutaneous fat loss in extremities, face, buttocks
Eyes	■ Purplish spots of Kaposi's syndrome in conjunctiva
	■ Petechiae
	■ Hemorrhages caused by cytomegalovirus retinitis
Oropharynx	■ Thrush
	■ Oral hairy leukoplakia
	■ Purplish spots or plaques on mucosal surfaces
Lymph nodes	■ Nontender or minimally tender generalized adenopathy, which may indicate HIV infection or lymphoma
Lungs	■ Fine, dry "cellophane" rales, diagnostic for *Pneumocystis carinii* pneumonia
Hepatosplenomegaly	■ Sign of disseminated infection with *Mycobacterium avium* complex, tuberculosis, histoplasmosis, or lymphoma
Pelvic	■ External genitalia: sores or ulcers indicative of herpes simplex or syphilis
	■ Condyloma acuminate
	■ Abnormal vaginal discharge from vaginitis or cervicitis
	■ Cervical motion and uterine and adnexal tenderness suggestive of pelvic inflammatory disease
Neurologic	■ Motor deficits
	■ Peripheral neuropathy, including symmetrical distal sensory deficits, more often of feet
	■ AIDS dementia complex: poor short-term memory, diminished concentration, sensorimotor retardation
Skin	■ Early manifestations: pruritic papular eruptions, bacterial folliculitis, scabies
	■ Molluscum contagiosum
	■ Shingles
	■ Seborrheic dermatitis
	■ Psoriasis
	■ Kaposi's syndrome

Note. From "Primary Medical Care," by J. Feinberg and J. Maenza, 2005, in J. R. Anderson (Ed.), *A Clinical Guide to the Clinical Care of Women with HIV* (pp. 91–166), Rockville, MD: Department of Health and Human Services, HIV/AIDS Bureau; *Sexually Transmitted Infections, Including HIV: Impact on Women's Reproductive Health*, by C. I. Fogel and B. Black, 2008, White Plains, NY: March of Dimes.

Based on the patient's history and physical and the laboratory findings, the health care team will devise a plan of follow-up care. Decisions related to the initiation of antiretroviral therapy, chemoprophylaxis against opportunistic infections, and follow-up evaluation may be deferred until all test results are received if the patient appears to be generally healthy at the time of the initial examination. Patients who are obviously immunocompromised with signs and symptoms of AIDS-related illness or opportunistic infection at the time of initial evaluation may be treated presumptively, with

further refinements and changes in treatments possible at the time all laboratory data are reviewed.

Two specific lab values that shape treatment decisions in persons with HIV are the viral load (HIV1 RNA) and the CD4+ count. With increasing emphasis in HIV care on maintaining viral load levels at an undetectable level, these lab values are important in ascertaining appropriate antiretroviral therapy and adherence to the medication regimen. The CD4 count is an important tool in assessing the overall status of the immune system. Also known as helper T-cells, CD4

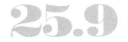

| Baseline HIV Lab Tests

Serology
- Confirm HIV diagnosis
- CD4 count lymphocyte count
- Viral load
- Complete blood count, including white blood cell count differential
- Chemistry panel, including liver and renal function
- Lipid profile
- Syphilis, toxoplasmosis, cytomegalovirus, varicella-zoster virus if no history of chicken pox or shingles
- Hepatitis A, B, C

Cultures
- Urinalysis
- Pap smear
- Chlamydia culture
- Gonorrhea culture
- Cervical human papillomavirus assay

Other
- Chest X ray
- Purified protein derivative

Note. From "Sexually Transmitted Disease Treatment Guidelines 2006," by Centers for Disease Control and Prevention, 2006, *Morbidity and Mortality Weekly Report, 55*(RR-11), pp. 1–94; "Primary Medical Care," by J. Feinberg and J. Maenza, 2005, in J. R. Anderson (Ed.), *A Clinical Guide to the Clinical Care of Women with HIV* (pp. 91–166), Rockville, MD: Department of Health and Human Services, HIV/AIDS Bureau; *Sexually Transmitted Infections, Including HIV: Impact on Women's Reproductive Health,* by C. I. Fogel and B. Black, 2008, White Plains, NY: March of Dimes.

cells signal other immune system cells to fight infection. Depletion of these cells is the hallmark of advancing HIV disease.

Antiretroviral Therapy

Effective antiretroviral therapy (ART) involves using a combination of medications that slow viral replication. The goals of ART are (1) to improve the patient's quality of life; (2) to reduce HIV-related morbidity and mortality; (3) maximal, durable suppression of viral load; and (4) restoration and/or preservation of immunologic function (Beal & Orrick, 2006a). ART is likely to involve complex dosage schedules and uncomfortable side effects.

Specific characteristics of HIV infection have important implications for antiretroviral therapy (Feinberg & Maenza, 2005):

- Between initial diagnosis and development of clinical disease, there is progressive immunosuppression evidenced by the decline in CD4 counts.

- Viral replication is extremely rapid; the half-life of HIV in plasma is less than 48 hours and a turnover of up to 1 billion virus per day.
- HIV has a high capacity for genetic mutability, and thus resistance to antiretroviral therapy can occur rapidly.

There is a rationale for beginning antiretroviral therapy prior to symptom onset to prevent immunosuppression. Further therapy must be continuous to prevent viral replication. Benefits and risks exist in initiating ART in treatment-naïve, asymptomatic patients (see Table 25.10) that must be considered prior to the initiation of ART. The risks and benefits of treatment of asymptomatic patients must be weighed carefully on a case-by-case basis to determine the appropriate course for any particular patient. The decision to initiate treatment in an asymptomatic patient must balance several competing factors that influence risk and benefit.

Asymptomatic patients considering the initiation of ART must receive thorough education and counsel regarding this decision. Patients must be fully informed

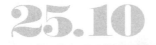

| Benefits and Risks of Antiretroviral Therapy

Benefits
- Control of viral replication and reduction of viral load
- Prevention of progressive immunosupression by control of viral load
- Delayed progression of clinical disease and progression to AIDS
- Prolongation of life
- Decreased risk of resistant virus
- Decreased risk of drug toxicity
- Possible decreased risk of viral transmission

Risks
- Reduction of quality of life from adverse drug effects and inconvenience of drug regimens
- Limitations of future options for therapy if drug resistance develops in current agents
- Potential for transmission of drug-resistant virus
- Limitation of future drug choices due to the development of resistance
- Potential long-term toxicity of therapy
- Unknown duration of effectiveness of current therapies

Note. From *Sexually Transmitted Infections, Including HIV: Impact on Women's Reproductive Health,* by C. I. Fogel and B. Black, 2008, White Plains, NY: March of Dimes; "Viral Load and Heterosexual Transmission of Human Immunodeficiency Virus Type 1," by T. C. Quinn, M. J. Wawer, N. Sewankambo, D. Serwadda, C. Chuanjun, F. Wabwire-Mangen, M. O. Meehan, Y. Lutalo, and R. H. Gray, 2000, *New England Journal of Medicine, 342*(13), pp. 921–929.

and willing to initiate therapy. Although this seems to be an obvious consideration in any therapeutic regimen, it is of particular importance in initiating ART. The patient must be reasonably likely to adhere to her regimen as prescribed, although no patient should automatically have ART withheld based on behaviors that some may assume are associated with a likelihood of nonadherence (Feinberg & Maenza, 2005). Thorough patient education and counsel and ongoing follow-up counsel and support increase the likelihood of effective adherence to ART.

The treatment guidelines put forth by the U.S. Department of Health and Human Services (Feinberg & Maenza, 2005) recommend deferring treatment on persons with CD4 counts greater than $350/mm^3$ (see Table 25.11). All patients who show signs of HIV disease progression should be offered ART. These signs can include thrush, wasting, unexplained fever for more than 2 weeks, and symptoms of opportunistic infection. Any patient with AIDS-defining criteria (see Table 25.12) should be offered ART. Patients who present with advanced HIV disease or AIDS can recover some degree of immune function after the initiation of ART. Patients with opportunistic infection must have it treated prior to or at the same time as the initiation of ART. Doing so, however, raises the issue of drug tolerance, interactions, and toxicities, in addition to the issues surrounding the complexities of scheduling multiple medications.

Specific Antiretroviral Therapies

The development of effective antiretroviral therapy represents one of the biggest scientific challenges in controlling and eventually eradicating HIV. A caveat is necessary before discussing ART therapy in the treatment of HIV infection: The research and development of new therapies and the testing of different combinations of therapies can quickly change the state of the science. Advanced practice nurses are encouraged to use reliable sources (e.g., the CDC and the National Institutes of Health) available on the Internet for the most current recommendations and practices in HIV care. A list of reliable Web sites is found at the end of this chapter.

Highly active antiretroviral therapy (HAART) consists of three or more antiretroviral agents used in combination to try to decrease an individual's plasma viral load to an undetectable level. Issues to be considered when choosing an antiretroviral regimen include (1) the patient's daily routines and social support as they influence her ability to adhere to a particular regimen; (2) the side effects of the medications, including evaluation of the patient's other medical conditions that may increase the risk of certain adverse effects; and (3) any drug interactions with other medications the woman may be taking (Beal & Orrick, 2006a). Currently, four classes of antiretroviral medications are available: *nucleoside reverse transcriptase inhibitors* (NRTIs), *nonnucleoside reverse transcriptase inhibitors* (NNRTIs; e.g., efavirenz, delavirdine, and nevirapine), *protease inhibitors* (PIs), and *fusion inhibitors* (enfuvirtide). NRTIs and NNRTIs work by disrupting the work of reverse transcriptase. Reverse transcriptase is an enzyme that changes the virus's chemical genetic message into a form that can be easily inserted inside the nucleus of an infected cell. This process occurs early in the viral

25.11 | Treatment Guidelines for HIV/AIDS

CLINICAL CATEGORY	CD4 CELL COUNT	PLASMA HIV RNA	RECOMMENDATIONS
Symptomatic (AIDS or severe symptoms	Any value	Any value	Treat
Asymptomatic AIDS	CD4 cells > $200/mm^3$	Any value	Treat
Asymptomatic	CD4 cells > $200/mm^3$ but < $350/mm^3$	Any value	Offer treatment; controversial
Asymptomatic	CD4 cells > $350/mm^3$	> 100,000	Some clinicians recommend initiating therapy; others recommend deferring and monitoring CD4 cell count and level of plasma HIV RNA more frequently
Asymptomatic	CD4 cells > $350/mm^3$	< 100,000	Defer treatment and monitor CD4 count

Note. From "Primary Medical Care," by J. Feinberg and J. Maenza, 2005, in J. R. Anderson (Ed.), *A Clinical Guide to the Clinical Care of Women with HIV* (pp. 91–166), Rockville, MD: Department of Health and Human Services, HIV/AIDS Bureau.

25.12 | AIDS-Defining Criteria

- CD4+ count below 200 cells/cubic millimeter
- Candidiasis, esophageal, tracheal, bronchi, or lungs
- Cervical cancer, invasive
- Coccidioidomycosis, disseminated or extrapulmonary
- Cryptococcosis, extrapulmonary
- Cryptosporidiosis with diarrhea for more than 1 month
- Cytomegalovirus of any organ other than liver, spleen, or lymph nodes
- HIV encephalopathy
- Herpes simplex infection: chronic ulcers of more than 1 month's duration; or bronchitis, pneumonitis, or esophagitis
- Histoplasmosis, disseminated or extrapulmonary
- Isosporiasis with diarrhea for more than 1 month
- Kaposi's sarcoma
- Lymphoma, Burkitt's, immunologic, primary central nervous system
- *Mycobacterium avium* complex or *M. kansasii,* disseminated
- *Mycobacterium,* other or unidentified species, disseminated or extrapulmonary
- *Pneumocystis carinii* pneumonia
- Pneumonia, recurrent bacterial with more than two episodes in 12 months
- Progressive multifocal leukoencephalopathy
- Salmonella septicemia
- Toxoplasmosis of internal organ or brain
- Wasting syndrome due to HIV

Note. From *The Complete HIV/AIDS Teaching Kit,* by J. J. Card, A. Amarillas, A. Conner, D. D. Akers, J. Solomon, and R. J. DiClemente, 2007, New York: Springer Publishing; "HIV Infection and AIDS, by G. Rieg, 2006, in A. L. Nelson and J. Woodward (Eds.), *Sexually Transmitted Diseases* (pp. 99–125), Totowa, NJ: Humana Press; *Varney's Midwifery* (4th ed.), by H. Varney, J. M. Kriebs, and C. L. Gegor, 2004, Sudbury, MA: Jones & Bartlett.

replication cycle. Reverse transcriptase inhibitors interrupt the duplication of genetic material necessary for the virus to replicate. PIs are an important class of antiviral medications that are currently in the forefront of treatment options. Prescribed with reverse transcriptase inhibitors, they work inside infected cells late in the HIV replication process. After HIV has infected a cell, it continues relentlessly to replicate itself. However, the newly produced genetic material, in the form of long chains of proteins and enzymes, is functional only after these long chains have been cut into shorter pieces by the HIV enzyme protease. By inhibiting the function of protease, PIs reduce the number of new infectious copies of HIV. Saquinavir, indinavir, and ritonavir are examples of PIs. Although antiretroviral therapy medications have demonstrated a high level of effectiveness

in reducing viral load in persons with HIV, they also have significant side effects that can adversely affect quality of life.

RTIs and PIs work together effectively to reduce the circulating viral load. With two different points of disruption of the replication cycle, concurrent use of these medications represents the best hope of managing HIV infection as a chronic illness. Regimens with the most experience in demonstrating serologic and immunologic efficacy are those composed of one NNRTI plus two NRTIs or one PI plus two NRTIs. The preferred NNRTI-based regimen (one NNRTI plus two NRTIs) is efavirez (except for during the first trimester of pregnancy or in women who are trying to conceive or who are not using effective, consistent contraception); the preferred alternative is nevirapine (DHHS Panel, 2006).

Highly active antiretroviral therapy is usually initiated in instances of failure of less potent ART, evidence of viral resistance, or in the case of serious immunocompromise requiring intense therapy and rapid viral reduction. HAART also may be initiated for treatment-naïve patients. Intense patient counseling to ensure maximal adherence to HAART is a crucial component of care for HIV-positive patients who are starting a HAART regimen in order to prevent early development of resistant virus and to maximize viral suppression.

Postexposure prophylaxis (PEP) with ART is recommended for health care workers who have an occupational exposure to HIV through a needle-stick injury or cut with a contaminated object, contact of a mucous membrane or nonintact skin with potentially infectious material or body fluids, or prolonged exposure (several minutes or more) of intact skin to potentially infectious materials (CDC, 2005a). The basic regimen is used when there is an exposure with a recognized risk of HIV transmission. This regimen includes 28 days of zidovudine 600 mg daily in divided doses and lamivudine 150 mg twice a day. For HIV exposures that pose an increased risk of transmission, such as a larger volume of blood or exposure to blood with a high viral load, the basic PEP regimen is initiated, plus indinavir 800 mg every 8 hours or nelfinavir 750 mg three times a day.

Patients on ART may have other chronic conditions requiring medications and frequent monitoring of lab values. For any patient for whom ART is initiated, the interactions between HIV medications and other medications the patient takes regularly must be examined. Furthermore, scheduling of medications to minimize untoward interactions is a critical component of care for these patients.

Adherence to Antiretroviral Therapy

Adherence to antiretroviral therapy is crucial. The complexities of these regimens, however, can be very difficult to understand for some patients and very difficult to follow over time. A critical nursing challenge is to teach and counsel HIV-positive patients in adhering to the prescribed medication regimen. Failure to adhere to an ART protocol results in the rapid increase in viral load with concurrent immune system damage. The likelihood of developing AIDS is directly related to viral load. Simply, the presence of more virus means more immune system damage and a worsening ability to fend off aggressive opportunistic infections.

The development of ART-resistant strains of virus is a primary concern in treatment failure and represents a serious sequela of nonadherence. Cross-resistance among treatment options limits the availability of effective therapy. Furthermore, the transmission of resistant strains complicates therapies for treatment-naïve patients, who may have few options available from the onset of the infection. Patients who fail to follow their ART regimen as prescribed face the risk of developing a resistant strain of virus. The danger of nonadherence is dual: First, an increased viral load with a resistant virus is an alarming clinical situation associated with a poor outcome for the patient. Second, additional treatments for opportunistic infections, with their concomitant side effects, will be necessary as symptoms of advancing disease manifest themselves.

Nurses have a distinct role in the preparation of patients as they begin ART. Effective nursing care must take into consideration the following issues related to the initiation of a treatment protocol that demands careful adherence:

- *What is the patient's understanding of HIV?* Nurses in settings that see HIV patients regularly may take for granted that patients have a more thorough understanding of HIV than they really do. With much of the knowledge about HIV filtered through rumor, innuendo, and incomplete or misleading media reports, patients may be woefully lacking in substantive knowledge of their disease. Recent developments in antiretroviral therapy have allowed the health care profession to understand HIV as a chronic and manageable disease; however, this understanding has not reached all segments of the general public. Emphasizing the chronic rather than fatal nature of the infection may help patients to reframe their understanding of the illness. Basic to the establishment of an effective nursing care plan is the thorough assessment of the patient's understanding of the disease, including its meaning to the patient.
- *Can the patient understand how the medications are to be taken?* The patient may have a limited ability to understand the issues surrounding ART and adherence. It is incumbent on the nurse to ensure that the patient or the patient's caregiver understands the importance of taking the medications as ordered. The nurse may have to be creative in devising charts, journals, pill boxes, or other reminders for the patient

and the caregiver to enhance the chances of successful adherence.

- *What is the patient's daily schedule, and how does ART fit into the schedule?* The nurse must consider shift work, sleep-wake patterns, meal times, and family responsibilities in assisting the patient in establishing a medication schedule to which the patient can adhere. If is it clear that the patient is likely to fail in following a complex schedule of medications in the context of a busy and active life, the nurse should consult with the physician or nurse practitioner in identifying alternative medications that may be more suitable for the patient.
- *Are there any social constraints on the patient related to taking ART?* Antiretroviral therapy represents the constant presence of HIV, an incurable infection that is fraught with social implications in addition to its health implications. Some persons find that the frequent reminder of the infection through taking ART is onerous and psychologically painful, lessening the likelihood of long-term adherence.

Many women keep their HIV infection a secret from their closest family members and friends. The presence of ART medications in the home increases the risk that someone will discover the patient's diagnosis. The patient must be counseled about that possibility and encouraged to think about the social implications if the HIV is discovered.

Beginning ART represents a small step in going public with the diagnosis. The patient must understand that the pharmacist filling the prescriptions will know the patient's diagnosis. The patient may prefer to have prescriptions filled in a place that is likely to offer more anonymity, such as a hospital pharmacy or a discount store pharmacy with a high volume of business. Finances may be an important consideration for the patient, who may have to seek outside sources of funds to enable the purchase of ART.

The goal for nurses is always the same: Patients will adhere to their antiretroviral therapy schedules as evidenced by decreasing, and ultimately nondetectable, viral loads, maintaining that level for as long as possible. Simply handing a patient several prescriptions for expensive medications requiring complicated schedules and having a number of uncomfortable and potentially serious side effects is likely to result in treatment failure. Nurses are in a unique position to make a substantial positive impact on the lives of persons living with HIV by spending time in careful assessment, planning, intervening, and goal setting.

Prevention of Opportunistic Infections

In the 25 years since the identification of HIV/AIDS, great improvements have been made in the prevention of opportunistic infections that ravaged the earliest victims of the HIV pandemic. Increasingly aggressive use of ART has helped in maintaining the immune systems of persons with HIV, therefore reducing the need for routine chemoprophylaxis against Opportunistic Infections. Further, infections such as *Pneumocystis carinii pneumonia*, toxoplasmosis, *Mycobacterium avium* complex disease, and other bacterial diseases have been effectively prevented in patients requiring chemoprophylaxis. A single daily dose of double-strength trimethoprim-sulfamethoxazole (Septra, Bactrim) has reduced the incidence of PCP, toxoplasmosis, and bacterial infections (Centers for Disease Control, 1999b). This is a particularly useful medication because it is effective, generally well tolerated, simple to take, and inexpensive. However, for those who are sensitive to or allergic to trimethoprim-sulfamethoxazole, dapsone is an effective alternative.

Persons with HIV should follow some specific, although not overly restrictive, guidelines regarding minimizing exposure to potential sources of opportunistic infection. For women who are likely to be managing the care of the home and children, understanding how to preserve and maintain her own health while fulfilling her household and parenting obligations is very important. Nurses should counsel women in basic good hygiene practices that can minimize the risk of many exposures. These practices include:

- Thorough hand washing with water and soap after toileting, after assisting children in toileting, and at intervals throughout the day. Paper towels in the bathroom provide a more sanitary means of drying hands than a hand towel that stays damp and may be used by others.
- Minimizing exposure to animal or human wastes by using disposable gloves. This includes wearing disposable gloves when doing yard work and when changing a baby's diaper.
- Drinking water only from sources known to be dependable and clean; avoiding ingestion of water from lakes, rivers, and recreational swimming pools.
- Avoiding contact with animals in specific circumstances:
  - □ pets younger than 6 months old (increased likelihood of exposure to parasites)
  - □ any animal with diarrhea
  - □ all reptiles: turtles, lizards, snakes, iguanas (risk of Salmonella exposure)
  - □ situations that may expose the patient to bird droppings
- Treating cats with special care:
  - □ adopting cats that are more than 1 year old (risk of exposure to bacteria and parasites)
  - □ daily cleaning of litter box, preferably by a person without HIV if possible
  - □ keeping the cat indoors, not allowing the cat to hunt
  - □ avoiding cat scratches or bites and washing scratches or bites thoroughly and immediately
  - □ controlling fleas on cats
- Avoiding raw or undercooked eggs, poultry, meat, or seafood, and preventing cross-contamination by using separate kitchen utensils and cutting boards when processing these foods. Cutting boards should be thoroughly scrubbed after each use. Careful kitchen and cooking practices can decrease greatly the risk of food-borne infection.

In addition, HIV-positive patients should be counseled to consult with a health care provider before traveling to developing countries that may result in exposure to opportunistic pathogens. The Centers for Disease Control and Prevention Web site provides travelers with up-to-date information regarding endemic diseases and recommendations regarding vaccinations prior to travel.

Basic health practices such as adequate sleep and rest, good nutrition, exercise, smoking cessation, and avoidance of stress should not be overlooked in counseling HIV-positive persons. Seven to 8 hours of sleep a night is ideal for most adults. This amount may be difficult to achieve; however, the nurse can assist the patient in developing a sleep schedule that allows adequate rest.

Principles of good nutrition apply to persons with HIV, and, in fact, are especially necessary to provide adequate vitamins, minerals, electrolytes, and protein. Persons with HIV who are significantly under- or overweight should be encouraged to improve their nutritional status through support groups, nutritional counseling, or other means of weight management. Persons with a high intake of alcohol should be counseled to decrease their intake, because alcohol does not have any significant nutritional value, can interfere with vitamin absorption, and contains excess calories. Furthermore, chronic alcohol abuse can exacerbate liver problems. And, importantly, excessive alcohol intake will impair one's ability to make good judgments regarding health and sexual behaviors and to adhere to the ART regimen.

Exercise improves muscle tone and cardiovascular health and reduces stress—all important factors in maintaining a state of health. HIV-positive persons should be encouraged to engage in some form of exercise on a regular basis. The nurse can assist the patient in identifying simple means of increasing activity, even if the patient is somewhat debilitated or reluctant to engage in regular workouts. Walking is a simple form of exercise that is within the abilities of most persons and can be incorporated into one's daily routine with little effort.

Patients should be encouraged and supported in their efforts to stop smoking. In addition to the well-documented negative effects of smoking on health, the propensity of HIV-positive persons to pulmonary infections makes smoking cessation imperative. The nurse should be cognizant of the difficulty of stopping smoking and support any efforts the patient makes to decrease the number of cigarettes per day. However, the nurse is also in an excellent position to help the patient find therapies, group support, and other means to stop smoking.

Stress reduction plays an important role in health maintenance. Nurse can assist patients in identifying changeable stressors and in developing strategies to decrease overall stress. Many persons with HIV have significant social stressors related to poverty and other sociocultural issues that may be difficult to ameliorate. Nurses can help these patients understand management of their HIV infection to lessen the effects of HIV on their lives. An important nursing intervention, then, is to help HIV patients understand the chronic, manageable aspects of the infection. Careful planning with patients in terms of making regular clinic visits, initiating and adhering to an antiretroviral therapy regimen, and improving general health behaviors can be an effective means of reducing some of the HIV-related stresses for these patients.

HIV-INFECTED WOMEN OF CHILDBEARING AGE

Special considerations must be taken into account when managing HIV in women of childbearing age. Goals of their treatment include improving overall health and quality of life; minimizing disease progression; minimizing unwanted pregnancies; preventing heterosexual transmission; and avoiding prescribing medical treatments with teratogenic potential. Contraception and safer sex counseling are essential for HIV-positive women. The benefits and drawbacks of various contraceptives are found in Table 23.13. Barrier methods are necessary for HIV and STI prevention. The effect of hormonal contraceptives on viral shedding is not clear, and the bioavailability of ethinyl estradiol in hormonal contraceptives may be significantly reduced by some antiretroviral medications, including ritonavir, nelfinavir, or ritonavir boosted lopinavirnevirapine. Women

25.13 | Contraception for HIV-Infected Women

METHOD	BENEFITS	DISADVANTAGES
Male condom	Protection against STIs and HIV Protects partner	Partner cooperation required
Female condom	Protection against STIs and HIV Protects partner	Partner cooperation helpful
Oral contraceptive	Effective when used consistently	No HIV protection for partner No STI protection Risk of cervical ectopy Possible interaction with antibiotics and antiretrovirals
Depo-provera	Effective Limited compliance needed	No STI protection No HIV protection for partner
Intrauterine device	Effective	No HIV protection for partner No STI protection
Diaphragm	Effective Female controlled	Leave in 6 to 8 hours after ejaculation May increase risk of urinary tract infection
Patch	Avoids first-pass metabolism Easy to use	No STI protection No HIV protection for partner
Tubal ligation	One-time procedure Permanent	No STI protection No HIV protection for partner

Note. From "Management of HIV/AIDS in Women," by A. Cotter, J. E. Potter, and N. Tessler, 2006, in J. Beal and J. J. Orrick (Eds.), *HIV/AIDS Primary Care Guide* (pp. 533–546), Norwalk, CT: Crown House.

using oral contraceptives methods, an intrauterine device, or tubal ligation should be counseled to use a barrier method as well to reduce the risk of contracting an STI or transmitting HIV or an STI to her partner. It is essential that advanced practice nurses be aware of the drug interactions between oral contraceptives and antiretroviral therapy, because some of the interactions may compromise the effectiveness of either the contraceptive method by lowering oral contraceptive drug levels (e.g., nevirapine, nelfinavir, ritonavir) or lowering the effectiveness of the ART (amprenavir) (Cotter et al., 2006).

HIV in Pregnancy

Childbearing in women with HIV is a complex issue to be addressed carefully and thoroughly by clinicians working with this population. Reproduction is a major life activity, and refusing to help someone based solely on their HIV status is considered illegal discrimination. The American College of Obstetricians and Gynecologists (ACOG, 2001) has stated that HIV-infected couples should not be denied assisted reproductive techniques based solely on their seropositive status (Cotter et al., 2006).

Preconception counseling for women known to have HIV is an important means of optimizing maternal health prior to pregnancy. Elements of preconception counseling for women with HIV should include appropriate contraceptive methods to reduce unintended pregnancy; safer sex practices; avoidance of alcohol, illicit drug use, and cigarette smoking; risk factors of perinatal transmission and effective strategies to reduce and prevent transmission; and potential effects of HIV on pregnancy and maternal health (Perinatal HIV Guidelines Working Group, 2007; Squires, 2007). Elements to be considered in providing care to HIV-infected women considering pregnancy include avoiding antiretroviral agents with a potential for teratogenicity; attaining a stable, maximally suppressed HIV-1 RNA; evaluating the need for prophylaxis or preconception immunizations (influenza, pneumococcal, hepatitis B); optimizing nutritional status and folic acid supplementation; evaluating for opportunistic infections and initiating appropriate treatments or prophylactic regimens; screening for psychiatric and substance abuse disorders and domestic violence; standard genetic and reproductive health screening; and planning for pediatric and perinatal consultation (Perinatal HIV Guidelines Working Group, 2007; Squires, 2007).

Protection of the health of the pregnant woman and the fetus is the primary therapeutic goal in all prenatal and perinatal care, and this goal is the same for all women regardless of their HIV status. For women with HIV, minimizing the risk of vertical transmission is an additional therapeutic goal. Without intervention, HIV is effectively transmitted from mother to child. Before antiretroviral prophylaxis use, vertical transmission rates ranged from 13% to 32% in industrialized countries (Dabis et al., 1993). Transmission can occur at any time during a pregnancy; however, without any prevention measures, most transmission occurs during the intrapartum period (Anderson, 2005). Factors affecting vertical transmission are found in Table 25.14. Perinatal transmission of HIV to the fetus has decreased significantly in the past decade due to the prophylactic administration of antiretroviral prophylaxis (zidovudine [ZDV, AZT, Retrovir]) to pregnant women in the prenatal and perinatal periods. Oral administration of ZDV 100 mg five times daily is initiated between 14 and 34 weeks

25.14 | Factors Affecting Vertical HIV Transmission

DISEASE-RELATED FACTORS	MATERNAL HEALTH AND SOCIAL FACTORS	OBSTETRICAL FACTORS	INFANT FACTORS
Maternal HIV-1 RNA (plasma and genital tract)	Clinical stage	Duration of ruptured membranes	Prematurity
Maternal CD4+ count	Sexually transmitted infections during pregnancy	Chrioamnionitis	Breast-feeding
Viral genotype	Vitamin A deficiency	Use of invasive antenatal procedures	
Viral resistance mutations	Ongoing Intra Uterine Device tobacco use	Mode of delivery	
	Multiple sexual partners during pregnancy		

Note. From *A Clinical Guide to the Clinical Care of Women with HIV,* by J. R. Anderson, 2005, Rockville, MD: U.S. Department of Health and Human Services, HIV/AIDS Bureau; "Management of Pregnancy in HIV-Infected Women," by K. E. Squires, 2007, in E. P. Seekins, E. King, K. Obholtz, and S. McGuire (Eds.), *HIV/AIDS Annual Update 2007* (pp. 151–169), Coronado, CA: Postgraduate Institute for Medicine and Clinical Care Options.

of pregnancy and continued throughout pregnancy. During labor, intravenous administration of ZDV in a 1-hour initial dose of 2 mg/kg body weight, followed by continuous infusion of 1 mg/kg body weight/hour until delivery. The newborn infant then receives oral ZDV (zidovudine syrup at 2 mg/kg body weight/dose every 6 hours) for the first 6 weeks of life, beginning at 8 to 12 hours after birth (Perinatal HIV Guidelines Working Group, 2007; Squires, 2007). The transmission rate of HIV to newborns using this protocol was associated with a two-thirds reduction after 18 months of follow-up (Squires, 2007). Newer data suggest that vertical transmission may be reduced to as low as 1.2% among women who receive combination therapy with protease inhibitors during pregnancy (Ioannidis et al., 2001).

Use of antiretroviral therapy during pregnancy involves two aims: (1) safeguarding maternal health and (2) reducing mother-to-child transmission. As with non-pregnant women, decisions regarding therapy initiation and selection should be based on standard clinical criteria (Table 25.10) applicable to all HIV-infected adults. Balancing potentially conflicting needs of mother and infant health may be challenging because data regarding the safety, efficacy, and pharmacokinetics of anti-retroviral therapy in pregnancy are limited, particularly with newer drugs. Women who are pregnant or considering pregnancy must be counseled regarding the potential short-term and long-term risks and benefits associated with antiretroviral management strategies. Given zidovudine's proven efficacy and the availability of longer-term safety data on this medication, the Perinatal HIV Guidelines Working Group (2007) recommends that zidovudine ideally be used in pregnancy, either with or without additional antiretrovirals.

Before the widespread use of HAART, elective cesarean was routinely recommended as the preferred delivery method for HIV-infected women. Whether cesarean delivery continues to be the optimal method of delivery today, given that current transmission rates are very low and multiagent chemoprophylaxis is the norm, has not been established (Squires, 2007). The American College of Obstetricians and Gynecologists (2001) advises that women with HIV-1 RNA > 1,000 copies/ml in the third trimester should be counseled regarding the potential benefits of elective cesarean delivery.

Breast-feeding has been implicated in the transmission of HIV. The current recommendation is that HIV-positive mothers in the United States formula-feed their infants to avoid possible transmission of the virus. However, in developing countries, women may not have access to safe alternatives to breast milk for their infants. Research suggests that subclinical mastitis in early breast-feeding may increase the risk of HIV transmission (Miotti, et al., 1999). Breast-feeding accounts for up to 50% of pediatric HIV infections throughout the world (Fowler, Bertolli, & Nieburg, 1999).

Mothers face the difficult issue regarding guardianship of their children in the event of their death. Women with HIV are more likely to be poor and may have limited financial and social support. A single mother may have little or no contact with the father of her children, or he may be a poor candidate for parenting the children full-time. Making choices regarding her children's welfare may be difficult at best, and impossible if she has severely limited familial or social support. She may face the possibility that her children will be placed into foster care if she becomes very ill or dies. Nurses can assist HIV-infected mothers in expressing fear and grief over this possible, if not likely, scenario. Furthermore, nurses can assist the woman in seeking community services dedicated to managing the legal affairs of persons with HIV if those services are available. HIV case managers at the local level can also assist HIV-infected women in making decisions about the eventual care of their children. Women who address this issue early after their diagnosis may feel relieved that the issue of guardianship is resolved and formalized.

SOCIAL CONCERNS RELATED TO HIV

Very few diseases in history have had the levels of stigma that accompany an HIV diagnosis. Many persons with HIV choose to keep their diagnosis a secret from family, friends, and coworkers. Although this means that they must hide clinic visits, medications, and HIV-related illnesses, they may feel this is preferable to experiencing the stigma that accompanies the diagnosis. Persons with HIV may face dissolution of important relationships when and if the diagnosis becomes known. Nurses can assist patients in identifying supportive others who can be helpful as the patient adapts to the diagnosis and ART when initiated. Nurses should respect the patient's decisions about disclosure of the diagnosis (Black & Miles, 2001).

The woman may also want to make explicit her wishes regarding end-of-life care by establishing advance directives and entrusting a friend or family member with power of attorney in the event she becomes incapacitated. Nurses can be useful in explaining the meanings of various levels of advanced care and the implications of aggressive care in advanced HIV disease and AIDS. Young women with children may want more aggressive therapies and interventions than older women whose children are grown. This is a personal decision based on a variety of considerations, including spiritual and theological issues. Nurses must be careful not to make assumptions about what is desirable and appropriate for each woman.

Nurses can help patients reframe their understanding of HIV, particularly in terms of understanding it as a chronic disease that can be managed, rather than the "death sentence" it once was. When a woman learns of her HIV diagnosis, she may become seriously depressed, expecting to die soon and in much pain. Intervening early with these patients may prepare them to live with the disease, rather than simply waiting to die. Furthermore, many persons with HIV are recognized as long-term nonprogressors who, although infected with HIV, do not progress to AIDS even years after infection. Researchers have found psychological and behavioral factors that may play a role in the continuing viral suppression of nonprogressors. These factors include: (1) viewing HIV as a manageable illness; (2) taking care of their physical health; (3) staying connected with others in supportive relationships; (4) taking care of their emotional and mental health; and (5) nurturing their spiritual well-being (Barroso, 1999). These means of adapting to the very serious diagnosis of HIV can assist the HIV-infected patient in regaining a sense of control and hope. Nurses are in a unique position to understand the multiplicity of factors and issues that face persons with HIV. Awareness of these factors can enhance nursing interventions to improve both the physical and mental health and the long-term health outcomes for their HIV-positive patients.

SUMMARY

HIV/AIDS is associated with multifaceted dimensions of morbidity, mortality, and societal costs that are often disproportionately experienced by women and their infants. The need for prevention is critical, and nurses must assume a primary role in helping women decrease risky behaviors and increase protective practices. To decrease the burden of HIV on women, screening and early detection are essential. Again, nurses are a first-line defense in providing these services. Finally, treatment of HIV can lessen the impact of the disease. Education and counseling are essential to ensure that women obtain the maximum benefit from treatment.

HIV-RELATED WEB SITES

AIDSinfo (a service of the U.S. Department of Health and Human Services), http://www.aidsinfo.nih.gov

The Body Pro, www.thebodypro.com

Centers for Disease Control and Prevention HIV, www.cdc.gov/hiv

International AIDS Society, www.iasociety.org

REFERENCES

American College of Obstetricians and Gynecologists. (2001). *Human immunodeficiency virus. Ethics in obstetrics and gynecology.* Retrieved November 2007, from http://www.acog.org

Anderson, J. R. (2005). *A clinical guide to the clinical care of women with HIV.* Rockville, MD: U.S. Department of Health and Human Services, HIV/AIDS Bureau.

Barroso, J. (1999). Long-term nonprogressors with HIV. *Nursing Research, 48*(5), 242–249.

Beal, J., & Orrick, J. J. (2006a). Antiretroviral therapy. In J. Beal & J. J. Orrick (Eds.), *HIV/AIDS primary care guide* (pp. 45–87). Norwalk, CT: Crown House.

Beal, J., & Orrick, J. J. (2006b). *HIV/AIDS primary care guide.* Norwalk, CT: Crown House.

Bennett, B. (2006). HIV testing. In J. Beal & J. J. Orrick (Eds.), *HIV/AIDS primary care guide* (pp. 9–16). Norwalk, CT: Crown House.

Black, B. P., & Miles, M. S. (2001). Calculating the risks and benefits of disclosure in African-American women who have HIV. *Journal of Family Psychology, 11,* 23–34.

Bradley-Springer, L. (2008). Women and HIV infection. *Journal of the Association of Nurses in AIDS Care, 19*(1), 1–2.

Brown, K. M. P. (2004). *Management guidelines for nurse practitioners working with women.* Philadelphia: F. A. Davis.

Bruckner, H., & Bearman, P. (2005). After the promise: The STD consequences of adolescent virginity pledges. *Journal of Adolescent Health, 36,* 271–278.

Burrage, J. W., Zimet, G. D., Cox, D. S., Cox, A. D., Mays, R. M., Fife, R. S., et al. (2008). The Centers for Disease Control and Prevention revised recommendations for HIV testing: Reactions of women attending community health centers. *Journal of the Association of Nurses in AIDS Care, 19*(1), 66–74.

Cagampang, H. H., Barth, R. P., Korpi, M., & Kirby, D. (1997). Education Now and Babies Later (ENABL): Life history of a campaign to postpone sexual involvement. *Family Planning Perspective, 29,* 109–114.

Card, J. J., Amarillas, A., Conner, A., Akers, D. D., Solomon, J., & DiClemente, R. J. (2007). *The complete HIV/AIDS teaching kit.* New York: Springer Publishing.

Centers for Disease and Control and Prevention. (1981). *Pneumocystis* pneumonia—Los Angeles. *Morbidity and Mortality Weekly Report, 30,* 250–252.

Centers for Disease and Control and Prevention. (1998). U.S. Public Health Service guidelines for the management of health-care worker exposures to HIV and recommendations for postexposure prophylaxis. *Morbidity and Mortality Weekly Report, 47*(RR-7), 3.

Centers for Disease Control and Prevention. (1999a). Guidelines for national human immunodeficiency virus case surveillance, including monitoring for human immunodeficiency virus and acquired immunodeficiency syndrome. *Morbidity and Mortality Weekly Report, 48*(RR-13), 1–28.

Centers for Disease Control and Prevention. (1999b). U.S. Public Health Service (USPHS) and Infectious Diseases Society of America (IDSA) guidelines for the prevention of opportunistic infections in persons infected with human immunodeficiency virus. *Morbidity and Mortality Weekly Report, 48*(RR-10), 1–59.

Centers for Disease Control and Prevention. (2004). Standard precautions. Retrieved November 2007, from http://www.cdc.gov/ncidod/dhqp/gl_isolation_standard.html

Centers for Disease Control and Prevention. (2005). Universal precautions for the prevention of transmission of HIV and other blood borne infections. Retrieved November 2007, from www.cdc.gov/ncidod/dhap/bp-universal_precautions.html

Centers for Disease Control and Prevention. (2006a). Sexually transmitted disease treatment guidelines 2006. *Morbidity and Mortality Weekly Report, 55*(RR-11), 1–94.

Centers for Disease Control and Prevention. (2006b). *HIV/AIDS among women who have sex with women.* Retrieved November 2007, from http://www.cdc.gov/hiv

Centers for Disease Control and Prevention. (2006c). Revised recommendations for HIV testing of adults, adolescents, and pregnant women in health-care settings. *Morbidity and Mortality Weekly Report, 55*(RR-14), 1–27.

Centers for Disease Control and Prevention. (2007a). *HIV/AIDS among women.* Retrieved November 2007, from http://www.cdc.gov/hiv

Centers for Disease Control and Prevention. (2007b). *HIV/AIDS Surveillance Report, 17,* 1–54.

Clark, R. A., Theall, K. P., Amdee, A. M., & Kissinger, P. J. (2007). Frequent douching and clinical outcomes among HIV-infected women. *Sexually Transmitted Diseases, 34*(12), 985–990.

Cohen, P. T. (1999). Understanding HIV disease: Hallmarks, clinical spectrum and what we need to know. In P. T. Cohen, M. A. Sande, & P. A. Volberding (Eds.), *AIDS knowledge base* (3rd ed., pp. 175–194). Philadelphia: Lippincott, Williams & Wilkins.

Constantine, N. (2003). HIV antibody assays. In L. Pierperl, S. Coffey, O. Bacon, & P. Volberding (Eds.), *HIV InSite Knowledge Base.* San Francisco: Center for HIV Information, University of California, San Francisco.

Cotter, A., Potter, J. E., & Tessler, N. (2006). Management of HIV/AIDS in women. In J. Beal & J. J. Orrick (Eds.), *HIV/AIDS primary care guide* (pp. 533–546). Norwalk, CT: Crown House.

Dabis, F., Msellati, P., Dunn, D., et al. (1993). Estimating the rate of mother-to-child transmission of HIV: Report of a workshop on methodological issues Ghent (Belgium), 17–20 February 1992. *AIDS, 7,* 1139–1148.

DeCarlo, P., & Gomez, C. (1997). *What are women who have sex with women's HIV prevention needs?* Center for AIDS Prevention Studies, University of California, San Francisco and Harvard AIDS Institute. Retrieved November 2007, from http://www.caps.ucsf.edu

DHHS Panel on Antiretoviral Guidelines for Adults and Adolescents. (2006). *Guidelines for the use of antiretroviral agents in HIV-1 infected adults and adolescents.* Retrieved November 2007, from http://www.AIDSinfo.nih.gov

Espinoza, L., Hall, I., Hardnett, F., Selik, R. M., Ling, Q., & Lee, L. M. (2007). Characteristics of persons with heterosexually acquired HIV infection, United States 1999–2004. *American Journal of Public Health, 97*(1), 144–149.

Feinberg, J., & Maenza, J. (2005), Primary medical care. In J. R. Anderson (Ed.), *A clinical guide to the clinical care of women with HIV* (pp. 91–166). Rockville, MD: U.S. Department of Health and Human Services, HIV/AIDS Bureau.

Fisher, J. D., Cornman, D. H., Osborn, C. Y., Amico, K. R., Fisher, W. A., and Friedland, G. A. (2004). Clinician-initiated HIV risk-reduction intervention for HIV-positive persons. *Journal of Acquired Immune Deficiency Syndromes, 37*(Suppl. 2), S78–S87.

Fogel, C. I., & Black, B. (2008). *Sexually transmitted infections, including HIV: Impact on women's reproductive health.* White Plains, NY: March of Dimes.

Fowler, M., Bertolli, J. & Nieberg, P. (1997). Women and HIV. *Obstetrics and Gynecology, 24*(4), 705–729.

Grella, C. E., Anglin, M. D., & Annon, J. J. (1996). HIV risk behaviors among women in methadone maintenance treatment. *Substance Abuse and Misuse, 31,* 277–301.

Harris, R. M., & Kavanaugh, K. H. (1995). Perception of AIDS risk and high-risk behaviors among women in methadone maintenance treatment. *AIDS Education and Prevention, 7*(5), 415–428.

Hatcher, R. M., Truessel, J., Stewart, F., Cates, W. Jr., Stewart, G., Guest, F., et al. (Eds.). (2004). *Contraceptive technology* (18th rev. ed.). New York: Springer Publishing.

Henderson, D. (1997, November). Transition to the community for incarcerated addicted women. Presented at the 49th Annual Meeting of the American Society of Criminology, San Diego, CA.

Hessol, N. A., Gandhi, M., & Greenblatt, R. M. (2005). Epidemiology and natural history of HIV infection in women. In J. R. Anderson (Ed.), *A clinical guide to the clinical care of women with HIV* (pp. 1–34). Rockville, MD: Department of Health and Human Services, HIV/AIDS Bureau.

Ioannidis, J. P., Abrams, E. J., Ammann, A., et al. (2001). Perinatal transmission of human immunodeficiency virus type 1 by pregnant women with RNA virus loads < 1000 copies/ml. *Journal of Infectious Diseases, 183,* 539–545.

Jacobson, M. A., & Hicks, M. L. (2000). *HIV treatment: A primer for primary care clinicians.* West Conshohocken, PA: Meniscus.

Jemmott, L. S., & Brown, E. J. (2003, January/February). Reducing HIV sexual risk among African American women who use drugs: Hearing their voices. *Journal of the Association of Nurses in AIDS Care,* 19–26.

Jemmott, L. S., Jemmott, J. B., & O'Leary, A. (2007). Effects on sexual risk behavior and STD rate of brief HIV/STD prevention interventions for African American women in primary care settings: Effects on sexual risk behavior and STD incidence. *American Journal of Public Health, 97,* 1034–1040.

Kaiser Family Foundation. (2006). *Women and HIV/AIDS in the United States.* Retrieved November 2007, from http://www.kff.org

Kalichman, S. C. (1998). *Preventing AIDS: A sourcebook for behavioral interventions.* Mahwah, NJ: Lawrence Erlbaum Associates.

Kearney, M. H. (2001). *Perinatal impact of alcohol, tobacco, and other drugs* (2nd ed.). White Plains, NY: March of Dimes.

Kurth, A. (1998). Promoting sexual health in the age of HIV/AIDS. *Journal of Nurse-Midwifery, 43*(30), 162–181.

Kwakwa, H. A., & Ghobrial, M. W. (2003). Female-to-female transmission of human immunodeficiency virus. *Clinical Infectious Diseases, 36*(1), 40–41.

Lichtenstein, B. (2004). Domestic violence, sexual ownership, and HIV risk in women in the Deep South. *Social Science and Medicine, 60*(4), 701–714.

Lifson, A., & Rybicki, S. (2007). Routine opt-out HIV testing. *Lancet, 369,* 539–540.

Long, E. M., Martin, H. L., & Kriess, J. K. (2006). Gender differences in HIV-1 diversity at time of infection. *Nature Medicine, 6*(1), 71–75.

Maman, S. C. (2000). The intersection of HIV and violence: Directions for future research and interventions. *Social Science and Medicine, 50,* 459–478.

Marrazzo, J. M. (2007). Sexually transmitted diseases in women who have sex with women. In J. D. Klausner & E. W. Hook III (Eds.), *Current diagnosis and treatment of sexually transmitted diseases* (pp. 177–180). New York: McGraw Hill Medical.

Mays, V. M., & Cochran, S. D. (1988, November). Issues in the perception of AIDS risk and risk reduction activities by Black and Hispanic/Latina women. *American Psychologist,* 949–957.

McCoy, H. V., McCoy, C. B., & Lai, S. (1998). Effectiveness of HIV interventions among women drug users. *Women and Health, 27*(1–2), 49–66.

Miotti, P. G., Taha, T. E., Kumwenda, N. I., Broadhead, R., Mtimavalye, L. A., Van der Hoeven, L., et al. (1999). HIV transmission through breastfeeding: A study in Malawi. *Journal of the American Medical Association, 282*, 744–749.

Miller, S., Exner, T. M., Williams, S. P., & Ehrhardt, A. A. (2000). A gender-specific intervention for at-risk women in the U.S.A. *AIDS Care, 13*(3), 603–612.

Nadler, J. P. (2006). Pathophysiology of HIV infection. In *HIV infection in women.*

National Institute of Allergy and Infectious Diseases. (2006). HIV Infection in Women. Washington, DC (NIH U.S. DHHS, NIAID).

Nelson, A. L. (2006). Introduction to sexually transmitted infections. In A. L. Nelson & J. Woodward (Eds.), *Sexually transmitted diseases: A practical guide for primary care.* Totowa, NJ: Human Press.

Perinatal HIV Guidelines Working Group. (2007). *Public Health Service Task Force recommendations for use of antiretroviral drugs in pregnant HIV-1 infected women for maternal health and interventions to reduce perinatal HIV-1 transmission in the United States.* Retrieved December 2007, from http://aidsinfo.nih.gov/Content Files/PerinatalGL.pdf

Quinn, T. C., Wawer, M. J., Sewankambo, N., Serwadda, D., Chuanjun, C., Wabwire-Mangen, et al. (2000). Viral load and heterosexual transmission of human immunodeficiency virus type 1. *New England Journal of Medicine, 342*(13), 921–929.

Rieg, G. (2006). HIV infection and AIDS. In A. L. Nelson & J. Woodward (Eds.), *Sexually transmitted diseases* (pp. 99–125). Totowa, NJ: Humana Press.

Squires, K. E. (2007). Management of pregnancy in HIV-infected women. In E. P. Seekins, E. King, K. Obholtz, & S. McGuire (Eds.), *HIV/AIDS annual update 2007* (pp. 151–169). London: Postgraduate Institute for Medicine and Clinical Care Options. Retrieved November 2007, from http://www.clinicaloptions.com/ccohiv2007

Stine, G. J. (2008). *AIDS update.* New York: McGraw-Hill.

Stratton, P., & Alexander, N. (1997). Heterosexual spread of HIV infection. In D. Cotton & D. Watts (Eds.), *The medical management of AIDS in women* (pp. 115–124). New York: Wiley-Liss.

Upchurch, D. M., & Kusunoki, Y. (2004). Associations between forced sex, sexual and protective practices and sexually transmitted diseases among a national sample of adolescent girls. *Women's Health Issues, 14*(3), 75–84.

Valdiserri, R. (2007). Late HIV diagnosis: Bad medicine and worse public health. *PLoS Medicine, 4*, 1–2.

Varney, H., Kriebs, J. M., & Gegor, C. L. (2004). *Varney's midwifery* (4th ed.). Sudbury, MA: Jones & Bartlett.

Wang, C., & Celum, C. (2001). Prevention of HIV. In J. R. Anderson (Ed.), *A guide to the clinical care of women with HIV.* HSRA/HAB. Retrieved December 15, 2007 from hab.hrsa.gov/womencare.htm

Wechsberg, W. M., Lam, W. K., Zule, W., & Bobashev G. V. (2004). Reemphasizing the context of women's risk for HIV/AIDS in the United States. *Women's Health Issues, 15*(4), 154–156.

Wechsberg, W. M., Lam, W. K., Zule, W., Hall, G., Middlesteadt, R., & Edwards, J. (2003). Violence, homelessness, and HIV risk among crack-using African-American women. *Substance Use and Misuse, 38*(3–6), 669–700.

Wohfeiler, D., & Ellen, J. (2007). The limits of behavioral intervention for HIV prevention. In L. Cohen, V. Chavez, & S. Chehimi (Eds.), *Prevention is primary: Strategies for community wellbeing.* Hoboken, NJ: Jossey-Bass.

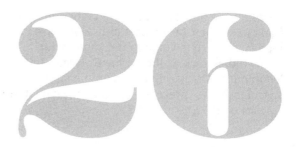

Cardiovascular Disease in Women

Susanna Garner Cunningham

Atherosclerotic cardiovascular disease (ASCVD) is the leading cause of death in the United States, Canada, and most industrialized nations. By 2020, it is projected to be the leading cause of death worldwide (Murray & Lopez, 1997). Despite these facts, many women and health care providers do not consider cardiovascular disease to be a major component of women's health.

Women need information on how to prevent, delay, and recognize cardiovascular disease. They need to learn that behaviors that prevent cardiovascular disease also reduce the occurrence of the other major chronic diseases that disable and kill women (LaCroix, Newton, LeVeille, & Wallace, 1997). Although women in industrialized countries tend to live longer than men, they spend more of their living years disabled (Mathers, Sadana, Salomon, Murray, & Lopez, 2001). Healthy lifestyles have been demonstrated to reduce disability; therefore, if women were supported in adopting these lifestyles, they would have the potential of more healthy and productive lives (Fries, 1980; Lloyd-Jones et al., 2006; Vita, Terry, Hubert, & Fries, 1998). Data from large prospective, cohort studies indicate that women who are physically active, do not smoke, have healthy diets, no obesity, and who consume small amounts of alcoholic beverages are at an approximately 80% lower risk of developing or dying from cardiovascular disease that women who do not have such healthy habits (Akesson, Weismayer, Newby, & Wolk, 2007; Daviglus et al., 2004; Hu, Li, Colditz, Willett, & Manson, 2003; Stampfer, Hu, Manson, Rimm, & Willett, 2000). Specifically, for optimal care, women and their care providers need to understand the following key factors related to cardiovascular disease in women. They need to know:

1. All women are at high risk for atherosclerotic cardiovascular disease.

2. The activities that reduce the risk of cardiovascular disease will work synergistically to reduce the risk of other chronic diseases.

3. How to identify risk, and which risk reduction strategies have been demonstrated to be effective in women.

4. How to recognize the signs and symptoms of myocardial infarction and stroke, the two manifestations of CVD with acute onset.

5. Which diagnostic strategies are recommended for women.

6. Treatment strategies for cardiovascular disease in women.

One challenge in assessing and managing cardiovascular disease and risk in women is the relative lack of randomized controlled trial data on the efficacy of diagnostic tools and interventions in women. Much of the information about risk in women comes from large prospective observational studies such as the Nurses Health Study, Women's Health Study, Iowa Women's Health Study in the United States, and the Million Women Study in the United Kingdom. As wonderful as it is to have the data from these ongoing epidemiologic studies, the data are primarily obtained by self-report, have a greater potential to be confounded than data from randomized controlled trials, and the women being studied are not necessarily representative of all the women in the country where the study was done. Some of the large risk factor reduction trials have included women, but the required inclusion of women in clinical trials is a relatively recent occurrence (Healy, 1991a, 1991b). The one topic on which we now have data from randomized controlled trials in women relates to the use of hormone replacement therapy for women after menopause. The results from studies such as the Women's Health Initiative have led to major changes in the recommendations for cardiovascular disease prevention and management in women (Mosca et al., 2007).

DEFINITIONS

The focus of this chapter is on atherosclerotic cardiovascular disease in women. Atherosclerosis results from an interaction of plaque accumulation with thrombotic and inflammatory pathologic processes that accelerate the accumulation of fatty deposits, foam cells, macrophages, T cells, smooth muscle cells, and a fibrous cap layer beneath the endothelium of large and medium sized arteries (Croce & Libby, 2007; Hansson & Libby, 2006; Ross, 1999). The most common vessels to be affected by atherosclerotic cardiovascular disease are the aorta, the coronary arteries, carotid arteries, renal arteries, and femoral arteries. The term coronary heart disease (CHD) refers to a subset of atherosclerotic disease in the coronary arteries. Typically, the term CHD refers to both the disease in the vessels and its manifestations that include myocardial infarction, stable and unstable angina pectoris, sudden cardiac death, and heart failure.

EPIDEMIOLOGY OF CARDIOVASCULAR DISEASE IN WOMEN

In the United States, the National Center for Health Statistics (NCHS) provides an annual analysis of the leading causes of death categorized by age, sex, and ethnicity. The data from 2004 confirm that, for women (and men), the first three leading causes of death, in order, are heart disease, cancer, and stroke (National Center for Health Statistics, 2006a). In addition, diabetes mellitus and kidney diseases, the fifth and ninth causes of death in women, respectively, are also closely linked with ASCVD.

To put the risk of cardiovascular disease in perspective, it is helpful to look at how the causes of death in women change over the life span. As discussed below, many women are more concerned about their risks of developing breast and ovarian cancer than they are about heart disease. Cancers (categorized as malignant neoplasms) are, in fact, the leading causes of death in women between the ages of 35 and 65, but, above age 65, heart disease is the leading cause of death. Even in the younger women, heart disease is the second leading cause of death in Black women and the third leading cause of death in White women ages 35 to 44, and then moves to second place for all women between the ages of 45 and 65 years

(Anderson, 2001). The importance of cancer as a cause of death in younger women is one of the reasons why care providers need to integrate their information about chronic disease risk prevention so that women will not feel that they are getting competing advice about healthy lifestyle choices (Cunningham, 1998).

Cardiovascular disease has been a greater cause of death for women than men in the United States since 1984 (American Heart Association, 2006b). It was estimated that, in 2004, CVD caused 461,152 deaths in women and that about 53 percent of the CVD deaths each year are in women. According to the American Heart Association (2006b), approximately 23% of women over age 40 who are aware they had had a myocardial infarction (MI) die within 1 year of the event compared to 18% of men. It is thought that the mortality rate following MI is higher in women because women are older when they have their MI (American Heart Association, 2006b).

Worldwide CVD morbidity and mortality rate estimates depend on a country's ability to collect, analyze, and publish vital statistics, with the result that the most information is available from industrialized countries, particularly Europe and the United Kingdom. In all the European countries, CVD is the leading cause of death in women (Stramba-Badiale et al., 2006). In Canada, CVD is responsible for 36% of deaths in women and 34% of deaths in men (American Heart Association, 2006a). The World Health Organization's Multinational Monitoring of Trends and Determinants in Cardiovascular Disease project has reported that death rates from CVD in women are highest in Glasgow, Scotland; Belfast, Northern Ireland; Newcastle, Australia; and Warsaw, Poland (Tunstall-Pedoe et al., 1999).

Women's Perceptions and Knowledge of Cardiovascular Risk

Despite this wealth of data indicating women's high probability of developing cardiovascular disease, surveys have indicated that many women are unaware of this risk (Biswas, Calhoun, Bosworth, & Bastian, 2002; Legato, Padus, & Slaughter, 1997; Mosca et al., 2000). The hopeful news is that awareness rates among women in the United States are increasing—30% of women surveyed in 1997 and 55% in 2005 were able to identify that CVD was the leading cause of death in women (Mosca et al., 2006). Unfortunately, there was large difference in CVD awareness between women of different ethnic backgrounds; awareness among Blacks and Hispanics was 38% and 34%, respectively, compared to 62% among White women. Women of all ethnic groups were less well informed about the risk factors for CVD, with less than half who knew the recommended risk factor levels (such as what their blood pressure should be).

A telephone survey of 1,002 women in the United States found that, even though most women felt they were knowledgeable about women's health, 44% of the respondents felt they were unlikely to have a heart attack (Legato et al., 1997). In addition, even though most of the women saw a physician yearly for a check-up, over half the women said their physicians did not talk to them about their risk of developing heart disease. A nonrandomized study reported the results from mailed a questionnaire returned by 328 women veterans over age 35 without heart disease who received care at a veterans hospital in North Carolina (Biswas et al., 2002). Among the women with at least one CVD risk factor, 66% were not worried about heart disease, while, among women with four or more risk factors, 41% were not worried.

Even women who have just been diagnosed with CHD are not well-informed about their risks. Oliver-McNeil and Artinian (2002) mailed a questionnaire to a small nonrandomly chosen group of women over age 18 who had been evaluated for CHD or who had experienced an MI in the prior week. Thirty-three women with a mean age of 66 years returned questionnaires. The results indicated that the women were unaware of their own risk factors; for example, although 17 of the women had hyperlipidemia noted in their records, only 4 women reported that they knew they had high cholesterol. Fourteen women had hypertension documented in their records, but only 6 reported they had high blood pressure. Although this study was small, with a convenience sample and untested data collection instruments, the results are consistent with the surveys of women without disease. These data raise the strong possibility that many women who have been diagnosed with heart disease are lacking the knowledge they need to manage their own care.

Overall, these data about women's perceptions and knowledge of their risks of heart disease expose a large problem with significant consequences. If women are not aware they are at risk, they will not be motivated to institute preventive behaviors and, perhaps even more importantly, they will not recognize a CVD event when it occurs and will therefore delay seeking care. Studies have reported that women may delay seeking medical care longer than men, and their reasons for delay may be different than men's (Ashton, 1999; Canto et al., 2000; Lefler & Bondy, 2004; Marrugat et al., 1998; Menon, Pandey, & Margenstern, 1998; Moser, McKinley, Dracup, & Chung, 2005).

RISK FACTORS AND RISK REDUCTION

Knowledge about the relationship between risk factors and the occurrence of clinical events related to ASCVD is critical to clinicians caring for women for four rea-sons. First, strategies for primary and secondary prevention of cardiovascular disease are grounded in the research on risk and risk reduction efficacy (Buse et al., 2007; Ebrahim & Smith, 1997; Grover, Paquet, Levinton, Coupal, & Zowall, 1998; Hu & Willett, 2002; Mosca et al., 2007; Nabel, 2000; Stampfer et al., 2000). Secondly, clinicians need to know the risk factors to ensure that their assessment and management of their clients is optimal. Third, information about risk factors and conditions can be used to stratify women according to their degree of risk. One challenge in this area is keeping up with the latest research and recommendations about what factors are not unique to CVD. Finally, favorable risk factor profiles are associated with lower mortality rates and health care costs (Daviglus et al., 1998; Lloyd-Jones et al., 2006).

Risk factors for ASCVD in women can be categorized on at least two dimensions. First, risk factors traditionally have been discussed according to whether it is possible to modify them. Age, gender, and family history are the three nonmodifiable risk factors. The list of potentially modifiable risk factor is long and growing. Second, for clinicians, these potentially modifiable risk factors can be divided into at least two sub-groups: (1) risk factors for which there are data showing that modification of the risk factors results in a reduction of both cardiovascular morbidity and mortality and also all-cause mortality (there is no benefit to not dying of heart disease if the treatment causes the patient to have an equal chance of dying of something else) and (2) risk factors for which we do not yet have data on the benefit of risk reduction or for which there may even be risks associated with risk reduction. Two good examples of risk factors whose modification has been shown to be associated with increased risk are the use of antioxidant vitamin supplements and hormone replacement therapy after menopause (Kris-Etherton, Lichtenstein, Howard, Steinberg, & Witztum, 2004; Mosca et al., 2007). Even though the literature usually discusses risk factors as being either modifiable or not modifiable, experienced clinicians are aware of the inherent difficulties in actually modifying some of them. Body weight management, for example, is a challenge for most, even when we are well aware of the risks associated with obesity. For this reason, it may be more realistic to refer to some risk factors as potentially modifiable.

Nonmodifiable Risk Factors

Although the three key nonmodifiable risk factors—age, gender, and family history—cannot be altered, it is important that clinicians note them and include the information in the client's risk assessment. Age as a risk factor is easy: the older you are, the greater the risk. In relation to gender, women can develop ASCVD signs or symptoms at any age; however, women in general tend to manifest disease about 10 years later than men—unless they are diabetic (diabetes mellitus is discussed in more detail later in this chapter). Data from a large Italian study known as the GISSI-2 Trial indicated that a family history of heart disease among first-degree relatives was important for women (Roncaglioni et al., 1992). Women who had a positive family history and who smoked were 14 times more likely to have a myocardial infarction, and women who had a positive family history plus dyslipidemia were 8 times more likely to have a myocardial infarction than women without these risk factors. Also, because research has indicated that the children of women with premature coronary heart disease have levels of CVD risk factors that are higher than is typically found in the general population, it is important to suggest that women presenting with heart disease risk factors or symptoms bring their children for assessment (Allen & Blumenthal, 1998; Lloyd-Jones et al., 2004).

Modifiable Risk Factors

There are four modifiable risk factors for which there are data demonstrating that risk reduction results in reduced morbidity and mortality: cigarette smoking, high blood pressure, dyslipidemia, and a sedentary lifestyle. Diabetes mellitus and obesity are also important risk factors for women because of their documented influence on the risk of adverse outcomes, so they will be discussed individually in the next section. Finally, some of the other factors and conditions that have been associated with increases in risk will be mentioned. Only future research will show the significance of these factors for the prevention and management of CVD. Table 26.1 summarizes the current recommended risk factor management goals for CVD prevention in women (Mosca et al., 2007).

The impact of risk factors on an individual's lifetime risk of CVD and survival has been examined using data from the Framingham study (Lloyd-Jones et al., 2006). The risk for CVD and survival were compared in persons aged 50 who did or did not have any of the following risk factors: obesity, smoking, hypertension, dyslipidemia, and diabetes. Women with no risk factors at age 50 were estimated to have a 39% risk of developing CVD by age 95, while women with two or more risk factors had a 50% risk. Women with optimal levels of risk factors had even less risk and longer predicted survivals than women with two or more risk factors, with the risks being 8% versus 50%, respectively, and the survival times 39 years compared to 31 years. Having diabetes mellitus at age 50 had the greatest impact of all the factors studied in increasing one's lifetime risk of CVD. Although the Framingham population is predominantly White and from one geographic area, the data are reflective of the White U.S. population, but may not be as representative of other ethnic populations (Lloyd-Jones et al., 2006).

Smoking

Smoking or exposure to second-hand smoke increases the accumulation of atherosclerotic plaque in women's arteries, and quitting smoking has been documented to reduce this risk and to improve survival of women who have CVD events (Burke et al., 1998; Caralis, Deligonul, Kern, & Cohen, 1992; Hermanson, Omenn, Kronmal, Gersh, & Study, 1988; Howard et al., 1994; Katz, Holmes, Power, & Wise, 1995; Kawachi et al., 1993; LaCroix et al., 1991; Otten, Teutsch, Williamson, & Marks, 1990; Palmer, Rosenberg, & Shapiro, 1989; Rosenberg, Palmer, Rao, & Adams-Campbell, 1999; Rosenberg, Palmer, & Shapiro, 1990; Tunstall-Pedoe, Woodward, Tavendale, A'Brook, & McCluskey, 1997; Wilson, Garrison, & Castelli, 1985; Witteman et al., 1993). Autopsy studies of children and young people (up to age 40) have revealed a correlation between aortic and coronary artery atherosclerosis and a history of smoking (Berenson et al., 1998; McGill et al., 2001). The challenge for policymakers, public health, and direct care providers is to convince girls and young women to not start smoking and to support quitting in those who are addicted. In 2006, the National Center for Health Statistics (2007) reported that 19% of women over age 18 were smokers.

High Blood Pressure

The higher an individual's systolic or diastolic blood pressure, the greater the risk of morbidity and mortality from cardiovascular or cerebrovascular disease (Glynn et al., 1995; Hsia et al., 2007; Lewington, Clarke, Qizilbash, Peto, & Collins, 2002). The National Center for Health Statistics (2007) currently estimates that approximately 32% of Americans have high blood pressure, making it the most prevalent of the CVD risk factors in women. NCHS also estimates that about 82% of women older than age 75 have hypertension. An analysis of data from the Atherosclerosis in Communities study indicated that hypertension markedly increased the risk of coronary heart disease for Black women (Jones et al., 2002). Among the Women's Health Initiative enrollees, the prevalence of hypertension was 38% (Oparil, 2006).

The National High Blood Pressure Program at the National Heart, Lung, and Blood Institute (NHLBI) produces the Joint National Committee Reports on the Prevention, Detection, Evaluation, and Treatment of High Blood Pressure at intervals dictated by the publication of relevant research. These documents, usually referred to as JNC reports, set the standard of practice for the care of persons with high blood pressure. The most recent JNC document can be obtained from the NHLBI Web site, which is www.nhlbi.nih.gov. All professionals providing care to women with high blood pressure must read the JNC-VII document if they wish to provide

26.1 | Guidelines for the Prevention of Cardiovascular Disease in Women: Clinical Recommendations

Lifestyle interventions	**Cigarette smoking**	Women should not smoke and should avoid environmental tobacco smoke. Provide counseling, nicotine replacement, and other pharmacotherapy as indicated with a behavioral program or formal smoking cessation program.
	Physical activity	Women should accumulate a minimum of 30 minutes of moderate-intensity physical activity (e.g., brisk walking) on most, and preferably all, days of the week. Women who need to lose weight or sustain weight loss should accumulate a minimum of 60 to 90 minutes of moderate-intensity physical activity (e.g., brisk walking) on most, and preferably all, days of the week.
	Rehabilitation	A comprehensive risk-reduction regimen—such as cardiovascular or stroke rehabilitation or a physician-guided home- or community-based exercise training program—should be recommended to women with a recent acute coronary syndrome or coronary intervention, new-onset or chronic angina, recent cerebrovascular event, or peripheral arterial disease.
	Dietary intake	Women should consume a diet rich in fruits and vegetables; choose whole-grain, high-fiber foods; consume fish, especially oily fish,[a] at least twice a week; limit intake of saturated fat to less than 10% of energy, and if possible to less than 7%, cholesterol to under 300 mg/d, alcohol intake to no more than one drink per day,[b] and sodium intake to less than 2.3 g per day (approximately 1 tsp salt). Consumption of trans-fatty acids should be as low as possible (e.g., < 1% of energy).
	Weight maintenance/reduction	Women should maintain or lose weight through an appropriate balance of physical activity, caloric intake, and a formal behavioral program when indicated to maintain or achieve a body mass index between 18.5 and 24.9 kg/m^2 and a waist circumference of 35 inches or less.
	Omega-3 fatty acids	As an adjunct to diet, omega-3 fatty acids in capsule form (approximately 850 to 1,000 mg of eicosapentaenoic acid and docosahexaenoic acid may be considered in women with CHF (Congestive heart failure), and higher doses (2 to 4 g) may be used for treatment of women with high triglyceride levels.
	Depression	Consider screening women with coronary heart disease for depression and refer or treat when indicated.
Major risk factor interventions	**Blood pressure: optimal level and lifestyle**	Encourage an optimal blood pressure of lower than 120/80 mm Hg through lifestyle approaches such as weight control, increased physical activity, alcohol moderation, sodium restriction, and increased consumption of fresh fruits, vegetables, and low-fat dairy products.
	Blood pressure: pharmacotherapy	Pharmacotherapy is indicated when blood pressure is 140/90 mm Hg or higher or at an even lower blood pressure in the setting of chronic kidney disease or diabetes (130/80 mm Hg or higher). Thiazide diuretics should be part of the drug regimen for most patients unless contraindicated or if there are compelling indications for other agents in specific vascular diseases. Initial treatment of high-risk women[c] should be with beta blockers and/or ACE inhibitors/ARBs, with the addition of other drugs such as thiazides as needed to achieve goal blood pressure.
	Lipid and lipoprotein levels: optimal levels and lifestyle	The following levels of lipids and lipoprotein in women should be encouraged through lifestyle approaches: LDL-C < 100mg/dl, HDL-C > 50 mg/dl, triglycerides < 150 mg/dl, and non-HDL-C (total cholesterol minus HDL cholesterol) < 130 mg/dl. If a woman is at high risk[c] or has hypercholesterolemia, intake of saturated fat should be < 7% and cholesterol intake < 200 mg/dl.
	Lipids: pharmacotherapy for LDL lowering, high-risk women	Utilize LDL-C-lowering drug therapy simultaneously with lifestyle therapy in women with coronary heart disease to achieve an LDL-C < 100 mg/dl and similarly in women with other atherosclerotic CVD or diabetes mellitus or 10-year absolute risk > 20%. A reduction to < 70 mg/dl is reasonable in very-high-risk women[d] with coronary heart disease and may require an LDL-lowering drug combination.

(continued)

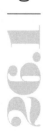

26.1 Guidelines for the Prevention of Cardiovascular Disease in Women: Clinical Recommendations (continued)

Major risk factor interventions (*continued*)	**Lipids: pharmacotherapy for LDL lowering, other at-risk women**	Utilize LDL-C-lowering therapy if LDL-C level is = 130 mg/dl with lifestyle therapy and there are multiple risk factors and 10-year absolute risk 10% to 20%.
		Utilize LDL-C-lowering therapy if LDL-C level is = 160 mg/dl with lifestyle therapy and multiple risk factors even if 10-year absolute risk is < 10.
		Utilize LDL-C-lowering therapy if LDL-C level is = 190 mg/dl regardless of the presence or absence of other risk factors or cardiovascular disease on lifestyle therapy.
	Lipids: pharmacotherapy for low HDL or elevated non-HDL, high-risk women	Utilize niacin[d] or fibrate therapy when HDL-C is low or non-HDL-C is elevated in high-risk women[c] after LDL-C goal is reached.
	Lipids: pharmacotherapy for low HDL or elevated non-HDL, other at-risk women	Consider niacin[d] or fibrate therapy when HDL-C is low or non-HDL-C is elevated after LDL-C goal is reached in women with multiple risk factors and a 10-year absolute risk 10% to 20%.
	Diabetes mellitus	Lifestyle and pharmacotherapy should be used as indicated in women with diabetes to achieve and HbA$_{1c}$ < 7% if this can be accomplished without significant hypoglycemia.
Preventive drug interventions	**Aspirin: high risk**	Aspirin therapy (75 to 325 mg/d)[f] should be used in high-risk[c] women unless contraindicated.
		If a high-risk woman[c] is intolerant of aspirin therapy, clopidogrel should be substituted.
	Aspirin: other at-risk or healthy women	In women 65 years of age and older, consider aspirin therapy (81 mg daily or 100 mg every other day) if blood pressure is controlled and benefit for ischemic stroke and myocardial infarction prevention is likely to outweigh risk of gastrointestinal bleeding and hemorrhagic stroke and in women younger than 65 years of age when benefit for ischemic stroke prevention is likely to outweigh adverse effects of therapy.
		Beta blockers should be used indefinitely in all women after myocardial infarction, acute coronary syndrome, or left ventricular dysfunction with or without heart failure symptoms, unless contraindicated.
	ACE inhibitors/ARBs	ACE (angiotension converting enzyme) inhibitors should be used (unless contraindicated) in women after myocardial infarction and in those with clinical evidence of heart failure or a left ventricular ejection fraction = 40% or with diabetes mellitus. In women after myocardial infarction and in those with clinical evidence of heart failure and a left ventricular ejection fraction = 40% or with diabetes mellitus who are intolerant of ACE inhibitors, ARBs (angiotension receptor blockers) should be used instead.
	Aldosterone blockade	Use aldosterone blockade after myocardial infarction in women who do not have significant renal dysfunction or hyperkalemia who are already receiving therapeutic doses of an ACE inhibitor and beta blocker, and have a left ventricular ejection fraction = 40% with symptomatic heart failure.

Note. From "Evidence-Based Guidelines for Cardiovascular Disease Prevention in Women: 2007 Update," by L. Mosca, C. L. Banka, E. J. Benjamin, K. Berra, C. Bushnell, R. J. Dolor, et al., 2007, *Circulation,* 115(11), pp. 1481–1501.

[a] Pregnant and lactating women should avoid eating fish potentially high in methylmercury (e.g., shark, swordfish, king mackerel, or tile fish) and should eat up to 12 oz/wk of a variety of fish and shellfish low in mercury and check the Environmental Protection Agency and the US Food and Drug Administration's Web sites for updates and local advisories about safety of local catch.

[b] A drink equivalent is equal to a 12-oz bottle of beer, a 5-oz glass of wine, or a 1.5 oz shot of 80-proof spirit.

[c] Criteria for high risk include established CHD, cerebrovascular disease, peripheral arterial disease, abdominal aortic aneurysm, end-stage or chronic renal disease, diabetes mellitus, and 10-year Framingham risk > 20%.

[c] Criteria for very high risk include established CVD plus any of the following: multiple major risk factors, severe and poorly controlled risk factors, diabetes mellitus.

[e] Dietary supplement niacin should not be used as a substitute for prescription niacin.

[f] After percutaneous interventions with stent placement or coronary artery bypass grafting within previous year and in women with noncoronary forms of CVD, use current guidelines for aspirin and clopidogrel.

quality care. Choice of initial therapy for blood pressure treatment is based on the individual's blood pressure stage and risk stratification, which is based on the presence of other CVD risk factors and the presence of target organ disease as shown in Table 26.2.

The National High Blood Pressure Program uses the concept of goal blood pressures to support the achievement of controlled pressure (< 140/90 mm Hg) for persons with hypertension. The current recommendations for blood pressure control in the United States state that normal blood pressure is ≤120/80 mm Hg. Persons are considered to be prehypertensive if their pressures are 120–139/80–89 mm Hg and definitely hypertensive if their pressures are ≥140/90 mm Hg (Chobanian et al., 2003). That these categories represent levels of risk was supported by an analysis of data from over 60,000 participants in the Women's Health Initiative. The results revealed that normotensive women had a 10-year incidence of CVD events that was 3.6%, compared to 7.1% in prehypertensive women and 14% in hypertensive women (Hsia et al., 2007). Goal setting was demonstrated to be an effective management strategy in the Hypertension Detection and Follow-up Program Clinical Trial (Daugherty, 1983; Hypertension Detection and Follow-up Program Cooperative Group, 1979, 1982). The JNC-VII report sets a lower data-based, goal blood pressure of < 130/80 mm Hg for persons with diabetes mellitus or renal insufficiency (Chobanian et al., 2003). Despite these recommendations, it is currently estimated that only 34% of persons with hypertension have their pressure controlled (Chobanian et al., 2003).

Clinical trials have demonstrated that nonpharmacologic interventions are effective for lowering blood pressure. The current recommendations for lifestyle control of blood pressure are listed in Table 26.3. The most effective lifestyle strategies are weight loss, physical activity, reduced sodium intake, and limited alcohol intake. Three dietary trials—the Dietary Approaches to Stop Hypertension (DASH) and OmniHeart trials—have shown that blood pressure can be lowered with a diet that is high in fruits, vegetables, and low-fat dairy products and has a low content of total fat, saturated fat, and sodium (2005; ALLHAT Collaborative Research Group, 2002; Appel et al., 1997; Sacks et al., 2001). The details of the DASH

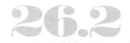

26.2	Cardiovascular Risk Factors and Target Organ Damage to Guide the Choice of Initial Therapy for Persons With Hypertension

Major risk factors	Hypertension
	Age (older than 55 years for men, 65 years for women)
	Diabetes mellitus
	Elevated LDL (or total) cholesterol or low HDL cholesterol
	Estimated glomerular filtration rate < 60 ml/min
	Family history of premature CVD (men younger than 55 years of age or women younger than 65 years of age)
	Microalbuminuria
	Obesity (body mass index 30 kg/m² or higher)
	Physical inactivity
	Tobacco use, particularly cigarettes
Target organ damage	Heart
	Left ventricular hypertrophy
	Angina, prior myocardial infarction
	Prior coronary revascularization
	Heart failure
	Brain
	Stroke or transient ischemic attack
	Dementia
	Chronic kidney disease
	Peripheral arterial disease
	Retinopathy

Note. Adapted from "The Seventh Report of the Joint National Committee on Prevention, Detection, Evaluation, and Treatment of High Blood Pressure: The JNC 7 Report," by A. V. Chobanian, G. L. Bakris, H. R. Black, W. C. Cushman, L. A. Green, J. L. Izzo, Jr., et al., 2003, *Journal of the American Medical Association,* 289(19), pp. 2560–2572. [Erratum in *Journal of the American Medical Association,* 2003, *290*(2), p. 197]

diets can be found at the DASH page on the NHLBI Web site: www.nhlbi.nih.gov/health/public/heart/hbp/dash. When individuals who had participated in one of the two Trials of Hypertension Prevention were studied 10 to 15 years later, those who decreased their sodium intake to between 33 and 44 mmol per day had 25% fewer cardiovascular events than persons who did not control their salt intake (Cook et al., 2007). There were also fewer cardiovascular deaths in the low salt group, but the difference was not significant ($p = 0.34$).

Randomized controlled trials of pharmacologic treatment of high blood pressure have shown that lowering the blood pressure results in a reduction in strokes, myocardial infarctions, and other cardiovascular endpoints (Collins et al., 1990; Hypertension Detection and Follow-up Program Cooperative Group, 1979, 1982; MacMahon et al., 1990; MacMahon & Rodgers, 1993; MRC Working Party, 1992). A variety of drug classes are recommended for use in blood pressure control: diuretics, beta blockers, calcium channel antagonists, angiotensin-converting enzyme inhibitors, angiotensin II receptor blockers, and direct vasodilators. The Antihypertensive and Lipid-Lowering Treatment to Prevent Heart Attack Trial (ALLHAT) was a randomized controlled trial comparing the efficacy of a diuretic, chlorthalidone, a calcium channel antagonist, amlodipine, and an angiotensin-converting enzyme inhibitor, lisinopril; the researchers found that the diuretic was equivalent to the other two drugs in preventing the primary endpoint of the study in preventing all-cause and cardiovascular mortality and that it was more effective in lowering blood pressure and preventing complications related to hypertension (ALLHAT Collaborative Research Group, 2002). An added benefit is that diuretics are much cheaper than most other antihypertensive medications. JNC-VII emphasizes that most individuals who do not respond to lifestyle interventions require a minimum of two antihypertensive medications to achieve blood pressure control (Chobanian et al., 2003). In the Women's Health Initiative participants, about 60% were on one medication, and control rates were low: 41% in women aged 50 to 59 years, 37% in women 60 to 69, and 29% in women aged 70 to 79 (Wassertheil-Smoller et al., 2000).

Dyslipidemia

Altered levels of blood lipids are associated with ASCVD. Specifically, an increased risk of ASCVD is associated with elevated levels of low-density lipoproteins

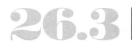 | LifeStyle Modification to Prevent and Manage Hypertension

MODIFICATION	RECOMMENDATION	APPROXIMATE SYSTOLIC BLOOD PRESSURE REDUCTION (RANGE)
Weight reduction	Maintain normal body weight (body mass index 18.5 to 24.9 kg/m²)	5–20 mm Hg/10kg
Adopt DASH eating plan (Dietary Approaches to Stop Hypertension)	Consume a diet rich in fruits, vegetables, and low-fat dairy products with a reduced content of saturated and total fat	8–14 mm Hg
Dietary sodium reduction	Reduce dietary sodium intake to no more than 100 mmol per day (2.4 g of sodium or 6 g sodium chloride)	2–8 mm Hg
Physical activity	Engage in regular aerobic physical activity such as brisk walking (at least 30 minutes per day, most days of the week)	4–9 mm Hg
Moderation of alcohol consumption	Limit consumption to no more than two drinks per day (e.g., 24 ounces beer, 10 ounces wine, or 3 ounces 80-proof whiskey) in most men, and to no more than one drink per day in women and lighter weight persons	2–4 mm Hg

Note. For overall cardiovascular risk reduction, stop smoking. The effects of implementing these modifications are dose and time dependent and could be greater for some individuals. From "The Seventh Report of the Joint National Committee on Prevention, Detection, Evaluation, and Treatment of High Blood Pressure: The JNC 7 Report," by A. V. Chobanian, G. L. Bakris, H. R. Black, W. C. Cushman, L. A. Green, J. L. Izzo, Jr., et al., 2003, *Journal of the American Medical Association, 289*(19), pp. 2560–2572. [Erratum in *Journal of the American Medical Association,* 2003, 290(2), p. 197]

(LDL), triglycerides, and total cholesterol and with lower than normal levels of high-density lipoprotein (HDL). The fact that low levels of HDL are associated with increased risk of ASCVD is the reason that the term dyslipidemia is more precise than the more frequently used terms hyperlipidemia or hypercholesterolemia. The National Center for Health Statistics (2006b) estimates that 17% of American women have high total cholesterol levels (> 200 mg per deciliter).

Although women have not been studied as extensively as men, there are sufficient data to establish that women with dyslipidemia are at increased risk for ASCVD and that treatment decreases this risk. A pooled analysis of data from 22 studies from around the world found that high levels of total cholesterol and LDL and low levels of HDL were associated with increased morbidity and mortality in women (Manolio et al., 1992). Numerous primary and secondary intervention studies have documented that women treated with a variety of lipid-lowering agents benefit as much or more than men (Aronow et al., 2001; Heart Protection Study Collaborative Group, 2002; Herrington et al., 2002; Kane et al., 1990; Sacks et al., 1996; Scandinavian Simvastatin Survival Study Group, 1994; Smilde et al., 2001; Waters et al., 1994). One review of 13 trials of lipid lowering in women found that the benefits were restricted to women with known cardiovascular disease (Walsh & Pignone, 2004).

The National Cholesterol Education Program at the National Heart, Lung, and Blood Institute develops and disseminates the consensus guidelines that outline the standard of care for the treatment of persons with dyslipidemia. The current guidelines on the detection, evaluation, and treatment of high blood cholesterol in adults are usually referred to by their acronym, ATP III, which stands for Adult Treatment Panel III (National Cholesterol Education Program Expert Panel on Detection, Evaluation, and Treatment of High Blood Cholesterol in Adults [Adult Treatment Panel III], 2001). To append the results of several clinical trials on cholesterol management, an update to the ATP III guidelines was published in 2004 (Grundy et al., 2004). According to ATP III, an adult who has a total cholesterol level of ≥ 200 mg per deciliter, an LDL level of ≥ 160 mg per deciliter, or an HDL level ≤ 40 has dyslipidemia. The guidelines emphasize that lowering the LDL cholesterol level is the primary target in lipid management therapy. Professionals caring for women should read at least the executive summary of the ATP III and the 2004 update. The 284-page full report is an outstanding resource for those wanting to learn about lipid management in depth. Both documents and clinical tools and charts can be found on the NHLBI Web site (www.nhbli.nih.gov). There is a special section in the ATP III that describes a constellation of CVD risk factors called the metabolic syndrome, and this syndrome is discussed later in this chapter.

The recommendations for lipid management include both lifestyle strategies and medications. The lifestyle strategies, termed *therapeutic lifestyle changes* in the ATP III Report, include dietary changes; an increased intake of plant stanols or sterols, which are found in some margarines; an increased intake of soluble fiber; weight loss; and increased physical activity as shown in Table 26.4 (National Cholesterol Education Program, 2001). The drug classes recommended for the treatment of dyslipidemia include HMG CoA reductase inhibitors, usually referred to as statins; bile acid sequestrants; nicotinic acid; and fibric acids. Women have been included in two large randomized controlled trials of statins, and the results found decreased cardiovascular morbidity and mortality as well as all-cause mortality (Heart Protection Study Collaborative Group, 2002; Shepherd et al., 2002). The American Heart Association; American College of Cardiology; and the National Heart, Lung, and Blood Institute have released a statement intended to guide clinicians in the safe use of statins; the statement is available on the Web sites of all three of the agencies (Pasternak et al., 2002). As with blood pressure, the presence of other CVD risk factors are used to stratify care, and the LDL level goals are lower for persons with more risk factors.

Despite the information that women experience dyslipidemia and that they would benefit from lifestyle and pharmaceutical intervention, studies has shown that women are inadequately treated for dyslipidemia. In an analysis of the baseline data for the Heart and Estrogen/Progestin Replacement Study (HERS), Schrott and colleagues (1997) found that 91% of the postmenopausal women with known coronary heart disease that were recruited for HERS did not have their lipid levels adequately controlled. In addition, the results showed that only one-third of the women with LDL levels above 160 mg per deciliter were on lipid-lowering medications. This information is a call to action for women's care providers: women need to be screened and treated appropriately for dyslipidemia. A nonrandomized post hoc comparison of the HERS participants who did or did not use statins revealed hazard ratios for heart disease of 0.79 (Confidence Interval [CI] 0.63–0.99) and total mortality of 0.67 (CI 0.51–0.87) in the users (Herrington et al., 2002). In the one randomized control of statin use in only women, the results showed no impact on the progression of coronary calcification, but the follow-up was for only 1 year (Raggi et al., 2005). We lack sufficient data to inform our care of women with dyslipidemia.

Sedentary LifeStyle and Physical Activity

The 1996 Surgeon General's report focused on physical activity and its critical importance in preventing diseases including ASCVD (U.S. Department of Health and

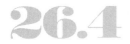

Essential Components of Therapeutic LifeStyle Changes for Lipid Management

COMPONENT	RECOMMENDATION
LDL-raising nutrients	
Saturated fats[a]	Less than 7 % of total calories
Dietary cholesterol	Less than 200 mg per day
Therapeutic options for LDL lowering	
Plant stanols/sterols	2 g per day
Increased viscous (soluble) fiber	10– 25 g per day
Total calories (energy)	Adjust total caloric intake to maintain desirable body weight and prevent weight gain
Physical activity	Include enough moderate exercise to expend at least 200 kcal per day

Note. From *Detection, Evaluation, and Treatment of High Blood Cholesterol in Adults (Adult Treatment Panel III)*, NIH Publication No. 02-5215, by National Cholesterol Education Program, 2002, National Heart, Lung and Blood Institutes, National Institutes of Health.
[a] Trans fatty acids are another LDL-raising fat that should be kept at a low intake.

Human Services, 1996). An analysis focused on the role of walking in preventing ASCVD in women participating in the Women's Health Initiative found that CVD risk increased with the number of hours spent sitting per day (Manson et al., 2002). Women who spent more than 16 hours per day sitting had a relative risk of 1.68 (95 % CI 1.07, 2.64) compared to women who spend 4 hours sitting. During a 6-year follow-up of women in the Nurses' Health Study, a positive correlation was found between hours of television watched and the occurrence of obesity and diagnosis of diabetes mellitus (Hu et al., 2003). For every 2 hours of television women watched, their risks for obesity and diabetes increased by 23 % and 14 %, respectively.

Several analyses from the prospective observational Nurses' Health Study have documented that brisk walking is associated with a decreased risk of ASCVD and also with decreased blood pressure, lipids, and the occurrence of diabetes mellitus (Hu, Manson, et al., 2001; Hu et al., 1999; Manson et al., 1991, 1999, 2002). A randomized controlled trial of moderate-intensity exercise in postmenopausal women demonstrated that brisk walking resulted in significant decreases in total body fat, intra-abdominal fat, sub-

cutaneous abdominal fat, and body weight (Irwin et al., 2003). In a prospective study of 9,518 White women older than age 65 living at home, the hazard rate ratio for mortality from all causes in the women who increased their activity levels between baseline and the 6-year follow-up was 0.52 (95 % CI 0.40, 0.69). The hazard rate ratios for death from CVD and cancer were 0.64 and 0.49, respectively (Gregg et al., 2003). For participants in the WISE study, all of whom underwent angiography to evaluate symptoms of possible heart disease, there was a significant inverse relationship between the amount of coronary artery disease and reported levels of physical activity (Wessel et al., 2004). In summary, being inactive is associated with an increased risk of ASCVD, while participating in moderate activity such as brisk walking reduces risk and waistlines simultaneously.

Despite the well-recognized benefits of exercise for longevity and well-being, in 2006, only 29 % of adult women met the national guidelines of 30 or more minutes on five or more days per week (National Center for Health Statistics, 2006b). The survey also revealed that, as women age, the prevalence of inactivity increases, so that 66 % of women older than age 65 reported no vigorous leisure-time physical activity of more than 10 minutes. Even more problematic is the finding of a disturbing trend in declining activity in adolescent girls (Kimm et al., 2002). In a sample of 1,213 Black girls and 1,166 White girls enrolled at age 9 to 10 years and followed to the age of 18 or 19, researchers found that activity declined by 64 % in the White girls and by 100 % in the Black girls. By the end of the observation period, 56 % of the Black girls and 31 % of the White girls reported no regular leisure-time physical activity. The girls in the study were recruited from schools near San Francisco, Pittsburgh, and Washington, DC, and, therefore, are probably not representative of all girls in the United States—but the trend is still disturbing.

The current recommendation from the American College of Sports Medicine, the Centers for Disease Control and Prevention, and from the Surgeon General is that adults should invest at least 30 minutes a day for days of the week in moderate-intensity physical activity (Pate et al., 1995; U.S. Department of Health and Human Services, 1996). This activity can be done all at once or, if more convenient, in two or three shorter time periods, such a three 10-minute walks. The message is clear: regular physical activity is important. Now the challenge is how to support women to be more active. A report of the Centers for Disease Control and Prevention (2001) summarizes research and recommendations on community strategies to support physical activity. Two of the recommended strategies are (1) point-of-decision signage, such as having a sign encouraging stair climbing next to a stair entrance and (2) having a buddy with whom to exercise. Another strategy is having health care providers ask clients about their physical activity. Data from national surveys indicate that older women are significantly less likely than older men to be asked about their physical activity and that, overall, only 31% of the U.S. population has been advised to exercise by their health care provider (Galuska, Serdula, Brown, & Kruger, 2002; Morrato, Hill, Wyatt, Ghushchyan, & Sullivan, 2006).

Overweight and Obesity

As women's body weight increases, so does the incidence of most of the other physiologic risk factors for ASCVD as well as CVD morbidity and mortality. Increased body weight and an increased waist circumference in women have been shown to be associated with hypertension, dyslipidemia, sedentary lifestyle, diabetes mellitus, cardiovascular morbidity, cardiovascular mortality, all-cause mortality, and the risk of many types of cancer (Berenson, Srinivasan, & Bao, 1997; Calle, Rodriguez, Walker-Thurmond, & Thun, 2003; Calle, Thun, Petrelli, Rodriguez, & Heath, 1999; Haarbo, Hassager, Riis, & Christiansen, 1989; Huang et al., 1998; Kannel, Brand, Skinner, Dawber, & McNamara, 1967; Larsson et al., 1992; Lissner et al., 1991; Manson et al., 1995; McTigue et al., 2006; Must, Jacques, Dallai, Bajema, & Dietz, 1992; National Institutes of Health, 1998; Van Horn et al., 1991; Willett et al., 1995; Wing et al., 1989). In the Bogalusa Heart Study, a longitudinal, cross-sectional study of CVD in children, the rela-

tionship between cardiovascular risk factors and body weight was observed to develop in girls followed from the ages of 5 to 6 years to 11 to 12 years (Tershakovec et al., 2002). Weight loss is known to decrease blood pressure levels, reduce total and LDL cholesterol levels, increase HDL, and reduce the incidence of diabetes (Hu, Manson, et al., 2001; Huang et al., 1998; Wood, Stefanick, Williams, & Haskell, 1991).

The National Heart, Lung, and Blood Institute at the National Institutes of Health has established the Obesity Education Initiative to support the public and professionals in preventing weight gain and managing overweight. In collaboration with the National Institute of Diabetes and Digestive and Kidney Diseases, the organizations have developed and distribute a variety of resources related to body weight, including *Clinical Guidelines on the Identification, Evaluation, and Treatment of Overweight and Obesity in Adults* (National Institutes of Health, 1998). The Web site for this project can be found at http://www.nhlbi.nih.gov/health/public/heart/obesity/lose_wt. The recommended classification system that relates body size and weight distribution to disease risk is shown in Table 26.5. Overweight and obesity are components of the metabolic syndrome that is discussed below.

Diabetes Mellitus

Women with type 2 diabetes have much greater risk of mortality and morbidity from cardiovascular disease than women without diabetes (Beckman, Creager, &

26.5 | Classification of Overweight and Obesity by Body Mass Index, Waist Circumference, and Associated Risk for Type 2 Diabetes, Hypertension, and Cardiovascular Disease

	BMI (kg/m²)	Obesity class	DISEASE RISK RELATIVE TO NORMAL WEIGHT AND WAIST CIRCUMFERENCE[a] Men 102 cm (= 40 inches) Women = 88 cm (= 35 inches)	Men > 102 cm (> 40 inches) Women > 88 cm (> 35 inches)
Underweight	< 18.5		——	——
Normal	18.5–24.9		——	——
Overweight	25.0–29.9		Increased	High
Obesity	30.0–34.9	I	High	Very high
	35–39.9	II	Very high	Very high
Extreme obesity	≥ 40	III	Extremely high	Extremely high

Note. From *Clinical Guidelines on the Identification, Evaluation, and Treatment of Overweight and Obesity in Adults: The Evidence Report,* NIH Publication No. 98-4083, by National Institutes of Health, 1998, Retrieved April 28, 2007, 2007, from http://www.nhlbi.nih.gov/guidelines/obesity/ob_gdlns.htm
[a] Increased waist circumference can also be a marker for increased risk even in persons of normal weight.

Libby, 2002; Hu, Stampfer et al., 2001; Huxley, Barzi, & Woodward, 2006; Jones et al., 2002; Kanaya, Grady, & Barrett-Connor, 2002; Kannel & Wilson, 1995; Thomas et al., 2003). In a meta-analysis of 16 studies, Kanaya, Grady, and Barrett-Connor (2002) found that the odds ratio for CHD mortality in diabetic women compared to women without diabetes was 2.9 (95% CI, 2.2–3.8). In the Nurses' Health Study, the age-adjusted relative risk of mortality in diabetic women was 3.38 (95% CI, 3.08, 3.73); if the women had both diabetes and a history of CHD, their risk was 6.84 (95% CI, 4.71, 9.95) compared to women with neither diabetes nor CHD at baseline (Hu, Stampfer, et al., 2001). Women who have had gestational diabetes mellitus (GDM) are at increased risk for developing diabetes (Cheung & Byth, 2003). A cross-sectional study of women with first-degree relatives with diabetes compared women with and without a history of GDM and found that those with a positive GDM history were more likely to have CVD risk factors and to have CVD events (Carr et al., 2006). Women who had a history of prior CHD and who had had diabetes for more than 15 years were at 30 times greater risk than women with neither condition at baseline. The Atherosclerosis Risk in Communities study found that the hazard rate ratio for CHD was 1.8 in diabetic Black women and 3.3 in diabetic White women (Jones et al., 2002). In a follow-up of participants in the first National Health and Nutrition Examination Survey, it was found that heart disease mortality in nondiabetic women decreased by 27% between 1971 and 1984, while, in the same period, it increased by 23% in women with diabetes (Gu, Cowie, & Harris, 1999).

In addition to increasing women's risk of CHD mortality, diabetes also is associated with a less favorable outcome in women who experience a CHD event such as myocardial infarction. The 28-day mortality rate of Finnish women hospitalized with a myocardial infarction was 2.6 times greater than in nondiabetic women (Miettinen et al., 1998). Studies have found that persons with diabetes also have a higher probability of having other risk factors of cardiovascular disease, including hypertension, increased triglyceride levels, decreased high density lipoprotein levels, and obesity (Bog-Hansen et al., 1998; Meigs et al., 1997). Impaired glucose tolerance also has been found to be associated with all-cause mortality, the incidence of cardiovascular disease, and an increased incidence of other cardiovascular risk factors (Barrett-Connor, Wingard, Criqui, & Suarez, 1984; Meigs, Nathan, Wilson, Cupples, & Singer, 1998; Tominaga et al., 1999). In light of the risk of ASCVD related to both impaired glucose tolerance and diabetes mellitus, women must be encouraged to choose lifestyles that reduce the likelihood of developing impaired glucose metabolism. Data from the Nurses' Health Study indicate that a diagnosis of diabetes is associated with excess body weight; lack of exercise; a low-fiber,

high-fat diet; and smoking (Hu, Manson, et al., 2001). Quitting smoking is associated with a marked reduction of risk in diabetic women (Al-Delaimy et al., 2002).

Metabolic Syndrome

Building on criteria proposed in the ATP III, an expert committee has defined the metabolic syndrome as including abdominal obesity, increased blood pressure, dyslipidemia, and an elevated fasting glucose level (Grundy et al., 2005). To make the criteria applicable worldwide, the International Diabetes Federation added waist circumference criteria specific to seven ethnic groups: Europids, South Asians, Chinese, Japanese, Central and South Americans, Sub-Saharan Africans, and Eastern Mediterranean and Middle East (Arab) populations (Alberti, Zimmet, & Shaw, 2005). The goal of these definitions is identification of those at risk for atherosclerotic cardiovascular disease and type 2 diabetes (Alberti et al., 2005). When all the definitions of metabolic syndrome were used to evaluate the risk of subsequently developing CVD and diabetes in participants of Phase 2 of the San Antonio Heart Study, all the definitions were found to be predictive in women age 55 and older (Lorenzo, Williams, Hunt, & Haffner, 2007).

An analysis of the third U.S. National Health and Nutrition Examination Survey (NHANES III) data revealed that 23% of women in the United States have metabolic syndrome. When the distribution was analyzed by body weight categories, the syndrome was noted to increase markedly with body weight and was seen in 6% of normal-weight women, 28% of overweight women, and 50% of obese women (Park et al., 2003). For the NHANES III analysis, the metabolic syndrome was defined as the presence of three or more of the following characteristics: abdominal obesity, elevated triglyceride level, a low HDL value, a high-normal or greater level of blood pressure (> 130/85 mm Hg), and a fasting glucose level greater than 110 mg/dl. When the associations of the metabolic syndrome and obesity with cardiovascular risk were compared among the participants of the WISE study, it was found that the presence of the metabolic syndrome was a better predictor of CVD risk than an elevated body mass index (Kip et al., 2004). Women aged 60 to 70 years with metabolic syndrome had a more rapid accumulation of atherosclerotic plaque in their carotid arteries over a 12-year period than those without the syndrome (Hassinen et al., 2006).

Although research on interventions that focus specifically on the management of all aspects of the metabolic syndrome is not yet available, lifestyle management of risk factors is the recommended first step (Grundy et al., 2005). Two randomized controlled trials offer some insight into therapy (Hill & Bessesen, 2003). These studies that enrolled women and men with impaired glucose tolerance with the goal of preventing the development of diabetes have shown that weight loss, a low-fat high-fiber diet, and physical activity reduced the incidence of diabetes (Knowler et al., 2002; Tuomilehto et al., 2001). The studies were similar in that about 67% of the subjects were women; the follow-up was for about 3 years, and each found that the lifestyle intervention reduced the incidence of diabetes in high-risk subjects by about 50%.

Menopause and Hormone Replacement Therapy

Because women experience ASCVD events about 10 years later than men, and typically after menopause, it had been hypothesized that hormone replacement therapy (HRT) would prevent or delay cardiovascular disease in postmenopausal women. Observational studies supported this hypothesis, but these results did not provide a sound basis for intervention because of the high likelihood of confounding factors such as selection bias. Selection bias means that, because the women who used hormones in these observational studies were not randomly selected from a representative population of women, it was likely that factors other than hormone replacement could influence the results. It was known that women who used HRT were more affluent and had more education and probably also more access to health care than the women who were not taking hormones. For an in-depth review of these studies, see Barrett-Connor and Bush (1991).

None of the major randomized controlled trials of hormone replacement therapy for primary or secondary prevention of cardiovascular disease events in postmenopausal women have shown positive results (Angeja et al., 2001; Angerer, Stork, Kothny, Schmitt, & von Schacky, 2001; Byington et al., 2002; Cherry et al., 2002; Clarke, Kelleher, Lloyd-Jones, Slack, & Schofiel, 2002; Grady et al., 2002; Grady & Sawaya, 1998; Herrington et al., 2000; Hsia et al., 2000; Hulley et al., 1998; Rossouw et al., 2002; Viscoli et al., 2001; Waters et al., 2002). In fact, most of these trials have shown increases in events such as strokes and thromboembolic disease in the early years of the studies as well as later increases in breast cancer (Curb et al., 2006; Hsia et al., 2006; Lemaitre et al., 2006; Rossouw et al., 2007). The prospective observational Million Women Study Collaborators have reported a 20% increase in ovarian cancer risk in women who chose to use hormone replacement therapy (Beral & Million Women Study Collaborators, 2007). The 7% reduction in breast cancer in 2003 following the report of the Women's Health Initiative randomized controlled trial of estrogen plus progestin replacement in postmenopausal women in 2002 has been interpreted as support for the causative role of hormone replacement therapy in some breast cancers (Ravdin et al., 2007). Based on an analysis of the data on hormone replacement, the American Heart Association now recommends that HRT not be used for either primary or secondary prevention of heart disease in postmenopausal women (Mosca et al., 2007).

Social Risk Conditions

Poverty, low levels of education, and disadvantageous social conditions are risk factors for CVD that are commonly omitted from lists of modifiable risk factors. In cross-sectional and case-control studies, women with lower socioeconomic status had increased levels of both CVD risk factors and a greater degree of carotid stenosis and CVD than women with more education and income (Cabrera et al., 2001; Hayes et al., 2006; Iscan, Uyanik, Vurgun, Ece, & Yigitoglu, 1996; Rosvall et al., 2002; Rutledge et al., 2003; Wamala, Mittleman, Schenck-Gustafsson, & Orth-Gomer, 1999; Wamala, Murray, et al., 1999). Single mothers in Sweden have been found to have a higher mortality rate than partnered mothers (Ringback Weitoft, Haglund, & Rosen, 2000). In an analysis of data from the NHANES III, mothers who experienced a CVD event were 3.3 (95% CI 3.24, 3.31) times more likely to be single rather than partnered mothers (Young, Cunningham, & Buist, 2005). Swedish women who lived in neighborhoods characterized by low levels of education and income, unemployment, and receipt of social welfare were 1.9 to 1.6 times as likely to experience coronary heart disease events and death, respectively, as women who lived in the least deprived neighborhoods (Winkleby, Sundquist, & Cubbin, 2007). Social policies to ensure that women have access to health care, child care, affordable housing, optimal employment, and opportunities for education and training need to be considered as management strategies to reduce CVD in women.

Other Risk Factors and Conditions

Although smoking, hypertension, dyslipidemia and lack of physical activity are the risk factors whose modification results in improved morbidity and mortality from ASCVD, many other risk factors have been found to be associated with the incidence of CVD in women. What is not available is research demonstrating that changing these other risk factors will result in either longer life or less disability for women. Some of these other risk factors include C-reactive protein levels, interleukin-6 levels, use of oral contraceptives, left ventricular hypertrophy, too much or too little sleep, marital stress, hostility, depression, and renal insufficiency (Ayas et al., 2003; Bermudez, Rifai, Buring, Manson, & Ridker, 2002; Chaput et al., 2002; Hackam & Anand, 2003; Liao, Cooper, Mensah, & McGee, 1995; Rosenberg, Palmer, Rao, & Shapiro, 2001; Rosvall et al., 2002; Rutledge et al., 2006; Shlipak et al., 2001; Wang et al.,

2002; Wassertheil-Smoller et al., 2004). Diseases with an inflammatory component such as rheumatoid arthritis and some autoimmune conditions also have been found to be associated with an elevated incidence of cardiovascular risk factors and disease (Chung et al., 2005; de Leeuw, Kallenberg, & Bijl, 2005).

PATHOPHYSIOLOGY OF ATHEROSCLEROTIC CARDIOVASCULAR DISEASE

The relationship between risk factors, the pathologic processes that contribute to the development of ASCVD, and the clinical manifestations of ASCVD are shown in Exhibit 26.1. These pathophysiologic processes include atherosclerosis, inflammation, and thrombosis. In industrialized cultures, the earliest pathologic signs of atherosclerosis—raised lesions and fatty streaks—are found in the aortas of infants and young children (Berenson et al., 1998; Wissler, Hiltscher, Oinuma, & and the PDAY Research Group, 1996). The clinical manifestations associated with ASCVD include myocardial infarction, stable and unstable angina, heart failure, stroke, peripheral vascular disease, and renal insufficiency and failure.

Atherosclerosis

Atherosclerotic lesions typically develop in medium- to large-sized musculoelastic arteries such as the aorta, coronary arteries, femoral arteries, and carotid arteries

(Stary, 1996; Stary et al., 1995). Musculoelastic arteries have three major layers: the adventitia (outermost layer), the media, and the intima. Atherosclerotic lesions form in the proteoglycan-rich layer of the intima that is located below the vascular endothelium and above the intimal smooth muscle layer. Early atherosclerotic lesions, such as raised streaks, are composed mainly of foam cells, which are macrophages containing lipid droplets. As lesions progress through life, they become more complex and may include smooth muscle cells—some of which also contain lipid droplets, extracellular lipid deposits, lymphocytes, fibrous connective tissue, and, in advanced lesions, there may be calcium deposits. As lesions progress, they develop a fibrous cap above the lesions and beneath the vascular endothelium. Recent research has focused on the influence that the thickness and stability of this cap has on whether an individual develops signs and symptoms of ASCVD. It is believed that persons with stable lesions (those with a thick fibrous cap) are less likely to experience signs and symptoms, while persons with a thin and vulnerable cap are believed to be at increased risk of events associated with ASCVD such as myocardial infarction and unstable angina.

In the early and middle stages of development, arteries with atherosclerotic lesions increase in size so that, even though the wall of the artery is becoming thicker, there is no change in the diameter of the vessel lumen (Glagov, Weisenberg, Zarins, Stankunavicius, & Kolettis, 1987). It is only in the late stages of atherosclerosis that the atherosclerotic plaque decreases the lumen diameter leading to stenosis or narrowing of the artery. Because the vessels in early to middle stages of disease development have this compensatory enlargement, an individual can have notable amounts of atherosclerosic plaque in the coronary or other vascular beds, but the lesions cannot be seen with angiography.

The vascular endothelium, which is considered by some scientists as a separate organ, plays a key role in vascular health and disease (DiCorleto & Gimbrone, 1996). The endothelium has a role in controlling:

- The movement of fluid, nutrients, and components of the immune and inflammatory system between the vascular and interstitial spaces.
- Coagulation and fibrinolysis—clot formation and breakdown.
- Vasomotion—contraction and dilation of the blood vessel wall.
- Growth of the cells that form the layers of the blood vessel.

The endothelium accomplishes these tasks by the production and release of regulatory cytokines and by up- and down-regulating the receptors on the blood side surface of the vascular endothelial cell walls.

EXHIBIT 26.1 RELATIONSHIP BETWEEN THE RISK FACTORS, PATHOLOGIC PROCESSES, AND CLINICAL

Risk Factors

Pathologic Processes

(Atherosclerosis, Inflammation, Thrombosis)

Clinical Manifestations

Manifestations of Atherosclerotic Cardiovascular Disease

Research indicates that dysfunction of the vascular endothelium is one of the factors that contributes to the formation of atherosclerotic plaque (Lerman, Cannan, Higano, Nishimura, & Holmes, 1998; Panza, 1997; Vogel, Corretti, & Gellman, 1998). In a healthy person, the endothelium is slightly anticoagulant; when atherosclerotic lesions are present, the endothelium becomes prothrombotic, which means the probability that clots will form in the atherosclerotic areas of the artery is increased. One example of the prothrombotic state is the expression of tissue factor by the vascular endothelial cells. Tissue factor has a critical role in initiating coagulation and is not expressed on the luminal surface of the endothelium of healthy vessels (Narahara, Enden, Wiiger, & Prydz, 1994).

Inflammation

The inflammatory process has been shown to have an important role in the development and presentation of ASCVD (Hansson & Libby, 2006; Ross, 1999). As mentioned earlier, macrophages, usually the coordinators of the inflammatory response in healthy individuals, become part of the problem in atherosclerosis when they take up LDL particles via their scavenger receptors and transform into foam cells. These foam cells are major contributors to the formation of atherosclerotic plaque, both as cells filled with lipid droplets and also after they die, when their lipid contents contribute to the lipid core found in advanced atherosclerotic lesions. The release of tissue-digesting enzymes, called matrix metalloproteases, by macrophages and T lymphocytes is thought to be an important factor that predisposes to the rupture of atherosclerotic plaque that precipitates acute coronary events such as myocardial infarction and unstable angina (Burke et al., 1997; Fuster, 1994; Kullo, Edwards, & Schwartz, 1998; Libby, Schoenbeck, Mach, Selwyn, & Ganz, 1998; Pasterkamp et al., 1999). These interactions between the inflammatory process and the stability of atherosclerotic lesions have fueled research about the role of inflammation in atherosclerosis (Maseri, 1997; Mehta, Saldeen, & Rand, 1998). Researchers are interested in determining whether the markers of inflammation such as interleukin-6 and C-reactive protein levels will be useful in predicting future incidence of coronary events and thus the management of CVD (Bermudez et al., 2002; Koenig et al., 1999; Levinson, 2005; Liuzzo et al., 1994; Ridker, 1998; Ridker, Buring, Shih, Matias, & Hennekens, 1998; Ridker, Cushman, Stampfer, Tracy, & Hennekens, 1998; Wang et al., 2002).

The usefulness of aspirin as treatment to prevent atherosclerotic events may be linked to aspirin's anti-inflammatory actions as well as its actions as an inhibitor of platelet aggregation (Husain, Andrews, Mulcahy, Panza, & Quyyumi, 1998; Patrono, 1994; Ridker, Cushman, Stampfer, Tracy, & Hennekens, 1997). Although aspirin has been demonstrated to be useful in the prevention of CVD in men, there is only one substantial randomized controlled trial of aspirin use in women. In the Women's Health Study, 39,876 healthy women older than age 45 were randomized to aspirin 100 mg every other day or to placebo and followed for 10 years (Ridker et al., 2005). There was no significant effect of aspirin treatment on the study's primary outcome, which was a first major cardiovascular event defined as a nonfatal myocardial infarction or stroke or death from CVD. There were significant decreases in three of the secondary endpoints: total strokes were decreased by 17%, ischemic strokes by 24%, and transient ischemic attacks by 22%. Women taking aspirin experienced significantly more peptic ulcers and gastrointestinal bleeding as well as more minor bleeding such as nosebleeds and bruising. The American Heart Association's *Evidence-Based Guidelines for CVD Prevention* does not recommend routine use of aspirin in healthy women younger than 65, and, in women older than 65, the possible benefits of aspirin use for ischemic stroke prevention must be weighed against the risks of gastrointestinal bleeding and hemorrhagic stroke (Mosca et al., 2007). Authors of a systematic review of clinical trials that evaluated the efficacy of long-term aspirin use to prevent CVD concluded that there is no evidence to support the use of daily doses of aspirin greater than 75 to 81 mg (Campbell, Smyth, Montalescot, & Steinhubl, 2007). Higher doses did not increase efficacy, but the risk of bleeding from the gastrointestinal tract increased.

Thrombosis

A prothrombotic tendency increases the likelihood of the occurrence of CVD events, including myocardial infarction, unstable angina, and stroke. Formation of a clot in the area of an atherosclerotic plaque is often the initiating cause of these events (Croce & Libby, 2007). It is postulated that matrix metalloproteases (tissue-digesting enzymes) released by macrophages within vulnerable plaques weaken the fibrous cap, which is then prone to breaking open or rupturing. Once the fibrous cap of an atherosclerotic plaque ruptures, the vascular endothelium is disrupted and the subendothelial tissues are exposed. Subendothelial tissues are rich in tissue factor, the physiological activator of the clotting cascade that, once exposed, initiates clotting. Also when the fibrous cap ruptures, hemorrhage into the plaque occurs, leading to an increase of the volume of the plaque and thus further local stenosis and diminution of blood flow.

Some, but not all, epidemiologic studies have documented an association between elevated levels of components of the clotting cascade plus decreased levels of fibrinolytic substances in women who have ASCVD events (Bielak et al., 2000; Eichner et al., 1996; Eriksson et al., 1999; Lindmark, Wallentin, & Siegbahn, 2001; Nielsen, Logander, & Swahn, 2001; Roest, Voorbij, Barendrecht, Peeters, & van der Schouw, 2007; Salomaa et al., 2002; Tunstall-Pedoe et al., 1997; Woodward, Lowe, Rumley, & Tunstall-Pedoe, 1998). One of the most consistent findings is a relationship between plasma fibrinogen levels and the risk of coronary heart disease morbidity and mortality (Bielak et al., 2000; Eichner et al., 1996; Eriksson et al., 1999; Roest et al., 2007; Tunstall-Pedoe et al., 1997). In a case-control study in which 292 women younger than age 65 who had been hospitalized for a coronary event were compared with matched controls picked from the city census, the adjusted odds ratio for having a coronary event among those in the highest quartile of fibrinogen levels was 3.0 (98% CI, 1.6 to 5.5). The prospective cohort Scottish Heart Health Study, which included 5,095 women between the ages of 40 and 59, also found a significant association between fibrinogen levels and the risk of a coronary event or death in women (Tunstall-Pedoe et al., 1997). It is not yet clear whether these findings will be most useful as predictors of future risk or whether they can be used as targets for treatment. Interestingly, physical activity has been shown to be associated with lower fibrinogen levels in pre- and postmenopausal women (DeSouza, Jones, & Seals, 1998; Geffken et al., 2001).

Signs and Symptoms of ASCHD in Women

Although the literature on women and heart disease includes an ongoing debate about whether women have different presenting symptoms than men, this discussion is basically more academic than practical (DeVon & Zerwic, 2002, 2003; Kudenchuk, Maynard, Martin, Wirkus, & Weaver, 1996; Miller, 2002; Milner, Funk, Arnold, & Vaccarino, 2002; Milner et al., 1999; Mosca et al., 1997; Penque et al., 1998). Women have the potential to experience all the signs and symptoms of CHD that men do, although the incidence of a specific sign or symptom may differ between genders. Women need to know all the possible signs and symptoms that might indicate that they are having an event and what to do if such symptoms occur. Clinicians need to know what symptoms in women indicate heart disease and thus need to be included in an assessment. They also need to include ASCVD in their differential diagnoses for women. There is no debate about gender differences in the signs and symptoms of stroke. Table 26.6 lists the warning signs for heart attack and stroke.

The two larger studies of CHD whose data were collected prospectively and in real time indicated that women and men have the potential to experience any of the symptoms shown in Table 26.7 that indicate an event related to myocardial infarction (Kudenchuk et al., 1996; Milner et al., 1999). In a prospective study in which nurse researchers observed all patients presenting with possible coronary heart disease, about 30% of men and women presented without chest pain, and the remaining 70% had chest pain or chest heaviness/pressure/tightness/squeezing (Canto et al., 2000; Milner et al., 1999). Of the non–chest pain symptoms, women were significantly more likely than men to experience mid-back pain, nausea/vomiting, dyspnea, palpitations, and indigestion ($p < 0.05$) and perhaps fatigue and arm/shoulder pain (p values between 0.05 and 0.10; Milner et al., 1999). In another study that included only persons who presented with an acute myocardial infarction, there were no differences in presenting signs and symptoms between men and women: 99% of both men and women experienced some form of chest pain (Kudenchuk et al., 1996). These researchers found that women were less likely to have Q waves (13% versus 25%) and intraventricular conduction abnormalities (16% versus 26%) in their prehospital electrocardiograms, which were done in the field by paramedics (Kudenchuk et al., 1996).

Although women who have chest pain are less likely than men to have abnormal angiograms, data from the WISE study indicate that the pain is prognostic of the risk of future events. When 412 women from the WISE study with normal coronary angiograms were compared over a 5-year period based on whether they also had persistent chest pain, it was found that the women with persistent chest pain were twice as likely as the women without such pain to have an adverse outcome such as a stroke or myocardial infarction (Johnson et al., 2006).

The data on angina and myocardial infarction in women also indicate that women are more likely to have events if they are older and have other CVD risk factors or events (DeVon & Zerwic, 2003; Kudenchuk et al., 1996; Milner et al., 1999). For these reasons, every woman who is postmenopausal or who has experienced a CVD event needs education about both the possible signs and symptoms of an event and the importance of immediately calling 911 (or its equivalent in other countries; Finnegan et al., 2000). Survey and focus group data indicate that women are more likely than men to delay before calling emergency help (Finnegan et al., 2000; Menon et al., 1998; Pancioli et al., 1998).

DIAGNOSIS

Diagnosing ASCVD, especially CHD, in women is more challenging than in men. Some of the reasons for this difference are related to women's anatomy and size. The presence of breast tissue on the chest wall makes

26.6 | The Warning Signs of Heart Attack, Stroke, and Cardiac Arrest

Heart attack warning signs

Some heart attacks are sudden and intense, like the "movie heart attack," where there is no doubt about what's happening. But most heart attacks start slowly, with mild pain or discomfort. Often people affected aren't sure what's wrong and wait too long before getting help. Here are signs that can mean a heart attack is happening:

As with men, women's most common heart attack symptom is chest pain or discomfort. But women are somewhat more likely than men to experience some of the other common symptoms, particularly shortness of breath, nausea/vomiting, and back or jaw pain.

- Chest discomfort
  Most heart attacks involve discomfort in the center of the chest that lasts more than a few minutes, or that goes away and comes back. It can feel like uncomfortable pressure, squeezing, fullness, or pain.
- Discomfort in other areas of the upper body
  Symptoms can include pain or discomfort in one or both arms, the back, neck, jaw, or stomach.
- Shortness of breath
  This feeling often accompanies chest discomfort. But it can occur before the chest discomfort.
- Other signs
  These may include breaking out in a cold sweat, nausea, or lightheadedness.

Stroke warning signs

- Sudden numbness or weakness of the face, arm, or leg, especially on one side of the body
- Sudden confusion, trouble speaking or understanding
- Sudden trouble seeing in one or both eyes
- Sudden trouble walking, dizziness, loss of balance or coordination
- Sudden, severe headache with no known cause

Cardiac arrest strikes immediately and without warning

- Sudden loss of responsiveness. No response to gentle shaking
- No normal breathing. The victim does not take a normal breath when you check for several seconds
- No signs of circulation. No movement or coughing

Note. If any of these warning signs occur, call 911. See the American Heart Association's Web site (www.americanheart.org) for specific action plans for each type of emergency. From *Heart Attack, Stroke & Cardiac Arrest Warning Signs,* by the American Heart Association, 2007. Retrieved April 27, 2007, from http://www.americanheart.org/presenter.jhtml?identifier=3053

---

electrocardiography, echocardiography, and imaging more challenging. Another reason is that women are generally smaller than men, for whom some of the equipment was designed. Overall, the same diagnostic tests are used in men and women even though the interpretation of the test results in women is less clear. Both the sensitivity and specificity of the diagnostic tests used for CHD are lower in women (Kwok, Kim, Grady, Segal, & Redberg, 1999). The tests that can be used to diagnose CHD are listed in Table 26.8. Another modality, transesophageal echocardiography, is being studied to determine its potential usefulness. A consensus statement on Noninvasive Testing in the Clinical Evaluation of Women With Suspected Coronary Artery Disease has been developed by several Councils of the American Heart Association and offers a detailed analysis of diagnostic strategies to detect CHD in women (Mieres et al., 2005). In addition, the investigators from the WISE study have published two papers summarizing their insights related to the presentation, diagnosis, and nature of coronary disease in women (Bairey Merz et al., 2006; Shaw et al., 2006).

As with any other condition, the clinician's assessment—including a complete history, assessment of risk factors, and consideration of the client's age—is the cornerstone of the diagnostic process for ASCVD (Douglas & Ginsburg, 1996; Kwok & Redberg, 2002). Experts have developed recommendations for further testing based on an estimation of the likelihood that the client has CHD. Typically, the proposed schema suggests categorizing the probability that a woman has CHD into three categories such as low, moderate, and high. This categorization is based on the woman's age, type of chest pain or angina, and the results of a noninvasive test such as an exercise electrocardiogram. If a woman has chest pain, there are three definitions (shown in Table 26.9) that the clinician can use to categorize it. Ridker and colleagues (2007) have published two algorithms for the assessment of women's CVD risk that were developed with and validated on the data from the 10-year Women's

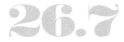

26.7 | Possible Symptoms of Acute Myocardial Infarction

Chest pain	Pain in center or left side of chest
	Chest heaviness, pressure, tightness, or squeezing
Non–chest pain symptoms	Dyspnea
	Diaphoresis
	Nausea or vomiting
	Epigastric discomfort or indigestion
	Mid-back pain
	Palpitations
	Fatigue
	Arm or shoulder pain
	Jaw pain
	Dizziness or fainting
	Neck or throat pain

Note. Based on "Comparison of Presentation, Treatment, and Outcome of Acute Myocardial Infarction in Men Versus Women (The Myocardial Infarction Triage and Intervention Registry)," by P. J. Kudenchuk, C. Maynard, J. S. Martin, M. Wirkus, and W. D. Weaver, 1996, *American Journal of Cardiology, 78*(1), pp. 9–14; "Typical Symptoms Are Predictive of Acute Coronary Syndromes in Women," by K. A. Milner, M. Funk, A. Arnold, and V. Vaccarino, 2002, *American Heart Journal, 143*(2), pp. 283–288.

26.8 | Diagnostic Tests for Coronary Heart Disease

Nonimaging	Electrocardiogram
	Exercise electrocardiogram
Imaging	Nuclear imaging using planar or single-photon emission computed tomography; can be used with stressors such as exercise
	Thallium-201
	Technetium-99m sestamibib
	Technetium-99m tetrofosmin
	Echocardiography
	Electron beam computed tomography
	Magnetic resonance imaging
	Positron emission tomography
	Coronary angiography

26.9 | Chest Pain Definitions

Definite angina	Substernal pressure that is precipitated by stress and exertion and relieved by rest or nitroglycerin in less than 10 minutes
Probable angina	Has most of the features of definite angina but is atypical in some aspect, such as radiation or duration
Nonspecific chest pain	Does not fit the patterns described for definite or probable angina

Note. From "Diagnostic Testing—Nonimaging and Imaging," by Y. Kwok and R. Redberg, 2002, in *Cardiovascular Health and Disease in Women* (2nd ed., pp. 342–356), by P. S. Douglas (Ed.), Philadelphia: Saunders.

Health Study. When these algorithms were used to classify women as low, moderate, or high risk, they were found to be more accurate than the Framingham or ATP III prediction scores for women. An online version of one of the two algoritms, the Reynolds Risk Score, can be found at www.reynoldriskscore.org.

A cost-effectiveness analysis by Kim and colleagues showed that women with definite angina, who therefore have a high probability of disease, should be sent directly for coronary catheterization, while women with moderate probability should first have a stress echocardiogram, and women with a low probability of disease should either receive a stress echocardiogram or no further testing (Douglas & Ginsburg, 1996; Kim, Kwok, Saha, & Redberg, 1999; Kwok & Redberg, 2002). Both cost and safety considerations constrain the use of coronary angiography. The American Heart Association and American College of Cardiology have collaborated to write guidelines on the appropriate use and conduct of coronary angiography as well as for other procedures such as exercise testing (Scanlon et al., 1999). The Web site of the American Heart Association (www.americanheart.org) posts the most recent versions of specific guidelines in the Statements and Guidelines section, which is in the Scientific Publications part of the site.

Management and Treatment of ASCVD

Once women have developed ASCVD, the treatment and management options include an increased focus on risk factor modification, often referred to as secondary prevention; use of anticoagulants, statins, beta blockers, and angiotensin-converting enzyme inhibitors; and a variety of more invasive interventions. The invasive interventions include angioplasty with or without stents, coronary artery bypass grafting, carotid endarterectomy, pacemakers, and implantation of a defibrillator. Although early studies indicated that women had a less favorable outcome after invasive interventions, studies that have adjusted the results for age and the presence of comorbid conditions have shown that the short- and long-term outcomes for women are similar to those for men (Gan et al., 2000; Glaser et al., 2002; Jacobs et al., 2002). What is most important is that women are offered all the treatment options that meet the current standard of care in a timely manner. As discussed in the previous section on risk factors, hormone replacement therapy is not recommended for either primary or secondary prevention of ASCVD.

Warning Signs of Heart Attack and Stroke

Because ASCVD is one of the major causes of death in women, one could argue that all women need to know how to identify whether they are having an event such as a heart attack or stroke. This need is particularly acute in women younger than age 55, in whom the diagnosis is often missed, and in women with known CVD risk factors, who are more likely to have events (Kannel, 2002; Pope et al., 2000). Clinicians must consider whether women in their care receive adequate information about their risks and appropriate actions if symptoms occur. Should any woman who is being treated for a CVD risk factor *not* receive information and periodic reminders about warning signs and actions? What education is appropriate for her family and friends? Now that this information is easy to access on the Internet and patient education literature can be printed at the point of care, we all need to be active in making sure women are knowledgeable about the importance of not delaying in seeking emergency care. Health care providers and emergency medical technicians must suspect ASCVD in women as well as in men.

REFERENCES

Akesson, A., Weismayer, C., Newby, P. K., & Wolk, A. (2007). Combined effect of low-risk dietary and lifestyle behaviors in primary prvention of myocardial infarction in women. *Archives of Internal Medicine, 167*(19), 2122–2127.

Alberti, K. G., Zimmet, P., & Shaw, J. (2005). The metabolic syndrome—a new worldwide definition. *Lancet, 366*(9491), 1059–1062.

Al-Delaimy, W. K., Manson, J. E., Solomon, C. G., Kawachi, I., Stampfer, M. J., Willett, W. C., et al. (2002). Smoking and risk of coronary heart disease among women with type 2 diabetes mellitus. *Archives of Internal Medicine, 162*(3), 273–279.

Allen, J. K., & Blumenthal, R. S. (1998). Risk factors in the offspring of women with premature coronary heart disease. *American Heart Journal, 135*(3), 428–434.

ALLHAT Collaborative Research Group. (2002). Major outcomes in high-risk hypertensive patients randomized to angiotensin-converting enzyme inhibitor or calcium channel blocker vs diuretic: The Antihypertensive and Lipid-Lowering Treatment to Prevent Heart Attack Trial (ALLHAT). *Journal of the American Medical Association, 288*(23), 2981–2997.

American Heart Association. (2006a). *Statistical fact sheet—Populations: International cardiovascular disease statistics.* Retrieved April 27, 2007, from http://www.americanheart. org/presenter.jhtml?identifier=3001008

American Heart Association. (2006b). *Statistical fact sheet—Populations: Women and cardiovascular diseases.* Retrieved April 27, 2007, from http://www.americanheart.org/presenter. jhtml?identifier=3000941

American Heart Association. (2007). *Heart attack, stroke & cardiac arrest warning signs.* Retrieved April 27, 2007, from http:// www.americanheart.org/presenter.jhtml?identifier=3053

Anderson, R. N. (2001). Deaths: Leading causes for 1999. *National Vital Statistics Report, 49*(11), 1–87.

Angeja, B. G., Shlipak, M. G., Go, A. S., Johnston, S. C., Frederick, P. D., Canto, J. G., et al. (2001). Hormone therapy and the risk of stroke after acute myocardial infarction in postmenopausal women. *Journal of the American College of Cardiology, 38*(5), 1297–1301.

Angerer, P., Stork, S., Kothny, W., Schmitt, P., & von Schacky, C. (2001). Effect of oral postmenopausal hormone replacement on progression of atherosclerosis: A randomized, controlled trial. *Arteriosclerosis, Thrombosis and Vascular Biology, 21*(2), 262–268.

Appel, L. J., Moore, T. J., Obarzanek, E., Vollmen, W. M., Svetkey, L. P., Sacks, F. M., et al. (1997). A clinical trial of the effects of dietary patterns on blood pressure. *New England Journal of Medicine, 336*, 1117–1124.

Aronow, H. D., Topol, E. J., Roe, M. T., Houghtaling, P. L., Wolski, K. E., Lincoff, A. M., et al. (2001). Effect of lipid-lowering therapy on early mortality after acute coronary syndromes: An observational study. *Lancet, 357*(9262), 1063–1068.

Ashton, K. C. (1999). How men and women with heart disease seek care: The delay experience. *Progress in Cardiovascular Nursing, 14*(2), 53–60, 74.

Ayas, N. T., White, D. P., Manson, J. E., Stampfer, M. J., Speizer, F. E., Malhotra, A., et al. (2003). A prospective study of sleep duration and coronary heart disease in women. *Archives of Internal Medicine, 163*(2), 205–209.

Bairey Merz, C. N., Shaw, L. J., Reis, S. E., Bittner, V., Kelsey, S. F., Olson, M., et al. (2006). Insights from the NHLBI-sponsored Women's Ischemia Syndrome Evaluation (WISE) Study: Part II: Gender differences in presentation, diagnosis, and outcome with regard to gender-based pathophysiology of atherosclerosis and macrovascular and microvascular coronary disease. *Journal of the American College of Cardiology, 47*(Suppl. 3), S21–S29.

Barrett-Connor, E., & Bush, T. L. (1991). Estrogen and coronary heart disease in women. *Journal of the American Medical Association, 265*, 1861–1867.

Barrett-Connor, E., Wingard, D. L., Criqui, M. H., & Suarez, L. (1984). Is borderline fasting hyperglycemia a risk factor for cardiovascular death? *Journal of Chronic Disease, 37*, 773–779.

Beckman, J. A., Creager, M. A., & Libby, P. (2002). Diabetes and atherosclerosis: Epidemiology, pathophysiology, and management. *Journal of the American Medical Association, 287*(19), 2570–2581.

Beral, V., & Million Women Study Collaborators. (2007). Ovarian cancer and hormone replacement therapy in the Million Women Study. *Lancet, 369*(9574), 1703–1710.

Berenson, G. S., Srinivasan, S. R., & Bao, W. (1997). Precursors of cardiovascular risk in young adults from a biracial (Black-White) population: The Bogalusa Heart Study. *Annals of the New York Academy of Sciences, 817,* 189–198.

Berenson, G. S., Srinivasan, S. R., Bao, W., Newman, W. P., III Tracy, R. E., Wattigney, W. A., et al. (1998). Association between multiple cardiovascular risk factors and atherosclerosis in children and young adults. *New England Journal of Medicine, 338,* 1650–1656.

Bermudez, E. A., Rifai, N., Buring, J., Manson, J. E., & Ridker, P. M. (2002). Interrelationships among circulating interleukin-6, C-reactive protein, and traditional cardiovascular risk factors in women. *Arteriosclerosis, Thrombosis and Vascular Biology, 22*(10), 1668–1673.

Bielak, L. F., Klee, G. G., Sheedy, P. F., 2nd, Turner, S. T., Schwartz, R. S., & Peyser, P. A. (2000). Association of fibrinogen with quantity of coronary artery calcification measured by electron beam computed tomography. *Arteriosclerosis, Thrombosis and Vascular Biology, 20*(9), 2167–2171.

Biswas, M. S., Calhoun, P. S., Bosworth, H. B., & Bastian, L. A. (2002). Are women worrying about heart disease? *Women's Health Issues, 12*(4), 204–211.

Bog-Hansen, E., Lindblad, U., Bengtsson, K., Ranstam, J., Melander, A., & Rastam, L. (1998). Risk factor clustering in patients with hypertension and non-insulin-dependent diabetes mellitus. The Skaraborg Hypertension Project. *Journal of Internal Medicine, 243*(3), 223–232.

Burke, A. P., Farb, A., Malcom, G. T., Liang, Y.-H., Smialek, J., & Virmani, R. (1997). Coronary risk factors and plaque morphology in men with coronary disease who died suddenly. *New England Journal of Medicine, 336,* 1276–1282.

Burke, A. P., Farb, A., Malcom, G. T., Liang, Y., Smialek, J., & Virmani, R. (1998). Effect of risk factors on the mechanism of acute thrombosis and sudden coronary death in women. *Circulation, 97,* 2110–2116.

Buse, J. B., Ginsberg, H. N., Bakris, G. L., Clark, N. G., Costa, F., Eckel, R., et al. (2007). Primary prevention of cardiovascular diseases in people with diabetes mellitus: A scientific statement from the American Heart Association and the American Diabetes Association. *Circulation, 115*(1), 114–126.

Byington, R. P., Furberg, C. D., Herrington, D. M., Herd, J. A., Hunninghake, D., Lowery, M., et al. (2002). Effect of estrogen plus progestin on progression of carotid atherosclerosis in postmenopausal women with heart disease: HERS B-mode substudy. *Arteriosclerosis, Thrombosis and Vascular Biology, 22*(10), 1692–1697.

Cabrera, C., Helgesson, O., Wedel, H., Bjorkelund, C., Bengtsson, C., & Lissner, L. (2001). Socioeconomic status and mortality in Swedish women: Opposing trends for cardiovascular disease and cancer. *Epidemiology, 12*(5), 532–536.

Calle, E. E., Rodriguez, C., Walker-Thurmond, K., & Thun, M. J. (2003). Overweight, obesity, and mortality from cancer in a prospectively studied cohort of U.S. adults. *New England Journal of Medicine, 348*(17), 1625–1638.

Calle, E. E., Thun, M. J., Petrelli, J. M., Rodriguez, C., & Heath, C. W., Jr. (1999). Body-mass index and mortality in a prospective cohort of U.S. adults. *New England Journal of Medicine, 341*(15), 1097–1105.

Campbell, C. L., Smyth, S., Montalescot, G., & Steinhubl, S. R. (2007). Aspirin dose for the prevention of cardiovascular disease: A systematic review. *Journal of the American Medical Association, 297*(18), 2018–2024.

Canto, J. G., Shlipak, M. G., Rogers, W. J., Malmgren, J. A., Frederick, P. D., Lambrew, C. T., et al. (2000). Prevalence, clinical characteristics, and mortality among patients with myocardial infarction presenting without chest pain. *Journal of the American Medical Association, 283*(24), 3223–3229.

Caralis, D. G., Deligonul, U., Kern, M. J., & Cohen, J. D. (1992). Smoking is a risk factor for coronary spasm in young women. *Circulation, 85,* 905–909.

Carr, D. B., Utzschneider, K. M., Hull, R. L., Tong, J., Wallace, T. M., Kodama, K., et al. (2006). Gestational diabetes mellitus increases the risk of cardiovascular disease in women with a family history of type 2 diabetes. *Diabetes Care, 29*(9), 2078–2083.

Centers for Disease Control and Prevention. (2001). Increasing physical activity. A report on recommendations of the Task Force on Community Preventive Services. *MMWR Recommendation Report, 50*(RR-18), 1–14.

Chaput, L. A., Adams, S. H., Simon, J. A., Blumenthal, R. S., Vittinghoff, E., Lin, F., et al. (2002). Hostility predicts recurrent events among postmenopausal women with coronary heart disease. *American Journal of Epidemiology, 156*(12), 1092–1099.

Cherry, N., Gilmour, K., Hannaford, P., Heagerty, A., Khan, M. A., Kitchener, H., et al. (2002). Oestrogen therapy for prevention of reinfarction in postmenopausal women: A randomised placebo controlled trial. *Lancet, 360*(9350), 2001–2008.

Cheung, N. W., & Byth, K. (2003). Population health significance of gestational diabetes. *Diabetes Care, 26*(7), 2005–2009.

Chobanian, A. V., Bakris, G. L., Black, H. R., Cushman, W. C., Green, L. A., Izzo, J. L., Jr., et al. (2003). The seventh report of the Joint National Committee on Prevention, Detection, Evaluation, and Treatment of High Blood Pressure: The JNC 7 report. *Journal of the American Medical Association, 289*(19), 2560–2572. [Erratum in *Journal of the American Medical Association,* 2003, *290*(2), 197]

Chung, C. P., Oeser, A., Raggi, P., Gebretsadik, T., Shintani, A. K., Sokka, T., et al. (2005). Increased coronary-artery atherosclerosis in rheumatoid arthritis: Relationship to disease duration and cardiovascular risk factors. *Arthritis and Rheumatism, 52*(10), 3045–3053.

Clarke, S. C., Kelleher, J., Lloyd-Jones, H., Slack, M., & Schofiel, P. M. (2002). A study of hormone replacement therapy in postmenopausal women with ischaemic heart disease: The Papworth HRT atherosclerosis study. *British Journal of Gynaecology, 109*(9), 1056–1062.

Collins, R., Peto, R., MacMahon, S., Hebert, P., Fiebach, N. H., Eberlein, K. A., et al. (1990). Blood pressure, stroke, and coronary heart disease. Part 2, short-term reductions in blood pressure: Overview of randomised drug trials in their epidemiological context. *Lancet, 335,* 827–838.

Cook, N. R., Cutler, J. A., Obarzanek, E., Buring, J. E., Rexrode, K. M., Kumanyika, S. K., et al. (2007). Long term effects of dietary sodium reduction on cardiovascular disease outcomes: Observational follow-up of the trials of hypertension prevention (TOHP). *British Medical Journal, 334*(7599), 885.

Croce, K., & Libby, P. (2007). Intertwining of thrombosis and inflammation in atherosclerosis. *Current Opinions in Hematology, 14*(1), 55–61.

Cunningham, S. G. (1998). Women's heart health—An integrated approach to prevention. *Canadian Journal of Cardiovascular Nursing, 9*(3), 28–37.

Curb, J. D., Prentice, R. L., Bray, P. F., Langer, R. D., Van Horn, L., Barnabei, V. M., et al. (2006). Venous thrombosis and conjugated equine estrogen in women without a uterus. *Archives of Internal Medicine, 166*(7), 772–780.

Daugherty, S. A. (1983). Hypertension detection and follow-up: Description of the enumerated and screened population. *Hypertension, 5*(Suppl. 4), 1–43.

Daviglus, M. L., Liu, K., Greenland, P., Dyer, A. R., Garside, D. B., Manheim, L., et al. (1998). Benefit of a favorable cardiovascular risk-factor profile in middle age with respect to Medicare costs. *New England Journal of Medicine, 339*, 1122–1129.

Daviglus, M. L., Stamler, J., Pirzada, A., Yan, L. L., Garside, D. B., Liu, K., et al. (2004). Favorable cardiovascular risk profile in young women and long-term risk of cardiovascular and all-cause mortality. *Journal of the American Medical Association, 292*(13), 1588–1592.

de Leeuw, K., Kallenberg, C., & Bijl, M. (2005). Accelerated atherosclerosis in patients with systemic autoimmune diseases. *Annals of the New York Academy of Sciences, 1051*, 362–371.

DeSouza, C. A., Jones, P. P., & Seals, D. R. (1998). Physical activity status and adverse age-related differences in coagulation and fibrinolytic factors in women. *Arteriosclerosis, Thrombosis and Vascular Biology, 18*(3), 362–368.

DeVon, H. A., & Zerwic, J. J. (2002). Symptoms of acute coronary syndromes: Are there gender differences? A review of the literature. *Heart Lung, 31*(4), 235–245.

DeVon, H. A., & Zerwic, J. J. (2003). The symptoms of unstable angina: Do women and men differ? *Nursing Research, 52*(2), 108–118.

DiCorleto, P. E., & Gimbrone, M. A., Jr. (1996). Vascular endothelium. In V. Fuster, R. Ross, & E. J. Topol (Eds.), *Atherosclerosis and coronary artery disease* (Vol. 1, pp. 387–399). Philadelphia: Lippincott-Raven.

Douglas, P. S., & Ginsburg, G. S. (1996). The evaluation of chest pain in women. *New England Journal of Medicine, 334*, 1311–1315.

Ebrahim, S., & Smith, G. D. (1997). Systematic review of randomised controlled trials of multiple risk factor interventions for preventing coronary heart disease. *British Medical Journal, 314*(7095), 1666–1674.

Eichner, J. E., Moore, W. E., McKee, P. A., Schechter, E., Reynolds, D. W., Qi, H., et al. (1996). Fibrinogen levels in women having coronary angiography. *American Journal of Cardiology, 78*(1), 15–18.

Eriksson, M., Egberg, N., Wamala, S., Orth-Gomer, K., Mittleman, M. A., & Schenck-Gustafsson, K. (1999). Relationship between plasma fibrinogen and coronary heart disease in women. *Arteriosclerosis, Thrombosis and Vascular Biology, 19*(1), 67–72.

Finnegan, J. R., Jr., Meischke, H., Zapka, J. G., Leviton, L., Meshack, A., Benjamin-Garner, R., et al. (2000). Patient delay in seeking care for heart attack symptoms: Findings from focus groups conducted in five U.S. regions. *Preventive Medicine, 31*(3), 205–213.

Fries, J. F. (1980). Aging, natural death, and the compression of morbidity. *New England Journal of Medicine, 303*, 130–135.

Fuster, V. (1994). Conner Memorial Lecture. Mechanisms leading to myocardial infarction: Insights from studies of vascular biology [Erratum in *Circulation*, 1995, *91*(1), 256]. *Circulation, 90*, 2126–2146.

Galuska, D., Serdula, M., Brown, D., & Kruger, J. (2002). Prevalence of health-care providers asking older adults about their physical activity levels—United States, 1998. *MMWR, 51*(19), 412–414.

Gan, S. C., Beaver, S. K., Houck, P. M., MacLehose, R. F., Lawson, H. W., & Chan, L. (2000). Treatment of acute myocardial infarction and 30-day mortality among women and men. *New England Journal of Medicine, 343*(1), 8–15.

Geffken, D. F., Cushman, M., Burke, G. L., Polak, J. F., Sakkinen, P. A., & Tracy, R. P. (2001). Association between physical activity and markers of inflammation in a healthy elderly population. *American Journal of Epidemiology, 153*(3), 242–250.

Glagov, S., Weisenberg, E., Zarins, C. K., Stankunavicius, R., & Kolettis, G. J. (1987). Compensatory enlargement of human atherosclerotic coronary arteries. *New England Journal of Medicine, 316*(22), 1371–1375.

Glaser, R., Herrmann, H. C., Murphy, S. A., Demopoulos, L. A., DiBattiste, P. M., Cannon, C. P., et al. (2002). Benefit of an early invasive management strategy in women with acute coronary syndromes. *Journal of the American Medical Association, 288*(24), 3124–3129.

Glynn, R. J., Field, T. S., Rosner, B., Hebert, P. R., Taylor, J. O., & Hennekens, C. H. (1995). Evidence for a positive linear relation between blood pressure and mortality in elderly people. *Lancet, 345*(8953), 825–829.

Grady, D., Herrington, D., Bittner, V., Blumenthal, R., Davidson, M., Hlatky, M., et al. (2002). Cardiovascular disease outcomes during 6.8 years of hormone therapy: Heart and Estrogen/Progestin Replacement Study follow-up (HERS II). *Journal of the American Medical Association, 288*(1), 49–57.

Grady, D., & Sawaya, G. (1998). Postmenopausal hormone therapy increases risk of deep vein thrombosis and pulmonary embolism. *American Journal of Medicine, 105*, 41–43.

Gregg, E. W., Cauley, J. A., Stone, K., Thompson, T. J., Bauer, D. C., Cummings, S. R., et al. (2003). Relationship of changes in physical activity and mortality among older women. *Journal of the American Medical Association, 289*(18), 2379–2386.

Grover, S. A., Paquet, S., Levinton, C., Coupal, L., & Zowall, H. (1998). Estimating the benefits of modifying risk factors of cardiovascular disease: A comparison of primary vs secondary prevention. *Archives of Internal Medicine, 158*(6), 655–662. [Erratum in *Archives of Internal Medicine*, 1998, *158*(11), 1228]

Grundy, S. M., Cleeman, J. I., Daniels, S. R., Donato, K. A., Eckel, R. H., Franklin, B. A., et al. (2005). Diagnosis and management of the metabolic syndrome: An American Heart Association/National Heart, Lung, and Blood Institute scientific statement. *Circulation, 112*(17), 2735–2752.

Grundy, S. M., Cleeman, J. I., Merz, C. N., Brewer, H. B., Jr., Clark, L. T., Hunninghake, D. B., et al. (2004). Implications of recent clinical trials for the National Cholesterol Education Program Adult Treatment Panel III guidelines. *Circulation, 110*(2), 227–239.

Gu, K., Cowie, C. C., & Harris, M. I. (1999). Diabetes and decline in heart disease mortality in US adults. *Journal of the American Medical Association, 281*(14), 1291–1297.

Haarbo, J., Hassager, C., Riis, B. J., & Christiansen, C. (1989). Relation of body fat distribution to serum lipids and lipoproteins in elderly women. *Atherosclerosis, 80*, 57–62.

Hackam, D. G., & Anand, S. S. (2003). Emerging risk factors for atherosclerotic vascular disease: A critical review of the evidence. *Journal of the American Medical Association, 290*(7), 932–940.

Hansson, G. K., & Libby, P. (2006). The immune response in atherosclerosis: A double-edged sword. *Nature Reviews of Immunology, 6*(7), 508–519.

Hassinen, M., Komulainen, P., Lakka, T. A., Vaisanen, S. B., Haapala, I., Gylling, H., et al. (2006). Metabolic syndrome and the progression of carotid intima-media thickness in elderly women. *Archives of Internal Medicine, 166*(4), 444–449.

Hayes, D. K., Denny, C. H., Keenan, N. L., Croft, J. B., Sundaram, A. A., & Greenlund, K. J. (2006). Racial/ethnic and socioeconomic differences in multiple risk factors for heart disease and stroke in women: Behavioral risk factor surveillance system, 2003. *Journal of Women's Health (Larchmt), 15*(9), 1000–1008.

Healy, B. (1991a). Women's health, public welfare. *Journal of the American Medical Association, 266*, 566–568.

Healy, B. (1991b). The Yentl syndrome. *New England Journal of Medicine, 325*(4), 274–276.

Heart Protection Study Collaborative Group. (2002). MRC/BHF Heart Protection Study of cholesterol lowering with simvastatin in 20,536 high-risk individuals: A randomised placebo-controlled trial. *Lancet, 360*(9326), 7–22.

Hermanson, B., Omenn, G. S., Kronmal, R. A., Gersh, B. J., & Participants in the Coronary Artery Surgery Study. (1988). Beneficial six-year outcome of smoking cessation in older men and women with coronary artery disease. *New England Journal of Medicine, 319*, 1365.

Herrington, D. M., Reboussin, D. M., Brosnihan, K. B., Sharp, P. C., Shumaker, S. A., Snyder, T. E., et al. (2000). Effects of estrogen replacement on the progression of coronary-artery atherosclerosis. *New England Journal of Medicine, 343*(8), 522–529.

Herrington, D. M., Vittinghoff, E., Lin, F., Fong, J., Harris, F., Hunninghake, D., et al. (2002). Statin therapy, cardiovascular events, and total mortality in the Heart and Estrogen/Progestin Replacement Study (HERS). *Circulation, 105*(25), 2962–2967.

Hill, J. O., & Bessesen, D. (2003). What to do about the metabolic syndrome? *Archives of Internal Medicine, 163*(4), 395–397.

Howard, G., Burke, G. L., Szklo, M., Tell, G. S., Eckfeldt, J., Evans, G., et al. (1994). Active and passive smoking are associated with increased carotid wall thickness. The Atherosclerosis Risk in Communities Study. *Archives of Internal Medicine, 154*(11), 1277–1282.

Hsia, J., Langer, R. D., Manson, J. E., Kuller, L., Johnson, K. C., Hendrix, S. L., et al. (2006). Conjugated equine estrogens and coronary heart disease: The Women's Health Initiative. *Archives of Internal Medicine, 166*(3), 357–365.

Hsia, J., Margolis, K. L., Eaton, C. B., Wenger, N. K., Allison, M., Wu, L., et al. (2007). Prehypertension and cardiovascular disease risk in the Women's Health Initiative. *Circulation, 115*(7), 855–860.

Hsia, J., Simon, J. A., Lin, F., Applegate, W. B., Vogt, M. T., Hunninghake, D., et al. (2000). Peripheral arterial disease in randomized trial of estrogen with progestin in women with coronary heart disease: The Heart and Estrogen/Progestin Replacement Study. *Circulation, 102*(18), 2228–2232.

Hu, F. B., Li, T. Y., Colditz, G. A., Willett, W. C., & Manson, J. E. (2003). Television watching and other sedentary behaviors in relation to risk of obesity and type 2 diabetes mellitus in women. *Journal of the American Medical Association, 289*(14), 1785–1791.

Hu, F. B., Manson, J. E., Stampfer, M. J., Colditz, G., Liu, S., Solomon, C. G., et al. (2001). Diet, lifestyle, and the risk of type 2 diabetes mellitus in women. *New England Journal of Medicine, 345*(11), 790–797.

Hu, F. B., Sigal, R. J., Rich-Edwards, J. W., Colditz, G. A., Solomon, C. G., Willett, W. C., et al. (1999). Walking compared with vigorous physical activity and risk of type 2 diabetes in women: A prospective study. *Journal of the American Medical Association, 282*(15), 1433–1439.

Hu, F. B., Stampfer, M. J., Solomon, C. G., Liu, S., Willett, W. C., Speizer, F. E., et al. (2001). The impact of diabetes mellitus on mortality from all causes and coronary heart disease in women: 20 years of follow-up. *Archives of Internal Medicine, 161*(14), 1717–1723.

Hu, F. B., & Willett, W. C. (2002). Optimal diets for prevention of coronary heart disease. *Journal of the American Medical Association, 288*(20), 2569–2578.

Huang, Z., Willett, W. C., Manson, J. E., Rosner, B., Stampfer, M. J., Speizer, F. E., et al. (1998). Body weight, weight change, and risk for hypertension in women. *Annals of Internal Medicine, 128*, 81–88.

Hulley, S., Grady, D., Bush, T., Furberg, C., Herrington, D., Riggs, B., et al. (1998). Randomized trial of estrogen plus progestin for secondary prevention of coronary heart disease in postmenopausal women. *Journal of the American Medical Association, 280*, 605–613.

Husain, S., Andrews, N. P., Mulcahy, D., Panza, J. A., & Quyyumi, A. A. (1998). Aspirin improves endothelial dysfunction in atherosclerosis. *Circulation, 97*, 716–720.

Huxley, R., Barzi, F., & Woodward, M. (2006). Excess risk of fatal coronary heart disease associated with diabetes in men and women: Meta-analysis of 37 prospective cohort studies. *British Medical Journal, 332*(7533), 73–78.

Hypertension Detection and Follow-up Program Cooperative Group. (1979). Five-year findings of the hypertension detection and follow-up program. I. Reduction in mortality of persons with high blood pressure, including mild hypertension. *Journal of the American Medical Association, 242*, 2562–2571.

Hypertension Detection and Follow-up Program Cooperative Group. (1982). The effect of treatment on mortality in "mild" hypertension. Results of the hypertension detection and follow-up program. *New England Journal of Medicine, 307*, 976–980.

Irwin, M. L., Yasui, Y., Ulrich, C. M., Bowen, D., Rudolph, R. E., Schwartz, R. S., et al. (2003). Effect of exercise on total and intra-abdominal body fat in postmenopausal women: A randomized controlled trial. *Journal of the American Medical Association, 289*(3), 323–330.

Iscan, A., Uyanik, B. S., Vurgun, N., Ece, A., & Yigitoglu, M. R. (1996). Effects of passive exposure to tobacco, socioeconomic status and a family history of essential hypertension on lipid profiles in children. *Japanese Heart Journal, 37*(6), 917–923.

Jacobs, A. K., Johnston, J. M., Haviland, A., Brooks, M. M., Kelsey, S. F., Holmes, D. R., et al. (2002). Improved outcomes for women undergoing contemporary percutaneous coronary intervention: A report from the National Heart, Lung, and Blood Institute Dynamic Registry. *Journal of the American College of Cardiology, 39*(10), 1608–1614.

Johnson, B. D., Shaw, L. J., Pepine, C. J., Reis, S. E., Kelsey, S. F., Sopko, G., et al. (2006). Persistent chest pain predicts cardiovascular events in women without obstructive coronary artery disease: Results from the NIH-NHLBI-sponsored Women's Ischaemia Syndrome Evaluation (WISE) study. *European Heart Journal, 27*(12), 1408–1415.

Jones, D. W., Chambless, L. E., Folsom, A. R., Heiss, G., Hutchinson, R. G., Sharrett, A. R., et al. (2002). Risk factors for coronary heart disease in African Americans: The atherosclerosis risk in communities study, 1987–1997. *Archives of Internal Medicine, 162*(22), 2565–2571.

Kanaya, A. M., Grady, D., & Barrett-Connor, E. (2002). Explaining the sex difference in coronary heart disease mortality among patients with type 2 diabetes mellitus: A meta-analysis. *Archives of Internal Medicine, 162*(15), 1737–1745.

Kane, J. P., Malloy, M. J., Ports, T. A., Phillips, N. R., Diehl, J. C., & Havel, R. J. (1990). Regression of coronary atherosclerosis during treatment of familial hypercholesterolemia with combined drug regimens. *Journal of the American Medical Association, 264*, 3007–3012.

Kannel, W. B. (2002). The Framingham Study: Historical insight on the impact of cardiovascular risk factors in men versus women. *Journal of Gender Specific Medicine, 5*(2), 27–37.

Kannel, W. B., Brand, N., Skinner, J. J., Jr., Dawber, T. R., & McNamara, P. M. (1967). The relation of adiposity to blood pressure and development of hypertension: The Framingham study. *Annals of Internal Medicine, 67,* 48–59.

Kannel, W. B., & Wilson, P. W. (1995). Risk factors that attenuate the female coronary disease advantage. *Archives of Internal Medicine, 155*(1), 57–61.

Katz, M. E., Holmes, M. D., Power, K. L., & Wise, P. H. (1995). Mortality rates among 15- to 44-year-old women in Boston: Looking beyond reproductive status. *American Journal of Public Health, 85*(8 Pt. 1), 1135–1138.

Kawachi, I., Colditz, G. A., Stampfer, M. J., Willett, W. C., Manson, J. E., Rosner, B., et al. (1993). Smoking cessation in relation to total mortality rates in women: A prospective study. *Annals of Internal Medicine, 119,* 992–1000.

Kim, C., Kwok, Y. S., Saha, S., & Redberg, R. F. (1999). Diagnosis of suspected coronary artery disease in women: A cost-effectiveness analysis. *American Heart Journal, 137*(6), 1019–1027.

Kimm, S. Y., Glynn, N. W., Kriska, A. M., Barton, B. A., Kronsberg, S. S., Daniels, S. R., et al. (2002). Decline in physical activity in Black girls and White girls during adolescence. *New England Journal of Medicine, 347*(10), 709–715.

Kip, K. E., Marroquin, O. C., Kelley, D. E., Johnson, B. D., Kelsey, S. F., Shaw, L. J., et al. (2004). Clinical importance of obesity versus the metabolic syndrome in cardiovascular risk in women: A report from the Women's Ischemia Syndrome Evaluation (WISE) study. *Circulation, 109*(6), 706–713.

Knowler, W. C., Barrett-Connor, E., Fowler, S. E., Hamman, R. F., Lachin, J. M., Walker, E. A., et al. (2002). Reduction in the incidence of type 2 diabetes with lifestyle intervention or metformin. *New England Journal of Medicine, 346*(6), 393–403.

Koenig, W., Sund, M., Frohlich, M., Fischer, H. G., Lowel, H., Doring, A., et al. (1999). C-reactive protein, a sensitive marker of inflammation, predicts future risk of coronary heart disease in initially healthy middle-aged men: Results from the MONICA (Monitoring Trends and Determinants in Cardiovascular Disease) Augsburg Cohort Study, 1984 to 1992. *Circulation, 99*(2), 237–242.

Kris-Etherton, P. M., Lichtenstein, A. H., Howard, B. V., Steinberg, D., & Witztum, J. L. (2004). Antioxidant vitamin supplements and cardiovascular disease. *Circulation, 110*(5), 637–641.

Kudenchuk, P. J., Maynard, C., Martin, J. S., Wirkus, M., & Weaver, W. D. (1996). Comparison of presentation, treatment, and outcome of acute myocardial infarction in men versus women (The Myocardial Infarction Triage and Intervention Registry). *American Journal of Cardiology, 78*(1), 9–14.

Kullo, I. J., Edwards, W. D., & Schwartz, R. S. (1998). Vulnerable plaque: Pathobiology and clinical implications. *Annals of Internal Medicine, 129*(12), 1050–1060.

Kwok, Y., Kim, C., Grady, D., Segal, M., & Redberg, R. (1999). Meta-analysis of exercise testing to detect coronary artery disease in women. *American Journal of Cardiology, 83*(5), 660–666.

Kwok, Y., & Redberg, R. (2002). Diagnostic testing—Nonimaging and imaging. In P. S. Douglas (Ed.), *Cardiovascular health and disease in women* (2nd ed., pp. 342–356). Philadelphia: Saunders.

LaCroix, A. Z., Lang, J., Scherr, P., Wallace, R. B., Coroni-Huntley, J., Berkman, L., et al. (1991). Smoking and mortality among older men and women in three communities. *New England Journal of Medicine, 324,* 1619–1625.

LaCroix, A. Z., Newton, K. M., LeVeille, S. G., & Wallace, J. (1997). Healthy aging: A women's issue. *Western Journal of Medicine, 167,* 220–232.

Larsson, B., Bengtsson, C., Bjorntorp, P., Lapidus, L., Sjostrom, L., Svordsudd, K., et al. (1992). Is abdominal body fat distribution a major explanation for the sex difference in the incidence of myocardial infarction. *American Journal of Epidemiology, 135,* 266–273.

Lefler, L. L., & Bondy, K. N. (2004). Women's delay in seeking treatment with myocardial infarction: A meta-synthesis. *Journal of Cardiovascular Nursing, 19*(4), 251–268.

Legato, M. J., Padus, E., & Slaughter, E. (1997). Women's perceptions of their general health, with special reference to their risk of coronary artery disease: Results of a national telephone survey. *Journal of Women's Health, 6,* 198.

Lemaitre, R. N., Weiss, N. S., Smith, N. L., Psaty, B. M., Lumley, T., Larson, E. B., et al. (2006). Esterified estrogen and conjugated equine estrogen and the risk of incident myocardial infarction and stroke. *Archives of Internal Medicine, 166*(4), 399–404.

Lerman, A., Cannan, C. R., Higano, S. H., Nishimura, R. A., & Holmes, D. R., Jr. (1998). Coronary vascular remodeling in association with endothelial dysfunction. *American Journal of Cardiology, 81*(9), 1105–1109.

Levinson, S. S. (2005). Brief review and critical examination of the use of hs-CRP for cardiac risk assessment with the conclusion that it is premature to use this test. *Clinica Chimica Acta, 356*(1–2), 1–8.

Lewington, S., Clarke, R., Qizilbash, N., Peto, R., & Collins, R. (2002). Age-specific relevance of usual blood pressure to vascular mortality: A meta-analysis of individual data for one million adults in 61 prospective studies. *Lancet, 360*(9349), 1903–1913.

Liao, Y., Cooper, R. S., Mensah, G. A., & McGee, D. L. (1995). Left ventricular hypertrophy has a greater impact on survival in women than in men. *Circulation, 92*(4), 805–810.

Libby, P., Schoenbeck, U., Mach, F., Selwyn, A. P., & Ganz, P. (1998). Current concepts in cardiovascular pathology: The role of LDL cholesterol in plaque rupture and stabilization. *American Journal of Medicine, 104*(2A), 14S–18S.

Lindmark, E., Wallentin, L., & Siegbahn, A. (2001). Blood cell activation, coagulation, and inflammation in men and women with coronary artery disease. *Thrombosis Research, 103*(3), 249–259.

Lissner, L., Odell, P. M., D'Agostino, R. B., Stokes, J., Kreger, B. E., Belanger, A. J., et al. (1991). Variability of body weight and health outcomes in the Framingham population. *New England Journal of Medicine, 324,* 1839–1844.

Liuzzo, G., Biasucci, L. M., Gallimore, J. R., Grillo, R. L., Rebuzzi, A. G., Pepys, M. B., et al. (1994). The prognostic value of C-reactive protein and serum amyloid A protein in severe unstable angina. *New England Journal of Medicine, 331,* 417–424.

Lloyd-Jones, D. M., Leip, E. P., Larson, M. G., D'Agostino, R. B., Beiser, A., Wilson, P. W., et al. (2006). Prediction of lifetime risk for cardiovascular disease by risk factor burden at 50 years of age. *Circulation, 113*(6), 791–798.

Lloyd-Jones, D. M., Nam, B. H., D'Agostino, R. B., Sr., Levy, D., Murabito, J. M., Wang, T. J., et al. (2004). Parental cardiovascular disease as a risk factor for cardiovascular disease in middle-aged adults: A prospective study of parents and offspring. *Journal of the American Medical Association, 291*(18), 2204–2211.

Lorenzo, C., Williams, K., Hunt, K. J., & Haffner, S. M. (2007). The National Cholesterol Education Program—Adult Treatment Panel III, International Diabetes Federation, and World Health Organization definitions of the metabolic syndrome as predictors of incident cardiovascular disease and diabetes. *Diabetes Care, 30*(1), 8–13.

MacMahon, S., Peto, R., Cutler, J., Collins, R., Sorlie, P., Neaton, J., et al. (1990). Blood pressure, stroke, and coronary heart disease. Part 1, prolonged differences in blood pressure: Prospective observational studies corrected for dilution bias. *Lancet, 335,* 765–774.

MacMahon, S., & Rodgers, A. (1993). The effects of blood pressure reduction in older patients: An overview of five randomized controlled trials in elderly hypertensives. *Clinical and Experimental Hypertension, 15*(6), 967–978.

Manolio, T. A., Pearson, T. A., Wenger, N. K., Barrett-Connor, E., Payne, G. H., & Harlan, W. R. (1992). Cholesterol and heart disease in older persons and women. Review of an NHLBI workshop. *Annals of Epidemiology, 2*(1–2), 161–176.

Manson, J. E., Greenland, P., LaCroix, A. Z., Stefanick, M. L., Mouton, C. P., Oberman, A., et al. (2002). Walking compared with vigorous exercise for the prevention of cardiovascular events in women. *New England Journal of Medicine, 347*(10), 716–725.

Manson, J. E., Hu, F. B., Rich-Edwards, J. W., Colditz, G. A., Stampfer, M. J., Willett, W. C., et al. (1999). A prospective study of walking as compared with vigorous exercise in the prevention of coronary heart disease in women. *New England Journal of Medicine, 341*(9), 650–658.

Manson, J. E., Rimm, E. B., Stampfer, M. J., Colditz, G. A., Willett, W. C., Krolewski, A. S., et al. (1991). Physical activity and incidence of non-insulin-dependent diabetes mellitus in women. *Lancet, 338*, 774–778.

Manson, J. E., Willett, W. C., Stampfer, M. J., Colditz, G. A., Hunter, D. J., Hankinson, S. E., et al. (1995). Body weight and mortality among women. *New England Journal of Medicine, 333*, 677–685.

Marrugat, J., Sala, J., Masia, R., Pavesi, M., Sanz, G., Valle, V., et al. (1998). Mortality differences between men and women following first myocardial infarction. *Journal of the American Medical Association, 280*, 1405–1409.

Maseri, A. (1997). Inflammation, atherosclerosis, and ischemic events—Exploring the hidden side of the moon. *New England Journal of Medicine, 336*, 1014–1015.

Mathers, C. D., Sadana, R., Salomon, J. A., Murray, C. J., & Lopez, A. D. (2001). Healthy life expectancy in 191 countries, 1999. *Lancet, 357*(9269), 1685–1691.

McGill, H. C., Jr., McMahan, C. A., Zieske, A. W., Malcom, G. T., Tracy, R. E., & Strong, J. P. (2001). Effects of nonlipid risk factors on atherosclerosis in youth with a favorable lipoprotein profile. *Circulation, 103*(11), 1546–1550.

McTigue, K., Larson, J. C., Valoski, A., Burke, G., Kotchen, J., Lewis, C. E., et al. (2006). Mortality and cardiac and vascular outcomes in extremely obese women. *Journal of the American Medical Association, 296*(1), 79–86.

Mehta, J. L., Saldeen, T. G., & Rand, K. (1998). Interactive role of infection, inflammation and traditional risk factors in atherosclerosis and coronary artery disease. *Journal of the American College of Cardiology, 31*(6), 1217–1225.

Meigs, J. B., D'Agostino, R. B., Sr., Wilson, P. W., Cupples, L. A., Nathan, D. M., & Singer, D. E. (1997). Risk variable clustering in the insulin resistance syndrome. The Framingham Offspring Study. *Diabetes, 46*(10), 1594–1600.

Meigs, J. B., Nathan, D. M., Wilson, P. W., Cupples, L. A., & Singer, D. E. (1998). Metabolic risk factors worsen continuously across the spectrum of nondiabetic glucose tolerance. The Framingham Offspring Study. *Annals of Internal Medicine, 128*(7), 524–533.

Menon, S. C., Pandey, D. K., & Margenstern, L. B. (1998). Critical factors determining access to acute stroke care. *Neurology, 51*, 427–432.

Mieres, J. H., Shaw, L. J., Arai, A., Budoff, M. J., Flamm, S. D., Hundley, W. G., et al. (2005). Role of noninvasive testing in the clinical evaluation of women with suspected coronary artery disease: Consensus statement from the Cardiac Imaging Committee, Council on Clinical Cardiology, and the Cardiovascular Imaging and Intervention Committee, Council on Cardiovascular Radiology and Intervention, American Heart Association. *Circulation, 111*(5), 682–696.

Miettinen, H., Lehto, S., Salomaa, V., Mahonen, M., Niemela, M., Haffner, S. M., et al. (1998). Impact of diabetes on mortality after the first myocardial infarction. The FINMONICA Myocardial Infarction Register Study Group. *Diabetes Care, 21*(1), 69–75.

Miller, C. L. (2002). A review of symptoms of coronary artery disease in women. *Journal of Advanced Nursings, 39*(1), 17–23.

Milner, K. A., Funk, M., Arnold, A., & Vaccarino, V. (2002). Typical symptoms are predictive of acute coronary syndromes in women. *American Heart Journal, 143*(2), 283–288.

Milner, K. A., Funk, M., Richards, S., Wilmes, R. M., Vaccarino, V., & Krumholz, H. M. (1999). Gender differences in symptom presentation associated with coronary heart disease. *American Journal of Cardiology, 84*(4), 396–399.

Morrato, E. H., Hill, J. O., Wyatt, H. R., Ghushchyan, V., & Sullivan, P. W. (2006). Are health care professionals advising patients with diabetes or at risk for developing diabetes to exercise more? *Diabetes Care, 29*(3), 543–548.

Mosca, L., Banka, C. L., Benjamin, E. J., Berra, K., Bushnell, C., Dolor, R. J., et al. (2007). Evidence-based guidelines for cardiovascular disease prevention in women: 2007 update. *Circulation, 115*(11), 1481–1501.

Mosca, L., Jones, W. K., King, K. B., Ouyang, P., Redberg, R. F., & Hill, M. N. (2000). Awareness, perception, and knowledge of heart disease risk and prevention among women in the United States. American Heart Association Women's Heart Disease and Stroke Campaign Task Force. *Archives of Family Medicine, 9*(6), 506–515.

Mosca, L., Manson, J. E., Sutherland, S. E., Langer, R. D., Manolio, T., & Barrett-Connor, E. (1997). Cardiovascular disease in women: A statement for healthcare professionals from the American Heart Association. *Circulation, 96*, 2468–2482.

Mosca, L., Mochari, H., Christian, A., Berra, K., Taubert, K., Mills, T., et al. (2006). National study of women's awareness, preventive action, and barriers to cardiovascular health. *Circulation, 113*(4), 525–534.

Moser, D. K., McKinley, S., Dracup, K., & Chung, M. L. (2005). Gender differences in reasons patients delay in seeking treatment for acute myocardial infarction symptoms. *Patient Education and Counseling, 56*(1), 45–54.

MRC Working Party. (1992). Medical Research Council trial of treatment of hypertension in older adults: Principal results. *British Medical Journal, 304*(6824), 405–412.

Murray, C. J., & Lopez, A. D. (1997). Alternative projections of mortality and disability by cause 1990–2020: Global Burden of Disease Study. *Lancet, 349*(9064), 1498–1504.

Must, A., Jacques, P. F., Dallai, G. E., Bajema, C. J., & Dietz, W. H. (1992). Long-term morbidity and mortality of overweight adolescents. *New England Journal of Medicine, 327*, 1350–1355.

Nabel, E. G. (2000). Coronary heart disease in women—An ounce of prevention. *New England Journal of Medicine, 343*(8), 572–574.

Narahara, N., Enden, T., Wiiger, M., & Prydz, H. (1994). Polar expression of tissue factor in human umbilical vein endothelial cells. *Arteriosclerosis and Thrombosis, 14*(11), 1815–1820.

National Center for Health Statistics. (2006a). *Faststats A to Z: Deaths/mortality*. Retrieved April 27, 2007, from http://www.cdc.gov/nchs/fastats/deaths.htm

National Center for Health Statistics. (2006b). *Health, United States, 2006 with chartbook on trends in the health of Americans*. Hyattsville, MD: Author.

National Center for Health Statistics. (2007). *Faststats: Women's health.* Retrieved April 28, 2007, from http://www.cdc.gov/nchs/fastats/womens_health.htm

National Cholesterol Education Program. (2002). *Detection, evaluation, and treatment of high blood cholesterol in adults (Adult Treatment Panel III).* NIH Publication No. 02-5215. National Heart, Lung and Blood Institutes, National Institutes of Health.

National Cholesterol Education Program Expert Panel on Detection, Evaluation, and Treatment of High Blood Cholesterol in Adults (Adult Treatment Panel III). (2001). Executive summary of the third report of the National Cholesterol Education Program (NCEP) Expert Panel on Detection, Evaluation, and Treatment of High Blood Cholesterol in Adults (Adult Treatment Panel III). *Journal of the American Medical Association, 285*(19), 2486–2497.

National Institutes of Health. (1998). *Clinical guidelines on the identification, evaluation, and treatment of overweight and obesity in adults: The evidence report.* NIH Publication No. 98-4083. Retrieved April 28, 2007, from http://www.nhlbi.nih.gov/guidelines/obesity/ob_gdlns.htm

Nielsen, N. E., Logander, E., & Swahn, E. (2001). Fibrinolytic variables in postmenopausal women with unstable coronary artery disease. *Journal of Thrombosis and Thrombolysis, 12*(3), 217–223.

Oliver-McNeil, S., & Artinian, N. T. (2002). Women's perceptions of personal cardiovascular risk and their risk-reducing behaviors. *American Journal of Critial Care, 11*(3), 221–227.

Oparil, S. (2006). Women and hypertension: What did we learn from the Women's Health Initiative? *Cardiology Reviews, 14*(6), 267–275.

Otten, M. W., Teutsch, S. M., Williamson, D. F., & Marks, J. S. (1990). The effect of known risk factors on the excess mortality of Black adults in the United States. *Journal of the American Medical Association, 263*, 845–850.

Palmer, J. R., Rosenberg, L., & Shapiro, S. (1989). "Low yield" cigarettes and the risk of nonfatal myocardial infarction in women. *New England Journal of Medicine, 320*, 1569–1573.

Pancioli, A. M., Broderick, J., Kothari, R., Brott, T., Tuchfarber, A., Miller, R., et al. (1998). Public perception of stroke warning signs and knowledge of potential risk factors. *Journal of the American Medical Association, 279*, 1288–1292.

Panza, J. A. (1997). Endothelial dysfunction in essential hypertension. *Clinical Cardiology, 20*(11 Suppl. 2), 26–33.

Park, Y. W., Zhu, S., Palaniappan, L., Heshka, S., Carnethon, M. R., & Heymsfield, S. B. (2003). The metabolic syndrome: Prevalence and associated risk factor findings in the US population from the Third National Health and Nutrition Examination Survey, 1988–1994. *Archives of Internal Medicine, 163*(4), 427–436.

Pasterkamp, G., Schoneveld, A. H., van der Wal, A. C., Hijnen, D. J., van Wolveren, W. J., Plomp, S., et al. (1999). Inflammation of the atherosclerotic cap and shoulder of the plaque is a common and locally observed feature in unruptured plaques of femoral and coronary arteries. *Arteriosclerosis, Thrombosis and Vascular Biology, 19*(1), 54–58.

Pasternak, R. C., Smith, S. C., Jr., Bairey-Merz, C. N., Grundy, S. M., Cleeman, J. I., & Lenfant, C. (2002). ACC/AHA/NHLBI clinical advisory on the use and safety of statins. *Journal of the American College of Cardiology, 40*(3), 567–572.

Pate, R. R., Pratt, M., Blair, S. N., Haskell, W. L., Macera, C. A., Bouchard, C., et al. (1995). Physical activity and public health. A recommendation from the Centers for Disease Control and Prevention and the American College of Sports Medicine. *Journal of the American Medical Association, 273*(5), 402–407.

Patrono, C. (1994). Aspirin as an antiplatelet drug. *New England Journal of Medicine, 330*, 1287–1294.

Penque, S., Halm, M., Smith, M., Deutsch, J., Van Roekel, M., McLaughlin, L., et al. (1998). Women and coronary disease: Relationship between descriptors of signs and symptoms and diagnostic and treatment course. *American Journal of Critical Care, 7*(3), 175–182.

Pope, J. H., Aufderheide, T. P., Ruthazer, R., Woolard, R. H., Feldman, J. A., Beshansky, J. R., et al. (2000). Missed diagnoses of acute cardiac ischemia in the emergency department. *New England Journal of Medicine, 342*(16), 1163–1170.

Raggi, P., Davidson, M., Callister, T. Q., Welty, F. K., Bachmann, G. A., Hecht, H., et al. (2005). Aggressive versus moderate lipid-lowering therapy in hypercholesterolemic postmenopausal women: Beyond Endorsed Lipid Lowering with EBT Scanning (BELLES). *Circulation, 112*(4), 563–571.

Ravdin, P. M., Cronin, K. A., Howlader, N., Berg, C. D., Chlebowski, R. T., Feuer, E. J., et al. (2007). The decrease in breast-cancer incidence in 2003 in the United States. *New England Journal of Medicine, 356*(16), 1670–1674.

Ridker, P. M. (1998). Inflammation, infection, and cardiovascular risk: How good is the clinical evidence? *Circulation, 97*(17), 1671–1674.

Ridker, P. M., Buring, J. E., Rifai, N., & Cook, N. R. (2007). Development and validation of improved algorithms for the assessment of global cardiovascular risk in women: The Reynolds Risk Score. *Journal of the American Medical Association, 297*(6), 611–619.

Ridker, P. M., Buring, J. E., Shih, J., Matias, M., & Hennekens, C. H. (1998). Prospective study of C-reactive protein and the risk of future cardiovascular events among apparently healthy women. *Circulation, 98*(8), 731–733.

Ridker, P. M., Cook, N. R., Lee, I. M., Gordon, D., Gaziano, J. M., Manson, J. E., et al. (2005). A randomized trial of low-dose aspirin in the primary prevention of cardiovascular disease in women. *New England Journal of Medicine, 352*(13), 1293–1304.

Ridker, P. M., Cushman, M., Stampfer, M. J., Tracy, R. P., & Hennekens, C. H. (1997). Inflammation, aspirin, and the risk of cardiovascular disease in apparently healthy men. *New England Journal of Medicine, 336*, 973–979.

Ridker, P. M., Cushman, M., Stampfer, M. J., Tracy, R. P., & Hennekens, C. H. (1998). Plasma concentration of C-reactive protein and risk of developing peripheral vascular disease. *Circulation, 97*(5), 425–428.

Ringback Weitoft, G., Haglund, B., & Rosen, M. (2000). Mortality among lone mothers in Sweden: A population study. *Lancet, 355*(9211), 1215–1219.

Roest, M., Voorbij, H. A., Barendrecht, A. D., Peeters, P. H., & van der Schouw, Y. T. (2007). Risk of acute ischemic heart disease in postmenopausal women depends on von Willebrand factor and fibrinogen concentrations, and blood group genotype. *Journal of Thrombosis and Haemostasis, 5*(1), 189–191.

Roncaglioni, M. C., Santoro, L., D'Avanzo, B., Negri, E., Nobili, A., Ledda, A., et al. (1992). Role of family history in patients with myocardial infarction. An Italian case-control study. GISSI-EFRIM Investigators. *Circulation, 85*(6), 2065–2072.

Rosenberg, L., Palmer, J. R., Rao, R. S., & Adams-Campbell, L. L. (1999). Risk factors for coronary heart disease in African American women. *American Journal of Epidemiology, 150*(9), 904–909.

Rosenberg, L., Palmer, J. R., Rao, R. S., & Shapiro, S. (2001). Low-dose oral contraceptive use and the risk of myocardial infarction. *Archives of Internal Medicine, 161*(8), 1065–1070.

Rosenberg, L., Palmer, J. R., & Shapiro, S. (1990). Decline in the risk of myocardial infarction among women who stop smoking. *New England Journal of Medicine, 322*, 213–217.

Ross, R. (1999). Atherosclerosis—An inflammatory disease. *New England Journal of Medicine, 340*(2), 115–126.

Rossouw, J. E., Anderson, G. L., Prentice, R. L., LaCroix, A. Z., Kooperberg, C., Stefanick, M. L., et al. (2002). Risks and benefits of estrogen plus progestin in healthy postmenopausal women: Principal results from the Women's Health Initiative randomized controlled trial. *Journal of the American Medical Association, 288*(3), 321–333.

Rossouw, J. E., Prentice, R. L., Manson, J. E., Wu, L., Barad, D., Barnabei, V. M., et al. (2007). Postmenopausal hormone therapy and risk of cardiovascular disease by age and years since menopause. *Journal of the American Medical Association, 297*(13), 1465–1477.

Rosvall, M., Ostergren, P. O., Hedblad, B., Isacsson, S. O., Janzon, L., & Berglund, G. (2002). Life-course perspective on socioeconomic differences in carotid atherosclerosis. *Arteriosclerosis, Thrombosis and Vascular Biology, 22*(10), 1704–1711.

Rutledge, T., Reis, S. E., Olson, M., Owens, J., Kelsey, S. F., Pepine, C. J., et al. (2003). Socioeconomic status variables predict cardiovascular disease risk factors and prospective mortality risk among women with chest pain. The WISE Study. *Behavior Modification, 27*(1), 54–67.

Rutledge, T., Reis, S. E., Olson, M., Owens, J., Kelsey, S. F., Pepine, C. J., et al. (2006). Depression is associated with cardiac symptoms, mortality risk, and hospitalization among women with suspected coronary disease: The NHLBI-sponsored WISE Study. *Psychosomatic Medicine, 68*(2), 217–223.

Sacks, F. M., Pfeffer, M. A., Moye, L. A., Rouleau, J. L., Rutherford, J. D., Cole, T. G., et al. (1996). The effect of pravastatin on coronary events after myocardial infarction in patients with average cholesterol levels. *New England Journal of Medicine, 335*, 1001–1009.

Sacks, F. M., Svetkey, L. P., Vollmer, W. M., Appel, L. J., Bray, G. A., Harsha, D., et al. (2001). Effects on blood pressure of reduced dietary sodium and the Dietary Approaches to Stop Hypertension (DASH) diet. DASH-Sodium Collaborative Research Group. *New England Journal of Medicine, 344*(1), 3–10.

Salomaa, V., Rasi, V., Kulathinal, S., Vahtera, E., Jauhiainen, M., Ehnholm, C., et al. (2002). Hemostatic factors as predictors of coronary events and total mortality: The FINRISK '92 Hemostasis Study. *Arteriosclerosis, Thrombosis and Vascular Biology, 22*(2), 353–358.

Scandinavian Simvastatin Survival Study Group. (1994). Randomised trial of cholesterol lowering in 4444 patients with coronary heart disease: The Scandinavian Simvastatin Survival Study (4S). *Lancet, 344*(8934), 1383–1389.

Scanlon, P. J., Faxon, D. P., Audet, A. M., Carabello, B., Dehmer, G. J., Eagle, K. A., et al. (1999). ACC/AHA guidelines for coronary angiography: Executive summary and recommendations. A report of the American College of Cardiology/American Heart Association Task Force on Practice Guidelines (Committee on Coronary Angiography) developed in collaboration with the Society for Cardiac Angiography and Interventions. *Circulation, 99*(17), 2345–2357.

Schrott, H. G., Bittner, V., Vittinghoff, E., Herrington, D. M., Hulley, S., & for the HERS Research Group. (1997). Adherence to National Cholesterol Education Program treatment goals in postmenopausal women: The Heart and Estrogen/Progestin Replacement Study (HERS). *Journal of the American Medical Association, 277*, 1281–1286.

Shaw, L. J., Bairey Merz, C. N., Pepine, C. J., Reis, S. E., Bittner, V., Kelsey, S. F., et al. (2006). Insights from the NHLBI-sponsored Women's Ischemia Syndrome Evaluation (WISE) Study: Part I. Gender differences in traditional and novel risk factors, symptom evaluation, and gender-optimized diagnostic strategies. *Journal of the American College of Cardiology, 47*(Suppl. 3), S4–S20.

Shepherd, J., Blauw, G. J., Murphy, M. B., Bollen, E. L., Buckley, B. M., Cobbe, S. M., et al. (2002). Pravastatin in elderly individuals at risk of vascular disease (PROSPER): A randomised controlled trial. *Lancet, 360*(9346), 1623–1630.

Shlipak, M. G., Simon, J. A., Grady, D., Lin, F., Wenger, N. K., & Furberg, C. D. (2001). Renal insufficiency and cardiovascular events in postmenopausal women with coronary heart disease. *Journal of the American College of Cardiology, 38*(3), 705–711.

Smilde, T. J., van Wissen, S., Wollersheim, H., Trip, M. D., Kastelein, J. J., & Stalenhoef, A. F. (2001). Effect of aggressive versus conventional lipid lowering on atherosclerosis progression in familial hypercholesterolaemia (ASAP): A prospective, randomised, double-blind trial. *Lancet, 357*(9256), 577–581.

Stampfer, M. J., Hu, F. B., Manson, J. E., Rimm, E. B., & Willett, W. C. (2000). Primary prevention of coronary heart disease in women through diet and lifestyle. *New England Journal of Medicine, 343*(1), 16–22.

Stary, H. C. (1996). The histological classification of atherosclerotic lesions in human coronary arteries. In V. Fuster, R. Ross, & E. J. Topol (Eds.), *Atherosclerosis and coronary artery disease* (Vol. 1, pp. 463–474). Philadelphia: Lippincott-Raven.

Stary, H. C., Chandler, A. B., Dinsmore, R. E., Fuster, V., Glagov, S., Insull, W., Jr., et al. (1995). A definition of advanced types of atherosclerotic lesions and a histological classification of atherosclerosis. A report from the Committee on Vascular Lesions of the Council on Arteriosclerosis, American Heart Association. *Circulation, 92*(5), 1355–1374.

Stramba-Badiale, M., Fox, K. M., Priori, S. G., Collins, P., Daly, C., Graham, I., et al. (2006). Cardiovascular diseases in women: A statement from the policy conference of the European Society of Cardiology. *European Heart Journal, 27*(8), 994–1005.

Tershakovec, A. M., Jawad, A. F., Stouffer, N. O., Elkasabany, A., Srinivasan, S. R., & Berenson, G. S. (2002). Persistent hypercholesterolemia is associated with the development of obesity among girls: The Bogalusa Heart Study. *American Journal of Clinical Nutrition, 76*(4), 730–735.

Thomas, R. J., Palumbo, P. J., Melton, L. J., 3rd, Roger, V. L., Ransom, J., O'Brien, P. C., et al. (2003). Trends in the mortality burden associated with diabetes mellitus: A population-based study in Rochester, Minn, 1970–1994. *Archives of Internal Medicine, 163*(4), 445–451.

Tominaga, M., Eguchi, H., Manaka, H., Igarashi, K., Kato, T., & Sekikawa, A. (1999). Impaired glucose tolerance is a risk factor for cardiovascular disease, but not impaired fasting glucose. The Funagata Diabetes Study. *Diabetes Care, 22*(6), 920–924.

Tunstall-Pedoe, H., Kuulasmaa, K., Mahonen, M., Tolonen, H., Ruokokoski, E., & Amouyel, P. (1999). Contribution of trends in survival and coronary-event rates to changes in coronary heart disease mortality: 10-year results from 37 WHO MONICA project populations. Monitoring trends and determinants in cardiovascular disease. *Lancet, 353*(9164), 1547–1557.

Tunstall-Pedoe, H., Woodward, M., Tavendale, R., A'Brook, R., & McCluskey, M. K. (1997). Comparison of the prediction by 27 different factors of coronary heart disease and death in men and women of the Scottish heart health study: Cohort study. *British Medical Journal, 315*, 722–729.

Tuomilehto, J., Lindstrom, J., Eriksson, J. G., Valle, T. T., Hamalainen, H., Ilanne-Parikka, P., et al. (2001). Prevention of type 2 diabetes mellitus by changes in lifestyle among subjects with impaired glucose tolerance. *New England Journal of Medicine, 344*(18), 1343–1350.

U.S. Department of Health and Human Services. (1996). *Physical activity and health: A report of the Surgeon General.* Atlanta, GA: U.S. Department of Health and Human Services, Centers for Disease Control and Prevention, National Center for Chronic Disease Prevention and Health Promotion.

Van Horn, L. V., Ballew, C., Liu, K., Ruth, K., McDonald, A., Hilner, J. E., et al. (1991). Diet, body size, and plasma lipids-lipoproteins in young adults: Differences by race and sex. *American Journal of Epidemiology, 133*, 9–23.

Viscoli, C. M., Brass, L. M., Kernan, W. N., Sarrel, P. M., Suissa, S., & Horwitz, R. I. (2001). A clinical trial of estrogen-replacement therapy after ischemic stroke. *New England Journal of Medicine, 345*(17), 1243–1249.

Vita, A. J., Terry, R. B., Hubert, H. B., & Fries, J. F. (1998). Aging, health risks, and cumulative disability. *New England Journal of Medicine, 338*, 1035–1041.

Vogel, R. A., Corretti, M. C., & Gellman, J. (1998). Cholesterol, cholesterol lowering, and endothelial function. *Progress in Cardiovascular Disease, 41*(2), 117–136.

Walsh, J. M., & Pignone, M. (2004). Drug treatment of hyperlipidemia in women. *Journal of the American Medical Association, 291*(18), 2243–2252.

Wamala, S. P., Mittleman, M. A., Schenck-Gustafsson, K., & Orth-Gomer, K. (1999). Potential explanations for the educational gradient in coronary heart disease: Apopulation-based case-control study of Swedish women [Erratum in *American Journal of Public Health,* 1999, *89*(5), 785]. *American Journal of Public Health, 89*(3), 315–321.

Wamala, S. P., Murray, M. A., Horsten, M., Eriksson, M., Schenck-Gustafsson, K., Hamsten, A., et al. (1999). Socioeconomic status and determinants of hemostatic function in healthy women. *Arteriosclerosis, Thrombosis and Vascular Biology, 19*(3), 485–492.

Wang, T. J., Nam, B. H., Wilson, P. W., Wolf, P. A., Levy, D., Polak, J. F., et al. (2002). Association of C-reactive protein with carotid atherosclerosis in men and women: The Framingham Heart Study. *Arteriosclerosis, Thrombosis and Vascular Biology, 22*(10), 1662–1667.

Wassertheil-Smoller, S., Anderson, G., Psaty, B. M., Black, H. R., Manson, J., Wong, N., et al. (2000). Hypertension and its treatment in postmenopausal women: Baseline data from the Women's Health Initiative. *Hypertension, 36*(5), 780–789.

Wassertheil-Smoller, S., Shumaker, S., Ockene, J., Talavera, G. A., Greenland, P., Cochrane, B., et al. (2004). Depression and cardiovascular sequelae in postmenopausal women. The Women's Health Initiative (WHI). *Archives of Internal Medicine, 164*(3), 289–298.

Waters, D. D., Alderman, E. L., Hsia, J., Howard, B. V., Cobb, F. R., Rogers, W. J., et al. (2002). Effects of hormone replacement therapy and antioxidant vitamin supplements on coronary atherosclerosis in postmenopausal women: A randomized controlled trial. *Journal of the American Medical Association, 288*(19), 2432–2440.

Waters, D., Higginson, L., Gladstone, P., Kimball, B., Le May, M., Boccuzzi, S. J., et al. (1994). Effects of monotherapy with an HMG-CoA reductase inhibitor on the progression of coronary atherosclerosis as assessed by serial quantitative arteriography: The Canadian Coronary Atherosclerosis Intervention Trial. *Circulation, 89*, 959–968.

Wessel, T. R., Arant, C. B., Olson, M. B., Johnson, B. D., Reis, S. E., Sharaf, B. L., et al. (2004). Relationship of physical fitness vs body mass index with coronary artery disease and cardiovascular events in women. *Journal of the American Medical Association, 292*(10), 1179–1187.

Willett, W. C., Manson, J. E., Stampfer, M. J., Colditz, G. A., Rosner, B., Speizer, F. E., et al. (1995). Weight, weight change, and coronary heart disease in women. *Journal of the American Medical Association, 273*, 461–465.

Wilson, P. W. F., Garrison, R. J., & Castelli, W. P. (1985). Postmenopausal estrogen use, cigarette smoking, and cardiovascular morbidity in women over 50: The Framingham Study. *New England Journal of Medicine, 313*, 1038–1043.

Wing, R. R., Kuller, L. H., Bunker, C. H., Matthews, K. A., Caggiula, A., Meilahn, E. N., et al. (1989). Obesity, obesity-related behaviors and coronary heart disease risk factors in Black and White premenopausal women. *International Journal of Obesity, 13*, 511–519.

Winkleby, M., Sundquist, K., & Cubbin, C. (2007). Inequities in CHD incidence and case fatality by neighborhood deprivation. *American Journal of Preventive Medicine, 32*(2), 97–106.

Wissler, R. W., Hiltscher, L., Oinuma, T., & the PDAY Research Group. (1996). The lesions of atherosclerosis in the young: From fatty streaks to intermediate lesions. In V. Fuster, R. Ross, & E. J. Topol (Eds.), *Atherosclerosis and coronary artery disease* (Vol. 1, pp. 475–489). Philadelphia: Lippincott-Raven.

Witteman, J. C. M., Grobbee, D. E., Valkenburg, H. A., van Hemert, A. M., Stijnen, T., & Hofman, A. (1993). Cigarette smoking and the development and progression of aortic atherosclerosis: A 9-year population-based follow-up study in women. *Circulation, 88*(Pt. 1), 2156–2162.

Wood, P. D., Stefanick, M. L., Williams, P. T., & Haskell, W. L. (1991). The effects on plasma lipoproteins of a prudent weight-reducing diet, with or without exercise, in overweight men and women. *New England Journal of Medicine, 325*, 461–466.

Woodward, M., Lowe, G. D., Rumley, A., & Tunstall-Pedoe, H. (1998). Fibrinogen as a risk factor for coronary heart disease and mortality in middle-aged men and women. The Scottish Heart Health Study. *European Heart Journal, 19*(1), 55–62.

Young, L. E., Cunningham, S. L., & Buist, D. (2005). Lone mothers are at higher risk for cardiovascular disease compared with partnered mothers. Data from the National Health and Nutrition Examination Survey III (NHANES III). *Health Care for Women International, 26*, 604–621.

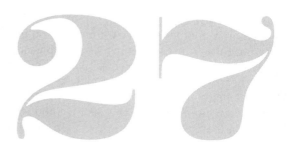

Chronic Illness and Women

Phyllis Christianson, Eleanor F. Bond, Anne Skelly, and Janet Primomo

Chronic diseases are biological malfunctions or pathological changes in body systems that persist for long periods of time, generally 6 months or longer. The term chronic derives from the Greek word *khronos*, meaning time. Chronic conditions usually develop slowly, insidiously, over months or years. Commonly, these diseases cannot be cured and persist for the duration of the person's lifetime. In contrast, acute diseases occur relatively abruptly, generally persisting for less than 3 months.

This chapter discusses general approaches to chronic disease monitoring and clinical management in women. Several common chronic diseases and symptom conditions are discussed in detail. Additional chronic diseases are discussed in other chapters.

ETIOLOGY OF CHRONIC DISEASE

The cause or etiology of a chronic disease is typically multifactorial. These factors might be environmental, genetic, behavioral (such as diet, activity), or a combination of the factors. There may be a long period of latency during which the disease process has begun, but symptoms have not yet appeared. An exposure (for example, to asbestos) can lead to symptomatic pathology (such as chronic obstructive pulmonary disease) many years later. A genetic predisposition to cancer or heart disease can lead to disease. Behavioral patterns such as dietary habits can increase the risk of diabetes or heart disease.

Causative factors may interact and combine in specific ways to place the individual at a higher risk for developing disease than if a single factor were present alone. For example, a smoker with an occupational exposure to certain industrial chemicals or asbestos is at greater risk for the development of lung cancer than a smoker without this work exposure. Therefore, a multiple cause/ multiple effect modeling approach is often used to guide investigations of chronic diseases (Dever, 1991).

THE EPIDEMIOLOGY OF CHRONIC DISEASE IN WOMEN

Chronic diseases are prevalent in the United States and are a significant cause of death and disability. This trend is a dramatic break from the past, when infectious disease and trauma were the primary causes of death and disease. The risk of developing a chronic disease increases with aging. Thus, increased longevity has resulted in increased prevalence of many chronic diseases. Women, partly because they are likely to live longer, are at risk for development of chronic diseases. Obesity increases the risk of chronic disease; this, too, puts many women at increased risk of chronic disease.

The Centers for Disease Control and Prevention (CDC) estimates that 90 million Americans suffer from chronic disease; 7 of every 10 deaths (1.7 million annually) in the United States are due to a chronic disease (CDC, 2007). Of the nine most common causes of death in the United States, seven are chronic diseases: heart disease, cancer, stroke, chronic obstructive pulmonary disease, diabetes, Alzheimer's disease, and renal failure (CDC, 2007). Chronic diseases cause major activity limitations for more than 10% of Americans (that is, 25 million people; National Center for Health Statistics, 2008). Arthritis, heart disease, lung disease, hypertension, and diabetes are among the most common causes of disability among Americans age 15 years or older (CDC, 2007). Depression is another relatively common and potentially disabling chronic disease among women. Breast cancer is a common cause of death and disability. Of those who die due to heart disease, more than half are women (CDC, 2007). Diabetes mellitus (type 2) is more prevalent among women than among men (CDC, 2007). Although women live longer than men, on average, women over the age of 70 are more likely to be disabled than are men of the same age (CDC, 2007). Several infectious diseases such as acquired immune deficiency syndrome (AIDS) and infectious hepatitis are emerging as significant chronic disease conditions. The National Center for Health Statistics tracks the prevalence of selected chronic conditions; their 2005 data regarding women 18 years of age and older are presented in Table 27.1. Among the most common conditions are arthritis, joint and back problems, high blood pressure, sinusitis, heart disease, and asthma (National Center for Health Statistics, 2008).

Chronic diseases result in substantial health care costs and significant loss of productivity. The CDC (2007) notes that chronic disease care services account for more than 75% of the medical care costs in the United States. The cost of chronic disease care is rising, contributing significantly to escalating health care costs in the United States. To generate data about health status, the National Center for Health Statistics conducts an annual National Health Interview Survey of the civilian noninstitutionalized U.S. population (about 29,000 households) using a wide range of questions about health and health practices. This survey demonstrates that a significant number of adult women experience substantial activity limitations, such as the inability to walk a quarter of a mile or climb 10 steps without resting. These data are given in Table 27.2.

THE TRAJECTORY OF CHRONIC ILLNESS

Chronic illness trajectory refers to the overall course of a person's experience as a result of the illness over time. This trajectory can describe not only pathological changes but also other aspects of the disease such as symptom experience, physical functioning, quality of life, social or role performance, and other variables (Corbin & Strauss, 1988). Each aspect of the disease progression is considered an outcome; its trajectory can be monitored.

Unlike acute conditions, which are often self-limiting, chronic conditions are generally not easily curable and

27.1 | Age-Adjusted Frequencies of Chronic Conditions Among Civilian Noninstitutionalized Women 18 Years of Age and Older, 2005

CONDITION	AGE-ADJUSTED PERCENTAGE
Heart disease	11.1
Hypertension	22.5
Stroke	2.5
Emphysema	1.5
Asthma	9.2
Sinusitis	17
Chronic bronchitis	5.3
Cancer	7.8
Breast cancer	2.2
Cervical cancer	1.1
Diabetes	7.1
Ulcers	7.1
Kidney disease	1.8
Liver disease	1.2
Arthritis	24.4
Chronic joint symptoms	28.2
Back pain	30.3
Feelings of sadness all or most of the time	3.7

Note. Data are based on National Center for Health Statistics, Centers for Disease Control and Prevention. (2007). *Summary health statistics for U.S. adults: National Health Interview Survey, 2005.* DHHS Publication PHS 2007-1560. Hyattsville, MD: U.S. Department of Health and Human Services.

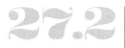

27.2 | Age-Adjusted Percentages of Difficulties Among Civilian Noninstitutionalized Women 18 Years of Age and Older

PHYSICAL ACTIVITY	PERCENTAGE OF WOMEN REPORTING DIFFICULTY
Any physical difficulty	17.4
Walk a quarter of a mile	8.2
Climb 10 steps without resting	6.7
Stand for 2 hours	10

Note. Data are based on National Center for Health Statistics, Centers for Disease Control and Prevention. (2007). *Summary health statistics for U.S. adults: National Health Interview Survey, 2005.* DHHS Publication PHS 2007-1560. Hyattsville, MD: U.S. Department of Health and Human Services.

generally are not self-limiting. A chronic disease can vary over time, sometimes transiently improving, often worsening. The course of a specific illness depends on the characteristics of the condition (e.g., relapsing, episodic), characteristics of the individual (e.g., age, gender), and psychological, family, and sociocultural factors.

Health care providers can use the concept of illness trajectory to identify and understand the specific needs of patients and families as the patient moves along the continuum of chronic disease. Many chronic diseases worsen over time, as illustrated in Figure 27.1. It is useful for providers to have a general understanding of the usual course of a disease. The patient and provider can then compare the patient's course of the disease with the usual progression. If the disease is characterized by general deterioration, then slowing the progression of the disease represents a major therapeutic success. On the other hand, if the patient's disease is progressing faster than is typical, this could invoke analysis and redesign of the treatment plan. More data are needed regarding the typical progression of the multiple outcomes of common chronic diseases so that providers and patients can evaluate the success of the treatment regimen.

MANAGING CHRONIC ILLNESS

Unlike acute care, in which the goal of treatment is typically to secure a cure, in chronic care, the goal is to manage the chronic disease and help the patient cope with its impact. In chronic care, an ideal outcome might be that nothing happens, the patient remains stable. In many ways, the health care system is geared more toward curing acute illness than managing chronic illness.

The impact of chronic disease on the individual is often substantial, affecting physical health, physical functioning, symptom experience, quality of life, and social and role performance. Chronic diseases such as diabetes, heart failure, hypertension, arthritis, and lung disease are associated with significant underlying pathology. Factors related to the disease itself, such as the type of organ damage, disease severity, treatment regime, personal factors (such as individual coping ability), and social support can influence whether the chronic disease is associated with altered physical functioning or disability. Chronic conditions frequently cause disabling symptoms such as pain and fatigue. Chronic diseases may have a profound influence on the individual and her family. All of these factors are considered in managing the patient.

The term chronic disease invokes the pathological manifestations of the disease. However, because the impact of the disease is generally much broader, the term chronic illness is used to refer to the individual's experience with the disease. Clinicians and researchers are increasingly aware of the influence of the person's experience with the disease on the course and outcomes of the disease. Therefore, in this chapter, aspects of both the chronic disease and the experience of having

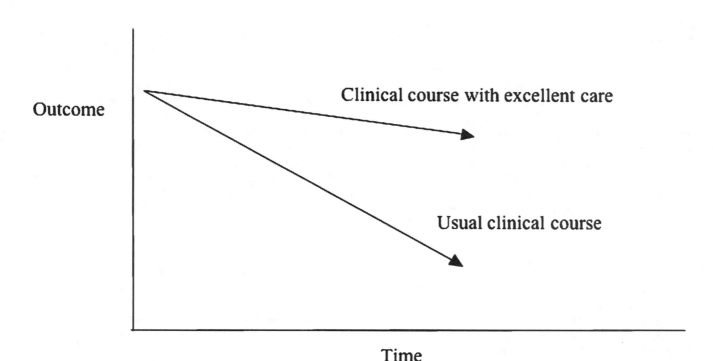

Figure 27.1   Illustration of chronic illness over time.
Adapted from Kane, R. L., Priester, R., & Totten, A. M. (2005). *Meeting the challenge of chronic illness.* Baltimore: Johns Hopkins University Press. 13.

this disease are addressed. For similar reasons, treatment is referred to as chronic care, not chronic disease care. Chronic care incorporates biological management with medical interventions for the broader range of suffering and symptoms. Chronic care requires significant emphasis on health promotion, to slow or reverse the progression of the disease. Chronic care services also address the woman's experience of the disease, the impact of the disease on her daily life and functioning, and the suffering caused by the disease.

The health care system is better tooled to respond to acute conditions. The Institute of Medicine has described a "quality chasm" to characterize the gap between the health care needs of patients with chronic conditions and the institutions delivering that care (Kane, Priester, & Totten, 2005). Goals of chronic care include slowing the rate of decline due to the disease, reducing the frequency of disease exacerbations or complications, mitigating the functional impairment, maximizing the quality of life, reducing trips to the emergency department, reducing hospitalizations, prolonging life, and maintaining a sense of normalcy.

In acute care situations, the patient experiences cure-directed care as advised by an expert care provider. With chronic care, the roles of the patient and physician are somewhat reversed. In chronic care, it is critical that the patient partner with the provider to plan her chronic care. The patient lives with her illness constantly, and sees the clinician only occasionally and then typically for brief visits. The patient must monitor her condition on a day-to-day basis and recognize deterioration or improvement. The clinician and the patient must share the responsibility for care decisions. Sometimes clinical management requires choosing between one of two undesirable outcomes. For example, there might be a trade-off between improving function versus relieving pain. Patient-centered care mandates that the patient be the primary decision maker in managing the disease and its effects. Chronic care requires developing skills in decision counseling and decision support. The care provider can make recommendations based on science and experience regarding surgical or medical pharmaceutical treatments. The well-informed patient will be able to choose among the options based on her own analysis. It is useful for patients to learn how to prepare for the clinician encounter, so that they are able to take an active role in monitoring, managing, and decision making.

The care paradigm for chronic care is very different from that for an acute medical problem. When a patient presents acutely with a problem such as a fractured bone, the health care provider, the expert, provides direct and immediate interventions to correct or cure the underlying problem and treat the related symptoms. The patient receives the care, often somewhat passively. With chronic care, the ideal circumstance involves the patient partnering with her care provider to design and implement a plan of care. This plan incorporates biological disease management with health promotion to slow deterioration. The plan of care includes supportive services such as counseling related to diet, exercise, lifestyle, and self-care. Psychological care services may be required to assist in the adjustment to the condition. The woman is educated to self-monitor and manage her condition. Women frequently utilize complementary and alternative health approaches to health care. These approaches can be integrated into the plan of care.

The growing body of literature on women's roles, development, and cognitive processes is helpful in considering how chronic illness may affect women's lives. Women value their connections to others and their interdependence with others. The family and social context become crucial in understanding how women are affected by, and manage, chronic illness. The impact of chronic illness on women's self-esteem, roles, and social support has been described (Foxall, Ekberg, & Griffith, 1985). Social support systems are important in adjustment to chronic disease and mitigating the intrapersonal, interpersonal, and environmental demands imposed on women by chronic disease.

Women with chronic illness must cope not only with their disease but with the day-to-day struggles of life as well. Haberman, Woods, and Packard (1990) reported a multidimensional construct of demands of illness for women that included physical symptoms, personal meaning, family functioning, social relationships, self-image, symptom monitoring, and treatment issue demands. It is important to note that, while women reported family functioning demands such as child care difficulties, they did not attribute these demands to their chronic illness. Although a body of knowledge to guide interventions with chronically ill women does not exist at this time, it is vital that health care professionals address changes in women's personal, family, and social lives as they attempt to help women manage their chronic disease.

Women with chronic illness live with symptoms and disabilities that they often must manage for their lifetime and that require collaborative partnerships with health care providers to assist them in integrating self-care into their daily activities. This requires that health care providers not only be knowledgeable about managing medical treatment regimens but also be able to provide emotional and tangible support, including ongoing patient and family education and counseling. The role of the woman with chronic disease has changed over the years paralleling the changing model of health and illness and the shift from morbidity and mortality related to the infectious etiologies of disease to the noninfectious (with the exception of human immunodeficiency virus). Due to the emphasis on lifestyle factors as risks for the development of many chronic diseases, a woman's role in prevention has become much more active than in the past, involving changing behaviors and environments to improve health outcomes.

FAMILIES AND CHRONIC ILLNESS

Chronic illness may require pervasive changes in every aspect of family life (Corbin & Strauss, 1988). Physical changes may necessitate the need for personal, social, financial, and health care assistance. Psychological adjustment to chronic illness may include changes in self-concept and self-image. The family may serve as a buffer in helping the woman with chronic illness derive a sense of purpose in life and feelings of self-worth.

Women with chronic illness may be concerned about their ability to maintain role expectations at home or at work. The treatment regimens for some chronic illnesses require major adjustments on the part of family members. If the woman with chronic illness has children, she may have a special set of concerns (Packard, Haberman, Woods, & Yates, 1991; Stetz, Lewis, & Primomo, 1986).

Exactly how families are affected by chronic illness is not known. It is likely that many factors affect adaptation by families to chronic illness (Lewis, 1986). Families may experience financial insecurity as a result of chronic illness. Because work is often associated with health insurance coverage, if an individual is not able to work and health care insurance is not financially affordable, access to health care may be limited.

Supporting families with chronic illness is a critical concern for all health care providers. The type, timing, nature, and source of support appropriate for families vary depending on the specific illness, the characteristics and needs of family members, and the sources of support available (Woods, Yates, & Primomo, 1989). The type of support needed is also determined by the phase in the trajectory of the illness. Emotional support may be needed during all phases of the illness due to uncertainty about the consequences of the illness. Emotional support from a partner may be most effective in preventing depression, maintaining marital quality, and enhancing family functioning (Primomo, Yates, & Woods, 1990). In contrast, tangible support may be crucial at the initial phase of an illness diagnosis and at the terminal phase. Informational support may be most important during transitional phases (Woods et al., 1989). To facilitate women's coping with chronic illness, health care professionals need to consider the various types, sources, and benefits of support.

CHRONIC DISEASE IN OLDER WOMEN

Both the number and proportion of adults who are over the age of 65 in the United States are increasing; by the year 2030, predictions estimate that 71 million older adults will live in the United States, double the number in 2000, and will represent 20% of the U.S. population. Worldwide estimates are similar. Currently, women comprise about 59% of the population, and that percentage is expected to remain fairly stable. The prevalence of chronic disease is higher among older people; in the United States, 80% of adults older than 65 have at least one chronic disease, and 50% have two (He, Sengupta, Velkoff, & DeBarros, 2005). Chronic diseases that are more prevalent in older adults include diabetes, Alzheimer's dementia, cancer, and arthritis—all of which can lead to disability, diminished quality of life, and increased health care costs for the individual. Older women are also more likely to have a higher prevalence of depression, again contributing to increased disability (Kasper & Simonsick, 1995). Older women are more likely to have incomes at poverty level or below, increasing the risk of limited access to health care and limited resources for assistance living with chronic disease and disability.

In addition to chronic diseases, several geriatric conditions contribute to disability of older adults. In a study by Cigolle and associates (2007), the authors defined geriatric conditions as those that occurred in older, vulnerable adults; were multifactorial in cause; episodic in nature; precipitated by a variety of acute insults; and often followed by a functional decline. They collected data on incidence of the following conditions: falls resulting in injury, incontinence requiring protective undergarments, low body mass index, dizziness, vision and hearing impairment (poor despite corrective aids), and cognitive impairment, as well as presence of chronic diseases. About 40% of participants aged 65 had at least one geriatric condition. Among participants who were 85, one-third had at least three geriatric conditions, and over one-half had at least two. The study found a strong and significant association between geriatric conditions and disability, when controlling for chronic diseases. This study suggests that chronic disease burden alone underestimates disability in the older population. It also underlines that assessment for the presence of these conditions is an important part of the health care provider's role in helping older women improve function and decrease disability.

The remainder of this chapter discusses selected chronic diseases seen in women, their major clinical manifestations, treatment, and implications for practice.

UPPER AND LOWER RESPIRATORY DISEASE

Sinusitis

The most common chronic health problem reported by women in 2005 was chronic sinusitis (National Center for Health Statistics, 2007). Sinusitis is an inflammation of one or more of the paranasal sinuses, usually caused by a bacterial infection such as *Streptococcus pneumoniae, Haemophilus influenzae,* and, less commonly, *Staphylococcus aureus* or *Moraxella catarrhalis* (Gwaltney, Scheld, Sande, & Sydor, 1992; Tierney, McPhee, & Papadakis, 2006). Viral infections account for 9% of cases. In chronic sinusitis, anaerobic organisms and staphylococci may be present. Fungal infections may be seen in immunocompromised patients.

Acute sinusitis may be precipitated by any agent that causes swelling of the nasal mucosa such as allergic or vasomotor rhinitis (the common cold). Other factors associated with an increased risk of developing sinusitis are nasal polyps, septal deviations, overuse of nasal decongestants, dental infections, air pollution, tobacco smoke, low humidity, nasal or facial trauma, and nasal or sinus tumors. Chronic sinusitis is diagnosed when a symptomatic sinus infection persists for longer than 3 weeks with adequate treatment. In an adult, the most commonly affected sites are the maxillary and frontal sinuses.

The most common presenting complaints of sinusitis are facial pain and pressure. The pain may be referred to the upper incisor and canine teeth via branches of the trigeminal nerve, which transverses the floor of the sinus. When obtaining the patient's health history, the health care provider should inquire about the duration of the symptoms, presence of fever, chills, color of drainage (serous, mucopurulent), sore throat, postnasal drip, cough, headache, toothache or facial pain, halitosis, and pain with mastication. The headaches associated with sinusitis are usually worse at night and early in the morning and worse if the patient bends over. Recent use of antibiotics, steroids, decongestants, nasal sprays, and antihistamines should be elicited. The health care provider should also ask about a family history of asthma, allergies, and chronic sinusitis, whether the woman is a smoker or a smoker resides in the home, and whether there are household pets. In the elderly, fever with associated cognitive changes and/or delirium may be the only presenting symptoms of sinusitis (Robinson, Kidd, & Rogers, 2000). In chronic sinusitis, chronic nasal congestion, headache, postnasal drip, and cough are present. The nasal drainage may vary in color and consistency, sense of taste and smell may be reduced, and halitosis may be present.

Periorbital edema, fever, and signs of acute toxicity in sinusitis are rare but warrant immediate referral, because they may indicate complications such as periorbital cellulitis, osteomyelitis, meningitis, or brain abscess. It is important to remember that paranasal sinus cancer is always part of the differential for sinusitis, particularly chronic sinusitis.

The physical examination of the patient with sinusitis should include vital signs, including temperature, the presence of allergic shiners (discoloration, darkening of the skin below the eyes) or periorbital edema,

examination of the nares for patency, color of the mucosa, presence/color of discharge, presence of polyps, septal deviations, and examination of the ears, mouth, and throat for signs of inflammation. The frontal and maxillary sinuses should be inspected for edema and erythema, percussed to elicit tenderness.

Transillumination of the sinuses may be helpful, although interpretation may be difficult due to variations in the thickness of soft tissue, and sensitivity and specificity are low. The teeth may be percussed to check for a dental source of maxillary sinusitis. The presence of lymphadenopathy should be assessed in the neck and the heart and lungs auscultated. The findings of chronic sinusitis are similar to those seen with acute sinusitis. The diagnosis of sinusitis is often made clinically. If symptoms have not resolved after 10 to 14 days of treatment, computerized tomography (CT) scan or sinus films are recommended. CT scans have largely replaced sinus films due to their increased sensitivity in detecting inflammatory changes and bone destruction (Robinson et al., 2000). Allergy testing is done as a third-line test in recurrent acute sinusitis or chronic sinusitis.

The management of uncomplicated sinusitis involves the use of oral decongestants (e.g., pseudoephedrine 60–120 mgm three or four times per day), nasal decongestants (e.g., oxymetazoline 0.05%, 1–2 sprays each nares every 6–8 hours for up to 3 days; xylometazoline, 0.05%–0.1%, 1–2 sprays per nares every 6–8 hours for up to 3 days), and oral antibiotics (amoxicillin 250—500 mgm three times a day for 14 days; trimethoprim/sulfamethoxazole twice a day for 14 days; Tierney et al., 2006). Failure of sinusitis to resolve after an adequate course of oral antibiotics may necessitate hospital admission. Patients should be instructed to contact their health care provider if symptoms worsen or do not significantly lessen with antibiotic treatment.

Patient education should stress the need for increasing fluid intake and humidifying the air in the household. The use of nasal irrigations with warm saline and application of warm compresses locally to the maxillary area are helpful in decreasing the viscosity of secretions and reducing local pain. Patients should be aware of the nature of the disease process, causes and risk factors, side effects of treatment, and changes warranting immediate evaluation and treatment (i.e., orbital or facial swelling).

Prevention of sinusitis includes the avoidance of known allergens and dry heat, avoidance of the use of antihistamines unless there is a known allergic component to a disease, and cessation of smoking or exposure to passive smoke.

Asthma

Asthma is a chronic, inflammatory disorder of the airways causing recurring episodes of wheezing, breathlessness, chest tightness, and cough, particularly at night and in the early morning (National Asthma Education and Prevention Program [NAEPP], 1997). More than 15 million people have been diagnosed with asthma in the United States, with asthma being a major cause of outpatient visits and hospitalizations among people of all ages (NAEPP, 1997). Asthma hospitalizations and death rates are highest among African Americans and inner city residents (Centers for Disease Control and Prevention, 1996). Underdiagnosis and inappropriate therapy are major factors influencing morbidity and mortality. Asthma prevalence, morbidity, and mortality appear to be increasing in the United States and many other Western countries. More than 5,000 deaths annually in the United States are attributed to asthma (Centers for Disease Control and Prevention, 1996).

Asthma requires the presence of both host and environmental factors. Host factors include a genetic component that determines an individual's response to allergens and the maturity and integrity of the lungs during fetal development and the immediate newborn period. Environmental factors include inhaled allergens, occupational exposures to chemicals or fumes, and exposure to airway irritants such as tobacco smoke, air pollution, or respiratory viruses. Additional host factors that may affect asthma severity include rhinitis/sinusitis; aspirin sensitivity; sensitivity to other nonsteroidal anti-inflammatory drugs (NSAIDs) and metabisulfites such as monosodium glutamate; and topical and systemic beta blockers. In a susceptible individual, these environmental factors trigger an inflammatory response involving mast cells, eosinophils, macrophages, and activated T cells, resulting in bronchospasm, airway hyperresponsiveness, and obstruction to airflow. Repeated exposure results in recurrent bronchoconstriction, airway edema, formation of mucous plugs, and airway remodeling. Since inflammation is an early and persistent manifestation of asthma, aggressive suppression of inflammation is the paramount goal of therapy.

The patient will report recurrent symptoms of wheezing, cough, chest tightness, and shortness of breath. Signs and symptoms vary from patient to patient and individually over time. Symptoms may be associated with exercise, changes in weather, emotion (stress-induced asthma), menses, or exposure to dust or allergens. Exercise-induced bronchospasm usually begins right after the end of exercise, peaks within 10 to 15 minutes, and resolves within 60 minutes. Cardiac asthma is a form of bronchospasm seen in patients with uncompensated congestive heart failure. Symptoms of asthma are usually worse at night or in the early morning. Questions regarding a history of childhood allergy and frequent respiratory infections and family history of allergic disorders or atopy (hay fever, allergic rhinitis, urticaria, atopic dermatitis, or eczema) help establish the probability of a diagnosis of asthma (Meredith & Horan, 2000). A history of allergy to aspirin or NSAIDs is also supportive. An additional factor known to trigger an asthma attack is gastroesophageal reflux. The effect of pregnancy on asthma is unpredictable. Premenstrual worsening of asthma symptoms is common and troublesome to the woman experiencing it, but usually of little clinical significance.

The physical examination of the patient includes vital signs with attention to respiratory rate and depth and length of inspiration and expiration. Use of the accessory muscles of respiration, retractions, and increased effort at breathing should be noted. Additional physical signs that suggest asthma are the presence of nasal polyps, nasal mucosal swelling, and nasal secretions. Hyperexpansion of the thorax, wheezing during normal breathing, and a prolonged phase of forced exhalation are supportive signs.

Wheezing during forced expiration is not diagnostic of asthma. Percussion of the thorax should be resonant. Auscultation of the chest may be normal between episodes in patients with mild asthma. With severe symptoms, airflow may be so reduced as to not produce wheezing (a critical finding). In this instance, the only diagnostic clue may be reduced breath sounds over the thorax with prolonged expiration (Tierney et al., 2006).

The differential diagnosis of asthma includes chronic obstructive pulmonary disease, laryngeal dysfunction, and mechanical obstruction of the airways by tumor and vocal cord dysfunction. The laboratory evaluation of asthma should include spirometry (FEV-1, FVC, FEV1/FVC ratio) before and after the administration of a bronchodilator. These measures will determine whether airflow obstruction exists and whether it is reversible. Airflow obstruction is indicated by a reduced FEV1/FVC ratio (less than 75%). When patients have symptoms of asthma but normal spirometry, use of a peak flow meter over the course of 1 to 2 weeks to assess the daily variation in peak expiratory flow (PEF) is recommended. PEF is usually lowest in the morning and highest 6 to 8 hours after rising. A 20% difference between the two measures is called PEF variability and supports a diagnosis of asthma (NAEPP, 1997). The diagnosis of asthma is based on the patient's pattern of symptoms, significant reversible airway obstruction (as measured by spirometry or PEF measures), and the exclusion of other possible diagnoses. Chest radiographs are not necessary unless pneumonia or a complication of asthma such as pneumothorax is suspected. Skin testing to identify sensitivity to specific environmental allergens may be useful in individuals with persistent asthma. Spirometry tests should be done at the time of diagnosis, after treatment is initiated and symptoms have stabilized (to document airway function), and every 1 to 3 years to assess airway function.

The Expert Panel of the National Asthma Education and Prevention Program of the National Heart, Lung, and Blood Institute (1997) has developed a classification system that helps to direct treatment and to identify persons at high risk for life-threatening asthma attacks (Table 27.3). The patient's clinical features before treatment are used to classify the patient. Patients are assigned to the most severe grade in which any feature occurs.

The therapeutic management of asthma is directed to preventing and/or resolving airway inflammation. This is accomplished through the use of environmental controls and drug therapy. Asthma medications can be divided into two categories: quick relief and long-term control. Quick relief medications are used to provide prompt reversal of acute airflow obstruction by direct relaxation of bronchial smooth muscle. Long-term control medications (or maintenance or preventive medications) are taken on a regular basis to attenuate airway inflammation, thus maintaining control of asthma symptoms. A stepwise approach to therapy has been endorsed by the NAEPP (1997) (Table 27.4). It is important to remember that these are general guidelines, and therapy needs to be tailored to the specific needs of the patient. A thorough assessment of patient technique in using asthma medications and devices is essential. Asthma medications (e.g., steroids) may aggravate conditions such as diabetes and osteoporosis, necessitating adjustments in the plan of care. Ongoing, periodic assessments of functional status and quality of life for individuals with asthma should be conducted, including monitoring of exacerbation of symptoms and use of pharmacotherapy (including use of over-the-counter treatments).

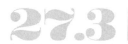 Classification of Asthma Severity

CLINICAL FEATURES BEFORE TREATMENT[a]			
	SYMPTOMS[b]	NIGHTTIME SYMPTOMS	LUNG FUNCTION
Step 1 Mild intermittent	■ Symptoms two or fewer times per week ■ Asymptomatic and normal PEF between exacerbations ■ Exacerbations brief (from a few hours to a few days); intensity may vary	■ Two or fewer times per month	■ FEV_1 or PEF ≥ 80% predicted ■ PEF variability < 20%
Step 2 Mild persistent	■ Symptoms more than times per week but less than once per day ■ Exacerbations may affect activity	■ More than two times per month	■ FEV_1 or PEF ≥ 80% predicted ■ PEF variability 20% to 30%
Step 3 Moderate persistent	■ Daily symptoms ■ Daily use of inhaled short-acting beta$_2$-agonist ■ Exacerbations affect activity ■ Exacerbations two or more times a week; may last days	■ More than once per week	■ FEV_1 or PEF 60% to 80% predicted ■ PEF variability > 30%
Step 4 Severe persistent	■ Continual symptoms ■ Limited physical activity ■ Frequent exacerbations	■ Frequent	■ FEV_1 or PEF ≤ 60% predicted ■ PEF variability > 30%

Note. PEF is peak expiratory flow. FEV_1 is forced expiratory volume in 1 second. Adapted from *Expert Panel Report 2: Guidelines for the Diagnosis and Management of Asthma,* by National Asthma Education and Prevention Program, 1997, National Institutes of Health Publication No. 97-4051. Bethesda, MD. Retrieved August 27, 2007, from http://www.nhlbi.nih.gov/guidelines/asthma/asthgdln.pdf
[a] The presence of one of the features of severity is sufficient to place a patient in that category. An individual should be assigned to the most severe grade in which any feature occurs. The characteristics noted in this table are general and may overlap because asthma is highly variable. Furthermore, an individual's classification may change over time.
[b] Patients at any level of severity can have mild, moderate, or severe exacerbations. Some patients with intermittent asthma experience severe and life-threatening exacerbations separated by long periods of normal lung function and no symptoms.

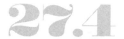

| Stepwise Approach for Managing Asthma in Adults and Children Older Than 5 Years of Age: Treatment |

	LONG-TERM CONTROL	QUICK RELIEF	EDUCATION
Step 1 Mild intermittent	■ No daily medication needed	■ Short-acting bronchodilator: inhaled beta$_2$-agonists as needed for symptoms ■ Intensity of treatment will depend on severity of exacerbation ■ Use of short-acting inhaled beta$_2$-agonists more than two times per week may indicate the need to initiate long-term-control therapy.	■ Teach basic facts about asthma ■ Teach inhaler/spacer/holding chamber technique ■ Discuss roles of medications ■ Develop self-management plan ■ Develop action plan for when and how to take rescue actions, especially for patients with a history of severe exacerbations ■ Discuss appropriate environmental control measures to avoid exposure to known allergens and irritants.
Step 2 Mild persistent	One-day medication ■ Anti-inflammatory: either inhaled corticosteroid (low doses) or cromolyn or nedocromil (children usually begin with a trial of cromolyn or nedocromil) ■ Sustained-release theophylline to serum concentration of 5–15 mcg/mL is an alternative, but not preferred, therapy. Zafirlukast or zileuton may also be considered for patients 12 years of age or younger, although their position in therapy is not fully established.	■ Short-acting bronchodilator: inhaled beta$_2$-agonists as needed for symptoms ■ Intensity of treatment will depend on severity of exacerbation ■ Use of short-acting inhaled beta$_2$-agonists on a daily basis, or increasing use, indicate the need for additional long-term-control therapy.	Step 1 action plus: ■ Teach self-monitoring ■ Refer to group education if available ■ Review and update self-management plan
Step 3 Moderate persistent	Daily medication ■ Either anti-inflammatory: inhaled corticosteroid (medium dose) or inhaled corticosteroid (low-medium dose) and add a long-acting bronchodilator, especially for nighttime symptoms; either long-acting inhaled beta$_2$-agonist, sustained-release theophylline, or long-acting beta$_2$-agonist tablets ■ If needed anti-inflammatory: inhaled corticosteroids (medium-high dose) and long-acting bronchodilator, especially for nighttime symptoms; either long-acting inhaled beta$_2$-agonist, sustained-release theophylline or long-acting beta$_2$-agonist tablets	■ Short-acting bronchodilator: inhaled beta$_2$-agonists as needed for symptoms ■ Intensity of treatment will depend on severity of exacerbation ■ Use of short-acting inhaled beta$_2$-agonists on a daily basis or increasing use indicates the need for additional long-term-control therapy.	Step 1 action plus ■ Teach self-monitoring ■ Refer to group education if available ■ Review and update self-management plan.

(continued)

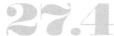

Stepwise Approach for Managing Asthma in Adults and Children Older Than 5 Years of Age: Treatment (*continued*)

LONG-TERM CONTROL		QUICK RELIEF	EDUCATION
Step 4 Severe persistent	Daily medications ■ Anti-inflammatory: inhaled corticosteroid (high dose) and ■ Long-acting bronchodilator: either long-acting inhaled beta$_2$-agonist, sustained-release theophylline, or long-acting beta$_2$-agonist tablets and ■ Corticosteroid tablets or syrup long term (make repeat attempts to reduce systemic steroids and maintain control with high-dose inhaled steroids).	■ Short-acting bronchodilator: inhaled beta$_2$-agonists as needed for symptoms ■ Intensity of treatment will depend on severity of exacerbation ■ Use of short-acting inhaled beta$_2$-agonists on a daily basis or increasing use indicates the need for additional long-term-control therapy.	Steps 2 and 3 actions plus ■ Refer to individual education/counseling

↑ **Step up**
If control is not maintained, consider step up. First, review patient medication technique, adherence, and environmental control (avoidance of allergens or other factors that contribute to asthma severity).

↓ **Step down**
Review treatment every 1 to 6 months; a gradual stepwise reduction in treatment may be possible.

Note. The stepwise approach presents general guidelines to assist clinical decision making; it is not intended to be a specific prescription. Asthma is highly variable; clinicians should tailor specific medication plans to the needs and circumstances of individual patients. Gain control as quickly as possible; then decrease treatment to the least medication necessary to maintain control. Gaining control may be accomplished by either starting treatment at the step most appropriate to the initial severity of the condition or starting at a higher level of therapy (e.g., a course of systemic corticosteroids or higher dose of inhaled corticosteroids). A rescue course of systemic corticosteroids may be needed at any time and at any step. Some patients with intermittent asthma experience severe and life-threatening exacerbations separated by long periods of normal lung function and no symptoms. This may be especially common with exacerbation provoked by respiratory infections. A short course of systemic corticosteroids is recommended. At each step, patients should control their environment or avoid or control factors that make their asthma worse (e.g., allergens, irritants); this requires specific diagnosis and education. Referral to an asthma specialist for consultation or co-management is *recommended* if there are difficulties achieving or maintaining control of asthma or if the patient requires step 4 care. Referral may be *considered* if the patient requires step 3 care. Adapted from *Expert Panel Report 2: Guidelines for the Diagnosis and Management of Asthma,* by the National Asthma Education and Prevention Program, 1997, National Institutes of Health Publication No. 97-4051. Bethesda, MD. Retrieved August 27, 2007, from http://www.nhlbi.nih.gov/guidelines/asthma/asthgdln.pdf

Patient education should include a written action plan detailing the actions a patient (or family) should take based on the signs and symptoms and/or PEF. Additional areas to include in the teaching plan are basic facts about asthma; how the medications work; skill training in the use of inhalers, symptom monitoring, peak flow monitoring, and recognizing early signs of deterioration; and identifying and preventing environmental exposures. Resources for families about asthma and allergies are shown in Table 27.5.

GASTROINTESTINAL DISORDERS

Chronic disorders of the gastrointestinal tract that commonly affect women are cholelithiasis (gallstones), gastroesophageal reflux disease, peptic ulcer disease, irritable bowel syndrome, and inflammatory bowel disease.

Cholelithiasis

Problems related to gallstones can present with a broad spectrum of symptoms from acute to chronic. Most patients with gallstones have mild symptoms that may be evaluated and treated in a primary care setting. However, under certain conditions, gallstones can result in serious complications requiring immediate hospitalization. Gallstones are the most common cause of hospitalization for gastrointestinal complaints (Ghiloni, 1993).

Gallstones are more common in women than in men, with an increasing incidence associated with aging in all races and both sexes. In the United States, by age 65, 10% to 20% of men and women will have gallstones. Risk factors for the development of gallstones in addition to gender and age are Native American ethnicity, obesity, rapid weight loss (particularly in

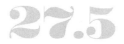

Resources for Patient and Families With Asthma and Allergies

- American Lung Association
  http://www.lungusa.org/
- Healthline: Allergic Rhinitis
  http://www.healthline.com/adamcontent/allergic-rhinitis
- American College of Allergy, Asthma and Immunology
  85 West Algonquin Road, Suite 550, Arlington Heights, IL 60005
  Phone: (847) 427-1200, Fax: (847) 427-1294
  http://www.acaai.org
- National Jewish Medical and Research Center
  1400 Jackson Street, Denver, CO 80206
  Phone: (800) 222-LUNG
  http://www.njc.org

obese individuals), exogenous estrogen, hypertriglyceridemia, and diagnoses of sickle cell anemia, diabetes, Crohn's disease, and cirrhosis. Pregnancy increases the risk of gallstones and symptomatic gallbladder disease (Tierney et al., 2006).

Gallstones are classified according to their chemical composition. There are two types of gallstones: cholesterol and pigmented stones. Cholesterol stones account for 70% to 80% of gallstones in developed countries. Three factors contribute to cholesterol stone formation: (a) supersaturation of the bile with cholesterol, (b) accelerated nucleation with formation of biliary sludge, and (c) hypomotility of the gall bladder. Hypomotility has been shown to be a prominent risk in pregnant patients, patients receiving total parenteral nutrition, patients with diabetes, and patients with spinal cord injuries (Johnston & Kaplan, 1993).

Most individuals with cholelithiasis are asymptomatic and do not develop symptoms. Stone-related symptoms, when present, are abdominal pain (which is often nonspecific and must be differentiated from that of gastritis), peptic ulcer disease, reflux esophagitis, pancreatitis, renal disease, diverticulitis, radicular pain, and angina (Giurgiu & Roslyn, 1996; Moscati, 1996). Therefore, the identification of stones in a patient should not preclude a careful evaluation for other etiologies of the presenting signs and symptoms.

Biliary pain (formerly called biliary colic) comes on quickly, builds to a plateau lasting for several hours, and then resolves. The usual time span for this pain is less than 3 hours. Pain lasting for more than 6 hours is more suggestive of acute rather than chronic cholecystitis (Singleton et al., 1999). The epigastrium is the most common location for this pain, followed by the right costal margin. Biliary pain may be localized in

those areas or referred to the right scapula and shoulder. Symptoms of belching, heartburn, early satiety, bloating, and fullness, although atypical, are extremely common, especially in the elderly. Research does not support the ingestion of a fatty meal as a precipitant of pain.

Many patients will not report any such association and will have symptoms at night (Moscati, 1996). Chronic cholecystitis is characterized by recurrent epsiodes of biliary pain without jaundice or fever, which tend to reoccur with increasing frequency and severity. Laboratory tests for white blood cell counts, liver enzymes, and bilirubin are normal. As a caveat, any patient who presents with fever, jaundice, or a positive Murphy's sign or who has leukocytosis and elevated liver function tests should be referred for immediate evaluation and probable hospitalization (Singleton et al., 1999).

The management of cholelithiasis includes both surgical and nonsurgical treatments. There is generally no need for a prophylactic cholecystectomy in an asymptomatic patient unless the gallbladder is calcified or gallstones are larger than 3 cm in diameter. Laparoscopic cholecystectomy is the treatment of choice for symptomatic gallbladder disease. Patients are usually able to leave the hospital in 2 days and return to work in 7 days. In selected cases, the procedure may be done on an outpatient basis.

Persistence of symptoms after the removal of the gallbladder, the postcholecystectomy syndrome, may be due to a mistake in the initial diagnosis, functional bowel disorder, retained or recurrent stones in the common bile duct, or spasm of the sphincter of Oddi (Tierney et al., 2006). In selected patients who refuse laparoscopic procedures or who are poor surgical candidates, bile salts (cheno and ursodeoxycholic acids) may be given orally for up to 2 years to dissolve cholesterol stones. These salts are most effective in patients with a functioning gallbladder and multiple, small, floating gallstones. Half of all patients will experience recurrence of stones within 5 years after treatment is stopped.

Extracorporeal shockwave lithotripsy with bile salts therapy is no longer generally used in the United States (Tierney et al., 2006). Table 27.6 reviews some of the common diseases of the biliary tract, their clinical presentation, diagnosis, laboratory features, and suggested treatment.

Primary prevention of asymptomatic gallstones is not recommended. Lifestyle modifications such as weight loss (but avoiding rapid weight loss), increased exercise, frequent meals, and high-fiber diets have been theorized to decrease the risk of gallstones, but empirical evidence is lacking (Hofmann, 1993). Special consideration should be given to older individuals and patients with diabetes mellitus who are at increased risk for complications related to symptomatic gallstone

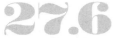 Diseases of the Biliary Tract

	CLINICAL FEATURES	DIAGNOSIS	LABORATORY FEATURES
Gallstones	Asymptomatic	Ultrasound	Normal
Gallstones	Biliary colic	Ultrasound	Normal
Acute cholecystitis	Epigastric or right upper quadrant pain, nausea, vomiting, fever, Murphy's sign	Ultrasound, HIDA scan[a]	Leukocytosis
Chronic cholecystitis	Biliary colic, constant epigastric or right upper quadrant pain, nausea	Ultrasound (stones), oral chole-cystography (nonfunctioning gallbladder)	Normal
Choledocholithiasis	Asymptomatic or biliary colic, jaundice, fever, gallstone pancreatitis	Ultrasound (dilated ducts), ERCP[b]	Liver function tests; leukocytosis and positive blood cultures in cholangitis; elevated amylase and lipase in pancreatitis

[a] HIDA = hepatobiliary, hydroxyl iminodiacetic acid, also known as cholescintigraphy.
[b] ERCP = endoscopic retrograde cholangiopancreatography.

disease. Patients with diabetes who are diagnosed with symptomatic gallstone disease should be treated promptly. Clinicians need to be aware that older individuals may present with atypical symptoms such as dyspepsia, heartburn, chest tightness, bloating, and nausea. Surgery is successful in healthy, older individuals with a mortality rate for nonemergent cholecystectomy of less than 4% (Gholson, Sittig, & McDonald, 1994). Patients who are taking estrogen, clofibrate, or gemfibrozil or who are pregnant should be educated about their increased risk for gallstones.

Gastroesophageal Reflux Disease

Gastroesophageal reflux disease (GERD) is a commonly seen problem in primary care caused by reflux of the acidic contents of the stomach into the esophagus. The major symptom is heartburn, and, although the exact incidence of GERD is unknown, approximately 35% to 50% of all Americans are reported to have some degree of heartburn (Meredith & Horan, 2000). The highest incidence of heartburn is seen in pregnant women (Baron & Richter, 1992).

Most individuals with GERD have mild disease without complications, but esophageal obstruction, esophageal perforation, bleeding, and adenocarcinoma can occur. Adenocarcinoma is increasing at a faster rate than any other cancer, and studies have shown a correlation between adenocarcinoma and reflux (Lagergren, Bergstrom, Lindgren, & Nyren, 1999). Barrett's esophagus is present in 10% of patients with chronic reflux and is thought to be linked with severe GERD.

The most serious complication of Barrett's esophagus is esophageal adenocarcinoma (Tierney et al., 2006).

Many patients presenting with symptoms of asthma also have GERD, which, when treated, will result in improvement of their asthma symptoms (Reynolds, 1996). Several pathophysiological factors, alone or in combination, may cause GERD. These include (a) an incompetent lower esophageal sphincter (LES), (b) gastric pH lower than 2, (c) abnormal esophageal clearance, and (d) delayed gastric emptying (e.g., gastroparesis). Patients with transient relaxation of the LES may experience symptoms of reflux during abdominal straining, bending, or lifting. Damage to the esophageal mucosa from reflux is related to the degree of acidity of the reflux and the amount of time it is in contact with the mucosa. Normally, the acid reflux is cleared and neutralized by esophageal peristalsis and salivary bicarbonate. Diminished peristalstic clearance is associated with Raynaud's phenomenon, CREST syndrome, and scleroderma. Conditions that are associated with impaired salivation such as the use of anticholinergic medications, oral radiation therapy, and Sjogren's syndrome may exacerbate GERD (Richter, 1996).

The typical symptom of GERD is heartburn that usually occurs 30 to 60 minutes after a meal. This symptom is often precipitated by reclining and relieved by baking soda or antacids. Nocturnal symptoms are important to elicit because of the supine position at bedtime that may exacerbate reflux. The severity of the symptoms is not correlated with the extent of esophageal tissue damage; some patients with severe esophagitis may be asymptomatic. Other symptoms reported include the regurgitation of sour or bitter stomach contents into the mouth and complaints of indigestion. Less common symptoms include dysphagia and epigastric pain. Atypical manifestations of GERD that are being recognized with increasing frequency include asthma, chronic cough (particularly if nocturnal), chronic laryngitis, hoarseness, sore throat, and atypical (noncardiac) chest pain. The diagnosis of GERD is often overlooked in these patients, because they may not present with the classic symptoms of heartburn or regurgitation (Tierney et al., 2006).

Patients with GERD can also present with symptoms of cardiac ischemia aggravated by the GERD. Complaints suggesting a cardiac etiology should receive a complete cardiac evaluation and referral. Dysphagia may also be suggestive of serious pathology that should be evaluated by a specialist. The physical examination is almost always normal in patients with GERD.

The differential diagnoses of heartburn include a number of disorders emanating from the gastrointestinal, cardiac, and other body systems. A brief list of these diagnoses is presented in Table 27.7. Numerous diagnostic studies can be used to evaluate the esophagus, including upper endoscopy, barium esophagography, esophageal manometry, and ambulatory esophageal pH monitoring. The barium swallow is usually the first test performed in patients presenting with persistent dysphagia and provides data to help in the differential diagnosis of mechanical versus motility disorders. Upper endoscopy is helpful in evaluating patients presenting with odynophagia (sensation of burning or squeezing pain when swallowing) or for further evaluation (and biopsy) of structural abnormalities noted on the barium swallow. The decision regarding which of these tests to use is based on indicators such as an acute onset of GERD after the age of 40, failure to improve with treatment, dysphagia, and a history of chronic heartburn for more than 5 years. Individuals who are 35 years of age or older with complaints of heartburn and a history of smoking and/or alcohol use are at greater risk for serious sequelae of GERD and should receive an earlier and more aggressive work-up (Meredith & Horan, 2000).

A stepwise approach is used in the treatment of GERD. Patients without complications and typical symptoms of heartburn may be treated empirically for 4 weeks without diagnostic studies and then reevaluated (Spechler, 1998). The first line of treatment is lifestyle modifications. These include weight loss (if indicated); a low-fat diet with smaller, more frequent meals; and elevation of the head while sleeping. Patients should be taught to avoid nighttime snacks, smoking, chocolate, acidic foods, and lying down after eating. They also should avoid the use of any medications that are known to decrease the tone of the LES (e.g., calcium channel blockers, beta adrenergic agonists, alpha adrenergic blockers, anticholinergics, levodopa, narcotics, nitrates, progestins, theophylline, and transdermal nicotine). Initially, antacids may be prescribed. If these lifestyle modifications are unsuccessful, histamine (H2) receptor antagonists may be added to reduce 24-hour gastric acid secretion or promotility agents to reduce reflux by increasing sphincter tone and enhancing esophageal acid clearance and gastric emptying.

Treatment twice daily with either an H2 receptor antagonist or a promotility agent will result in symptomatic improvement in about two-thirds of patients with heartburn (Spechler, 1998). Dosages should be reduced to the lowest level that maintains effective symptom control. If the second line of treatment fails, patients may be treated with higher doses of H2 receptor antagonists or use an 8- to 12-week course of proton pump inhibitors such as omeprazole or lansoprazole.

Patients and families should be counseled about the importance of lifestyle modifications, including diet, in both the initial treatment of GERD and the prevention of relapse. Smoking cessation should be stressed as well as the avoidance of alcohol. The side effects of all medications should be reviewed and the patient instructed in signs and symptoms indicating a call to their health care provider, such as unexplained weight loss associated with GERD and persistence of symptoms despite treatment.

27.7 Differential Diagnosis of Heartburn

Gastrointestinal	Cardiac
Gastroesophageal reflux disease	Angina
Esophagitis	Myocardial infarction
Gastritis/malignancy	Heart failure
Peptic ulcer disease	Pericarditis
Pancreatitis	
Hepatitis	
Appendicitis/peritonitis	
Crohn's disease	
Drug induced—Aspirin, nonsteroidal anti-inflammatory drugs, other	
Other: pregnancy, systemic lupus erythematosus, scleroderma, irritable bowel syndrome, Raynaud's phenomenon, sarcoidosis	

Peptic Ulcer Disease

Peptic ulcer disease (PUD) occurs when there is a break in the gastric or duodenal mucosa arising from impairment of the normal mucosal defense system or overwhelming of this system by aggressive luminal factors such as acid or pepsin. Peptic ulcers can be classified as either gastric or duodenal. The clinical picture of PUD, including approaches to treatment, has changed over the years with the recognition of an infectious etiology of PUD in 1982. In addition, the prevalence of duodenal ulcer disease has been declining in the United States since 1955, possibly related to the decreased incidence of *Helicobacter pylori* infection secondary to improved water supply, sanitation, widespread use of antibiotics, decreases in cigarette smoking, and improved dietary habits (McCarthy, 1996). However, the incidence of gastric ulcers appears to be increasing, possibly related to the widespread use of NSAIDs (Smalley & Griffin, 1996).

In the United States, there are about 500,000 new cases of PUD and 4 million ulcer recurrences yearly. Duodenal ulcers are more common than gastric ulcers, affecting both sexes almost equally. Although ulcers are common in any age group, duodenal ulcers usually occur between the ages of 30 and 55 and gastric ulcers between the ages of 55 and 70.

H. pylori is the major cause of PUD. This is a gram-negative rod found in the antrum of the stomach; it secretes urease and other enzymes into the mucous layer of the gastric mucosa. This damages the protective barrier and causes ulceration. *H. pylori* infection is associated with 65% to 70% of gastric ulcers and 90% to 95% of duodenal ulcers. In the United States, *H. pylori* infection is more prevalent in older adults, African Americans, Hispanics, and lower socioeconomic groups. Infected individuals have a two to six times greater risk for gastric cancer (Singleton et al., 1999). The importance of *H. pylori* in duodenal and gastric ulcers is undeniable, and evidence of this infection should be an important part of the patient work-up.

Patients who chronically ingest aspirin or other NSAIDs, for example, to treat a chronic pain condition such as arthritis are at risk for development of PUD. Other reversible risk factors include cigarette smoking, which may alter intestinal mucosal blood flow, causing hypoxic damage to the mucosa and ulcer formation. Dietary factors such as caffeine, alcohol, and spicy foods were once thought to be linked with ulcer formation, but are no longer implicated in the development of the disease.

The most common complication of PUD is bleeding. Other complications include gastric outlet obstruction (secondary to scarring), perforation, and penetration into the viscous of an adjacent organ such as the liver or pancreas. If these complications are suspected, the patient should be immediately referred to a surgeon or gastroenterologist. Bleeding in the elderly can be fatal. Ulcer perforation, a surgical emergency, is more common in the elderly and in patients using NSAIDs, aspirin, corticosteroids, and cocaine (Meredith & Horan, 2000).

The typical patient with a duodenal ulcer presents with epigastric pain relieved by food or antacids; pain reoccurs about 2 to 4 hours after eating. Ulcer symptoms have a rhythmicity and periodicity. The pain of a duodenal ulcer classically wakes the patient in the middle of the night. The pain of gastric ulcers differs in that it is decreased or absent with fasting, occurs about 5 to 15 minutes after eating, and resolves when the stomach empties. Patients with gastric ulcers often avoid food and lose weight.

Although gastric ulcer pain may awaken the patient at night, it is much less common than duodenal ulcer pain. Perforation of an ulcer may present as persistent radiation of pain to the back or generalization of pain over the abdomen. A history of nonspecific epigastric pain with a variable relationship to meals is present in 80% to 90% of patients, with 10% to 20% of patients presenting with ulcer complications without any antecedent symptoms; 30% to 50% of ulcers caused by NSAIDs are asymptomatic.

The physical examination in mild PUD is often unremarkable. On deep palpation, mild epigastric tenderness may be elicited. Positive fecal blood testing is present in one-third of patients. Laboratory tests are typically normal in patients with uncomplicated mild disease, but they are necessary to rule out complications or confounding diseases. These include a CBC, serum creatinine, serum calcium, and stool for occult fecal blood. A CBC is useful to rule out anemia. An elevated serum amylase in the presence of severe epigastric pain may indicate penetration of the ulcer into the pancreas. A fasting serum gastrin level may be used to screen for Zollinger-Ellison syndrome.

The upper endsocopy is considered the gold standard for the diagnosis of duodenal and gastric ulcers because it provides better diagnostic accuracy than barium radiography and the opportunity to biopsy for the presence of malignancy and *H. pylori* infection. The double barium contrast (upper gastrointestinal) study is considered somewhat safer and less expensive. Barium studies and endoscopy should be avoided if perforation is suspected. If symptoms resolve with treatment, duodenal ulcers require no further work-up (unless Crohn's disease is suspected). Gastric ulcers require endoscopic biopsy initially in order to rule out gastric malignancy and reevaluation after 3 months of therapy to document complete healing. *H. pylori* testing is indicated in patients with active ulcer disease, recurrence of ulcer disease, and those who have had a gastric resection. Testing methods for *H. pylori* include urea breath testing, serologic testing, and endoscopic biopsy (CDC, 1997; Soll, 1996).

The differential diagnosis for PUD includes GERD, cholecystitis, pancreatitis, biliary obstruction, ruptured aortic aneurysm, and cancers of the stomach and pancreas. Consultation with, or referral to, a physician is recommended for the diagnosis of these patients.

The therapeutic management of PUD involves the potential use of three categories of medications: (a) acid antisecretory agents, (b) mucosal protective agents, and (c) agents to eradicate *H. pylori*. Clinicians need to be familiar with the most up-to-date recommendations for the treatment of *H. pylori* that can be obtained from the Food and Drug Administration. Many patients can be managed without referral to a specialist.

Indications for referral include situations where there is no (or little) response to treatment or there is development of complications. Patients should be encouraged to eat balanced meals at regular intervals, avoiding foods that are known to aggravate symptoms, as well as to avoid the use of aspirin, NSAIDs, and alcohol. There is no justification for bland or restrictive diets. Patients who are smoking should be counseled to stop, because smoking not only retards the rate of healing of ulcers but also increases the frequency of reoccurrence. Patients should be instructed to take medications correctly, for the time prescribed, and should know the side effects of their medications. One of the primary difficulties with the treatment of *H. pylori* is the long-term treatment regimen that is required to eradicate the infection.

Ulcers that are truly refractory to treatment are now uncommon, with only 10% of ulcers unhealed after 8 to 12 weeks of treatment with H2 receptor antagonists of sucralfate (Tierney et al., 2006). Noncompliance is the most common cause of failure to respond to therapy.

Among the complementary and alternative medicine treatments sometimes used, licorice root is one of the most common remedies. This product has a long history of being used to soothe inflamed digestive tract mucous membranes; it may increase production of mucin, protective to the mucosal lining.

Irritable Bowel Syndrome

Irritable bowel syndrome (IBS) is a common, chronic, functional disorder characterized by alterations in bowel habits and abdominal pain. The onset of symptoms is usually in late adolescence with approximately half of all patients being between the ages of 30 and 50. The incidence of IBS is greater in women and higher in Whites than in non-Whites (Verne & Cerda, 1997). Up to 20% of the adult population may experience these symptoms, but most will not seek medical treatment.

The definition of IBS is based on the following criteria, known as the Rome II criteria (in the absence of a structural or biochemical explanation for the symptoms). The patient should demonstrate at least 12 weeks (need not be consecutive) in the preceding 12 months with abdominal discomfort or pain that has at least two of the following three features: (a) it is relieved with defecation; (b) the onset is associated with a change in frequency of stool; (c) the onset is associated with a change in form (appearance) of stool.

Irritable bowel syndrome is characterized by a variable combination of recurrent gastrointestinal symptoms that are not related to any identifiable structural or biochemical abnormalities. There is no definitive diagnosis or test. The diagnosis is based on recognition of a typical profile and exclusion of other organic disorders. The most plausible model of causation of IBS suggests a dysregulation in intestinal, motor, sensory, and central nervous system functions that result in pain and discomfort due to disturbances in intestinal motility and enhanced visceral sensitivity (Dalton & Drossman, 1997; Meredith & Horan, 2000). Additional theories on the role of stress, diet, and infection in IBS may be relevant to the etiology of this disorder. Symptoms of IBS have been known to be exacerbated by extended periods of increased stress (Carlson, 1998). Some patients develop IBS after an episode of bacterial gastroenteritis.

Patients present with symptoms of abdominal pain and altered bowel habits. Many complain of overly acute sensory ability with respect to the gastrointestinal tract. Often there is an associated psychiatric diagnosis such as anxiety or depression. The condition is more common among women who have experienced physical abuse.

A thorough physical examination should be performed to identify any organic pathology. In IBS, the physical examination is usually unremarkable except for some mild distention and tenderness in the lower abdomen, especially in the area of the sigmoid colon. A gynecological examination to rule out endometriosis and a rectal examination should be performed. They are usually unremarkable. Laboratory studies are used to rule out other possible etiologies for symptoms. Suggested baseline studies include a complete blood count and serum chemistries. A urinalysis is used to rule out urinary tract infections, which can mimic the symptoms of IBS. Additional diagnostic studies may be suggested by the history and physical examination. These might include thyroid function tests, stool for ova and parasites, stool for occult blood, and erythrocyte sedimentation rate. Patients younger than 40 should receive a flexible sigmoidoscopy. Patients over the age of 40 who have not had a previous test should be considered for a barium enema or colonoscopy (American Gastroenterological Association, 1997). All suspicious or unclear diagnostic results should be evaluated by a gastroenterologist.

The differential diagnoses for IBS are shown in Table 27.8. To assist in the diagnosis of IBS, which can often be difficult because many of the symptoms are present in other disorders, the Rome II criteria are used to facilitate a diagnosis of IBS in a cost-effective manner (Meredith & Horan, 2000).

The management of IBS involves diet and pharmacotherapy. Lifestyle modifications such as stress reduction are important to reduce the hypersensitive response of the colon and promote general well-being. Because this is a functional disorder, the emphasis should move away from finding the cause of the symptoms to successful ways of coping with them.

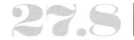

Selected Differential Diagnoses for Irritable Bowel Syndrome

Bacterial infection

Biliary or gastric disease

Chronic pancreatitis

Depression, anxiety, panic disorders

Diverticulitis

Drugs—for example, laxatives, magnesium-containing antacids, cholinergics, diuretics, prostaglandins, opiate analgesics

Food intolerance—for example, lactase deficiencies, fermentable carbohydrates, certain artificial sweeteners

Inflammatory bowel disease

Malabsorption

Neoplasia

Neoplasms

Thyroid disease

Diet is a first-line therapy. Patients may report dietary intolerances, although the role of dietary triggers in IBS has never been established. The use of a food diary in which patients report food intake and its correlation with symptoms and life events may provide insights on dietary and psychosocial factors that precipitate symptoms. All patients with IBS should be screened for lactose intolerance because IBS and lactose intolerance can coexist. Patients with lactose intolerance can experience symptomatic improvement with a lactose-free diet. Eating smaller, more frequent meals may help control symptoms, as will avoidance of known troublesome foods such as caffeine, alcohol, fats, brown beans, Brussels sprouts, cabbage, sugar, dairy, yeast, onions, gluten, and sorbitol (which is found in many diet drinks and foods). Recommendations on supplementation with fiber should be individualized to the patient situation.

More than two-thirds of patients with IBS will respond to education, reassurance, and dietary interventions. Pharmacotherapy should target specific symptoms such as pain, constipation, and diarrhea and should be reserved for patients with more severe symptoms (Camilleri & Choi, 1997). In this situation, these agents can be viewed as adjunctive rather than curative. Examples of classes of drugs used in IBS are antispasmodic, antidiarrheal, anticonstipation, and psychotropic agents. Behavioral modification, relaxation techniques, and hypnotherapy also have been found to be successful.

Patients and families require information about the disease and its treatment. The importance of a trusting, open, therapeutic provider-patient alliance is essential to the successful management of this disorder and has been shown to reduce the number of follow-up visits required by patients. Patients need to be reassured that the disorder is neither life-threatening nor a known precursor to cancer. Realistic goals for symptom control need to be mutually established and the patient informed that symptoms may take months to improve and may reoccur periodically. If medications are used, patients need to be counseled on when and how they should be used and potential side effects.

Inflammatory Bowel Disease

Inflammatory bowel disease (IBD) describes chronic immunologic diseases that cause inflammation of the gastrointestinal tract. The two chronic diseases in this category are ulcerative colitis (UC) and Crohn's disease (CD). Ulcerative colitis and Crohn's disease share certain clinical findings; however, they have important differences that influence their management. Ulcerative colitis is a chronic, recurrent disease characterized by diffuse mucosal inflammation of the colon. Crohn's disease is a chronic, recurrent disease characterized by patchy, transmural inflammation of any part of the gastrointestinal mucosa from the mouth to the anus. Inflammatory bowel disease is a lifelong illness with profound psychosocial, emotional, and economic impacts.

The prevalence of IBD ranges from 20 to 200 per 100,000 of the population in the United States. The incidence of CD has been increasing over the past 50 years, while the incidence of UC has remained stable (Singleton et al., 1999). Both are diseases of young people affecting both sexes equally.

Whites are more likely to have IBD than Asians or African Americans; IBD is more common in those of Jewish ancestry. The cause of IBD is unknown, although a variety of bacterial, viral, and dietary agents have been suggested. A genetic predisposition is likely. Although only 15% of cases are familial, genes associated with IBD have been found on chromosomes 16, 10, and 7. These genes encode for cell-to-cell interactions in epithelial tissue. The role of the immune system as a factor in the inflammatory response continues to be investigated. Smoking has been positively associated with CD; however, smoking is linked with disease mitigation in ulcerative colitis (Singleton et al., 1999).

Patients with IBD can present with a variety of symptoms that need to be differentiated from other gastrointestinal diseases as well as differentiated between UC and CD. Patients with mild UC present with frequent loose bowel movements associated with cramping; often there is blood and mucus in the stool. With more severe UC, the patient experiences more defecations per day and more blood and mucus in the stool. The patient could have tachycardia, fever, weight loss, and signs of undernutrition such as hypoproteinemia and peripheral edema. The patient with CD commonly presents with abdominal cramping and tenderness, fever, anorexia, weight loss, and pain. There is intermittent blood loss in the stool. The loss of mucosa could be sufficient to interfere with bile salt absorption, producing steatorrhea. If the bowel perforates, peritonitis will occur.

On examination, the patient with IBD may have abdominal tenderness. A digital rectal exam is performed to assess for perianal inflammation and blood in the stool. The patient with CD could have extraintestinal symptoms such as erythema nodosum and nondeforming peripheral arthritis. Clinical features of both of these disorders and their laboratory findings are shown in Table 27.9.

There are no established tests to diagnose IBD. Instead, the diagnosis is made based on the history and physical examination as well as supportive laboratory data. Laboratory studies may demonstrate the nutritional consequences of the disease as well as inflammatory activity or be nonspecific. All patients with symptoms suggestive of IBD, or diagnosed cases with an acute exacerbation, should be referred to a gastroenterologist for further diagnostic procedures such as sigmoidoscopy and colonoscopy with biopsy (Pardi & Tremaine, 1998; Taylor & DiPalma, 1998). Colonoscopy with biopsy is useful to differentiate between UC and CD, to define the sites and extent of involvement, and to identify any premalignant lesions. Stool culture for ova and parasites should be performed before the use of barium or colonoscopy. The differential diagnoses for CD include irritable bowel syndrome (IBS), appendicitis, diverticulitis, enteric infections such as *Yersinia enterocolitica*, intestinal lymphoma or carcinoma, celiac sprue, and undiagnosed AIDS. The diagnosis of idiopathic UC is made after excluding all other known causes of colitis such as CD involving the colon, cancer of the colon, pseudomembranous or antibiotic-associated colitis, infectious colitis (salmonella, shigella, campylobacter, amebiasis, *C. difficile*), proctitis (gonorrhea, syphilis, chlamydia, herpes), cytomegalovirus colitis (in immunocompromised patients), and ischemic colitis (Marion, George, & Ware, 1997).

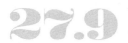 | Clinical Characteristics of Ulcerative Colitis and Crohn's Disease

	CROHN'S DISEASE	**ULCERATIVE COLITIS**
History	■ Insidious onset ■ Intermittent low-grade fever, diarrhea, and right left quadrant pain ■ Watery diarrhea; malabsorption ■ Steatorrhea	■ Bloody diarrhea (hallmark) ■ Lower abdominal cramps and fecal urgency ■ Tenesmus
Physical examination	■ Right lower quadrant tenderness and mass ■ Perianal disease with abscess, fistula ■ Fever, oral ulcerations ■ Extraintestinal signs ■ Volume depletion	■ Fever ■ Variable tenderness ■ Extraintestinal signs ■ Dermal manifestations; arthritis ■ Volume depletion (check orthostatics)
Laboratory	■ Evidence of ulceration, stricturing, or fistulas of the small intestine or colon ■ Same as for ulcerative colitis, but also hypocalcemia and vitamin B_{12} deficiency ■ On radiograph/endoscope: discontinuous disease, skin lesions, rectum often spared; aphthous ulcerations; "cobble-stoning"	■ Anemia; low serum albumin ■ Sigmoidoscopy—key to diagnosis ■ Leukocytosis with left shift ■ Elevated erythrocyte sedimentation rate ■ Hypokalemia; hypomagnesia ■ On radiograph and endoscope, continuous disease involving rectum, no small bowel disease ■ Fine ulcerations ■ Friable mucosa ■ Toxic dilitation
Other	■ Patients with Crohn's disease are at increased risk for colon cancer ■ Cigarette smoking exacerbates disease	■ Cigarette smoking protective

Note. Adapted from *Current Medical Diagnosis and Treatment 2006,* by L. M. Tierney, S. J. McPhee, and M. A. Papadakis, 2006, New York: Lange Medical Books/ McGraw Hill.

Patients with UC disease proximal to the sigmoid colon have a markedly increased risk of developing colon carcinoma; risk is related to the extent and duration of the disease (Meredith & Horan, 2000). Therefore, it is recommended that patients with UC undergo routine colonoscopy every 1 to 2 years. Although this association has not been found with CD, it is considered prudent to periodically screen those patients with long-standing disease.

The mainstays of treatment of IBD are 5-aminosalicylic acid derivatives (e.g., sulfasalazine, oral and topical mesalamine, olsalazine), corticosteroids, and mercaptopurine and azathioprine (Sandborn, 1996; Tierney et al., 2006). The goal of therapy is to resolve acute exacerbations and prevent relapse through suppression of the inflammatory response. Although antibiotics have not been proven to be effective in UC, metronidazole may be used in CD and in those who have not responded to mesalamine or sulfasalazine (Meredith & Horan, 2000). Mild disease may require only symptomatic measures (e.g., control of diarrhea) and dietary changes such as low-fiber diets with avoidance of raw fruits and vegetables in patients with acute symptoms. Patients with chronic disease should be encouraged to eat a well-balanced diet with few restrictions. Lactose restriction may be necessary in patients with a lactose intolerance. Folate and vitamin deficiencies such as vitamin B_{12} deficiencies, may be seen in patients with CD and will require supplementation. Iron-deficiency anemia may result from blood loss, requiring iron supplementation.

For patients with refractory CD, immunosuppression with 6MP is sometimes tried. Cyclosporine is also sometimes used experimentally in patients with steroid refractory CD. Infliximab is an IgG anti-TNF antibody also sometimes helpful in patients with moderate CD.

There are several complementary and alternative medicine approaches to IBD. Because it is an inflammatory disease, anti-inflammatory omega 3 fatty acids such as fish oil are sometimes prescribed; there is some evidence that these approaches can be effective (Belluzzi et al., 1996; Lorenz-Meyer et al., 1996). Probiotics have had mixed results. Because the inflammatory cytokine TNF-alpha is often elevated in IBD, the botanical curcumin has been used. Curcumin is derived from turmeric and inhibits TNF-alpha. An in vitro study found that TNF-alpha was associated with increased intestinal permeability; curcumin inhibited the TNF-alpha-stimulated increase in intestinal permeability (Ma et al., 2004). *Boswellia serrata* and berberine are botanicals with anti-inflammatory activity that have been suggested for use in IBD. Experimental studies are needed. Because stress sometimes exacerbates IBD, there may be a role for relaxation therapies such as yoga and meditation in the treatment. Again, systematic studies are needed. The provider and patient can work together to test the effect of these interventions. As with all chronic diseases, it is

likely to be helpful for the provider and patient to partner together to design therapeutic approaches and test their efficacy in the individual case.

Surgery is indicated for patients who do not respond to treatment or develop side effects, or if serious complications such as hemorrhage, perforation, fibrostenosis, or toxic megacolon develop. Surgery is also the treatment of choice where evidence of dysplasia exists or if malignancy is suggested (Pardi & Tremaine, 1998). Approximately 60% to 70% of patients with CD will require surgery for abscess, fistula, or obstruction, with 50% requiring surgery again at some later point in their disease.

Health care providers need to be sensitive to the psychosocial and economic burden of a chronic illness like IBD and strive to establish a supportive relationship with the patient through active listening, involving the patient and family in all aspects of the treatment plan, identifying sources of support and successful coping strategies, and encouraging an optimistic outlook. Most patients with IBD can lead a normal, active life.

However, fears about cancer, complications, and issues regarding self-image (particularly those with a colectomy or ileostomy) need to be discussed openly. Patients should be routinely screened for signs and symptoms of depression and increased stress and referred appropriately. Persons with IBD need to be informed about the disease, its potential complications, and the possible side effects of medications. In CD, where malabsorption can be a serious problem, ongoing nutritional counseling and weight maintenance are essential. Web resources for individuals and families with gallbladder disease, GERD, peptic ulcer disease, and IBD are shown in Table 27.10.

RHEUMATIC AND MUSCULOSKELETAL DISORDERS

More than 100 different types of rheumatic disorders have been identified that affect joints, the tissues surrounding the joints, and other connective tissue. As a group, these disorders affect more than 46 million adults in the United States, more than one-third of whom have limitation in activity related to the disease. Women have a higher prevalence than men in every age group, and the prevalence increases with age (National Center for Chronic Disease Prevention and Heath Promotion, 2006). With the predicted aging of the U.S. population, rheumatic disorders may affect as many as 67 million adults by 2030, and about two-thirds will be women. The most common rheumatic disorders affecting women are osteoarthritis, rheumatoid arthritis, and fibromyalgia. Systemic lupus erythematosus (SLE) is a less prevalent rheumatologic disease, but occurs predominantly in women. Osteoporosis, characterized

27.10 | Web Resources for Selected Gastrointestinal Disorders

Gall bladder
- National Digestive Diseases Information Clearinghouse: http://digestive.niddk.nih.gov/ddiseases/pubs/gallstones

Gastroesophageal reflux disease (GERD)
- Healthtouch: http://www.emedicinehealth.com/heartburn/article_em.htm
- GERD Information Resource Center: http://www.gerd.com
- American College of Gastroenterologists: http://www.acg.gi.org/acghome.html

Inflammatory bowel disease
- Crohn's and Colitis Foundation of Canada, 21 St. Clair Avenue East, Suite 301, Toronto, Ontario M4T IL9, 1 (800) 387-1479; http://www.ccfc.ca
- National Digestive Diseases Information Clearinghouse, Crohn's information page: http://digestive.niddk.nih.gov/ddiseases/pubs/crohns/index.htm

Peptic ulcer disease
- MedicineNet.com Stomach and Duodenal Ulcers page: http://www.medicinenet.com/peptic_ulcer/article.htm
- Mayo Health Oasis: http://www.mayohealth.org/mayo/askphys/qa970402.html
- Aetna U.S. Health Care Peptic Ulcer Page: http://www.intelihealth.com/IH/ihtIH/WSIHW000/9339/10799.html

by low bone mass and increased bone fragility, is also more predominant in women. The epidemiology, symptom description, and management of these disorders are presented in this section.

Osteoarthritis

Osteoarthritis (OA) is a chronic arthropathy characterized by degradation of the articular cartilages and subchondral bone and the subsequent reactive remodeling of cartilage and bone. Inflammatory cytokines also contribute to the cartilage destruction. It is generally considered to be progressive; however, studies have shown individual variance in progression rates, with some individuals stable over long periods of time. Osteoarthritis is the most common of all joint disorders, affecting more than 20 million people in the United States. The incidence increases with age, and more than 80% of adults older than 75 years are affected (Harris, 2005). However, it is not an inevitable consequence of aging.

The precise etiology of OA is unknown, but factors that predispose to its development include older age, obesity (primarily in the weight-bearing joints), female gender, joint injury or repetitive overuse, genetic predisposition, and joint malalignment. After age 50, women have a marked increase in prevalence of OA compared to men, especially in the knee. Women also tend to have more severe symptoms and more joints involved. The primary modifiable risk factor for OA is obesity. Research has shown that a modest weight loss has been associated with a decrease in symptoms (Ling & Rudolph, 2006).

Symptoms are typically insidious, progress slowly, and usually do not appear before the age of 40 to 45. The joints commonly affected by OA include the distal interphalangeal (DIP) and proximal interphalangeal (PIP) joints of the hand, the carpometacarpal joint at the base of the thumb, the hips, knees, and the cervical and lumbosacral spine. Joint pain is the most common symptom of OA. Pain initially occurs after strenuous activity and then may progress to pain after moderate activity and then pain at rest. Other symptoms may include joint stiffness after sleep or prolonged inactivity, changes in joint range of motion, and a perception that the knees lock or give way with ambulation. In contrast to rheumatoid arthritis, the morning stiffness of OA usually lasts less than 30 minutes.

On physical examination, bony enlargement and deformities may be seen especially in the hands and knees. In the hands, Heberden's nodes may be seen at the DIPs and Bouchard's nodes at the PIPs. The gait of the patient should be carefully evaluated to identify problems related to OA of the hip and knee. In the later stages of the disease, muscle wasting may be observed. Although not usual, signs of inflammation such as an effusion, erythema, heat, and tenderness may signal an acute exacerbation. Passive or active range of motion may elicit pain or crepitus in the affected joints.

The most common disorders to consider in the differential diagnosis of OA are rheumatoid arthritis (RA), gout, pseudogout, fibromyalgia, polymyalgia rheumatica, and, with a monoarticular presentation, infectious arthritis. The diagnosis of OA is based on symptoms, physical findings, and radiographic studies. Laboratory studies may be helpful to rule out other diagnoses and should be selected carefully following a thorough history and exam. Tests that may be used to differentiate OA from other rheumatologic disorders include CBC, erythrocyte sedimentation rate, C-reactive protein, rheumatoid factor (RF), antinuclear antibody, urinalysis, blood urea nitrogen (BUN), and creatinine. Many of the laboratory tests used to differentiate rheumatologic diseases have a low specificity, and, especially in the elderly, may have a high false positive rate (Goroll & Mulley, 2006). Additional laboratory synovial fluid analysis is used when an infection is suspected. Normal synovial fluid is noninflammatory with a normal viscosity and few leukocytes. Joint radiographs alone are not sufficient to make the diagnosis but are helpful in classifying the stage of OA because the changes seen are pathognomonic. Radiographic changes include narrowing of the joint space, formation of subchondral cysts and osteophytes, and bone remodeling. The radiologic changes do not necessarily correlate with the patient's clinical symptoms.

The goals of therapy for OA include control or reduction of pain and swelling and maintenance or improvement of joint mobility and function. Disease-modifying modalities have not yet been identified for OA, although ongoing research is promising (Ling & Rudolph, 2006). The American College of Rheumatology (2000) recommends that nonpharmacologic modalities be the cornerstone of management of OA, with pharmacologic agents used as an adjunct. Nonpharmacologic therapies include patient education, self-management programs (such as the Arthritis Foundation Self-Help Program or Stanford University's Chronic Disease Self-Management Program), social support, weight loss, exercise (both self-directed and those prescribed by physical and occupational therapists), assistive devices for ambulation and other activities of daily living, alterations in living environment, bracing, supportive footwear, and heat and/or cold applications. Exercise programs have been shown to improve pain and function for individuals with knee OA (American College of Rheumatology, 2000; Talbot, Gaines, Huynh, & Metter, 2003). Exercises need to be chosen to enhance strengthening while not increasing stress on the affected joints, and gradual increase of intensity is recommended. Patient education should include information about the disease process, therapeutic options (including alternative therapies), and access to additional resources such as the Arthritis Foundation.

Medications are used in OA primarily for pain relief. Capsaicin is a nonprescription topical agent that is effective for relieving pain. It needs to be applied two to four times daily to be effective and may cause a localized sensation of burning and heat for several days. Other topical agents such as menthol, salicylate-based products, or topical NSAIDs may be helpful, although evidence of benefit is not available. Acetaminophen is recommended as an initial choice for treatment of the pain of OA. Dosing can be as needed or scheduled based on the pattern of pain, in doses up to 4 g per day, with adjustments for renal or hepatic impairment or with chronic alcohol use. NSAIDs are effective in relieving pain in adults with OA and may be appropriate for those who do not respond to acetaminophen, those who have moderate to severe pain, and those with evidence of inflammation. However, these medications can have serious gastrointestinal, cardiac, and renal effects, and providers need to assess patient risks and prescribe and monitor appropriately. Doses should be titrated to the lowest effective dose. Older adults are at higher risk of side effects from NSAIDs. Opioids are also used to manage pain of OA, sometimes with other medications such as acetaminophen or NSAIDs. Risks of side effects must be assessed and dosing adjusted or monitored as appropriate. Glucosamine and chondroitin sulfate, both together and individually, have been studied for efficacy in pain relief and disease modification in OA, with contradictory results and differing recommendations by rheumatology experts (Reginster, 2007; Vlad, LaValley, McAlindon, & Felson, 2007). They are considered safe and are generally well tolerated.

Intraarticular injections are used for select patients with more severe pain, or who do not respond to oral medications. Surgical procedures such as osteotomy and total joint arthroplasty are reserved for those cases of OA that are refractory to medical management.

Rheumatoid Arthritis

Rheumatoid arthritis is a chronic, progressive, systemic disorder characterized primarily by inflammation of the synovial joints. It is an autoimmune disorder and has periods of remission and exacerbation. The progressive joint destruction typically leads to significant disability in 10 to 20 years from onset, increased medical costs, hospitalization rates, and work disability (American College of Rheumatology, 2002). Rheumatoid arthritis is most common in women 40 to 50 years old, although it can occur at any age. The overall prevalence of RA is 1% to 2% of the general population in the United States and is three times higher in women than in men. African Americans and Whites have a similar rate of disease, while Native American populations have a higher prevalence of RA (Harris et al., 2005).

The signs and symptoms of RA may begin abruptly or develop insidiously. Typically, the patient complains of joint pain and morning stiffness in the joints lasting for more than 30 minutes. This pain and stiffness subsides during the day with moderate joint use, reoccurs following inactivity, and may worsen with strenuous activity. The patient may also complain of fatigue, malaise, anorexia, loss of weight, and low-grade fever. These systemic symptoms may precede the onset of joint pain by weeks or months. The joint involvement is usually symmetrical and polyarticular on exam, with swelling, warmth, and tenderness causing limitation in range of motion. The swelling may feel boggy (due to synovial hypertrophy) or fluctuant (due to an effusion; Gornisiewicz & Moreland, 2001). Joints primarily affected are the proximal interphalangeal and metacarpophalangeal joints of the fingers, wrists, elbows, knees, and ankles and the metatarsophalangeal joints in the feet. Less frequently, the temporomandibular joint may be involved. RA also causes inflammatory changes in the connective tissue of the skin, eyes, lungs, heart, muscles, kidney, nervous system, hematological system, blood vessels, and pleurae.

Atrophy of the muscle and skin surrounding the joints may develop, as well as subcutaneous nodules over pressure points such as the elbows. Characteristic deformities of the fingers and joints may develop after months or years of the disease. These include ulnar deviation, swan neck, and boutonniere deformities. Patients with RA are also prone to the development of flexion contractures, Baker's cysts, and carpal tunnel syndrome.

Current theories suggest a genetic susceptibility with active disease possibly triggered by a variety of agents and environmental factors. Risk factors other than genetic predisposition associated with an increased chance of developing RA in certain populations include female gender and cigarette smoking, although the reasons are not clear. Certain Native American populations also have higher prevalence of RA. Bacterial, viral, or retroviral triggers have been suspected and investigated, but no clear link has yet been found. Hormonal factors may be associated with susceptibility or modulation; during pregnancy, up to 75% of women with RA have a remission, and flares are common after pregnancy. Low testosterone levels have been reported in men with RA. Studies exploring the effect of exogenous estrogen have had contradictory results, providing no clear understanding of the relationship (Hannan, 2001).

The differential diagnosis for RA includes systemic lupus erythematosus; osteoarthritis; gout; acute viral polyarthritis; Sjogren's syndrome; fibromyalgia; late Lyme disease; and reactive, psoriatic, and infectious arthritis. Similarly to OA, the diagnosis of RA is made on the basis of the history and clinical examination. Differentiation among the possible disorders can be challenging, and a referral to a health care provider with expertise in rheumatology for work-up and management is recommended. Initial laboratory tests that help to establish a diagnosis of RA include a C-reactive protein, rheumatoid factor, erythrocyte sedimentation rate, and antinuclear antibody (American College of Rheumatology, 2002). None of these tests are diagnostic in themselves. Aspiration of synovial fluid is used to rule out an infectious etiology, especially in monoarticular presentations. Radiographic studies early in the disease process show only soft tissue swelling, but are useful as a baseline for monitoring disease progression and response to treatment (American College of Rheumatology, 2002). As the disease progresses, radiographic changes include narrowing of the joint spaces, periarticular osteoporosis, and juxtaarticular erosions (Gornisiewicz & Moreland, 2001).

The goals of management for RA are to prevent or control joint damage, preserve function, and decrease or relieve pain. The therapeutic management of RA is multifactorial, including nutrition, rest and exercise, medications, physical and occupational therapy to preserve joint function and promote independence in activities of daily living, surgery to correct deformities, and patient and family education about the disease process, self-management strategies, and sources of support.

Formal education programs have been shown to improve knowledge and coping behavior, at least in the short term (Niedermann, Fransen, Knols, & Uebelhart, 2004). Self-management programs aim to give patients strategies to cope with their disease on a daily basis and can impact behaviors and improve coping and psychological status (Vliet Vlieland, 2007). Exercise programs can improve symptoms of pain, fatigue, and depression (Neuberger et al., 2007), as well as muscle strength and functional ability (Vliet Vlieland, 2007). Exercise has not been shown to have detrimental effects on function, pain, or disease progression. Additional nonpharmacologic interventions used by individuals include thermotherapy (hot and cold applications), electrotherapy (i.e., TENS unit), spa therapy, massage, and adaptive and orthotic devices. For many therapies, there are limited controlled studies evaluating effectiveness, but adverse events are rare. Herbal therapies are also used by individuals with RA. Herbals are generally well tolerated, although studies of their efficacy are limited. The use of gamma-linolenic acid is associated with decreased pain, morning stiffness, and joint tenderness in several studies (Little & Parsone, 2000).

Surgery is used in all stages of RA to correct deformity and improve function and comfort; it involves a variety of surgical techniques such as carpal tunnel release, synovectomy, resection of metatarsal heads, joint fusion, and arthroplasties.

Two general types of medications may be employed: those that relieve symptoms and those that prevent or alter the progression of the disease. Research supports early and aggressive treatment with disease-modifying drugs to control inflammation and minimize disease progression and joint destruction, optimally within 3 months of onset of symptoms. The three major drug categories used in the treatment of RA are (a) NSAIDs, (b) disease-modifying antirheumatic drugs, and (c) corticosteroids (oral and injected). Patients need to be aware of the purpose of each medication in their treatment plan, as well as the expected outcomes and potential side effects. They should be encouraged to be active participants in their treatment plan and discuss their suggestions and concerns freely with members of the treatment team. The complexity of management options and potential toxicities of therapies warrant the active involvement of a health care provider with expertise in RA in the ongoing care. Disease progress is monitored using symptom assessment (pain, stiffness, fatigue, mood), functional assessment, exam findings (joint inflammation, limitation in motion, instability, malalignment, deformity), laboratory markers of disease, and radiographs.

Community-based and national organizations for patients and families with RA include local departments of vocational rehabilitation, social service agencies, and the Arthritis Foundation, which provides educational materials and also sponsors lay support groups.

Systemic Lupus Erythematosus (SLE)

Systemic lupus erythematosus (SLE) is a chronic, systemic, inflammatory autoimmune disease that primarily affects the skin, kidneys, joints, and central nervous and hematologic systems, although all organ systems can be involved. It occurs predominantly in females between 15 and 40 years old. The occurrence of SLE in women is about nine times greater than in men (Harris, 2005). In the United States, SLE is more common among women of African American descent and suspected to be more common in women of Hispanic, Asian, and Native American descent. Incidence and prevalence among African American women is about three times greater than among White women. The first symptoms usually appear between ages 15 and 25 but may occur at any age. The severity of the disease ranges from fairly benign with mild, treatable symptoms to severe, life-threatening renal or central nervous system damage. More than half of individuals with SLE develop permanent organ damage, either from the disease or the treatment.

SLE can be difficult to diagnose initially, because it can present in multiple systems, and symptoms may be similar to other diseases, such as joint pain and swelling similar to RA. The diagnosis of SLE should be considered in any patient presenting with characteristic symptoms in two or more organ systems (see Table 27.11; American College of Rheumatology, 1999). The ACR has developed specific criteria for the diagnosis of SLE incorporating laboratory findings, primarily to correctly classify patients enrolled in research studies as having SLE, but the criteria can also be useful in clinical practice (American College of Rheumatology, 1999). Primary care providers need to recognize characteristic symptoms of SLE and refer early to a provider with expertise in this disease, such as a rheumatologist, for diagnosis and treatment planning. Patients with mild or stable symptoms may be managed by their primary provider but should be referred when symptoms of the disease change or worsen or complications develop.

The exact cause of SLE is not known. Individuals may have a genetic predisposition, and environmental factors have been associated with disease onset and disease flares. These include ultraviolet light, medications (trimethoprim/sulfa, Echinacea, oral contraceptives, and hormone replacement therapy), smoking, infections, and toxins (silica and mercury; Petri, 2006).

Medications used in the treatment of SLE include NSAIDs, topical and oral glucocorticoids, antimalarial drugs such as hydroxychloroquine, and immunosuppressive or cytotoxic drugs. Nonpharmacological management of SLE includes patient education (about disease process, treatment, monitoring, and possible environmental triggers) as well as self-management strategies,

27.11 | Clinical Features of Systemic Lupus Erythematosus

SYSTEM	FEATURES
Cardiac	Endocarditis Myocarditis Pericarditis
Constitutional	Fatigue Fever Weight loss
Gastrointestinal	Abdominal pain Nausea, vomiting
Hematologic	Anemia Leukopenia Thrombocytopenia
Musculoskeletal	Arthralgia, arthritis Myositis
Neuropsychiatric	Cognitive impairment Cranial neuropathies Peripheral neuropathies Psychosis Seizures Transverse myelitis
Pulmonary	Pleurisy Pulmonary hypertension Pulmonary parenchyma
Renal	Casts Hematuria Nephrotic syndrome Proteinuria
Reticuloendothelial	Hepatomegaly Lymphadenopathy Splenomegaly
Skin	Alopecia Butterfly rash Mucous membrane lesion Photosensitivity Purpura Raynaud's phenomenon Urticaria Vasculitis

Note. Adapted from "Guidelines for Referral and Management of Systemic Lupus Erythematosus in Adults," by the American College of Rheumatology Ad Hoc Committee on Systemic Lupus Erythematosus Guidelines, 1999, *Arthritis and Rheumatism, 42*(9), pp. 1785–1796.

including symptoms that should be reported to the provider. Exercise may help decrease symptoms such as fatigue and pain and is an important part of treatment. Exercise and diet modification also may help decrease the risk of obesity and osteoporosis, especially for those managed with glucocorticoid therapy. Both the disease and treatment may increase risk of infections, and preventative immunizations should be provided. Ongoing counseling and support are also important.

Organizations that provide educational material and sources of support include the Arthritis Foundation (www.arthritis.org), the Lupus Foundation of America (www.lupus.org), Lupus Canada (www.lupuscanada.org), and the National Institute of Arthritis and Musculoskeletal and Skin Diseases (www.niams.nih.gov).

Fibromyalgia

Fibromyalgia is a chronic syndrome characterized by diffuse musculoskeletal pain with localized areas of tenderness, sleep disturbance, morning stiffness, and fatigue. The tender points are symmetrical points that, when palpated, trigger an exaggerated pain response (see Figure 27.2). Prevalence is estimated at 3% to 5% in adult women, typically between the ages of 30 and 50, as opposed to 0.5% in adult men. Fibromyalgia is chronic, may fluctuate in severity, and can be debilitating but is not progressive or fatal.

The diagnosis of fibromyalagia is made on the basis of history and the physical examination. The American College of Rheumatology standard for the diagnosis of fibromyalgia is the presence of both of the following criteria for the musculoskeletal pain:

1. A history of widespread pain that has been present for at least 3 months; widespread meaning that it occurs above and below the waist, on both the right and left side of the body, and also involves the axial skeleton, such as the cervical, thoracic, or lumbar spine or anterior chest.

2. Localized pain, elicited by palpation just firm enough to blanch the examiner's fingernail, present in at least 11 of the 18 specific tender point sites (see Figure 27.2; Pertusi, Patel, & Rubin, 2006; Wolfe et al., 1990).

In addition to the above signs and symptoms, patients with fibromyalgia also may have major depression, forgetfulness or difficulty concentrating, Raynaud's phenomena, dysphagia, and irritable bowel and irritable bladder symptoms. Symptoms may be exacerbated by time of day, changes in weather and temperature, and stress. The exact etiology of this syndrome is unknown. Diagnostic work-up is typically normal, unless another disease coexists.

As with other rheumatic disorders, the management of fibromyalgia is multifactorial; it includes patient education, pain management, exercise, psychosocial support, and sleep restoration. Strategies that include the patient as an active participant are encouraged, to promote self-management and increase control of the disease. Low-dose antidepressants (tricyclics or serotonin reuptake inhibitors) may be used to improve sleep and to reduce fatigue and depression. Mixed reuptake inhibitors (venlaxafine and duloxetine) may also help. NSAIDs and glucocorticoids are generally not indicated, because this is a noninflammatory disorder. If NSAIDs are tried, pain should be monitored closely and NSAIDs discontinued in 1 to 2 weeks if not effective due to the risk of side effects. Nonopioid choices such as acetaminophen are preferred for pain relief. Pramipexole and gabapentin have been shown to reduce pain (Pertusi et al., 2006). Exercise is the best studied treatment for fibromyalgia and has documented efficacy (Goroll & Mulley, 2006). Regularly scheduled low-impact aerobic exercise can reduce pain and improve sleep and mood. A physical therapist can individualize cardiovascular exercise programs to promote better posture and flexibility. Cognitive-behavioral therapy has been used with demonstrated improvement in pain and function. Many patients with fibromyalgia use chiropractic or massage therapy, and studies, though limited, suggest improvement in pain with these modalities also. Although no evidence of efficacy exists, many patients report using herbals such as glucosamine and chondroitin, green tea, Echinacea, St. John's wort, ginkgo biloba, garlic, valerian, and ma huang, as well as vitamin supplements. Some of these herbals have the potential for adverse effects (Goroll & Mulley, 2006). Questions about the use of herbals and vitamins are important to include during the patient visit.

Resources for patients with fibromyalgia include the Arthritis Foundation (www.arthritis.org), the Arthritis Society (www.arthritis.ca), Mayo Clinic (www.mayoclinic.com/health/DiseasesIndex), Stanford self-help programs (patienteducation.stanford.edu/programs), and the Fibromyalgia Network (www.healthfinder.gov/orgs/HR2439.htm).

Osteoporosis

Osteoporosis is a chronic, progressive disease of decreasing bone strength, which significantly increases the risk of fracture. The decline in strength is due to both a decrease in the density of the bone (bone mineral density or BMD) and a deterioration in bone architecture. The greatest decline occurs in the trabecular bone of the femoral neck and lumbar vertebrae. Bone density is easier to assess than bone architecture, and BMD measurements are used to diagnose osteoporosis. The World Health Organization has defined osteoporosis as a BMD of 2.5 or greater standard deviations below the mean BMD for a healthy young White woman. (Goroll & Mulley, 2006). The National Osteoporosis Foundation (2003) estimates that osteoporosis affects 20% of postmenopausal women in the United States, and an additional 52% have low hip bone density. The risk of hip fracture in women rises exponentially after the age of 45, at the time of increasing estrogen deficiency (Maricic, 2006). Although men can develop osteoporosis, women have a higher prevalence than men because they typically have a lower level of peak bone mass (achieved by ages 20 to 35) and lose bone mass at a faster rate. The prevalence in Asian American women is similar to that of White women; in Hispanic women prevalence is slightly lower and is lowest in African American women (about 6%, based on BMD values at the hip; U.S. Department of Health and Human Services, 2004).

Osteoporosis has a major impact both medically and economically. About 1.5 million osteoporotic frac-

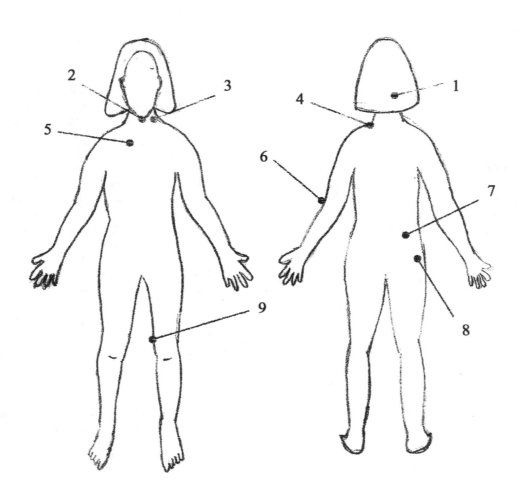

1. Occiput: at the suboccipital muscle insertions
2. Low Cervical: at anterior aspects of the intertransverse spaces C5-C7
3. Trapezius: at midpoint of upper border
4. Supraspinatus: at origin, above scapula spine near medial border
5. Second rib: just lateral to second costochondral junction on upper surface
6. Lateral epicondyle: 2 cm distal to epicondyle
7. Gluteal: in upper outer quadrant of buttock in anterior muscle fold
8. Greater trochanter: posterior to the trochanteric prominence
9. Knee: at medial fat pad proximal to joint line

Figure 27.2 "Tender points" palpated with pain response.
From American College of Rheumatology 1990 Criteria, in Wolfe, F. et al. (1990). *Arthritis and Rheumatism 33*(2), pp. 160–172.

tures occur each year in the United States, typically involving the hip, spine, and distal radius (U.S. Department of Health and Human Services, 2004). Hip fractures lead to about 300,000 hospitalizations every year and 180,000 nursing home admissions, and are associated with an increased risk of death within the first year (U.S. Department of Health and Human Services, 2004). Hip fractures also lead to a decline in functional ability, and as many as 60% of those individuals may not return to previous function after healing (National Osteoporosis Foundation, 2003). Vertebral fractures can cause chronic pain, loss of height, kyphosis, alterations in balance and mobility, and restrictive lung disease. The psychological impact of osteoporosis and subsequent fractures can include depression, low self-esteem, anxiety, anger, and increased dependency.

An individual's peak bone mass is primarily influenced by genetic factors but can be impacted by health and lifestyle practices. Factors that increase the risk of bone loss include older age; low weight; chronic alcohol use; smoking; prolonged calcium deficiency; immobilization; and medications such as glucocorticoids, anticonvulsants, excess thyroid supplementation, excess vitamin A, and lithium (Goroll & Mulley, 2006; Maricic, 2006). Diseases that are associated with osteoporosis include HIV/AIDS, hyperparathyroidism, hyperthyroidism, hyperprolactinemia, celiac disease, IBS, renal failure, RA, ankylosing spondylitis, and bone marrow disease.

Screening for osteoporosis and fracture risk includes questions about history of a fracture as an adult, early-onset menopause, and a fragility fracture in a first-degree relative. The term *fragility fracture* is used to describe a fracture resulting from trauma that would not break normal bone (Miller, 2007). In addition, BMD testing is recommended (if it will influence treatment decisions) on all women older than 65, postmenopausal women with one or more risk factors, and postmenopausal women who present with a fracture. BMD results of −1.0 to −2.4, while not diagnostic of osteoporosis, indicate lower than normal bone mass (osteopenia). Several osteoporosis studies have shown a significant number of fragility fractures occurring in women who have low bone mass but not osteoporosis. National Osteoporosis Foundation (2003) treatment guidelines reflect a concern about fracture risk in women with osteopenia. They recommend initiation of pharmacological therapy for women with BMD lower than −1.5 and at least one risk factor for osteoporosis, women with BMD below −2.0 even without risk factors, and those with a prior vertebral or hip fracture.

Several preventative measures have been shown to decrease the risk of osteoporosis, and/or decrease the risk of future fracture. These include adequate calcium and vitamin D intake, weight-bearing and muscle-strengthening exercises, avoidance or cessation of tobacco use, and avoidance of excess alcohol. Prevention should begin as early as adolescence to promote higher peak bone mass. Educating patients about osteoporosis and prevention strategies from adolescence to old age and supporting them in lifestyle and dietary modifications is a critical role for providers in decreasing the morbidity and mortality of this disease.

Elemental calcium intake of at least 1,200 to 1,500 mg per day is recommended starting in adolescence, and increasing to 2 g per day in older women. Vitamin D improves calcium absorption, reduces calcium excretion, and helps to maintain muscle strength. It has been shown to decrease the risk of falls in the elderly through the effect on muscle (Goroll & Mulley, 2006). An intake of 400 to 800 IU per day is recommended, and, for those at high risk of deficiency, at least 800 IU is recommended. Recent studies using 25-hydroxyvitamin D serum concentrations suggest that vitamin D deficiency is common in older adults, even in individuals taking supplements, and recommend doses up to 1,000 IU per day. However, the level of 25-hydroxyvitamin D used to identify deficiency varies across studies (Linnebur, Vondracek, Vande Griend, Ruscin, & McDermott, 2007). In the older adult population, the combination of adequate calcium and vitamin D intake reduces the risk of hip fractures.

Aerobic, weight-bearing, and muscle-strengthening exercises may increase bone density and have been shown to decrease the risk of falling (Bonaiuti et al., 2002). The studies reported vary in type of exercise and in intensity, frequency, and duration of the exercise, so no clear prescription for exercise is supported by evidence. However, walking is frequently recommended for exercise, because it has been shown to decrease risk of hip fracture, does not require special equipment or location, can be easily regulated in intensity, and may have a higher compliance rate. Tai-chi has also has been recommended for improving balance and potentially decreasing fall risk.

The goal of pharmacological treatment is to reduce fracture risk. Current treatment options, in addition to measures mentioned above, include biphosphonates, calcitonin, parathyroid hormone, selective estrogen receptor modulators, and estrogen replacement. Although estrogen therapy is effective in fracture risk reduction, alternate treatment is generally recommended due to the risks of estrogen use. Biphosphonates are antiresorptive agents. Two currently in use, alendronate and risedronate, are dosed daily or weekly and can reduce the risk of vertebral and hip fracture by about 35% to 50% (National Osteoporosis Foundation, 2003). Weekly dosing is as efficacious as daily dosing and often is preferred, because the dose must be taken on an empty stomach upon awakening and upright, followed by a full glass of water and staying in the upright position for 30 minutes to decrease the risk of esophageal irritation or trauma. Alendronate is also available as a solution for feeding tube administration. Ibandronate, another biphosphonate, is dosed monthly with similar administration precautions (except upright for 60 minutes), and has been shown to reduce vertebral fracture risk but not hip fracture risk. Parathyroid hormone (teriparatide) is an anabolic agent that is administered in daily subcutaneous injections. Teriparatide has been shown to reduce risk of both vertebral and nonvertebral fracture in osteoporosis by about 50% to 60% and may reduce risk earlier than other agents. Currently, it is the most expensive therapy option. Raloxifene (a selective estrogen receptor modulator) reduces the risk of vertebral fracture but not hip fracture. It also increases the risk of thromboembolic events. Calcitonin is given as a nasal inhaler and reduces vertebral fracture risk after 3 to 5 years, but has no evidence of hip fracture risk reduction.

Resources for patients with osteoporosis include the National Osteoporosis Foundation (www.nof.org) and the American College of Rheumatology (www.rheumatology.org/public/factsheets/osteopor_new.asp). Resources for fall prevention strategies include the National Center for Injury Prevention and Control (www.cdc.gov/ncipc/duip/spotlite/falls.htm) and the American Academy of Family Physicians (www.aafp.org/afp/20000401/2173ph.html).

NEUROLOGICAL DISORDERS

Headache is a frequently encountered complaint in primary care. The World Health Organization ranks migraine headaches 19th worldwide among health problems causing disability (International Headache Society, 2007). In one study of about 700 randomly selected individuals, 99% of the women reported a headache sometime in their life, and more than 85% had had a headache within the last year (Rasmussen, 1991). Migraine and tension headaches disproportionately affect women and are one of the most common neurological disorders seen in women. Seizure disorders, although seen less commonly in women, have important health implications for women, especially those in the childbearing years.

Headaches

Most headaches seen in primary care settings are primary headaches and are considered to be benign (in reference to prognosis, not a reflection of the level of disability). A primary headache is one that is not directly related to a specific underlying cause or secondary to another problem. Primary headaches include migraine, cluster, and tension-type headaches. Some patients may have both migraine and tension headaches. Secondary headaches are headaches that arise from an identifiable structural or pathological process, such as changes in intracranial pressure, meningeal irritation, or brain lesions. Secondary headaches can also have facial, cervical, systemic, or traumatic causes. Patients with suspected secondary headaches need referral to an appropriate specialist for further assessment.

A thorough, detailed history is critical to determine the type of headache, especially since the exam will usually be completely normal. Identifying correctly the type of headache will guide appropriate treatment, which may include referral. A complete exploration of the pain is diagnostically important, especially details about the course and progression of the headache, both the individual headache pattern and the headache syndrome (Rakel & Bope, 2005). This would include the age at onset of first headache; the frequency of headaches; the pattern within the day, week, or month; anything associated with the headache such as menses or pregnancy; and the duration range of the headaches (shortest and longest). Factors that seem to trigger the headache, those that abort or relieve it, and other symptoms or signs that occur along with the headache can differentiate specific type, as can a description of the perception of the pain (quantity and quality). After the initial visit, asking the patient to keep a log of each headache and other occurrences at the time of the headache can be helpful to give the provider more accurate detail. Additional questions include medication use, caffeine intake, sleep patterns and disturbances, and symptoms of depression, which can accompany headaches (Goroll & Mulley, 2006).

A thorough neurological exam is necessary for a patient with a new headache, when ongoing headaches have never been evaluated by a health care provider, or have changed in character since the last evaluation. A complete head and neck exam should also be included.

The provider during the encounter should be alert for any of the following signs that might indicate a potentially life-threatening cause of headache and prompt referral and a more urgent assessment: very sudden onset of the headache or severe and persistent pain; worst headache ever; progressively worsening pattern of headaches over time; focal neurological findings; accompanying fever; change in level of consciousness, personality, or mental status; rapid onset during strenuous exercise; pain spreading into lower neck and between the shoulders; new headache in someone older than 50; and a new headache with history of Lyme's disease, HIV, or during pregnancy.

Migraine headaches affect about 10% of adults, and are three times more common in women. They typically begin in childhood or in young adults, although about 16% of women have onset at menopause (Goroll & Mulley, 2006). The etiology is currently considered to be neurovascular, with components of vasodilation and neurogenic inflammation involving the trigeminal and meningeal vascular systems (Silberstein, 2004).

Many patients with migraine have a long personal history of headaches and may have a family history of migraine, especially patients who have migraine with aura. They also may report a history of motion sickness and vertigo as a child. Migraines occur in well-delineated attacks, and the patient feels completely well between headaches. Often patients can identify specific factors that precipitate a headache, such as stress, lack or excess of sleep, menses, certain foods or food additives, or irregular eating habits. Migraine headaches can be further classified as migraine without aura and migraine with aura. This differentiation replaces the older terms common and classic migraines. The headache seen in a patient with migraine without aura may last anywhere from 4 to 72 hours. At least two of the following four characteristics will be present: (a) moderate to severe intensity, (b) a unilateral location, (c) a pulsating quality, and (d) aggravation of symptoms by routine physical activity such as climbing stairs. During the headache, at least one of the following accompanying symptoms will also be experienced: nausea or vomiting, phonophobia, and photophobia (Goroll & Mulley, 2006; International Headache Society, 2007).

In migraine with aura, the same clinical picture of a recurrent, unilateral, throbbing or pulsating headache is seen, preceded by distinct neurological symptoms that are known as auras. An aura may be a visual disturbance, vertigo, aphasia, or hemiplegia and indicates focal cerebral, cortical, or brainstem involvement. The aura should be at least one symptom, or two or more in succession, is fully reversible, and lasts less than 60 minutes. The headache may follow the aura or may begin before and occur simultaneously with the aura. Auras may vary from episode to episode and may occur without headache. The identification of an aura can be helpful in establishing the diagnosis of migraine.

Tension-type headaches (TTHs) are the most common type of headache, with a lifetime prevalence varying from 30% to 78% in studies (International Headache Society, 2007) and are more common in women than men (about a five-to-four ratio). Despite the much higher prevalence of TTHs than migraines, they are much less frequently seen and treated in a primary care setting, because many people do not seek treatment. The exact etiology is unknown; in the past, this type of headache was often believed to be psychogenic, but evidence suggests that there is a neurobiological basis. However, stress, anxiety, or depression may precipitate a tension headache. Typically, a TTH has a gradual onset, and may occur daily, waxing and waning over

a period of years. The pain is usually described as bilateral, vise or band-like, and a steady ache, most prominent in the occipital and upper neck area but also may occur in the frontal and temporal area. The intensity of the pain is described as mild to moderate and may inhibit, but not prevent, activity. Tension headaches may last from minutes to days, weeks, or months. They can be triggered by stress, noise, and glare and may be accompanied by depression and anxiety. However, symptoms should not be aggravated by walking or climbing stairs or other physical activity, and there should be no nausea or vomiting. On physical examination, muscle tension, such as cervical muscle tension, may or may not be palpable.

As mentioned, the assessment of a patient with a headache includes differentiating between the primary causes as well as ruling out secondary causes. For the patient with migraine and aura, an important differential, especially in older persons, is that of transient ischemic attacks and cerebral vascular accidents. In younger patients, seizure disorders should be considered, particularly temporal lobe epilepsy. Other possible diagnoses include temporal arteritis, trigeminal neuralgia, sinusitis, cervical spine osteoarthritis, and meningitis. Acute causes should be considered even in a patient with known chronic primary headaches if something about the presentation has changed.

The management of chronic headaches includes both preventive and abortive therapies specific to the type of headache. Complete elimination of pain or headaches may be difficult to achieve, so the goal is to decrease frequency, duration, and intensity; improve quality of life; reduce distress and disability; and enable patients to control their disease (Silberstein, 2000).

Classes of medications used for aborting tension headaches include analgesics such as acetaminophen, aspirin, or NSAIDs. Tricyclic antidepressants may be effective as preventative therapy, as can selective serotonin reuptake inhibitors. Effective nonmedication approaches include avoidance of known precipitants, proper nutrition and rest, relaxation techniques, and a regular exercise regimen. Cognitive-behavioral therapy has also been shown to be effective.

For migraine headaches, based on the frequency of the headaches and the degree of impairment caused by them, the clinician must decide whether to use prophylactic or abortive medications or both. Many different classes of drugs are used for abortive therapy for migraine patients. The earlier the treatment is started, the more likely it will be effective. Choice of agents is determined by the individual patient situation, prior response to treatment, patient preference, and concomitant symptoms that may restrict the use of certain agents or routes of administration. Abortive medication classes include analgesics (aspirin, acetaminophen, NSAIDs), dihydroergotamine, and triptans. Metoclopramide or prochlorperazine may be used for nausea accompanying the headache. Caution is advised when analgesics, or analgesics and sedative combinations, are used to avoid consistent frequent use (e.g., more than two times per week), which can lead to habituation or rebound headaches. Preventive therapy should be considered if frequent abortive therapy is needed. The use of prophylactic medications is indicated for patients who have at least one migraine headache a week that is interfering with their daily activities. Similarly to abortive agents, the clinician has many prophylactic medication options. These include beta blockers, tricyclic antidepressants, calcium channel blockers, NSAIDs, and anticonvulsants. The American Academy of Neurology lists feverfew and vitamin B_2 as treatment options that have evidence of effectiveness. Cognitive-behavioral therapy, relaxation training, thermal biofeedback, and electromyographic feedback may also be effective for the prevention of migraines (Silberstein, 2000).

Patients and families need good information about their illness and self-care strategies, including how to recognize headache triggers, how to intervene early using both medical and nonmedical therapies, and when to seek consultation from their health care providers. Additional community resources for headache patients include:

- National Headache Foundation (www.headaches.org)
- American Council for Headache Education (800-255-ACHE or www.achenet.org)
- U.S. National Library of Medicine: Medline Plus (www.nlm.nih.gov/medlineplus/headache.html)
- American College of Physicians (www.doctorsforadults.com/index.html)

Seizure Disorders

Seizures result from abnormal paroxysmal neuronal discharges in the brain and cause an involuntary change in body movement or function, sensation, awareness, or behavior (CDC, 2007; Rakel & Bope, 2005). These behaviors can be a loss of consciousness, a staring episode, a short period of confusion, a recurring thought, a peculiar feeling, an emotional outburst, a strange sensation, an odd posturing, or uncontrolled movements. The seizure is a symptom. Seizure disorder, or epilepsy, involves recurrent seizure activity. A single seizure does not mean an individual has epilepsy. The worldwide prevalence of epilepsy (those who have had at least one seizure in the last 5 years) is 4 to 8 per 1,000 (World Health Organization, 2006). Fifty million people have epilepsy, approximately 2.7 million in the United States, and more are men than women. Many are not seizure free, even while on treatment. The diagnosis of epilepsy can affect the individual's employment security, educational options, driving status, and insurance.

Epilepsy carries a significant stigma due to misconceptions about the disease, which contribute to social and workplace discrimination, lower self-esteem, and lower quality of life.

Seizures can be divided into two groups according to their etiology: primary, for which a probable cause can be determined, and secondary, for which multiple causes have been identified—including cerebral hypoxia, trauma (most common cause in young adults), brain tumor, scar tissue, metabolic disturbances such as hypoglycemia, central nervous system infections, toxic agents such as ethyl alcohol, lead, drugs, and neurocirculatory disorders. The International League Against Epilepsy classification is based on distinctive behaviors, symptoms, and characteristic electroencephalogram (EEG) changes and describes two major subclasses of seizures: (a) partial seizures and (b) generalized seizures (Rakel & Bope, 2005). Partial seizures (focal seizures) begin in one area of the cortex (focus) and produce EEG abnormalities in that area. Generalized seizures begin in the brain bilaterally and show diffuse EEG abnormalities. The appearance of the seizure (ictus), what is observed behaviorally and on the EEG, is determined by the area of the cerebral cortex from which the seizure originates and to which it spreads. Using this classification system to establish the type of seizure helps direct the choice of medication and treatment plan for the person with seizures.

The patient history is the single most important factor in the establishment of the diagnosis, particularly a complete description of a witnessed seizure. Information should be obtained on age of seizure onset, any precipitating factors (e.g., fever, light, noise), the frequency and duration of the episode, loss of consciousness, presence of an aura, and description of the postictal state. Complete prenatal, familial, and developmental histories should be obtained as well as a past medical history to identify any neurological or medical etiologies. Medications should be reviewed to rule out their role in either lowering the threshold for seizures or directly contributing to seizure activity (e.g., stimulants, antipsychotics, drug or alcohol withdrawal).

The neurological examination is usually normal in a patient with seizures. The identification of focal abnormalities on a neurological exam helps to establish the location of cerebral pathology. These focal abnormalities may be most evident immediately after a seizure. Older persons presenting with seizures should also be evaluated for a cardiac etiology.

The most important diagnostic test for epilepsy is the electroencephalogram, which helps to establish the diagnosis of epilepsy and also the specific type of seizure; however, a normal EEG does not rule out epilepsy. An abnormal EEG with interictal epileptiform discharges recorded supports the diagnosis of epilepsy; however, many EEGs of seizure patients are normal because they are not conducted during a seizure. A sleep EEG is obtained when partial complex seizures are suspected. An MRI or CT scan can help identify structural brain pathology. An MRI is considered substantially more sensitive than a CT scan and is indicated for evaluation of new onset seizures, and patients with refractory seizures. Positron emission tomography and single photon emission computed tomography scans may also be part of the diagnostic evaluation.

Baseline blood tests should be obtained (electrolytes, CBC, liver and renal functions, Venereal Disease Research Laboratory), including a toxicology screen for individuals presenting with unexplained generalized seizures. An electrocardiogram should be obtained on all individuals with a family history of arrhythmia, sudden unexplained death, episodic unconsciousness, and a personal history of cardiac arrhythmia or valvular disease.

The most common differential diagnoses for an adult with new onset seizures are syncope and cardiac arrhythmia, ethyl alcohol blackouts, transient ischemic attacks, and behavioral/psychiatric disorders such as rage and panic attacks. Patients with new onset seizures, patients who do not adequately respond to therapy, and patients with an acute episode of status epilepticus should be referred to a neurologist.

The goal for the treatment of epilepsy is to prevent seizures and minimize the side effects of therapy. The choice of medications is dictated by the type of seizure and is individualized to the patient situation. A single medication is used initially for treatment and is successful for most patients. Therapy is started at a low dose, which is gradually increased until (a) seizures are controlled, (b) blood levels reach the upper limits of the therapeutic range, or (c) side effects prevent further increases. If a second drug is added to the regimen, it is gradually increased until within therapeutic range, and then the first drug is gradually withdrawn. About 50% of patients will have a therapeutic response to the second drug. Side effects are usually seen when a drug is first started or when the dosage is increased. The therapeutic ranges of drugs should be used as guidelines; optimal levels for some patients may fall above or below the recommended levels, and side effects may occur at low therapeutic levels. Therefore, therapeutic blood levels alone are not the goal of treatment. Instead, the clinician needs to also monitor the patient's clinical progress and frequency of seizure activity and evaluate for the presence of drug-related side effects or toxicity symptoms.

More than half of persons with epilepsy will be seizure free within 10 years of diagnosis. Discontinuance of antiepileptic medications may be considered under the supervision of a neurologist when the patient has been seizure free for 2 to 5 years. Patients who had generalized seizures and were diagnosed before age 10 have the best probability of remaining seizure free off medication. One drug is withdrawn at a time, with gradual reduction in dosage over a period of weeks and months. Abrupt withdrawal of seizure medications may precipitate status epilepticus.

Epileptic patients in the childbearing years present special challenges. The use of antiepileptic medication may interact with some contraceptives, lowering protection against pregnancy. Women contemplating pregnancy require special attention and care before, during, and after pregnancy. Although there are no contraindications to becoming pregnant, patients are advised to consult a physician preconceptually, because the fetus can be damaged from seizure activity, high concentrations of antiepileptic drugs, and the use of polytherapy to control seizures. Folic acid supplementation is provided, because some antiepileptic medications can impair folate absorption. Women who have been seizure free for 2 to 5 years, have a single type of seizure, and a normal neurological exam and EEG may be candidates for withdrawal of antiepileptic medication before pregnancy. Risk of seizure recurrence is greatest in the first 6 months, so optimally the medication would be discontinued more than 6 months before conception (American Academy of Neurology, 1998). Risks and benefits should be clearly communicated so the patient and provider can partner in the decision about discontinuation of medication.

Patients with epilepsy and their families need to be educated regarding the nature of the disease, the importance of compliance with the medication regimen, the potential side effects of the medications, and over-the-counter medications that can affect seizure control. They need to be aware of stimuli that can trigger seizures in otherwise well-controlled individuals, such as stress, lack of sleep, use of alcohol, and emotional upset. Patients need to be aware of their own seizure triggers (and aura, if present) so they can safeguard themselves. Families need to understand how to care for a patient during a seizure.

Patients with epilepsy should be counseled about state laws regarding driving and the best way to obtain life, automobile, and health insurance. Because certain occupations are contraindicated for the person with seizures, patients may need vocational counseling and may benefit from the assistance of local support groups. Optimally, epilepsy is treated on an outpatient basis with an interdisciplinary team of primary care provider, neurologist, nurse, social worker, and vocational counselor.

Nationally, the Epilepsy Foundation (www.epilepsyfoundation.org) provides patient education materials and networking to state and local resources.

ENDOCRINE DISORDERS

The most common endocrine disorders seen in women are Type 2 diabetes and thyroid disorders. Obesity, a metabolic disorder, can occur as a result of endocrine dysfunction, but only in a minority of cases. The prevalence of obesity in the United States is increasing; the most recently published data from the National Health and Nutrition Examination Survey indicate that approximately 31% of adults age 20 and older are obese, compared to 13.3% in 1962 (National Center for Health Statistics, 2004). Approximately 61% of adult women are overweight, and over half of those are considered obese (defined as a body mass index or of equal to or greater than 30). Obesity is recognized as a risk factor for the development of type 2 diabetes, coronary artery disease, hypertension, dyslipidemia, stroke, gallbladder disease, osteoarthritis, sleep apnea and breathing disorders, and certain forms of cancer (CDC, 2006). Disorders of the thyroid are common in women and include hyperthyroidism, hypothyroidism, and, less commonly, thyroiditis.

Diabetes Mellitus

Diabetes mellitus (DM) is a metabolic disorder characterized by hyperglycemia resulting from inadequate secretion of insulin, defective insulin action (insulin resistance), or both. An estimated 21 million people in the United States have diabetes, about one-third of whom are not aware that they have the disease (Saaddine et al., 2006). Slightly more than half of those 21 million are women. About another 40 to 50 million Americans have what is called prediabetes, which gives them a significantly increased risk for developing diabetes and cardiovascular disease. This presents primary care clinicians with the challenge of identifying both those with increased risk and those with undiagnosed diabetics. Diabetes disproportionately affects minority populations in the United States; the risk of diabetes for Hispanics, African Americans, and Native Americans is almost twice that for Whites (CDC, 2005).

The Expert Committee on the Diagnosis and Classification of Diabetes (1997) of the American Diabetes Association established new criteria for the diagnosis and classification of diabetes mellitus. The classification of diabetes is by etiology rather than type of treatment.

Type 1 diabetes mellitus (formerly known as insulin-dependent diabetes mellitus) accounts for 5% to 10% of all diagnosed cases of diabetes. The etiology of type 1 DM is autoimmune beta cell destruction resulting in an absolute deficiency of insulin. This disease usually first appears in youth and has a rapid onset of symptoms that may culminate in diabetic ketoacidosis. Patients with type 1 diabetes are ketosis prone and require insulin replacement for survival. Risk factors for type 1 diabetes have not been determined, although both genetic and environmental factors have been implicated.

Type 2 diabetes (formerly known as non–insulin-dependent diabetes mellitus), the most common form,

accounts for 90% to 95% of all cases and usually occurs after the age of 40, although increasing cases are being diagnosed in young people, including children and teens. Persons with type 2 diabetes typically have normal or high levels of circulating insulin, yet a relative deficiency due to insulin resistance. The onset of type 2 diabetes is gradual, and patients may be completely asymptomatic at the time of diagnosis or present with symptoms such as polyuria, polydipsia, weight loss, blurred vision, and frequent infections such as candidiasis or urinary tract infection. They may present with signs and symptoms of complications (e.g., impotence or stroke), having had the disease for years. Patients with type 2 diabetes are not ketosis prone (because of the available insulin) and may be controlled with diet, exercise, weight loss, oral medications, and/or insulin. Risk factors for the development of type 2 diabetes include obesity, ethnicity, genetic predisposition, physical inactivity, use of corticosteroids, and history of gestational diabetes, with obesity contributing the majority of risk.

Gestational diabetes (GDM) develops due to insulin resistance during pregnancy. African American, Hispanic, and Native American women are at higher risk for GDM, as well as women who are obese or have a first-degree relative with diabetes mellitus. About 3% of pregnant women in the United States are diagnosed with gestational diabetes, 5% to 10% of whom will be diagnosed with type 2 DM after delivery, and 20% to 50% will develop type 2 DM in the next 5 to 10 years (CDC, 2005).

Individuals with prediabetes have glucose intolerance, either measured by an elevated fasting glucose level or an elevated postprandial glucose level (see Table 27.12). About one-third will progress to type 2 DM. They are also at higher risk of developing cardiovascular disease than people with normal glucose levels, even without progressing to diabetes (Rakel & Bope, 2005). In this population, both modest weight loss and regular physical activity have been shown to delay and sometimes prevent the onset of diabetes, and studies suggest that lipid and blood pressure control may benefit cardiovascular health. This potential for morbidity and mortality reduction, given both the individual and health care system burden of diabetes, makes screening and lifestyle modification counseling a critical component of the visit for the health care provider.

Secondary prevention, or early detection and treatment of diabetes, involves screening for type 2 diabetes in asymptomatic individuals according to the new American Diabetes Association (2007) guidelines. These guidelines recommend screening all individuals over the age of 45 at least every 3 years. More frequent or earlier testing should be considered for anyone with one of the following characteristics: overweight (body mass index ≥ 25); a first-degree relative with type 2

27.12 | Diagnostic Criteria for Nonpregnant Adults

		Fasting plasma glucose (FPG) (no caloric intake for 8 hours)	Casual (random) glucose	Oral glucose tolerance test (glucose load = 75 g anhydrous glucose dissolved in water)
Prediabetes	Impaired fasting glucose	100–125 mg/dl		
	Impaired glucose tolerance			2-hour plasma glucose 140–199 mg/dl
Diabetes (any one test diagnostic)		≥ 126	Plasma glucose ≥ 200 and symptoms of diabetes mellitus	2-hour plasma glucose ≥ 200 mg/dl

Note. Results using any of the three types of tests above must be confirmed on a subsequent day unless unequivocal symptoms of hyperglycemia exist. From "Standards of Medical Care in Diabetes, 2007," by the American Diabetes Association, 2007, *Diabetes Care, 30*(Suppl. 1), pp. S4–S41.

diabetes; high-risk ethnic descent (African American, Native American, Latino, Asian American, Pacific Islander); history of delivering a baby weighing more than 9 pounds; having GDM; hypertensive (≥ 140/90); history of vascular disease; history of polycystic ovarian syndrome; HDL cholesterol < 35 mg/dl and/or a triglyceride level > 250 mg/dl; or the presence of impaired fasting glucose (IFG) or impaired glucose tolerance (IGT). The American Diabetes Association recommends a fasting plasma glucose as the test of choice because of its low cost, ease of use, and better tolerance by patients. Criteria for diagnosing diabetes are presented in Table 27.12.

Although the etiology of the hyperglycemia differs in type 1 and type 2 diabetes, the pathological consequences are similar. Complications of diabetes include microvascular disease involving the small blood vessels of the body (retinopathy, nephropathy), macrovascular disease involving the large blood vessels (accelerated cerebrovascular and coronary atherosclerosis, accelerated peripheral vascular disease), and neuropathic disease (gastroparesis and peripheral neuropathy). These complications have significant effects on patient morbidity, mortality, and quality of life.

Several studies such as the Diabetes Control and Complications Trial Research Group (1993) with patients with type 1 diabetes and the United Kingdom Prospective Diabetes Study (1998) with patients with type 2 diabetes have demonstrated that these complications can be prevented or delayed by achieving and maintaining glycemic control at the recommended target goals (see Table 27.13).

The history for a patient with diabetes should include a review of the acute symptoms of diabetes (polyuria, polyphagia, polydipsia, fatigue, weight loss); a review of the results of their home glucose monitoring as well as testing technique; frequency and severity of episodes of hyperglycemia and hypoglycemia (including identification and documentation of hypoglycemic unawareness); challenges with adhering to the treatment plan; a complete review of the diet, exercise, and foot care regimens; review of symptoms suggesting complications of diabetes; status of comorbidities; review of all medications and patient satisfaction with regimen; family issues and issues affecting quality of life; and maintenance care (e.g., podiatry, dental care, immunizations). Laboratory data should be reviewed with the patient and interpreted as needed. Patients need to be aware of their target glycemic goals and the clinical implication of tests such as glycosylated hemoglobin and micro albuminuria. An ongoing log book of laboratory values (e.g., HbA1C, urine microalbumin, HDL/LDL) is often useful to patients in tracking their control as are written goals.

The physical examination should include measurements of weight, height (for body mass index calculation), blood pressure, and resting pulse and any areas indicated by the interim history. Weight gain or weight loss should be noted and addressed in the treatment plan. Areas of importance in the physical examination of a person with diabetes are the integumentary system, mouth (because of the high incidence of dental caries and periodontal disease), eyes, neck (evaluation of the carotids and thyroid gland), the cardiac and peripheral

27.13 | Monitoring Components and Therapeutic Goals for Adults With Diabetes Mellitus

	FREQUENCY	GOAL
Weight	At each visit	
Blood pressure	At each visit	< 130/80
Eye exam (dilated fundoscopy)	Initially, then yearly	
Distal sensation (feet) and inspection	Initially, then at least yearly Insensate feet: every 3 months	
Glycosylated hemoglobin	Twice a year, more frequent if not meeting goals or when treatment changes	< 7.0 % (based on normal upper limit of 6.0%)
Fasting blood glucose	Self-monitored, results reviewed at each visit	90–130 mg/dl
Postprandial glucose	Self-monitored, results reviewed at each visit	< 180 mg/dl
Urine microalbumin	Yearly until positive	
Lipid profile	Initially, then yearly	LDL < 100 mg/dl LDL < 70 option if overt cardiovascular disease Triglygerides < 150 mg/dl HDL > 40 mg/dl in men HDL > 50 mg/dl in women
Serum creatinine and glomerular filtration rate	Initially, then at least yearly[a]	
Nutrition	Initially, then at each visit	
Activity and exercise	Initially, then at each visit	

Note. Based on "Standards of Medical Care in Diabetes, 2007," by the American Diabetes Association, 2007, *Diabetes Care, 30*(Suppl. 1), pp. S4–S41.
[a] Increased frequency based on renal function, change in condition, or change in medication.

vascular systems, the neurological system, including sensation of the feet and lower extremity reflexes. The American Diabetes Association (2007) has established clinical guidelines for the initial visit and the follow-up visit for a person with diabetes. These recommendations are updated annually and include the following recommendations for laboratory testing during periodic visits (see Table 27.13 for frequency): glycosylated hemoglobin (HbA1C), fasting lipid profile, and urine for microalbumin. In addition, serum creatinine with estimation of glomerular filtration rate should be done at frequencies dictated by renal function, changes in condition, or changes in therapy. Fasting and 2-hour postprandial glucose values are helpful in evaluating control, especially in patients with normal fasting plasma values but elevated HbA1C. Additional laboratory tests recommended for the initial visit are thyroid-stimulating hormone (TSH) and liver function profile.

The management of diabetes is directed toward (a) glycemic control, (b) prevention and management of complications of the disease, and (c) minimizing the risk of adverse events related to therapy. An essential component of disease management is the active participation of the patient. This can only be accomplished through a patient-provider relationship in an environment of mutual trust and acceptance, where the clinician acts as a guide and resource (Kaplan, Greenfield, Gandek, Rogers, & Ware, 1996). Self-management education will help the patient become active in the daily control of the disease, and facilitate coping with the lifestyle modifications necessitated by the disease and disease treatment. The treatment plan needs to be individualized based on age, health risks and comorbidities, daily schedule, activity and eating patterns, social and family support, and cultural and economic factors.

The American Diabetes Association goals for glycemic control are shown in Table 27.13. Tight glycemic control (or treating to target) is the gold standard of diabetes management. To achieve these goals, a treatment plan involving nutritional therapy, exercise, self-monitoring of blood glucose (SMBG), and pharmacological agents (oral and insulin) are utilized. Minimizing cardiovascular risk is equally as important in achieving glycemic control. Control of the systolic and diastolic blood pressure and lipid levels, smoking cessation, and vascular protection with a daily aspirin are recommended as part of routine diabetes care (American Diabetes Association, 2007). Improvement in control of lipids can decrease the incidence of cardiovascular events by 22% to 24% (American College of Physicians, 2007). Similarly, the United Kingdom Prospective Diabetes Study (1998) found that each decrease in systolic blood pressure of 10 mmHg decreased complications of DM by 12%. Systolic goals vary slightly by source from 130 to 135; as with other aspects of patient management, providers can be guided in recommendations for patients by individual variance or characteristics, such as comorbidities and life expectancy. In older adults, the presence of dizziness or orthostatic hypotension and fall risk should be assessed when treating hypertension. All diabetic patients should take an angiotensin-converting enzyme inhibitor or an angiotensin receptor blocker to delay the onset or progress of nephropathy, except during pregnancy or if unable to tolerate. The strength of evidence for reduction in cardiovascular risk and complications of DM through lifestyle modifications and the use of medications offers hope for both providers and patients and an opportunity for the individual to have greater control over the disease.

Nutrition

Nutrition therapy remains a cornerstone of care in both type 1 and type 2 diabetes and should be individualized to the person's lifestyle and customary food intake, including ethnic preferences. Emphasis is placed on a healthy balanced diet. Current recommendations include 10% to 35% of calories from protein, 20% to 35% from fat (with less than 7% from saturated fat and limited trans fat), and the remaining 45% to 65% of calories from carbohydrates. Carbohydrates high in fiber are preferable (American Diabetes Association, 2007). The area of nutrition and the appropriate balance of nutrients to facilitate safe weight loss and improved glycemic control is the focus of increasing public and scientific interest, and guidelines may change based on ongoing studies. Sodium restriction is recommended in patients who also have hypertension or heart failure. Dietary lifestyle modifications are often the most difficult part of the diabetes treatment regimen. Patients may benefit from the assistance of a registered dietician or other certified diabetic educator, especially at the time of diagnosis and when difficulties with metabolic control arise. For individuals with type 2 diabetes who are overweight or obese, emphasis is on achieving a *reasonable* weight rather than a *normal* weight, with achievable goals. For these individuals, weight loss is a part of their therapeutic regimen, and often a small loss of 5 to 10 pounds can result in significant improvements in metabolic control.

Exercise

Physical activity and exercise are often the missing link in the diabetes plan of care and can have positive effects on glucose control across the life span (Clark, 1997; Eriksson, Taimela, & Koivisto, 1997). Exercise reduces insulin resistance and increases glucose uptake by the cells for as long as 48 to 72 hours (Manson et al., 1991). Other benefits of regular exercise include weight loss, increased sense of well-being, and reduction in cardiovascular risk factors such as lipid levels. Like nutritional therapy, a physical activity or exercise plan should be tailored to the individual's lifestyle and preferences and should consider other comorbidities that may influence activity. Persons with long-term complications of diabetes such as retinopathy, neuropathy, nephropathy, or autonomic symptoms require specialized activity plans and physician consultation before beginning an exercise program. For example, a patient with peripheral neuropathy may require special shoes and will be safer using a treadmill indoors than running outside. A sedentary or rarely exercising person, without complications, should be encouraged to approach exercise in a stepwise progression. Walking is an excellent exercise that is low in cost and easy to begin. Patients should exercise a minimum of 3 days per week or on an every-other-day schedule with a goal of 150 minutes a week at a moderate level to achieve cardiovascular conditioning and improved glycemic control. Patients should be taught to always inspect their feet for cuts and blisters after exercise, and avoid exercising during extremes of temperature (Horton, 1998).

Meal planning must be linked to daily activity; medication doses may need to be adjusted if activities vary widely. Exercise can alter the rate of absorption of insulin; therefore, patients should not inject into an anatomic site that will be exercised, such as the thigh if the patient is running. Patients who take insulin will need to perform additional SMBG to determine whether extra calories are needed before activity. Blood glucoses should be checked after exercise to prevent hypoglycemia and several hours after exercise when a late-onset postexercise hypoglycemic response may occur (e.g., 6 to 15 hours after exercising; Horton, 1998). In this way, individuals will learn their own responses to exercise and will be able to plan proactively. All persons should be encouraged to carry a fast-acting source of carbohydrate and medic-alert information that identifies them as having diabetes.

Self-Monitoring

Self-monitoring of blood glucose by the patient provides excellent information on short-term glycemic control and is necessary if the target goals for glycemia are to be met. The term *self-monitoring* instead of glucose *testing* supports the concept of SMBG as a guide to treatment, instead of being a test that the patient passes or fails (Meredith & Horan, 2000). Self-monitoring is an excellent tool for patient motivation; patients can immediately see the effects of dietary change, exercise, or changes in their medications and make the necessary adjustments. For SMBG to be effective, patients must be educated about not only how to use their blood glucose meters, but also the meaning of the blood glucose values seen and how to use this feedback to improve their glycemic control. They also need to understand when and how to communicate their data to their health care providers (e.g., critical low and high values; sick day rules), the implications of the time that SMBG is done (i.e., relationship to meals, activity), and the proper use of their meters, including how to troubleshoot problems with their meters. Most blood glucose meters have toll-free numbers printed (albeit in tiny print) on the reverse side of the machine, which can be used for technical assistance.

Critical to patient adherence with self-monitoring is a reasonable schedule for testing and consideration of the cost of testing supplies. The SMBG needs to be negotiated with the patient based on the type of information that is needed. Although many meters have a memory capacity, the use of a written log helps patients and clinicians visualize patterns more readily.

Pharmacologic Agents

When diet and exercise do not provide adequate control in type 2 diabetes, a pharmacological agent is initiated based on the individual's profile and blood glucose values. Most patients with type 2 DM will need at least an oral medication for adequate glycemic control. Since the mid-1990s, the therapeutic options in treating type 2 diabetes have vastly expanded, providing opportunities for improved control through the use of monotherapy, combinations of oral agents, and oral agents and insulin. Oral agents are selected on the basis of their mode of action, side effects, cost, and dosing.

The most common types of oral agents currently in use for persons with type 2 diabetes are shown in Table 27.14. Over time, beta cell function in type 2 DM will decline, requiring adjustments in treatment such as combinations of oral agents, use of oral agents plus insulin, or the use of insulin alone.

All individuals with type 1 diabetes require insulin therapy. Insulin regimens should be negotiated with the patient and should be based on their glycemic fluctuations, lifestyle, and ability to carry through the regimen. The advantages and disadvantages of each regimen should be discussed with the patient as well as a plan for dosage adjustments made on the basis of SMBG results. Various types of insulin, combinations of insulin, and modes of administration are available (see Table 27.15).

Patient and Family Education

Patients and families need to be knowledgeable about all aspects of the diabetes self-care regimen and be active participants in decision making regarding their care. Diabetes education is an ongoing process; as the state of the art and science of diabetes care changes, patients need to be updated and learn where to access information. Traditionally, patients receive diabetes education when they are first diagnosed and when their metabolic control deteriorates. Ongoing diabetes education (i.e., the exchange of information between the health care provider and patient) and troubleshooting can often prevent this deterioration and identify problems earlier.

Older adults with diabetes should be assessed for hearing, visual, or cognitive loss, and teaching about the disease and management plans should be adjusted as needed. Inclusion of family and other care providers in education is even more critical. Glycemic control goals may need to be readjusted on the basis of life expectancy or frailty and risk of harm. The elderly are at increased risk of hyperglycemia after eating, so self-monitoring needs to include postprandial testing. Risks are similar to younger adults, but comorbidities and polypharmacy may increase the likelihood of adverse events.

Resources

Numerous resources are available to both clinicians and patients that include diabetes information for special populations such as the elderly, visually impaired, and members of ethnic minorities. National organizations that provide information about diabetes include:

- American Diabetes Association (1-800-DIABETES, 1-800-342-2383, www.diabetes.org)
- American College of Physicians Clinical Practice Guidelines (www.acponline.org/clinical/guidelines/index.html)
- American Dietetic Association (www.eatright.org)
- American Association of Diabetes Educators (www.aadenet.org)
- Centers for Disease Prevention and Health Promotion (www.cdc.gov/diabetes)
- Diabetes Action Research and Education Foundation (www.diabetesaction.org)

27.14 | Oral Agents for Glycemic Control in Type 2 Diabetes Mellitus

CLASS	GENERIC NAME (TRADE NAME)	DOSING	RENAL ADJUSTMENT	HEPATIC ADJUSTMENT	SITE AND MECHANISM
Sulfonylureas	Glipizide (Glucotrol)[a]	2.5–20 mg once to twice per day Start at 2.5–5 mg once per day	Yes	Yes	Beta cell, increase insulin secretion
	Glypizide (Glucotrol XL)[a]	5–10 mg once per day Start at 5 mg once per day	Yes	Yes	
	Glyburide (DiaBeta, Micronase)	1.25–20 mg once per day Start at 1.25–5 mg once per day	Yes	Yes	
	Glimepiride (Amaryl)[a]				
Biguanide	Metformin (Glucophage)	850–1,000 mg twice per day Start at 850 mg once per day or 500 mg twice per day	Yes	Yes	Reduce hepatic glucose production; reduce intestinal glucose absorption; increase insulin sensitivity
Alpha glucosidase inhibitors	Acarbose (Precose)	50–100 mg three times per day	Yes	Yes	Beta cell, increase insulin secretion
	Miglitol (Glyset)	Start at 25 mg three times per day	Yes	No	
Glitazones	Pioglitazone (Actos)	15–30 mg once per day	No	Yes	Increase insulin sensitivity
	Rosiglitazone (Avandia)	4–8 mg daily divided once or twice Start at 4 mg once per day or 2 mg twice per day	No	Yes	
Glinides	Repaglinide (Prandin)	0.5–4 mg three times per day before meals Start at 0.5–2 mg before meals	Yes	Yes	Beta cell, increase insulin secretion
	Natelinide (Starlix)	60–120 mg three times per day before meals	No	Yes	

[a] Preferred agents due to risk of hypoglycemia.

27.15 | Types of Insulin

	AGENT	ONSET OF ACTION	PEAK (IN HOURS)	DURATION (IN HOURS)
Rapid acting	Lispro			
	Aspart			
	Glulisine	10–15 minutes	1–2	3–5
	Exubera (inhaled)			
Short acting	Regular	20–60 minutes	1–4	4–10
Intermediate acting	Isophane suspension (NPH)	1–3 hours	5–7	13–18
	Lente	1–4 hours	4–8	13–20
Long acting	Ultralente	1–4 hours	8–12	18–30
	Glargine	About 2 hours	None	About 24
Intermediate and short acting	70 NPH/30 Reg	See individual components		

Note. Data about pharmacokinetics and dynamics of insulin types differ slightly across sources. Adapted from *Conn's Current Therapy 2005,* by R. E. Rakel and E. T. Bope, 2005, Philadelphia: Elsevier Saunders.

- Indian Health Service Diabetes Program (www.ihs.gov/MedicalPrograms/diabetes)
- Joslin Diabetes Center (www.joslin.org)
- National Diabetes Information Clearinghouse (diabetes.niddk.nih.gov)
- Office of Minority Health (www.omhrc.gov)

Disorders of the Thyroid

Hyperthyroidism (including Graves' disease), hypothyroidism, and thyroiditis are disorders of the thyroid seen in primary care settings. Hyperthyroidism is a clinical condition characterized by the presence of excessive thyroid hormone, either due to increased production, increased release of hormone through inflammation or destruction of thyroid tissue, or addition of thyroid hormone from outside the thyroid gland. Hyperthyroidism occurs in about 19 per 1,000 women in North America as compared to 1.6 per 1,000 men (Goroll & Mulley, 2006). There are several causes of hyperthyroidism. Graves' disease is the most common, accounting for 70% to 90% of cases, and is most prevalent in younger women. It is an autoimmune process also known as diffuse toxic goiter. The differential diagnoses of hyperthyroidism include Graves' disease, thyroiditis, multinodular goiter, hyperfunctioning adenoma, and TSH-secreting pituitary tumor. Thyroid carcinoma must be considered and ruled out in any person presenting with a nodular gland. Acute psychosis and severe systemic illnesses can also present with transient elevations of serum T4 and the free T4 index.

Hypothyroidism is a clinical condition characterized by decreased thyroid hormone production. Hypothyroidism may be primary (caused by thyroid disease) or secondary (resulting from disease of the pituitary or hypothalamus). Primary hypothyroidism accounts for about 95% of the cases and occurs in about 1% to 3% of the population; it is eight times more common in women than men. The prevalence increases in women in the postmenopausal years; about 10% of women at age 65 are hypothyroid, and about 15% by age 75 (Rakel & Bope, 2005). Chronic autoimmune (Hashimoto's) thyroiditis is the most common cause. The prevalence of postpartum thyroiditis is about 9% following pregnancy (Dayan & Daniels, 1996; Lazarus, 1996) and as high as 25% in women with type 1 diabetes. It is a painless, transient form of thyroiditis.

Risk factors for the development of hypothyroidism are destruction of thyroid tissue due to an autoimmune process (chronic autoimmune thyroiditis); external radiation to the neck (for treatment of acne, tonsillitis, lymphoma); subtotal or total thyroidectomy; infiltrative disease (amyloidosis, sarcoidosis); defective synthesis of thyroid hormone (iodine deficiency or use of medications that block synthesis); or transient thyroiditis (postpartum thyroiditis, subacute thyroiditis). Patients presenting with myalgias, asthenia, unexplained weight changes, menstrual disorders, problems with fertility, carpal tunnel syndrome, depression, and cognitive impairment should be screened for hypothyroidism.

When evaluating patients, symptoms of hyperfunctioning and hypofunctioning of the thyroid should be reviewed. These include fatigue, weight gain or loss, heat and cold intolerance, changes in texture of the hair and skin, sweating, palpitations, angina, tremors, diarrheal constipation, menstrual irregularities, myalgias, arthralgias, and changes in mood (depression, irritability), concentration, and memory. Individuals presenting with goiter should be evaluated for compression symptoms, such as difficulty swallowing (e.g., sensation of food sticking in throat), airway obstruction, hoarseness, or changes in the size of the neck (e.g., collars fitting more tightly, necklaces tighter). The effect of these changes on the patient's self-image should be evaluated. A careful medication history and history of other nonthyroidal illnesses should be obtained because many nonthyroidal illnesses may mimic thyroid disease. A complete review of systems is needed because many symptoms of thyroid disorders are subtle and may involve many different systems of the body.

The physical examination should include evaluation of vital signs, including weight changes, pulse pressure, and resting heart rate. Resting tachycardia is seen in hyperthyroidism, and bradycardia may be seen in hypothyroidism. In hyperthyroidism, the skin is often moist and smooth; in hypothyroidism, the skin is often dry and scaly. Similar changes are seen in the hair and nails. Examination of the eyes may reveal periorbital puffiness in patients with hypothyroidism and loss of the lateral half of the eyebrow. Patients with hyperthyroidism may exhibit lid lag and lid retraction. Proptosis and limited range of the extraocular eye muscles may also be seen in hyperthyroidism and should be assessed for unilateral versus bilateral occurrence. Examination of the neck may reveal enlargement of the thyroid (either focal or diffuse), tenderness over the gland, nodularity, or the presence of a bruit or a venous hum. In hyperthyroidism, signs of a hyperdynamic heart may be auscultated such as tachycardia, flow murmur, and extracardiac sounds. In hypothyroidism, the heart sounds may be quiet, with bradycardia and signs of pericardial effusion present in advanced states. The patient with hyperthyroidism may appear gaunt, with atropy and weakness of the muscles due to excessive muscle catabolism. They may have difficulty walking, climbing stairs, and rising from a chair due to proximal muscle weakness. They may also have emotional lability, anxiety, and fine tremors of the hand on extensions and hyperactive deep tendon reflexes with brisk relaxation. In hypothyroidism, proximal muscle weakness may also be seen, as may slowness of speech and decreases in the deep tendon reflexes with delayed recovery ("hung-up reflexes").

About 20% to 40% of individuals with Graves' disease may also have Graves' opthalmopathy (Rakel & Bope, 2005). Risks for opthalmopathy include female gender, smoking, use of radioactive iodine therapy (may worsen already present opthalmopathy), and possibly age older than 60. Symptoms include blurred vision, a sensation of grittiness in the eyes, increased lacrimation, photophobia, or sensation of pressure within the orbit. Signs of ophthalmopathy include proptosis (exophthalmos), which is usually bilateral, as well as limited ocular movements especially upward gaze, and periorbital or conjunctival edema. Rarely, increased intraocular pressure may develop which can cause optic nerve damage and vision loss (Singer et al., 1995).

Elderly patients may not present with the typical signs and symptoms of hyperthyroidism. Their presenting features may be weakness and depression or apathy. This is referred to as apathetic hyperthyroidism. These patients may not have a goiter, and proptosis is rare. Atrial fibrillation and heart failure as a consequence of hyperthyroidism are more common and may be the presenting symptom.

The common laboratory tests used in primary care for the evaluation of thyroid functioning are presented in Table 27.16. Knowledge of the feedback loop helps in interpreting laboratory findings. A basic review of thyroid testing and the feedback loop can be accessed at http://www.endocrineweb.com/tests.html. Some patients may be asymptomatic but have a TSH below normal on testing; this is called subclinical hyperthyroidism if other possible causes of low TSH are excluded.

The management of thyroid disorders is directed toward relief of symptoms and restoration of the euthyroid state. The methods used in hyperthyroidism vary according to the cause of the hyperthyroidism and the severity of symptoms. In Graves' disease, the treatment choices are antithyroid therapy (such as with methimazole or propylthiouracil), thyroid ablation with radioactive iodine, and thyroidectomy. Beta adrenergic blockers such as propranolol can be used for the symptomatic relief of tachycardia, tremor, diaphoresis, and anxiety until the hyperthyroidism responds to therapy. Because fetal irradiation is harmful, radioactive iodine should not be given to pregnant women (Rakel & Bope, 2005). Antithyroid drugs achieve euthyroidism more rapidly, are inexpensive, do not cause permanent damage to the thyroid, and are often used initially outside the United States (Rakel & Bope, 2005). However, due to more risk of side effects and low remission rate (about 50%), radioactive iodine is more commonly used now in the United States. Radioactive iodine almost always results in hypothyroidism, occurring any time after treatment. The treatment of hypothyroidism is replacement with levothyroxine (thyroxine T4). Thyroid replacement in the elderly and those with cardiac disease is begun at low doses and increased slowly to prevent complications. Patients must understand that thyroid replacement

27.16 | Commonly Used Laboratory Tests of Thyroid Function

NORMAL RANGE[a]	TSH 0.4–6.0	FREE T4 0.7–1.9	T3 80–180 NG/DL
Subclinical hypothyroidism	High	Normal	Normal
Hypothyroidism	High	Low	Normal or low
Hyperthyroidism	Low	Normal or high	High
Subclinical hyperthyroidism	Low	Normal	Normal
Thyroiditis	Low	High	High

Note. TSH = thyroid stimulating hormone: sensitivity of assay has improved markedly; best test for diagnosis of both hypothyroidism and hyperthyroidism; used alone to screen for hypothyroidism and to monitor therapy for hypothyroidism. Free T4 = unbound thyroxine, used with TSH to confirm hyper- or hypothyroidism or if patient is clearly symptomatic and TSH normal. Free T3—not useful in hypothyroidism—is used to detect hyperthyroidism if Free T4 is normal and patient appears thyrotoxic; may be used to monitor therapy for hyperthyroidism.
[a] Varies among laboratories.

is for life with periodic reassessments of dosages and thyroid status required.

Thyroiditis is generally transient, and the treatment is symptom management. Beta adrenergic blockers are often used, as well as analgesics or corticosteroids for the pain of subacute thyroiditis.

Hyperthyroidism can be difficult to recognize and treat in pregnant patients (Burman, 1995) because normal pregnancy may mimic some of the signs of hyperthyroidism. Thyroid enlargement should not occur in pregnant women with an adequate iodine intake. Screening for hyperthyroidism in pregnancy should be done in patients presenting with hyperemesis gravidarum, patients with weight loss, severe nausea and vomiting, tachycardia, muscle weakness, and thyroid enlargement.

Community resources for individuals and families with thyroid disease include the American Thyroid Association (www.thyroid.org), the National Graves' Disease Foundation (www.ngdf.org), and the Thyroid Foundation of America (www.tsh.org).

SUMMARY

Chronic diseases are very common among women, affecting not only physical health but also physical functioning, symptom experience, quality of life, and role performance for at least 6 months and often for a lifetime. The U.S. health care system is designed to respond promptly and effectively to cure and manage acute problems. However, in chronic disease, a different paradigm is needed. The goals of treatment are to mitigate the disease progression and limit the impact of the disease on the woman's physical functioning, symptoms, quality of life, and role performance. These

goals are best accomplished when the woman partners with the care provider, the latter providing information relating to treatment options. The woman herself is the primary monitor for the disease progression and the decision maker. Health care providers need to be sensitive to the long-term implications of chronic disease, especially the effects of concurrent chronic diseases, which present challenges in the form of complex regimens and competing requirements.

"No one can live perfectly with a chronic disease. To live in partnership with a chronic disease requires a habit of forgiveness—forgiving yourself for not being perfect, for making mistakes, for not giving it your best all of the time" (Poirier & Coburn, 2000, p. 5).

REFERENCES

American Academy of Neurology. (1998). *Practice parameter management issues for women with epilepsy (Summary statement)*. Retrieved February 23, 2008, from http://aan.com/professionals/practice/pdfs/pdf_1995_thru_1998/1998.51.944.pdf

American College of Physicians. (2007). *ACP diabetes care guide*. Philadelphia: Author.

American College of Rheumatology Ad Hoc Committee on Systemic Lupus Erythematosus Guidelines. (1999). Guidelines for referral and management of systemic lupus erythematosus in adults. *Arthritis and Rheumatism, 42*(9), 1785–1796.

American College of Rheumatology Subcommittee on Osteoarthritis Guidelines. (2000). Recommendations for the medical management of osteoarthritis of the hip and knee. *Arthritis and Rheumatism, 43*(9), 1905–1915.

American College of Rheumatology Subcommittee on Rheumatoid Arthritis Guidelines. (2002). Guidelines for the management of rheumatoid arthritis 2002 update. *Arthritis and Rheumatism, 46*(2), 328–346.

American Diabetes Association. (2007). Standards of medical care in diabetes, 2007. *Diabetes Care, 30*(Suppl. 1), S4–S41.

American Gastroenterological Association. (1997). Medical position statement: Irritable bowel syndrome. *Gastroenterology, 112,* 2118–2119.

Baron, T., & Richter, J. (1992). Gastroesophageal reflux disease in pregnancy. *Gastroenterology Clinics of North America, 21*(4), 777–791.

Belluzzi, A., Brignola, C., Campieri, M., Pera, A., Boschi, S., Migliolo, M., et al. (1996). Effect of an enteric-coated fish-oil preparation on relapses in Crohn's disease. *New England Journal of Medicine, 334*(24), 1557–1560.

Bonaiuti, D., Shea, B., Iovine, R., Negrini, S., Robinson, V., Kemper, H. C., et al. (2002). Exercise for preventing and treating osteoporosis in postmenopausal women. *Cochrane Database of Systematic Reviews, 2,* Art. No. CD000333.

Burman, K. (1995). Hyperthyroidism. In K. I. Becker (Ed.), *Principles and practices of endocrinology and metabolism* (2nd ed., pp. 367–385). Philadelphia: Lippincott.

Camilleri, M., & Choi, M. (1997). Irritable bowel syndrome. *Alimentary Pharmacology and Therapeutics, 11,* 3.

Carlson, E. (1998). Irritable bowel syndrome. *Nurse Practitioner, 23,* 82–91.

Centers for Disease Control and Prevention. (1996). Asthma mortality and hospitalization among children and young adults—United States, 1980–1993. *MMWR, 45*(17), 350–353.

Centers for Disease Control and Prevention. (1997). FDA approved treatment options. In *Helicobacter pylori fact sheet for physicians* (p. 3). Atlanta, GA: Author.

Centers for Disease Control and Prevention. (2005). *National diabetes fact sheet: General information and national estimates on diabetes in the United States.* Atlanta, GA: U.S. Department of Health and Human Services, Centers for Disease Control and Prevention.

Centers for Disease Control and Prevention. (2006). State-specific prevalence of obesity among adults—United States, 2005. *MMWR, 55*(36), 985–988.

Centers for Disease Control and Prevention. (2007). *Targeting epilepsy: One of the nation's most common disabling neurological conditions 2007.* Atlanta, GA: U.S. Department of Health and Human Services, Centers for Disease Control and Prevention.

Cigolle, C. T., Langa, K. M., Kabeto, M. U., Tian, Z., & Blaum, C. S. (2007). Geriatric conditions and disability: The Health and Retirement Study. *Annals of Internal Medicine, 147*(3), 156–164.

Clark, D. (1997). Physical activity efficacy and effectiveness among older adults and minorities. *Diabetes Care, 20*(7), 1176–1182.

Corbin, J., & Strauss, A. (1988). *Unending work and care: Managing chronic illness at home.* San Francisco: Jossey-Bass.

Dalton, C., & Drossman, D. (1997). Diagnosis and treatment of irritable bowel syndrome. *American Family Physician, 55*(3), 875–880.

Dayan, C., & Daniels, G. (1996). Chronic autoimmune thyroiditis. *New England Journal of Medicine, 335*(2), 99–107.

Dever, G. E. A. (1991). *Community health analysis* (2nd ed.). Gaithersburg, MD: Aspen.

Diabetes Control and Complications Trial Research Group. (1993). The effect of intensive treatment of diabetes on the development and progression of long-term complications in insulin-dependent diabetes mellitus. *New England Journal of Medicine, 329,* 977–986.

Eriksson, J., Taimela, S., & Koivisto, V. (1997). Exercise and the metabolic syndrome. *Diabetologia, 40*(2), 125–135.

Expert Committee on the Diagnosis and Classification of Diabetes Mellitus. (1997). Report of the expert committee on the diagnosis and classification of diabetes mellitus. *Diabetes Care, 20*(7), 1183–1197.

Foxall, M., Ekberg, J., & Griffith, N. (1985). Adjustment patterns of chronically ill middle-aged persons and spouses. *Western Journal of Nursing Research, 7,* 425–444.

Ghiloni, B. W. (1993). Cholilithiasis: Current treatment options. *American Family Physician, 48*(5), 762–768.

Gholson, C., Sittig, K., & McDonald, J. C. (1994). Research advances in the management of gallstones. *The American Journal of Medical Sciences, 307*(4), 2293–2304.

Giurgiu, D., & Roslyn, J. (1996). Treatment of gallstones in the 1990's. *Primary Care, 23*(3), 497–513.

Gornisiewicz, M., & Moreland, L. W. (2001). Rheumatoid arthritis. In L. Robbins, C. S. Burkhardt, M. T. Hannan, & R. J. DeHoratius (Eds.), *Clinical care in the rheumatic diseases* (2nd ed., pp. 89–96). Atlanta, GA: American College of Rheumatology Health Professionals.

Goroll, A. H., & Mulley, A. G. (2006). *Primary care medicine* (5th ed.). Philadelphia: Lippincott Williams & Wilkins.

Gwaltney, J., Scheid, W., Sande, M., & Sydor, A. (1992). The microbial etiology and antimicrobial therapy of adults with acute community-acquired sinusitis. *Journal of Allergy and Clinical Immunology, 90*(3), 457–461.

Haberman, M. R., Woods, N. F., & Packard, N. J. (1990). Demands of chronic illness: Reliability and validity assessment of the demands of illness inventory. *Holistic Nursing Practice, 5*(1), 25–35.

Hannan, M. T. (2001). Epidemiology of rheumatic diseases. In L. Robbins, C. S. Burckhardt, M. T. Hannan, & R. J. DeHoratius (Eds.), *Clinical care in the rheumatic diseases* (2nd ed., pp. 9–14). Atlanta, GA: Association of Rheumatology Health Professionals.

Harris, E. D. Jr., Budd, R. C., Firestein, G. S., Genovese, M. C., Sergent, J. S., Ruddy, S., et al. (2005). *Kelly's textbook of rheumatology* (7th ed.). Philadelphia: Elsevier Saunders.

He, W., Sengupta, M., Velkoff, V. A., & DeBarros, K. A. (2005). 65 + in the United States. Washington, DC: U.S. Department of Health and Human Services, National Institutes of Health, National Institute on Aging, and U.S. Department of Commerce, Economics and Statistics Administration, U.S. Census Bureau. Retrieved February 23, 2008, from http://www.census.gov/prod/2006pubs/p23-209.pdf

Hofmann, A. F. (1993). Primary and secondary prevention of gallstone disease: Implications for patient management and research priorities. *American Journal of Surgery, 165*(4), 541–548.

Horton, E. (1998). Exercise. In H. E. Lebovitz (Ed.), *Therapy for diabetes mellitus and related disorders* (3rd ed.). Alexandria, VA: American Diabetes Association.

International Headache Society. (2007). *IHS classification ICHD-II: Migraine and tension-type headache.* Retrieved August 29, 2007, from http://www.ihs-classification.org/en

Johnston, D., & Kaplan, M. (1993). Pathogenesis and treatment of gallstones. *New England Journal of Medicine, 328*(6), 412–421.

Kane, R. L., Priester, J. D., & Totten, A. M. (2005). *Meeting the challenge of chronic illness.* Baltimore: Johns Hopkins University Press.

Kaplan, S. H., Greenfield, S., Gandek, B., Rogers, W. H., & Ware, J. E. Jr. (1996). Characteristics of physicians with participatory decision-making styles. *Annals of Internal Medicine, 124*(5), 497–504.

Kasper, J. D., & Simonsick, E. M. (1995). Mental health and general well-being. In J. M. Guralnik, L. P. Fried, E. M. Simonsick, J. D. Kasper, & M. E. Lafferty (Eds.), *The women's health and aging study: Health and social characteristics of older women with disability* (NIH Pub. No. 95-4009). Bethesda, MD: National Institute on Aging.

Lagergren, J., Bergstrom, R., Lindgren, A., & Nyren, O. (1999). Symptomatic esophageal reflux as a risk factor for esophageal adenocarcinoma. *New England Journal of Medicine, 340,* 825–831.

Lazarus, J. H. (1996). Silent thyroiditis and subacute thyroiditis. In I. E. Braverman & R. D. Utiger (Eds.), *Werner and Ingbar's the thyroid: A fundamental and clinical text* (7th ed., pp. 577–591). Philadelphia: Lippincott.

Lewis, F. (1986). The impact of cancer on the family: A critical analysis of the research literature. *Patient Education and Counseling, 8,* 269–289.

Ling, S. M., & Rudolph, K. (2006). Osteoarthritis. In S. J. Bartlett, C. O. Bingham III, M. J. Maricic, M. D. Iverson, & V. Ruffing (Eds.), *Clinical care in the rheumatic diseases* (3rd ed.). Atlanta, GA: Association of Rheumatology Health Professionals. 127–134.

Linnebur, S. A., Vondracek, S. F., Vande Griend, J. P., Ruscin, J. M., & McDermott, M. T. (2007). Prevalence of vitamin D insufficiency in elderly ambulatory outpatients in Denver, Colorado. *American Journal of Geriatric Pharmacotherapy, 5*(1), 1–8.

Little, C. V., & Parsone, T. (2000). Herbal therapy for treating rheumatoid arthritis. *Cochrane Database of Systematic Reviews, 4,* Art. No. CD002948.

Lorenz-Meyer, H., Bauer, P., Nicolay, C., Schulz, B., Purrman, J., Fleig, W. E., et al. (1996). Omega-3 fatty acids and low carbohydrate diet for maintenance of remission in Crohn's disease. A randomized controlled multicenter trial. Study Group Members. *Scandinavian Journal of Gastroenterology, 31,* 778–785.

Ma, T. Y., Iwamoto, G. K., Hoa, N. T., Akotia, V., Pedram, A., Boivin, M. A., et al. (2004). TNF alpha-induced increase in intestinal epithelial tight junction permeability requires NF-kappa B activation. *American Journal of Physiology: Gastrointestintal and Liver Physiology, 286,* G367–G376.

Manson, J. E., Rimm, E. B., Stampfer, M. J., Colditz, G. A., Willett, W. C., Krolewski, A. S., et al. (1991). Physical activity and incidence of non-insulin-dependent diabetes mellitus in women. *Lancet, 338*(8770), 774–778.

Maricic, M. J. (2006) Osteoporois. In S. J. Bartlett, C. O. Bingham III, M. J. Maricic, M. D. Iverson, & V. Ruffing (Eds.), *Clinical care in the rheumatic diseases* (3rd ed.). Atlanta, GA: Association of Rheumatology Health Professionals, 135–140.

Marion, J., George, L., & Ware, J. (1997). Crohn's disease. In A. J. Dimarino & S. B. Benjamin (Eds.), *Gastrointestinal disease, an endoscopic approach.* London: Blackwell.

McCarthy, D. (1996). Diseases of the stomach and small intestine: Peptic ulcer disease. In J. H. Grendell, K. R McQuaid, & S. I. Friedman (Eds.), *Current diagnosis and treatment in gastroenterology.* Norwalk, CT: Appleton-Lange.

Meredith, P., & Horan, N. (2000). *Adult primary care.* Philadelphia: Saunders.

Miller, R. G. (2007) Osteoporosis in postmenopausal women: Therapy options across a wide range of risk of fracture. *Geriatrics, 61*(1), 24–30.

Moscati, R. (1996). Cholelithiasis and cholecystitis, and pancreatitis. *Emergency Medicine Clinics of North America, 14*(4), 719–737.

National Asthma Education and Prevention Program. (1997). *Expert panel report 2: Guidelines for the diagnosis and management of asthma.* National Institutes of Health Publication No. 97-4051. Bethesda, MD: National Institutes of Health, National Heart, Lung, and Blood Institute. Retrieved August 27, 2007, from http://www.nhlbi.nih.gov/guidelines/asthma/asthgdln.pdf

National Center for Chronic Disease Prevention and Health Promotion. (2006). *Arthritis.* Retrieved August 26, 2007, from http://www.cdc.gov/arthritis/data_statistics/national_data_nhis.htm#specific

National Center for Health Statistics. (2004). *Health, United States, 2004 with chartbook on trends in the health of Americans.* Hyattsville, MD: U.S. Department of Health and Human Services.

National Center for Health Statistics, Centers for Disease Control and Prevention. (2007). *Summary health statistics for U.S adults: National Health Interview Survey, 2005.* DHHS Publication PHS 2007-1560. Hyattsville, MD: U.S. Department of Health and Human Services.

National Center for Health Statistics, Centers for Disease Control and Prevention. (2008). *Summary health statistics for the U.S. population: National Health Interview Survey, 2006.* DHHS Publication PHS 2008-1564. Hyattsville, MD: U.S Department of Health and Human Services. Retrieved January 23, 2008, from http://www.cdc.gov/nccdphp/index.htm

National Osteoporosis Foundation. (2003). *Physician's guide to prevention and treatment of osteoporosis.* Washington, DC: Author.

Neuberger, G. B., Aaronson, L. S., Gajewski, B., Embretson, S. E., Cagle, P. E., Loudon, J. K., et al. (2007). Predictors of exercise and effects of exercise on symptoms, function, aerobic fitness, and disease outcomes of rheumatoid arthritis. *Arthritis and Rheumatology, 57*(6), 943–952.

Niedermann, K., Fransen, J., Knols, R., & Uebelhart, D. (2004). Gap between short- and long-term effects of patient education in rheumatoid arthritis patients: A systematic review. *Arthritis and Rheumatology, 51*(3), 388–398.

Packard, N. J., Haberman, M. R., Woods, N. F., & Yates, B. C. (1991). Demands of illness among chronically ill women. *Western Journal of Nursing Research, 13*(4), 434–457.

Pardi, D., & Tremaine, W. (1998). Inflammatory bowel disease: Keys to diagnosis and treatment. *Consultant, 38*(1), 87–97.

Pertusi, R. M., Patel, R. K., & Rubin, B. R. (2006). Fibromyalgia. In S. J. Bartlett, C. O. Bingham III, M. J. Maricic, M. D. Iversen, & V. Ruffing (Eds.), *Clinical care in the rheumatic diseases* (3rd ed., pp. 103–107). Atlanta, GA: Association of Rheumatology Health Professionals.

Petri, M. A. (2006). Systemic lupus erythematosus. In S. J. Bartlett, C. O. Bingham III, M. J. Maricic, M. D. Iversen, & V. Ruffing (Eds.), *Clinical care in the rheumatic diseases* (3rd ed., pp. 187–191). Atlanta, GA: Association of Rheumatology Health Professionals.

Poirier, L. & Coburn, K. (2000). *Women and diabetes (2nd edition).* Alexandria, VA: American Diabetes Association.

Primomo, J., Yates, B., & Woods, N. (1990). Social support for women during chronic illness: The relationship among sources and type to adjustment. *Research in Nursing and Health, 13*(3), 153–161.

Rakel, R. E., & Bope, E. T. (2005). *Conn's current therapy 2005.* Philadelphia: Elsevier Saunders.

Rasmussen, B. K. (1991). Epidemiology of headache in a general population—a prevalence study. *Journal of Clinical Epidemiology, 44*(11), 1147–1157.

Reginster, J. (2007). The efficacy of glucosamine sulfate in osteoarthritis: Financial and nonfinancial conflict of interest. *Arthritis and Rheumatolgy, 56*(7), 2105–2110.

Reynolds, J. (1996). Influence of pathophysiology, severity, and cost on the medical management of gastroesophageal reflux disease. *American Journal of Health-System Pharmacy, 53*(22 Suppl. 3), S5–12.

Richter, J. E. (1996). Typical and atypical presentations of gastroesophageal reflux disease: The role of esophageal testing in diagnosis and management. *Gastroenterology Clinics of North America, 25*(1), 75–102.

Robinson, D. L., Kidd, P. S., & Rogers, K. M. (2000). *Primary care across the lifespan.* St. Louis, MO: Mosby.

Saaddine, J. B., Cadwell, B., Gregg, E. W., Ebeglgau, M. M., Vinicor, F., Imperatore, G., et al. (2006). Improvements in diabetes processes of care and intermediate outcomes: United States, 1988–2002. *Annals of Internal Medicine, 144,* 465–474.

Sandborn, W. J. (1996). A review of immune modifier therapy for inflammatory bowel disease: Azathioprine, 6-mercaptopurine, cyclosporine, and methotrexate. *American Journal of Gastroenterology, 91*(3), 423–433.

Silberstein, S. D. (2000). Practice parameter: Evidence based guidelines for migraine headache (an evidence based review): Report of the quality standards subcommittee of the American Academy of Neurology. *Neurology, 55,* 754–762.

Silberstein, S. D. (2004). Migraine pathophysiology and its clinical implications. *Cephalgia, 24*(Suppl. 2), 2–7.

Singer, P., Cooper, D., Levy, E., et al. (1995). Treatment guidelines for patients with hyperthyroidism and hypothyroidism. *Journal of the American Medical Association, 273*(10), 808–812.

Singleton, J., Sandowski, S., Green-Hernandez, C., Horvath, T., DiGregorio, R., & Holzemer, S. (1999). *Primary care.* Philadelphia: Lippincott.

Smalley, W., & Griffin, M. (1996). The risks and costs of upper gastrointestinal disease attributable to NSAIDs. *Gastroenterology Clinics of North America, 25*(2), 373–396.

Soll, A. (1996). Medical treatment of peptic ulcer disease. *Journal of the American Medical Association, 275*(8), 622–629.

Spechler, S. (1998). Gastroesophageal reflux disease. *Current Treatment Options in Gastroenterology, 1*(1), 40–48.

Stetz, K., Lewis, F., & Primomo, J. (1986). Family coping strategies and chronic illness in the mother. *Family Relations, 35,* 515–522.

Talbot, L. A., Gaines, J. M., Huynh, T. N., & Metter, E. J. (2003). A home based pedometer driven walking program to increase physical activity in older adults with osteoarthritis of the knee: A preliminary study. *Journal of Applied Gerontology, 51,* 387–392.

Taylor, B., & DiPalma, J. (1998). Colitis: Key components of the evaluation. *Consultant, 38*(2), 375–384.

Tierney, L. M., McPhee, S. J., & Papadakis, M. A. (2006). *Current medical diagnosis and treatment, 2006.* New York: Lange Medical Books/McGraw-Hill.

United Kingdom Prospective Diabetes Study. (1998). Intensive blood-glucose control with sulfonylureas or insulin compared with conventional treatment and risk of complications in patients with type 2 diabetes. *Lancet, 352*(9131), 837–853.

U.S. Department of Health and Human Services. (2004). *Bone health and osteoporosis: A report of the Surgeon General (2004).* Retrieved October 31, 2007, from http://www.surgeongeneral.gov/library/bonehealth/content.html

Verne, G. N., & Cerda, J. J. (1997). Irritable bowel syndrome: Streamlining the diagnosis. *Postgraduate Medicine, 102*(3), 197–198, 201–204, 207–208.

Vlad, S. V., LaValley, M. P., McAlindon, T. E., & Felson, D. T. (2007). Glucosamine for pain in osteoarthritis: Why do trial results differ? *Arthritis and Rheumatology, 56*(7), 2267–2277.

Vliet Vlieland, T. P. (2007). Non-drug care for RA: Is the era of evidence-based practice approaching? *Rheumatology* (Oxford), 46(9), 1397–1404.

Wolfe, F., Smythe, H. A., Yunus, M. B., et al. (1990). The American College of Rheumatology 1990 criteria for the classification of fibromyalgia. *Arthritis and Rheumatology, 33*(2), 160–172.

Woods, N., Yates, B., & Primomo, J. (1989). Supporting families during chronic illness: What, who, when, and why. *Image, the Journal of Nursing Scholarship, 21*(1), 46–50.

World Health Organization. (2006). *Neurological disorders: Public health challenges.* Geneva, Switzerland: Author.

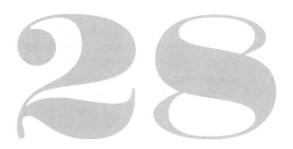

Problems of the Breast

Barbara B. Cochrane

Breast problems may range from concerns about normal maturational changes and minor skin changes or lumps to more serious problems, such as breast cancer. Breast health is focused on maintaining an awareness of normal and abnormal changes so that early evaluation and treatment can be sought before abnormal changes have more profound effects on a woman's health. This chapter describes current knowledge about breast health, changes women experience in their breasts, benign breast problems, and breast cancer. As a defining feature of the female body and a focus of female nurturing and sexuality, the breast, throughout time, has carried important meanings and value for women and men alike.

SOCIOCULTURAL CONTEXTS

The meanings attributed to women's breasts throughout history can be seen in written documents and images and reflected in women's clothing. Breasts have been hidden, bound, supported, enhanced, uncovered, and adorned. Although the sexualized view of the female breast is not universal across cultures (Yalom, 1997), the notion of women's breasts as nurturing is universal. In the United States, breast-feeding in public is more common now than in decades past. However, mothers are still expected to be discrete and keep the breast (and the infant's face) covered as much as possible.

The meanings women give to their breasts will always be bound with societal values and cultural norms—and women both inform and are informed by those values and norms (Yalom, 1997). For example, women who are identified as being at risk because of uncontrollable factors, such as hereditary breast cancer, may have an ambivalent relationship with their bodies because their breasts provide them with their feminine identity at the same time that they expose a woman to risk (Hallowell, 2000).

More recently, meanings attributed to women's breasts are being informed by the voices and experiences of women and not just by outsider awareness. We are experiencing a stage of transition in which many women see through the sociocultural constructions of the female breast and the obsession with the breast as both nurturing and sexual, but women are still not immune to social influences (Latteier, 1998).

Breast cancer is a disease that affects so many women that it is a social concern, not just a medical problem. Breast cancer is unusual among illnesses, especially other cancers, because of the specific way that the site of the cancer—a woman's breast—is socially constructed (Yalom, 1997). Breast health, as represented in the popular and medical literature, focuses almost exclusively on breast cancer, such that the idea of breast cancer has become a lived reality for women from puberty on (Potts, 2000a).

Many lives are at stake in the process of constructing knowledge about breast health and breast cancer. The media constitute a rich source of information for exploring representations of breast cancer, particularly as women's health issues have become increasingly newsworthy in recent years. Much of the popular and professional discourse on breast cancer has shaped the manner in which women experience the illness—with media focusing on such issues as identity, body image, and self-worth in women with breast cancer (Andsager, Hust, & Powers, 2000). However, the popular texts and images of breast cancer that have survived to date do not necessarily represent the experiences of women from different cultures (Thorne & Murray, 2000).

Breast cancer awareness and a sense of urgency around this issue have increased in the 1990s, in part because of the political activism of breast cancer survivors. Until the women's movement of the 1960s, breast cancer, and women's experience with the disease, remained largely silent in the popular press. Recent decades have seen a burgeoning cultural awareness of breast cancer, with the voices of women who have experienced the disease being heard in poetry and literature, the visual arts, the performing arts, and the national press. Media coverage of breast cancer provides a useful window into the ways that sociocultural constructions of breast health and breast cancer have varied over time. Today, October is recognized as Breast Cancer Awareness Month, with national campaigns and local events focused on breast cancer screening, breast cancer survivorship, and memorializing women who have died from this illness. For example, breast cancer coverage in general women's, fashion and beauty, and news magazines in the 1970s compared to the 1990s indicates that such articles are less fatalistic, more frequent, and discuss a much broader range of issues (e.g., economic costs, social issues) than ever before (Andsager et al., 2000). Images in magazine articles are becoming more representative of the demography and epidemiology of breast cancer, some even with images of older women and women of color. Over the last two decades, personal accounts of the breast cancer experience have been published, many by women who would not have previously identified themselves as writers (Potts, 2000b). These accounts give voice to the experience of breast cancer and its sociocultural constructions.

BIOMEDICAL APPROACHES TO BREAST HEALTH: THE ILLNESS PARADIGM

Just as sociocultural constructions of the female breast have resulted in an omnipresent commercialization of breast support, enhancement, and exposure, so have biomedical constructions of breast health and illness expanded into a women's health care industry focused on the female breast (Fosket, 2000). In the name of breast health and breast cancer awareness, women take on the biomedical discourse of breast cancer with a clinical vigilance and personal attention to changes in their breasts. In this climate, the 1990s saw an expansion of mammography centers across the country, many of which were identified as women's health care centers.

Breast health and illness care encompass big industry (pharmaceuticals, prosthetics, and biotechnology), general and specialized health care, research funding agendas, political activism, and national news. Lactation, management of breast changes (e.g., tumors),

and, more recently, cosmetic surgery largely encompass the breast-related concerns of the medical profession (Yalom, 1997). This focus has resulted in important progress in breast health and the possibility that we may live to see a cure for breast cancer in our lifetime. However, the dominant biomedical knowledge about breast cancer can fall short of articulating the experiential truths that women come to know (Fosket, 2000).

Breast cancer activism has taken on the character of a national movement, and advocates have made enormous strides in getting public dollars dedicated to breast cancer research and ensuring that women who have experienced breast cancer are "at the political and funding tables," speaking for themselves and for all women threatened with the disease (Yalom, 1997). However, the predominant focus of these efforts has been biomedical research on cure and early detection, with less attention to prevention.

BREAST HEALTH

Breast health involves much more than breast cancer, and breast health maintenance is enhanced by an understanding of breast anatomy, physiology, development, and changes through the life span. The female breast consists of three major components: (a) glandular tissue, consisting of 15 to 25 breast lobes that drain into lactiferous ducts and subsequently empty onto the surface of the nipple; (b) fibrous or connective tissue; and (c) adipose tissue (Givens & Luszczak, 2002). The pigmented areola and nipple are the most richly innervated portions of the breast, with Montgomery's tubercles or small protuberances on the areola that serve as the opening of sebaceous glands that lubricate the breasts. The breasts receive a rich blood supply from branches of the internal mammary, lateral thoracic, and subscapular arteries and venous drainage that starts in the subareolar plexus that empties into the intercostals, internal mammary, and axillary veins. Lymphatic drainage from the breast primarily goes to the axilla, with a small portion also going to the internal mammary nodes and other areas.

Breast Changes Throughout the Life Span

Breast Development

Breast development and function is controlled by both the anterior lobe of the pituitary and the ovaries. Follicle stimulating hormone (FSH) and luteinizing hormone (LH) released by the anterior pituitary stimulate ovarian function and cause the release of estrogen and progesterone that stimulate breast changes.

Breast development begins at about 5 weeks' gestation. Primitive breast tissue, known as the mammary ridge, develops in the thorax and regresses elsewhere. Incomplete regression of this mammary ridge may result in accessory nipples (polythelia) or even extra breasts, which rarely cause any problems but may become engorged and produce milk (Osborne, 1991). From about 20 weeks' gestation, mammary ducts and lobes develop under the influence of estrogen and progesterone. The newborn's breasts may be enlarged due to hormonal stimulation during fetal life, such that colostrum can be expressed from a neonate's breasts during the first few days after birth. Between infancy and puberty, while estrogen levels are low and relatively noncyclic, there are few developmental changes in the breast.

About a year before menarche, breast tissue begins to grow, beginning with a swelling subareolar bud that may feel itchy, then the areola and nipple become more darkly pigmented and the nipple enlarges (Whitaker-Worth, Carlone, Susser, Phlean, & Grant-Kels, 2000). Breast development is one of the earliest visible signs of puberty. The hormonal influences of the menstrual cycle are responsible for waxing and waning breast size and tactile sensitivity during puberty, although the exact mechanism by which this occurs remains unclear. Some women have vivid memories of pubertal breast development and their adolescent feelings about their breasts; sharing these with their daughters can be affirming to both. By about 20 years of age, a woman's breasts have reached their full development. The anatomy of the mature breast and breast changes in the sexual response cycle are described in chapter 4, on "Women's Bodies."

Pregnancy and Lactation

Prolactin released from the anterior pituitary acts in conjunction with estrogen and progesterone directly on breast development during pregnancy and in the process of milk production after pregnancy. During pregnancy, both the areola and nipples become more darkly pigmented and the nipples enlarge (Whitaker-Worth et al., 2000). Breast problems, particularly nipple irritation and soreness, are common in lactating women, and clinical examination of the breasts should include an evaluation for signs of engorgement, infection, or nipple problems. In many cases, breast problems related to lactation can be managed by positioning of the infant during feedings, encouraging shorter or more frequent feedings, allowing the nipples to air dry between feedings, and avoiding the use of soaps and other irritants.

Postlactation involution occurs within about 3 months after cessation of nursing and results in loss of the glandular hypertrophy of pregnancy and lactation (Givens & Luszczak, 2002). Although the nipples may lighten in the postpartum period, they usually do not return to their original prepartum color (Whitaker-Worth et al., 2000).

Menopause and Aging

Unlike the involution of the breast seen when lactation ends, postmenopausal involution, as hormonal cycles cease, involves a loss of glandular tissue, which is replaced by fat and connective tissue (Givens & Luszczak, 2002). Therefore, as women age, their breasts tend to shrink and may become more pendulous. The postmenopausal breast is less dense, breast lumps needing further evaluation are easier to palpate, and malignant changes are easier to visualize on mammogram, unless a woman is taking menopausal hormone therapy (Barton, Harris, & Fletcher, 1999).

Common Breast Problems

Benign breast conditions constitute nearly 90% of the breast problems that cause women to enter the clinical setting (Marchant, 2002). The most common breast problems include breast pain, palpable masses, and nipple discharge, which usually turn out to be benign on further evaluation (Morrow, 2000). Problems that vary with the menstrual cycle are also likely to be benign.

Nevertheless, the goal of evaluation for breast symptoms is to rule out breast cancer, with appropriate management after cancer is ruled out. The *triple test*, consisting of a clinical breast examination, imaging (ultrasound and/or mammogram, particularly in women over 40), and cytology or histology via biopsy or aspiration, is commonly regarded as the optimal approach for evaluating breast problems in that it has been associated with low false-positive and false-negative rates (less than 1%) (Foxcroft, Evans, Hirst, & Hicks, 2001). These diagnostic strategies help identify the specific characteristics of the breast problem and are described in more detail later in this chapter.

A strategy for organizing and evaluating common breast problems in the context of normal growth and development has been developed. Aberrations of Normal Development and Involution facilitate the evaluation of benign breast problems, particularly in terms of those most commonly seen at an early reproductive phase, mature reproductive phase, and during involution (Hughes, 2002). It is important to note that this system is useful for understanding and categorizing benign breast problems but does not classify risk of malignancy.

Pain and Nodularity

Breast pain (mastalgia or mastodynia) is the most common breast problem for which women consult a health care provider (Morrow, 2000). Breast pain alone is rarely the initial symptom of cancer, although localized breast pain is more indicative of an underlying malignancy than is generalized pain (Whitaker-Worth et al., 2000). Breast pain is more common in premenopausal women, although breast tenderness or pain may also be associated with postmenopausal hormone therapy. Cyclical breast pain accounts for about two-thirds of patients with breast pain (Marchant, 2002). It is usually bilateral and poorly localized, often described as a heaviness or soreness radiating to the axillae and arm, and often resolves after menses (Morrow, 2000). The cyclic nature of FSH and LH would indicate that breast engorgement and tenderness is more common before the menstrual period. Although pain and nodularity are most commonly associated with the reproductive years, these types of symptoms are still seen in postmenopausal women, particularly those who have recently lost weight or are taking menopausal hormone therapy (Marchant, 2002).

Noncyclical pain may be either true breast pain arising from the breast tissue or musculoskeletal pain from the ribs or chest wall, as with costochondritis (Mansel & Bundred, 1995). Noncyclical pain is more common in women over 40 or 50. Noncyclic pain that is localized in one breast and is sharp or burning may be caused by a breast fibroadenoma or cyst (Morrow, 2000). In the absence of a palpable mass, mammogram may still be an appropriate tool for evaluating breast pain, particularly if a woman is older than 35 years and the physical examination is equivocal.

Once specific masses or other underlying causes are ruled out, breast pain can usually be treated with nonsteroidal anti-inflammatory medications (Givens & Luszczak, 2002). Other treatments for breast pain associated with fibrocystic changes are largely untested, although progestins and vitamin therapy have been tried (Marchant, 2002). Although clinical trials have not shown significant benefit, women with benign breast pain are usually cautioned to stop smoking and decrease food or drinks containing methylxanthines (e.g., caffeine, chocolate), which may increase the pain.

Normal glandular tissue is nodular, and this nodularity is usually most pronounced in the upper outer quadrant of the breast and in the area of the inframammary ridge (Morrow, 2000). Nodularity, particularly when it waxes and wanes during the menstrual cycle, is a physiological process and not an indication of specific breast pathology. Fibrocystic changes, the term often applied to this nodularity, is, therefore, more of a diagnostic problem than a specific disease state. In fact, fibrocystic changes have been noted in up to 90% of premenopausal women, regardless of whether they are symptomatic (Morrow, 2000). To date, no clear hormonal abnormality has been associated with these types of changes. This nonspecific term is used to describe a wide spectrum of benign breast changes that are commonly noted in women during their reproductive years, when breast tissue is more dense and responsive to hormonal changes (Whitaker-Worth et al., 2000). Physical findings and symptoms of fibrocystic breast changes are less common with increasing parity and more frequently noted in more than one family member (Marchant, 2002).

Palpable Masses

Although breast lumps and masses may be noted throughout a woman's life, the type of lumps normally seen changes over time. In younger women, up to age 25 or 35, most palpable breast lumps are fibroadenomas (Whitaker-Worth et al., 2000). From ages 35 to 55, most palpable lumps turn out to be breast cysts. Over age 55, it is much more likely that a palpable breast lump will turn out to be cancerous, and more extensive evaluation (e.g., diagnostic mammogram or other imaging studies) should be carried out (Morrow, 2000). Tumors of the breast most commonly present as palpable masses that are usually discovered by the patient. Benign lumps should be examined and measured every 3 to 4 months during the first year to assess their stability.

Fibroadenomas. A common abnormality during the pubertal years, fibroadenomas are discrete, smooth, firm, solitary, and usually painless masses that may grow quite large and are almost never malignant (Foxcroft et al., 2001). Fibroadenomas differ from juvenile hypertrophy, which is more of a diffuse enlargement of the entire breast without a specific, palpable mass. Ultrasound, rather than mammography, is more useful for diagnosing fibroadenomas, and, particularly in juveniles, biopsy or fine needle aspiration is not appropriate. Although rarely necessary, a fibroadenoma can be removed if it becomes very large.

Cysts. Simple breast cysts are primarily seen in perimenopausal women and more commonly in cigarette smokers; they are much less common in premenopausal or postmenopausal women (unless they are taking menopausal hormone therapy) (Marchant, 2002). A macrocyst, which is a clinically evident breast cyst, is formed by accumulating fluid in the terminal ductal lobular unit of the breast or from an obstructed or ectatic duct. The cyst is usually firm and mobile and will flatten on compression, but it is also often tender and may show cyclic changes in size, particularly during times of hormone irregularity (Marchant, 2002). The risk of breast cancer in such gross cysts is very small (Whitaker-Worth et al., 2000).

Most breast cysts are palpable rather than visible. On ultrasound, a breast cyst appears as a clear, rounded lesion with no internal echoes or acoustic shadows; occasionally, a fluid level will be seen. Nonpalpable cysts identified by screening mammogram in an otherwise asymptomatic patient, and confirmed to be simple cysts by ultrasound, usually do not require treatment (Morrow, 2000). Treatment of symptomatic breast cysts usually involves aspiration by either fine needle aspiration or ultrasound-guided aspiration; it is critical that a cyst be aspirated dry (Marchant, 2002). The conventional wisdom regarding cysts, to wait for fluctuance, does not apply to breast cysts and abscesses. Blood-tinged fluid or fluid containing tissue debris is usually sent for cytological evaluation and women are reexamined 4 to 6 weeks after aspiration to ensure that the cyst has not recurred (Morrow, 2000).

Nipple Changes

Nipple changes are more common than one would think, even in nonlactating women, but they are usually due to benign processes (Morrow, 2000). A nipple discharge that is evident with compression only; is bilateral; involves multiple ducts; and is whitish-yellow, green, or blue-black is usually benign. Cytological examination of such discharge is often uninformative, because the absence of malignant cells does not necessarily exclude cancer, and a positive result cannot differentiate carcinoma in situ from invasive cancer (Morrow, 2000). Galactorrhea, rarely a sign of breast cancer, is common in lactating women or may be a side effect of certain medications (e.g., oral contraceptives), but should be evaluated if a milky discharge is noted in nonlactating women (Morrow, 2000). Although a blood-tinged nipple discharge should be evaluated carefully, particularly if it is unilateral and not associated with a mass or menstrual cycle changes, it will still usually be associated with a benign process such as intraductal papilloma (wart-like growths of glandular and fibrovascular tissues involving the milk ducts near the nipple), rather than malignancy, particularly among women in their 40s (Givens & Luszczak, 2002). Careful evaluation with ultrasound or magnetic resonance imaging (MRI) may be diagnostic when mammograms are not, and excision of the papilloma is usually indicated (Whitaker-Worth et al., 2000).

Benign nipple changes are usually bilateral, including nipple eczema (a sign of dermatitis or psoriasis); changes associated with candidiasis (usually seen during lactation and associated with oral thrush in a breast-feeding infant); or signs of nipple irritation, which may result from vigorous rubbing, chronic abrasion, or lactation, particularly when an infant is switching over to solid food (Whitaker-Worth et al., 2000). Benign nipple inversion needs to be distinguished from nipple retraction, which may be a sign of cancer. Benign nipple changes are usually not associated with axillary lymphadenopathy. Such changes, however, may be a sign of Paget's disease of the breast, a cancerous condition. Even when cancer is ruled out, the probable cause for nipple changes should be determined because treatment may vary. Application of lubricants or protective pads may be helpful if the cause is irritation, but such substances may also be triggers for atopic or contact dermatitis, in which case they should be avoided.

Mastitis and Duct Ectasia

Inflammation of the breast (mastitis) is often misdiagnosed and treated inadequately (Marchant, 2002). Periductal mastitis is an inflammatory condition seen in women in their early 30s and has been associated with cigarette smoking in up to 90% of cases (Whitaker-Worth et al., 2000). Pain associated with this condition can increase before menses. The nipple discharge is present in up to 20% of women with this condition and may be spontaneous, varying in color from a straw- or cream-colored thick discharge to a green or brown color. It may cause secondary eczematous changes on the surface of the areolar region and may be chronic. The nipple aspirate is rarely blood-tinged or positive for occult blood. Surgical treatment is indicated only if an abscess forms. Mastitis may be associated with lactation (puerperal or lactational mastitis), particularly during the first 2 to 3 weeks postpartum in a small percentage of nursing mothers. This condition is associated with persistent pain and swelling and, at times, erythema in the obstructed area (Marchant, 2002). With improvements in nutrition and prenatal care over the last several decades, however, early lactational mastitis, seen in the first few days following delivery and more consistently associated with an infectious process, is rarely seen, as is its progression to abscess. Risk factors for lactational mastitis include problems with positioning of the infant for attachment, milk stasis (due to interrupted or erratic feeding schedules or sudden weaning), maternal or infant illness, or other lifestyle or demographic factors. Although mastitis is not always associated with an infective process, pathogenic organisms, such as *Staphylococcus aureus*, may be isolated and fever along with localized erythema, tenderness, and warmth may occur in the affected breast. Infectious processes of the breast in nonlactating women should prompt a surgical consultation and careful evaluation for inflammatory cancer (Givens & Luszczak, 2002). If benign, antibiotic treatment with penicillinase-resistant penicillins or cephalosporins should be started early to treat the pathogenic organism associated with the infectious process (Whitaker-Worth et al., 2000). However, it is important to carefully evaluate the underlying cause before prescribing an antibiotic. In the case of benign periductal mastitis, breast-feeding should continue to promote incomplete emptying of the breast. Increasing fluids, massage, moist heat applied before nursing, more frequent feedings or use of a breast pump and, when necessary, analgesics such as acetaminophen may be helpful (Whitaker-Worth et al., 2000).

Duct ectasia or nonpuerperal mastitis often begins and ends with a bilateral nipple discharge—usually black or green—that occurs from multiple ducts on compression, but may also be asymptomatic (Whitaker-Worth et al., 2000). It is typically a chronic problem associated with the mature, aging breast and associated with minimal inflammation and dilatation of the subareolar ducts in postmenopausal women (Marchant, 2002). It may evolve from a simple discharge to periductal inflammation and mastitis to a subareolar abscess or periareolar fistula if left untreated. Duct ectasia is seen more commonly in women who smoke cigarettes, and the condition may be recurrent.

Other Problems

Mondor's disease is a rare, benign condition associated with a superficial phlebitis of the veins of the anterior chest, usually appearing as a dimpling or retraction along the lateral breast and a firm, red, slightly tender cord that is not associated lymphadenopathy (Marchant, 2002). This condition is more common among women between the ages of 30 and 60 and may be associated with breast trauma (including biopsy or mammoplasty), resulting in a painful thrombosed vein, usually palpable as a fibrous cord. The painful symptoms may last from 1 to 6 weeks, and the cord may be palpable for up to 7 months. Treatment, other than with analgesic or anti-inflammatory medications and application of cold or heat, is rarely needed (Marchant, 2002).

Fat necrosis, hematomas, or ecchymoses associated with a painful breast mass may be seen following breast trauma (or after breast surgery), such as blunt injury or a motor vehicle accident (Marchant, 2002). However, malignancy should be ruled out, and domestic violence as a cause of breast trauma should be considered.

Cosmetic Breast Surgery

There are essentially two feminist perspectives on cosmetic surgery: (a) women who elect to have their bodies surgically altered are victims of a false consciousness associated with sociocultural constructions of feminine beauty, and (b) women who undergo cosmetic surgery are exercising free choice and control over their own bodies and lives (Gagné & McGaughey, 2002). For the purposes of activism and social change, the first perspective may be more useful, but the second may be more consistent with the thoughts and feelings of women who seek cosmetic surgery. For the clinician, a synthesis of both perspectives may be most useful.

Augmentation

Breast augmentation, for cosmetic enhancement as well as mastectomy reconstruction, has been taking place for over a century. Various materials have been used in breast augmentation, including fat, ivory, glass balls, acrylic resins, sponges, Teflon, rubber, and silicone (Grigg, Bondurant, Ernster, & Herdman, 2003; Musick, 1997). In 1962, silicone gel breast implants were introduced and grew in popularity in the 1980s, when the feminine ideal of the sleek, firm body with large breasts became difficult to achieve without cosmetic enhancement (Latteier, 1998; Yalom, 1997). Although saline implants were developed in the 1960s, their use was dwarfed by that of silicone gel, which had a more natural look and feel (Grigg et al., 2003). Estimates are that up to 2 million women have had breast implant surgery since the 1960s, with about 20% to 25% of those replacing a breast lost to breast cancer (Musick, 1997).

As medical devices, over 240 different types of breast implants by at least 10 manufacturers have been developed since the 1960s. As of the 1980s, breast implants are in their third generation of development, with thinner but stronger shells, more flexible gels, and a textured shell surface that discourages the formation of capsular contractures (an often painful distortion and shrinkage of fibrous tissue around the implant; Grigg et al., 2003). However, even modern implants are not permanent, and up to 20% may rupture within the first 10 years—more obvious to women with saline than with silicone implants (Hölmich et al., 2003). Important questions about implants have arisen, and the Food and Drug Administration has issued regulations about their use and required safety evaluation.

Studies of women with breast implants have shown a great deal of dissatisfaction with the decision-making process that led to their choice. Most women report that the mass media are important sources of information about augmentation surgery (Didie & Sarwer, 2003), although that information may be sensationalized and not always accurate. Many women who have had augmentation surgery indicate that they feel vulnerable and need more information about situations that may pose a risk to the integrity of the implant (including mammograms and air bag deployment in relation to rupture; Byram, Fischhoff, Embrey, de Bruin, & Thorne, 2001). Specifically, mammograms can and should still be performed even in women with implants, although the mammographer should be told of the implants so that more appropriate maneuvers that decrease the risk of rupture can be carried out.

Silicone Breast Implants. The issue of breast implants is a complicated one, colored by insufficient information, strongly held interests, and conflicting opinions and beliefs (Latteier, 1998). Insurance coverage for breast augmentation not associated with reconstruction after breast cancer surgery is rare, and, in particular, many insurance companies will not cover later complications (Musick, 1997). Controversies over breast implants have largely focused on silicone implants, which have been implanted in more than 1.5 million women in the United States, with approximately two-thirds being used for breast augmentation (rather than reconstruction after breast cancer surgery; Grigg et al., 2003). Although most women were apparently satisfied with their implants, some experienced complications, such as implant rupture, capsular contracture, and pain, necessitating additional surgery or removal of the implant (Grigg et al., 2003). In addition, there have been concerns that the silicone gel can cause connective tissue or other autoimmune disease, such as rheumatoid arthritis or systemic lupus erythematosus.

In 1997, the Institute of Medicine was asked to carry out an extensive study of silicone breast implants to produce recommendations regarding research needs and information for women who have or are considering breast implant surgery (Grigg et al., 2003). Major findings of this special Institute of Medicine committee included: (a) there is no evidence that silicone implants are responsible for any major disease of the whole body; (b) there is no evidence of a novel autoimmune disease caused by implants; (c) there is no increase in either primary or recurrent breast cancer in women with breast implants; (d) there is no danger in breast-feeding; (e) major complications with implants are local and not life-threatening; (f) implants do not last forever, and many women should expect to have more than one implant in their lifetime; and (g) although some women with breast implants are very ill, there was no evidence that these illnesses were due to their implants (Grigg et al., 2003). Although silicone-gel implants were previously banned, in 2006, the Food and Drug Administration (FDA) approved the use of selected implants for breast augmentation in women 22 years or older and breast reconstruction in women of any age.

Saline Breast Implants. Although less cosmetically appealing, saline implants are generally thought to be safer than silicone-gel implants. Rupture or leakage of the implant remains a problem, but the substance leaked is harmless and readily absorbed. Saline implants appear to have lower rates of capsular contracture, although additional studies are needed (Grigg et al., 2003). In 1993, the FDA notified saline implant manufacturers that they, too, needed to submit safety and effectiveness data, although saline implants could stay on the market.

Reduction

Although breast augmentation and reconstruction has been performed since the late 1800s, the plastic surgery literature, up until the 1930s and 1940s, was focused on breast reduction (Jacobson, 1998). Today, fewer women have breast reduction surgery compared to those who have breast augmentation surgery, perhaps because large breasts are a deeply entrenched American ideal (Yalom, 1997). Reduction mammoplasty may be performed because the weight of large breasts can produce postural and neck and shoulder deformities, as well as skin irritation and increased self-consciousness and discomfort during sports and exercise and while trying to properly fit clothes (Marchant, 2002). Reduction mammoplasty is a more involved procedure (in-hospital surgery with general anesthesia) with a more prolonged recovery than breast augmentation.

BREAST CANCER

Breast cancer, the most common cancer diagnosed in women, can begin in the ducts (approximately 85% of breast cancers) or lobules (approximately 10% to 12% of cancers), rarely in the surrounding tissue. The cancer may be described as noninvasive (carcinoma in situ, which is localized within the ducts) or invasive (when it has spread to surrounding tissue). Probably due to improved screening techniques and increased screening in general over the last several decades, today more than half of the breast cancers are localized (rather than regional or metastatic), with the majority being noninvasive (Dow, 2004). Cancer occurs when there is abnormal cell growth, with poorly differentiated cells being more aggressive than those that are well differentiated or normal-appearing.

Epidemiology

Based on a 90-year life span, one in eight women in the United States will be diagnosed with breast cancer in their lifetime. Women in the United States have one of the highest breast cancer rates in the world, with the overall incidence increasing in the early 1970s to 1990s and then leveling off. Although the incidence of breast cancer has increased over the years, mortality rates began to decline in the early 1990s, in part because of earlier detection and improved treatment, and, therefore, better chance of cure (Jatoi, Becher, & Leake, 2003). Breast cancer is the second leading cause of cancer death in the United States overall, but it is the leading cause of cancer death for Filipino and Hispanic women.

Ethnicity and culture can have an important impact on the diagnosis, treatment, and outcomes of women with breast cancer, and racial/ethnic differences are reported across many research studies (Dow, 2004). Although breast cancer incidence is higher in White women, women from most racial/ethnic minority groups have lower breast cancer survival rates and tend to present at an advanced stage of disease with more aggressive tumors (Henson, Chu, & Levine, 2003; Jemal et al., 2007). These survival and clinical differences have multiple explanations, such as limited access to routine breast cancer screening and diagnostic services, inadequate treatment, and specific social and economic disparities (e.g., insurance and access to care).

Breast Cancer Risk

Risk is probably one of the most familiar and commonly used terms in discussions regarding breast cancer prevention. It is a word that typically connotes fear or anxiety, implying that someone is, in a sense, in danger. Women tend to overestimate their risk of breast cancer and risk of death from breast cancer, often viewing this risk as being greater than their risk for coronary heart disease or their risk of dying from lung or colorectal cancer (Morris, Wright, & Schlag, 2001). In fact, women are more accurate in their knowledge of men's disease mortality than their own (Wilcox & Stefanick, 1999).

Risk Factors

Women's understanding of breast cancer risk is often confused by the increased media attention to current known genetic mutations and family history (associated with less than 20% of breast cancers) and the fact that 70% of women diagnosed with breast cancer have no known risk factors (Cristofanilli, Newman, & Hortobagyi, 2000). Most lifestyle risk factors associated with breast cancer are thought to contribute to breast cancer etiology via hormonal mechanisms, with increased levels of endogenous hormones being associated with breast cancer risk, particularly in postmenopausal women (Cristofanilli et al., 2000; McTiernan, 2003).

Age. The strongest risk factor for breast cancer is age; incidence is extremely rare in women before age 30, and up to 75% of new breast cancer cases occur in women 50 years of age and older (Dow, 2004). Only 13% of breast cancers occur in women ages 40 to 49, although younger women are thought to experience a more aggressive form of breast cancer with higher mortality.

Family History. Much information is available in the popular press these days regarding breast cancer genetics. When talking with women about their risk of breast cancer, it is important to differentiate between their family history of breast cancer and the proportion of women with a family history who actually have hereditary breast cancer confirmed by genetic testing. Hereditary breast cancer is usually associated with early-onset disease and increased incidence of bilateral disease (Cristofanilli et al., 2000). Additionally, some mutations are not hereditary. For women who are found to have a breast cancer (BRCA) genetic mutation, their risk of breast cancer by age 70 is about 85%, regardless of family history (Keitel & Kopala, 2000). Cancer detection rates in women with

first-degree relatives with breast cancer are similar to those of women who are decades older without such family history (Kerlikowske et al., 2000).

Reproductive History. Many risk factors for breast cancer have a final, common endocrine pathway, with estrogen appearing to be the major risk factor associated with all of these variables (Levy, Ewing, & Lippman, 1988). Having a first full-term pregnancy by age 20, increased parity, late-onset menarche, early menopause, and breast-feeding (in a dose-dependent manner) have all been identified as factors that decrease a woman's risk for breast cancer (but do not delay onset of breast cancer), presumably by limiting the number of ovulatory estrogen cycles over a woman's life time (Collaborative Group on Hormonal Factors in Breast Cancer, 2002; Hamilton & Mack, 2003; Hulka & Moorman, 2002). These factors, along with decreased access to supportive health care, have been cited as influencing the increased risk of breast cancer seen in lesbians.

The relationship between induced abortion and breast cancer has been controversial and problematic to understand. Although some studies have shown an increased risk of breast cancer associated with induced abortion, other studies have shown no effect or increased risk associated with spontaneous abortion but not with induced abortion (Paoletti, Clavel-Chapelon, & the E3N group, 2003). These differences in findings may depend on the age of women studied (e.g., induced abortion may be associated with decreased risk of breast cancer in premenopausal women but not postmenopausal women). Other studies of reproductive history and breast cancer in African American women have shown that, if they are younger than 45 years of age, parity is associated with increased risk of breast cancer. However, African American women 45 years and older have a decreased risk of breast cancer associated with increased parity (Palmer, Wise, Horton, Adams-Campbell, & Rosenberg, 2003).

Hormones. The effects of exogenous hormone use in relation to development of breast cancer have been studied primarily in observational or cohort studies, with clinical implications being made more difficult by changes in both oral contraceptive and menopausal hormone therapy dosages and formulations over time (Cristofanilli et al., 2000). Although some studies have shown oral contraceptive use may be associated with an increased risk of breast cancer, particularly lobular carcinoma, this increased risk has not been statistically significant in all studies, and risk seems to decrease steadily after stopping birth control pills (and to disappear completely after 10 years; Collaborative Group on Hormonal Factors in Breast Cancer, 1996; Marchbanks et al., 2002; Newcomer, Newcomb, Trenthan-Dietz, Longnecker, & Greenberg, 2003). Long-term use of certain fertility drugs (e.g., human menopausal gonadotropin) may also increase breast cancer risk, although overall use of infertility drugs has not been associated with increased risk (Burkman et al., 2003).

Current postmenopausal hormone use, particularly with combined oral estrogen plus progestin (but also with estrogen alone, tibilone, and other forms of estrogen such as transdermal and implanted formulations), has been associated with increased risk of breast cancer (Million Women Study Collaborators, 2003). Observational studies of postmenopausal hormone use, again primarily with combination therapy and use over 5 years, have shown such use to be associated with an increased incidence of lobular carcinoma, which, although accounting for less than 10% of invasive breast cancers, is also a more aggressive form of breast carcinoma (Chen, Weiss, Newcomb, Barlow, & White, 2002; Li, Malone, et al., 2003; Newcomer, Newcomb, Potter, et al., 2003). In a randomized clinical trial, breast cancers associated with estrogen plus progestin use were similar histologically to those in other women, but were larger and discovered at a more advanced stage, possibly because the increased breast density associated with menopausal hormone use may hinder diagnosis of breast cancer (Chlebowski et al., 2003). As with past oral contraceptive use, past use of menopausal hormone therapy is not associated with increased risk of incident or fatal breast cancer (Million Women Study Collaborators, 2003).

Dietary Factors. Based on international studies of diet and breast cancer, as well as studies of changes in risk in immigrants to the United States, diets high in fat—particularly animal fats—may have high potential for increasing women's risk of breast cancer (Prentice, 2000). These international differences in breast cancer rates are particularly great for postmenopausal women (Willett, 1990). Case-control studies have shown that increased vegetable consumption and decreased consumption of red meat are associated with decreased breast cancer risk (Cho et al., 2003). More recently, increased consumption of isoflavone-containing soy foods—particularly miso soup—and increased intake of green tea (even after adjusting for other risk factors) have also been associated with a decreased risk of breast cancer (Wu, Yu, Tseng, Hankin, & Pike, 2003; Yamamoto et al., 2003). Higher consumption of fish, in one study, was only weakly associated with decreased breast cancer risk (Terry, Rohan, Wolk, Maehle-Schmidt, & Magnusson, 2002). Although considerable scientific disagreement and controversy exist about the relationship between dietary fat and breast cancer, to date, low-fat dietary patterns have not been consistently associated with decreased breast cancer risk (Prentice et al., 2006; Willett, 1990).

Alcohol. An increased alcohol intake (more than two drinks per day, regardless of type of alcoholic beverage) has been associated with a dose-dependent increase in a woman's risk of breast cancer by more than 70% to 80% (Cristofanilli et al., 2000; Longnecker, Berlin, Orza, & Chalmers, 1988; Tjønneland et al., 2003). It is thought that alcohol consumption increases estrogen levels in postmenopausal women, particularly those on menopausal hormone therapy (Dorgan et al., 2001). The risk of breast cancer associated with alcohol intake may be minimized by ensuring an adequate folate intake, although these conclusions still need additional study (Feigelson et al., 2003; Zhang et al., 1999).

Anthropometric Factors. Up to 25% of breast cancer cases worldwide are due to being overweight or obese and having a sedentary lifestyle (McTiernan et al., 2003). Even in women who had never used menopausal hormone therapy, an increased body mass index, adult weight gain after age 18, and increased height have been associated with an increased risk of breast cancer (Endogenous Hormones and Breast Cancer Collaborative Group, 2003; Lawlor, Okasha, Gunnell, Smith, & Ebrahim, 2003). This association is stronger in women with a family history of breast cancer (Carpenter, Ross, Paganini-Hill, & Bernstein, 2003). Type 2 diabetes, also seen more often in obese women, may be associated with a slightly higher risk of breast cancer (Michels et al., 2003).

Exercise. Women who engage in 3 to 4 hours of moderate to vigorous exercise each week have a 30% to 40% lower risk for breast cancer compared to sedentary women (McTiernan, 2003). It is not clear whether increases in intensity or duration of physical activity have a progressively increased impact on reducing breast cancer risk or whether a specific level of activity (and no more) is protective (Drake, 2001; Patel, Calle, Bernstein, Wu, & Thun, 2003). Family history may reduce the protective effect of exercise on breast cancer risk.

Environmental Exposures. Beyond exposure to ionizing radiation (associated with nuclear weapons), no specific environmental carcinogens for breast cancer have been identified. Although there are some conflicting results, exposure to DDT, PCBs, vehicle exhaust, contaminated drinking water, electric blankets, and residential electromagnetic fields have not been definitively linked to breast cancer risk (Kabat et al., 2003; Schoenfeld et al., 2003). Studies of the relationship between night-shift work or rotating shifts and increased risk of breast cancer have not been conclusive, but indicate an increased risk among women who do not sleep during the period at night when melatonin production is at its highest (Davis, Mirick, & Stevens, 2001; Schernhammer et al., 2001).

Other. Growing research in the area of psychoneuroimmunology has evaluated the relationship between stress and decreased immune function. However, research has shown only "modest" associations at best between depression or stress and breast cancer risk (Butow et al., 2000; Price, Tennant, Butow, et al., 2001; Price, Tennant, Smith, et al., 2001). In some studies, major life events or severely threatening life events, rather than accumulated stress, have been associated with increased breast cancer risk (Butow et al., 2000; Lillberg et al., 2003).

Other than exogenous hormones, medications such as antidepressants, antihistamines, and aspirin have not been associated with increased breast cancer risk (Bahl, Cotterchio, & Kreiger, 2003; Desai, Bruce, & Kasl, 1999; Johnson, Anderson, Lazovich, & Folsom, 2002; Moorman, Grubber, Millikan, & Newman, 2003; Nadalin, Cotterchio, & Kreiger, 2003). Bone mineral density has also been studied for its association with breast cancer risk. Older women with a high bone mineral density have been found to have an increased risk of breast cancer, especially advanced breast cancer, compared to women with low bone mineral density—again, probably because of hormonal mechanisms (Zmuda et al., 2001).

Risk Assessment

The two types of risk assessment are risk assessment models that calculate risk estimates on an individual woman's risk factors and genetic testing that evaluates a woman's blood for the presence of the two currently known breast cancer gene mutations, BRCA1 and BRCA2. Communications about risk must be carefully considered but offered at all appropriate clinical encounters. Women tend to overestimate, rather than underestimate, risk (Lynch et al., 1999). A strictly fact-based discussion of breast cancer risk information may correct inaccurate risk perceptions but may not effectively address associated breast cancer anxiety (Meiser et al., 2001; van Dijk et al., 2003). Instead, effective risk communication involves an assessment of information needs, a collaborative exchange of information and concerns between a woman and the clinician, and nonpersuasive communication techniques (Nekhlyudov & Partridge, 2003).

Risk Assessment Models

Quantification of disease risk is usually estimated using statistical models from epidemiological research to project risk over a specific period of time (Cristofanilli et al., 2000). The two models most frequently used for breast cancer risk appraisal clinically and in research are the Gail model, developed from data collected in the Breast Cancer Detection Demonstration Project (Gail et al., 1989), and the Claus model, developed from data collected in the Cancer and Steroid Hormone study conducted by the Centers for Disease Control (Claus, Risch, & Thompson, 1994).

Health care professionals can access an Internet-based, scientifically validated breast cancer risk assess-

ment tool, based on the Gail model, developed by the National Cancer Institute and the National Surgical Adjuvant Breast and Bowel Project, to calculate a woman's estimated risk for invasive breast cancer over a 5-year period as well as over her lifetime (to age 90) at http://bcra.nci.nih.gov/brc. Variables included in this model are outlined in Exhibit 28.1. Although a full discussion of breast cancer risk appraisal models is beyond the scope of this chapter, it is important to understand the strengths and limitations of each model—particularly in terms of their relevance to specific racial/ethnic groups—because no model fully incorporates research to date on breast cancer risk (Bondy & Newman, 2003; Bucholtz, 2004; McTiernan et al., 2001). Additionally, because these models provide a "predicted" risk, women already diagnosed with breast cancer will not necessarily have a higher calculated risk estimate (Bucholtz, 2004). It may be most meaningful to present more than one model's risk estimate summary to a woman, along with appropriate explanations.

Genetic Risk Counseling and Testing

Hundreds of different BRCA1 and BRCA2 germline mutations have been identified, and hereditable breast cancer, due to BRCA1 and BRCA2 genetic mutations and other genetic syndromes, accounts for about 10% of diagnosed breast cancers (de Sanjosé et al., 2003; Lynch & Lynch, 2000). Even in women with breast cancer, more than 60% overestimate their chances of having such a mutation (Bluman et al., 1999) and choose to have genetic testing. Over 40% of women without diagnosed breast cancer who had an earlier screening mammogram indicated that they would probably or definitely pursue genetic testing (Gwyn, Vernon, & Conoley, 2003).

The BRCA1 and BRCA2 mutations are not connected, except that both are associated with an increased hereditable risk of breast cancer. The BRCA1 mutation accounts for approximately 45% of all hereditable breast

---

EXHIBIT 28.1 VARIABLES INCLUDED IN THE BREAST CANCER RISK ASSESSMENT TOOL BASED ON THE GAIL MODEL

- Age
- Number of first-degree relatives with breast cancer
- Age at menarche
- Nulliparity or age at first birth
- Number of breast biopsies
- Presence or absence of atypical hyperplasia on breast biopsy

Note: From Gail et al. 1989.

cancer–prone families (Cristofanilli et al., 2000; Lynch & Lynch, 2000). Carriers of this mutation have an estimated lifetime risk for breast cancer of 85% and a risk for ovarian cancer of between 40% and 60%. The BRCA1 mutation is present in approximately 1% of Ashkenazi Jewish women, contributing to a lifetime risk of breast cancer of over 20% in Jewish women (Cristofanilli et al., 2000; Lynch & Lynch, 2000).

The BRCA2 mutation is associated with early-onset breast cancer and accounts for approximately 30% of all hereditable breast cancers. Carriers of this mutation also have a lifetime risk for breast cancer of approximately 85%, but the risk for ovarian cancer is much lower compared to the risk associated with the BRCA1 mutation (approximately 10% to 20%) (Lynch & Lynch, 2000). Male breast cancer is associated with the BRCA2 genetic mutation, which is also associated with an increased lifetime risk for prostate cancer (Lynch & Lynch, 2000). The BRCA2 mutation is also associated with an increased risk of pancreatic and colon cancer, as well as malignant melanoma (Clark, 2004).

Genetic counseling, regardless of whether testing is carried out, can help women with a positive family history of breast cancer develop a more accurate sense of their risk and more realistic views about genetic testing (Burke et al., 2000). Breast cancer risk assessment and evaluation of a woman's family pedigree of breast and ovarian cancer are usually carried out during an initial genetic counseling session (Khabele & Runowicz, 2002). Genetic counseling should take place before a sample of DNA is obtained as well as at the time that results are disclosed (Lynch & Lynch, 2000). In fact, genetic testing is usually not offered as an option until after extensive counseling and analysis of the family pedigree indicate a likelihood of hereditary breast cancer. About 50% to 60% of women who undergo such counseling choose to have genetic testing (Armstrong et al., 2000). Genetic testing is usually not recommended until a woman is over 18 years of age (Lynch & Lynch, 2000).

Although some researchers have found that women have increased distress after obtaining positive genetic test results (Tercyak et al., 2001), others document both negative (e.g., sadness, anger) and positive (relief, acceptance) reactions to receiving positive genetic test results, regardless of pretesting emotions (Lynch & Lynch, 2000). Regardless of whether test results are positive or negative, women are more likely to communicate these results to a sister and least likely to communicate them to a young child (Hughes, 1982). Concerns have been raised about life insurance discrimination as a result of genetic testing (e.g., decreasing or refusing coverage if results are positive). One study of 636 women who had genetic testing and/or counseling showed that none of the women had life insurance denied or canceled, although 4% sought an increase in their life insurance coverage after testing (Armstrong et al., 2003).

If genetic test results are positive for a BRCA genetic mutation, available preventive strategies (e.g., chemoprevention and bilateral prophylactic mastectomy) and testing as many family members as possible are discussed. Women from families in which there is a known BRCA1 mutation have a 50% chance of having the mutation themselves (Khabele & Runowicz, 2002). Women who undergo genetic testing have shown increased adherence to breast cancer screening guidelines after testing (Lynch et al., 1999).

Risk Management—Prevention

Many people consider breast cancer screening as a form of breast cancer prevention in that increased surveillance can promote earlier detection of breast cancer, and thereby a better chance of cure. Indeed, although the causes for breast cancer have yet to be clearly identified, biomedical knowledge about breast cancer treatment and early detection far exceeds knowledge about prevention (Potts, 2000a; Thorne & Murray, 2000). Risk management is based on three predominant themes: (a) an emphasis on promoting personal or individual responsibility for health; (b) a belief in technological and pharmacological solutions to problems; and (c) a social ideology that shifts responsibilities from the individual to the social, economic, and political realms (Simpson, 2000). Current prevention strategies, therefore, primarily involve risk management, including modification of known risk factors and more extreme measures, such as chemoprevention (using chemical agents to inhibit or reverse carcinogenesis before development of a clinically evident malignancy) and bilateral prophylactic mastectomy (surgical removal of the breasts).

Chemoprevention

The ideal breast cancer chemopreventive agent would be one that is easy to administer, has a low toxicity profile, is effective in both low- and high-risk patients, and produces only beneficial estrogen effects (including decreased vasomotor symptoms; Bucholtz, 2004). To date, there is no such agent. In 1998, with the early conclusion of the large national Breast Cancer Prevention Trial (BCPT; also known as the Tamoxifen Trial), tamoxifen was approved by the Food and Drug Administration for breast cancer prevention. Before the BCPT, tamoxifen had been used for over 30 years as adjuvant therapy following surgery for estrogen-sensitive breast cancer (Bucholtz, 2004). The BCPT found that administration of tamoxifen for 5 years decreased the risk of invasive breast cancer by 51% and noninvasive breast cancer (i.e., carcinoma in situ) by 30% in women over 50 (Fisher et al., 1998). Tamoxifen was also associated with a decreased risk for osteoporosis in these older women and an increased risk for stroke, pulmonary embolus, deep vein thrombosis, endometrial hyperplasia, and cancer. In women 35 to 50 years, tamoxifen resulted in a similar decreased risk for invasive breast cancer and a decreased risk of noninvasive breast cancer by 73%, with no added risk of endometrial cancer or venous thromboemboli. The BCPT findings indicated that tamoxifen was not effective in preventing estrogen-receptor negative tumors.

Tamoxifen is classified as a selective estrogen receptor modulator (SERM) in that it acts as an estrogen antagonist in some tissues (e.g., breast) and as a partial estrogen agonist in others (e.g., increasing bone mineral density and decreasing cholesterol), particularly in postmenopausal women (Fisher et al., 1998). Tamoxifen is contraindicated if a woman is pregnant or has a history of problems with blood clots. Its use for breast cancer chemoprevention is generally covered by insurance plans (Bucholtz, 2004). Recommended follow-up while women are taking tamoxifen includes yearly gynecological examinations and careful attention to prevention of venous thromboemboli (e.g., avoiding prolonged immobilization).

Promising research indicates that another SERM, raloxifene, currently approved for osteoporosis prevention and treatment, may decrease invasive breast cancer risk without the increased endometrial cancer risk associated with tamoxifen (although the risk of venous thromboemboli remains; Cummings et al., 1999). The Study of Tamoxifen and Raloxifene is ongoing at over 400 centers across the United States to compare the effects of tamoxifen and raloxifene on decreasing risk of breast cancer (Chlebowski et al., 2002). Aromatase inhibitors, currently used as adjunct therapy for breast cancer, are also being studied as breast cancer chemo-preventive agents.

Bilateral Prophylactic Mastectomy

Prophylactic mastectomy, although considered by many to be an overly radical strategy for preventing breast cancer, is viewed as a viable and important option for some women at high risk for the disease, either because of increased hereditable risk or biopsy findings indicating increased risk (Bucholtz, 2004). In one study of 95 women over 25 years of age who had genetic testing, 62% said they would consider prophylactic mastectomy (Lynch & Lynch, 2000). One year after genetic testing, 3% of women who tested positive for a BRCA genetic mutation had a bilateral prophylactic mastectomy (Lerman et al., 2000). In addition, some women with diagnosed cancer in one breast will elect to have the contralateral breast surgically removed as a prophylactic measure. Although microscopic amounts of breast tissue may still remain after such surgery, generally risk is reduced by 90% to 100%, with a several-

year gain in life expectancy (Hartmann et al., 1999; Meijers-Heijboer et al., 2001).

The decision to undergo a prophylactic mastectomy is a difficult one. Women who have the surgery often have undergone several previous breast biopsies and report increased worry about developing breast cancer as well as increased perceived risk (Stefanek, Helzlsouer, Wilcox, & Houn, 1995; van Dijk et al., 2003). Many women choose to have immediate reconstruction during the surgery. Most women who undergo a prophylactic mastectomy report they are satisfied with their decision (Frost, Vockley, et al., 2000; Stefanek et al., 1995), although older women are more likely to be satisfied than younger women (Metcalfe, Esplen, Goel, & Narod, 2004).

Breast Cancer Screening

Breast cancer screening with resulting earlier detection of cancer may be the most important factor explaining recent declines in overall mortality from breast cancer in the United States (Cristofanilli et al., 2000; Winchester, 2000). To date, breast cancer screening has involved primarily three strategies: breast self-examination, clinical breast examination, and mammography (see Table 28.1). However, promising new imaging techniques and serum biomarker studies are underway.

Breast Self-Examination—New Focus on Awareness of Changes

The utility of breast self-examination (BSE) as a screening strategy has been reevaluated recently in light of research, including a large clinical trial in Shanghai, China, showing that intensive BSE teaching does not decrease mortality from breast cancer and may increase the likelihood of having benign breast biopsies (i.e., more benign breast lesions were diagnosed in the treatment group; Hackshaw & Paul, 2003; Thomas et al., 2002). Other studies indicate that many women are not confident in their ability to detect a problem, that BSE makes them anxious, and that they are not performing it regularly (Millar & Millar, 1992). Although monthly BSE is no longer recommended by some organizations and agencies, others still recommend BSE teaching as a strategy for enhancing breast cancer awareness (see Table 28.1). Women should be aware of physical changes that warrant further evaluation for breast cancer or other conditions. These changes include nipple retraction or discharge, obvious changes in size or shape of the breast (particularly if changes are unilateral), scaliness, dimpling, or puckering. During BSE teaching, it is helpful for women to see illustrations of physical changes to look for and to practice BSE on breast models that simulate both normal and abnormal tissue (Machia, 2004). Numerous resources are available from

28.1 | Breast Cancer Screening Guidelines

SUSAN G. KOMEN FOR THE CURE	AMERICAN CANCER SOCIETY	NATIONAL CANCER INSTITUTE	U.S. PREVENTIVE SERVICES TASK FORCE
Mammography			
Every year beginning at age 40	Every year beginning at age 40	Every 1 to 2 years beginning at age 40	Every 1 to 2 years beginning at age 40
Clinical Breast Exam			
At least every 3 years between ages 20–39	About every 3 years between ages 20–39	No specific recommendation	Not enough evidence to recommend for or against
Every year beginning at age 40	Every year beginning at age 40		
Breast Self-Exam			
Breast Self-Exam can be a tool to both increase awareness of breast cancer and to learn about what changes in the breast should be reported.	Beginning in 20s, review benefits and limitations of self-exam with health care provider. Choice to perform self-exam is up to individual.	No specific recommendation	Not enough evidence to recommend for or against

Note. Women at higher risk may need to get screened earlier and more frequently than recommended here. Adapted from Recommendations for Mammography, by the Susan G. Komen Foundation. Reprinted with permission from www.komen.org

breast cancer organizations for teaching BSE, including shower cards, pamphlets, and Web pages such as the Susan G. Komen Foundation Web site (www.komen.org), which includes downloadable BSE cards for various racial/ethnic groups in many different languages.

Clinical Breast Examination

An annual clinical breast examination (CBE) in a health care provider's office is consistently recommended by most scientific authorities and breast cancer organizations. The sensitivity of the CBE to detect cancers increases with increasing lump size (Baker, 1982). In one large medical center, 8% of diagnosed breast cancers were found by CBE alone (i.e., mammogram was negative; Green & Taplin, 2003). The CBE encounter should include a thorough medical history, an evaluation of breast cancer risk factors, and a discussion of any breast changes or symptoms. The clinician performing such exams should develop a standardized, systematic approach to performing the clinical breast exam in a detailed and unhurried manner, with sufficient proficiency to detect subtle physical changes and differentiate probably benign findings from suspicious findings warranting additional evaluation. Women's breasts vary in the amount of background nodularity (Barton et al., 1999). In older women not taking post-

menopausal hormones, the breast becomes more fatty, and breast lumps are easier to palpate. The sensitivity of CBE to detect lumps may be slightly lower in women with larger breasts (Barton et al., 1999).

Based on a careful evaluation of the research literature, Barton and colleagues (1999) have identified a preferred technique for carrying out a systematic CBE, which can detect at least 50% of asymptomatic cancers (see Figure 28.1a, Figure 28.1b, and Figure 28.1c). The technique involves proper positioning to ensure that the breast tissue can be flattened against the woman's chest during palpation, a thorough search extending fully to the midaxillary line and breast boundaries, use of a vertical-strip search pattern such that the rows are overlapping, proper positioning and movement of the fingers, and a duration of at least 3 minutes per breast. The value of inspection with multiple maneuvers (raising hands over the head, hands on hips and bearing down, leaning forward and allowing breasts to hang out from the chest) remains unproved, although inspection remains a part of the CBE for many practitioners (Barton et al., 1999). The value of compressing the nipples for discharge is also questioned by some but still practiced by many. An abnormal nipple discharge is more likely to be spontaneous, whereas a discharge noted only on squeezing the nipples is most likely benign.

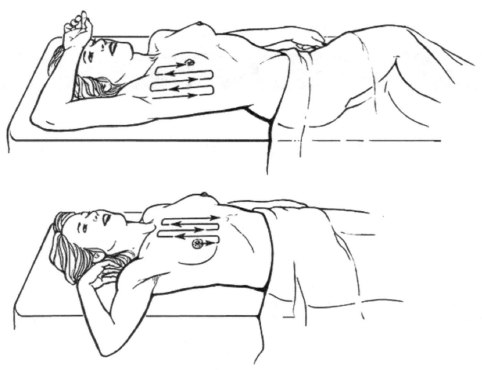

Figure 28.1a   Clinical breast examination technique.

A. Positioning and direction of palpation: The top figure shows appropriate positioning to flatten the lateral part of the breast (woman rolled onto contralateral hip and shoulders rotated back with ipsilateral hand on the forehead). The bottom figure shows positioning to flatten the medial portion of the breast (woman lying flat on her back with elbow level with the shoulder). Arrows show the vertical strip pattern of examination.

From Barton et al., 1999. *JAMA*, October 6, 1999, Vol 282, p. 1276. Copyright © 1999, American Medical Association. All rights reserved.

Physical Signs of Breast Cancer

Breast cancer is rarely visible on inspection of the breast. However, changes associated with breast cancer may include nipple flattening or retraction or skin thickening or retraction, which may appear as shallow or deep skin dimples or as shrinkage of the entire breast. These changes are more worrisome if they are of recent onset, progressive, or unilateral (Whitaker-Worth et al., 2000). Nipple discharge associated with breast cancer is usually bloody or serous, associated with a mass, unilateral, and confined to one duct (Givens & Luszczak, 2002; Morrow, 2000). Cancerous lumps detected on palpation will usually be hard, solitary, fixed to adjacent tissue, painless, and of irregular shape (Barton et al., 1999; Whitaker-Worth et al., 2000). Axillary lymph node enlargement may also be palpated. The upper outer quadrant of the breast is an area that warrants careful attention; 48% of cancers are found in this area (Whitaker-Worth et al., 2000). In women who have had previous breast surgery (whether for cosmetic reasons or for breast cancer), the clinician should look for signs of edema, inflammation, or infection at the site of the scar, and, if breast implants are in place, for contracture formation or deviation of the implant (Givens & Luszczak, 2002).

Mammography

Screening Mammograms. Regular mammography has been identified as the primary strategy available for detecting breast cancer at a stage that is early enough to cure, minimizing treatment-associated morbidity (e.g., breast conservation rather than mastectomy), and decreasing mortality (Freedman et al., 2003; Tabar et al., 2003). Some experts estimate that the increased incidence of noninvasive breast cancer in the 1990s can be partially attributed to increased use of mammogram screening (Dow, 2004).

A screening mammogram is used to detect breast changes, such as tumors that cannot be felt and microcalcifications (calcium deposits in the breast) that may indicate the presence of breast cancer in women who do not show signs or symptoms of the disease. However, up to 20% of breast cancers may not be seen on a mammogram (Morrow, 2000). Detection of breast cancer by mammogram may depend on the equipment used, the technician's skill in performing the procedure, the radiologist's skill in reading the films, and individual characteristics of the woman. Women should inform the mammogram technician about their personal and family history of breast cancer, any history of breast biopsies, current use of menopausal hormone

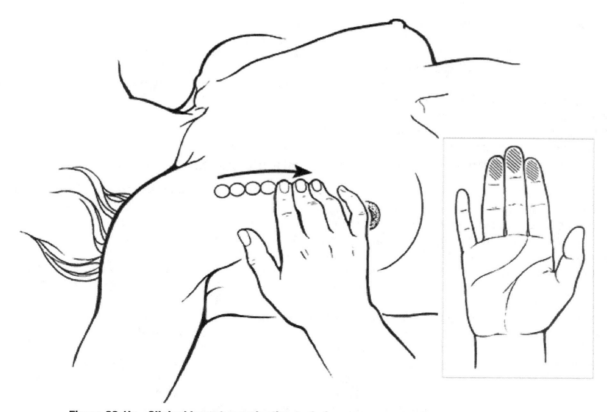

Figure 28.1b   Clinical breast examination technique.

B. Palpation technique. Pads of the three middle fingers move in a circular motion down and up along the vertical strip pattern.

From Barton et al., 1999. *JAMA*, October 6, 1999, Vol 282, p. 1276. Copyright © 1999, American Medical Association. All rights reserved.

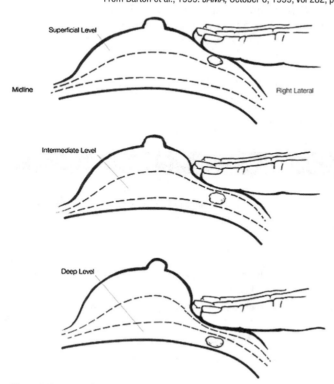

Figure 28.1c   Clinical breast examination technique.

C. Levels of pressure for palpation of breast tissue. Finger pads make 3 small circles (as if circling around the edge of a dime), increasing the level of pressure with each circle. From Barton et al., 1999. *JAMA,* October 6, 1999, Vol 282, p. 1276. Copyright © 1999, American Medical Association. All rights reserved.

therapy, or presence of breast implants (Greendale et al., 2003).

The mammogram equipment uses very low radiation, and the procedure usually involves two x-ray views of each breast compressed between two plates to flatten and spread out the breast tissue as much as possible. Although the compression is uncomfortable, particularly for smaller breasts with less surface area, it usually lasts only a few seconds, with the whole procedure taking about 20 minutes. The mammogram technician's skill and sensitivity can have an important impact on the ability of the procedure to detect breast cancer with minimal distress for the woman. Younger women and women taking menopausal hormone therapy may have less accurate mammograms because their breasts are denser and may, therefore, obscure abnormalities. In addition, specific positioning strategies and special implant displacement views are required for women who have breast implants in order to visualize tissue behind the implant.

Digital mammography is an x-ray technique that stores breast images digitally and, therefore, involves less time between image acquisition and display and allows computer analysis of the entire breast and identification of suspicious areas, based on specific algorithms, for the radiologist to evaluate areas of concern. From the woman's perspective, the imaging procedure is similar to a standard film mammogram. Because the image is digital, the radiologist can magnify and adjust the contrast of specific sections of the breast to enhance visualization and can share the images with specialists to obtain appropriate consultation about suspicious findings. Therefore, women may not need to return as often for additional imaging. Digital mammogram use is increasing, but the equipment and procedure are more expensive, and many mammogram centers still use primarily standard mammogram x-ray imaging (Fraker, 2004).

Interpreting the Mammogram. Radiologists are often able to differentiate benign from possibly malignant findings on mammogram, based on the appearance of masses, calcifications, and architectural distortion of breast tissue. Benign masses (e.g., cysts or fibroadenomas) usually appear round or oval-shaped, with well-defined margins, are not dense (i.e., are not radio-opaque), may be associated with fatty tissue, and do not disrupt surrounding breast architecture (Jeske, Bernstein, & Stull, 2000). Malignant masses are more asymmetrical and dense, with irregular margins, associated microcalcifications, and distortion of surrounding breast tissue. The Breast Imaging Reporting and Database System (see Table 28.2) was established by the American College of Radiology in collaboration with many other federal agencies and professional organizations to facilitate uniform reporting of mammogram findings (Jeske et al., 2000). The reporting system uses a lexicon or standard language for describing lesions and specific reporting categories of negative, benign, probably benign, suspicious abnormality, and highly suggestive of malignancy to summarize the findings. Each category is associated with a specific follow-up plan that helps radiologists and health care providers appropriately manage ongoing care.

Supporting Breast Health and Breast Cancer Screening

Current recommendations about mammogram screening are outlined in Table 28.1. In general, women 40 years and older should have a screening mammogram every 1 to 2 years. Women under 40 who are at higher than average risk may also need regular screening mammograms. Recent scientific debates about the appropriate scheduling for screening mammograms, particularly for women 40 to 49 years, has prompted some confusion for health care providers and women alike (Meissner, Rimer, Davis, Eisner, & Siegler, 2003) and has significantly predicted women being off schedule for having mammography (Rimer, Halabi, Strigo, Crawford, & Lipkus, 1999). Guidelines are clearer for older women, and Medicare and other health insurance providers now support annual mammograms in women over 50. Although less than 50% to 60% of older women get annual screening mammograms, regardless of racial/ethnic group, the percentage of older women who have never had a mammogram has declined significantly in recent years (Harrison et al., 2003; Tu et al., 2003).

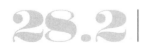 | Breast Imaging Reporting and Database System (BI-RADS®)

CATEGORY	ASSESSMENT	FOLLOW-UP
0	Need additional imaging evaluation and/or prior mammograms for comparison	Additional imaging or prior images are needed before a final assessment can be assigned
1	Negative	Continue annual screening mammography (for women older than age 40)
2	Benign finding(s)	Continue annual screening mammography (for women older than age 40)
3	Probably benign finding—initial short-interval follow-up suggested	Initial short-term follow-up (6-month) examination
4	Suspicious abnormality—biopsy should be considered	May require biopsy
5	Highly suggestive of malignancy—appropriate action should be taken	Requires biopsy or surgical treatment
6	Known biopsy–proven malignancy—appropriate action should be taken	Category reserved for lesions identified on imaging study with biopsy proof of malignancy prior to definitive therapy

Overcoming Barriers to Screening

Reminders from health care providers have been shown to be one of the most effective strategies for promoting mammogram adherence in studies of women, regardless of their age or ethnicity (Lukwago et al., 2003; Schwartz, Taylor, & Willard, 2003; Tu et al., 2003). Other factors shown to predict mammogram adherence include having previous mammograms; engaging in other healthy behaviors; and having health insurance, better access to health care, and higher education (Bastani, Maxwell, Bradford, Das, & Yan, 1999; Holm, Frank, & Curtin, 1999; Qureshi, Thacker, Litaker, & Kippes, 2000).

Addressing Breast Cancer Worries

Breast cancer worries and psychological distress associated with risk perceptions are thought to affect adherence to breast cancer screening. Although the research evidence is not fully consistent, when anxiety is low there may be little motivation to be screened, and when anxiety is high and a woman is very fearful of a breast cancer diagnosis, avoidance of screening may occur (Andersen, Smith, Meischke, Bowen, & Urban, 2003; Diefenbach, Miller, & Daly, 1999; McCaul, Schroeder, & Reid, 1996). Women with a family history of breast cancer may overestimate their risk of developing breast cancer, which can increase their anxiety and worry (Gilbar, 1998; Lerman et al., 1995; Meiser et al., 2001). Therefore, additional support and follow-up may be appropriate for women with a positive family history, as well as women who have experienced false-positive screening results (Absetz, Aro, & Sutton, 2003). Fatalism, or a belief that if cancer is present, death will occur, has also been associated with nonadherence (Mayo, Ureda, & Parker, 2001). For these reasons, high-risk breast cancer clinics, in addition to providing genetic counseling and testing, often offer psychosocial support services to women (Gilbar, 1998).

Patterns of Seeking Care

Breast cancer worry can affect a woman's adherence to screening recommendations as well as care seeking when breast cancer symptoms or other breast problems develop. Women who have had a friend or relative with breast cancer may seek help promptly once problems are noticed, but up to 25% of women delay seeking care for 2 to 3 months after becoming aware of breast problems (Lauver, 1994; Meechan, Collins, & Petrie, 2003). Health care providers may be able to circumvent such delays by using routine health screening visits as an opportunity to confirm women's awareness of the signs and symptoms of breast cancer, as well as assess women's beliefs about outcomes of seeking care for breast problems (Grunfeld, Hunter, Ramirez, & Richards, 2003; Lauver & Angerame, 1993).

Addressing Myths About Breast Cancer

It is important for health care providers to be aware of health myths and rumors, so that they can offer clarification and reassurance to women. There are a surprising number of myths about breast cancer risk factors. Examples of factors that have been claimed as breast cancer risk factors—but not supported by research—include fibrocystic disease, trauma (including aggressive fondling of the breast), ill-fitting bras, and the use of certain antiperspirants (Keitel & Kopala, 2000).

Diagnosis of Breast Cancer

In adult women with breast symptoms, interval changes, or suspicious findings on screening examinations, the triple test is usually considered an appropriate diagnostic evaluation (Foxcroft et al., 2001). The triple test is not an actual test, but instead a way of confirming benign changes using diagnostic techniques—namely, physical examination, —diagnostic mammogram or other imaging techniques, and biopsy.

Diagnostic Mammograms

Diagnostic mammograms are usually performed based on a routine screening mammogram or physical signs or symptoms that are probably benign or suspicious of breast cancer. These mammograms usually involve additional views of the breast, focused on the area of concern. Women who are recalled for diagnostic mammograms often experience increased levels of anxiety and depression, regardless of the outcome (Ekeberg, Skjauff, & Kåresen, 2001; Thorne, Harris, Hislop, & Vestrup, 1999), indicating a need for open communication and support from health care providers about the need for and anticipated outcomes of appropriate follow-up. This procedure usually takes longer than a screening mammogram because more X rays are obtained to view the breast in more detail or from several angles.

Other Imaging Techniques

Breast ultrasonography uses high-frequency sound waves that bounce off of tissues and other internal structures to produce a two-dimensional image of the breast. It has recently been approved to provide a more detailed picture of suspicious findings and lesions identified on mammogram or for evaluating palpable masses in younger women who have denser breasts or may be pregnant or breast-feeding. A breast ultrasound is an excellent way to identify benign findings, because it allows the radiologist to visualize the margins of a mass as well as determine whether it is cystic or solid (which may indicate the need for a biopsy). However, its effectiveness depends in part on technician skill, and it is associated with a high false-negative rate. Ultrasonography is being used increasingly in women with breast implants to evaluate implant integrity, with suspected breast cancer to look for other areas of involvement (e.g., axillary), and following breast cancer surgery to monitor and manage seromas and hematomas and evaluate the area for breast cancer recurrence (Fine, 2000).

Magnetic resonance imaging (MRI) using contrast enhancement techniques is becoming an important adjunct to other diagnostic techniques for the evaluation of suspicious findings on mammogram (particularly in women with dense breasts), preoperative characterization of tumors, and postoperative monitoring of breast cancer (National Comprehensive Cancer Network, 2007). MRIs create hundreds of detailed images of the breast, which is imaged within a depression with surrounding coils on the scanning table while the patient lies prone and the scanning table moves through a tube-like machine that contains a magnet. Fatty tissue can be excluded from the digital images, and contrast enhancement supports visualization of areas of vascularity, which may be increased around areas of cancer. MRI is also used to evaluate breast implant integrity and can differentiate implant complications from other inflammatory lesions. However, it is associated with a higher false-positive rate than traditional mammogram (and therefore additional testing), in that it identifies as suspicious findings that turn out later to be benign. Its widespread use is primarily limited by its high cost and the availability of appropriate equipment (e.g., coils) dedicated to breast imaging.

Nuclear medicine studies, such as scintimammography and positron emission tomography, involve intravenous injection of a radioactive substance (e.g., technetium sestamibi, fluorodeoxyglucose) followed by special visualization of the radioactive signal as it travels to breast tissue that is more vascular or metabolically active, depending on the type of substance. These studies are not currently in wide use for breast cancer screening or diagnosis, but may be useful in women with dense breasts and in evaluating breast cancer metastasis (Fraker, 2004). Current research is ongoing to improve these technologies and their ability to characterize smaller, malignant tumors.

Breast Biopsies

Suspicious findings on physical examination, screening or diagnostic mammogram, or other radiological exams may indicate the need for a breast biopsy. Overall, 80% of breast biopsies prove to be benign (Keitel & Kopala, 2000), which explains why clinicians and re-

searchers continue to try to identify more sensitive and specific noninvasive imaging techniques. However, the rate of malignancy does increase with age, with over 75% of breast masses in older women being cancerous (Whitaker-Worth et al., 2000). Some women, particularly those with fibrocystic breasts, may go through repeated breast biopsies. Pathologic evaluation of the breast biopsy tissue can determine whether a mass is benign or malignant and provide more specific information about the breast cancer cells (e.g., type of cancer, how aggressive it is). Although the goal of a breast biopsy is to limit discomfort and prevent breast tissue scarring (which can complicate future mammogram follow-up), biopsies may be more or less invasive, depending on the size of the biopsy needle or surgical excision (Fine, 2000). The choice of biopsy technique is often guided by the characteristics of the breast problem but may also be determined by the availability of equipment, the physician's skill with the technique, the patient's preferences (e.g., to fully remove the abnormality), or insurance coverage. Generally, when a breast biopsy is performed, a woman is given the results and then further treatment, if needed, is discussed; the decision to carry it out is made at a later time. However, on rare occasions, rather than this two-step approach, a woman will give consent before the biopsy to have a mastectomy or breast-conserving surgery if cancer is detected.

Periareolar *fine-needle aspiration biopsy* (FNAB) has been used to obtain fluid and tissue from clinically palpable breast masses and is the least invasive of the breast biopsy techniques. In brief, local anesthetic is injected before a very thin needle is inserted in multiple directions in the area of breast change while fluid is aspirated. This procedure is generally faster and less painful than other types of biopsies, but it may result in insufficient sampling in the area of concern (Fine, 2000). The lump is usually palpated during the procedure, or, if the lump is difficult to palpate, needle placement may be guided by ultrasonography or mammographic techniques. If the fluid withdrawn through the needle is clear, the lump is more likely a benign cyst. Cloudy or bloody fluid or fluid with small tissue fragments warrants careful pathological evaluation.

Stereotactic core or tru-cut needle biopsy involves the removal of a small cylinder of tissue using a slightly larger needle and guided by three-dimensional mammographic, ultrasound, or MRI views of the breast. This procedure is associated with fewer false-negative results compared to FNAB (Fine, 2000). Two new stereotactic techniques—the Mammotome® vacuum-assisted system and Advanced Breast Biopsy Instrument—involve insertion of a probe through which a slightly larger core of breast tissue can be removed. A core needle biopsy may involve some bruising and minimal scarring. Sedation may be used during the procedure to minimize the discomfort of positioning.

Excisional or surgical biopsy generally involves the removal of an entire lesion and surrounding margins under local anesthesia and usually with intravenous sedation. Although only a portion of a lesion may be removed, with newer stereotactic and sampling techniques, a core biopsy will generally be performed if full excision is not the goal. An excisional biopsy allows for a more complete pathological evaluation, including size, histology, and receptor status. Wire localization of the abnormality may be used, in which a thin needle is guided into the lesion by multiple X rays, and a thin wire is passed through the needle into the site. Once the needle is removed, the wire remains as a surgical guide for the area to be removed. Some minimal scarring of the breast may result from a surgical biopsy.

Diagnostic Findings

Hyperplasia

Hyperplasia or proliferative breast disease may be associated with an increased risk of breast cancer. Approximately 20% of women with diagnostic findings of proliferative breast disease have atypical hyperplasia, which is associated with a four-fold or greater increased risk for breast cancer (Cristofanilli et al., 2000; Dupont & Page, 1985).

Calcifications

Although many women have some calcifications in the breast, most of them are benign. Calcifications that are larger, clustered, higher in volume (number in a defined area), and irregular are more indicative of malignancy (Jeske et al., 2000). Up to 90% of diagnosed, nonpalpable ductal carcinoma in situ cases and 70% of other breast cancers are identified on the basis of microcalcifications (Jeske et al., 2000).

Breast Carcinoma

Breast cancer is the most common form of cancer in women, and their second most common cause of cancer death (Jemal et al., 2007). Estimates are that the average breast cancer remains occult (not clinically manifested) for 5 to 8 years before it is diagnosed (Brewster & DiSaia, 2000).

Carcinoma In Situ. Carcinoma in situ is considered a noninvasive, rather than invasive, form of breast cancer—a distinction that may be confusing and anxiety producing for some women, who are still usually advised to undergo surgical and medical treatment regimens (Dow, 2004). Lobular carcinoma in situ is sometimes classified as a noninvasive breast cancer, but it is more often considered a high-risk condition rather than a true cancer and

may be followed by observation (e.g., routine, diagnostic mammograms) alone (Fraker, 2004; Whitaker-Worth et al., 2000). Ductal carcinoma in situ (DCIS) is a true noninvasive breast cancer lesion, usually discovered on mammogram, and it accounts for 10% to 20% of breast cancer diagnoses (Fraker, 2004; Whitaker-Worth et al., 2000). It is often associated with more adverse pathological factors in younger compared to older women (Vicini & Recht, 2002). The cumulative, 10-year risk of developing an invasive breast cancer after carcinoma in situ has been estimated to be four times that of the general population, with the risk slightly higher for women diagnosed before age 55 than for older women (Crocetti, Miccinesi, Paci, & Zappa, 2001). Carcinoma in situ is often treated by breast-conserving surgery.

Invasive Carcinoma. Invasive breast cancers can be broadly divided into ductal and lobular carcinomas. Ductal or infiltrating ductal carcinoma is the most common form of breast cancer, accounting for up to 85% of invasive breast carcinomas with the remaining 15% coming from the lobular structures (Fraker, 2004; Jeske et al., 2000).

Although both the ductal and lobular types of breast cancer usually involve a dense mass with spiculated or irregular margins, lobular carcinoma is less distinct and more difficult to palpate clinically or diagnose on mammogram, particularly in women with dense breasts (Fraker, 2004; Goldschmidt, 2000; Li, Anderson, Daling, & Moe, 2003). Invasive carcinomas may also be associated with areas of DCIS, which, if extensive, may require a total mastectomy (Winchester, 2000). Poorly differentiated invasive carcinomas are considered more aggressive and associated with a poorer prognosis. Prognosis is thought to be better for women with tumors in the upper lateral quadrant of the breast than for those located elsewhere and worse for tumors located greater distances from the axilla (e.g., medial quadrant; Kroman, Wohlfahrt, Mouridsen, & Melbye, 2003).

Inflammatory Breast Cancer. Inflammatory breast cancer is a rare and very aggressive cancer that involves widespread lymph node involvement, a peau d'orange (erythematous and dimpled) appearance to the skin, and, at times, nipple retraction. The breast may be tender, warm, and edematous, and there is an underlying mass in 30% to 65% of cases (Whitaker-Worth et al., 2000). This type of cancer generally involves initial treatment with combination chemotherapy, which may then allow surgical resection (Jeske et al., 2000).

Paget's Disease. Paget's disease of the nipple is rare but may be diagnosed by cytological smear from nipple discharge or needle biopsy (and not to be confused with Paget's disease of the bone). It often appears as a thickening, scaling, itching, or excoriation of the skin on or around the nipple and areola that does not heal with topical medications (Jeske et al., 2000). Nipple retraction and serous or bloody discharge from the nipple may be accompanied by pain, crusting, and pruritis. These surface manifestations usually reflect an underlying breast malignancy that is ductal in origin (Whitaker-Worth et al., 2000). Prognosis is generally excellent with surgical treatment and chemotherapy, depending on the degree of invasion into the breast.

Other Breast Cancers.   Papillary tumors, which may be noninvasive or invasive, are found in approximately 1% to 2% of breast cancers, usually in older women, and occur more often in the central portion of the breast, associated with nipple discharge (Brenin, Hibshoosh, & Kinne, 2000). Papillary tumors generally have a more favorable prognosis, are rarely associated with axillary spread, and can be removed using breast-conserving surgery. Phyllodes tumor is a very rare, but usually benign, breast tumor that develops in the breast's connective tissue rather than the ducts or lobules. Both benign and malignant phyllodes tumors are treated by surgical excision, although surgical management of the malignant form usually involves removal of a wide margin of normal tissue or mastectomy, if normal margins cannot be obtained (National Comprehensive Cancer Network, 2007). Sarcomas, primary lymphoma or melanoma of the breast, Bowen's disease, and basal cell carcinoma are all cancerous conditions of the breast, but are extremely rare. Metastasis of other cancers to the breast is rare but may appear as lesions on the anterior chest wall that mimic shingles (herpes zoster; Whitaker-Worth et al., 2000).

Determining Breast Cancer Stage and Tumor Behavior

Determining cancer stage and tumor characteristics are critical steps in the process of diagnosing any cancer. Staging usually defines the extent and severity of a cancer, thereby providing information about a patient's prognosis, and, more importantly, guides appropriate surgical and medical treatment and short- and long-term clinical follow-up. There are many systems for staging cancers; however, the TNM system is used most widely and is accepted by the American Joint Committee on Cancer and the International Union Against Cancer (Fraker, 2004).

TNM Staging System

The TNM staging system categorizes cancers based on the size of the tumor (T), its spread to the lymph nodes (N), and the presence of any metastasis (M). A number is added to each letter to indicate extent (e.g., of spread). For breast cancer, and many other cancers, the TNM combinations are categorized into one of five

stages, indicating a progressively worsening 5-year prognosis (from 100% 5-year survival at stage 0 to approximately 20% survival at stage IV):

- Stage 0: Carcinoma in situ or noninvasive breast cancer; Paget's disease of the nipple is usually classified at this stage.
- Stage I: Local involvement only; the tumor measures up to 2 cm and there is no lymph node involvement.
- Stage II: The tumor measures 2 to 5 cm or there is some axillary lymph node involvement (one to three lymph nodes).
- Stage III: Regional involvement (e.g., other parts of the breast or nearby lymph nodes); the tumor size is greater than 5 cm; there is extensive lymph node involvement; or the cancer has spread to the breast skin, chest wall, or internal mammary lymph nodes; inflammatory breast cancer is usually classified at this stage.
- Stage IV: Advanced breast cancer, distant metastasis, or spread beyond the breast, underarm, and internal mammary lymph nodes, and to other organs (e.g., bones, liver, lungs, or brain).

Tumor Characteristics

Estrogen and Progesterone Receptors.   Breast cancers are also classified based on whether the tumor is sensitive to hormones. Hormone receptor assays are used to guide treatment—particularly the use of hormone therapies—and can indicate the tumor's aggressiveness. Estrogen receptor positive tumors are more commonly seen in postmenopausal women, are slower growing, and can be treated with hormone or endocrine therapy (a cancer therapy not to be confused with menopausal hormone therapy). Estrogen receptor negative tumors proliferate more rapidly and are associated with an overall poorer prognosis, in part because they are rarely responsive to (and may be worsened by) hormonal therapy (Keitel & Kopala, 2000). Women who carry the BRCA1 mutation often have estrogen receptor negative tumors (Clark, 2004). Progesterone receptor positive tumors may benefit from adjuvant hormonal therapy (Bardou, Arpino, Elledge, Osborne, & Clark, 2003).

HER2/neu Positive Tumors.   About one of every four breast cancers has too much HER2/neu, a growth-promoting protein, or oncogene. Testing a tumor's HER2/neu status is now standard practice (Ross et al., 2003). In the past, HER2/neu-positive tumors (which are more likely to be ER negative and PR negative) were associated with a less favorable outlook than those that were HER2/neu-negative. However, trastuzumab (Herceptin®), a newer synthetic antibody, can be used to prevent the HER2/neu protein from stimulating breast cancer cell growth.

Lymph Node Dissection and Sentinel Node Biopsy

Because lymph node status is a critical component of breast cancer staging systems, removal and pathological evaluation of lymph nodes are a high priority for guiding treatment. Axillary lymph node dissection at the time of surgery, with the removal of at least 10 nodes, has been associated with significant morbidity (e.g., pain and swelling, chronic lymphedema; Fraker, 2004). Because lymph node dissection in women older than 70 is not associated with increased survival, some surgeons recommend deferring the procedure to prevent postsurgical axillary complications (Newlin, Reiling, & Nichols, 2002).

A technique known as sentinel node biopsy (SNB) is being used increasingly to spare women the more extensive axillary lymph node dissection and its resultant morbidity. SNB typically involves the preoperative injection of a dye into the breast tumor to determine the first node that malignant cells would encounter as they leave the breast. The sentinel lymph node (or nodes, depending on the size of the tumor) to be stained by the dye can then be visualized, removed surgically, and evaluated pathologically. If the sentinel node is positive for cancer, axillary lymph nodes are removed during surgery. If the sentinel node is cancer free, it is likely (with up to 98% accuracy) that all other axillary nodes are cancer free as well (Fraker, 2004). SNB is often carried out as an accompaniment to breast-conserving surgery or mastectomy (Lyman et al., 2005; Veronesi et al., 2003). Although it is associated with a high detection rate and a low false-negative rate (less than 5%), its success depends on the clinical team's experience and skill with the procedure (Schwartz, Ciuliano, Veronesi, & the Consensus Conference Committee, 2002). SNB is not expected to result in better survival, but it has been associated with significantly less morbidity than axillary lymph node dissection (Schijven et al., 2003).

Breast Cancer Treatments

Treatment for breast cancer, based on its stage and tumor characteristics, currently involves one or more of the following strategies: surgery, radiation therapy, chemotherapy, or hormonal therapy. The National Comprehensive Cancer Network maintains free, online (www.nccn.org), evidence-based clinical practice guidelines on breast cancer treatment, based on the consensus of a panel of experts in the field.

Surgical Treatment

Breast surgery for cancer, including cutting of the breast, cauterization of bleeding, and removal of tumors as well as swellings under the armpit, has been documented since the first century (Thorne & Murray, 2000; Yalom, 1997). In the 1880s, the Halsted procedure was developed, involving not only the removal of the breast, but also the muscles of the chest wall, the lymph glands, and all surrounding fat tissue (Thorne & Murray, 2000). This technique, including, at times, bilateral oophorectomy, became the surgical standard for breast cancer for over 60 years (Thorne & Murray, 2000; Yalom, 1997). To this day, most patients with early-stage disease will have surgical intervention as the first phase of their breast cancer treatment (see Figure 28.2). Over the last several decades—particularly as breast cancer is being detected at earlier stages—surgical management has shifted from radical mastectomy to modified radical mastectomy to breast-conserving surgery (Sener & Lee, 2000).

Breast-Conserving Surgery. The treatment of choice for women with DCIS and smaller tumors confined to one area is breast-conserving surgery (BCS)—accompanied by radiation therapy and, rarely, axillary lymph node assessment if the cancer is located in an area that would make future SNB difficult—which allows a satisfactory cosmetic outcome and comparable distant metastasis and survival rates to those of more extensive surgeries (National Comprehensive Cancer Network, 2007). BCS with axillary lymph node staging and radiation therapy (with or followed by adjuvant therapy) also may be appropriate for women with early-stage breast cancer. A quadrantectomy or partial or segmental mastectomy is a special type of BCS that may be carried out if removal of more breast tissue than a lumpectomy (up to one-quarter of the breast) is needed. Women diagnosed with breast cancer in the early months of pregnancy are not good candidates for BCS if postoperative radiation therapy is indicated (Winchester, 2000). Even with early-stage breast cancer, a woman and her surgeon may choose mastectomy over BCS (Apantaku, 2002) if the radiation therapy schedule will be problematic or if a woman has two or more affected areas on the breast, a larger tumor relative to her breast size, a tumor that does not shrink much with neoadjuvant (preoperative) chemotherapy, had previous radiation therapy to the affected breast, scleroderma, or positive surgical margins during BCS (Fenner & Mustoe, 2000; National Comprehensive Cancer Network, 2007; Winchester, 2000). Women can usually go home the day of or the day after BCS, and recovery is usually rapid, although decreased sensation in the breast and a change in the size and shape of the breast may be noted (Keitel & Kopala, 2000). For most women with early-stage breast cancer, BCS is associated with survival rates comparable to other breast surgeries. However, local (i.e., in-breast) recurrence associated with BCS is slightly higher in some studies (Poggi et al., 2003; Vrieling et al., 2003).

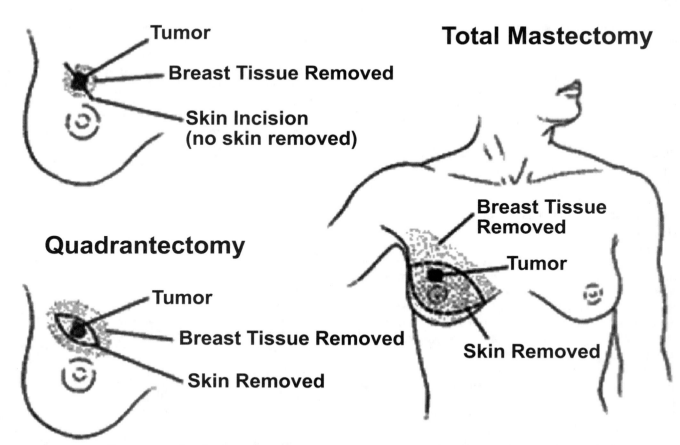

Figure 28.2 Surgical treatments for breast cancer; the extent of breast tissue and skin removed during the most common types of breast cancer surgeries.
From American Cancer Society, 2007. Reprinted by the permission of the American Cancer Society, Inc. from www.cancer.org

Mastectomy. Despite the dramatic increase in the use of BCS since the 1990s, mastectomy is still commonly performed, particularly in later-stage cancers. Radical mastectomy is rarely done today, because the modified radical mastectomy has been shown to be just as effective and is now the most commonly performed mastectomy procedure, involving the removal of the breast and some axillary lymph nodes only. A total or simple mastectomy with removal of the entire breast, but not axillary lymph nodes or muscle tissue, may be performed for multicentric DCIS; if SNB is negative; or, prophylactically, in high-risk women. Most women who have a modified radical mastectomy can go home the day after surgery. Drains, which may stay in place for up to 2 weeks, are often placed to remove blood and lymph fluid and decrease the changes of a seroma. Women may have little pain in the breast area, but they may experience new sensations (e.g., numbness, pinching, pulling) and other possible side effects in the axillary region.

Radiation Therapy

Radiation therapy is frequently used to treat the intact breast after BCS and postmastectomy patients at high risk for local or regional recurrence. If radiation therapy is indicated, it will generally be started within approximately 12 weeks of surgery, after the breast cancer has been removed, the surgical wound has healed, and comfortable arm movement is restored. Postmastectomy radiation therapy may be indicated following adjuvant chemotherapy in women with larger tumors and/or positive axillary lymph nodes who are at high risk for local or regional recurrence (National Comprehensive Cancer Network, 2007). Radiation therapy involves a substantial time commitment over the short term; it is usually scheduled for 5 days a week for approximately 6 weeks.

The goal of radiation therapy is to destroy any remaining cancer cells in the breast area but minimize radiation to healthy surrounding tissue. A standard course of external beam radiation therapy may include "boost" radiation, delivered during the final week of therapy specifically to the site of the tumor (Perun, 2004). Brachytherapy (internal or interstitial radiation), rather than external beam radiation, is sometimes used to deliver the radiation boost and involves placing a small radioactive seed or pellet directly into the area of the breast cancer and allowing it to dwell for a 24- to 48-hour hospital stay. In recent years, more women have had MammoSite, a special type of brachytherapy, in which a balloon is passed into the lumpectomy area and filled with saline (Perun, 2004; Shah & Wazer, 2005). The radioactive material is placed temporarily into the balloon twice daily for 5 days. Other new techniques are currently undergoing clinical trial evaluation. Partial breast irradiation more specifically focuses the radiation therapy and may shorten the amount of time needed for radiation therapy to 5 days or less (Arthur & Vicini, 2005).

Although modern radiotherapy techniques minimize adverse effects seen in the past (e.g., cardiac injury), some effects may last for several weeks after the treatment period is over. Side effects may include asymptomatic rib fractures, severe rash, fatigue, edema, thickening or darkening of the skin, as well as an increased risk of lymphedema (LaCombe & Bloomer, 2000; Wengström, Häggmark, Strander, & Forsberg, 2000). Careful attention to skin care recommendations (e.g., avoid direct sunlight, direct cold, irritating soaps, and tight clothing) can be helpful in preventing or minimizing these side effects (Perun, 2004).

Neoadjuvant Therapy

Neoadjuvant therapy for breast cancer refers to chemotherapy or hormonal therapy administered preoperatively to reduce tumor size. It also may be used to minimize the amount of surgical intervention that is needed or to ensure that the tumor can be better managed with radiation therapy. A good response to neoadjuvant therapy will sometimes allow BCS to be carried out, even though initial tumor size might indicate that a mastectomy should be considered (Geddie, 2004b; Kaufmann et al., 2003). Neoadjuvant therapy (or preoperative systemic therapy) is typically considered for women with inflammatory breast cancer or those who wish to delay surgery for some reason (Kaufmann et al., 2003). Neoadjuvant therapy, however, has not been shown to be more effective than postoperative adjuvant therapy (Kaufmann et al., 2003; Locker, 2000).

Adjuvant Therapy

The goals of surgery, radiation therapy, and neoadjuvant therapy for breast cancer are local and regional treatment. The goal of adjuvant therapy, which generally involves cytotoxic chemotherapeutic agents or the use of hormonal therapy, is systemic treatment. Adjuvant therapy is deemed appropriate when concerns about clinically occult micrometastases or systemic spread of the cancer are raised because of a particularly large tumor or findings of positive axillary lymph nodes (Geddie, 2004b). For most women with intermediate or high risk of recurrence, these benefits of adjuvant therapy far exceed the risks or side effects (Hortobagyi, 2001). Various prognostic and predictive factors are used to determine appropriate adjuvant therapy, including TNM stage, tumor characteristics (e.g., hormone receptor status), the individual woman's situation (e.g., menopausal status), and, more recently, genomic/gene expression microarray techniques to characterize the cancer (e.g., Oncotype DX™, MammaPrint®; National Comprehensive Cancer Network, 2007). In some situations (e.g., selected older women with comorbid disease), systemic therapy alone (without surgery) may be considered (Enger et al., 2006). Evidence indicates that high-dose treatment regimens (with stem cell or bone marrow transplant) are not associated with a clear survival advantage over standard adjuvant therapy, so these regimens are not offered outside of a randomized clinical trial, but research is ongoing (NIH Consensus Conference, 1991). A discussion of the various adjuvant therapy medications and regimens is beyond the scope of this chapter. However, some key considerations are identified below.

Chemotherapy. Adjuvant chemotherapy regimens may be administered orally, intravenously, or intramuscularly. Combination (or poly-) chemotherapy is generally appropriate for most women with locally invasive breast cancer, regardless of lymph node, menopausal, or hormone receptor status (NIH Consensus Conference, 1991). It is usually begun on an outpatient basis approximately 4 to 12 weeks after surgery and lasts 3 to 6 months or longer, depending on the patient's response to treatment (Geddie, 2004b). Chemotherapy cycles are often spaced so that the woman's body can recover before the next treatment cycle.

Hormonal Therapy. Hormonal (endocrine) therapy includes selective estrogen receptor modulators, aromatase inhibitors, and antiestrogens. Available agents and their indications are continually evolving as new clinical trial results become available. The goal of adjuvant hormonal therapy (not to be confused with menopausal hormone therapy) is to limit hormonal stimulation of cancer cells and therefore reduce the risk of recurrence or new primary breast cancer (National Comprehensive Cancer Network, 2007). The decision about adjuvant hormonal therapy is based on the tumor's stage, a woman's menopausal status, and the presence of estrogen or progesterone receptor proteins in the tumor (Tallman et al., 2003).

The most firmly established adjuvant hormonal therapy for both premenopausal and postmenopausal women with estrogen receptor positive tumors is tamoxifen, given for up to 5 years, generally following any adjuvant chemotherapy (Cummings, 2002). Newer aromatase inhibitors (e.g., anastrozole, letrozole, exemestane) have been shown to be highly effective in the adjuvant setting for postmenopausal women and may be given as sole hormonal therapy or following tamoxifen therapy (National Comprehensive Cancer Network, 2007). Except in the context of a randomized clinical trial, aromatase inhibitors are not appropriate for premenopausal women, even if they become amenorrheic postoperatively, because current agents are not likely to suppress estrogen levels sufficiently to be of benefit if some ovarian function still exists (Winer et al., 2002). Both tamoxifen and aromatase inhibitors can cause menopausal-like symptoms, consistent with estrogen withdrawal (Dienger, 2004). Aromatase inhibitors are also associated with musculoskeletal symptoms and osteoporosis, while tamoxifen is associated with an increased risk of uterine cancer and deep venous thrombosis (National Comprehensive Cancer Network, 2007).

Although tamoxifen and aromatase inhibitors are often described as antiestrogens, ovarian suppression with other types of antiestrogen agents (e.g., fulvestrant, toremifene) or surgical or radiation-induced ovarian ablation may be appropriate to limit hormonal stimulation of cancer cells in premenopausal breast cancer patients with hormone-receptor positive tumors (National Comprehensive Cancer Network, 2007). For women who undergo ovarian suppression or ablation, hormonal therapy is a consideration if postmenopausal status can be firmly established.

Immunotherapy. Trastuzumab (Herceptin®) is a monoclonal antibody developed to specifically bind to the HER2/neu protein, a protein that is normally present on the extracellular surface of breast cells but is overexpressed in some breast cancers, causing them to grow more quickly. Intravenous trastuzumab is used to prevent the HER2/neu protein from making breast cancer cells grow in women whose tumors overexpress HER2/neu and may also stimulate the immune system to more effectively attack cancers that overexpress the HER2/neu protein, which makes it useful in preventing or containing breast cancer metastasis in some women. The combination of trastuzumab with chemotherapy (either concurrently or sequentially) may be more effective than chemotherapy alone in women with HER2-positive breast cancer tumors (National Comprehensive Cancer Network, 2007). HER2 status, however, does not guide the choice of hormonal therapy (National Institutes of Health Consensus Development Panel, 2001). Trastuzumab may be associated with cardiac side effects, so its use with other cardiotoxic chemotherapeutic agents is not advised, and cardiac status should be monitored.

Stem Cell Transplantation. The use of stem cell or bone marrow transplantation has been proposed as a breast cancer treatment that allows the use of much higher doses of adjuvant therapy than used conventionally. Although transplantation has been shown to be effective with other cancers, research to date has shown no survival advantage in advanced breast cancer, and this procedure continues to be evaluated primarily in clinical trials (Keitel & Kopala, 2000). Although some studies of stem cell transplant have shown a longer time to recurrence, transplant-related complications have developed at a higher rate such that conventional-dose adjuvant chemotherapy remains the standard treatment of choice (Tallman et al., 2003).

Complementary and Alternative Medicine Therapies

A diagnosis of breast cancer and its treatment is a profound psychosocial and physical experience for women, which makes complementary and alternative medicine (CAM) therapies, with their focus on the mind-body connection, of special interest to women affected by this disease. Some of these therapies have strong roots in ancient healing practices, such as Chinese medicine and traditional folk practices. Others have developed in recent years as some women have felt dissatisfied and, at times, dehumanized by their clinical experience with breast cancer. Up to half of women with breast cancer may choose one or more CAM therapies to make conventional therapies more tolerable (e.g., relaxation and meditation techniques) or to directly impact cancer cells (Henderson & Donatelle, 2003; Ishida, 2004; Keitel & Kopala, 2000). Although the research evidence basis for these therapies lags far behind that of more conventional therapies for breast cancer, there is a growing recognition of the potential value for such therapies and the need to be aware of and stay informed about their risks and benefits. Such awareness on the part of women and their health care providers can enhance open communication, mutual respect, and continued engagement during the course of a woman's breast cancer experience.

Clinical Trials

Newer treatments for breast cancer—whether surgical, radiological, or medical—are being tested in ongoing clinical trials. For women whose breast cancer is not responsive to conventional treatments or who have special circumstances that make conventional treatment problematic, referral to a clinical trial regimen is an appropriate consideration. Oncologists are generally aware of clinical trials currently open to recruitment and can refer patients to appropriate centers. In addition, the Clinicaltrials.gov database, a service of the

National Institutes of Health, can be searched by condition, treatment, and location for current clinical trials.

Follow-Up Care

Follow-up care after the acute phase of breast cancer treatment focuses primarily on more frequent monitoring for the recurrence of breast cancer as well as long-term side effects of some cancer therapies (e.g., cardiac toxicity, skin healing, lymphedema). Generally, the first posttreatment (new baseline) mammogram after BCS is carried out 3 to 6 months after completion of treatment and repeated on at least an annual basis thereafter (Jeske et al., 2000). Clinical follow-up with physical examination is generally carried out every 3 to 6 months for the first 3 years, and then on a semiannual basis until 5 years postdiagnosis, after which annual follow-up is reinstituted (Apantaku, 2002). The physical examination focuses on evaluation of the tumor site and incision, where most recurrences are located. Additional assessment of regional lymph nodes, along with a standard physical examination and review of systems are done to monitor for resolution of side effects and any long-term effects of treatment.

Women report being very anxious about follow-up visits; some reexperience the emotions and distress of the early breast cancer experience (Allen, 2002; Loveys & Klaich, 1991), so it is critical that sufficient time is scheduled to discuss and process psychosocial as well as physical concerns. Another key component of breast cancer follow-up is education. Women may appreciate reminders about community resources for psychosocial counseling and peer support, in addition to the usual discussion about ongoing monitoring for physical changes, pain and wound management, and lymphedema precautions (which are appropriate even for women who have undergone sentinel lymph node biopsy, because a very small percentage may still experience some axillary symptoms; Lynn, 2004).

Impact of Breast Cancer

A diagnosis of breast cancer may represent a major turning point in a woman's life, with a myriad of emotional and physical implications that can have a profound impact on her family and friends as well. The diagnosis and treatment may be the first time a woman has had to relinquish control of her physical health and daily life to others. The treatment and its side effects can result in permanent changes in her body. Many women describe a process of reevaluating themselves and their relationships with others during the experience, as the demands of the illness are experienced in every aspect of their lives—daily routines; family and social experiences; and their perspectives on the past, present, and future (Loveys & Klaich, 1991).

Information Gathering and Decision Making

The many decisions that must be made once a woman receives a diagnosis of breast cancer can be overwhelming, because she must decide about treatment, reconstruction, choosing appropriate health care providers, facilities, and arranging insurance coverage, among others (Sepucha, Belkora, Mutchnick, & Esserman, 2002). Most women prefer to have as many details as possible and to participate in decision making (Jahraus, Sokolosky, Thurston, & Guo, 2002). However, there is some variability in the amount of information a woman wants about breast cancer, her particular situation, and the extent to which she can participate in decision making about treatment, but most prefer to be informed and involved (Keitel & Kopala, 2000). Studies of decision making about breast cancer treatment indicate that perceptions of having no choice in treatment were associated with increased physical symptoms and psychosocial distress (Mandelblatt et al., 2003; Morris & Royle, 1988). Although enhanced communication may be associated with a sense of having more choices about treatment (Liang et al., 2002), clinical encounters are typically time limited, making it difficult for the health care provider to fully determine and address a woman's needs and overwhelming for the woman who is trying to understand new content and jargon. Sometimes, having a caring family member or friend along or taping the clinical encounter can help women to absorb more fully the information being discussed. There is also a great deal of information about breast cancer and its treatment options available on the Internet, in magazines, and in books, but the volume of this information, some of which is targeted for more clinically trained audiences, can be overwhelming—particularly if one seeks guidance that is up to date, accurate, meaningful, and unbiased. Exhibit 28.2 identifies several excellent Internet sources of information for patients and their loved ones.

Side Effects of Treatment

Treatment-related side effects are largely due to the fact that chemotherapeutic agents attack cells that are rapidly turning over, including bone marrow, gastrointestinal, and hair follicle cells. The result is increased fatigue, nausea, and hair loss (Keitel & Kopala, 2000).

Fatigue. Women with breast cancer report that fatigue is one of the more universal physical changes they experience as the treatment course progresses (de Jong, Candel, Schouten, Abu-Saad, & Courtens, 2004). It is a multidimensional phenomenon, and there are many possible explanations for this profound fatigue, including recovery from the initial surgery, neutropenia or anemia induced by the adjuvant treatment regimen, side effects of radiation therapy, side effects of other medications, decreased nutritional intake during

EXHIBIT 28.2 INTERNET RESOURCES ON BREAST CANCER

For Health Care Professionals
- National Cancer Institute (pages for health professionals): www.cancer.gov
- American Cancer Society (pages for health professionals): www.cancer.org
- National Comprehensive Cancer Network: www.nccn.org
- ClinicalTrials.gov: www.clinicaltrials.gov

For Women With Breast Cancer and Their Families
- National Cancer Institute (pages for patients): www.cancer.gov
- American Cancer Society (pages for patients, including Reach to Recovery): www.cancer.org
- Susan G. Komen Foundation: www.komen.org
- Breastcancer.org: www.breastcancer.org
- Y-Me National Breast Cancer Organization: www.y-me.org
- National Lymphedema Network: www.lymphnet.org

periods of nausea and vomiting, emotional distress, or poor sleep quality (Denison et al., 2003; Velez-Barone, 2004). Sleep disturbances may be related to adjuvant therapy, physical discomforts, or emotional distress. Management of sleep problems and insomnia may help minimize fatigue and other concerns, such as cognitive changes (Quesnel, Savard, Simard, Ivers, & Morin, 2003; Velez-Barone, 2004). Fatigue may be particularly problematic for older women and those who have had prior cancer treatments or bone metastasis (Geddie, 2004a). Energy-conserving strategies are usually recommended for coping with cancer-related fatigue—scheduling activities (including rest), delegating, arranging the environment to minimize extra steps and effort, and setting appropriate priorities (Velez-Barone, 2004). Although women should discuss exercise plans with their physician, a regular exercise schedule has been associated with reduced fatigue, even during the acute phase of breast cancer (Schwartz, Mori, & Jao, 2001).

Nausea and Vomiting. Nausea and (sometimes) vomiting associated with chemotherapy may be mild to highly problematic, depending on the agent used. Some women experience anticipatory nausea just approaching the outpatient clinic for their treatments (Tomoyasu, Bovbjerg, & Jacobsen, 1996). Newer antiemetic agents are available to help with the nausea associated with the acute phase of chemotherapy. Some CAM therapies such as relaxation training, guided imagery, and hypnosis also have been used to cope with these side effects (Geddie, 2004a). Changing to a bland diet or foods that do not have strong odors or a spicy taste may help.

Hair Loss. Alopecia as a side effect of some chemotherapeutic agents is usually temporary; and hair grows back several months after treatment is completed. However, women may notice some changes in the color, texture, and pattern of the hair that grows back. Many women use scarves, hats, and wigs and will cut long hair to minimize the amount of perceived hair loss. The benefits of preventive strategies such as scalp cooling have been marginal at best (MacDuff, Mackenzie, Hutcheon, Melville, & Archibald, 2003).

Cognitive Changes. Breast cancer treatment can have a noticeable impact on cognitive function, particularly in the short term, as measured by standard neuropsychiatric tests and women's reports of having difficulty with concentration, short-term memory, word-finding, and problem solving (sometimes described as "chemobrain"; Ahles et al., 2002; Loerzel, 2004; Partridge, Burstein, & Winer, 2001). Some patients (e.g., older women or those receiving specific regimens) experience long-term cognitive deficits following systemic chemotherapy.

Lymphedema and Other Upper Extremity Changes. When surgical scarring prevents lymph fluid from draining, problems with lymphedema or arm swelling and pain occur due to an abnormal accumulation of protein-rich fluid in the affected area (Armer, 2004; Keitel & Kopala, 2000). Approximately 20% to 40% of women treated for breast cancer experience lymphedema in their lifetime (Armer, 2004; Kornblith et al., 2003), with an increased risk when they have had both surgical removal of axillary lymph nodes and radiation therapy to the axilla. The risk of lymphedema is greatly reduced but still exists in women who have had sentinel node biopsy and no axillary node dissection (Armer, 2004; Blanchard, Donohue, Reynolds, & Grant, 2003). On occasion, temporary arm swelling lasts for a few weeks and then goes away. Other times, the swelling is long-lasting and may involve the trunk and scapular area with associated heaviness, pain, and limitations in arm and shoulder

EXHIBIT 28.3 LYMPHEDEMA PRECAUTIONS FOR WOMEN FOLLOWING BREAST SURGERY (SUSAN G. KOMEN FOUNDATION, 2007A)

1. Have blood draws, injections, and blood pressure measurements on the unaffected arm.
2. Wear gloves when doing house- or yardwork.
3. Keep the affected arm clean and dry, and moisturize skin after bathing.
4. Protect skin with sunscreen (at least SPF 15) and protective clothing.
5. Avoid lifting or carrying heavy bags or other objects with the affected arm.
6. Avoid wearing tight jewelry or clothing.
7. Avoid cutting cuticles during manicures.
8. Use an electric razor to shave the underarm area.
9. Avoid any type of injury, including scratches and bruises, to the at-risk arm.
10. Rest your arm in an elevated position (above your heart or shoulder).
11. When flying in an airplane, wear a compression sleeve and drink lots of fluids during the flight.
12. Use insect repellent when outdoors, but wash it off when inside.

movement. In the clinical setting, arm circumference is usually measured at selected points and compared with the unaffected arm to ensure that there is no more than a 2-cm difference between the two arms (Armer, 2004; Lynn, 2004).

Lymphedema may not occur for years after breast cancer treatment, but, once it develops, its impact on quality of life can be extensive (e.g., difficulty with sleeping, carrying things, clothing comfort and fit), so prevention and early detection are usually emphasized (Armer, 2004; Keitel & Kopala, 2000). Prevention strategies are outlined in Exhibit 28.3. Treatment involves the use of analgesics and other strategies to address pain and discomfort, properly fitting compression sleeves to support the arm, manual lymph drainage (e.g., limb elevation), exercise (e.g., swimming in moderate, not hot, water temperatures), maintaining an optimal weight, and meticulous skin care. If lymphedema is left untreated, cellulitis, lymphadenitis, open wounds, and life-threatening septicemia can develop.

Menopausal Changes. Hormonal therapy and ovarian suppression and ablation may induce menopausal symptoms such as hot flashes in premenopausal women or exacerbate symptoms in some postmenopausal women (Carpenter & Elam, 2004). Other menopausal symptoms may be experienced by up to one-half of women receiving breast cancer treatment (Keitel & Kopala, 2000; McPhail & Smith, 2000). Treatment of these symptoms can follow guidelines for women who are experiencing normal menopausal changes of aging, except that menopausal hormone therapies should be avoided. Endometrial hyperplasia and an increased risk for endometrial cancer have been associated with tamoxifen therapy,

and endometrial monitoring and prompt follow-up of unexpected vaginal bleeding during therapy are warranted. Although many premenopausal women report menopausal symptoms associated with adjuvant breast cancer treatment, younger women are more likely than older premenopausal women to resume periods and retain their fertility (Keitel & Kopala, 2000).

Other Physical Changes. As described above, radiation therapy may result in a variety of skin changes (Whitaker-Worth et al., 2000). Dry mouth or mucositis and stomatitis can be problematic with some types of chemotherapy. Arthralgias and myalgias can occur as a result of tumor involvement, metastasis, or treatment. Some women experience phantom pain after a mastectomy, particularly if they had breast pain before surgery (Velez-Barone, 2004). Pain management involves a comprehensive assessment of the pain and appropriate pharmacological and nonpharmacological (e.g., CAM) therapies. Acute and long-term cardiac and pericardial adverse effects may be associated with some chemotherapeutic agents or radiation therapy near the mediastinum (Loerzel, 2004; Partridge et al., 2001).

Dealing With Changes in Appearance

Changes in appearance and body image vary depending on the type of surgery a woman has had and the side effects she may have experienced from radiation and adjuvant therapy. However, many women describe their concerns about body image as less troublesome than other concerns related to the breast cancer experience (Figueiredo, Cullen, Hwang, Rowland, & Mandelblatt, 2004).

Prostheses

As one might expect, women who have had a mastectomy, particularly those without reconstructive surgery, identify more changes in their physical appearance and more body image issues than women with BCS or mastectomy with reconstruction (Avis, Crawford, & Manuel, 2004). Women who do not have reconstructive surgery can be fitted with a prosthesis 4 to 6 weeks postoperatively (Lynn, 2004). Many different choices exist for prostheses, and the costs will vary, but most insurance plans cover at least a portion of the expense, particularly if the prosthesis is prescribed by a physician (Lynn, 2004; Mahon & Casey, 2003). A careful fitting can take an hour or more, but it is necessary so that women will have a satisfactory cosmetic result with a breast prosthesis (Mahon & Casey, 2003). A breast prosthesis can take some time to get used to, and some women initially have a negative reaction to the result, but this response will probably improve over time (Roberts, Livingston, White, & Gibbs, 2003).

Reconstruction

Postmastectomy breast reconstruction has been carried out since the late 1800s, when a part of the woman's healthy breast was used to rebuild the mastectomy side (Musick, 1997). Advances in breast reconstruction have paralleled advances in surgical techniques for breast cancer and reflect women's increased involvement and freedom of choice during diagnosis and treatment. Although two-stage surgery is the norm for breast cancer diagnosis and treatment, immediate reconstruction during surgical treatment (typically, a skin-sparing mastectomy) is also fairly common and is associated with less psychological distress due to body image changes (Fenner & Mustoe, 2000). Reconstruction may be delayed if the woman is likely to receive chest wall radiation therapy (Winchester, 2000). Decisions about breast reconstruction are highly personal. Factors that are associated with women deciding to forgo reconstruction include older age, significant comorbidity, concerns about additional surgery or anesthesia, or concerns about achieving an appropriate cosmetic result (Baron & Vaziri, 2004).

Rather than having reconstruction with breast implants, more and more women are choosing to use autologous tissue from other parts of their body. Autologous reconstruction can be a complicated surgery, but it results in a breast with a more natural look and feel (Baron & Vaziri, 2004; Fenner & Mustoe, 2000; Grigg et al., 2003). The trans-rectus abdominis muscle flap is the usual choice for autologous reconstruction because of the associated enhanced vascular reliability, versatility, and ease of recovery (Fenner & Mustoe, 2000). If reconstruction is done using implants, tissue expanders are often inserted under the pectoralis major muscle to allow a gradual increase over 6 to 8 weeks to the desired breast size (Baron & Vaziri, 2004; Mansel & Bundred, 1995). Regardless of the reconstructive technique chosen, nipple reconstruction is usually delayed until recovery from breast reconstruction (e.g., tissue expansion) is completed. Nipple reconstruction may involve nipple tattooing or reconstruction from transplanted tissue. Some women choose to use polyurethane removable nipples, rather than go through another surgical procedure.

Emotional Responses and Support Needs

Breast cancer has long been recognized as having a profound emotional impact for a woman as she is confronted with her mortality and the need to make lifestyle changes to accommodate the demands of the illness (Landmark, Strandmark, & Wahl, 2001). Emotional distress, particularly depression, can be a significant problem for some women and can exacerbate other side effects, such as fatigue and difficulty concentrating (Badger, Braden, & Mishel, 2001; Haghighat, Akbari, Holakouei, Rahimi, & Montazeri, 2003). Although most women do not experience clinical levels of psychological distress and depression (Ganz et al., 2002; Kornblith et al., 2003), women with recurrent disease sometimes experience greater difficulties with well-being than women experiencing their first diagnosis of breast cancer (Frost, Suman, et al., 2000). In addition, consistent with other research on women's moods, younger women report higher levels of depression and anxiety and slower resolution of emotional distress than older women, but older women experience a greater impact on physical aspects of quality of life (Cimprich, 1999; Cimprich, Ronis, & Martinez-Ramos, 2002; Vacek, Winstead-Fry, Secker-Walker, Hooper, & Plante, 2003; Wang, Cosby, Harris, & Liu, 1999). Research is somewhat conflicting about patterns of depression and distress throughout the course of the treatment and follow-up, with emotions changing as women confront new phases in their experience (Broeckel, Jacobsen, Balducci, Horton, & Lyman, 2000; Keitel & Kopala, 2000). For many women, finding positive meaning from the experience, spirituality, or what has been described as self-transcendence may be a personal coping strategy for minimizing the emotional impact of the experience (Coward, 1991; Loveys & Klaich, 1991; Taylor, 2000).

Although some women experience major disruptions in the physical and psychosocial dimensions of their lives during the acute phase of the breast cancer experience, many regain balance and a new equilibrium during the first year (Badger, Braden, Longman, & Mishel, 1999; Shimozuma, Ganz, Petersen, & Hirji, 1999). Women may experience changes in their friendship circles, which can then affect their ability to feel supported (Rabinowitz, 2002). A lack of social support and poor quality of interpersonal relationships have been associated with increased psychosocial morbidity during the first year after a breast cancer diagnosis (Nosarti, Roberts, Crayford, McKenzie, & David, 2002). A small percentage of women continue to need psychosocial support with the breast cancer for many years beyond the acute phase—particularly as medical follow-up becomes less intensive—and may benefit from psychosocial or peer group counseling as well as medication on an ongoing basis (Holzner et al., 2001; Kornblith et al., 2003; Lethborg, Kissane, Burns, & Snyder, 2000; Rustøen & Begnum, 2000).

Sexuality

Most women indicate that their interest in sex and their sexual relationships are largely unchanged after a diagnosis of breast cancer, but some women report some impact on their sexual function (Avis et al., 2004; McPhail & Wilson, 2000). Some couples have difficulty with the woman's changing physical appearance and body image issues. However, menopausal changes, such as vaginal dryness, may have more of an impact on sexual function and pleasure. Mood disturbances in the woman or her partner may cause some couples to emotionally withdraw from each other (Rabinowitz, 2002; Zarcone, Smithline, Koopman, Kraemer, & Spiegel, 1995).

Family Issues

The impact of breast cancer is experienced not only by the diagnosed woman, but also by her family (Lewis, 1986). During the acute phase of the breast cancer diagnosis and treatment, family routines and home management activities are often profoundly disrupted, even while family members are concerned about and try to support the diagnosed woman's health needs. Partnered women, in particular, identify increased concerns about their family and express increased needs for family counseling and support than single women (Wang et al., 1999). Many partners and spouses show evidence of increased anxiety and depression similar to and sometimes greater than the women experience, even beyond the acute phase of the illness (Compas et al., 1994; Given & Given, 1992; Lewis, Woods, Hough, & Bensley, 1989; Northouse, 1989a, 1989b; Zahlis & Shands, 1993). Marital tension may increase as partners feel overwhelmed by the experience of trying to support their loved one through many physical and psychosocial changes, maintain family routines and responsibilities, and deal with their own fears and distress (Lewis, Hammond, & Woods, 1993; Samms, 1999; Zahlis & Shands, 1991). These feelings and concerns are often only heightened when a woman is diagnosed with recurrent breast cancer (Northouse, 1996). Despite research indicating that partners have specific information needs and are sometimes uncomfortable approaching health care providers for this information, services and resources specifically for partners are often lacking in the clinical setting, and intervention research in this area is inadequate (Cochrane, Fletcher, & Lewis, 2005; Holmberg, Scott, Alexy, & Fife, 2001).

Most women have discussions with their children about their illness, surgery, and treatment, but some will not use the word *cancer*, and most are concerned about how to manage such discussions (Barnes et al., 2002). Shands, Lewis, and Zahlis (2000) found that mothers tend to assume more of a teacher/educator role rather than an interactive, emotive-expressive parenting role in talking with their children about the breast cancer. Children report a number of worries about their mother's breast cancer; chief among these is worrying that she will die (Zahlis, 2001)—yet one of the more common reasons given for not communicating with a child about the mother's cancer was to avoid such questions (Barnes et al., 2002). Women are rarely offered help with talking to their children about the cancer, but parents may benefit from assistance on ways to openly, but appropriately, discuss the mother's breast cancer with their children (Barnes et al., 2002; Davis Kirsch & Brandt, 2002).

No significant differences have been found in terms of mood, behavior problems, and social functioning in children of women diagnosed with breast cancer compared to those of women whose breast biopsy results were benign (Hoke, 2001). Adolescents whose mothers had breast cancer in this same study did better in social and academic activities, even when their mothers were distressed.

Breast Cancer Recurrence

Although the prognosis for early-stage breast cancer is excellent, up to 40% of women with breast cancer will experience a recurrence at some time after completing their initial course of treatment (Donegan, 2002). Treatment of recurrent breast cancer involves the same basic therapies as those used for an initial diagnosis—surgery, radiation therapy, and systemic medical therapy. Women with recurrent advanced breast cancer may be candidates for newer experimental therapies in the context of a clinical trial. Although recurrent disease may be curable, for many women the diagnosis of breast cancer recurrence is overwhelming and a further reminder of their mortality (Northouse et al., 2002). If the cancer progresses, therapeutic efforts will emphasize symptom and pain management and enhancement of quality of life and psychosocial support.

SUMMARY

The identification of problems of the breast and breast health considerations have expanded beyond sociocultural representations of female sexuality and nurturing and a biomedical view of breast health as breast cancer diagnosis and treatment. An awareness of normal and abnormal changes in the breast is important for evaluating breast problems, and regular clinical screening with clinical breast exams and mammograms is critical for ensuring that breast cancer is detected early, while it is still at a curable stage. Although surgical, radiation, and medical treatments have become more effective at curing breast cancer, a key area for research in the future is breast cancer prevention.

REFERENCES

Absetz, P., Aro, A. R., & Sutton, S. R. (2003). Experience with breast cancer, pre-screening perceived susceptibility and the psychological impact of screening. *Psycho-Oncology, 12*, 305–318.

Ahles, T. A., Saykin, A. J., Furstenberg, C. T., Cole, B., Mott, L. A., Skalla, K., et al. (2002). Neuropsychologic impact of standard-dose systemic chemotherapy in long-term survivors of breast cancer and lymphoma. *Journal of Clinical Oncology, 20*(2), 485–493.

Allen, A. (2002). The meaning of the breast cancer follow-up experience for the women who attend. *European Journal of Oncology Nursing, 6*(3), 155–161.

American Cancer Society. (2007). *How is breast cancer treated?* Retrieved February 23, 2008, from http://www.cancer.org/docroot/CRI/content/CRI_2_2_4X_How_Is_Breast_Cancer_Treated_5.asp?rnav = cri

Andersen, M. R., Smith, R., Meischke, H., Bowen, D., & Urban, N. (2003). Breast cancer worry and mammography use by women with and without a family history in a population-based sample. *Cancer Epidemiology, Biomarkers & Prevention, 12*, 314–320.

Andsager, J. L., Hust, S. J. T., & Powers, A. (2000). Patient-blaming and representation of risk factors in breast cancer images. *Women & Health, 31*(2/3), 57–79.

Apantaku, L. M. (2002). Breast-conserving surgery for breast cancer. *American Family Physician, 66*(12), 2271–2278.

Armer, J. (2004). Lymphedema. In K. H. Dow (Ed.), *Contemporary issues in breast cancer: A nursing perspective* (2nd ed., pp. 209–229). Sudbury, MA: Jones and Bartlett.

Armstrong, K., Calzone, K., Stopfer, J., Fitzgerald, G., Coyne, J. C., & Weber, B. (2000). Factors associated with decisions about clinical BRCA1/2 testing. *Cancer Epidemiology, Biomarkers & Prevention, 9*, 1251–1254.

Armstrong, K., Weber, B., FitzGerald, G., Hershey, J. C., Pauly, M. V., Lemaire, J., et al. (2003). Life insurance and breast cancer risk assessment: Adverse selection, genetic testing decisions, and discrimination. *American Journal of Medical Genetics, 120A*, 359–364.

Arthur, D. W., & Vicini, F. A. (2005). Accelerated partial breast irradiation as a part of breast conservation therapy. *Journal of Clinical Oncology, 23*(8), 1726–1735.

Avis, N. E., Crawford, S., & Manuel, J. (2004). Psychosocial problems among younger women with breast cancer. *Psycho-Oncology, 13*, 295–308.

Badger, T. A., Braden, C. J., Longman, A. J., & Mishel, M. M. (1999). Depression burden, self-help interventions, and social support in women receiving treatment for breast cancer. *Journal of Psychosocial Oncology, 17*(2), 17–35.

Badger, T. A., Braden, C. J., & Mishel, M. H. (2001). Depression burden, self-help interventions, and side effect experience in women receiving treatment for breast cancer. *Oncology Nursing Forum, 28*(3), 567–574.

Bahl, S., Cotterchio, M., & Kreiger, N. (2003). Use of antidepressant medications and the possible association with breast cancer risk. *Psychotherapy and Psychosomatics, 72*, 185–194.

Baker, L. H. (1982). Breast cancer detection demonstration project: Five-year summary report. *CA: A Cancer Journal for Clinicians, 32*, 194–225.

Bardou, V. J., Arpino, G., Elledge, R. M., Osborne, C. K., & Clark, G. M. (2003). Progesterone receptor status significantly improves outcome prediction over estrogen receptor status alone for adjuvant endocrine therapy in two large breast cancer databases. *Journal of Clinical Oncology, 21*(10), 1973–1979.

Barnes, J., Kroll, L., Lee, J., Burke, O., Jones, A., & Stein, A. (2002). Factors predicting communication about the diagnosis of maternal breast cancer to children. *Journal of Psychosomatic Research, 52*, 209–214.

Baron, R., & Vaziri, N. (2004). Reconstructive surgery. In K. H. Dow (Ed.), *Contemporary issues in breast cancer: A nursing perspective* (2nd ed., pp. 90–109). Sudbury, MA: Jones and Bartlett.

Barton, M. B., Harris, R., & Fletcher, S. W. (1999). Does this patient have breast cancer? The screening clinical breast examination: Should it be done? How? *Journal of the American Medical Association, 282*(13), 1270–1280.

Bastani, R., Maxwell, A. E., Bradford, C., Das, I. P., & Yan, K. X. (1999). Tailored risk notification for women with a family history of breast cancer. *Preventive Medicine, 29*, 355–364.

Blanchard, D. K., Donohue, J. H., Reynolds, C., & Grant, C. S. (2003). Relapse and morbidity in patients undergoing sentinel lymph node biopsy alone or with axillary dissection for breast cancer. *Archives of Surgery, 138*, 482–488.

Bluman, L. G., Rimer, B. K., Berry, D. A., Borstelmann, N., Iglehart, J. D., Regan, K., et al. (1999). Attitudes, knowledge, and risk perceptions of women with breast and/or ovarian cancer considering testing for BRCA1 and BRCA2. *Journal of Clinical Oncology, 17*(3), 1040–1046.

Bondy, M. L., & Newman, L. A. (2003). Breast cancer risk assessment models: Applicability to African-American women. *Cancer, 95*(1 Suppl.), 230–235.

Brenin, D. R., Hibshoosh, H., & Kinne, D. W. (2000). Unusual breast pathology. In D. J. Winchester & D. P. Winchester (Eds.), *Breast cancer: Atlas of clinical oncology* (pp. 99–112). Lewiston, NY: B. C. Decker.

Brewster, W. R., & DiSaia, P. J. (2000). Estrogen replacement therapy and breast cancer survivors. In D. J. Winchester & D. P. Winchester (Eds.), *Breast cancer: Atlas of clinical oncology* (pp. 253–262). Lewiston, NY: B. C. Decker.

Broeckel, J. A., Jacobsen, P. B., Balducci, L., Horton, J., & Lyman, G. H. (2000). Quality of life after adjuvant chemotherapy for breast cancer. *Breast Cancer Research and Treatment, 62*, 141–150.

Bucholtz, J. (2004). Prevention strategies. In K. H. Dow (Ed.), *Contemporary issues in breast cancer: A nursing perspective* (2nd ed., pp. 25–44). Sudbury, MA: Jones and Bartlett.

Burke, W., Culver, J. O., Bowen, D., Lowry, D., Durfy, S., McTiernan, A., et al. (2000). Genetic counseling for women with an intermediate family history of breast cancer. *American Journal of Medical Genetics, 90*, 361–368.

Burkman, R. T., Tang, M. T. C., Malone, K. E., Marchbanks, P. A., McDonald, J. A., & Folger, S. G. (2003). Infertility drugs and the risk of breast cancer: Findings from the National Institute of Child Health and Human Development Women's Contraceptive and Reproductive Experiences Study. *Fertility and Sterility, 79*(4), 844–851.

Butow, P. N., Hiller, J. E., Price, M. A., Thackway, S. V., Kricker, A., & Tennant, C. C. (2000). Epidemiological evidence for a relationship between life events, coping style, and personality factors in the development of breast cancer. *Journal of Psychosomatic Research, 49*, 169–181.

Byram, S., Fischhoff, B., Embrey, M., de Bruin, W. B., & Thorne, S. (2001). Mental models of women with breast implants: Local complications. *Behavioral Medicine, 27*, 4.

Carpenter, C. L., Ross, R. K., Paganini-Hill, A., & Bernstein, L. (2003). Effect of family history, obesity and exercise on breast cancer risk among postmenopausal women. *International Journal of Cancer, 106*, 96–102.

Carpenter, J. S., & Elam, J. L. (2004). Menopausal symptoms. In K. H. Dow (Ed.), *Contemporary issues in breast cancer: A nursing perspective* (2nd ed., pp. 230–262). Sudbury, MA: Jones and Bartlett.

Chen, C.-L., Weiss, N. S., Newcomb, P. A., Barlow, W., & White, E. (2002). Hormone replacement therapy in relation to breast cancer. *Journal of the American Medical Association, 287*(6), 734–741.

Chlebowski, R. T., Col, N., Winer, E. P., Colyar, D. E., Cummings, S. R., Vogel, V. G., et al. (2002). American Society of Clinical Oncology technology assessment of pharmacologic interventions for breast cancer risk reduction including tamoxifen, raloxifene, and aromatase inhibition. *Journal of Clinical Oncology, 20*(15), 3328–3343.

Chlebowski, R. T., Hendrix, S. L., Langer, R. D., Stefanick, M. L., Gass, M., Lane, D., et al. (2003). Influence of estrogen plus progestin on breast cancer and mammography in health postmenopausal women: The Women's Health Initiative Randomized Trial. *Journal of the American Medical Association, 289*(24), 3243–3253.

Cho, E., Spiegelman, D., Hunter, D. J., Chen, W. Y., Stampfer, M. J., Colditz, G. A., et al. (2003). Premenopausal fat intake and risk of breast cancer. *Journal of the National Cancer Institute, 95*(14), 1079–1085.

Cimprich, B. (1999). Pretreatment symptom distress in women newly diagnosed with breast cancer. *Cancer Nursing, 22*(3), 185–194.

Cimprich, B., Ronis, D. L., & Martinez-Ramos, G. (2002). Age at diagnosis and quality of life in breast cancer survivors. *Cancer Practice, 10*(2), 85–93.

Clark, P. M. (2004). Nongenetic and heritable risk factors. In K. H. Dow (Ed.), *Contemporary issues in breast cancer: A nursing perspective* (2nd ed., pp. 10–24). Sudbury, MA: Jones and Bartlett.

Claus, E. B., Risch, N., & Thompson, W. D. (1994). Autosomal dominant inheritance of early-onset breast cancer: Implications for risk prediction. *Cancer, 73*, 643–651.

Cochrane, B. B., Fletcher, K. A., & Lewis, F. (2005). Partner adjustment to breast cancer: Patterns over time. *Psycho-Oncology, 14*(Suppl.), S53–S54.

Collaborative Group on Hormonal Factors in Breast Cancer. (1996). Breast cancer and hormonal contraceptives: Collaborative reanalysis on data from 53,297 women with breast cancer and 100,239 women without breast cancer in 54 epidemiological studies. *Lancet, 347*(9017), 1713–1727.

Collaborative Group on Hormonal Factors in Breast Cancer. (2002). Breast cancer and breastfeeding: Collaborative reanalysis of individual data from 47 epidemiological studies in 30 countries, including 50,302 women with breast cancer and 96,973 women without the disease. *Lancet, 360*, 187–195.

Compas, B. E., Worsham, N. L., Epping-Jordan, J. E., Grant, K. E., Mireault, G., Howell, D. C., et al. (1994). When mom or dad has cancer: Markers of psychological distress in cancer patients, spouses, and children. *Health Psychology, 13*(6), 507–515.

Coward, D. D. (1991). Self-transcendence and emotional well-being in women with advanced breast cancer. *Oncology Nursing Forum, 18*(5), 857–863.

Cristofanilli, M., Newman, L., & Hortobagyi, G. N. (2000). Breast cancer risk and management: Chemoprevention, surgery, and surveillance. In D. J. Winchester & D. P. Winchester (Eds.), *Breast cancer: Atlas of clinical oncology* (pp. 19–40). Lewiston, NY: B. C. Decker.

Crocetti, E., Miccinesi, G., Paci, E., & Zappa, M. (2001). Incidence of second cancers among women with in situ carcinoma of the breast. *The Breast, 10*, 438–441.

Cummings, F. J. (2002). Evolving uses of hormonal agents for breast cancer. *Clinical Therapeutics, 24*(Suppl. C), C3–C25.

Cummings, S. R., Eckert, S., Krueger, K. A., Grady, D., Powles, T. J., Cauley, J. A., et al. (1999). The effect of raloxifene on risk of breast cancer in postmenopausal women: Results from the MORE randomized trial. *Journal of the American Medical Association, 281*(23), 2189–2197.

Davis Kirsch, S. E., & Brandt, P. A. (2002). Telephone interviewing: A method to reach fathers in family research. *Journal of Family Nursing, 8*(1), 73–84.

Davis, S., Mirick, D. K., & Stevens, R. G. (2001). Night shift work, light at night, and risk of breast cancer. *Journal of the National Cancer Institute, 93*(20), 1557–1562.

de Jong, N., Candel, M. J. J. M., Schouten, H. C., Abu-Saad, H. H., & Courtens, A. M. (2004). Prevalence and course of fatigue in breast cancer patients receiving adjuvant chemotherapy. *Annals of Oncology, 15*, 896–905.

Denison, U., Baumann, J., Peters-Engle, C., Samonigg, H., Krippl, P., Lang, A., et al. (2003). Incidence of anaemia in breast cancer patients receiving adjuvant chemotherapy. *Breast Cancer Research and Treatment, 79*, 347–353.

Desai, M. M., Bruce, M. L., & Kasl, S. V. (1999). The effects of major depression and phobia on stage at diagnosis of breast cancer. *International Journal of Psychiatry in Medicine, 29*(1), 29–45.

de Sanjosé, S., Léone, M., Bérez, V., Izquierdo, A., Font, R., Brunet, M. J., et al. (2003). Prevalence of BRCA1 and BRCA2 germline mutations in young breast cancer patients: A population-based study. *International Journal of Cancer, 106*, 588–593.

Didie, E. R., & Sarwer, D. B. (2003). Factors that influence the decision to undergo cosmetic breast augmentation surgery. *Journal of Women's Health, 12*(3), 241–253.

Diefenbach, M. A., Miller, S. M., & Daly, M. B. (1999). Specific worry about breast cancer predicts mammography use in women at risk for breast and ovarian cancer. *Health Psychology, 18*(5), 532–536.

Dienger, M. J. (2004). Hormonal therapy in advanced and metastatic disease. In K. H. Dow (Ed.), *Contemporary issues in breast cancer: A nursing perspective* (2nd ed., pp. 175–186). Sudbury, MA: Jones and Bartlett.

Donegan, W. L. (2002). Local and regional recurrence. In W. L. Donegan & J. S. Spratt (Eds.), *Cancer of the breast* (5th ed., pp. 825–839). Philadelphia: Saunders.

Dorgan, J. F., Baer, D. J., Albert, P. S., Judd, J. T., Brown, E. D., Corle, D. K., et al. (2001). Serum hormones and the alcohol-breast cancer association in postmenopausal women. *Journal of the National Cancer Institute, 93*(9), 710–715.

Dow, K. H. (2004). Incidence, epidemiology, and survival. In K. H. Dow (Ed.), *Contemporary issues in breast cancer: A nursing perspective* (2nd ed., pp. 3–10). Sudbury, MA: Jones and Bartlett.

Drake, D. A. (2001). A longitudinal study of physical activity and breast cancer prediction. *Cancer Nursing, 24*(5), 371–377.

Dupont, W. D., & Page, D. (1985). Risk factors for breast cancer in women with proliferative breast disease. *New England Journal of Medicine, 312*(3), 146–151.

Ekeberg, Ø., Skjauff, H., & Kåresen, R. (2001). Screening for breast cancer is associated with a low degree of psychological distress. *The Breast, 10,* 20–24.

Endogenous Hormones and Breast Cancer Collaborative Group. (2003). Body mass index, serum sex hormones, and breast cancer risk in postmenopausal women. *Journal of the National Cancer Institute, 95*(16), 1218–1226.

Enger, S. M., Thwin, S. S., Buist, D. S. M., Field, T., Frost, F., Geiger, A. M., et al. (2006). Breast cancer treatment of older women in integrated health care settings. *Journal of Clinical Oncology, 24*(27), 4377–4383.

Feigelson, H. S., Jonas, C. R., Roberston, A. S., McCullough, M. L., Thun, M. J., & Calle, E. E. (2003). Alcohol, folate, methionine, and risk of incident breast cancer in the American Cancer Society Cancer Prevention Study II nutrition cohort. *Cancer Epidemiology, Biomarkers & Prevention, 12,* 161–164.

Fenner, G. C., & Mustoe, T. A. (2000). Breast reconstruction. In D. J. Winchester & D. P. Winchester (Eds.), *Breast cancer: Atlas of clinical oncology* (pp. 171–200). Lewiston, NY: B. C. Decker.

Figueiredo, M. I., Cullen, J., Hwang, Y.-T., Rowland, J. H., & Mandelblatt, J. S. (2004). Breast cancer treatment in older women: Does getting what you want improve your long-term body image and mental health? *Journal of Clinical Oncology, 22*(19), 4002–4009.

Fine, R. E. (2000). Image-directed breast biopsy. In D. J. Winchester & D. P. Winchester (Eds.), *Breast cancer: Atlas of clinical oncology* (pp. 65–87). Lewiston, NY: B. C. Decker.

Fisher, B., Costantino, J. P., Wickerham, D. L., Redmond, C. K., Kavanah, M., Cronin, W. M., et al. (1998). Tamoxifen for prevention of breast cancer: Report of the National Surgical Adjuvant Breast and Bowel Project P-1 study. *Journal of the National Cancer Institute, 90*(18), 1371–1388.

Fosket, J. (2000). Problematizing biomedicine: Women's constructions of breast cancer knowledge. In L. K. Potts (Ed.), *Ideologies of breast cancer: Feminist perspectives* (pp. 15–36). New York: St. Martin's Press.

Foxcroft, L. M., Evans, E. B., Hirst, C., & Hicks, B. J. (2001). Presentation and diagnosis of adolescent breast disease. *The Breast, 10,* 399–404.

Fraker, T. (2004). Diagnosis and staging. In K. H. Dow (Ed.), *Contemporary issues in breast cancer: A nursing perspective* (2nd ed., pp. 58–77). Sudbury, MA: Jones and Bartlett.

Freedman, G. M., Anderson, P. R., Goldstein, L. J., Hanlon, A. L., Cianfrocca, M. E., Millenson, M. M., et al. (2003). Routine mammography is associated with earlier stage disease and greater eligibility for breast conservation in breast carcinoma patients age 40 years and older. *Cancer, 98*(5), 918–925.

Frost, M. H., Suman, V. J., Rummans, T. A., Dose, A. M., Taylor, M., Novotny, P., et al. (2000). Physical, psychological and social well-being of women with breast cancer: The influence of disease phase. *Psycho-Oncology, 9,* 221–231.

Frost, M. H., Vockley, C. W., Suman, V. J., Greene, M. H., Zahasky, K., & Hartmann, L. (2000). Perceived familial risk of cancer: Health concerns and psychosocial adjustment. *Journal of Psychosocial Oncology, 18*(1), 63–82.

Gagné, P., & McGaughey, D. (2002). Designing women: Cultural hegemony and the exercise of power among women who have undergone elective mammoplasty. *Gender & Society, 16*(6), 814–838.

Gail, M. H., Brinton, L. A., Byar, D. P., Corle, D. K., Green, S. B., Schairer, C., et al. (1989). Projecting individualized probabilities of developing breast cancer for White females who are being examined annually. *Journal of the National Cancer Institute, 81,* 1879–1886.

Ganz, P. A., Desmond, K. A., Leedham, B., Rowland, J. H., Meyerowitz, B. E., & Belin, T. R. (2002). Quality of life in long-term, disease-free survivors of breast cancer: A follow-up study. *Journal of the National Cancer Institute, 94*(1), 39–49.

Geddie, P. I. (2004a). Acute side effect management. In K. H. Dow (Ed.), *Contemporary issues in breast cancer: A nursing perspective* (2nd ed., pp. 189–197). Sudbury, MA: Jones and Bartlett.

Geddie, P. I. (2004b). Adjuvant therapy. In K. H. Dow (Ed.), *Contemporary issues in breast cancer: A nursing perspective* (2nd ed., pp. 134–145). Sudbury, MA: Jones and Bartlett.

Gilbar, O. (1998). Coping with threat: Implications for women with a family history of breast cancer. *Psychosomatics, 39*(4), 329–339.

Given, B., & Given, C. W. (1992). Patient and family caregiver reaction to new and recurrent cancer. *Journal of the American Medical Women's Association, 47,* 201–206.

Givens, M. L., & Luszczak, M. (2002). Breast disorders: A review for emergency physicians. *Journal of Emergency Medicine, 22*(1), 59–65.

Goldschmidt, R. A. (2000). Histopathology of malignant breast disease. In D. J. Winchester & D. P. Winchester (Eds.), *Breast cancer: Atlas of clinical oncology* (pp. 89–98). Lewiston, NY: B. C. Decker.

Green, B. B., & Taplin, S. H. (2003). Breast cancer screening controversies. *Journal of the American Board of Family Practice, 16,* 233–241.

Greendale, G. A., Reboussin, B. A., Slone, S., Wasilauskas, C., Pike, M. C., & Ursin, G. (2003). Postmenopausal hormone therapy and change in mammographic density. *Journal of the National Cancer Institute, 95*(1), 30–37.

Grigg, M., Bondurant, S., Ernster, V. L., & Herdman, R. (Eds.). (2003). *Information for women about the safety of silicone breast implants.* Washington, DC: National Academy Press.

Grunfeld, E. A., Hunter, M. S., Ramirez, A. J., & Richards, M. A. (2003). Perceptions of breast cancer across the lifespan. *Journal of Psychosomatic Research, 54,* 141–146.

Gwyn, K., Vernon, S. W., & Conoley, P. M. (2003). Intention to pursue genetic testing for breast cancer among women due for screening mammography. *Cancer Epidemiology, Biomarkers & Prevention, 12,* 96–102.

Hackshaw, A. K., & Paul, E. A. (2003). Breast self-examination and death from breast cancer: A meta-analysis. *British Journal of Cancer, 88,* 1047–1053.

Haghighat, S., Akbari, M. E., Holakouei, K., Rahimi, A., & Montazeri, A. (2003). Factors predicting fatigue in breast cancer patients. *Supportive Care in Cancer, 11,* 533–538.

Hallowell, N. (2000). Reconstructing the body or reconstructing the woman? Problems of prophylactic mastectomy for hereditary breast cancer risk. In L. K. Potts (Ed.), *Ideologies of breast cancer: Feminist perspectives* (pp. 153–180). New York: St. Martin's Press.

Hamilton, A. S., & Mack, T. M. (2003). Puberty and genetic susceptibility to breast cancer in a case-control study in twins. *New England Journal of Medicine, 348,* 2313–2322.

Harrison, R. V., Janz, N. K., Wolfe, R. A., Tedeschi, P. J., Huang, X., McMahon, L. F. Jr., et al. (2003). 5-year mammography rates and associated factors for older women. *Cancer, 97,* 1147–1155.

Hartmann, L. C., Schaid, D. J., Woods, J. E., Crotty, T. P., Myers, J. L., Arnold, P. G., et al. (1999). Efficacy of bilateral prophylactic mastectomy in women with a family history of breast cancer. *New England Journal of Medicine, 340*(2), 77–84.

Henderson, J. W., & Donatelle, R. J. (2003). The relationship between cancer locus of control and complementary and alternative medicine use by women diagnosed with breast cancer. *Psycho-Oncology, 12,* 59–67.

Henson, D. E., Chu, K. C., & Levine, P. H. (2003). Histologic grade, stage, and survival in breast cancer: Comparison of African American and Caucasian women. *Cancer, 98*(5), 908–917.

Hoke, L. A. (2001). Psychosocial adjustment in children of mothers with breast cancer. *Psycho-Oncology, 10,* 361–369.

Holm, C. J., Frank, D. I., & Curtin, J. (1999). Health beliefs, health locus of control, and women's mammography behavior. *Cancer Nursing, 22*(2), 149–156.

Holmberg, S. K., Scott, L. L., Alexy, W., & Fife, B. L. (2001). Relationship issues of women with breast cancer. *Cancer Nursing, 24*(1), 53–60.

Hölmich, L. R., Friis, S., Fryzek, J. P., Vejborg, I. M., Conrad, C., Sletting, S., et al. (2003). Incidence of silicone breast implant rupture. *Archives of Surgery, 138*(7), 801–806.

Holzner, B., Kemmler, G., Kopp, M., Moschen, R., Schweigkofler, H., Dünser, M., et al. (2001). Quality of life in breast cancer patients—Not enough attention for long-term survivors? *Psychosomatics, 42,* 117–123.

Hortobagyi, G. N. (2001). Progress in systemic chemotherapy of primary breast cancer: An overview. *Journal of the National Cancer Institute Monographs, 30,* 72–79.

Hughes, J. (1982). Emotional reactions to the diagnosis and treatment of early breast cancer. *Journal of Psychosomatic Research, 26*(2), 277–283.

Hughes, L. E. (2002). A unifying concept for benign disorders of the breast: ANDI. In W. L. Donegan & J. S. Spratt (Eds.), *Cancer of the breast* (5th ed., pp. 57–66). Philadelphia: Saunders.

Hulka, B. S., & Moorman, P. G. (2002). Breast cancer: Hormones and other risk factors. *Maturitas, 42*(Suppl. 1), S95–S108.

Ishida, D. (2004). Asian women and breast cancer. In K. H. Dow (Ed.), *Contemporary issues in breast cancer: A nursing perspective* (2nd ed., pp. 299–310). Sudbury, MA: Jones and Bartlett.

Jacobson, N. (1998). The socially constructed breast: Breast implants and the medical construction of need. *American Journal of Public Health, 88*(8), 1254–1261.

Jahraus, D., Sokolosky, S., Thurston, N., & Guo, D. (2002). Evaluation of an education program for patients with breast cancer receiving radiation therapy. *Cancer Nursing, 25*(4), 266–275.

Jatoi, I., Becher, H., & Leake, C. R. (2003). Widening disparity in survival between White and African-American patients with breast carcinoma treated in the U.S. Department of Defense Healthcare System. *Cancer, 98*(5), 894–899.

Jemal, A., Siegel, R., Ward, E., Murray, T., Xu, J., & Thun, M. J. (2007). Cancer statistics, 2007. *CA: A Cancer Journal for Clinicians, 57*(1), 43–66.

Jeske, J. M., Bernstein, J. R., & Stull, M. A. (2000). Screening and diagnostic imaging. In D. J. Winchester & D. P. Winchester (Eds.), *Breast cancer: Atlas of clinical oncology* (pp. 41–63). Lewiston, NY: B. C. Decker.

Johnson, T. W., Anderson, K. E., Lazovich, D., & Folsom, A. R. (2002). Association of aspirin and nonsteroidal anti-inflammatory drug use with breast cancer. *Cancer Epidemiology, Biomarkers & Prevention, 11,* 1586–1591.

Kabat, G. C., O'Leary, E. S., Schoenfeld, E. R., Greene, J. M., Grimson, R., Henderson, K., et al. (2003). Electric blanket use and breast cancer on Long Island. *Epidemiology, 14*(5), 514–520.

Kaufmann, M., von Minckwitz, G., Smith, R., Valero, V., Gianni, L., Eiermann, W., et al. (2003). International Expert Panel on the Use of Primary (Preoperative) Systemic Treatment of Operable Breast Cancer: Review and recommendations. *Journal of Clinical Oncology, 21*(13), 2600–2608.

Keitel, M. A., & Kopala, M. (2000). *Counseling women with breast cancer: A guide for professionals.* Thousand Oaks, CA: Sage.

Kerlikowske, K., Carney, P. A., Geller, B., Mandelson, M. T., Taplin, S. H., Malvin, K., et al. (2000). Performance of screening mammography among women with and without a first-degree relative with breast cancer. *Annals of Internal Medicine, 133,* 855–863.

Khabele, D., & Runowicz, C. D. (2002). Genetic counseling, testing, and screening for breast and ovarian cancer: Practical and social considerations. *Current Women's Health Reports, 2,* 163–169.

Kornblith, A. B., Herndon, J. E., II, Weiss, R. B., Zhang, C., Zuckerman, E. L., Rosenberg, S., et al. (2003). Long-term adjustment of survivors of early-stage breast carcinoma, 20 years after adjuvant chemotherapy. *Cancer, 98*(4), 679–689.

Kroman, N., Wohlfahrt, J., Mouridsen, H. T., & Melbye, M. (2003). Influence of tumor location on breast cancer prognosis. *International Journal of Cancer, 105,* 542–545.

LaCombe, M. A., & Bloomer, W. D. (2000). Breast cancer and radiation therapy. In D. J. Winchester & D. P. Winchester (Eds.), *Breast cancer: Atlas of clinical oncology* (pp. 219–238). Lewiston, NY: B. C. Decker.

Landmark, B. T., Strandmark, M., & Wahl, A. K. (2001). Living with newly diagnosed breast cancer—The meaning of existential issues: A qualitative study of 10 women with newly diagnosed breast cancer, based on grounded theory. *Cancer Nursing, 24*(3), 220–226.

Latteier, C. (1998). *Breasts: The women's perspective on an American obsession.* New York: Haworth Press.

Lauver, D. (1994). Care-seeking behavior with breast cancer symptoms in Caucasian and African-American women. *Research in Nursing & Health, 17*(6), 421–431.

Lauver, D., & Angerame, M. (1993). Women's expectations about seeking care for breast cancer symptoms. *Oncology Nursing Forum, 20*(3), 519–525.

Lawlor, D. A., Okasha, M., Gunnell, D., Smith, G. D., & Ebrahim, S. (2003). Associations of adult measures of childhood growth with breast cancer: Findings from the British Women's Heart and Health Study. *British Journal of Cancer, 89,* 81–87.

Lerman, C., Hughes, C., Croyle, R. T., Main, D., Durham, C., Snyder, C., et al. (2000). Prophylactic surgery decisions and surveillance practices one year following BRCA1/2 testing. *Preventive Medicine, 31,* 75–80.

Lerman, C., Lustbader, E., Rimer, B., Daly, M., Sands, C., & Rimer, B. (1995). Effects of individualized breast cancer risk counseling: A randomized trial. *Journal of the National Cancer Institute, 87,* 286–292.

Lethborg, C. E., Kissane, D., Burns, W. I., & Snyder, R. (2000). "Cast adrift": The experience of completing treatment among women with early stage breast cancer. *Journal of Psychosocial Oncology, 18*(4), 73–90.

Levy, S. M., Ewing, L. J., & Lippman, M. E. (1988). Gynecological cancers. In E. A. Blechman & K. D. Brownell (Eds.), *Handbook of behavioral medicine for women* (pp. 126–139). New York: Pergamon Press.

Lewis, F. M. (1986). The impact of cancer on the family: A critical analysis of the research literature. *Patient Education and Counseling, 8,* 269–289.

Lewis, F. M., Hammond, M. A., & Woods, N. F. (1993). The family's functioning with newly diagnosed breast cancer in the mother: The development of an explanatory model. *Journal of Behavioral Medicine, 16*(4), 351–370.

Lewis, F. M., Woods, N. F., Hough, E. E., & Bensley, L. S. (1989). The family's functioning with chronic illness in the mother: The spouse's perspective. *Social Science & Medicine, 29*(11), 1261–1269.

Li, C. I., Anderson, B. O., Daling, J. R., & Moe, R. E. (2003). Trends in incidence rates of invasive lobular and ductal breast carcinoma. *Journal of the American Medical Association, 289,* 1421–1424.

Li, C. I., Malone, K. E., Porter, P. L., Weiss, N. S., Tang, M.-T. C., Cushing-Haugen, K. L., et al. (2003). Relationship between long durations and different regimens of hormone therapy and risk of breast cancer. *Journal of the American Medical Association, 289*(24), 3254–3263.

Liang, W., Burnett, C. B., Rowland, J. H., Meropol, N. J., Eggert, L., Hwang, Y.-T., et al. (2002). Communication between physicians and older women with localized breast cancer: Implications for treatment and patient satisfaction. *Journal of Clinical Oncology, 20*(4), 1008–1016.

Lillberg, K., Verkasalo, P. K., Kaprio, J., Teppo, L., Helenius, H., & Koskenvuo, M. (2003). Stressful life events and risk of breast cancer in 10,808 women: A cohort study. *American Journal of Epidemiology, 157*(5), 415–423.

Locker, G. Y. (2000). Adjuvant systemic therapy of early breast cancer. In D. J. Winchester & D. P. Winchester (Eds.), *Breast cancer: Atlas of clinical oncology* (pp. 201–218). Lewiston, NY: B. C. Decker.

Loerzel, V. W. (2004). Late physical effects of cancer treatment. In K. H. Dow (Ed.), *Contemporary issues in breast cancer: A nursing perspective* (2nd ed., pp. 263–280). Sudbury, MA: Jones and Bartlett.

Longnecker, M., Berlin, J., Orza, M., & Chalmers, T. (1988). A meta-analysis of alcohol consumption in relation to the risk for breast cancer. *Journal of the American Medical Association, 260,* 652–656.

Loveys, B. J., & Klaich, K. (1991). Breast cancer: Demands of illness. *Oncology Nursing Forum, 18*(1), 75–80.

Lukwago, S. N., Kreuter, M. W., Holt, C. L., Steger-May, K., Bucholtz, D. C., & Skinner, C. S. (2003). Sociocultural correlates of breast cancer knowledge and screening in urban African American women. *American Journal of Public Health, 93*(8), 1271–1274.

Lyman, G. H., Giuliano, A. E., Somerfield, M. R., Benson, A. B., III, Bodurka, D. C., Burstein, H. J., et al. (2005). American Society of Clinical Oncology guideline recommendations for sentinel lymph node biopsy in early-stage breast cancer. *Journal of Clinical Oncology, 23,* 7703–7720.

Lynch, H. T., & Lynch, J. F. (2000). Genetics, natural history, and DNA-based genetic counseling in hereditary breast cancer. In D. J. Winchester & D. P. Winchester (Eds.), *Breast cancer: Atlas of clinical oncology* (pp. 1–18). Lewiston, NY: B. C. Decker.

Lynch, H. T., Watson, P., Tinley, S., Snyder, C., Durham, C., Lynch, J., et al. (1999). An update on DNA-based BRCA1/BRCA2 genetic counseling in hereditary breast cancer. *Cancer Genetics and Cytogenetics, 109,* 91–98.

Lynn, J. (2004). Surgery techniques. In K. H. Dow (Ed.), *Contemporary issues in breast cancer: A nursing perspective* (2nd ed., pp. 81–90). Sudbury, MA: Jones and Bartlett.

MacDuff, C., Mackenzie, T., Hutcheon, A., Melville, L., & Archibald, H. (2003). The effectiveness of scalp cooling in preventing alopecia for patients receiving epirubicin and docetaxel. *European Journal of Cancer Care, 12,* 154–161.

Machia, J. (2004). Screening and early detection. In K. H. Dow (Ed.), *Contemporary issues in breast cancer: A nursing perspective* (2nd ed., pp. 45–57). Sudbury, MA: Jones and Bartlett.

Mahon, S. M., & Casey, M. (2003). Patient education for women being fitted for breast prostheses. *Clinical Journal of Oncology Nursing, 7*(2), 194–199.

Mandelblatt, J. S., Edge, S. B., Meropol, N. J., Senie, R., Tsangaris, T., Grey, L., et al. (2003). Predictors of long-term outcomes in older breast cancer survivors: Perceptions versus patterns of care. *Journal of Clinical Oncology, 21,* 855–863.

Mansel, R. E., & Bundred, N. J. (1995). *Color atlas of breast diseases.* Baltimore: Mosby-Wolfe.

Marchant, D. J. (2002). Benign breast disease. *Obstetrics and Gynecology Clinics, 29*(1), 1–20.

Marchbanks, P. A., McDonald, J. A., Wilson, H. G., Folger, S. G., Mandel, M. G., Daling, J. R., et al. (2002). Oral contraceptives and the risk of breast cancer. *New England Journal of Medicine, 346*(26), 2025–2032.

Mayo, R. M., Ureda, J. R., & Parker, V. G. (2001). Importance of fatalism in understanding mammography screening in rural elderly women. *Journal of Women & Aging, 13*(1), 57–72.

McCaul, K. D., Schroeder, D. M., & Reid, P. A. (1996). Breast cancer worry and screening: Some prospective data. *Health Psychology, 15*(6), 430–433.

McPhail, G., & Smith, L. N. (2000). Acute menopause symptoms during adjuvant systemic treatment for breast cancer. *Cancer Nursing, 23*(6), 430–443.

McPhail, G., & Wilson, S. (2000). Women's experience of breast conserving treatment for breast cancer. *European Journal of Cancer Care, 9,* 144–150.

McTiernan, A. (2003). Behavioral risk factors in breast cancer: Can risk be modified? *Oncologist, 8,* 326–334.

McTiernan, A., Kuniyuki, A., Yasui, Y., Bowen, D., Burke, W., Culver, J. B., et al. (2001). Comparisons of two breast cancer risk estimates in women with a family history of breast cancer. *Cancer Epidemiology, Biomarkers & Prevention, 10,* 333–338.

McTiernan, A., Rajan, K. B., Tworoger, S. S., Irwin, M., Bernstein, L., Baumgartner, R., et al. (2003). Adiposity and sex hormones in postmenopausal breast cancer survivors. *Journal of Clinical Oncology, 21*(1), 1961–1966.

Meechan, G., Collins, J., & Petrie, K. J. (2003). The relationship of symptoms and psychological factors to delay in seeking medical care for breast symptoms. *Preventive Medicine, 36,* 347–378.

Meijers-Heijboer, H., van Geel, B., van Putten, W. L. J., Henzen-Logmans, S. C., Seynaeve, C., Menke-Pluymers, M. B. E., et al. (2001). Breast cancer after prophylactic bilateral mastectomy in women with a BRCA1 or BRCA2 mutation. *New England Journal of Medicine, 345*(3), 159–164.

Meiser, B., Butow, P., Barratt, A., Gattas, M., Gaff, C., Haan, E., et al. (2001). Risk perceptions and knowledge of breast cancer genetics in women at increased risk of developing hereditary breast cancer. *Psychology and Health, 16,* 297–311.

Meissner, H. I., Rimer, B. K., Davis, W. W., Eisner, E. J., & Siegler, I. C. (2003). Another round in the mammography controversy. *Journal of Women's Health, 12*(3), 261–276.

Metcalfe, K. A., Esplen, M. J., Goel, V., & Narod, S. A. (2004). Psychosocial functioning in women who have undergone bilateral prophylactic mastectomy. *Psycho-Oncology, 13,* 14–25.

Michels, K. B., Solomon, C. G., Hu, F. B., Rosner, B. A., Hankinson, S. E., Colditz, G. A., et al. (2003). Type 2 diabetes and subsequent incidence of breast cancer in the Nurses' Health Study. *Diabetes Care, 26*(6), 1752–1758.

Millar, M. G., & Millar, K. U. (1992). Feelings and beliefs about breast cancer and breast self-examination among women in three age groups. *Family and Community Health, 15*(3), 30–37.

Million Women Study Collaborators. (2003). Breast cancer and hormone-replacement therapy in the Million Women Study. *Lancet, 362,* 419–427.

Moorman, P. G., Grubber, J. M., Millikan, R. C., & Newman, B. (2003). Antidepressant medications and their association with invasive breast cancer and carcinoma in situ of the breast. *Epidemiology, 14,* 307–314.

Morris, C. R., Wright, W. E., & Schlag, R. D. (2001). The risk of developing breast cancer within the next 5, 10, or 20 years of a woman's life. *American Journal of Preventive Medicine, 20*(3), 214–218.

Morris, J., & Royle, G. T. (1988). Offering patients a choice of surgery for early breast cancer: A reduction in anxiety and depression in patients and their husbands. *Social Science & Medicine, 26*(6), 583–585.

Morrow, M. (2000). The evaluation of common breast problems. *American Family Physician, 61*(8), 2371–2378.

Musick, K. G. (1997). The politics of implants for breast cancer survivors: Feminist issues for counsel and action. *Women & Therapy, 20*(3), 39–50.

Nadalin, V., Cotterchio, M., & Kreiger, N. (2003). Antihistamine use and breast cancer risk. *International Journal of Cancer, 106,* 566–568.

National Comprehensive Cancer Network. (2007). The NCCN Breast Cancer Clinical Practice Guidelines in Oncology (Version 2.2007). Retrieved August 15, 2007, from http://www.nccn.org

National Institutes of Health Consensus Development Panel. (2001). National Institutes of Health Consensus Development Conference Statement: Adjuvant therapy for breast cancer, November 1–3, 2000. *Journal of the National Cancer Institute, 93*(13), 979–989.

Nekhlyudov, L., & Partridge, A. (2003). Breast cancer risk communication: Challenges and future research directions: Workshop report (United States). *Cancer Causes and Control, 14,* 235–239.

Newcomer, L. M., Newcomb, P. A., Potter, J. D., Yasui, Y., Trentham-Dietz, A., Storer, B. E., et al. (2003). Postmenopausal hormone therapy and risk of breast cancer by histologic type (United States). *Cancer Causes and Control, 14,* 225–233.

Newcomer, L. M., Newcomb, P. A., Trenthan-Dietz, A., Longnecker, M. P., & Greenberg, E. R. (2003). Oral contraceptive use and risk of breast cancer by histologic type. *International Journal of Cancer, 106,* 961–964.

Newlin, M. E., Reiling, R., & Nichols, K. (2002). Necessity of axillary dissection in elderly women with early breast cancer. *World Journal of Surgery, 26,* 1239–1242.

NIH Consensus Conference. (1991). Treatment of early-stage breast cancer. *Journal of the American Medical Association, 265*(3), 391–395.

Northouse, L. L. (1989a). The impact of breast cancer on patients and husbands. *Cancer Nursing, 12*(5), 276–284.

Northouse, L. (1989b). A longitudinal study of the adjustment of patients and husbands to breast cancer. *Oncology Nursing Forum, 16*(4), 511–516.

Northouse, L. L. (1996). Sharing the cancer experience: Husbands of women with initial and recurrent breast cancer. In L. Baider, C. L. Cooper, & A. Kaplan De-Nour (Eds.), *Cancer and the family* (pp. 304–317). New York: Wiley.

Northouse, L. L., Mood, D., Kershaw, T., Schafenacker, A., Mellon, S., Walker, J., et al. (2002). Quality of life of women with recurrent breast cancer and their family members. *Journal of Clinical Oncology, 20*(19), 4050–4064.

Nosarti, C., Roberts, J. V., Crayford, T., McKenzie, K., & David, A. S. (2002). Early psychological adjustment in breast cancer patients: A prospective study. *Journal of Psychosomatic Research, 53,* 1123–1130.

Osborne, M. P. (1991). Breast development and anatomy. In J. R. Harris, S. Hellman, I. C. Henderson, & D. W. Kinne (Eds.), *Breast diseases* (2nd ed., pp. 1–13). Philadelphia: Lippincott.

Palmer, J. R., Wise, L. A., Horton, N. J., Adams-Campbell, L. L., & Rosenberg, L. (2003). Dual effect of parity on breast cancer risk in African-American women. *Journal of the National Cancer Institute, 95*(6), 478–483.

Paoletti, X., Clavel-Chapelon, F., & the E3N group. (2003). Induced and spontaneous abortion and breast cancer risk: Results from the E3N cohort study. *International Journal of Cancer, 106,* 270–276.

Partridge, A. H., Burstein, H. J., & Winer, E. P. (2001). Side effects of chemotherapy and combined chemohormonal therapy in women with early-stage breast cancer. *Journal of the National Cancer Institute Monographs, 30,* 135–142.

Patel, A. V., Calle, E. E., Bernstein, L., Wu, A. H., & Thun, M. J. (2003). Recreational physical activity and risk of postmenopausal breast cancer in a large cohort of US women. *Cancer Causes and Control, 14,* 519–529.

Perun, J. (2004). Radiation therapy. In K. H. Dow (Ed.), *Contemporary issues in breast cancer: A nursing perspective* (2nd ed., pp. 110–133). Sudbury, MA: Jones and Bartlett.

Poggi, M. M., Danforth, D. N., Sciuto, L. C., Smith, S. L., Steinberg, S. M., Liewehr, D. J., et al. (2003). Eighteen-year results in the treatment of early breast carcinoma with mastectomy versus breast conservation therapy: The National Cancer Institute randomized trial. *Cancer, 98*(4), 697–702.

Potts, L. K. (2000a). Introduction: Why ideologies of breast cancer? Why feminist perspectives? In L. K. Potts (Ed.), *Ideologies of breast cancer: Feminist perspectives* (pp. 1–11). New York: St. Martin's Press.

Potts, L. K. (2000b). Publishing the personal: Autobiographical narratives of breast cancer and the self. In L. K. Potts (Ed.), *Ideologies of breast cancer: Feminist perspectives* (pp. 98–127). New York: St. Martin's Press.

Prentice, R. L. (2000). Review: Future possibilities in the prevention of breast cancer: Fat and fiber and breast cancer research. *Breast Cancer Research, 2,* 268–276.

Prentice, R. L., Caan, B., Chlebowski, R. T., Patterson, R. E., Kuller, L. H., Ockene, J. K., et al. (2006). Low-fat dietary pattern and risk of invasive breast cancer: The Women's Health Initiative Randomized Controlled Dietary Modification Trial. *Journal of the American Medical Association, 295*(6), 629–642.

Price, M. A., Tennant, C. C., Butow, P. N., Smith, R. C., Kennedy, S. J., Kossoff, M. B., et al. (2001). The role of psychosocial factors in the development of breast carcinoma: Part II. Life event stressors, social support, defense style, and emotional coping and their interactions. *Cancer, 91*(4), 686–697.

Price, M. A., Tennant, C. C., Smith, R. C., Butow, P. N., Kennedy, S. J., Kossoff, M. B., et al. (2001). The role of psychosocial factors in the development of breast carcinoma: Part I. The cancer prone personality. *Cancer, 91*(4), 679–685.

Quesnel, C., Savard, J., Simard, S., Ivers, H., & Morin, C. M. (2003). Efficacy of cognitive-behavioral therapy for insomnia in women treated for nonmetastatic breast cancer. *Journal of Consulting and Clinical Psychology, 71*(1), 189–200.

Qureshi, M., Thacker, H. L., Litaker, D. G., & Kippes, C. (2000). Differences in breast cancer screening rates: An issue of ethnicity or socioeconomics? *Journal of Women's Health & Gender-Based Medicine, 9*(9), 1025–1031.

Rabinowitz, B. (2002). Psychosocial issues in breast cancer. *Obstetrics and Gynecology Clinics, 29*(1), 233–247.

Rimer, B. K., Halabi, S., Strigo, T. S., Crawford, Y., & Lipkus, I. M. (1999). Confusion about mammography: Prevalence and consequences. *Journal of Women's Health & Gender-Based Medicine, 8*(4), 509–520.

Roberts, S. B., Livingston, P., White, V., & Gibbs, A. (2003). External breast prosthesis use: Experiences and views of women with breast cancer, breast care nurses, and prosthesis fitters. *Cancer Nursing, 26*(3), 179–186.

Ross, J. S., Fletcher, J. A., Linette, G. P., Stec, J., Clark, E. J., Ayers, M., et al. (2003). The HER-2/neu gene and protein in breast cancer 2003: Biomarker and target of therapy. *Oncologist, 8*, 307–325.

Rustøen, T., & Begnum, S. (2000). Quality of life in women with breast cancer: A review of the literature and implications for nursing practice. *Cancer Nursing, 23*(6), 416–421.

Samms, M. C. (1999). The husband's untold account of his wife's breast cancer: A chronologic analysis. *Oncology Nursing Forum, 26*(8), 1351–1358.

Schernhammer, E. S., Laden, F., Speizer, F. E., Willett, W. C., Hunter, D. J., Kawachi, I., et al. (2001). Rotating night shifts and risk of breast cancer in women participating in the Nurses' Health Study. *Journal of the National Cancer Institute, 93*(20), 1563–1568.

Schijven, M. P., Vingerhoets, A. J. J. M., Rutten, H. J. T., Nieuwenhuijzen, G. A. P., Roumen, R. M. H., van Bussel, M. E., et al. (2003). Comparison of morbidity between axillary lymph node dissection and sentinel node biopsy. *European Journal of Surgical Oncology, 29*, 341–350.

Schoenfeld, E. R., O'Leary, E. S., Henderson, K., Grimson, R., Kabat, G. C., Ahnn, S., et al. (2003). Electromagnetic fields and breast cancer on Long Island: A case-control study. *American Journal of Epidemiology, 158*(1), 47–58.

Schwartz, A., Mori, M., & Jao, R. (2001). Exercise reduces chemotherapy fatigue in breast cancer patients. *Physician & Sports Medicine, 29*, 5–6.

Schwartz, G. F., Ciuliano, A. E., Veronesi, U., & the Consensus Conference Committee. (2002). Proceedings of the Consensus Conference on the Role of Sentinel Lymph Node Biopsy in Carcinoma of the Breast, April 19–22, 2001, Philadelphia, PA, USA. *Breast Journal, 8*(3), 126–138.

Schwartz, M. D., Taylor, K. L., & Willard, K. S. (2003). Prospective association between distress and mammography utilization among women with a family history of breast cancer. *Journal of Behavioral Medicine, 26*(2), 105–117.

Sener, S. F., & Lee, L. H. (2000). Surgical management of ductal carcinoma in situ. In D. J. Winchester & D. P. Winchester (Eds.), *Breast cancer: Atlas of clinical oncology* (pp. 131–138). Lewiston, NY: B. C. Decker.

Sepucha, K. R., Belkora, J. K., Mutchnick, S., & Esserman, L. J. (2002). Consultation planning to help breast cancer patients prepare for medical consultations: Effect on communication and satisfaction for patients and physicians. *Journal of Clinical Oncology, 20*, 2695–2700.

Shah, N. M., & Wazer, D. E. (2005). The MammoSite balloon brachytherapy catheter for accelerated partial breast irradiation. *Seminars in Radiation Oncology, 15*, 100–107.

Shands, M. E., Lewis, F. M., & Zahlis, E. H. (2000). Mother and child interactions about the mother's breast cancer: An interview study. *Oncology Nursing Forum, 27*(1), 77–85.

Shimozuma, K., Ganz, P. A., Petersen, L., & Hirji, K. (1999). Quality of life in the first year after breast cancer surgery: Rehabilitation needs and patterns of recovery. *Breast Cancer Research and Treatment, 56*, 45–57.

Simpson, C. (2000). Controversies in breast cancer prevention: The discourse of risk. In L. K. Potts (Ed.), *Ideologies of breast cancer: Feminist perspectives* (pp. 131–152). New York: St. Martin's Press.

Stefanek, M. E., Helzlsouer, K. J., Wilcox, P. M., & Houn, F. (1995). Predictors of and satisfaction with bilateral prophylactic mastectomy. *Preventive Medicine, 24*, 412–419.

Susan G. Komen Foundation. (2007a). *Facts for life: Lymphedema.* Retrieved August 15, 2007, from http://cms.komen.org/stellent/groups/public/documents/komen_document/aftertreatlymphedema.pdf

Susan G. Komen Foundation. (2007b). *Recommendations for mammography.* Retrieved August 15, 2007, from http://cms.komen.org/Komen/AboutBreastCancer/EarlyDetectionScreening/EDS3-3-1-1?ssSourceNodeId=292&ssSourceSiteId=Komen

Tabar, L., Yen, M. F., Vitak, B., Chen, H. H. T., Smith, R. A., & Duffy, S. W. (2003). Mammography service screening and mortality in breast cancer patients: 20-year follow-up before and after introduction of screening. *Lancet, 361*, 1405–1410.

Tallman, M. S., Gray, R., Robert, N. J., LeMaistre, C. F., Osborne, C. K., Vaughan, W. P., et al. (2003). Conventional adjuvant chemotherapy with or without high-dose chemotherapy and autologous stem-cell transplantation in high-risk breast cancer. *New England Journal of Medicine, 349*(1), 17–26.

Taylor, E. J. (2000). Transformation of tragedy among women surviving breast cancer. *Oncology Nursing Forum, 27*(5), 781–788.

Tercyak, K. P., Lerman, C., Peshkin, B. N., Hughes, C., Main, D., Isaacs, C., et al. (2001). Effects of coping style and BRCA1 and BRCA2 test results on anxiety among women participating in genetic counseling and testing for breast and ovarian cancer risk. *Health Psychology, 20*(3), 217–222.

Terry, P., Rohan, T. E., Wolk, A., Maehle-Schmidt, M., & Magnusson, C. (2002). Fish consumption and breast cancer risk. *Nutrition and Cancer, 44*(1), 1–6.

Thomas, D. B., Gao, D. L., Ray, R. M., Wang, W. W., Allison, C. J., Chen, F. L., et al. (2002). Randomized trial of breast self-examination in Shanghai: Final results. *Journal of the National Cancer Institute, 94*(19), 1445–1457.

Thorne, S. E., Harris, S. R., Hislop, T. G., & Vestrup, J. A. (1999). The experience of waiting for diagnosis after an abnormal mammogram. *Breast Journal, 5*(1), 42–51.

Thorne, S. E., & Murray, C. (2000). Social constructions of breast cancer. *Health Care for Women International, 21*, 141–159.

Tjønneland, A., Thomsen, B. L., Stripp, C., Christensen, J., Overvad, K., Mellemkjær, L., et al. (2003). Alcohol intake, drinking patterns and risk of postmenopausal breast cancer in Denmark: A prospective cohort study. *Cancer Causes and Control, 14*, 277–284.

Tomoyasu, N., Bovbjerg, D. H., & Jacobsen, P. B. (1996). Condition reactions to cancer chemotherapy: Percent reinforcement predicts anticipatory nausea. *Physiology & Behavior, 59*(2), 273–276.

Tu, S. P., Yasui, Y., Kunihuki, A. A., Schwartz, S. M., Jackson, J. C., Hislop, T. G., et al. (2003). Mammography screening among Chinese-American women. *Cancer, 97*, 1293–1302.

Vacek, P. M., Winstead-Fry, P., Secker-Walker, R. H., Hooper, G. J., & Plante, D. A. (2003). Factors influencing quality of life in breast cancer survivors. *Quality of Life Research, 12,* 527–537.

van Dijk, S., Otten, W., Zoeteweij, M. W., Timmermans, D. R. M., van Asperen, C. J., Bruening, M. H., et al. (2003). Genetic counselling and the intention to undergo prophylactic mastectomy: Effects of a breast cancer risk assessment. *British Journal of Cancer, 88,* 1675–1681.

Velez-Barone, G. (2004). Fatigue, sleep disturbance, and pain. In K. H. Dow (Ed.), *Contemporary issues in breast cancer: A nursing perspective* (2nd ed., pp. 198–208). Sudbury, MA: Jones and Bartlett.

Veronesi, U., Paganelli, G., Viale, G., Luini, A., Zurrida, S., Galimberti, V., et al. (2003). A randomized comparison of sentinel-node biopsy with routine axillary dissection in breast cancer. *New England Journal of Medicine, 349*(6), 546–553.

Vicini, F. A., & Recht, A. (2002). Age at diagnosis and outcome for women with ductal carcinoma-in-situ of the breast: A critical review of the literature. *Journal of Clinical Oncology, 20*(11), 2736–2744.

Vrieling, C., Collette, L., Fourquet, A., Hoogenraad, W. J., Horiot, J. C., Jager, J. J., et al. (2003). Can patient-, treatment- and pathology-related characteristics explain the high local recurrence rate following breast-conserving therapy in young patients? *European Journal of Cancer, 39,* 932–944.

Wang, X., Cosby, L. G., Harris, M. G., & Liu, T. (1999). Major concerns and needs of breast cancer patients. *Cancer Nursing, 22*(2), 157–163.

Wengström, Y., Häggmark, C., Strander, H., & Forsberg, C. (2000). Perceived symptoms and quality of life in women with breast cancer receiving radiation therapy. *European Journal of Oncology Nursing, 4*(2), 78–88.

Whitaker-Worth, D. L., Carlone, V., Susser, W. S., Phlean, N., & Grant-Kels, J. M. (2000). Dermatologic diseases of the breast and nipple. *Journal of the American Academy of Dermatology, 43*(5), 733–751.

Wilcox, S., & Stefanick, M. L. (1999). Knowledge and perceived risk of major diseases in middle-aged and older women. *Health Psychology, 18*(4), 346–353.

Willett, W. (1990). *Nutritional epidemiology.* New York: Oxford University Press.

Winchester, D. J. (2000). Evaluation and surgical management of stage I and II breast cancer. In D. J. Winchester & D. P. Winchester (Eds.), *Breast cancer: Atlas of clinical oncology* (pp. 139–151). Lewiston, NY: B. C. Decker.

Winer, E. P., Hudis, C., Burstein, H. J., Chlebowski, R. T., Ingle, J. N., Edge, S. B., et al. (2002). American Society of Clinical Oncology technology assessment on the use of aromatase inhibitors as adjuvant therapy for women with hormone receptor-positive breast cancer: Status report 2002. *Journal of Clinical Oncology, 20,* 3317–3327.

Wu, A. H., Yu, M. C., Tseng, C.-C., Hankin, J., & Pike, M. C. (2003). Green tea and risk of breast cancer in Asian Americans. *International Journal of Cancer, 106,* 574–579.

Yalom, M. (1997). *A history of the breast.* New York: Ballantine Books.

Yamamoto, S., Sobue, T., Kobayashi, M., Sasaki, S., Tsugane, S., & for the Japan Public Health Center-Based Prospective Study on Cancer and Cardiovascular Diseases (JPHC Study) Group. (2003). Soy, isoflavones, and breast cancer risk in Japan. *Journal of the National Cancer Institute, 95*(12), 906–913.

Zahlis, E. H. (2001). The child's worries about the mother's breast cancer: Sources of distress in school-age children. *Oncology Nursing Forum, 28*(6), 1019–1025.

Zahlis, E. H., & Shands, M. E. (1991). Breast cancer: Demands of the illness on the patient's partner. *Journal of Psychosocial Oncology, 9*(1), 75–93.

Zahlis, E. H., & Shands, M. E. (1993). The impact of breast cancer on the partner 18 months after diagnosis. *Seminars in Oncology Nursing, 9*(2), 83–87.

Zarcone, J., Smithline, L., Koopman, C., Kraemer, H. C., & Spiegel, D. (1995). Sexuality and spousal support among women with advanced breast cancer. *Breast Journal, 1*(1), 52–57.

Zhang, S., Hunter, D. J., Hankinson, S. E., Giovannucci, E. L., Rosner, B. A., Colditz, G. A., et al. (1999). A prospective study of folate intake and the risk of breast cancer. *Journal of the American Medical Association, 281*(17), 1632–1637.

Zmuda, J. M., Cauley, J. A., Ljung, B.-M., Bauer, D. C., Cummings, S. R., Kuller, L. H., et al. (2001). Bone mass and breast cancer risk in older women: Differences by stage at diagnosis. *Journal of the National Cancer Institute, 93*(12), 930–936.

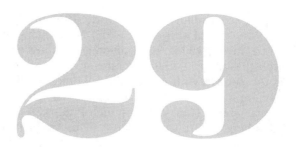

Care of Women With Disabilities

Kathleen J. Sawin and Janet C. Horton

Women with disabilities report a wide range of negative experiences when seeking care from their health care providers. Negative attitudes, stereotypes, physical barriers to care, discriminatory language, lack of knowledge about specific medical condition and lack of sensitivity to sexuality issues may be present in the practice from which a woman seeks care. Often nurses are well meaning but are uninformed. This chapter will address critical knowledge needed by health care providers. The chapter is organized by the ACCESS curriculum developed for health care providers (Sawin & Metzger, 2007). The components of this curriculum include:

Awareness: of unique issues and potential discrimination

Choices: individually, choice-centered approach to care

Consultation: with a colleague with expertise in women with disabilities

Expectations: normalcy for women with disabilities

Sensitivity: in language, inclusion, sexuality, well-women and environmental issues

Specific: considerations related to management knowledge for effective contraception choices, labor, delivery, parenting, and child care issues

In addition, there are groups of women whose unique needs are addressed in this curriculum. Adolescent women with disability face unique challenges in the development of independence skills, dealing with emerging sexuality, and achieving social competence. The challenges exist whether these young women grow up with their disability or acquire a disability during adolescence, but the nature of the challenge may vary somewhat. Women aging with disability face the interaction of their condition and aging. Women with disabilities in diverse cultures must deal not only with the illness experience but also from the definition of self that is divergent from the societal norm of the referent culture group. Finally, lesbian women report unique issues.

The ACCESS approach can be useful for health care providers wishing to increase both their sensitivity and knowledge of the evidence available in the care of women with disability. A critical team member for all intervention teams is a consumer member who herself has a disability. The ACCESS organization addresses issues, content and personnel needed to provide the learner with information needed for effective and sensitive care. Women with disabilities cannot and should not be defined (physically or psychologically) by their disability. All too often it is forgotten that an individual with a disability is an ordinary person who does ordinary things in a somewhat different or unique way.

AWARENESS

The discrimination that women with disability and chronic illness face are twofold: first, they are women, and second, they are individuals with disabilities. Women experience greater effects from disability than men in that they earn less, work less, and are studied less (Kane, 2005; McCauley Ohannessian, Lerner, Lerner, & von Eye, 1999). Further, the concerns of women are different than those of men in terms of self-image and the impact of disability on self-worth (Brownridge, 2006; Copel, 2006; Martin et al., 2006; Nosek, Hughes, Taylor, & Taylor, 2006). High divorce rates are associated with disability; the highest rates are when the woman is the spouse with a disability. Women with disabilities are at increased risk for emotional, physical, and sexual abuse (Curry, Hassouneh-Philips, & Johnston-Silverberg, 2001; Groce, 2003). This problem can be compounded by the societal attitudes toward disability, including discrimination and stereotyping (Crawford & Ostrove, 2003). Women with disabilities are frequently treated as if physical disability means mental retardation, especially if their speech is impaired. Frequently, inebriation is assumed in addition to low IQ. Specific disabilities (spinal cord injury, cerebral palsy, multiple sclerosis, or disabling arthritis) prevent women, it is thought, from meeting society's major functions. Narrow negative social attitudes set unnecessary barriers to the optimal growth and development of these women and the health care they obtain.

For African American women with disabilities, there may be issues of role conflict, employment and sexuality (Alston, Bell, & Feist-Price, 1996). African American women may experience greater difficulty with multiple role conflict. They tend to have more roles, more children, greater environmental stress and may be more likely to be single parents. Employment is a challenge for African American women. Women of color with disabilities have lower employment income levels than all other men and women. They earn $.22 for every dollar earned by a White nondisabled man (Anderson, 1991). The evidence indicates that many African American women are traditional in their sexual practices. If the woman is hesitant to participate in oral sex behaviors, masturbation, or experiment with alternative methods of sexual intimacy she may be at risk for sexual dissatisfaction. Health professionals need to assess the woman for the discrepancy between their ideal and real experiences. Assistance that helps decrease the discrepancy will optimize the woman's adjustment. Further, emphasis needs to placed on conditions that unequally affect African American women, such as sickle cell. Lupus strikes most during the childbearing years and African American women are overrepresented. For women who are immigrants, the experience is more difficult because the woman must deal with her marginality, social isolation, and alienation in a foreign culture (Howland & Rintala, 2001). The devaluation of self is not only rooted in the chronic illness experience but also from the definition of self that is constructed in dealing with the migration experience.

Many health care providers have negative attitudes toward women with disabilities, expect less of them, and overestimate the negative impact of disability on family life. Women are seen as more dependent, asexual, and less able to care for themselves or a child (Becker, Stuifbergen, & Tinkle, 1997; Iezzoni, McCarthy, Davis, & Siebens, 2000). Conflict is perceived between carrying out the responsibilities of parenthood and complying with a medical regimen. Mothers report that health care providers seem unable to recognize the profound interrelationship between their mothering responsibilities and chronic illness or disability (Nosek et al., 1994). Many women hold the opinion that it is a contradiction to be both an effective mother and a good patient. The perception of women as sexual beings is often linked to appearance and desirability to men. These attitudes affect how women perceive their sexuality and ability to attain their sexual potential. Many health care professionals are misinformed about the sexual potential of women with disabilities and focus only on the disabling condition (Di Giulio, 2003; Nosek et al., 1994, 1996).

The unmet needs of women with physical disabilities include accessibility to well-women care, gynecological care, sexuality and birth control counseling, pregnancy, birth, parenting care, and accessibility to professionals with knowledge of how disability impacts primary care. Too often, women with disabilities are not offered the recommended health care screenings that have been found to help with early detection and treatment of certain diseases (Hughes, 2006). Disability-related barriers often discourage women from participating in health-promoting activities (Hassouneh-Phillips, McNeff, Powers, & Curry, 2005; Mele, Archer, & Pusch, 2005). Women with disabilities often feel devalued and feel that their symptoms are overlooked by health care providers (Crow, 2003; Piotrowski & Snell, 2007). A lack of equipment and facilities for women with physical limitations and lack of assistance during health care visit present physical barriers to women with disabilities seeking health care. Bias on the part of health care providers that all health problems are due to the disabling condition or the failure of health care providers to deal with sexual or reproductive health in women with disabilities because of their focus only on the disabling condition are examples of the attitudinal barriers that must be overcome to meet the health care needs of women with disability.

Our understanding of disability has changed significantly during the past several decades. However, the most important change in the understanding of disability is recognizing that the lives of women with disability are usually far more limited by existing social, cultural, and economic constraints than by specific physical, sensory, psychological, or intellectual impairments (Groce, 1999). The development of cultural competence—sensitivity, knowledge and skills around cultural issues—has been identified as a priority in today's health care environment (Institute of Medicine, 2002). It is acknowledged that behaviors, attitudes, and policies across the health care spectrum must respect and act in response to the cultural diversity of the people it serves. In defining culture, all groups that have special needs by virtue of their cultural beliefs and values, social class, ethnicity, language, gender, sexual orientation, or marginalization are included (Institute of Medicine, 2002). The next logical step is to recognize those with disabilities as a legitimate cultural minority. Activists and scholars writing about the civil rights movement of individuals with disabilities reject the traditional view of disability as physically defective and needing to be fixed. Instead, these activists are asserting that most of the problems faced by individuals with disabilities are not caused by the body but by a society that refuses to accommodate our differences. This philosophy proposes that medical needs are only a small part of the disability experience, with the larger, more pressing problems being social and political (Gill & Brown, 2000). Providing culturally competent care for those with disabilities therefore requires awareness of the intrinsic relationship between the physical and emotional barriers that shape their response to events and situations that relate to health and illnesses and that health care providers examine their own views, attitudes, and behaviors and the impact they have on others.

Culture shapes women's experience with disability. The more the disability experience is divergent from the societal norm of the referent group, however, the more issues the woman will face. As long as women with disability are viewed as different from the norm based only on disability, they will continue to be invisible (Asgharian & Anie, 2003; Aulagnier et al., 2005; Baker, 2003; Li & Yau, 2006; McKay-Moffat & Cunningham, 2006; Nosek et al., 1994; Singh & Sharma, 2005; Sze, 2003). Health care providers have strong influence on knowledge, beliefs, and expectations of women with physical disabilities and chronic illness. In-service training sessions for health care providers and women's centers are needed to address access and attitudinal barriers. Health care providers must provide consumer-driven, culturally competent outreach, education, and accessible health care for women with disability. More research and collaboration with other health care professionals can determine ways to help women with disability overcome physical and emotional barriers to sexual functioning. More importantly, women with disability can be reassured of their self-worth, and the inclusion of sexuality can be encouraged as an important aspect of their lives.

CHOICES

Navigating the ever-changing health care system can be challenging to women with disability and their families. Although autonomy and choices are critical to adult functioning, the low level of knowledge and a high degree of uncertainty among health care professionals about best practice for women with disability may limit their autonomy. Best practice demands that the health care provider be knowledgeable regarding a wide variety of individual considerations such as contraceptives, pregnancy, labor and delivery, parenting, child care, and individual life issues such as adolescence, aging, and women who partner with women. Women with disability should be equal partners in all aspects and phases of health care planning, implementation, and ongoing development of wellness and disease prevention strategies. Health care providers have a responsibility to aggressively pursue current best-practice options for women with disability and enter into a partnership with women to assist them in making health care choices. Suggestions for improving care include involving women with disability in teaching health care providers about their special needs and self-advocacy training to help disabled women become more knowledgeable partners in their own health care. Disabled women should be encouraged to be proactive and advocate for their own health and health care needs. Each woman with a disability is unique and must carefully weigh all options and evaluate the choices in relation to her own personal goals and lifestyle. Women with disability should be prepared to ask questions about options and assume responsibility for making choices. Table 29.1 lists suggestions for women with disability in seeking the information they need to make informed decisions. Knowledgeable and sensitive health care providers need to be ever vigilant for ways to facilitate choice for women with disability.

CONSULTATION

Health care providers who provide care for women with disabilities and have no disability-related experience must consult with others. Developing relationships with people with expertise in various fields is needed to develop creative ways to adapt treatment procedures for people with disabilities. For example, consideration should be given to speaking with a lactation consultant to find ways to prevent fatigue in a nursing mother with multiple sclerosis. Professionals in rehabilitation nursing; advanced practice nurses with a specialty practice in chronic conditions of children or adults; lactation consultants; physicians with a specialty in physical medicine and rehabilitation; physical and occupational therapists; mental health, vocational, rehabilitation counselors' consumer organizations such as the Independent Living Centers; and specific disability-related organizations and support groups may all be potential consultants. The most effective consultant may be an experienced, active consumer with disabilities. A truly accessible environment regards women with disabilities

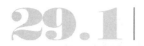

SUGGESTIONS FOR MAKING INFORMED HEALTH CARE DECISIONS

- Find reliable and knowledgeable resources and providers for your health care needs and issues.
- Speak up regarding your needs; explain what type of help you need.
- Be prepared to ask questions regarding your treatment options
- Ask for explanations, in terms you understand, about your health care options
- Ask for discussion regarding your health care concerns, do not allow the health care provider to ignore or dismiss your concerns.
- Do not allow yourself to be pressured into making a decision, take your time to consider all the options.

SPECIFIC LANGUAGE GUIDELINES

Disability. General term used for a (semi) permanent condition that interferes with a person's ability to do something independently—walk, see, hear, learn, lift. It may refer to a physical, mental or sensory condition. Preferred usage is a descriptive noun or adjective, as in a person who is disabled, people with disabilities, or disabled persons. Terms such as the disabled, crippled, deformed and invalid are inappropriate.

Limitation. Preferred term to be used in place of disability, emphasis is on functional abilities and limitations rather than the individuals health status or condition.

Handicap. Often used as a synonym for disability. Usage, however, has become less acceptable. Except when citing laws or regulations, handicap should not be used to describe a disability.

Mute or Person Who Cannot Speak. Preferred term to describe persons who cannot speak. Terms such as deaf-mute and deaf and dumb are not appropriate.

Nondisabled. In a media portrayal of persons with and without disabilities, nondisabled is the appropriate term for people without disabilities. Able-bodied should not be used, as it implies that persons with disabilities are less than normal. Normal is appropriate only in reference to statistical norms.

Seizure. Describes an involuntary muscular contraction symptomatic of the brain disorder epilepsy. Rather than saying "epileptic," say "person with epilepsy" or "person with seizure condition." The term *convulsion* should be reserved for seizures involving contractions of the entire body. The term *fit* is used in England but it has strong negative connotations.

Spastic. Describes a muscle with sudden, abnormal, involuntary spasms. It is not appropriate for describing a person with cerebral palsy. Muscles are spastic; people are not.

Speech Impaired. Describes a person with limited or difficult speech patterns.

Cesarean Birth. Should be used to describe a surgical birth. Avoid "section" Grapefruits get sectioned; women give birth.

ETIQUETTE GUIDELINES

- After an initial greeting, sit down so that a person using a wheelchair won't have to crane his/her neck to make eye contract.
- Always speak directly to a person with a disability. Don't assume a companion is a conversational go-between
- Shake whatever a person offers in greeting—a hand, prosthesis or elbow.
- When speaking with a person with speech difficulty, talk normally. Don't pretend to understand when you don't. If necessary, ask the person to repeat. They've experienced this before and know problems can arise.
- When speaking with a person with a hearing loss, try to keep your face out of the shadows and your hands away from your mouth as you speak.
- If sign language is used in relating issues of sexuality and sexual intercourse, it should be remembered that sign communication is easily interpreted "across the room"; therefore, attention must be given to interview area
- If you are speaking to someone and a sign-language interpreter is present, remember to took at and talk to the person, not the interpreter
- When someone with a disability enters your clinic, don't assume she needs your help. Greet the person and tell them you're available for assistance.
- When you offer to assist someone who is visually impaired, allow the person to take your arm so you can guide, rather than propel them.
- Act naturally. Do not be afraid to use expressions such as "Would you like to see that?" or "Let me run over there." On the other hand don't ask personal questions you wouldn't ask someone without a disability
- Ask permission from the client before sitting or leaning on the equipment or moving it particularly when the client is in it or on the examination table, where she may want her equipment close by.
- Service animals are working when they are with their owners. Don't touch the animal without the owner's permission.

Note. Adopted in part from: Center for Health Promotion for Women with Disabilities at Villanova University. (2003). Health-Related Rights. Retrieved October 19, 2007, from http://nurseweb.villanova.edu/womenwithdisabilities//other/Rights.html; Cohen, 1998.

Adapted from *Guidelines for reporting and writing about people with disabilities.* Media Project, Research and Training Center on Independent Living (348 Haworth Hall, University of Kansas, Lawrence, KS, 66045); *Disability Etiquette: Tips on interacting with people with disabilities.* Eastern Paralyzed Veterans Association publications (75-20 Astoria Boulevard, Jackson Heights, NY 11370) as experts in how their bodies function and promotes peer and mentoring relationships. Women with disabilities want to interact with and learn from their peers. One study found that women with rheumatoid arthritis depended on lay resources rather than health professionals for guidance in nutrition; use of alcohol, tobacco, and nonprescription drugs; sexuality; consequences of a pregnancy on their disability or disease; and infant care techniques, equipment, and devices (Hatcher et al., 1994). Numerous resources exist for the exploration of current and emerging treatment options for individuals with disabilities (see the resource list at the end of the chapter). In addition, multiple Internet resources have been developed; one study found that using Web sites aimed at women with disabilities was effective in increasing knowledge (Pendergrass, Nosek, & Holcomb, 2001). The value of these diverse resources should not be overlooked by the health care professional.

EXPECTATIONS

Many women with disabilities lead active and satisfying sex lives while others have not explored their sexuality. A variety of economic, social, psychological, and cultural barriers influence the sexual functioning of these women. Some authors propose that the primary barriers to full expression of sexuality are the negative attitudes of others, especially family members and medical and rehabilitation professionals (Becker et al., 1997; Broderick & Krause, 2003). The attitude that the disability has somehow "neutered" the woman interferes with her belief in her right to sexual feelings and expression (Nosek et al., 1994, 1995, 1996; Welner, 1993). Many health care professionals often send the message that a woman's body is unacceptable. In addition, health care providers may incorrectly assume that women with disabilities are not sexually active, especially if their disability is severe or disfiguring (Howland & Rintala, 2001). They may not screen these women for sexually transmitted infections (STIs) or even perform a gynecological examination. Screening for breast cancer detection—that is, performing monthly breast self-exams (BSE), annual clinical breast exams (CBE), and mammograms—are not routinely offered to women with disabilities even when they present for gynecological examinations (Capriotti, 2006; Piotrowski & Snell, 2007). Although many women with disabilities have heard the guidelines for breast cancer detection, most of those who want to have mammograms or clinical breast exams often cannot do so because of barriers unique to their functional limitations. Further, women with disabilities have markedly fewer cardiovascular disease prevention screenings (body mass index, baseline electrocardiograms, family history, and smoking history) and lower cardiovascular disease knowledge when compared to women without disability (Diab & Johnston, 2004). Women with mobility problems were unlikely to get immunizations for pneumonia and influenza) and were less likely to receive pap tests (Diab & Johnston, 2004). Although disability is not a contraindication to responsible parenting, family members and health care providers often discourage women with disability from childbearing. In fact, a significant factor in whether young women with disability have active social lives was their parent's expectations. Unfortunately, although these parents had educational goals for their daughters, only a small percentage expected their daughters to be socially active (Drench, 1992). Many women with disability report that they did not receive adequate education about sexuality and reproductive health (Nosek et al., 1995; Piotrowski & Snell, 2007). In a study of adolescents with disabilities, school nurses given the same vignette about young adolescents with and without disabilities starting their menstrual period for the first time at school held different expectations for knowledge, self-care, and independence based only on the adolescents' use of a wheelchair for mobility (Blackwell-Stratton, Breslin, Mayerson, & Bailey, 1988).

A study of women with spinal cord injuries (Persuad, 2000) indicated three barriers to preventive health: (1) inadequate knowledge regarding health risk, (2) reliance on caregivers to facilitate preventative health practices, and (3) perceived problems with access to competent health care providers. The characteristics of medical systems sometimes constitute barriers to women with physical disabilities. Several women report dissatisfaction with services they receive from their provider, such as a different provider each time, procedures in some offices that prohibit staff from offering assistance to women in mounting an exam table, staff unwilling to offer assistance with dressing, and appointments denied because the women use wheelchairs (Thomas & Cohn, 2006). In a recent study investigating the relationships between health care providers and women with sickle cell, the women reported that they felt negatively labeled and were unwilling to trust the provider (Hughes, Nosek, Howland, Groff, & Mullen, 2003; Smeltzer, 2006). However, women with disabilities have indicated that when a trusting relationship with a health care provider (HCP) who has appropriate expectations is established, it is a powerful tool in their empowerment.

In addition to attitudes, and even in the era of the Americans with Disabilities Act, physical access remains an issue for many women with disabilities seeking health care. Health care clinics that have architectural barriers limit the independence of women with mobility limitations. Access to buildings via appropriately constructed ramps and to elevators is critical to quality care, as is easy access to bathrooms, examination rooms, and accessible scales. Most medical facilities have numerous architectural barriers such as nonelevating exam tables and lack of accessible scales to weigh persons who use a wheelchair. Even if the facility is architecturally accessible, furniture placement can make the examination room functionally inaccessible. Little attention has been given to determining whether access issues for women are different than for men. For mothers, day care access, school, public playgrounds and affordable housing are all fundamental access issues that are usually not on the list for "assessing accessibility" for most organizations (Reinelt & Fried, 1993).

An additional access issue may be geographical. Rural women with disabilities make up more than 25% of women with disability (Hughes, Nosek, & Robinson-Whelen, 2007). Rural women with disabilities can be at risk for a number of issues including depression, economic challenges, and access to health care (Hughes, Robinson-Whelen, Taylor, Petersen, & Nosek, 2005). In a study of rural women with disability with depression were younger, had more pain, limited mobility, and less perceived social support. In addition, even though most in the study had moderate to severe depression, more than 33% had not been treated for their depression.

Women with disabilities who are depressed, especially minority women, are less likely to report depression and less likely to get treatment when depressed. This is a complex problem but is at least somewhat the result of HCP and societal expectations that assume that disability and depression are logically linked. Because depression may be viewed as a normal response to disability, the HCP may assume that treatment is not warranted. In contrast, disability is not necessarily the primary factor in depression for women with disabilities. Regardless of the cause, HCPs need to be as vigilant in screening for depression in women with disabilities as for other patients. The HCP may need to pay special attention to screening for depression in minority women with disabilities, especially Hispanic women, who have been reported to be the most hesitant to reveal depression (Hughes et al., 2005).

In summary, women with disabilities are women first and deserve acceptance of their sexuality. This includes the right to marry, parent, and care for children and to have access to accurate health information, including information about safe sex practices, STIs, and planning a healthy pregnancy—all of which will enable them to make informed choices and take appropriate actions. HCP knowledge regarding health promotion services, nutrition and eating disorders, physical activity and prevention of abuse are critical in providing women with disabilities with the same preventive health care as their counterparts without disabilities. Health promotion for women with disabilities should embrace not only all services offered in traditional health promotion programs but also may include treatments and programs aimed at specific disabilities.

Health Promotion

None of the Healthy People 2010 goals addressing individuals with disabilities have been met (U.S. Department of Health and Human Services, 2006a). Women with disabilities continue to receive less preventative care than women without disabilities and in most cases, less than the recommended guidelines. Preventative care for almost all services and groups remained below the targeted goals with women with greater disabilities receiving less screenings than those with mild or moderate disabilities (Diab & Johnston, 2004; Gordon, Sawin, & Basta, 1996; Stuifbergen, Becker, Rogers, Timmerman, & Kullberg, 1999). In Healthy People 2010 increasing the proportion of health and wellness programs and facilities accessible to women with disabilities remains a priority as does combating the perception that women with disabilities do not need prevention services and education. The health promotion and disease prevention needs of people with disabilities are not nullified because they were born with an impairing condition or have experienced a disability or injury that has long-term consequences. Having a long-term condition increases the need for health promotion (U.S. Department of Health and Human Services, 2006a).

There is a growing emphasis from both clinicians/researchers and the U. S. Department of Health and Human Services (2006a) to generate knowledge about health promotion and wellness needs of women with disabilities and chronic illnesses. The Center for the Study of Women with Disabilities (CROWD) has been created at Baylor University (www.bcm.tmc.edu/crowd). The National Institutes of Health held a consensus conference on the Health of Women with Disabilities, The "Health Promotion for Women with Disabilities Program" at Villanova University that specifically addressed health promotion for women with disabilities (www.nursing.villanova.edu/WomenWith Disabilities/html) and organizations such as the Spina Bifida Association and the American Epilepsy Society have created an organizational committee or task force to address the unique needs of this population. Nosek and colleagues (1994) interviewed 31 women about wellness issues. The concepts of coherence, self-regulation, competence, resilience, empowerment, and health awareness have been cited in existing models of wellness. These women's experiences indicated that resilience was the relevant concept in their lives. Their lines of defense emerged as an important part of this resilience because their boundaries were continually threatened by insensitive behaviors of medical professionals and overwhelming overprotectiveness by family. Maintaining a sense of sexual identity for women with disabilities is a critical component of wellness and health. Women who were identified as high in wellness tended to be assertive, resourceful and proactive in their search for knowledge and ways to overcome the barriers they experienced. The following wellness perspective of sexuality for women with physical disabilities conveys expectations that empower these women (Nosek et al., 1994).

1. *Positive sexual self-image.* She is accepting and not ashamed of her body. She appreciates her own value and asserts her right to make a choice. She is able to restrict the limitations resulting from her disability to physical functioning only and does not impose those limitations to her sexual self.

2. *Sexual information.* She actively seeks credible and reliable information about sexuality and is able to apply it to herself. She has knowledge about how her disability affects her sexuality.

3. *Positive, productive relationships.* She feels generally satisfied with her relationships and is able to communicate effectively with others. She feels stability in her relationships. She is able to control the amount and nature of contact with others

4. *Managing barriers.* She is able to recognize psychological, physical and sexual abuse and exploitation and take action to reduce it, eliminate it, or neutralize its impact. She has learned to reduce her vulnerability. She understands her disability-related environmental needs and seeks information on how to meet these needs. She recognizes her right to live in a barrier-free environment and takes action to achieve it. She confronts societal barriers by using good communication skills to educate her partner, friends and family

5. *Optimal health and sexual functioning.* She participates in health maintenance activities and engages in health promoting behaviors. She feels congruity between her values/desires and her sexual behaviors. She manages her environment to optimize privacy for intimate activities. She is satisfied with the frequency and quality of sexual activity. She is able to communicate freely with her partner about limitations and devices and about what pleases her sexually.

Health care providers need to better understand the health promotion practices of women with disability that we may assist them in dealing with their chronic conditions. In addition to wellness issues regarding sexuality and reproductive health, optimal health promotion, including adequate nutrition and exercise, is essential for women with chronic conditions.

Nutrition and Eating Disorders

Women with multiple sclerosis were found to consume inadequate (10% lower than recommended) carbohydrates, fiber, calcium, and zinc and higher than recommended vitamin C, A, fat, protein, and iron (Timmerman & Stuifbergin, 1999). In a survey identifying that over 50% of at-risk women are not taking a multivitamin, women acknowledged that they would be more likely to take the multivitamin if recommended by their health care provider (March of Dimes, 2005). Evidence (Centers for Disease Control and Prevention, 1998) supports that 0.4 mg (400 micrograms) per day of folic acid will significantly reduce the number of cases of neural tube defects (NTDs). Because NTDs occur in the early days of pregnancy before women are even aware of being pregnant, the U.S. Public Health Service recommends that all women of childbearing age who are capable of becoming pregnant should take a multivitamin containing 0.4 mg of folic acid once a day to reduce the risk of having a pregnancy affected with spina bifida or other NTDs. Women who have had a prior pregnancy affected by NTDs are considered high risk, should be placed on higher daily doses of folic acid (4 mg) and should plan with their health care provider for any anticipated pregnancies because supplementation needs to be taken for at least one month before pregnancy (Smeltzer, 2007). Providers need to be aware that high doses of folic acid may mask vitamin B12 deficiency (Centers for Disease Control and Prevention, 1991). Obesity may put women at two to four times higher risk for NTDs despite folic acid supplementation (Shaw, Rozen, Finnell, Wasserman, & Lammer, 1998; Shaw, Velie, & Schaffer, 1996). Thus, preconception counseling for weight reduction has even more impact if the client seeks conception (Murphy, 1996).

There is an increasing focus on the nutrition of women with disabilities. Women with disabilities face numerous barriers to good nutrition: physical barriers to shopping or cooking, limited financial resources, and fatigue contribute to less than adequate nutrition (Hall, Colantonio, & Yoshida, 2003). Data suggest that living with chronic illness or disability may adversely affect eating attitudes and behaviors and may increase susceptibility to the development of eating disorders (Antisdel & Chrisler, 2000; Neumark-Sztainer, Story, Resnick, & Blum, 1998). Eating disorder (ED) research studies suggest that 3%–42% of institutionalized adults with cognitive impairment and 1–19% of adults with cognitive impairment in the community have diagnosable EDs (Antisdel & Chrisler, 2000). Diabetes research found a prevalence of eating disorders of 5.9% (lifetime prevalence of 10%), regardless of gender and type of diabetes (Herpertz et al., 1998). A cross-sectional survey of 71 women (mean age = 23 years) with spina bifida or rheumatologically related illnesses was conducted to assess the symptoms of eating disorders. Of the participants, 8% reported a sufficient number of ED symptoms to indicate probable clinical disorder. More than 20% of the respondents scored at or above the clinical cut point on at least one of the eight ED subscales (Gross, Ireys, & Kinsman, 2000). Such data and case reports suggest that women with disabilities are at risk for poor psychological adjustment and unhealthy weight and mental comorbidities, especially obesity (Piotrowski & Snell, 2007). Eating disorders arise from a variety of physical, emotional, and social issues and have serious consequences for health, productivity, and relationships. All women with disabilities should be screened for EDs. Emergent clinical issues are the development of appropriate diagnostic criteria and multidisciplinary and clinically effective treatment approaches (Antisdel & Chrisler, 2000).

Nutrition issues related to osteoporosis can be especially important for women with disabilities who develop osteoporosis at an earlier age, especially if they have a disability that effects mobility (e.g., spinal cord injury, spina bifida, arthritis, or multiple sclerosis) or a specific condition (e.g., downs syndrome or epilepsy) that is known to put them at risk for osteoporosis. These women may need calcium and vitamin D supplementation as well as earlier screening (Harden, 2003; Schrager, 2004).

Physical Activity

Exercise may be a crucial component of wellness in individuals with disabilities (Yoshida & Li, 1999) but self-reported physical activity is generally low in women with disabilities, especially in African American women. These low levels of physical activity expose women with disabilities to higher risks of secondary conditions (Rimmer, 2001; Rimmer, Rubin, Braddock, & Hedman, 1999). Individuals with disabilities have demonstrated physiological responses to exercise similar to women without disabilities. In addition, exercise has been shown to yield positive overall fitness and psychological outcomes (Ashton-Shaeffer, Gibson, Autry, & Hanson, 2001; Goodwin & Compton, 2004; Rimmer et al., 1999). Although most of the studies have been done on men, the data suggest normal wheelchair propulsion is not sufficient to maintain physical condition and training programs yield positive changes in physical conditioning (DePauw, 1996). Research that explores the responses of women with disability to a variety of recreational and sports programs and the interaction of women's health status with these programs is needed. The opportunities for physical activity for women with disabilities need to be expanded. A recent evaluation of instruments measuring fitness and recreation accessibility—called AIMFREE—may offer HCPs useful aids in assisting women with disabilities to determine the appropriateness of fitness facilities (Rimmer, Riley, Wang, & Rauworth, 2004).

Abuse

Access to accurate sexuality materials is very important for women with disabilities, their families, and health care providers. Because people who are disabled are vulnerable to sexual abuse, prevention information should be readily accessible. In addition, health care providers need to include sexual assertiveness skills in sex education or family life curricula. Women with physical and cognitive disabilities may be at particularly high risk of abuse (Curry & Hassouneh-Phillips, 2002; Curry et al., 2001; Gill & Brown, 2000; Walsh & LeRoy, 2004; Young, Nosek, Howland, Chanpong, & Rintala, 1997). Women with disabilities may not report abuse because of fear of not being believed due to their devalued status (Cole, 1993; Hassouneh-Phillips et al., 2005) or due to feeling less worthy (Hassouneh-Phillips & McNeff, 2005). There is combined cultural devaluation of women based on age and disability. Women with disabilities often experience overprotection and have internalized social expectations. Combine this with a lack of knowledge, limited social opportunity, constant negative feedback (women with disability are ugly, worthless etc), low self-esteem, and limited or no assertiveness skills, and it is understandable that this population has a high incidence of abuse (Brownridge, 2006; Cohen, Forte, Du Mont, Hyman, & Romans, 2005; Copel, 2006; Hassouneh-Phillips, 2005; Martin et al., 2006; Nosek, Hughes, Taylor et al., 2006). In a landmark national survey of over 800 women, Nosek, Howland, Rintala, Young, and Chanpong (1997) found that women with disabilities are four times more likely to have been abused than their nondisabled peers (50% of women with disability and 34% women without disability reported abuse). These results suggest that women who receive little information regarding sexuality are vulnerable to exploitation. In a qualitative study of 31 women with disabilities, the disability itself did not seem to be related to the abuse experience (Nosek, 1995). The report concluded that it is the asexual, dependent passive stereotype of women with disabilities that causes vulnerability to sexual abuse rather than the disability itself. Children with disabilities are several times as likely to have a history of abuse as children without disabilities. Almost one-third of children with a wide variety of disabilities have confirmed histories of abuse and it is expected that many others have experienced unreported abuse (Murphy & Elias, 2006). Abuse is a significant barrier to achievement regardless of the disability or whether abuse was a factor in the child's primary diagnosis. Similarly, abuse contributes substantially to behavior problems and depression. To be effective in addressing learning and behavior problems, health care providers and educators must identify and respond to child abuse and its effects. Health care providers must learn to recognize signs of abuse, listen to the patient and act on reports of abuse. Assessment of abuse and treatment interventions for women with disabilities will be the same as for their peers without disabilities. However prevention is the key. Educational programs need to be developed to address skill building in coping with potential or real abuse and orientation to sexuality rights and responsibilities (Elvik, Berkowitz, Nicholas, Lipman, & Inkelis, 1990).

SENSITIVITY

Each woman with a disability is unique. It is the individual's level of ability and functioning—not the disability—that must be assessed to determine an effective treatment plan. Providers need to assess their assumptions. They may be surprised to learn that the severity of physical impairment is not a good predictor of the impact of the disability on women (Bellin, Sawin, Roux, Buran, & Brei, 2007; DePauw, 1996; Mudrick, 1988; Sawin, Brei, Buran, & Fastenau, 2002; Stengel, 1996). Individuals may have the same disability without having the same functional abilities or limitations. Further, even those who have limited functional abilities may perceive their quality of life as high. Functioning and disability are perceived as the complex interaction between the health of the individual and the background factors of the environment and personal dynamics. This combination of factors and dimensions is of "the person in his or her world" (World Health Organization, 2001). On May 22, 2001, the World Health Assembly approved the International Classification of Functioning, Disability and Health (ICF). The ICF classification enhances the WHOs International Classification of Diseases—10th Revision (ICD), which provides information on diagnosis and health condition, but not on functional status (World Health Organization, 2001). The ICF is designed to be relevant across cultures as well as age groups and genders, regardless of their health condition. The language of the ICF is neutral, placing emphasis on function rather than condition or disease. The ICF is structured according to the following components:

- Body functions and structure.
- Activities (related to tasks and actions by an individual).
- Participation (involvement in a life).
- Additional information on severity and environmental factors.

The ICF terminology allows for an assessment of the degree of disability and treats these dimensions as interactive and dynamic rather than linear or static (World Health Organization, 2001). Achieving optimal health and well-being requires an understanding of the effects of people's health status on their basic abilities to participate in the activities of life. Functional limitations occur when an individual's ability to participate in these activities is hampered by health status or condition and means of compensation are not made available. A functional assessment is applicable to every person regardless of condition and is integral to the development of appropriate care (World Health Organization, 2001). Health care providers must evaluate the individual's need when determining the level and type of service needed rather than developing a plan of care based solely on the disability. Examiners should look at their own attitudes and expectations before eliciting a history from women with disabilities to determine potential problems. The history protocol should not be varied or altered to omit certain issues. If providers usually ask about first sexual experiences, birth control, episodes of unwanted intercourse, or satisfaction with intimate relationships, then they also should ask women with disabilities. In doing so, it is important to watch one's so-called handicapism terms and use inclusive and sensitive language (see Table 29.1 for language guidelines). Language is a powerful communicator of negative attitudes. Using inclusive language is an important strategy to convey respect and empower women. Limiting, stereotypical terms must be avoided. Sometimes, health care providers speak without sensitivity (Kirshbaum, 1996; Muir & Ogden, 2001). Characteristically, clinic and hospital personnel talk to the person who is accompanying the individual with a disability, not to the individual herself. In addition, they frequently talk down or use language patterns appropriate for a child (Nosek, 1992). When talking about people with disabilities, providers should choose words that convey nonjudgmental implications and are accurate descriptions of the disability. As a general rule, one should always put people first, before their disabilities, referring to *persons with disabilities* rather than *disabled people*. Avoid using emotional descriptors such as *unfortunate* or *brave* that imply that people with disabilities are to be pitied, feared, or ignored or that they are somehow more heroic, courageous, patient, or special than others. Never use the term *normal* in contrast. Don't assume that, because someone has a disability, she needs help: people with disabilities want to be treated as independent people. Women with disabilities are the best judge of what they can and cannot do: if they need help, they will ask for it. Finally, remember that a person with a disability is just an ordinary person who does ordinary things in a somewhat different or unique way. If you don't know what to say or do, let the person who has the disability help set the pace for talking. See Table 29.1 for etiquette guidelines.

SPECIFIC ISSUES: SEXUALITY, UNIQUE POPULATIONS, AND REPRODUCTIVE HEALTH WITH SPECIFIC CONDITIONS

Sexuality and the Assessment of Reproductive Health

Women's sexuality and reproductive capacity plays a crucial role in shaping their lives and health experiences. Communicating and obtaining information about sexuality are among a woman's greatest concerns. The subject of sexuality and disabled women has been studied little, perhaps because of the erroneous assumption that among clients with a disability, sexuality adjustment is less an issue for women than for men (Drew, 1990). Women with disabilities face multiple barriers to quality reproductive health care services (Becker et al., 1997) and receive fewer services (Centers for Disease Control and Prevention, 1998). Women report that professionals rarely initiate discussion of sexuality issues (Meeropol, 1991; Nosek et al., 1996). Health care providers need to take responsibility for initiating discussions of sexuality, but also important is offering assistance rather than avoiding or overemphasizing the issue. Assumptions should not be made at either extreme: such as none of these women have sexuality issues, or all of them do. Instead, assess each individual.

Reproductive health screening such as mammogram and pap smears for women with disabilities may mean additional planning. Women with more severe disabilities may need to be especially targeted as they get screened less than their peers with mild or moderate disability (Smeltzer, 2006). Women with disabilities report fiscal constraints, inaccurate information, poor transportation, inaccessible facilities and equipment, and assistance barriers to getting to the mammography service and, difficulties with communication, physical limitations and attitudes of staff as barriers at the facility (McCarthy et al., 2006; Poulos, Balandin, Llewellyn, & Dew, 2006). Researchers call for both better training of HCP as well as adaptation of the mammography technique to meet the needs of women with disabilities. Further, they indicate it is important to identify women with disabilities for whom a mammogram is not an option and who need alternative breast screening methods (Poulos et al., 2006).

Sexuality and Sexual History

The woman's knowledge of sexuality is pertinent. What was her family life like while she was in school? Does she understand what implications her disability has for sexuality, contraception, birth control, and routine health needs? Ask whether the sexual information she was given either in adolescence or during rehabilitation was sufficient (Verhoef et al., 2000). Women with disabilities may have low sexual knowledge and less sexual experience (Vansteenwegen, Jans, & Revell, 2003). From discussions with the client, determine her knowledge deficits. In addition, identify unmet sexual and health needs. Include review of condition-specific issues such as dysreflexia for women with spinal cord injury, latex allergy for women with spina bifida, or spasticity issues for women with cerebral palsy. Ask all women about any allergy-type reactions to latex products (e.g., balloons, rubber products, condoms). Do not omit condition issues, such as incontinence, or psychosocial issues, such as self-confidence, that impact sexuality (Verhoef et al., 2000). Physical barriers such as weakness, vaginal dryness, lack of balance, and hip or knee pain, can present problems with sexual activity for women with disabilities (Dormire & Becker, 2007). Ask the client what problems the disability has presented and how she has overcome these barriers. More medical research and collaboration with health professionals can discover ways to help women with disabilities overcome physical barriers to sexual functioning.

Accessibility

It has been suggested that the client may find it more difficult to gain psychological accessibility to the health care provider than physical accessibility to the clinic. Providers must limit stereotypes, actively pursue optimal communication procedures, value mutual problem solving and goal setting, and use every opportunity to reaffirm normalcy. When communication is effective women with disabilities report less anxiety and more positive experiences (McKay-Moffat & Cunningham, 2006). In a clinical setting, guidelines are needed to enhance accessibility, beginning with the first telephone contact. Proposed guidelines have been delineated by the Task Force on Concerns of Physically Disabled Women (1978). When the first appointment is made, clients should be asked:

Do you have a physical disability? If so, ask the client to specify whether it is difficult getting around, hearing, or seeing, and so on.

What accommodations will be necessary for your visit to the clinic? Arrangements may need to be made that will allow for a longer visit.

The Americans With Disabilities Act, enacted in 1990, mandates that all new buildings meet minimal accessibility standards. Section 504 of the Persons With Disabilities Act of 1978 applies to all facilities receiving any federal funds. The regulations do not require that a facility have special programs or services. The regulations do, however, require that the same services offered to women without disabilities must be offered to women with disabilities (U.S. Department of Health and Human Services, 2006b). For example, if women without disabilities are weighed, accurate mechanisms are needed to weigh women with disabilities. Wheelchair-accessible scales can be used to weigh ambulating women as well. If the clinic offers Pap smears and pelvic examinations, it needs to offer women with disabilities the same services and to make necessary accommodations.

Accessible Supportive Examination Table

A table at wheelchair height facilitates transfer of women with motor disabilities. One such table (see resources) adjusts to wheelchair height to facilitate transfer to the table; it provides arm rests to support women with cerebral palsy and spasticity who may fear falling off the table when severe or unexpected spasms occur. The absence of leg support, however, may be a major drawback for women with leg weakness or paralysis. Examination tables that have leg support but are not at wheelchair height may be preferred in some settings. Each setting needs to assess its target population for services and provide the most accessible examination table.

Altered Pelvic Examination

A health care provider must be aware that a client with disabilities may need an altered pelvic examination. Discussion with the client should attempt to solve problems she might have had during previous pelvic exams. Ask what positions caused problems and what worked best for her. For example, women with cerebral palsy report spasms, especially adductor spasms, which may be controlled if the woman takes the knee-chest position, with an assistant hugging her, or the side-lying position, with the bottom leg flexed and upper leg on the examiner's shoulder (similar to left lateral delivery position) (Carty, Conine, Holbrook, & Riddell, 1993; Carty, Conine, & Hall, 1990). Keeping the woman's extremities close to the body decreases movement that may stimulate additional spasms. Additional personnel may be needed to assist in supporting the client (e.g., holding legs) during the exam. The client should collaborate in deciding the need. She may prefer to bring a family member or friend with her to the exam.

Amputation and Decreased Range of Motion

The client may be examined in a semi-sitting position. She may choose to hold the stump herself and place the other leg on the examiner's shoulder or she may choose to have assistance with holding her stump so she can hold a mirror and participate in the examination.

Specific Examination

Examination of the genitalia must include inspection of the vaginal walls for atrophic changes, determination of intravaginal tone, and assessment of hair distribution in the genital region to help rule out possible endocrinopathies (Dormire & Becker, 2007; Zasler, 1991). Some examiners find a "handle-up" technique helpful for women with limited range of motion. This handle-up technique may also make viewing a mid-position or anteverted cervix easier. In patients who have a history of autonomic dysreflexia, spasticity, or pain on insertion of the speculum, xylocaine gel applied generously to the perineal area can make the exam more effective and comfortable, as long as the gel will not interfere with any specimens needed. All movements in the examination should be gradual to allow patient accommodation. Some authors suggest select use of the cotton swab Pap smear for the rare woman with disabilities who is unable to tolerate a speculum examination. This technique is much less accurate, however, and every effort should be made to assist the client and her family to understand the implications of its use (Ware, Muram, & Gale, 1992). In contrast, a vaginal swab using a G-tips® is now an acceptable option for STI screening (Schachter et al., 2005). During the pelvic examination, reaffirm the client's identified normalcy and healthy status. This makes a strong positive impact on her perception of self.

Breast Self-Examination

Women with intact manual dexterity and sensation can be taught breast self-examination: however various physical limitations may affect women's ability to perform BSE according to recommended procedures. Some women with impaired sensation can perform a modified examination or an attendant or partner can perform it. If neither of these plans is acceptable, more frequent examination by a health care provider should be considered (Piotrowski & Snell, 2007).

Menarche and Menstruation

Some variations in menarche occur among women with select disabilities. For example, girls with Down syndrome and spina bifida experience menarche 11 months earlier than a comparison group of girls without disability; however, others with genetic disabilities may have delayed menarche (Accardo, 2008; Furman & Mortimer, 1994). Girls with blindness may experience menarche earlier than other girls. Children with spina bifida and hydrocephalus are more likely to have precocious puberty, which can result in additional problems with stature and psychosocial development (Liptak, 2001). Health care providers should be aware of these differences and be available to reassure and counsel clients appropriately.

Some conditions such as epilepsy, asthma, rheumatoid arthritis, irritable bowel syndrome, and diabetes have menstrual-related changes. Medical suppression of ovulation using gonadotropin-releasing hormone agonists may be useful for diagnosis and treatment of severe, recurrent menstrual cycle-related disease exacerbations (Case & Reid, 1998).

Secondary Conditions

Although women with disabilities generally have a primary condition, recent data indicate that they also have a range of secondary conditions. A vast majority (more than 90%) in a recent study of 443 women reported pain and fatigue as secondary conditions interfering with function (Nosek, Hughes, Petersen et al., 2006). In addition, the majority of these women also reported issues such as spasticity, weakness, sleep problems, vision impairment, and circulatory problems. These women reported experiencing from 0 to 20 secondary conditions with the majority having an average of 5.7 conditions. Race, disability type, functional limitations, and lower levels of mental health were factors explaining 33% of the variance in the interference of these secondary conditions in independence.

Unique Populations

Adolescents

Adolescents with disabilities or chronic conditions often face barriers accessing the traditional rites, roles, and rituals of adulthood not encountered by their peers without disabilities (Jordan & Dunlap, 2001; Sawin, Cox, & Metzger, 2004). Unfortunately, misconceptions are prevalent about the sexuality of children with disabilities. Blum and colleagues (2001) identify the following five myths related to sexuality and disability in adolescents.

1. Young people with disabilities are not sexually active.
2. The social and sexual aspirations of adolescents with disabilities and chronic conditions are different from their peers.
3. Parents of teenagers with disabilities provide sufficient sex education.
4. Young people with chronic conditions are not sexually vulnerable.
5. Problems of sexual expression are a function of the chronic condition or disability.

Unfortunately, over the past 15 years findings persist that adolescents with disabilities tend to lack basic sexual information such as information related to reproduction and contraceptive options and knowledge of sexually transmitted diseases (STIs) (Meeropol, 1991; Murphy & Young, 2005). Many people also think that individuals with disabilities will not marry or have children, so they do not have to learn about sexuality. In a study of adolescents with disabilities, Meeropol found few of the adolescents or their parents ever talked to a nurse or a physician for sexuality information, and one-quarter of the adolescents and 40% of their parents wished that a health care professional had offered this information (Blackford, Richardson, & Grieve, 2000). Parents report insufficient and inadequate information in prenatal education (Sawin, Buran, Brei, & Fastenau, 2002; Verhoef et al., 2005). Furthermore few adolescents receive their sexuality education from professionals, and, even when they do, they report deficits in specific information (Murphy & Young, 2005). At a minimum, adolescents need information regarding body parts, changes to expect in puberty, menstrual hygiene and other personal care, social skills, abuse prevention, sexual expression, their rights and responsibilities, birth control options, and STI prevention (Shah, Norlin, Logsdon, & Samson-Fang, 2005). Providers report poor comfort levels in addressing gynecological care for adolescents with disabilities due to time and reimbursement constraints, lack of knowledge, and disability related issues (Murphy & Young, 2005). At the same time, schools often focus only on the dangers of sex and fail to educate about the human sexual response and potential for sexual pleasure from many sources. To prove that they are normal, some adolescents with chronic illness or disability often increase their sexual behavior. Consequently, they are at increased risk of pregnancy, STIs, and abuse. Adolescent girls with, and without, disabilities are at risk for unintended pregnancy and STIs. For those with disabilities the consequences of an unwanted pregnancy may carry additional risks to both the mother and infant. As a consequence of increased choice and wider opportunity, adolescents with disabilities have an essential need to learn about sexuality and the responsibilities that go along with exploring and experiencing one's sexuality. Health care of all adolescent women with chronic illness and disability must include assessment of the potential for sexual activity or actual sexual activity and guidance regarding contraception, sexually transmitted diseases, and sexual exploitation (National Information Center for Children and Youth with Disabilities, 1992). Providers who wait for adolescent women with disabilities to initiate discussions of sexuality issues will often miss important opportunities. In addition, for adolescent women with disabilities in school, sexuality education should be included in their individual education plan (Cremer, Hoppe, Kleine-Diepenbruck, & Blaker, 1998; Murphy & Young, 2005). As adolescent women with disabilities transition into adulthood, additional opportunities and challenges emerge. It is critical that the adolescent get support for increasing self-management and decision making from both family and HCP (Sawin et al., 2004). In a qualitative study, three types of support were described by adults who grew up with chronic health conditions: (a) emotional (valuing and acceptance), (b) instrumental (guidance and provision of strategies leading to self-efficacy), and (c) cognitive support (affirmation, confirmation, and providing new perspectives). These findings help HCP understand women with disabilities need for different kinds of support, especially during periods of transition (King, Willoughby, Specht, & Brown, 2006). Adolescent women with disabilities may report a positive sense of self, strong family support, an inconsistent larger social network and lack of independent life skills (Bellin et al., 2007; Roux, Sawin, Bellin, Buran, & Brei, 2007; Sawin, Bellin, Roux, Buran, & Brei, in press). Several assessment tools exist that can assist the HCP in either assessing specific skills (California Healthy and Ready to Work Transition Assessment Tool) (Betz, Redcay, & Tan, 2003) or evaluating outcomes (AMIS II) (Sawin, Buran, Brei, Cashin, & Webb, 2007).

Issues Related to Aging

Gynecological health is not only an important component of women's health during their reproductive years, but throughout the course of their lives. Many of the changes that occur as a result of aging often have a direct or indirect effect on the disability. Women with disability may experience unique changes in addition to or independently of the customary aging processes (Nosek, 1992). For example, people with certain conditions such as spina bifida, spinal cord injuries, or polio survivors can begin to show the signs of aging earlier than those without disabilities. A woman with multiple sclerosis may experience an increase in fatigue, while a woman with epilepsy may find her medication for seizure control not as effective during perimenopause but may have fewer seizures after menopause (Harden, 2003). Children or young women who survived polio may experience postpolio syndrome characterized by increased joint weakness and joint stiffness when they reach midlife (40 to 60 years of age). Women with Down syndrome may experience sensory, adaptive or cognitive losses earlier than other women (Brown & Murphy, 1999). Unfortunately it is not always clear whether these changes are a direct result of the disabling condition or the result of aging with a disability. Health care providers who are not familiar with the effects of aging on a disability may dismiss vague and nonspecific

complaints as natural or as a normal course of events. women with disabilities need to monitor symptoms and become more informed about themselves, menopause and their conditions so that changes can be knowledgeably discussed with health care providers. Further research is needed to explore how the aging trajectory differs for people with disabilities since childhood or young adulthood. In addition we know little about the impact of lifelong disability or chronic illness on menopause nor about sexuality issues in those aging with disability (Dormire & Becker, 2007; Pitzele, 1995).

Even though most persons with disabilities are female there is very little research that examines the impact of aging on women with disabilities (Pentland, Tremblay, Spring, & Rosenthal, 1999). Individuals with disabilities and chronic illness are asking: What are the implications of aging to 60 if you have had osteoarthritis since 20? What is menopause like for women with disabilities (Capriotti, 2006; Welner, Foley, Nosek, & Holmes, 1999)? What are the implications on joint health of walking for many years with altered gait or of the early transition to wheelchair as primary source of mobility?

The long-term use of steroids in women with lupus may compound osteopenia and that calcium supplementation with vitamin D needs to be included unless creatinine clearance or calcium excretion is impaired (Julkunen, Kaaja, & Friman, 1993). Further, women with physical disabilities are less likely to ambulate, participate in physical exercise, and are more likely to have a history of phlebitis. They enter menopause with less years of weight bearing and little or no participation in aerobic activity, thus they are at risk for obesity and cardiovascular illnesses (Smeltzer, 2006; Smeltzer, Zimmerman, & Capriotti, 2005) and osteoporosis and related fractures (Dormire & Becker, 2007; Schrager, 2004). Women on seizure medication and who have Down syndrome are at especially high risk (Havercamp, Scandlin, & Roth, 2004; Parkes, 2006). In a study of women with multiple sclerosis, 35% were osteopenic and 20% osteoporotic; only 31% had been tested. Forty-seven percent with positive findings were not advised by their HCP to be tested (Smeltzer, Zimmerman, Capriotti, & Fernandes, 2002). Similarly, almost 50% of women with mobility impairment had never had bone density tests. Unique problems with typical testing that make assessment difficult include problems with positioning due to mobility problems and lack of norms for bone density under age 30 (Dormire & Becker, 2007). Treatment options are also complex. Nonmedical treatment may also be important. Resistance training has been shown to be effective in mainlining bone health and exercise can impact balance, decrease muscle mass, and reduce stress (Dormire & Becker, 2007).

Menopause can also bring decreased skin turgor and strength, loss of elasticity and decreased blood supply. This can put a woman with disability at increased risk for skin breakdown (Welner, 1996). Women who would benefit from estrogen replacement are usually eliminated from consideration due to concerns about the risk of thrombotic events. However, the transdermal estrogen therapy may be a safe option for many, especially if history of thrombosis is old (Stampfer et al., 1991). Management in collaboration with gynecologist, geriatric and psychiatrist consultants may optimize care for elderly women with disabilities. However, women with disabilities are women first, and the same healthy interventions addressing nutrition, exercise, and weight management are critical for women with disabilities.

The impact on mortality of aging with disability is unknown. The major causes of death to persons with spinal cord injuries are respiratory infections, urinary tract infections, and external causes such as suicide. However, there is little data explaining why other people with life-long disabilities die. Women with cognitive impairments face unique challenges to growing old and often need substantial supports to remain functional in the community (Walsh & LeRoy, 2004). Health care providers need to continually monitor emerging evidence that needs to be integrated into the care of ageing women with disabilities.

Women Who Partner With Women

Women with disabilities are not more or less likely to partner with women. However, lesbians have been totally excluded from the few studies that have explored the lives of women with disabilities. The literature exploring experiences of lesbians with disabilities reveals discrimination in the work place, a sense of being voiceless in social and political arenas, anger at public ignorance and injustice and a pervasive able-bodyism in the feminist movement that excludes lesbians with disabilities (Stevens, 1994). The family, a source of support for many individuals, may not be a positive factor for some women because they report the overwhelming feelings of powerlessness being both disabled and a lesbian within the traditional family. Women report both negative and positive experiences when relating to health care providers, although the overwhelming reaction is one of not being listened to and not feeling safe or respected. Women report how powerful the acceptance is when they can introduce their partner to their healthcare provider and feel that it's ok. However, many lesbian women with disabilities experience negative repercussions when they come out with their health care providers. Unapproachable health care providers add to the unaddressed health care needs of this population. For example more than half of lesbian women have not had a Pap smear in the last 12 months (Stevens, 1994). The interventions addressed for all lesbian women are

core to establishing a message of effective communication, approachability and effectiveness when working with women with disability.

Reproductive Health and Specific Conditions

Contraceptive Needs and Choices

Information on contraception is typically not offered to women with disabilities (Meeropol, 1991; Nosek et al., 1996; Piotrowski & Snell, 2007). It is important, however, for health care providers to examine the options with clients. The choice may be a balance of risk factors—for example, the risk of pregnancy versus the risk of the contraceptive method. If oral contraception or an intrauterine device (IUD) is considered and the method carries risk, consultation with or referral to a gynecological specialist needs to be initiated. Discussion of alternatives needs to take place with women who are allergic or whose partners are allergic to latex. Contraceptive options may be significantly restricted for women with mobility impairment or with a latex allergy. Joint management with a physician colleague is indicated.

It is not clear what impact the timing of disability onset has on a woman's satisfaction with contraception and sexuality information. Women whose onset of disability is after menarche are identified by some as having special needs for contraception and sexuality. Other data suggest that women who grow up with their disability do not have adequate sexuality and contraception counseling (Harrison, Glass, Owens, & Soni, 1995; Jackson & Sipski, 2005; Murphy & Elias, 2006; Sawin, Buran et al., 2002; Valtonen, Karlsson, Siosteen, Dahlof, & Viikari-Juntura, 2006; Verhoef et al., 2005). The need for sexuality and contraception counseling must be assessed regardless of the time of onset.

Barrier Methods

Barrier methods are often an optimal choice for women with disabilities. If a client has manual limitations and, consequently, difficulty manipulating a barrier device, it is important to determine the availability of a partner or personal care attendant and their roles. A client may need to explore ways to ask her partner to assist with a barrier method. Many women have not considered asking a personal care attendant to assist with placement of a contraceptive device before sexual activity.

Condoms. Condoms, which also provide protection against AIDS and other sexually transmitted diseases, are an option. Water-soluble lubricants can ease vaginal dryness. Caution should be taken to identify women who have or whose partners have latex allergies. A nonlatex condom (Avante) made by Durex is now available. Manufacturer's lab tests demonstrates that Avante stops sperm and small viruses, but the FDA requires that its labeling indicate that testing is still underway to determine effectiveness against STIs and HIV and that FDA approval is pending for these purposes. Trojan's nonlatex polyurethane condom, Trojan Supra, is a polyurethane condom available with Nonoxynol-9 spermicidal lubricant. Trojan Naturalamb skin is also latex free, but natural pores measure up to 1.5 microns across, or about 0.00006 inch—small enough to stop sperm cells but not HIV or the viruses that cause herpes and hepatitis B. So these condoms are labeled for contraception only, not disease prevention. Other nonlatex condoms (Tactylon) are currently under development and are being tested; their release is expected in the near future.

Female Condom. The Reality condom is a loose polyurethane sheath, lubricated inside and out, that lines the vagina. The Reality condom is inserted like a diaphragm, with a flexible ring at its closed end and a ring at the open end that remains outside, partly covering the labia. It appears to be a strong if somewhat awkward barrier.

Cervical Cap. For some women, a cervical cap is an attractive option, because it can be inserted in the morning by a personal care attendant and removed 24 hours later, eliminating the need for assistance during lovemaking.

Diaphragm. An increase in urinary infections is associated with the arch diaphragm. It may present particular problems and not be appropriate for women with urinary stasis. Caution should be taken to identify women who have or whose partners have latex allergies.

Implanted and Injected Hormonal Contraceptives

Norplant, or *Implanon,* may be an option for some women if memory or manual dexterity is an issue. However, the presence of erratic bleeding may be problematic for these women. This contraceptive has been prescribed for women, including adolescents, with cognitive impairment; 594 woman-months of experience were reported without pregnancy or side effects. Parents of youth with cognitive impairment reported high satisfaction with this method (Neinstein & Katz, 1986a). The World Health Organization has found no evidence that Depo-Provera is harmful. For teens with moderate or severe retardation, the benefits probably outweigh the risks. Women with severe mobility restrictions derive an additional benefit of injected hormones. If these women are dependent on others for menstrual hygiene care, the possible lack or decreased frequency

of menstrual periods may increase their functional status (Welner, 1993). Depo-Provera can be associated with decreased circulating estradiol and thus may cause vaginal dryness. More serious is the hypothetical concern about the effect of decreased estradiol on bone mass (Dangoor & Florian, 1994).

Sexually Transmitted Infections

Little is written about how women with disabilities experience STIs. Health care providers may mistakenly assume that women with disabilities are not sexually active and therefore not at risk for STIs. One study invalidates this myth of asexuality in that most (94%) of the women with disability studied had been sexually active, suggesting that they are as vulnerable to STIs as women without disabilities (Nosek et al., 1996). In Nosek, Howland, Rintala, and colleagues' (2001) study, the incidence of STIs was similar in the two groups, slightly more than one-fifth of the sample. Women with and without disabilities were just as likely to have had syphilis (.4% vs. .5%), gonorrhea (4% vs. 5%), chlamydia (7% each), Trichomonas (11% each), genital warts (8% vs. 10%), and pubic lice (11% each) (Nosek, Howland, Rintala et al., 2001). However, women with disabilities were significantly less likely to have had genital herpes (3% vs. 7%) or a nonspecific STD (3% vs. 5%) (Nosek, Howland, Rintala et al., 2001). There was no report of HIV/AIDS in either group. The rates reported in this study may be higher for both groups because STIs are often under-reported. Women with disabilities may have lower incidence than reported because they may be less likely to report symptoms and are less frequently screened for STIs. Women with disabilities may be less likely to be aware of symptoms suggesting an STD because of mobility and sensory impairments. For example, if women with disabilities have herpes simplex virus, they may have limited abilities to promptly respond to a prodrome if it is tingling or itching in the affected area. Inability to identify developing painful lesions may have severe consequences for these women. Undetected and untreated STIs puts them at risk for getting pelvic inflammatory disease, increasing their risk of cervical cancer, contracting HIV, ectopic pregnancy, and infertility. Getting information about STIs and safe sex practices is as important for women with disabilities as it is for any sexually active woman. Women with disabilities will need to learn to identify and monitor more subtle clues such as including the genital area in routine visual skin checks. It is important that health care provides acknowledge the sexuality of the women with disabilities and initiate discussions of sexuality issues such as STIs and safe sex. The optimal time for this education is in childhood or adolescence through family life education curricula. It is of interest that studies of parents of children with disabilities that the parents report that they are comfortable discussing STIs with their children, but only half of them actually do. Sixty-eight percent of the half that do initiate discussions of STIs included information only on HIV/AIDS, leaving their children vulnerable to other more prevalent STIs. Education regarding safe sex and screening for STIs should be offered to women with disabilities just as it is to their peers without disabilities. Professionals need to seek out opportunities to act as a consultant to schools and community groups that serve this population (independent living centers, local school districts, and schools). Examples and illustrations in literature about STIs should include women with disabilities to help dispel misconceptions and increase awareness (Nosek, Howland, Rintala, et al., 2001).

Pregnancy

Pregnancy is a time for change and preparation for all women. This is even more important for women with disabilities. Each woman and her condition are unique. Not all conditions affect pregnancy and pregnancy doesn't always affect every condition. Some conditions seem to improve during pregnancy while others may get worse during or after pregnancy. Some disabilities may require special considerations and others need no additional care. In some women, problems associated with a normal pregnancy—such as frequent urination—may increase because of the disability. For most women thinking about pregnancy, issues for consideration include getting appropriate health care, the possible impact of pregnancy on the body, concerns for labor and delivery, and care for the child following birth. Although a disability does not alter the ability of most women to be successful in all of the above areas, the disability does provide additional concerns for the expectant mother. Much of that success depends on the care and information the women receive to help them through pregnancy and the postpartum period. Most (81%) registered nurses, nurse practitioners, and occupational and physical therapists indicate their experience, education, and training have not prepared them adequately for this high-risk population (Carty et al., 1990). Unfortunately, this problem continues today (Smeltzer, 2007). Programs such as the ACCESS curriculum must be developed to address health care providers' lack of information about the needs of mothers with disabilities. Information that is modified to answer questions about the unique situation of women with disability is needed. What are the emotional and physical changes of pregnancy? Can the client identify her stressors and fears, both general and specific that are related to her disability? What are the special demands of labor and delivery? If cesarean birth is a possibility, discuss the options available, including the father's participation. Smeltzer (2007) reports that many women

fear that a cesarean birth will be assumed because they have a disability and providing reality data is essential. What are the condition-adaptive parenting skills and equipment necessary for responsible parenting? *The Disabled Woman's Guide to Pregnancy and Birth* (Rogers, 2005), for example, provides an excellent guide for women with disabilities, answering questions throughout each phase. It is important that the clinician be knowledgeable about specific issues for pregnancy and individual conditions. The descriptions of conditions later in this chapter contain condition-specific information.

Preconceptual and Prenatal Care

It is important for the HCP not to convey directly or indirectly to women with disabilities seeking preconceputal counseling or prenatal care that she is unfit to be a mother, should have genetic testing to avoid passing on her own condition, or to assume that she is considering a termination of the pregnancy (Smeltzer, 2007). Preconceputal counseling and prenatal care should focus on strategies to optimize health including nutrition, exercise, sleep, smoking cessation if applicable, and managing any symptoms or secondary conditions that could make pregnancy more complicated. While all women should take 0.4 mg of folic acid before and after conception, it is important that a woman who has had a child with NTD or a woman who has spina bifida, diabetes, or epilepsy, take an increased dose of folic acid by prescription for 4–12 weeks before becoming pregnant (Centers for Disease Control and Prevention, 1991; Smeltzer, 2007) After pregnancy, all women should continue 0.4 mg folic acid indefinitely as long as pregnancy is a possibility.

Case Management

During pregnancy and the postpartum period, case management may be indicated for a woman with disabilities. The case manager is responsible for assuring that the client's unique health care needs are being met, especially if numerous agencies are involved. If a woman's dependency increases during pregnancy, her specific level of function will need to be assessed. Generally, in perinatal management, a health care provider needs to determine whether a woman with a disability has access to a role model who has the same disability as she or whether the client needs case management services. The client should be able to identify her stressors and fears, both general and specific that are related to her disability. Community-based independent living centers may be useful referral resources for the woman with disabilities and HCP. In addition, prenatal referral to occupational therapy may assist the woman with disabilities in planning for care needs.

Partner Preparation

It is important for the health care provider to assess whether a woman's partner needs preparation. The partner may require information from the HCP about the woman's special needs in order to give realistic support and avoid unnecessary restrictions. A typical concern of any couple experiencing pregnancy—hesitancy to have sexual relations for fear of hurting the baby—may be expanded for couples in which the woman has a disability; they may be afraid of hurting the woman (Carty et al., 1990). Although it is especially important for health care providers to interact with partners, data indicate that women with disabilities feel their partners are unwanted by health care providers during labor and delivery (Craig, 1990; Wasser, Killoran, & Bansen, 1993). A prenatal care provider or case manager may need to initiate educational sessions to discuss attitudinal barriers. These activities should be organized well before delivery. If the partner also has a disability, special considerations may be needed to facilitate his involvement.

Specific Adaptive Needs of the Client

Determine what the client needs with respect to her condition. Is a pressure-relief mattress or raised toilet seat needed? Does she want to bring equipment from home? Plan a tour of the hospital during the fifth or sixth month of pregnancy so the need for special equipment can be identified and the equipment can be ordered. Having necessary equipment within reach is critical to the client's well-being and comfort (Carty et al., 1990). A home assessment by an occupational therapist may be helpful.

Education for All Staff

Housekeeping personnel may need to know that a wheelchair positioned in a particular way next to a bed allows a woman to be independent. To move the chair essentially makes the woman a prisoner, because it removes her independence. Nursing staff may need to review prevention of skin shearing, management of dysreflexia, and implications of contraction monitoring.

Specific Conditions and Reproductive Health

Although research is limited, available data for the most frequent disabilities and chronic illnesses are reported here and may be presented in discussions with clients. Generally, in prenatal management, a health care provider needs to determine if a woman with a disability has access to a role model who has the same disability as she or if the client needs case management services (Rogers, 2005). Because most women with disabilities are considered high risk medically, close pregnancy management with a physician colleague or specialist in women's health is recommended.

Cerebral Palsy

The effect of cerebral palsy on contraception varies greatly. If the client is paralyzed or has decreased mobility, hormonal contraception is risky. Independent use of barrier methods, especially the diaphragm or cervical cap, may be troublesome for women with spasticity; however, these methods are viable with partner participation. Cerebral palsy usually has no physical effect on sexual desire. Genital arousal and function are not directly affected although spasticity may need to be addressed if it interferes with positioning or gratification. The effects of cerebral palsy vary significantly so it is important that prospective mothers consult obstetricians who specialize in high-risk pregnancies.

Cognitive Impairment

Women with cognitive impairment and related developmental disabilities, like all people, have basic sexual rights and human needs. Fertility is not affected yet women with cognitive impairments are often denied effective contraception based on the erroneous assumption that they do not have or act upon sexual desires. Women with severe cognitive impairments are frequently seen as nonadults and as unequal to their peers without disabilities (Di Giulio, 2003; Dotson, Stinson, & Christian, 2003; Havercamp et al., 2004; Walsh & LeRoy, 2004). A qualitative study of sexuality in women with cognitive impairment found variation but most reported knowledge of STIs; ability to pleasure themselves; interest in sexuality; and lack of control over sexual health experiences (Dotson et al., 2003). Many people have an unfounded fear that parents with mental retardation cannot raise or support children and will require additional financial and government support (The Arc, 2005). The presence of cognitive impairment and related developmental limitations, regardless of their severity, does not validate loss of sexuality and reproductive rights. This loss affects an individual's development in gender identity, self-esteem, body image, emotional growth, and social behavior. In addition, forced participation in sexual activity continues to be an issue for people with cognitive limitations.

Choices related to birth control, including the decision to have and raise children; to accept personal responsibility for these decisions; and to have control over their own bodies remains the right of all women regardless of the severity of their cognitive impairment (The Arc, 2004). With the use of contraception, informed consent is a critical aspect. For many women with cognitive impairment, the choice of contraception is affected by mobility, chronic illness, and cognitive factors.

- Oral hormonal contraception requires that a woman's memory skills be adequate for the regimen.
- Women who have multiple disabilities (motor and cognitive) may not be able to manage a diaphragm.
- Implanted or injected hormonal contraceptives are often a good option for some women (see section on contraception).

Understanding the needs of young women who grow up with cognitive delay or developmental disabilities is crucial to provision of effective care (Alonso, Jick, Olek, Ascherio, Jick, et al., 2005; Jordan & Dunlap, 2001). Adolescents and young women with cognitive impairment need comprehensive ongoing sex education regarding safe sexual practices, sexual orientation, sexual abuse, and sexually transmitted diseases and accessible adults to assist with problem solving and skill development.

Although women with cognitive impairment often report friendships, meaningful work, and positive well being, they also report decreased social support, isolation, and financial stress and may need significant supports to live fully in the community. Risk factors for impaired health include inadequate nutrition, lack of exercise (especially cardiovascular), lack of screening for preventable conditions, and undertreatment of health issues. In addition, aging with cognitive impairment is accompanied with increase in cardiovascular disease, the major cause of death in this population (Walsh & LeRoy, 2004).

Cystic Fibrosis

Women with cystic fibrosis now live into their 30s or later, and with increasing technology, the age of survival may increase even further in the next few years. There is little evidence that fertility is impaired in healthy women with cystic fibrosis (CF). Pregnancy can be a significant risk for both mother and infant. Data on hormonal contraception are conflicting. The method may cause bronchial mucus to become scant, and it may support the development of endocervical polyps (Neinstein & Katz, 1986b). Pulmonary function and respiratory symptoms were not affected in a small study of 10 young women aged 15 to 24 years. Nevertheless, hormonal contraception should be used only with extreme caution and with very close monitoring of pulmonary status. There is no contraindication to the use of barrier methods among women with cystic fibrosis (Neinstein & Katz, 1986b). Although pregnancy is well tolerated in women with mild disease, those with poor lung function, severe disease and diabetes have

increased risk of prematurity and decline after delivery (Edenborough, 2001). Pregnancy in severe disease is often complicated by pulmonary exacerbations and by poor weight gain. In Edenborough's (2001), study of pregnant women with cystic fibrosis 81% of pregnancies progress after 20 weeks although one-fourth of these delivered prematurely. Breast milk secreted by women with CF appears to be safe for the infant, and breast-feeding by mothers with CF should be encouraged. Women with mild CF disease can maintain their own weight and support growth in healthy infants. Variations in the nutrient content of breast milk may necessitate routine monitoring of the mother and the breast-fed infant, especially during pulmonary exacerbations (Shiffman, Seale, Flux, Rennert, & Swender, 1989). Enlisting the aid of a dietitian as a member of the health care team is invaluable in assessing, monitoring, and managing women with cystic fibrosis during their childbearing years.

Diabetes

The major factor that impacts pregnancy outcomes for women with diabetes is prepregnancy glucose control. With current health care advances, women with diabetes who maintain prepregnancy glucose control for an extended period have similar potential for an uncomplicated pregnancy and a healthy baby, as women without diabetes. However, if a women has poorly controlled diabetes, she has two to four times more risk of having a baby with a serious birth defect as well as an increased risk of miscarriage and stillbirth. Preconception control is critical in women with diabetes. Unfortunately two-thirds of pregnancies in this population are unplanned. In the Charron-Prochownik and colleagues' (2006) study of adolescents with diabetes, 65% were unaware of the importance of preconception counseling and the risk of pregnancy-related complications in women with DM (Diabetes mellitus). All women of childbearing age should be carefully counseled, take folic acid at all times, and pursue effective contraception (American Diabetes Association, 2002). A different trajectory is generally common for women with gestational diabetes which generally develops later in pregnancy and generally does not increase the risk of having a baby with a birth defect. Some studies suggest that gestational diabetes severe enough to require treatment with insulin may result in increased risk of birth defects. Most women with blood sugar control begun before pregnancy reduce their risk of birth defects, miscarriage, stillbirth and complications in the newborn period (March of Dimes, 2007).

Epilepsy

Estrogen levels are related to seizure threshold in one-third to one-half of women with epilepsy (Morrell,

1999). In addition, women with epilepsy (WWE) are at risk for increased incidence of several gynecological problems including polycystic ovary syndrome (PCOS), hypothalamic amenorrhea, premature menopause, and hyperprolactinemia. This may be due to the antiepileptic drugs (AEDs) or the epilepsy itself (Isojarvi, 2003). Seizures vary during the menstrual cycle; incidence is highest during the estradiol spike before ovulation and during the rapid drop in progesterone immediately before and during menstruation. Women with epilepsy more frequently have anovulatory menstrual cycles and polycystic ovaries with some decrease in fertility (Morrell, 1999). The relationship between oral hormonal therapy and seizures is less evident; however, no strong evidence has been found against the use of hormonal contraception (Altman, 1996; Hatcher et al., 1998; Hatzichristou, 1996). Most reports of interaction between hormonal agents and seizure medication indicate accelerated breakdown of estrogens and recommend the use of 50 mg estrogen (Altman, 1996; Hatcher et al., 1998; Hatzichristou, 1996; LaVaccare & Bergen, 2000). This phenomenon is most likely to occur with the use of enzyme-inducing antiepileptic drugs (AEDs) such as phenobarbital, primidone, phenytoin, carbamazepine, topiramate, and valproate. For valproate these changes may be increased if the WWE gains weight during treatment or has polycystic ovaries and menstrual disorders (Isojarvi, 2003). The second-generation AEDs, gabapentin and lamotrigine, do not alter steroid hormones and do not interfere with the effectiveness of hormonal contraceptives (Morrell, 1999). Breakthrough bleeding is a common sign that the AED is lowering the effect of the birth control pill and a signal that a higher dose pill needs to be considered (Hatcher et al., 1998). After the start of AEDs, there should be close monitoring of weight and any changes in the menstrual cycle. Transvaginal ultrasounds of the ovaries may be indicated with changes in cycle, serum testertosne levels, and increased weight (Isojarvi, 2003).

Levonorgestral implants (Norplant) have a similar efficacy with antiepileptic inducers and are not a good option for women on these AEDs, while IM medroxyprogesterone (Depo-Provera) has not been evaluated to determine interaction (LaVaccare & Bergen, 2000). The World Health Organization does not recommend restricting the use of copper bearing intrauterine devices because of epilepsy (Hatcher et al., 1998), however, infection potentially caused by an IUD may decrease medication control. In addition, carbamazepine (CBZ) has been shown to decrease bioactivity of estradiol even for those not on contraceptives. This decrease may cause menstrual alterations in select women on long-term CBZ treatment (Isojarvi, 2003). A common issue for young adult women with a history of epilepsy in adolescence is the advantages and disadvantages of stopping AEDs. The risk–benefit needs

to be carefully considered by the young woman and her neurologist. A recent study did find that females who stopped AEDs before adulthood had no long-term effects on endocrine status. However, those that continued on AEDs (especially VPA) until adulthood had increased endocrine disorders (Mikkonen et al., 2004). In addition, WWE are at higher risk for osteoporosis due to a combination of AEDs and factors associated with epilepsy such as balance issues and falls (Harden, 2003). Perimenopause can be associated with an increase in seizures potentially because of its impact on the estrogen to progesterone ratio but menopause may bring a reduction of seizures (Harden, 2003).

Women often mistakenly believe that decreasing their AEDs will protect their baby against birth defects when, in fact, it may increase the risk if they have a breakthrough seizure due to low levels of AED. Women with epilepsy who wish to become pregnant need to be stable on the lowest dose of AEDs for at least 6 months before conception. Changing to an AED with a better risk profile during pregnancy is contraindicated. During the change, the fetus is exposed to two drugs and seizures might occur. Efforts to wean the woman off AEDs, change to an AED with a better profile for the mother, or attempt to achieve monotherapy in those with complex histories need to be accomplished well before pregnancy (LaVaccare & Bergen, 2000).

Up to 75% of women with epilepsy who are pregnant have increased seizures during pregnancy. AED levels need to be monitored before and during pregnancy by the women's neurologist. In addition, the American Association of Neurology (1998) recommends that free antiepileptic drug levels are the more stable measure and should be monitored at the beginning of each trimester, in the last month of pregnancy, and for the first 8 weeks postpartum. Many women may need an increase in their AEDs during pregnancy, and some will decrease their need in the postpartum period. However, clinical data (increased seizures or adverse effects) remain the major factor in management of AEDs in pregnancy.

Women taking multiple AEDs are most at risk for teratogenic impact (Pennell, 2005); the incidence of birth defects with individual drugs differs by drug, with valproac acid and carbamazephine having the highest risk. Less is known about the second-generation AEDs, but lamotrigine, gabapentin, and vigabatrin are not teratogenic in animals. It was thought some years ago that folic acid might potentiate seizure activity but that fear has been reputed. Indeed, there is good evidence now that low serum and red blood cell levels of folic acid in WWE are associated with an increase in birth defects. Routine supplementation for all women on AEDs is recommended. Some experts recommend the typical 0.4 mg contained in a multivitamin and others recommend the higher dose of 0.8 mg found in over-the-counter prenatal vitamins or 1.0 mg found in prescription prenatal vitamins, although, in practice supplementation is not common (Morrell, 2002). In addition, with the increasing use of AEDs for other conditions such as migraine headaches, bipolar disorders, and pain management, the HCP need to be diligent regarding the impact of these AEDs on the women's reproductive health and potential pregnancies (Kaplan, 2004). Choice of AEDs in women of childbearing age should always include consideration of unplanned pregnancy and be made in collaboration with a neurologist.

Epilepsy appears to alter the clotting factor of the infants born to mothers taking enzyme-inducing AEDs. Although further research is needed, at this time the American Association of Neurology (AAN) recommends that in the last month of pregnancy these mothers need to take 10 mg of vitamin K orally each day. If no prenatal Vitamin K is given, 10 mg IV can be given before delivery. The AAN recommendation that all neonates receive vitamin K1 at birth is not changed by maternal medication. Breast feeding is a option for women with epilepsy and the benefits for the baby and mother outweigh the small risk of problems caused by AEDs (American Association of Neurology, 1998). It is useful to understand that the AEDs with the lowest protein binding characteristics (i.e. phenobarbital or primidone) pass more readily into breast milk. Infants should be observed closely for sedation and failure to thrive.

Adolescents and young women with epilepsy need careful and continual teaching to prepare them to participate in decisions regarding AED management, contraception, pregnancy and breast-feeding. The situations are complex and education should begin early in adolescence. It is of interest that in a large study of women ages 16 to 55, 51% reported that they did not receive any advice about possible interactions between contraception and antiepileptic drug therapy, 34% reported that they had not received any advice regarding pregnancy, and 25% had not discussed pregnancy with anyone (Crawford & Lee, 1999). All health care providers have the opportunity to increase awareness of these issues in women with epilepsy and should do so aggressively.

Inflammatory Bowel Disease

Fertility is usually normal, although may be decreased in women with active Crohn's disease. Menstrual abnormalities are present in 50% of women with Crohn's disease (Feller, Ribaudo, & Jackson, 2001). Malabsorption or side effects of some medications may affect menstrual cycle or fertility. Data is limited on the relationship between inflammatory bowel disease and use of contraception. It is, however, known that most women with inflammatory bowel disease (IBD) worsen with pregnancy (Neinstein & Katz, 1986b). It is therefore important that the disease be stable for a year before

pregnancy is considered. Barrier methods are recommended for contraception. A review of the literature indicates that the use of oral hormonal contraceptives is advised only with reservations; low-dose estrogen or progestin-only oral contraceptives may be taken with close monitoring of the disease by the consulting physician. With active disease or in the presence of malabsorption, hormonal therapy may be ineffective or dangerous (Neinstein & Katz, 1986b). Women with inactive IBD who become pregnant do not have increased complications compared with women without the disease. In some women with IBD it may be necessary to continue drug therapy during pregnancy to control disease activity. Most medications used for IBD are safe in pregnancy and while nursing (Friedman & Regueiro, 2002). Methlytrexate should be avoided due to its antiabortifacient effects (Ferrero & Ragni, 2004; Friedman & Regueiro, 2002). Women with active IBD (especially Crohn's disease) are at risk of having small and premature babies (Alstead, 2002). Optimum disease control before and during pregnancy is essential for both maternal and infant health.

Multiple Sclerosis

The menstrual and fertility patterns of women with multiple sclerosis rarely change (Boston Women's Health Book Collective, 2005). Oral contraceptive use has no negative effect on the risk of developing multiple sclerosis and may provide a short-term protective effect (Alonso et al., 2005; Vukusic & Confavreux, 2006; Vukusic et al., 2004). However, smoking may be a risk factor (Cook, Troiano, Bansil, & Dowling, 1994). Significant evidence exists that hormonal therapy alters the course of multiple sclerosis. Such therapy is contraindicated only for women with paralysis or restricted mobility (Neinstein & Katz, 1986b). Of concern is an older study that reported that 54% of subjects used no contraception because of fear of side effects (Task Force on Concerns of Physically Disabled Women, 1978).

Pregnancy and postpregnancy stress may increase symptoms but do not worsen the long-term prognosis, in fact there is some evidence that pregnancy may slow the progression of the disease and that for some symptoms abate during pregnancy (Charlifue, Gerhart, Menter, Whiteneck, & Manley, 1992; Jackson, Lindsey, Klebine, & Poczatek, 2004; Westgren & Levi, 1998). Risk for exacerbation of symptoms may be greater in the postpartum, especially for those women whose symptoms improved during pregnancy. In first 3 months postpartum, 20%–40% of patients may have exacerbations. Women who have been on long-term corticosteroids at the time of delivery may have relative adrenal insufficiency and should be given supplemental corticosteroids for 24 hours. There is no contraindication to breastfeeding unless drugs are toxic to the baby.

Breastfeeding does not correlate to postpartum relapse (Vukusic et al., 2004). Limb weakness or gait disturbances may necessitate assistance with childcare. Infants born of mothers with multiple sclerosis experience no adverse effects (Lorenzi & Ford, 2002). The major issue in infant care is fatigue, especially if the mother has a postpartum relapse.

Rheumatoid Arthritis

Some evidence indicates that the onset of arthritis may be delayed by hormonal contraceptives (Hatcher et al., 1994). Hormonal therapy, however, has not been shown to affect active disease. Barrier methods may be difficult for some women to use if they experience weakness and decreased manual dexterity (Neinstein & Katz, 1986a). An intrauterine device may worsen existing anemia.

Rheumatoid arthritis (RA) is known to improve during pregnancy; 75% of women will experience remission of the disease with a 90% postpartum exacerbation rate (Queenan & Hobbins, 1996). Several studies suggest that postpartum flare may be induced by breastfeeding (Barrett, Brennan, Fiddler, & Silman, 2000; Jorgensen, Picot, Bologna, & Sany, 1996). Pregnant women who have remissions have significantly greater disparity in maternal-fetal antigens than do those with active disease, which suggests that a maternal immune response may be responsible for pregnancy-induced remission. There appears to be no increased rate of spontaneous abortion, perinatal mortality, or intrauterine growth restriction in the presence of uncomplicated RA. Activities of daily living are easier to perform due to decreased joint stiffness and swelling and increase in grip strength. Women who have overwhelming fatigue, may need to continue a supervised exercise routine. For those with hand/shoulder involvement, dressing may become difficult. Joint contracture may limit positioning. Pain needs to be carefully assessed. Initial treatment of joint pain and stiffness during pregnancy may include local steroid injections into the joint. If the response is inadequate, prednisone may be used in low doses. Acetaminophen remains the analgesic of choice. Nonsteroidal anti-inflammatory drugs should be avoided after 20 weeks gestation. Intramuscular gold salts may cross the placenta, creating a theoretical risk, but they may be useful postpartum to reduce exacerbations. Breast-feeding is not contraindicated.

Sickle Cell Disease

Contraception for women with sickle cell disease is important for two reasons. (1) women with this condition can get pregnant and (2) their pregnancies are high risk and need careful planning. All barrier methods, most low-dose oral contraceptives and injectable hormone contraceptives are options to consider for women with this condition. An IUD is contraindicated because of its association with infections and the complications of infections in women with sickle cell condition (Earles, Lessing, & Vichinsky, 1994). Women with this condition need to consider genetic counseling before pregnancy is attempted. The transmission risk may be as high as 100% or as low as 0%. All children of women with sickle cell disease will have the sickle cell trait (Earles et al., 1994).

Some women have no change in their disease during pregnancy. However, sickle cell crises may still occur in pregnancy. Preexisting kidney disease and congestive heart failure may worsen during pregnancy. Risks in pregnancy depend on whether the mother has sickle cell disease or sickle cell trait. Although pregnant women with sickle cell trait are not at higher risk for pregnancy complications, the infant may be affected if the father also carries the trait. Early and frequent prenatal care is critical for pregnant women with sickle cell disease. Because sickle cell disease affects many organs and body systems, women with the disease are more likely to have severe complications in pregnancy. General pregnancy care includes prenatal vitamins, folic acid supplements, preventing dehydration, and careful screening for signs of infection (particularly lung and urinary tract), as well as symptoms of vaso-occlusive crisis. Some women may benefit from partial prophylactic exchange transfusions to replace the sickled cells with fresh blood, which decrease the number of sickled cells and increases the blood's ability to carry oxygen. Women with sickle cell disease are not at greater risk for infertility and miscarriage than other women, but are more likely to experience preterm labor and growth restriction. Stillbirths also occur more frequently and are probably caused by severe vaso-occlusive crises. Most women with sickle cell can carry an infant to term and deliver vaginally unless there are complications. After delivery, these women should be observed closely for crisis and thrombosis. Emotional support as well as aggressive treatment of acute events will optimize their outcomes (Queenan & Hobbins, 1996). Breast-feeding is generally not recommended for women with sickle cell disease (Earles et al., 1994).

Sight and Hearing Impairment

Many women who are deaf-blind enter adulthood sexually unaware but with normal curiosities, drives, and interests. They usually lack basic sexual information such as physical differences between the sexes, information related to reproduction and contraceptive options and knowledge of STIs. This lack of sexual and reproductive education created by parents' and health care providers' deficiency in sign language skills and alternative methods of communication are compounded by the deaf-blind youth's inability to learn about sexuality by watching and hearing others express appropriate and inappropriate sexual behaviors (Ingraham, Vernon, Clemente, & Olney, 2000). Women who are deaf-blind should be provided sexuality education to help them attain a life with more personal fulfillment and to protect them from exploitation, unplanned pregnancy, and STIs.

Change in the body during pregnancy may affect the ability of women with sight impairments to function (change in center of gravity may alter her relation to object). Lack of educational material in Braille or audiotape necessitates increased individual teaching. Birth rehearsal in the labor room will help the woman orient herself to the room, bed, and bathroom. Use of tactile models and labeling of people and equipment are helpful. It's very important to describe the baby and his or her specific behaviors, reactions, and facial expressions. Women with sight impairment may need adaptive equipment or counseling about specific strategies to make breast-feeding successful.

For women with hearing impairment visual interaction is crucial. Talk to the woman even if an interpreter is present. Assess need for light and whether the woman will need to be in a room where the nurse's station can be seen.

Spinal Cord Injury

The fertility of women with spinal cord injury (SCI) is unaffected. Their decreased mobility and the increased incidence of deep vein thrombosis place them at high risk with respect to hormonal contraceptives, especially those containing estrogen. Birth control pills and injectable hormonal contraceptives are absolutely contraindicated if the woman is receiving antihypertensive medication or if she is known to have circulatory problems (Boston Women's Health Book Collective, 2005). Intrauterine devices pose a risk because of the woman's decreased sensation and ability to determine warning signs of infection. Some women, however, indicate that their partners could check the IUD string placement. Others with high SCI lesion indicate that autonomic dysreflexia (increased blood pressure, flushing above the level of lesion, headache) is triggered by "pain" that the patient is unable to perceive. The women may thus be able to identify infection with the occurrence of autonomic dysreflexia. In a large follow-up study of women with SCI, the IUD was actually the preferred method (Charlifue et al., 1992). Most women with paraplegia can usually manage barrier methods with no or minimal assistance in positioning their legs for effective insertion. Women with higher spinal cord lesions require assistance from a partner or an attendant.

Pregnant women with SCI are generally followed by a clinician that specializes in high-risk pregnancies. These women tend to have increased urinary tract infections, spasticity, impaired lower extremity circulation, constipation, respiratory function, and may have problems with increased skin breakdowns. Further, they may experience a change in self-care skills if their mobility is reduced due to center of gravity changes. Women with SCI may not be aware of labor onset and are at risk for an unattended delivery (Smeltzer, 2007). There is some evidence that premature labor is more likely for these women (Crosby, St-Jean, Reid, & Elliott, 1992). Weekly medical exams may be necessary late in the pregnancy. Other safety precautions may include use of a contraction monitor at home. Delivery for the most part is similar to that for able-bodied women and vaginal deliveries predominate. In women with higher spinal cord lesions, forceps may be used to assist in the delivery. Women with high lesions often experience autonomic dysreflexia with labor and birth. It is important to be aware of this potentially dangerous condition in women whose SCI is at T6 or above. These women have interrupted communication between the peripheral nerves, the spinal cord and the central nervous system. Contractions, skin pain, full bladder, catherizations, enema, insertion of fetal monitoring devices or any other noxious stimulation causes a reflexic physiological reaction that can be confused with toxemia. Increased blood pressure in both conditions needs to be treated urgently. Autonomic dysreflexia is treated by sitting the person up, removing the noxious stimuli, and by giving hypotensive medications. Because contractions cannot be removed, the BP may need to be treated with medications or an epidural might need to be used. Women with a history of autonomic dysreflexia should be in a sitting position during labor. The blood pressure needs to be taken during contractions because this is when it generally rises. Unlike with preeclampsia, with autonomic dysreflexia the blood pressure falls between contractions and mothers no not respond to magnesium sulfate. Close monitoring of respiratory status, skin status, perineal status, and urinary and bowel status are critical throughout labor. Early postpartum mobilization is recommended to prevent deep vein thrombosis. Breast-feeding is possible. Women with high lesions may need special assistance with positioning and feeding. Women with SCI above T-6 may experience decreased milk production 6 weeks after delivery (Crosby et al., 1992; Verhoef et al., 2005; Westgren, Hultling, Levi, & Westgren, 1993). Use of a rehabilitation consultant to evaluate the delivery and postpartum environment is useful (i.e., delivery table may need to be padded, room furniture may need to be rearranged to increase the woman's independence).

Spina Bifida

Most issues discussed for acquired SCI also apply to spina bifida (SB), a congenital SCI. Women with SB

(WWSB) report receiving general sexuality information but little that pertains to their disability (Mazon, Nieto, Linana, Montoro, Estornell, et al., 2000; Sawin, Buran et al., 2002; Szepfalusi, Seidl, Bernert, Dietrich, Spitzauer, et al., 1999). Individuals with SB have the highest incidence of latex allergies, varying from 12% to 50% (Cremer et al., 1998). Reactions vary from mild wheal to anaphylactic reactions. Health care workers should be alert to the possibilities of latex sensitivities in their patients. Staff in hospitals, clinics and doctors' offices should be well versed in latex precautions and all WWSB should be treated with latex precautions (Cass, Bloom, & Luxenberg, 1986). Avoidance of latex materials such as gloves, condoms and diaphragms is recommended for all individuals with spina bifida (see the SBA Web site for a list of latex materials).

Evidence regarding sexual function in WWSB is sparse. One older small study of 35 adult WWSB reported vulvar sensation that varies dependent on the level of their lesion. While more than one-half of sexually active women in one report with sacral or lower lumbar lesions (L3–5) report vulval sensation, only one-third with lesions above L2 report such sensation (Verhoef et al., 2000). More recent evidence in a slightly larger sample of 44 WWSB indicated that 81% reported sexual excitement with intercourse or masturbation, 77% reported lubrication, and over one-third of the women reported orgasms (Jackson & Sipski, 2005).

Although women with SB do not experience infertility more often than other women, there can be physical problems that interfere with becoming pregnant or delivering a baby. Women with spina bifida may have structural reproductive tract differences such as bicornate uterus. However, the information on the frequency or impact of these differences is so limited that no definitive guidelines can be proposed (Jackson & Sipski, 2005). In a study of pregnant WWSB, those who use wheelchairs required more prenatal admissions than those without; urinary tract infections, stomal problems and mobility changes were common, and, if pressure ulcers were present prenatally, they got worse during pregnancy (Arata, Grover, Dunne, & Bryan, 2000). As with other conditions, it is important to have an obstetrician who specializes in high-risk pregnancies and is familiar with SB and its effects on the body, especially if the woman has had a bladder augmentation or an appendicovesicostomy for bladder control. In the latter surgery, the appendix is used to create a catheterizable stoma usually hidden in the umbilicus. Relatively large numbers of young women undergo this procedure, so its implications on pregnancy will need to be evaluated as the young women grow up. For those who wish to become parents some adaptations may be necessary, such as the use of a wheelchair during pregnancy for some who do not

normally need one. Orthopedic complications of SB, such as scoliosis, kyphosis, hip dislocations, pelvic obliquity, and contractures, may impact reproductive anatomy and can increase the complexity of infant care. Pregnancy issues for women with SB and SCI are similar. Although many women with spina bifida can deliver vaginally, some with altered anatomy may need to deliver by cesarean birth (Jackson & Sipski, 2005). The few women whose SB is at T-6 or above need to be assessed for autonomic dysreflexia discussed in the section on spinal cord injury. It is only recently that WWSB have lived past age 50 so little is known about menopause for this population. However, SB can involve issues with skin integrity, urological status, and osteoporosis. These problems are all potentially exacerbated by menopause. Increased bone loss in an already comprised woman can lead to worsening scoliosis and fractures. As estrogen decreases urinary function can be further changed and a functional bladder program can be altered. Thinning skin can put a WWSB at further risk for skin breakdown. Close monitoring of these conditions during menopause will be needed.

In addition, a large number of WWSB who have normal cognition also have learning disabilities that may challenge their self-management. Executive functioning challenges, slower processing speed, and challenges with multiple-part, complicated directions are common. Verbal skills are usually a strength for these women with disabilities. These learning disabilities can be an issue in contraceptive decision making, pregnancy, and child care. Individual assessment and accommodations can usually address these issues, but times of high stress such as childbirth may be accompanied with loss of normal coping mechanisms and need for increased professional support.

While all women should take 0.4 mg of folic acid before conception and thereafter, it is important that a women who has had a child with NTD or a women who has spina bifida begin taking 4.0 mg of folic acid by prescription for 4 to 12 weeks before becoming pregnant and continue through the first 3 months of pregnancy (Centers for Disease Control and Prevention, 1991; Smeltzer, 2007). After pregnancy, all women should continue 0.4 mg folic acid indefinitely as long as pregnancy is a possibility. Women with SB need to carefully plan their pregnancies so they are on the increased dose of folic acid at conception.

Systemic Lupus Erythematosus

Because systemic lupus erythematosus or lupus is primarily a disease of young women, contraception and pregnancy often become crucial issues. For women with lupus oral contraceptives increase risk of hypertension, thrombosis, and disease exacerbation.

A barrier method in combination with spermicide is the safest form of contraception. Permanent sterilization may be an option chosen by some women. Although no longer advised not to have children, all lupus pregnancies should be considered high-risk with appropriate fetal monitoring, including ultrasounds to monitor growth and placental development, and biophysical profiles, usually from the 26th week. Pregnant women with lupus, especially those taking corticosteroids, are more likely to develop high blood pressure, diabetes, hyperglycemia (high blood sugar), and kidney complications. Approximately 20% to 25% of pregnancies in women with lupus end in miscarriage, compared to 10% to 15% of pregnancies in women without the disease (Clowse, Magder, Witter, & Petri, 2006; Lockshin, 2002). Inactive disease rather than controlled disease may play a more significant factor in determining preterm birth (Clark, Spitzer, Nadler, & Laskin, 2003). Careful management and close monitoring have substantially improved fetal outcomes. All women with lupus, even if they do not have a previous history of miscarriage, should be screened for antiphospholipid antibodies, both the lupus anticoagulant (the RVVT and sensitive PTT are the best screening battery) and anticardiolipin antibody. Twenty percent of preterm births are associated with antiphospholipid antibodies: most preterm births in women with lupus are due to pre-eclampsia and premature rupture of membranes (Lockshin, 2002; Petri, 1994). Risk factors for preterm birth in general include active lupus, high-dose prednisone, and renal disease.

Some women with lupus experience a mild to moderate flare during or after their pregnancy. The most common symptoms of these flares are arthritis, rashes and fatigue. Women who conceive after 5 to 6 months of remission are less likely to experience a lupus flare than those who get pregnant while their lupus is active. Women in remission have much less trouble than do women with active disease (Chakravarty et al., 2005; Petri, 1994). Most medications commonly taken by women with lupus are safe to use during pregnancy but care should be taken with dexamethasone and betamethasone. Cyclophosphamide (Cytoxan) should not be taken during the first trimester and only if necessary during the remainder of the pregnancy. Discontinuation of hydroxychloroquine (HCQ) during pregnancy has been associated with increased lupus activity (Clowse et al., 2006). Cesarean birth is needed only for obstetrical issues. Intensive nursing care for 24 to 48 hours may be necessary due to postpartum exacerbation. Infant care is often complicated by fatigue. Plaquenil and the cytotoxic drugs (Cytoxan, Imuran) are passed through breast milk to the baby, and some medications, such as prednisone, may interfere with milk production (Petri, 1994). Women with active lupus taking immunosuppressive medications should not breast-feed. Women with lupus who are not taking these medications need to have close monitoring of their child's growth while breast-feeding.

Lupus rarely occurs in children whose mothers have lupus but 10% of infants will have Neonatal lupus which is significantly different than lupus. Neonatal lupus causes a rash, blood count abnormalities, and infrequently irregular heartbeat (Lockshin, 2002).

Conditions Resulting From War, Traumatic Brain Injury, Amputations, and Posttraumatic Stress Disorder

Emerging as new disabilities for women are war-related traumatic brain injury (TBI), which can occur from blast as well as actual contact with flying material; amputations; and posttraumatic stress disorder (PTSD). Women in combat zones have experienced these disabilities in large numbers for the first time. Health care providers need to screen all female veterans for any war-related secondary conditions. The *Diagnostic and Statistical Manual of Mental Disorders* delineates symptoms such as depression, insomnia, or feeling constantly threatened as indicators of PTSD. In addition, intrusive, graphic memories and nightmares are common. Symptoms may appear or become exacerbated months after return from combat.

PARENTING WITH DISABILITIES

Mothers with disabilities and their children have the same ability for forming nurturing relationships as mothers without disabilities. Health care providers unfamiliar with the adaptive skills of women with disabilities sometimes question the ability of these women to care for their babies. In fact there are over 8 million families with children in which one or both parents has a disability (Farber, 2000; O'Toole & D'aoust, 2000). Most parents with disabilities are capable of raising happy and healthy children. The availability of a role model with a disability similar to the woman's can be very helpful to both the health care provider and the client. The roles of the parents and other caregivers must be assessed. Mothers with disabilities may have special needs that must be considered for them to be able to care for their children; special accommodations may be needed. Moreover, for providers without expertise in infant care issues, consultation with a pediatric nurse practitioner, pediatrician, occupational therapist, rehabilitation consultant, or rehabilitation engineer may be helpful. In addition, an independent living center or a program that focuses on promoting positive parenting for women with disabilities, such as Through the Looking Glass, may be consulted.

Assessment Needed

A woman's muscle strength, activities of daily living, and child care skills must be assessed. Determinations may be made by direct observation, reports of activities, and a child care activity assessment tool (Connie, 1988; Kirshbaum, 1988), or referral may be made to a physical or occupational therapist, depending on resources and the severity of the woman's limitations. Assessment needs to be made early in pregnancy in order to design adaptive equipment. For example, one woman with minimal distal muscle strength who wished to breastfeed was able to place the child at the breast and initiate nursing but did not have the strength to hold the child throughout nursing. Believing that she could not breastfeed, she switched to formula. If she had been assessed early in pregnancy, her strength deficiency might have been identified and referral made to a rehabilitation engineer to design or modify a fabric infant carrier that would support the child during nursing. Most women with a disability are able to nurse their newborn. Indeed, the convenience of breastfeeding can be an advantage for women with mobility limitations.

Parents With Disabilities

A videotape study of parents with disabilities was conducted and several findings were reported (Kirshbaum, 1988):

■ Infants adapt extremely early to their mothers who have physical disabilities.
■ Mothers develop the ability to read their infants' states and teach them to assist with necessary movement.
■ Children differentiate between care providers. For example, an active toddler lies still during a long diapering by the blind father, but resists and struggles from the outset with the sighted mother.

Equipment as Part of the Environment

It is common for children to consider a parent's equipment, such as wheelchairs and reachers, as ordinary parts of their environment without negative connotations. A toddler was overheard talking with her mom during a basketball tournament in which there was a wheelchair division. While observing a game played by nondisabled college students, she said, "Mom, what are they doing?" "Playing basketball, Honey." "But Mom, where are their wheelchairs?" Frequently, support services in both the health and social service arena are uninformed about resources that would make parenting and caretaking more effective for women with disability. Consultation with agencies that are knowledgeable in this area is critical to success.

Service Animals

Service animals can facilitate relationship skills in individuals who use them as well as provide assistance with activities. By law, service animals and those in training can accompany their owner to any location (Modlin, 2000, 2001). Because the match and training process can take time and energy, women are encouraged to plan ahead for requests. Modlin (2001) has developed a useful guide for those seeking more information. If a woman with a disability uses a guide dog or other animal to assist with impaired mobility, close assessment must be made of its impact on child care (Modlin, 2000, 2001).

Equipment Adaptation for Child Care

A woman with impaired mobility can alter equipment or procedures to assist with child care

■ Women with mobility impairment have special adaptation needs as parents (Carty et al., 1990). Women who previously used a manual wheelchair may choose to use an electrical wheelchair to free hands for child care.
■ Furniture may need to be altered so that the woman can wheel up to the crib, changing table, or reclined stroller and be able to change the baby without moving it. Furniture may also be altered to create firm raised edges for infant safety and to assist the woman with decreased hand or arm strength.
■ Hook-and-loop fasteners (VELCRO®) can be sewn on the clothes of both mother and baby for necessary alterations. For example, breastfeeding may be made easier if the mother's bra and blouse have fasteners. Also, fasteners on the infant's clothes assist the mother in dressing her baby (Earles et al., 1994).
■ Bottle holders and bottle devices, such as a tactile calibrated bottle, may be helpful, as may adapting a breastfeeding position in the wheelchair (Carty et al., 1990).

A woman with impaired vision or hearing also can adapt procedures for child care (Carty et al., 1990). The provider may need to facilitate the mother's interaction with her infant. The Brazelton tool is used to teach mothers about the states of the infant (Brazelton, 1973). For a woman with impaired vision, the focus is on her hearing and touching and how they increase interaction with the infant. On the other hand, for women with hearing impairment, a visual role model, tactile stimulation, and musical toys are used. If both parents have sensory impairment, referral to an infant stimulation program should be considered. Monitoring devices in a room or on a child can be helpful. Audiovisual resources may be useful.

SUMMARY

Sexuality and parenting are issues that have been largely ignored for women with disabilities. As people with disabilities and their advocates continue to break down barriers the unmet needs of women must be addressed. Researchers must call for major initiatives in several focus areas such as sexuality education, sexually transmitted disease, fertility, marriage, pregnancy and delivery, and parenting. The near future, it is hoped, will bring answers to many of the questions currently being raised.

RESOURCES

Internet Resources

CROWD, The Center for Research on Women with Disabilities: (Fact Sheet, Research Summary and Bibliography), www.bem.tmc.edu/crowd

National Clearinghouse on Women and Girls with Disabilities, www.edequity.org/welcome.html

National Women's Health Information Center, Women with Disabilities. Information and referral services, www.4women.gov/wwd

Parents with Disabilities Online: Information on products and solutions for making independent parenting more possible for people with disabilities, www.disabledparents.net

Siecus: Multiple annotated bibliographies on sexuality issues including disability, www.seicus.org

Through the Looking Glass: Information for parents with disabilities, www.lookingglass.org

General

Parenting and Infant Care

Breast Health and Beyond for Women with Disabilities: A Provider's Guide to the Examination and Screening of Women with Disabilities. Berkely, CA: Breast Health Access for Women with Disabilities (BHAWD), http://www.bhawd.org/sitefiles/index2.html

Conine, T. A., Carty, E., & Safarik, P. (1988). Aids and adaptations for disabled parents: An illustrated manual for service providers and parents with physical or sensory disabilities (2nd ed.). Vancouver: School of Rehabilitation Medicine, University of British Columbia.

Family Challenges: Parenting with a disability. 25 minute video that explores family relationships when a parent has a disability, for children, teens, and adults. Available from Aquarious Health Care Videos, 1-888-440-2963; E-mail: aqvideo@tiac.et

Kaufman, M. (1995). Easy for you to say: Questions and answers for teens living with chronic illness or disability. Toronto, Ontario, Canada: Key Porter Books, Ltd. A frank and explicit question and answer book addressing issues teens with disabilities or chronic illness and their families face. Includes sections on overprotection, sexuality, coping with medical personnel, work, school, and peers.

Kriegsman, K. H., Zaslow, E. L., & D'Zmura-Rechsteiner, M. A. (1992). Taking charge: Teenagers talk about life and physical disability. Bethesda, MD: Woodbine House. Available from the American Spina Bifida Association. Much acclaimed primer for older school-age and teenage patients.

Kroll, K., & Klein, E. L. (1992). Enabling romance: A guide to love, sex, and relationships for the disabled (and the people who care about them). New York: Harmony Books.

Rogers, J. (2005). The disabled woman's guide to pregnancy and birth. New York: Demos Medical Publishing.

Simpson, K. M., & Lankasky, K. (2001). Table manners: The gynecological exam for women with developmental disabilities and other functional limitations for teens and their families. Wellness Initiative of the California Department of Developmental Services.

Smeltzer, C. S., & Shart-Hopko, S. (2005). A providers guide for the care of women with physical disabilities and chronic health conditions. Chapel Hill: North Carolina Office of Disability and Health Sexuality and Women's Health Education.

Equipment/Latex Free Products

Avanti brand polyurethane condom (Schmid Laboratories). Has had limited testing that support the prevention of pregnancies and STIs. A 1995 Consumer Reports article questioned how much protection is offered. To date the FDA has not allowed the manufacturer to make any effectiveness claims.

Latex Allergy [video]. Available from the Spina Bifida Association of America, 4590 MacArthur Blvd NW, Suite 250, Washington, DC, 20007-4226. Twelve-minute video suitable for professional and lay audiences. For an extensive list of products updated every six months contact Spina Bifida Association of America, www.spinabifidaassociation.org

Latex Allergy List. A very useful list, updated yearly, www.spinabifidaassociation.org

Mammography for Women with Disabilities. Training for the Mammography Technologist, http://www.bhawd.org/sitefiles/index2.html

Patented wheelchair accessible Powermate (exam table, model #4450, 4453. Hausmann Industries, Model 4460, 4465 Inc. 103 Union Street, Northvale, NJ, 07647, Tel: 201-767-0255; Fax: 201-767-1369; Toll free 1-888-Hausman. Information on accessible GYN exam table, www.hausmann.com

Reality Female Condom (The Female Health Company). Made of polyurethane. Laboratory testing showed that Reality was an effective barrier to HIV and also to the smallest virus known to cause an STI. May be covered by Medicaid. Call to check in your state (1-800-643-0844), www.femalehealth.com

Organizations

Antiepileptic Drug Pregnancy Registry, 888-233-2334, http://www.epilepsyfoundation.org/research/aedpregreg.cfm

Breast Health and Beyond for Women with Disabilities (BHAWD), http://www.bhawd.org/sitefiles/index2.html

Epilepsy Society, http://www.aesnet.org/

National Dissemination Center for Children with Disabilities (NICHCY), 800-695-0285, www.nichcy.org

National Organization on Disability (DOD), 800-248-2253, www.nod.org

Spina Bifida Association of America, 800-621-3141, www.spinabifidaassociation.org

There are national groups for most chronic illness or disability conditions. Contact your local library or 1-800-555-1212 for current addresses or toll free numbers.

REFERENCES

Accardo, P. J. (Ed.). (2008). *Capute and Accardo's neurodevelopmental disabilities in infancy and childhood* (Vol. 2). Baltimore, MD: Brooks Publishing Co.

Alonso, A., Jick, S. S., Olek, M. J., Ascherio, A., Jick, H., & Hernan, M. A. (2005). Recent use of oral contraceptives and the risk of multiple sclerosis. *Archives of Neurology, 62*(9), 1362–1365.

Alstead, E. M. (2002). Inflammatory bowel disease in pregnancy. *Postgraduate Medical Journal, 78*(915), 23–26.

Alston, R. J., Bell, T. J., & Feist-Price, S. (1996). Racial identity and African Americans with disabilities: Theoretical and practical considerations. *Journal of Rehabilitation, 62*(2), 11–15.

Altman, B. M. (1996). Causes, risks and consequences of disability among women. In D. M. Krotoski, M. A. Nosek, & M. A. Turk (Eds.), *Women with physical disabilities* (pp. 17–34). Baltimore, MD: Brookes Publishing Co.

American Association of Neurology. (1998). Practice parameter: Management issues for women with epilepsy. *Neurology, 51*(4), 944–948.

American Diabetes Association. (2002). Preconception care of women with diabetes. *Diabetes Care, 25*(Suppl 1), S82–S84.

Anderson, J. M. (1991). Immigrant women speak of chronic illness: The social construction of the devalued self. *Journal of Advanced Nursing, 16*(6), 710–717.

Antisdel, J. E., & Chrisler, J. C. (2000). Comparison of eating attitudes and behaviors among adolescent and young women with type 1 diabetes mellitus and phenylketonuria. *Journal of Developmental and Behavioral Pediatrics, 21*(2), 81–86.

Arata, M., Grover, S., Dunne, K., & Bryan, D. (2000). Pregnancy outcome and complications in women with spina bifida. *Journal of Reproductive Medicine, 45*(9), 743–748.

Asgharian, A., & Anie, K. A. (2003). Women with sickle cell trait: Reproductive decision-making. *Journal of Reproductive and Infant Psychology, 21*(1), 323–334.

Ashton-Shaeffer, C., Gibson, H. J., Autry, C. E., & Hanson, C. S. (2001). Meaning of sport to adults with physical disabilities: A disability sport camp experience. *Sociology of Sport Journal, 18*(1), 95–114.

Aulagnier, M., Verger, P., Ravaud, J. F., Souville, M., Lussault, P. Y., Garnier, J. P., et al. (2005). General practitioners' attitudes towards patients with disabilities: The need for training and support. *Disability and Rehabilitation, 27*(22), 1343–1352.

Baker, S. (2003). Beating disability, embracing motherhood. *Practicing Midwife, 6*(7), 16–17.

Barrett, J. H., Brennan, P., Fiddler, M., & Silman, A. (2000). Breast-feeding and postpartum relapse in women with rheumatoid and inflammatory arthritis. *Arthritis and Rheumatism, 43*(5), 1010–1015.

Becker, H., Stuifbergen, A., & Tinkle, M. (1997). Reproductive health care experiences of women with physical disabilities: A qualitative study. *Archives of Physical Medicine and Rehabilitation, 78*(12 Suppl 5), S26–S33.

Bellin, M. H., Sawin, K. J., Roux, G., Buran, C. F., & Brei, T. J. (2007). The experience of adolescent women living with spina bifida part I: Self-concept and family relationships. *Rehabilitation Nursing, 32*(2), 57–67.

Betz, C. L., Redcay, G., & Tan, S. (2003). Self-reported health care self-care needs of transition-age youth: A pilot study. *Issues in Comprehensive Pediatric Nursing, 26*(3), 159–181.

Blackford, K. A., Richardson, H., & Grieve, S. (2000). Prenatal education for mothers with disabilities. *Journal of Advanced Nursing, 32*(4), 898–904.

Blackwell-Stratton, M., Breslin, M. L., Mayerson, A. B., & Bailey, S. (1988). Smashing icons: Disabled women and the disability women's movements. In M. Eine & A. Asch (Eds.), *Women with disabilities: Essays in psychology, culture, and politics* (pp. 306–332). Philadelphia: Temple University Press.

Blum, R. W., Kelly, A., & Ireland, M. (2001). Health-risk behaviors and protective factors among adolescents with mobility impairments and learning and emotional disabilities. *Journal of Adolescent Health, 28*(6), 481–490.

Boston Women's Health Book Collective. (2005). *Our bodies, ourselves: Updated and expanded for the 90s.* Gloucester, MA: Peter Smith Pub Inc.

Brazelton, T. B. (1973). *Neonatal behavioral assessment scale.* Philadelphia: J. B. Lippincott.

Broderick, L. E., & Krause, J. S. (2003). Breast and gynecologic health-screening behaviors among 191 women with spinal cord injuries. *Journal of Spinal Cord Medicine, 26*(2), 145–149.

Brown, A. A., & Murphy, L. (1999). *Aging with developmental disabilities: Women's health issues.* Arlington, TX: The Arc of the United States and the Rehabilitation Research and Training Center.

Brownridge, D. A. (2006). Partner violence against women with disabilities: Prevalence, risk, and explanations. *Violence Against Women, 12*(9), 805–822.

Capriotti, T. (2006). Inadequate cardiovascular disease prevention in women with physical disabilities. *Rehabilitation Nursing, 31*(3), 94–101.

Carty, E. M., Conine, T. A., & Hall, L. (1990). Comprehensive health promotion for the pregnant woman who is disabled. The role of the midwife. *Journal of Nurse-Midwifery, 35*(3), 133–142.

Carty, E. M., Conine, T., Holbrook, A., & Riddell, L. (1993, Autumn). Guidelines for serving disabled women. *Midwifery Today and Childbirth Education* (27), 28–37.

Case, A. M., & Reid, R. L. (1998). Effects of the menstrual cycle on medical disorders. *Archives of Internal Medicine, 158*(13), 1405–1412.

Cass, A. S., Bloom, B. A., & Luxenberg, M. (1986). Sexual function in adults with myelomeningocele. *Journal of Urology, 136*(2), 425–426.

Centers for Disease Control and Prevention. (1991). Use of folic acid for prevention of spina bifida and other neural tube defects: 1983–1991. *Morbidity and Mortality Weekly Report, 40*(30), 513–516.

Centers for Disease Control and Prevention. (1998). Use of cervical and breast cancer screening among women with and without functional limitations: United States, 1994–1995. *Morbidity and Mortality Weekly Report, 47*(40), 853–856.

Chakravarty, E. F., Colon, I., Langen, E. S., Nix, D. A., El-Sayed, Y. Y., Genovese, M. C., et al. (2005). Factors that predict prematurity and preeclampsia in pregnancies that are complicated by systemic lupus erythematosus. *American Journal of Obstetrics and Gynecology, 192*(6), 1897–1904.

Charlifue, S. W., Gerhart, K. A., Menter, R. R., Whiteneck, G. G., & Manley, M. S. (1992). Sexual issues of women with spinal cord injuries. *Paraplegia, 30*(3), 192–199.

Charron-Prochownik, D., Sereika, S. M., Wang, S., Hannan, M. F., Fischl, A. R., Stewart, S. H., et al. (2006). Reproductive health and preconception counseling awareness in adolescents with diabetes: What they don't know can hurt them. *Diabetes Educator, 32*(2), 235–242.

Clark, C. A., Spitzer, K. A., Nadler, J. N., & Laskin, C. A. (2003). Preterm deliveries in women with systemic lupus erythematosus. *Journal of Rheumatology, 30*(10), 2127–2132.

Clowse, M. E., Magder, L., Witter, F., & Petri, M. (2006). Hydroxychloroquine in lupus pregnancy. *Arthritis and Rheumatism, 54*(11), 3640–3647.

Cohen, M. M., Forte, T., Du Mont, J., Hyman, I., & Romans, S. (2005). Intimate partner violence among Canadian women with activity limitations. *Journal of Epidemiology and Community Health, 59*(10), 834–839.

Cole, S. S. (1993). Facing the challenges of sexual abuse in persons with disabilities. In M. Nagler (Ed.), *Perspectives in disability* (2nd ed., pp. 273–282). Palo Alto, CA: Health Markets Research.

Connie, T. A. (1988). *Aids and adaptations for disabled parents: An illustrated manual for service providers and parents with physical or sensory disabilities* (2nd ed.). Vancouver: School of Rehabilitation Medicine, University of British Columbia.

Cook, S. D., Troiano, R., Bansil, S., & Dowling, P. C. (1994). Multiple sclerosis and pregnancy. *Advances in Neurology, 64*, 83–95.

Copel, L. C. (2006). Partner abuse in physically disabled women: A proposed model for understanding intimate partner violence. *Perspectives in Psychiatric Care, 42*(2), 114–129.

Craig, D. I. (1990). The adaptation to pregnancy of spinal cord injured women. *Rehabilitation Nursing, 15*(1), 6–9.

Crawford, D., & Ostrove, J. M. (2003). Representations of disability and the interpersonal relationships of women with disabilities. *Women & Therapy, 26*(3/4), 179–194.

Crawford, P., & Lee, P. (1999). Gender difference in management of epilepsy: What women are hearing. *Seizure, 8*(3), 135–139.

Cremer, R., Hoppe, A., Kleine-Diepenbruck, U., & Blaker, F. (1998). Longitudinal study on latex sensitization in children with spina bifida. *Pediatric Allergy and Immunology, 9*(1), 40–43.

Crosby, E., St-Jean, B., Reid, D., & Elliott, R. D. (1992). Obstetrical anaesthesia and analgesia in chronic spinal cord-injured women. *Canadian Journal of Anaesthesia, 39*(5 Pt 1), 487–494.

Crow, L. (2003). Invisible and centre stage: A disabled woman's perspective on maternity services. *RCM Midwives, 6*(4), 158–161.

Curry, M. A., & Hassouneh-Phillips, D. (2002). Abuse of women with disabilities: State of the science. *Rehabilitation Counseling Bulletin, 45*(2), 96–104.

Curry, M. A., Hassouneh-Philips, D., & Johnston-Silverberg, A. (2001). Abuse of women with disabilities: An ecological model and review. *Violence Against Women, 7*(1), 60–79.

Dangoor, N., & Florian, V. (1994). Women with chronic physical disabilities: Correlates of their long-term psychosocial adaptation. *International Journal of Rehabilitation Research, 17*(2), 159–168.

DePauw, K. P. (1996). Adapted physical activity and sport. In D. M. Krotoski, M. A. Nosek, & M. A. Turk (Eds.), *Women with physical disabilities* (pp. 419–430). Baltimore: Brookes, Publishing Co.

Diab, M. E., & Johnston, M. V. (2004). Relationships between level of disability and receipt of preventive health services. *Archives of Physical Medicine and Rehabilitation, 85*(5), 749–757.

Di Giulio, G. (2003). Sexuality and people living with physical or developmental disabilities: A review of key issues. *Canadian Journal of Human Sexuality, 12*(1), 53–68.

Dormire, S., & Becker, H. (2007). Menopause health decision support for women with physical disabilities. *Journal of Obstetric, Gynecologic, and Neonatal Nursing, 36*(1), 97–104.

Dotson, L. A., Stinson, J., & Christian, L. (2003). "People tell me I can't have sex": Women with disabilities share their personal perspectives on health care, sexuality, and reproductive rights. *Women & Therapy, 26*(3/4), 195–209.

Drench, M. E. (1992). Impact of altered sexuality and sexual function in spinal cord injury: A review. *Sexuality and Disability, 10*(1), 3–14.

Drew, J. (1990). *Implications for nursing practice: A five-year review of recent spinal injury research.* Paper presented at the 16th Annual Conference, Association of Rehabilitation Nursing, Phoenix, AZ.

Earles, A., Lessing, S., & Vichinsky, E. (Eds.). (1994). *A parents' handbook for sickle cell disease, Part II.* Sacramento, CA: State of California Department of Health Services, Genetic Disease Branch.

Edenborough, F. P. (2001). Women with cystic fibrosis and their potential for reproduction. *Thorax, 56*(8), 649–655.

Elvik, S. L., Berkowitz, C. D., Nicholas, E., Lipman, J. L., & Inkelis, S. H. (1990). Sexual abuse in the developmentally disabled: dilemmas of diagnosis. *Child Abuse and Neglect, 14*(4), 497–502.

Farber, R. S. (2000). Mothers with disabilities: In their own voice. *American Journal of Occupational Therapy, 54*(3), 260–268.

Feller, E. R., Ribaudo, S., & Jackson, N. D. (2001). Gynecologic aspects of Crohn's disease. *American Family Physician, 64*(10), 1725–1728.

Ferrero, S., & Ragni, N. (2004). Inflammatory bowel disease: Management issues during pregnancy. *Archives of Gynecology and Obstetrics, 270*(2), 79–85.

Friedman, S., & Regueiro, M. D. (2002). Pregnancy and nursing in inflammatory bowel disease. *Gastroenterology Clinics of North America, 31*(1), 265–273, xii.

Furman, L., & Mortimer, J. C. (1994). Menarche and menstrual function in patients with myelomeningocele. *Developmental Medicine and Child Neurology, 36*(10), 910–917.

Gill, C. J., & Brown, A. A. (2000). Overview of health issues of older women with intellectual disabilities. *Physical & Occupational Therapy in Geriatrics, 18*(1), 23–36.

Goodwin, D. L., & Compton, S. G. (2004). Physical activity experiences of women aging with disabilities. *Adapted Physical Activity Quarterly, 21*(2), 122–138.

Gordon, D. L., Sawin, K. J., & Basta, S. M. (1996). Developing research priorities for rehabilitation nursing. *Rehabilitation Nursing Research, 5*(2), 60–66.

Groce, N. E. (1999). Disability in cross-cultural perspective: Rethinking disability. *Lancet, 354*(9180), 756–757.

Groce, N. E. (2003). HIV/AIDS and people with disability. *Lancet, 361*(9367), 1401–1402.

Gross, S. M., Ireys, H. T., & Kinsman, S. L. (2000). Young women with physical disabilities: Risk factors for symptoms of eating disorders. *Journal of Developmental and Behavioral Pediatrics, 21*(2), 87–96.

Hall, L., Colantonio, A., & Yoshida, K. (2003). Barriers to nutrition as a health promotion practice for women with disabilities. *International Journal of Rehabilitation Research, 26*(3), 245–247.

Harden, C. L. (2003). Menopause and bone density issues for women with epilepsy. *Neurology, 61*(6 Suppl 2), S16–S22.

Harrison, J., Glass, C. A., Owens, R. G., & Soni, B. M. (1995). Factors associated with sexual functioning in women following spinal cord injury. *Paraplegia, 33*(12), 687–692.

Hassouneh-Phillips, D. (2005). Understanding abuse of women with physical disabilities: An overview of the abuse pathways model. *Advances in Nursing Science, 28*(1), 70–80.

Hassouneh-Phillips, D., & McNeff, E. (2005). "I thought I was less worthy": Low sexual and body esteem and increased vulnerability to intimate partner abuse in women with physical disabilities. *Sexuality and Disability, 23*(4), 227–240.

Hassouneh-Phillips, D., McNeff, E., Powers, L., & Curry, M. A. (2005). Invalidation: A central process underlying maltreatment of women with disabilities. *Women and Health, 41*(1), 33–50.

Hatcher, R. A., Trussel, J., Stewart, F., Stewart, G. K., Kowal, D., Guest, F., et al. (1994). *Contraceptive technology* (16th rev. ed.). New York: Irvington.

Hatcher, R. A., Trussel, J., Stewart, F., Stewart, G. K., Kowal, D., Guest, F., et al. (1998). *Contraceptive technology* (17th rev. ed.). New York: Irvington.

Hatzichristou, D. G. (1996). Preface to the special issue: Management of voiding, bowel and sexual dysfunction in multiple sclerosis: Towards a holistic approach. *Sexuality & Disability, 14*(1), 3–6.

Havercamp, S. M., Scandlin, D., & Roth, M. (2004). Health disparities among adults with developmental disabilities, adults with other disabilities, and adults not reporting disability in North Carolina. *Public Health Reports, 119*(4), 418–426.

Herpertz, S., Wagener, R., Albus, C., Kocnar, M., Wagner, R., Best, F., et al. (1998). Diabetes mellitus and eating disorders: A multicenter study on the comorbidity of the two diseases. *Journal of Psychosomatic Research, 44*(3–4), 503–515.

Howland, C. A., & Rintala, D. H. (2001). Dating behaviors of women with physical disabilities. *Sexuality & Disability, 19*(1), 41–70.

Hughes, R. B. (2006). Achieving effective health promotion for women with disabilities. *Family and Community Health, 29*(1 Suppl), 44S–51S.

Hughes, R. B., Nosek, M. A., Howland, C. A., Groff, J. Y., & Mullen, D. (2003). Health promotion for women with physical disabilities: A pilot study. *Rehabilitation Psychology, 48*(3), 182–188.

Hughes, R. B., Nosek, M. A., & Robinson-Whelen, S. (2007). Correlates of depression in rural women with physical disabilities. *Journal of Obstetric, Gynecologic, and Neonatal Nursing, 36*(1), 105–114.

Hughes, R. B., Robinson-Whelen, S., Taylor, H. B., Petersen, N. J., & Nosek, M. A. (2005). Characteristics of depressed and nondepressed women with physical disabilities. *Archives of Physical Medicine and Rehabilitation, 86*(3), 473–479.

Iezzoni, L. I., McCarthy, E. P., Davis, R. B., & Siebens, H. (2000). Mobility impairments and use of screening and preventive services. *American Journal of Public Health, 90*(6), 955–961.

Ingraham, C. L., Vernon, M., Clemente, B., & Olney, L. (2000). Sex education for deaf-blind youths and adults. *Journal of Visual Impairment & Blindness, 94*(12), 756–761.

Institute of Medicine. (2002). *Unequal treatment: Confronting racial and ethnic disparities in health care.* Washington, DC: The National Academies Press.

Isojarvi, J. I. T. (2003). Reproductive dysfunction in women with epilepsy. *Neurology, 61*(6 Suppl 2), S27–S34.

Jackson, A. B., Lindsey, L. L., Klebine, P. L., & Poczatek, R. B. (2004). Reproductive health for women with spinal cord injury: Pregnancy and delivery. *SCI Nursing, 21*(2), 88–91.

Jackson, A. B., & Sipski, M. L. (2005). Reproductive issues for women with spina bifida. *Journal of Spinal Cord Medicine, 28*(2), 81–91.

Jordan, B., & Dunlap, G. (2001). Construction of adulthood and disability. *Mental Retardation, 39*(4), 286–296.

Jorgensen, C., Picot, M. C., Bologna, C., & Sany, J. (1996). Oral contraception, parity, breast feeding, and severity of rheumatoid arthritis. *Annals of the Rheumatic Diseases, 55*(2), 94–98.

Julkunen, H. A., Kaaja, R., & Friman, C. (1993). Contraceptive practice in women with systemic lupus erythematosus. *British Journal of Rheumatology, 32*(3), 227–230.

Kane, S. (2005). Gender issues in the management of irritable bowel syndrome. *International Journal of Fertility and Women's Medicine, 50*(2), 79–82.

Kaplan, P. W. (2004). Reproductive health effects and teratogenicity of antiepileptic drugs. *Neurology, 63*(10 Suppl 4), S13–S23.

King, G., Willoughby, C., Specht, J. A., & Brown, E. (2006). Social support processes and the adaptation of individuals with chronic disabilities. *Qualitative Health Research, 16*(7), 902–925.

Kirshbaum, M. (1988). Parents with physical disabilities and their babies. *Zero to Three, 8*(15), 8–15.

Kirshbaum, M. (1996). Mothers with physical disabilities. In D. M. Krotoski, M. A. Nosek, & M. A. Turk (Eds.), *Women with physical disabilities* (pp. 125–134). Baltimore: Brooks Publishing Co.

LaVaccare, J. A., & Bergen, D. (2000). Women with epilepsy. *Clinical Neuropharmacology, 23*(2), 63–68.

Li, C. M., & Yau, M. K. (2006). Sexual issues and concerns: Tales of Chinese women with spinal cord impairments. *Sexuality and Disability, 24*(1), 1–26.

Liptak, G. S. (2001). Precocious puberty in children who have spina bifida with hydrocephalus. Retrieved September 1, 2007, from http://www.sbaa.org/site/c.gpILKXOEJqG/b.2021297/k.651/SBAA_Fact_Sheet_Precocious_Puberty_in_Children_Who_Have_Spina_Bifida_with_Hydrocephalus.htm

Lockshin, M. D. (2002). Pregnancy and lupus. Lupus Foundation of America, Inc. Retrieved December 2002, from http://www.lupus.org

Lorenzi, A. R., & Ford, H. L. (2002). Multiple sclerosis and pregnancy. *Postgraduate Medical Journal, 78*(922), 460–464.

March of Dimes. (2005). Only one-third of women take vitamin to help prevent serious birth defects, survey finds. Retrieved October 19, 2007, from http://www.marchofdimes.com/aboutus/14458_17299.asp

March of Dimes. (2007). Gestational Diabetes. Retrieved October 22, 2007, from http://www.marchofdimes.com/pnhec/188_1025.asp

Martin, S. L., Ray, N., Sotres-Alvarez, D., Kupper, L. L., Moracco, K. E., Dickens, P. A., et al. (2006). Physical and sexual assault of women with disabilities. *Violence Against Women, 12*(9), 823–837.

Mazon, A., Nieto, A., Linana, J. J., Montoro, J., Estornell, F., & Garcia-Ibarra, F. (2000). Latex sensitization in children with spina bifida: Follow-up comparative study after two years. *Annals of Allergy, Asthma, and Immunology, 84*(2), 207–210.

McCarthy, E. P., Ngo, L. H., Roetzheim, R. G., Chirikos, T. N., Li, D., Drews, R. E., et al. (2006). Disparities in breast cancer treatment and survival for women with disabilities. *Annals of Internal Medicine, 145*(9), 637–645.

McCauley Ohannessian, C., Lerner, R. M., Lerner, J. V., & von Eye, A. (1999). Does self-competence predict gender differences in adolescent depression and anxiety? *Journal of Adolescence, 22*(3), 397–411.

McKay-Moffat, S., & Cunningham, C. (2006). Services for women with disabilities: Mothers' and midwives' experiences. *British Journal of Midwifery, 14*(8), 472–477.

Meeropol, E. (1991). One of the gang: Sexual development of adolescents with physical disabilities. *Journal of Pediatric Nursing, 6*(4), 243–250.

Mele, N., Archer, J., & Pusch, B. D. (2005). Access to breast cancer screening services for women with disabilities. *Journal of Obstetric, Gynecologic, and Neonatal Nursing, 34*(4), 453–464.

Mikkonen, K., Vainionpaa, L. K., Pakarinen, A. J., Knip, M., Jarvela, I. Y., Tapanainen, J. S., et al. (2004). Long-term reproductive endocrine health in young women with epilepsy during puberty. *Neurology, 62*(3), 445–450.

Modlin, S. J. (2000). Service dogs as interventions: State of the science. *Rehabilitation Nursing, 25*(6), 212–219.

Modlin, S. J. (2001). From puppy to service dog: Raising service dogs for the rehabilitation team. *Rehabilitation Nursing, 26*(1), 12–17.

Morrell, M. J. (1999). Epilepsy in women: The science of why it is special. *Neurology, 53*(4 Suppl 1), S42–S48.

Morrell, M. J. (2002). Folic acid and epilepsy. *Epilepsy Currents, 2*(2), 31–34.

Mudrick, N. R. (1988). Predictors of disability among midlife men and women: Differences by severity of impairment. *Journal of Community Health, 13*(2), 70–84.

Muir, E. H., & Ogden, J. (2001). Consultations involving people with congenital disabilities: Factors that help or hinder giving care. *Family Practice, 18*(4), 419–424.

Murphy, F. A. (1996). Commentary. *APNSCAN: Literature Review for the Advanced Practice Nurse, 12*, 3.

Murphy, N., & Young, P. C. (2005). Sexuality in children and adolescents with disabilities. *Developmental Medicine and Child Neurology, 47*(9), 640–644.

Murphy, N. A., & Elias, E. R. (2006). Sexuality of children and adolescents with developmental disabilities. *Pediatrics, 118*(1), 398–403.

National Information Center for Children and Youth with Disabilities. (1992). Sexuality education for children and youth with disabilities. *NICHCY News Digest, 1*(3), 2–23.

Neinstein, L. S., & Katz, B. (1986a). Contraceptive use in the chronically ill adolescent female. Part II. *Journal of Adolescent Health Care, 7*(5), 350–360.

Neinstein, L. S., & Katz, B. (1986b). Contraceptive use in the chronically ill adolescent female: Part I. *Journal of Adolescent Health Care, 7*(2), 123–133.

Neumark-Sztainer, D., Story, M., Resnick, M. D., & Blum, R. W. (1998). Lessons learned about adolescent nutrition from the Minnesota Adolescent Health Survey. *Journal of the American Dietetic Association, 98*(12), 1449–1456.

Nosek, M. A. (1992). Point of view: Primary care issues for women with severe physical disabilities. *Journal of Women's Health, 1*(4), 245–248.

Nosek, M. A. (1995). Sexual abuse of women with physical disabilities. *Physical Medicine & Rehabilitation: State of the Art Reviews, 9*(2), 487–502.

Nosek, M. A., Howland, C. A., Rintala, D. H., Young, M. E., & Chanpong, G. F. (1997). *National study of women with physical disabilities: Final report.* Houston: Center for Research on Women with Disabilities.

Nosek, M. A., Howland, C. A., Rintala, D. H., Young, M. E., & Chanpong, G. F. (2001). National Study of Women with Physical Disabilities: Final report. *Sexuality & Disability, 19*(1), 5–39.

Nosek, M. A., Howland, C. A., Young, M. E., Georgiou, D., Rintala, D. H., Foley, C. C., et al. (1994). Wellness models and sexuality among women with physical disabilities. *Journal of Applied Rehabilitation Counseling, 25*(1), 50–58.

Nosek, M. A., Hughes, R. B., Petersen, N. J., Taylor, H. B., Robinson-Whelen, S., Byrne, M., et al. (2006). Secondary conditions in a community-based sample of women with physical disabilities over a 1-year period. *Archives of Physical Medicine and Rehabilitation, 87*(3), 320–327.

Nosek, M. A., Hughes, R. B., Taylor, H. B., & Taylor, P. (2006). Disability, psychosocial, and demographic characteristics of abused women with physical disabilities. *Violence Against Women, 12*(9), 838–850.

Nosek, M. A., Rintala, D. H., Young, M. E., Howland, C. A., Foley, C. C., Rossi, D., et al. (1996). Sexual functioning among women with physical disabilities. *Archives of Physical Medicine and Rehabilitation, 77*(2), 107–115.

Nosek, M. A., Young, M. E., Rintala, D. H., Howland, C. A., Foley, C. C., & Bennett, J. (1995). Barriers to reproductive health maintenance among women with physical disabilities. *Journal of Women's Health, 4*(5), 505–518.

O'Toole, C. J., & D'aoust, V. (2000). Fit for motherhood: Towards a recognition of multiplicity in disabled lesbian mothers. *Disability Studies Quarterly, 20*(2), 145–154.

Parkes, N. (2006). Sexual issues and people with a learning disability. *Learning Disability Practice, 9*(3), 32–37.

Pendergrass, S., Nosek, M. A., & Holcomb, J. D. (2001). Design and evaluation of an internet site to educate women with disabilities on reproductive health care. *Sexuality and Disability, 19*(1), 71–83.

Pennell, P. B. (2005). Using current evidence in selecting antiepileptic drugs for use during pregnancy. *Epilepsy Currents, 5*(2), 45–51.

Pentland, W., Tremblay, M., Spring, K., & Rosenthal, C. (1999). Women with physical disabilities: Occupational impacts of ageing. *Journal of Occupational Science, 6*(3), 111–123.

Petri, M. (1994). Systemic lupus erythematosus and pregnancy. *Rheumatic Diseases Clinics of North America, 20*(1), 87–118.

Piotrowski, K., & Snell, L. (2007). Health needs of women with disabilities across the lifespan. *Journal of Obstetric, Gynecologic, and Neonatal Nursing, 36*(1), 79–87.

Pitzele, S. K. (1995). Chronic illness, disability and sexuality in people older than fifty. *Sexuality & Disability, 13*(4), 309–325.

Poulos, A. E., Balandin, S., Llewellyn, G., & Dew, A. H. (2006). Women with cerebral palsy and breast cancer screening by mammography. *Archives of Physical Medicine and Rehabilitation, 87*(2), 304–307.

Queenan, J. T., & Hobbins, J. C. (Eds.). (1996). *Protocols for high-risk pregnancies* (3rd ed.). Boston: Blackwell Science.

Reinelt, C., & Fried, M. (1993). "I am this child's mother": A feminist perspective on mothering with a disability. In M. Nagler (Ed.), *Perspectives on Disability* (pp. 195–202). Palo Alto, CA: Health Markets Research.

Rimmer, J. H. (2001). Physical fitness levels of persons with cerebral palsy. *Developmental Medicine and Child Neurology, 43*(3), 208–212.

Rimmer, J. H., Riley, B., Wang, E., & Rauworth, A. (2004). Development and validation of AIMFREE: Accessibility Instruments Measuring Fitness and Recreation Environments. *Disability and Rehabilitation, 26*(18), 1087–1095.

Rimmer, J. H., Rubin, S. S., Braddock, D., & Hedman, G. (1999). Physical activity patterns of African-American women with physical disabilities. *Medicine and Science in Sports and Exercise, 31*(4), 613–618.

Rogers, J. (2005). *The disabled woman's guide to pregnancy and birth.* New York: Demos Medical Publishing.

Roux, G., Sawin, K. J., Bellin, M. H., Buran, C. F., & Brei, T. J. (2007). The experience of adolescent women living with spina bifida. Part II: Peer relationships. *Rehabilitation Nursing, 32*(3), 112–119.

Sawin, K. J., & Metzger, S. G. (2007). *Optimizing health care for women with disabilties: The ACCESS curriculum for health care providers.* Unpublished manuscript.

Sawin, K. J., Bellin, M. H., Roux, G., Buran, C. F., & Brei, T. J. (in press). The experience of self-management in adolescent women with spina bifida. *Rehabilitation Nursing.*

Sawin, K. J., Brei, T. J., Buran, C. F., & Fastenau, P. S. (2002). Factors associated with quality of life in adolescents with spina bifida. *Journal of Holistic Nursing, 20*(3), 279–304.

Sawin, K. J., Buran, C. F., Brei, T. J., Cashin, S., & Webb, T. (2007). *Development of the Self Management Independence Scale (AMIS II): Psychometric properties.* Unpublished manuscript.

Sawin, K. J., Buran, C. F., Brei, T. J., & Fastenau, P. S. (2002). Sexuality issues in adolescents with a chronic neurological condition. *The Journal of Perinatal Education, 11*(1), 22–34.

Sawin, K. J., Cox, A., & Metzger, S. G. (2004). Transition to adulthood. In J. Jackson & J. Vessey (Eds.), *Primary care of children with chronic conditions* (4th ed.). St. Louis: Mosby.

Schachter, J., Chernesky, M. A., Willis, D. E., Fine, P. M., Martin, D. H., Fuller, D., et al. (2005). Vaginal swabs are the specimens of choice when screening for Chlamydia trachomatis and Neisseria gonorrhoeae: Results from a multicenter evaluation of the APTIMA assays for both infections. *Sexually Transmitted Diseases, 32*(12), 725–728.

Schrager, S. (2004). Osteoporosis in women with disabilities. *Journal of Women's Health, 13*(4), 431–437.

Shah, P., Norlin, C., Logsdon, V., & Samson-Fang, L. (2005). Gynecological care for adolescents with disability: Physician comfort, perceived barriers, and potential solutions. *Journal of Pediatric and Adolescent Gynecology, 18*(2), 101–104.

Shaw, G. M., Rozen, R., Finnell, R. H., Wasserman, C. R., & Lammer, E. J. (1998). Maternal vitamin use, genetic variation of infant methylenetetrahydrofolate reductase, and risk for spina bifida. *American Journal of Epidemiology, 148*(1), 30–37.

Shaw, G. M., Velie, E. M., & Schaffer, D. (1996). Risk of neural tube defect-affected pregnancies among obese women. *JAMA, 275*(14), 1093–1096.

Shiffman, M. L., Seale, T. W., Flux, M., Rennert, O. R., & Swender, P. T. (1989). Breast-milk composition in women with cystic fibrosis: report of two cases and a review of the literature. *American Journal of Clinical Nutrition, 49*(4), 612–617.

Singh, R., & Sharma, S. C. (2005). Sexuality and women with spinal cord injury. *Sexuality and Disability, 23*(1), 21–33.

Smeltzer, S. C. (2006). Preventive health screening for breast and cervical cancer and osteoporosis in women with physical disabilities. *Family and Community Health, 29*(1 Suppl), 35S–43S.

Smeltzer, S. C. (2007). Pregnancy in women with physical disabilities. *Journal of Obstetric, Gynecologic, and Neonatal Nursing, 36*(1), 88–96.

Smeltzer, S. C., Zimmerman, V., & Capriotti, T. (2005). Osteoporosis risk and low bone mineral density in women with physical disabilities. *Archives of Physical Medicine and Rehabilitation, 86*(3), 582–586.

Smeltzer, S. C., Zimmerman, V., Capriotti, T., & Fernandes, L. (2002). Osteoporosis risk factors and bone mineral density in women with MS. *International Journal of MS Care, 4*, 17–23, 29.

Stampfer, M. J., Colditz, G. A., Willett, W. C., Manson, J. E., Rosner, B., Speizer, F. E., et al. (1991). Postmenopausal estrogen therapy and cardiovascular disease: Ten-year follow-up from the nurses' health study. *New England Journal of Medicine, 325*(11), 756–762.

Stengel, P. J. (1996). *A train the trainer project on preconceptional counseling the role of folate in the prevention of neural tube defects.* Unpublished thesis, Virginia Commonwealth University, Richmond.

Stevens, P. E. (1994). Lesbians' health-related experiences of care and noncare. *Western Journal of Nursing Research, 16*(6), 639–659.

Stuifbergen, A., Becker, H., Rogers, S., Timmerman, G., & Kullberg, V. (1999). Promoting wellness for women with multiple sclerosis. *Journal of Neuroscience Nursing, 31*(2), 73–79.

Sze, M. B. (2003). Dating and intimate relationships involving women with early-onset physical disabilities. *Dissertation Abstracts International: Section B: The Sciences and Engineering, 63*(12-B), 6109.

Szepfalusi, Z., Seidl, R., Bernert, G., Dietrich, W., Spitzauer, S., & Urbanek, R. (1999). Latex sensitization in spina bifida appears disease-associated. *Journal of Pediatrics, 134*(3), 344–348.

Task Force on Concerns of Physically Disabled Women. (1978). *Within reach: Providing family planning services to physically disabled women.* New York: Human Sciences Press.

The Arc. (2004). Position statement on sexuality. Retrieved October 22, 2007, from http://www.thearc.org/NetCommunity/Page.aspx?&pid = 1375&srcid = 405

The Arc. (2005). Parents with intellectual disabilities. Retrieved October 22, 2007, from http://www.thearc.org/NetCommunity/Document.Doc?&id = 151

Thomas, V. J., & Cohn, T. (2006). Communication skills and cultural awareness courses for healthcare professionals who care for patients with sickle cell disease. *Journal of Advanced Nursing, 53*(4), 480–488.

Timmerman, G. M., & Stuifbergin, A. K. (1999). Eating patterns in women with multiple sclerosis. *Journal of Neuroscience Nursing, 31*(3), 152–158.

U.S. Department of Health and Human Services. (2006a). *Healthy people 2010 midcourse review.* Washington, DC: U.S. Government Printing Office.

U.S. Department of Health and Human Services. (2006b). Your rights under section 504 of the rehabilitation act. Retrieved October 19, 2007, from http://www.hhs.gov/ocr/504.pdf

Valtonen, K., Karlsson, A., Siosteen, A., Dahlof, L., & Viikari-Juntura, E. (2006). Satisfaction with sexual life among persons with traumatic spinal cord injury and meningomyelocele. *Disability and Rehabilitation, 28*(16), 965–976.

Vansteenwegen, A., Jans, I., & Revell, A. T. (2003). Sexual experience of women with a physical disability: A comparative study. *Sexuality and Disability, 21*(4), 283–290.

Verhoef, M., Barf, H. A., Vroege, J. A., Post, M. W., van Asbeck, F. W., Gooskens, R. H., et al. (2000). The ASPINE study: Preliminary results on sex education, relationships and sexual functioning of Dutch adolescents with spina bifida. *European Journal of Pediatric Surgery, 10*(Suppl 1), 53–54.

Verhoef, M., Barf, H. A., Vroege, J. A., Post, M. W., Van Asbeck, F. W., Gooskens, R. H., et al. (2005). Sex education, relationships, and sexuality in young adults with spina bifida. *Archives of Physical Medicine and Rehabilitation, 86*(5), 979–987.

Vukusic, S., & Confavreux, C. (2006). Pregnancy and multiple sclerosis: The children of PRIMS. *Clinical Neurology and Neurosurgery, 108*(3), 266–270.

Vukusic, S., Hutchinson, M., Hours, M., Moreau, T., Cortinovis-Tourniaire, P., Adeleine, P., et al. (2004). Pregnancy and multiple sclerosis (the PRIMS study): Clinical predictors of post-partum relapse. *Brain, 127*(Pt 6), 1353–1360.

Walsh, P. N., & LeRoy, B. (2004). *Women with Disabilities aging well: A global view.* Baltimore, MD: Brookes Publishing Co.

Ware, L., Muram, D., & Gale, C. L. (1992). Q-tip pap smear: Should it be done routinely in patients who have developmental disabilities? *Sexuality and Disability, 10*(3), 189–192.

Wasser, A. M., Killoran, C. L., & Bansen, S. S. (1993). Pregnancy and disability. *AWHONNS Clinical Issues in Perinatal and Women's Health Nursing, 4*(2), 328–337.

Welner, S. (1996). Contraception, sexually transmitted diseases and menopause. In D. M. Krotoski, M. A. Nosek, & M. A. Turk (Eds.), *Women with disabilities* (pp. 81–90). Baltimore, MD: Brooks Publishing Co.

Welner, S. L. (1993). Gynecologic care of the disabled woman. *Contemporary OB/GYN, 38*(1), 55–67.

Welner, S. L., Foley, C. C., Nosek, M. A., & Holmes, A. (1999). Practical considerations in the performance of physical examinations on women with disabilities. *Obstetrical and Gynecological Survey, 54*(7), 457–462.

Westgren, N., Hultling, C., Levi, R., & Westgren, M. (1993). Pregnancy and delivery in women with a traumatic spinal cord injury in Sweden, 1980–1991. *Obstetrics and Gynecology, 81*(6), 926–930.

Westgren, N., & Levi, R. (1998). Quality of life and traumatic spinal cord injury. *Archives of Physical Medicine and Rehabilitation, 79*(11), 1433–1439.

World Health Organization. (2001). *The international classification of functioning, disability and health.* New York: Author.

Yoshida, K. K., & Li, A. (1999). Cross-cultural views of disability and sexuality: Experiences of a group of ethno-racial women with physical disabilities. *Sexuality & Disability, 17*(4), 321–337.

Young, M. E., Nosek, M. A., Howland, C., Chanpong, G., & Rintala, D. H. (1997). Prevalence of abuse of women with physical disabilities. *Archives of Physical Medicine and Rehabilitation, 78*(12 Suppl 5), S34–S38.

Zasler, N. D. (1991). Sexuality in neurologic disability: An overview. *Sexuality and Disability, 9*(1), 11–27.

MONUMENTAL
VERSES

by J. Patrick Lewis

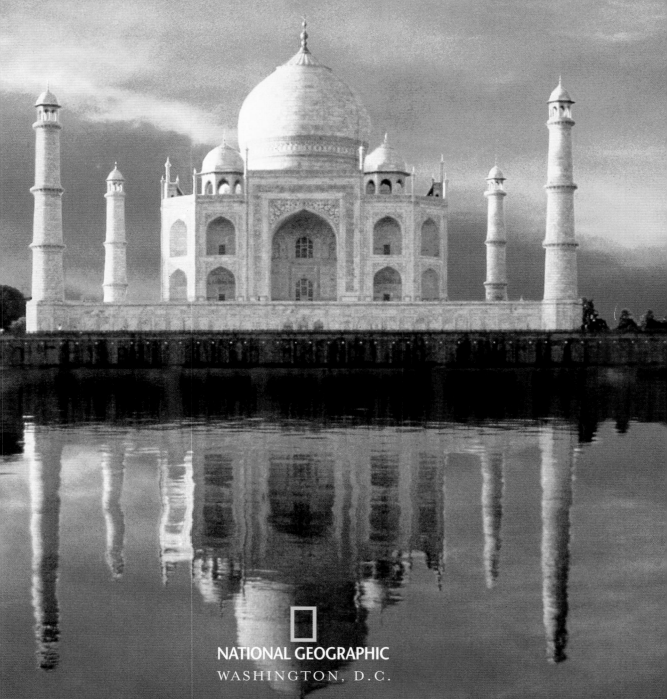

NATIONAL GEOGRAPHIC
WASHINGTON, D.C.

A bow to all who hoist the spirit high
And carve imagination into stone
By fire and forge, thrown hugely to the sky.
Whether they be well- or little-known,

The buildings in this picture book cement
A thought: No matter who the builders were,
They gave to time a timeless monument—
A human star-chitecture signature.

I cannot say what others make of this,
The mystery of Stonehenge, a Taj Mahal,
And yet I know how much the world would miss
Majesty at a glance if they should fall.

This book is for the curious at heart,
Startled at sights they seldom get to see
Or even dream of—science born of art,
Such works of genius these were meant to be.

TABLE OF CONTENTS

STONEHENGE

DATE: BUILT FROM 2800-1800 B.C.
LOCATION: SALISBURY PLAIN, WILTSHIRE, ENGLAND
BUILDER: THE BEAKER PEOPLE
PHYSICAL FACT: BLUESTONES AND SANDSTONES WERE HAULED IN FROM MARLBOROUGH DOWNS,
20 MILES (32 KM) AWAY. EVEN TODAY YOU CAN SEE THE DRAG MARKS.

Five thousand years ago, a star-struck night blinked down at them, huddled by twig fires among towering pines and hazel wood. Some spoke of weather, some of game, others told of death or heartbreak. Just as dawn sealed the envelope of night, someone uttered, for what was the first time in prehistory, a word for *monument*. A hush so deafening fell across that place that even tree moan and leaf fall stopped. Then, the earliest Timekeeper said, It must create shadows if Sun and Moon are to speak to us of their travels. Let stones be circular in praise, cried the first Priest, alive to prayer. Smooth out the chalk downland, said the first Henge-ineer. From the far north, drag giants of sandstone and bluestone to water, float them by raft, haul them over land. It will take us one hundred full moons to move a stone, the first Mathematician said. The Rope-weaver cautioned, We can expect no sympathy from the sea. Fifty generations from now, mused the old Philosopher, our ancestors might see it finally finished. Every one of the Beaker folk spoke in turn until only a small child was left to ask, How are you ever going to stand ten-ton stones upright? The wind carried away the answer before it was ever heard.

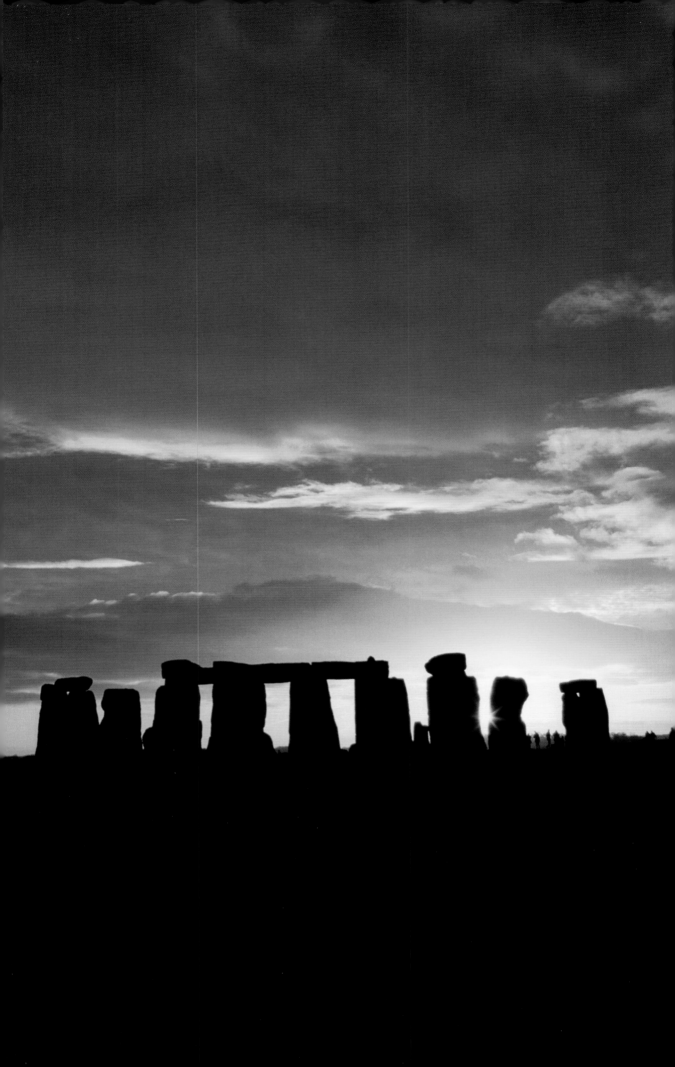

EASTER ISLAND

DATE: BUILT FROM A.D.1400 TO A.D.1600 A.D.
LOCATION: 2,300 MILES OFF THE COAST OF CHILE
BUILDER: INDIGENOUS PEOPLES
PHYSICAL FACT: THERE ARE NEARLY 900 GIANT STATUES ON THE ISLAND.

Volcanic ash carved into men,
Whose backs are turned against the sea—
The ancients show us now and then
A sense of mad nobility.

Dark heroes gazing at a sky
That never heeds our human cares
Are images that magnify
The possibilities of prayer,

Or high-flown hope, or an *homage*
Of people who cast their beliefs
Into this stone-faced entourage
Of big men, ancestors, and chiefs

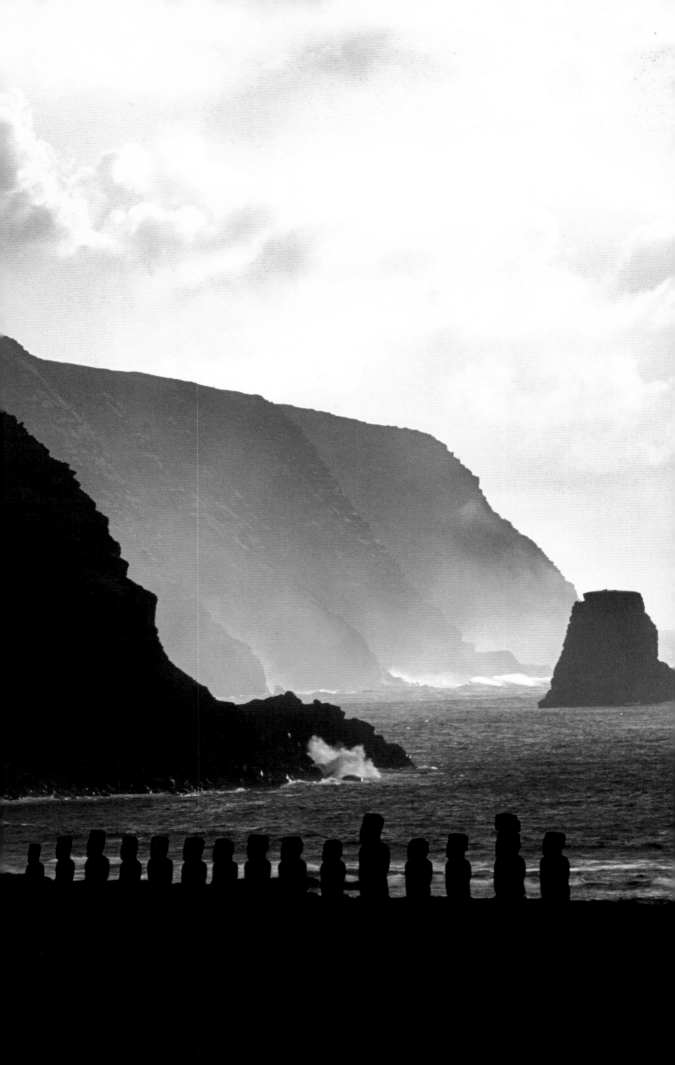

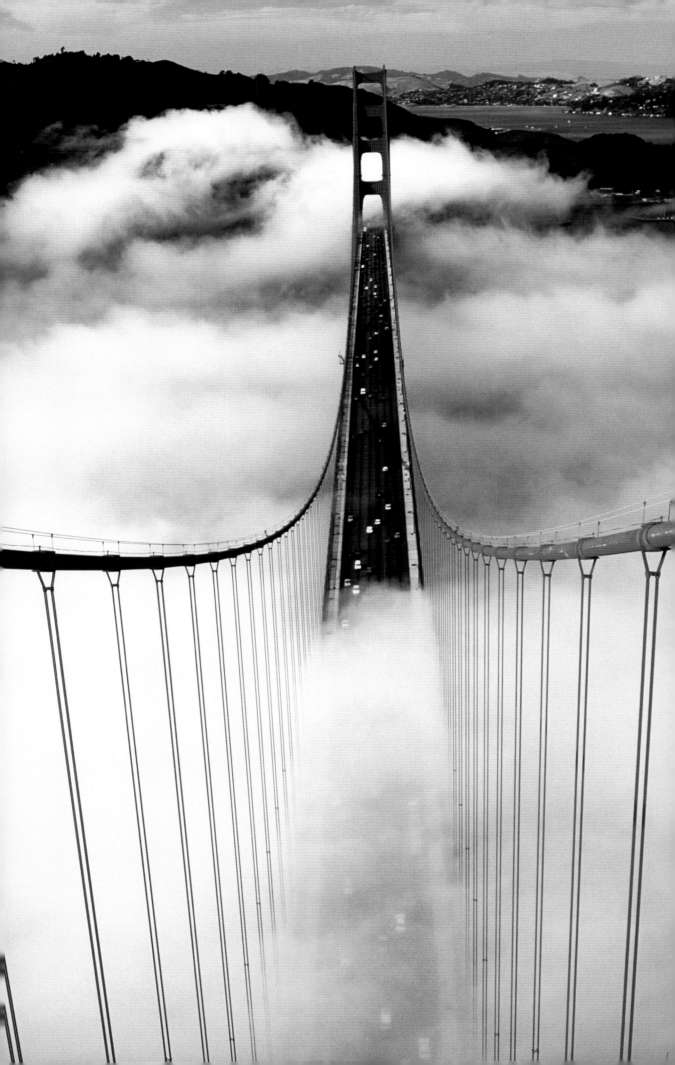

GOLDEN GATE BRIDGE

DATE: BUILT 1933-1937
LOCATION: SAN FRANCISCO, CALIFORNIA
ARCHITECT: JOSEPH B. STRAUSS
PHYSICAL FACT: TOTAL LENGTH = 1.7 MILES

If I had to choose a
Nifty color
To cover a whole bridge with,
Especially one that
Reminded me of a sunset
Neighborhood in a sunshine country
And made people think, Oh
That's span-tastic, just right,
I wouldn't choose black and white
Or yellow stripes—
Not polka dots either!—
Although such colors do look
Lovely on zebras, tigers, and Dalmatians.

Once I had stirred ten truckloads of
Red raspberries, I'd
Add a couple of tons of squeezed California
Nectarines, and hefty barrels of golden
Grape juice in the sweetest coat that
Ever bedazzled a bridge over a bay.

DATE: BUILT 2589-2566 B.C.

LOCATION: GIZA, EGYPT

BUILDER: ESTIMATED 100,000 SLAVES

PHYSICAL FACT: 2,300,000 BLOCKS OF STONE, AVERAGE WEIGHT OF 2.5 TONS EACH

The
story of
this ancient
land, where wind's
a glove designing sand,
is told by ghosts in silent
rooms beneath the most enormous
tombs of granite fame. Some thirty years
the peasants came, gaunt brigadiers of stone
by rope. Without the wheel, their only
hope was grim ordeal. Where Pharaohs lie, a
Pyramid should glorify what others did.

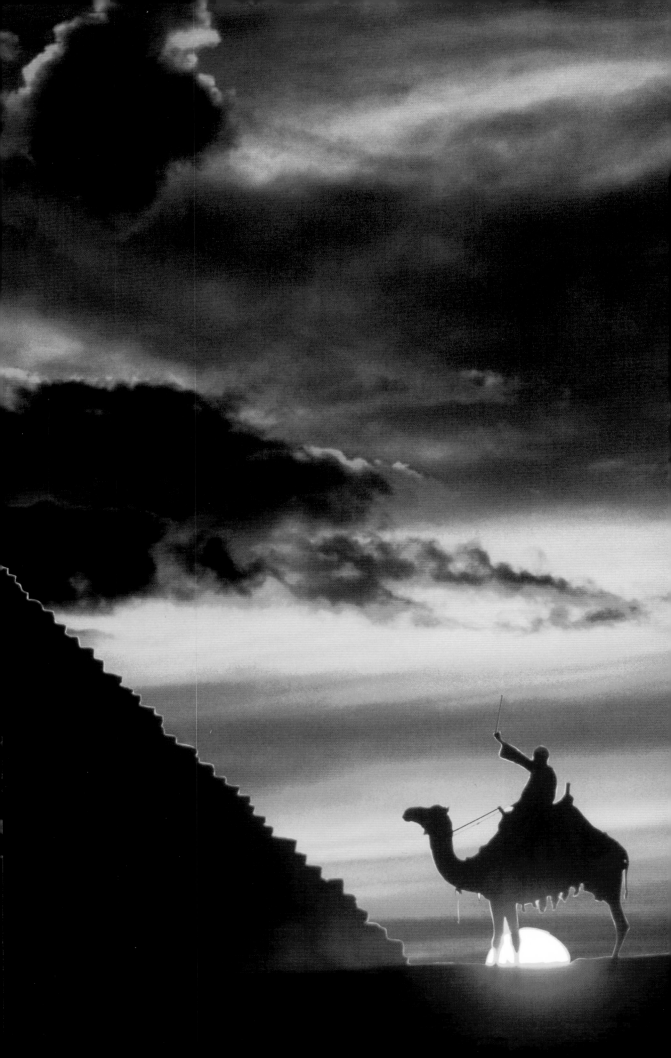

EMPIRE STATE BUILDING

DATE: BUILT 1929-1931
LOCATION: NEW YORK, NEW YORK
DESIGNERS: SHREVE, WILLIAM LAMB & HARMON
PHYSICAL FACT: CONSTRUCTED IN ONE YEAR AND FORTY-FIVE DAYS

I am an American boy, standing up to the world.
I sleep, the city sleeps. We dream
    the riveter's dream, held island-fast.
I wake to taxi alarms.
I am a 102-stop elevator ride to heaven.
I am ten million bricks of unshakable faith.
I capture imagination at its peak.
I hugged King Kong, he hugged me back.
I look down Broadway for a work of art,
    the Fulton Fish Market for a slice of life,
    United Nations Headquarters for a little peace.
It's lonely up here without my big twin brothers,
    the World Trade Center Towers.
Wait here on my doorstep, Central Park,
    while I look over Harlem.
I am an American boy, face to face with the world.

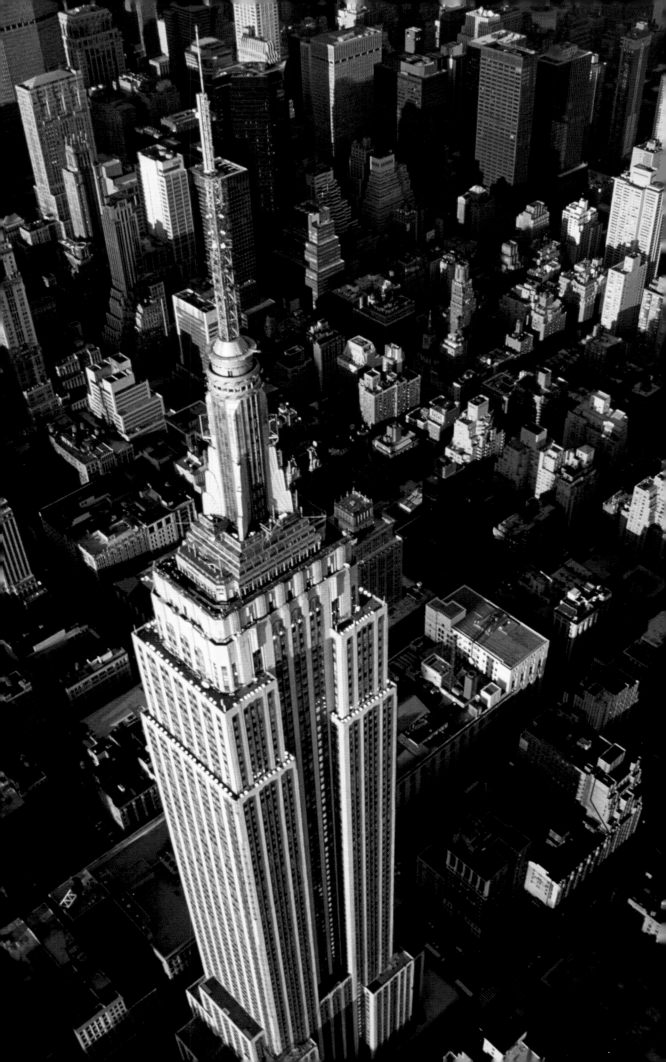

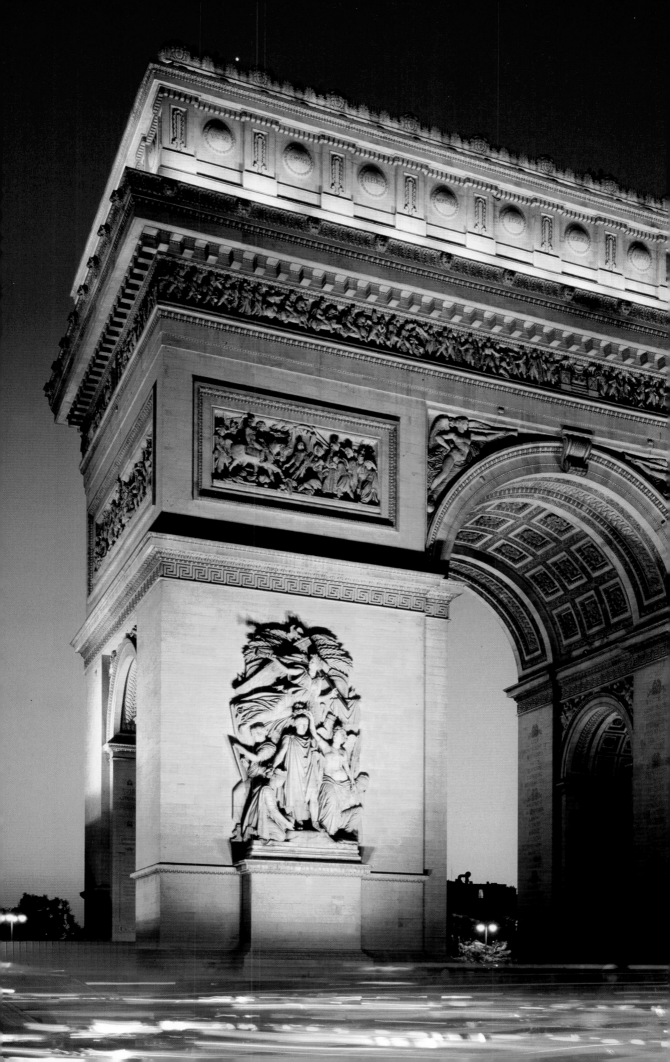

ARC DE TRIOMPHE

DATE: BUILT 1806-1836
LOCATION: PARIS, FRANCE
BUILDERS: JEAN-FRANÇOIS-THÉRÈSE CHALGRIN AND JEAN-ARMAND RAYMOND
PHYSICAL FACT: 164 FT (50 M) HIGH AND 148 FT (45 M) WIDE

Triumphal Roman arcs
Were magic doors
For ancient soldiers who,
Surviving wars,
Resumed their lives
As ordinary men
By merely passing through
Them once again.

And now where these
Twelve avenues converge,
Napolean, DeGaulle,
And history merge
Into the Arc of what
We know as France—
Tradition, culture,
Paris, and romance.

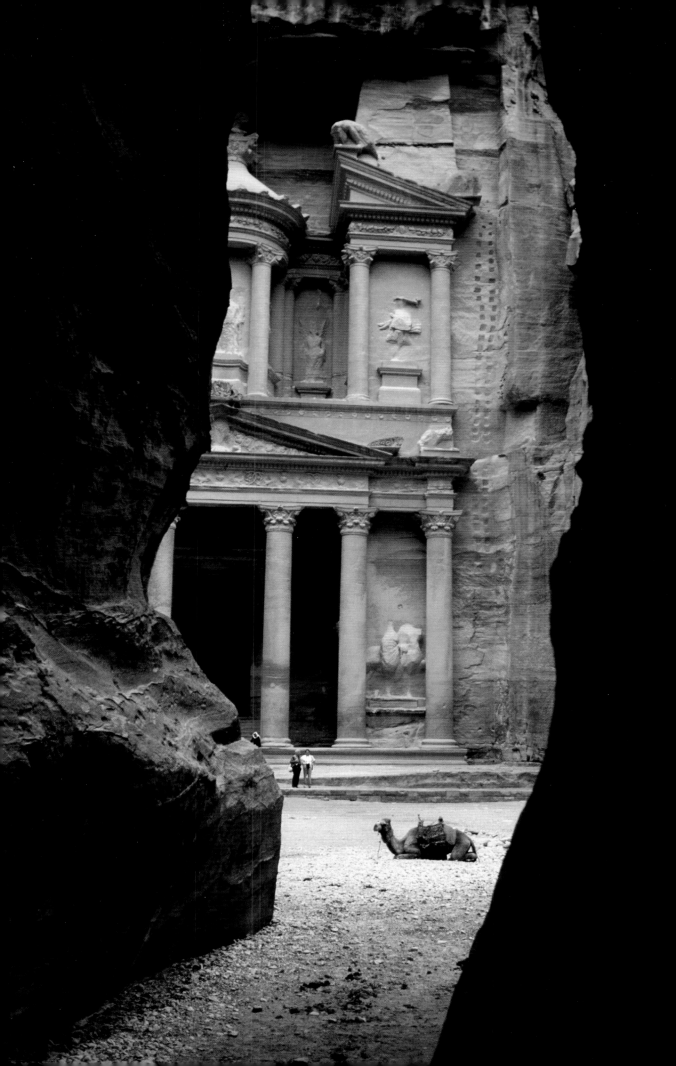

ROSE CITY OF PETRA

DATE: MORE THAN 2,000 YEARS OLD
LOCATION: SOUTH JORDAN
BUILDER: NABATAEAN ARABS
PHYSICAL FACT: REDISCOVERED IN 1812 AFTER BEING "LOST" FOR THREE HUNDRED YEARS.

In pink and salmon-colored rock,
Arabs from a distant past
Carved what remains a future shock—

This city built of canyons lives
In mystic beauty, glory, and
Awe beyond superlatives.

Four hundred years the mountain home
Of traders who touched every land,
Petra, too soon sacked by Rome,

Is now a sandstone-rich archive
For climbers and the curious,
Like bees upon a honeyed hive.

No other cliffs, no canyon view
Recalls to mind or calls to man
Such genius as the world once knew.

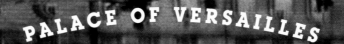

PALACE OF VERSAILLES

DATE: 1661-1710
LOCATION: FRANCE
ARCHITECTS: LOUIS LE VAU AND JULES HARDOUIN MANSART
PHYSICAL FACT: ITS HALL OF MIRRORS IS 44 YARDS (40 M) LONG WITH 578 MIRRORS.

A King, who thought himself the Sun,
Reclined in bed and said to Moon,
"If you look after Everynight,
Then I will be in charge of Noon."

And every day Noon came along,
According to the King's command.
His brilliance radiated far,
From peasant field to foreign land.

When later, though the King was dead,
Noon reappeared and filled the sky,
The peasants knew what glittered Noon—
It was the splendor of Versailles.

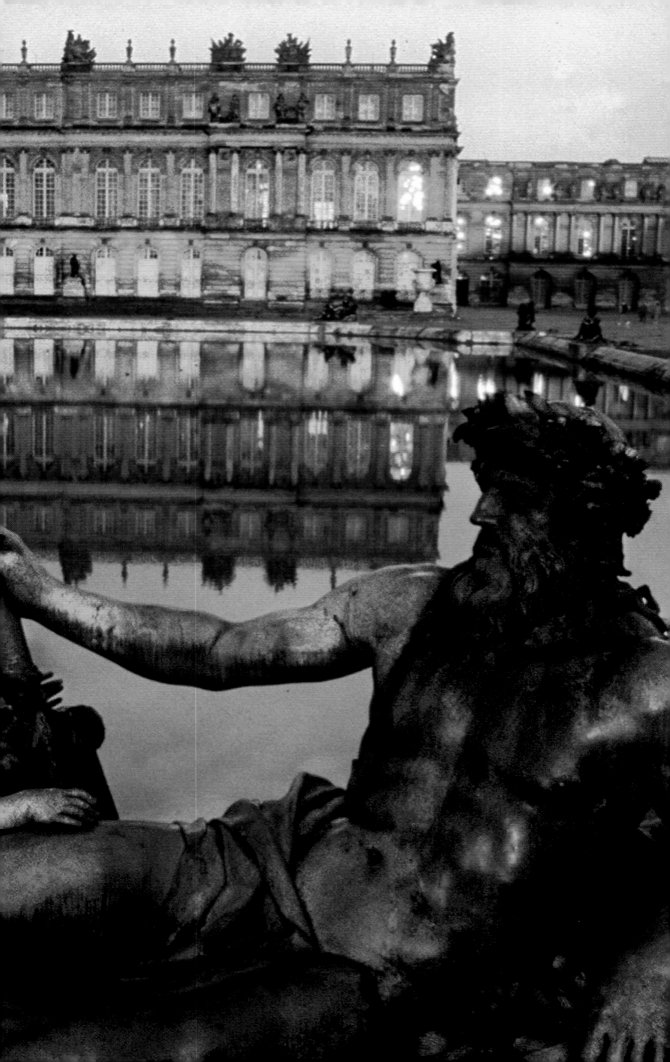

STATUE OF LIBERTY

DATE: ARRIVED FROM FRANCE ON JULY 4, 1884
LOCATION: NEW YORK, NEW YORK
ARCHITECT: FRÉDÉRIC AUGUSTE BARTHOLDI
PHYSICAL FACT: THE FOUNDATION ALONE REQUIRED 24,000 TONS OF CONCRETE.
IT TOOK SIX MONTHS TO MOUNT THE STATUE TO HER BASE.

My nose is four and a half feet long,
My mouth is three feet wide,
My head's ten feet from ear to ear...
I'm a gal you can step inside.

My hand is over sixteen feet,
I'm the first stop on the tour.
My index finger's eight feet long.
I'm America's signature.

My waist is thirty-five feet thick.
In tons, I'm two twenty-five—
I'm the biggest lady ever known
To keep freedom alive.

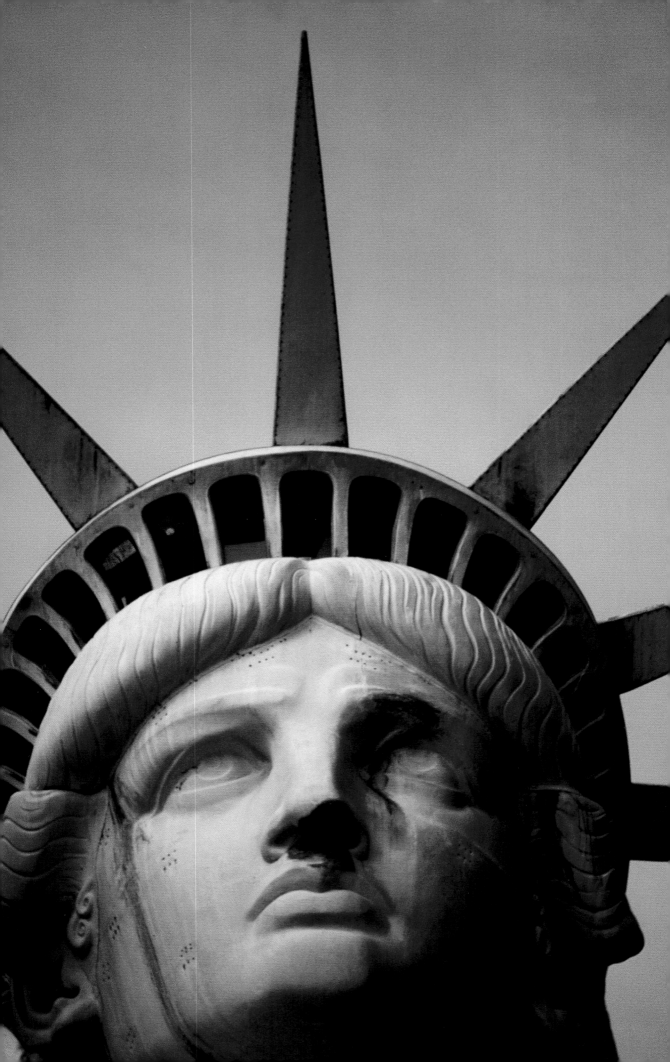

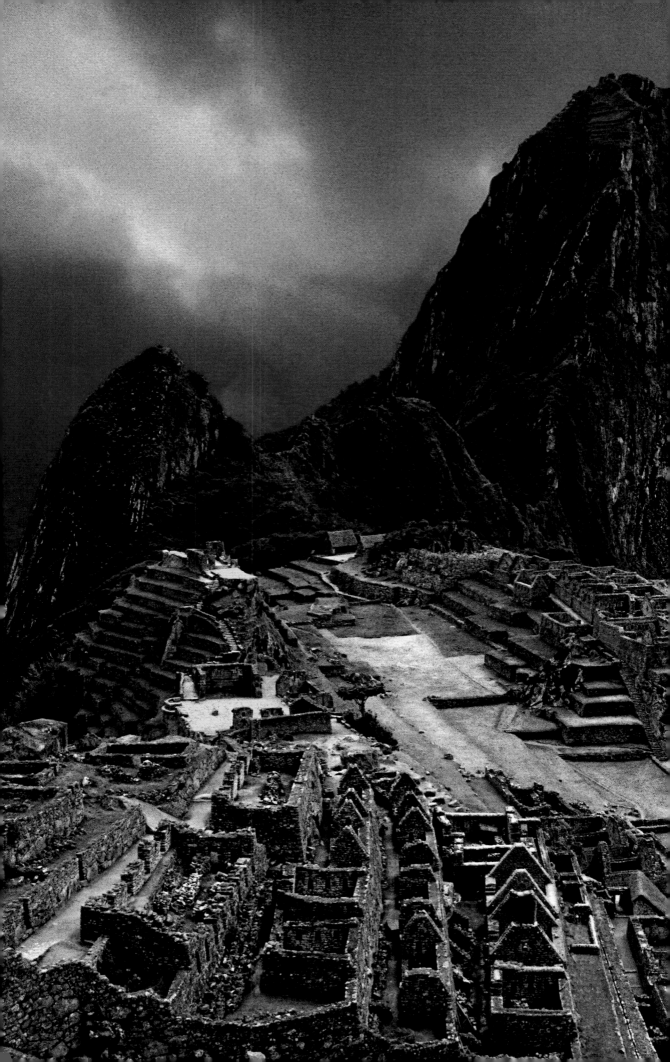

MACHU PICCHU

DATE: BUILT A.D. 1460-1470
LOCATION: PERU
BUILDER: THE INCA
PHYSICAL FACT: AT AN ALTITUDE OF 8,000 FEET (2400 M), THIS REALM
WAS FORGOTTEN AFTER THE INCA DIED OF SMALLPOX AND WAS
REDISCOVERED IN 1911 BY A YALE PROFESSOR.

Above the raintree country of their birth,
In ancient days the Inca hid from earth
A testament—"Old Peak"—in massive stone,
A secret sacred city all their own,
Invisible to enemies below.
    That sky, abandoned centuries ago,
        Where people gazed at each celestial gem
           As if the teeming stars were watching them,
              Remains as green and veiled a mist-ery
                  As humankind is privileged to see.

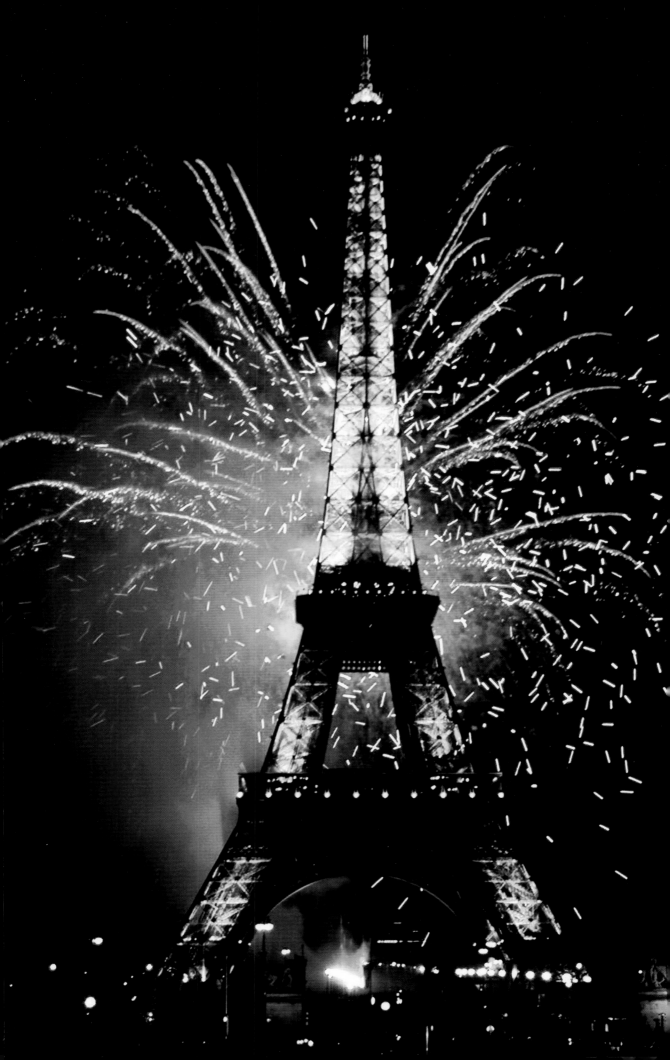

THE EIFFEL TOWER

DATE: BUILT 1887-1889
LOCATION: PARIS, FRANCE
ARCHITECT: GUSTAVE EIFFEL
PHYSICAL FACT: THE PANORAMIC VIEW FROM THE TOP IS BEST ONE HOUR BEFORE SUNSET.

Three hundred workers nailed you,
The Prince of Wales unveiled you.
Your countrymen have hailed you a star.

A mountaineer has scaled you,
Two parachutists sailed you,
A million postcards mailed you afar.

Gustave Eiffel intended you
To be so sleek and splendid, you
Know nothing has transcended you, *mon cher.*

We tourists recommended you,
Ascended and descended you,
And all of us befriended you...up there!

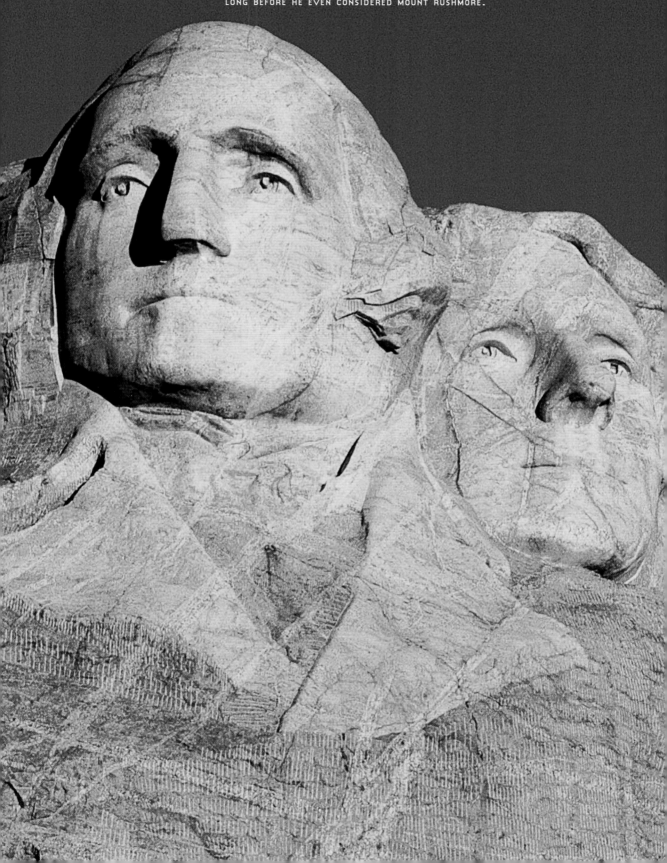

MOUNT RUSHMORE

DATE: BUILT 1927-1941
LOCATION: SOUTH DAKOTA, USA
CHIEF ENGINEER: GUTZON BORGLUM
PHYSICAL FACT: BORGLUM WAS ONE OF AMERICA'S MOST SUCCESSFUL PAINTERS
LONG BEFORE HE EVEN CONSIDERED MOUNT RUSHMORE.

Gutzon Borglum designed four faces
that trumpeted American history
across the western skyline.
Four hundred miners built roads,
blasted stone, sharpened drill bits,
ran the hoists and generated power.

Norman "Happy" Anderson, a skilled
powderman, earned $1.25 an hour,
more than mines were paying at the time.
Describing his presidential task, Happy's
dynamite words were worthy of a bonus:

> *I put the curl in Lincoln's beard,*
> *the part in Teddy's hair,*
> *and the twinkle in Washington's eye.*

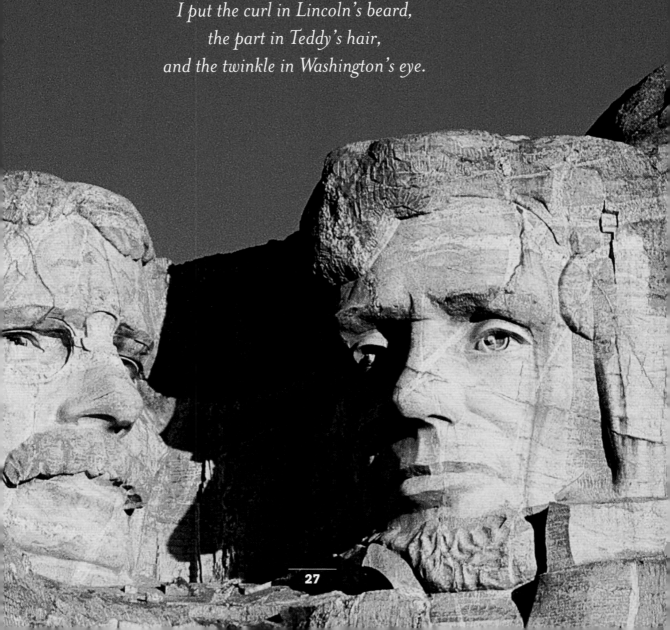

GREAT WALL OF CHINA

DATE: BUILT FROM 3RD CENTURY B.C. TO 20TH CENTURY A.D.
LOCATION: JINSHANLING, CHINA
BUILDER: ABOUT HALF A MILLION PEOPLE
PHYSICAL FACT: 1,500 MILES LONG (2,400 KM)

This
fabled
monument
of earth
and brick
and stone,
designed
by nothing
more than
bucket,
cup, and
spoon,
is still
the
only
structure
built
by human
hands
some
thought
you'd
see if
you
were
standing
on the
moon.

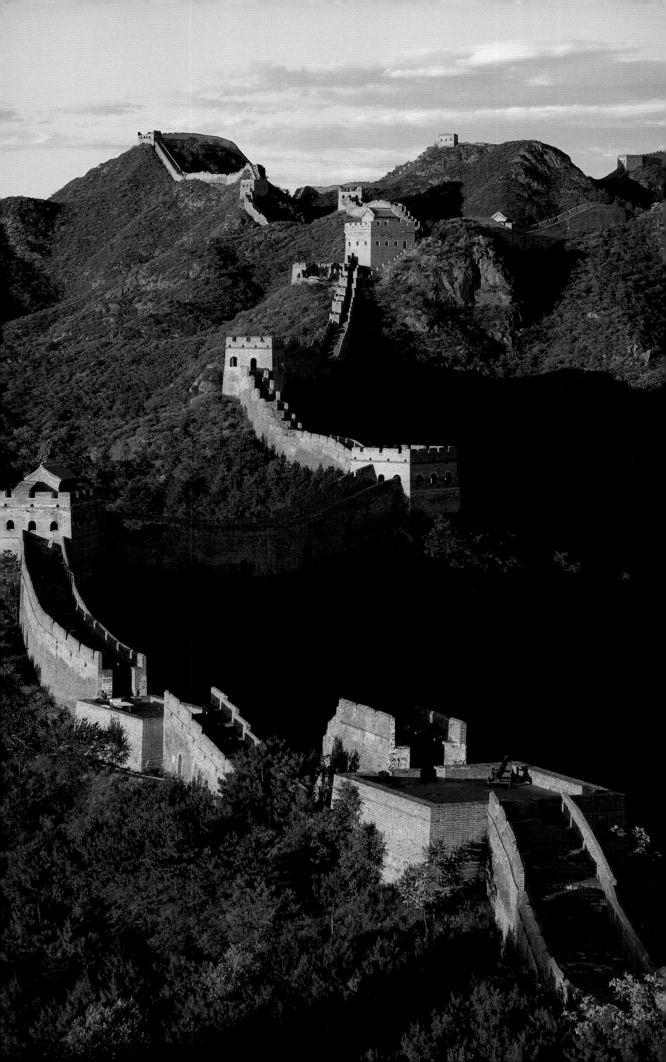

EPILOGUE

If, as the poet Dante Gabriel Rossetti once wrote, a poem is a "moment's monument," then perhaps a monument is a timeless poem. When I first thought about honoring some of the world's enduring man-made constructions, I was humbled by wonder, subdued by such towering greatness.

How to begin? Once I overcame awe, the difficult task of selection arose. It will be obvious to any reader that the subjects in this book are only a few of the finest architectural achievements of humankind. If your favorite is missing—the Leaning Tower of Pisa, the Taj Mahal, Japan's Imperial Palace?—I invite you to write a poem about it.

Try any poetic form that appeals to you: free verse, ballad, acrostic, shaped poem. I tried to make the form match the building itself in some small, indirect way that spoke to me. Pretend your pen is a camera: Take a picture of the monument, but only with your words. And who knows? The word picture you capture may turn out to be as captivating and satisfying as the the image that inspired you.

JPL

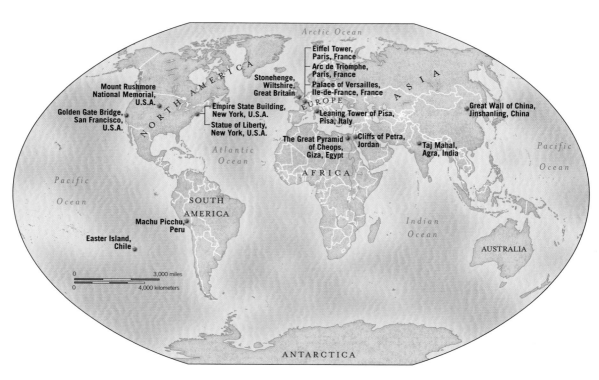

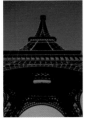

EIFFEL TOWER

PARIS, FRANCE

(COVER) The City of Paris owns this 10,100 ton structure. Six million visitors annually travel up its 1,665 steps and nine elevators to reach the top. The elevators travel the equivalent of two and half times around the world each year.

DALLAS AND JOHN HEATON/CORBIS

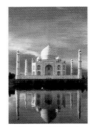

TAJ MAHAL

AGRA, UTTAR PRADESH, INDIA

(TITLE PAGE) In 1630 the Emperor Shah Jehan lost his wife as she gave birth to their 14th child. The Taj Mahal, her tomb, took 23 years to build. It is covered in white marble and surrounded by four minarets.

GEORGINA BOWATER/CORBIS

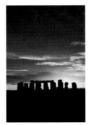

STONEHENGE

WILTSHIRE, ENGLAND

Speculation on the reasons Stonehenge was built range from human sacrifice to astronomy. It seems to have been designed to allow for observation of astronomical phenomena—summer and winter solstices, eclipses, and more.

DAVID PATERSON/GETTY IMAGES

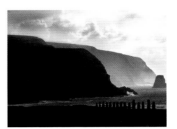

EASTER ISLAND

EASTER ISLAND, CHILE

No written record remains of those who built nearly 900 giant stone "maoi" averaging 13 feet (4m) and 14 tons each, but they might represent the spirits of famous ancestors—or simply the human imagination set in stone.

THOMAS HOEPKER/MAGNUM.

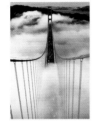

GOLDEN GATE BRIDGE

SAN FRANCISCO, CALIFORNIA

Rumor has it that the U.S. Navy wanted to paint the Golden Gate Bridge black with yellow stripes to make it more visible to passing ships. Architects chose international orange to blend with California's beauty and natural surroundings.

ROGER RESSMEYER/CORBIS

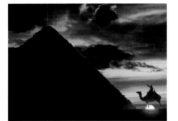

GREAT PYRAMID OF CHEOPS

GIZA, EGYPT

Many have guessed how the Great Pyramid was built; none have provided a definitive answer. Not much is known about the pharaoh Cheops. His tomb had been robbed long before archaeologists came upon it. LARRY LEE/CORBIS

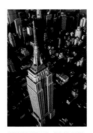

EMPIRE STATE BUILDING

MANHATTAN, NEW YORK

How many millions of Earth's tourists have visited the 86th and 102nd floor observatories of the Empire State Building? Constructed in just one year and 45 days, this legendary structure opened on May 1, 1931. ALAN SCHEIN/CORBIS

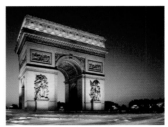

ARC DE TRIOMPHE

PARIS, FRANCE

This famous structure, the largest triumphal arch in the world, was begun in 1806 at the whim of Napoleon Bonaparte to glorify himself, his army, and his military victories. Beneath this national war memorial lies the tomb of the unknown soldier. DAVID HIGGS/CORBIS

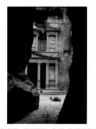

ROSE CITY OF PETRA

PETRA, TURKEY

The very success of Petra as a caravan crosssroads attracted the attention of the Roman Empire, which annexed it. Its glory waned, and the sandstone cliff paradise fell into disuse, to be "rediscovered" by a Swiss adventurer in 1812.

ANDY CHADWICK/GETTY IMAGES

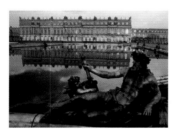

PALACE OF VERSAILLES

ILE-DE-FRANCE, FRANCE

In 1668 France's Louis the 14th, who thought himself divine, decided to build a palace outside Paris away from the boisterous crowds but close to prime hunting grounds. The French Revolution of 1789 deposed King Louis the 16th. BRUNO BARBEY, MAGNUM

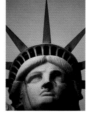

STATUE OF LIBERTY

LIBERTY ISLAND, NEW YORK HARBOR

One hundred years after America's War of Independence, which the French did so much to help win, France presented the U.S. with a lasting monument to commemorate the two countries' abiding friendship and love of freedom.CORBIS

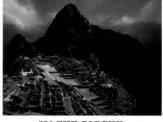

MACHU PICCHU

MACHU PICCHU, PERU

Most likely a religious retreat or royal estate, Machu Picchu was known to few people, even among the Inca. When Pizarro and the Spanish conquistadors arrived, much of the Inca population had died of smallpox. It was rediscoved in 1911. ED FREEMAN/GETTY IMAGES

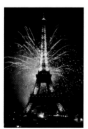

THE EIFFEL TOWER

PARIS, FRANCE

The Eiffel Tower was built to honor the 100th anniversary of the French Revolution. Among its statistics: 40 tons of paint, 1,652 steps to the top, and a sway of up to 4.8 inches (12 cm) in high winds. REUTERS/CORBIS

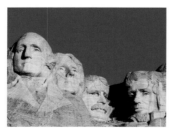

MOUNT RUSHMORE

MOUNT RUSHMORE NATIONAL MEMORIAL, SOUTH DAKOTA

Between 1927 and 1941, Gutzon Borglum and his team chiseled those four famous presidential faces by removing some 450,000 tons of granite, most of it with dynamite. CORBIS

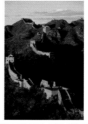

GREAT WALL OF CHINA

JINSHANLING, CHINA

Astronauts assure us that the Great Wall cannot be seen from the moon: nothing man-made can. The Great Wall of China is not continuous. It is a collection of short walls that often follow the crest of hills on the southern edge of the Mongolian plain. LIU LIQUN/CORBIS

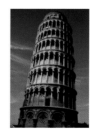

LEANING TOWER OF PISA

TUSCANY REGION, ITALY

(BACK COVER) This circular bell tower began its famous lean during construction. After extensive studies of the plans and testing of the subsoil, the cause of the lean is still a mystery. O. LOUIS MAZZATENTA / NG IMAGE COLLECTION

FOR LEE BENNETT HOPKINS, GRAMMAGABOODLE
ANTHOLOGIST AND SWELLIFFILASTICAL FRIEND
JPL

Text copyright © 2005 J. Patrick Lewis

Published by the National Geographic Society.
All rights reserved. Reproduction of the whole or any part of the contents
without written permission from the National Geographic Society is strictly prohibited.

Book Designers: Bea Jackson and David M. Seager
Illustrations Editor: Janet Dustin
Titles in this book are set in ITC Lubalin Bold.
The text is set in Mrs. Eaves and captions are set in Citizen, both fonts by Emigre.

Library of Congress Cataloging-in-Publication Information is available
from the Library of Congress upon request.

Trade Edition ISBN 0-7922-7135-1   Library Edition ISBN 0-7922-7139-4

The world's largest nonprofit scientific and educational organization,
the National Geographic Society was founded in 1888
"for the increase and diffusion of geographic knowledge."
Since then it has supported scientific exploration and spread information
to its more than eight million members worldwide.

The National Geographic Society educates and inspires millions every day through magazines, books,
television programs, videos, maps and atlases, research grants, the National Geographic Bee, teacher
workshops, and innovative classroom materials. The Society is supported through membership dues,
charitable gifts, and income from the sale of its educational products. Members receive
NATIONAL GEOGRAPHIC magazine—the Society's official journal—discounts on Society products
and other benefits. For more information about the National Geographic Society,
its educational programs and publications, and ways to support its work,
please call 1-800-NGS-LINE (647-5463) or write to the following address:

NATIONAL GEOGRAPHIC SOCIETY
1145 17th Street N.W.
Washington, D.C. 20036-4688 U.S.A.
Visit the Society's Web site: www.nationalgeographic.com

PRINTED IN BELGIUM

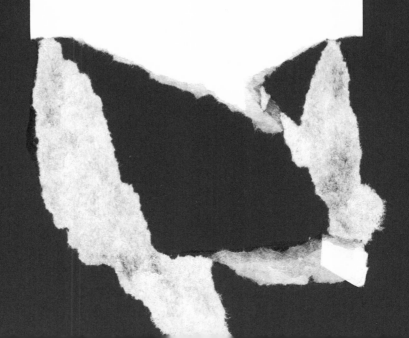